Assistive Technologies in Care and Rehabilitation: Research, Developments, and International Initiatives

Assistive Technologies in Care and Rehabilitation: Research, Developments, and International Initiatives

Guest Editor

Daniele Giansanti

MDPI

Basel • Beijing • Wuhan • Barcelona • Belgrade • Novi Sad • Cluj • Manchester

Guest Editor
Daniele Giansanti
Centre Tisp
Istituto Superiore di Sanità
Rome
Italy

Editorial Office
MDPI AG
Grosspeteranlage 5
4052 Basel, Switzerland

This is a reprint of the Special Issue, published open access by the journal *Technologies* (ISSN 2227-7080), freely accessible at: https://www.mdpi.com/journal/technologies/special_issues/3JP949711D.

For citation purposes, cite each article independently as indicated on the article page online and as indicated below:

Lastname, A.A.; Lastname, B.B. Article Title. *Journal Name* **Year**, *Volume Number*, Page Range.

ISBN 978-3-7258-5535-3 (Hbk)
ISBN 978-3-7258-5536-0 (PDF)
https://doi.org/10.3390/books978-3-7258-5536-0

Contents

About the Editor

Daniele Giansanti

Daniele Giansanti is a professor at Sapienza University and the Catholic University in Rome, Italy. His research interests span biomedical engineering, medical physics, and e-Health, with a focus on developing wearable medical devices, advancing telemedicine and mHealth applications, and studying the acceptance of robotics and artificial intelligence in healthcare. He currently leads research as Research Director at the Italian National Institute of Health (ISS), where his projects include technology assessment for telerehabilitation and domiciliary monitoring, as well as investigating cybersecurity challenges in the health domain. Dr. Giansanti is the holder of three national patents for portable medical devices, has authored over 200 Scopus-indexed publications, and serves as a board editor and reviewer for several scientific journals.

Preface

This Special Issue addresses recent developments and promising innovations in the field of assistive technologies for assistance and rehabilitation. It presents 24 contributions, plus a concluding Editorial, highlighting advances that are shaping research, clinical practice, and technology implementation. Among these, 18 are original research articles, while the remaining 6 contributions are reviews and systematic reviews.

The original research articles introduce novel solutions, including neuro-visual adaptive control for robot-assisted surgery, foot-controlled prosthetic arms, smart systems supporting daily activities for people with intellectual disabilities, and sensor-based rehabilitation interventions for chronic conditions. These studies demonstrate how robotics, AI, sensors, and virtual reality can enhance precision, autonomy, and patient engagement in rehabilitation and care.

The review studies complement these contributions by analyzing existing technologies and interventions. They cover assistive devices for synovial joints, virtual reality for mobility rehabilitation, robotic systems for hand recovery, remote rehabilitation for chronic low back pain, stress-reducing technologies for children with autism, and indoor air quality monitoring for chronic respiratory diseases. Together, these reviews provide insights into design, effectiveness, usability, and research gaps, guiding future development and implementation.

Collectively, the articles in this Special Issue illustrate the synergy between technological innovation, clinical practice, and research synthesis, offering valuable perspectives for scientists, engineers, and healthcare professionals working to advance assistive and rehabilitative solutions.

I would like to sincerely thank all the authors, reviewers, and contributors whose outstanding work made this Special Issue possible. I also extend my gratitude to the editorial team for their dedication and support, and to the Managing Editor, Juicy Yang, for her exceptional guidance and continued commitment. Their combined efforts have been essential in bringing this Special Issue to fruition.

Daniele Giansanti

Guest Editor

technologies

MDPI

Editorial

Empowering Independence: The Role of Assistive Technologies in Enhancing Quality of Life

Daniele Giansanti

Centro TISP, Istituto Superiore di Sanità, Vi Regina Elena 299, 00161 Roma, Italy; daniele.giansanti@iss.it

Assistive technologies are increasingly central to improving quality of life across various settings, from rehabilitation to ongoing care [1]. They are transforming how we address complex needs [2,3], ranging from communication support—such as augmentative and alternative communication (AAC) systems [4,5]—to solutions for neuromotor disabilities [6]. Continuous research advances drive the development of innovative, high-performance technologies, including robotics, wearable devices, and implantable prostheses, which enhance physical abilities, support mobility, and facilitate communication. These technologies also extend care beyond traditional settings through telemedicine and networked medical applications [7].

Despite significant progress, key challenges remain, including person-centered care, personalized assistive solutions, and improved accessibility [8]. Regulatory frameworks like the International Classification of Functioning, Disability, and Health (ICF) [9] and global initiatives led by the World Health Organization (WHO) [10] play a crucial role in raising awareness, monitoring developments, and promoting access to assistive technologies worldwide [8,9].

The Special Issue Assistive Technologies in Care and Rehabilitation: Research, Developments, and International Initiatives [11] explore topics such as the integration of robotics and artificial intelligence in rehabilitation, the role of wearable devices in enhancing autonomy, the impact of telemedicine on remote care, international standards and regulations, the personalization of assistive solutions, ambient assistive technologies, advances in virtual and augmented reality, ethical and economic considerations, user experience, training, and collaboration among healthcare providers, developers, and patients.

The editorial project produced 24 contributions (contributions 1 to 24) plus the present editorial. The contributions include 18 research studies, consisting of 17 scientific articles (contributions 1–5, 7–18), 1 communication (contribution 6), and 6 review studies (contributions 19–24), of which 3 are systematic reviews (contributions 22–24).

Overall, about 75% of the contributions are research studies (18 out of 24) and 25% are review studies (6 out of 24), with half of the reviews being systematic reviews (3 out of 6).

Common message

The collection of contributions (contribution 1–24) presents significant progress in assistive and rehabilitative technologies aimed at improving independence, functionality, and quality of life for diverse populations. The research articles (contribution 1–18) explore innovations such as real-time tactile feedback for speech assistance (contribution 1), socially assistive robots (contribution 3, 7), vision-based activity recognition (contribution 8), and AI-powered personalized rehabilitation programs (contribution 12). These studies emphasize user-centered design and the integration of advanced technologies into everyday and clinical settings.

Supporting these findings, the reviews (contribution 19–24) synthesize current knowledge on various assistive devices, virtual reality applications, robotic rehabilitation systems, and environmental monitoring technologies. They provide critical evaluations of effectiveness, trends, and knowledge gaps, guiding future research and development efforts.

Together, these contributions reflect a multidisciplinary approach where technology, clinical practice, and patient needs intersect to create accessible, effective, and sustainable healthcare solutions (contribution 1–24).

Key Scientific Contributions of the Articles

A total of 18 original research articles present innovative advancements across various fields, including healthcare, assistive technologies, rehabilitation, and human–technology interactions. Each contribution offers novel solutions or insights that enhance quality of life, improve clinical practices, and support independent living for diverse populations such as individuals with disabilities, the elderly, and patients undergoing medical treatment. Together, these studies demonstrate the growing impact of technology-driven research in addressing complex challenges and fostering personalized, effective interventions.

Contribution 1 addresses a wearable haptic feedback system designed to assist speech training for individuals with speech and hearing impairments. Unlike previous methods, this system offers real-time, phoneme-level tactile cues that empower users to independently improve their pronunciation through a multimodal interface combining audio, visual, and vibrotactile feedback. Validation studies demonstrated significant improvements in articulation accuracy and user engagement, highlighting its potential as an accessible tool for speech rehabilitation and language learning.

Contribution 2 focuses on the integration of advanced assistive technologies—such as socially assistive robots, virtual reality, and conversational AI—into Speech and Language Therapy (SLT) for children with communication disorders. This work presents the "ATLog" platform, a user-friendly software enabling therapists to design personalized interactive learning scenarios without programming expertise. Evaluations by SLT experts show high acceptance and usability, suggesting the platform effectively supports the practical adoption of these innovative technologies in therapy.

Contribution 3 explores the role of social robots within Ambient Assisted Living (AAL) environments aimed at enhancing elderly care. The proposed framework positions a social robot as the central coordinator of smart home devices, facilitating natural interaction and real-time recognition of gestures and moods to support seniors' independence. This paper discusses the technical aspects and scenarios demonstrating how this integration can improve quality of life and reduce caregiver burden.

Contribution 4 presents a novel approach to assess neck pain by using a virtual reality (VR) environment simulating an apple-harvesting task. By continuously tracking head movement kinematics, this study identifies functional limitations in patients with neck pain that traditional range-of-motion measurements might miss. The VR-based assessment shows promise for remote evaluation and personalized telerehabilitation strategies.

Contribution 5 introduces a non-contact system leveraging a Microsoft Azure Kinect depth camera to evaluate physical function and postural stability in older adults. Through motion capture during squats and balance stances, the platform detects biomechanical differences associated with aging and fall risk. The findings support the feasibility of using low-cost depth-camera technology for ongoing risk assessment and fall prevention.

Contribution 6 details an innovative in vivo device for dynamic mechanical analysis (DMA) of plantar soft tissue, enabling multidimensional characterization under physiological conditions. This device overcomes limitations of conventional testing by providing real-time measurements of viscoelastic properties such as tensile, compressive, shear, and torsional behaviors. The open-source design facilitates further research and has applications in diagnostics and personalized orthopedic treatments.

Contribution 7 investigates changes in elderly residents' perceptions of a humanoid social robot (HSR) following direct interaction. Using the Godspeed Questionnaire Series, this study found positive shifts in views on anthropomorphism, animation, likeability, and perceived intelligence after hands-on experience. Results emphasize the importance of real interaction in developing social robots tailored to older adults' needs.

Contribution 8 proposes a computer vision-based activity monitoring system for elderly care environments, combining cameras and infrared sensors to detect daily activities and anomalies without extensive labeled data. Real-world deployment demonstrated improved emergency response and respect for privacy via anonymized views. The system supports continuous, unobtrusive monitoring to enhance safety and independence.

Contribution 9 analyzes the impact of emerging technologies on the quality of life for individuals with autism spectrum disorder (ASD) and comorbid chronic anxiety or depression. Using large-scale survey data, this study identifies communication and learning challenges as significant factors affecting well-being. It suggests that technological interventions, potentially evaluated through quantum computing methods, could improve emotional regulation and social skills in this population.

Contribution 10 explores the optimization of sensor types, locations, and models for high-accuracy Human Activity Recognition (HAR) in fall prevention. By analyzing four multimodal HAR datasets (USC-HAD, HuGaDB, Camargo et al., CSL-SHARE), it identifies that window sizes between 2 and 5 s and models such as Support Vector Machines (SVMs) and Artificial Neural Networks (ANNs) achieve the best performance. This study further reveals that Inertial Measurement Units (IMUs) placed on the thigh yield optimal classification accuracy, while Electromyography (EMG) sensors show inconsistent results.

Contribution 11 proposes a study on the usability of no-code (NC) platforms by individuals with disabilities. Conducted in a German sheltered workshop, this study involved targeted training enabling participants to develop workplace chatbots. Results demonstrate that participants successfully created multiple chatbots that were well received by their peers, confirming that, with appropriate support, people with disabilities can leverage NC tools to build effective, accessible workplace applications.

Contribution 12 evaluates the feasibility of using large language models (LLMs) to generate personalized postoperative rehabilitation plans for head and neck surgery patients. Four LLMs (ChatGPT-4o, DeepSeek V3, Gemini 2, and Copilot) were compared across clinical scenarios, with ChatGPT-4o producing the most clinically relevant plans. This study highlights that AI-generated rehabilitation programs have potential to complement existing protocols but require further clinical validation.

Contribution 13 introduces a Neuro-Visual Adaptive Control (NVAC) architecture for enhanced precision in robot-assisted surgery. Combining a YOLO11n-based vision system, Model Reference Adaptive Control with Proportional-Derivative terms (MRAC-PD), and Closed-Form Continuous-Time Neural Networks (CfC-mmRNNs), the system achieves sub-millimeter tracking accuracy in laparoscope guidance under dynamic disturbances, demonstrating a scalable framework for increasing surgical robot autonomy.

Contribution 14 investigates a novel technology system designed to assist individuals with intellectual disabilities and blindness in handling and transporting boxes within a facility. Using RFID tags, a smartphone interface, and audio prompts with preferred music, the system significantly increased the frequency of correct box handling without human guidance, suggesting potential benefits for supporting autonomy in this population.

Contribution 15 presents improvements in the "Infinity" foot controller for prosthetic arm operation and introduces the "Persistence Arm," a novel transradial prosthesis prototype. The new system enables barefoot foot control with low latency, and the arm features advanced direct-drive wrist actuation and tendon-driven fingers. Tests demonstrate effective grip strength and adaptability, indicating the promise of foot control and 3D-printed prosthetics as cost-effective alternatives to traditional upper limb prostheses.

Contribution 16 applies a technology assessment framework and key performance indicators (KPIs) to evaluate telemedicine services within the Telemechron project. This study confirms the framework's effectiveness in measuring telemedicine improvements and stresses the need for KPI customization to fit diverse contexts. It advocates for further development of adaptable evaluation metrics to support telemedicine performance nationally and internationally.

Contribution 17 proposes an original rehabilitation device for passive mobilization of the neck joint using pneumatic muscle actuators. Designed for patients with work-related musculoskeletal disorders, the device adapts to individual pain tolerance and provides controlled mobilization in sagittal and frontal planes. This paper details the device's construction, mechanical properties, and offers recommendations for optimal clinical use.

Contribution 18 examines the relationships between technology readiness/acceptance, exercise motivation, sensation seeking, and the use of Smart Sport Watches (SSWs) in adolescents. This study finds that SSW users display higher positive technology readiness and lower negative readiness, while exercise motivation is more related to physical activity (walking/running) than to SSW usage. The findings highlight the role of technology acceptance in wearable adoption and suggest tailored measures for deeper understanding.

Key Scientific Contributions of the review studies

The following review studies provide valuable insights into the advancement of assistive technologies and rehabilitation interventions across various medical conditions. Contributions range from comprehensive analyses of assistive devices for joint mobility (Contribution 19) and virtual reality applications in physical rehabilitation (Contribution 20) to detailed examinations of hand rehabilitation devices for neurological disorders (Contribution 21). Additionally, systematic reviews explore sensor-based remote rehabilitation for chronic low back pain (Contribution 22), assistive technologies aimed at stress reduction in autism spectrum disorder (Contribution 23), and the role of indoor air quality monitoring in managing chronic respiratory diseases (Contribution 24). Collectively, these reviews highlight technological progress, clinical effectiveness, challenges, and emerging research needs in their respective fields.

Contribution 19 presents a comprehensive review of assistive devices for synovial joints, focusing on their definitions, classifications, and technological evolution. This work analyzes artificial exoskeletons, orthoses, prostheses, and splints, clarifying terminology and biomechanical principles. It emphasizes the need for a systematic approach to design and categorization to enhance rehabilitation and human mobility across medical, industrial, and military applications.

Contribution 20 presents a scoping review of virtual reality (VR) interventions aimed at improving mobility in both adults and children, based on studies from 2010 to 2023. It highlights significant clinical research demonstrating VR's effectiveness, primarily in inpatient settings, with many studies showing statistically significant motor improvements. This review underlines VR's transition from proof of concept to clinical translation in physical rehabilitation.

Contribution 21 provides an extensive review of hand rehabilitation devices for neurological conditions such as stroke, Parkinson's disease, and multiple sclerosis. Categorizing devices by design, mobility, and actuation, it identifies key trends like the predominance of electric actuation and dorsal placement. This review notes challenges like incomplete data and limited clinical validation but underscores opportunities for improving device functionality and therapeutic efficacy.

Contribution 22 offers a systematic review of sensor-based remote rehabilitation and VR interventions for chronic low back pain (CLBP). Analyzing randomized controlled trials and observational studies from 2015 to 2025, it reports positive outcomes in pain reduction, functional mobility, adherence, and quality of life. This review highlights gamification and biofeedback as critical to enhancing patient engagement but calls for more long-term and economic evaluations.

Contribution 23 presents a systematic review investigating assistive and emerging technologies aimed at reducing stress and neurophysiological distress in children and adolescents with autism spectrum disorder (ASD). Using PRISMA guidelines, this study found beneficial impacts of these technologies on stress reduction and identified limitations affecting replicability and generalizability.

Contribution 24 offers a systematic review on indoor air quality (IAQ) monitoring and its role in managing chronic respiratory diseases such as COPD and asthma. This review highlights significant research gaps including standardization issues, geographic and patient heterogeneity, and the need for long-term studies. It also points to the emerging potential of integrating IAQ monitoring with machine learning to improve respiratory health outcomes.

Conclusions

The collection of 24 scientific articles reviewed herein—including 18 original research contributions and 6 comprehensive reviews—demonstrates significant innovative advancements across healthcare, assistive technologies, rehabilitation, and human–technology interactions. Together, these works highlight the accelerating impact of technology-driven research in addressing complex health challenges, improving clinical practices, and enhancing quality of life for diverse populations such as individuals with disabilities, elderly people, and patients undergoing specialized medical care. The original studies present novel solutions ranging from wearable feedback systems and AI-supported therapy platforms to advanced prosthetics and intelligent monitoring frameworks. The review articles further contextualize these advances by synthesizing current evidence on assistive devices, virtual reality in rehabilitation, sensor-based remote therapies, stress-reducing technologies in autism, and environmental health monitoring. Collectively, the body of work underscores the critical importance of user-centered design, clinical validation, and interdisciplinary collaboration in fostering effective and personalized interventions.

Future Directions

Future efforts should focus on longitudinal clinical validation and real-world implementation to ensure the efficacy, safety, and scalability of these emerging technologies. Enhancing personalization through AI and adaptive systems, improving accessibility via no-code and user-friendly platforms, and emphasizing inclusive design for vulnerable and underserved populations will be essential. Cross-disciplinary partnerships among clinicians, engineers, data scientists, and users are crucial to accelerate translation from research to practice. Furthermore, proactive attention to ethical considerations, data privacy, and regulatory frameworks will support responsible technology deployment. By integrating these priorities, ongoing research can fully harness technological innovation to transform healthcare and rehabilitation, ultimately improving patient outcomes and autonomy.

Acknowledgments: The author acknowledges the assistance of GPT-5 mini (OpenAI, free version) for English language editing.

Conflicts of Interest: The author declares no conflicts of interest.

List of Contributions:

1. Sharon, A.; Yozevitch, R.; Holdengreber, E. Touch to Speak: Real-Time Tactile Pronunciation Feedback for Individuals with Speech and Hearing Impairments. *Technologies* **2025**, *13*, 345. https://doi.org/10.3390/technologies13080345.
2. Lekova, A.; Tsvetkova, P.; Andreeva, A.; Dimitrov, G.; Tanev, T.; Simonska, M.; Stefanov, T.; Stancheva-Popkostadinova, V.; Padareva, G.; Rasheva, K.; et al. A Design-Based Research Approach to Streamline the Integration of High-Tech Assistive Technologies in Speech and Language Therapy. *Technologies* **2025**, *13*, 306. https://doi.org/10.3390/technologies13070306.
3. Sanchez-Torres, C.E.; Lozano, E.A.; López-Nava, I.H.; Garcia-Macias, J.A.; Favela, J. A Socially Assistive Robot as Orchestrator of an AAL Environment for Seniors. *Technologies* **2025**, *13*, 260. https://doi.org/10.3390/technologies13060260.
4. Santos-Paz, J.A.; Sánchez-Picot, Á.; Bocos-Corredor, E.; Moggioli, F.; Martin-Pintado-Zugasti, A.; García-Carmona, R.; Otero, A. Neck Functional Status Assessment Using Virtual Reality Simulation of Daily Activities. *Technologies* **2025**, *13*, 248. https://doi.org/10.3390/technologies13060248.
5. Sobrino-Santos, A.; Anuarbe, P.; Fernandez-Viadero, C.; García-García, R.; López-Higuera, J.M.; Rodríguez-Cobo, L.; Cobo, A. Non-Contact Platform for the Assessment of Physical Function in Older Adults: A Pilot Study. *Technologies* **2025**, *13*, 225. https://doi.org/10.3390/technologies13060225.
6. Wu, L.; Huang, R.; Zhu, J.; Ma, X. A Dynamic Mechanical Analysis Device for In Vivo Material Characterization of Plantar Soft Tissue. *Technologies* **2025**, *13*, 191. https://doi.org/10.3390/technologies13050191.
7. Tobis, S.; Piasek-Skupna, J.; Suwalska, A.; Wieczorowska-Tobis, K. The Impact of Real-World Interaction on the Perception of a Humanoid Social Robot in Care for Institutionalised Older Adults. *Technologies* **2025**, *13*, 189. https://doi.org/10.3390/technologies13050189.
8. Ullah, R.; Asghar, I.; Akbar, S.; Evans, G.; Vermaak, J.; Alblwi, A.; Bamaqa, A. Vision-Based Activity Recognition for Unobtrusive Monitoring of the Elderly in Care Settings. *Technologies* **2025**, *13*, 184. https://doi.org/10.3390/technologies13050184.
9. Benedicto-Rodríguez, G.; Zorrilla-Muñoz, V.; Garcia-Aracil, N.; Fernandez, E.; Ferrández, J. M. Understanding Technology Perception in Autism with Separate Analyses for Anxiety and Depression Using Quantum Circuit Simulation Approach. *Technologies* **2025**, *13*, 165. https://doi.org/10.3390/technologies13040165.
10. Mitchell, J.C.; Dehghani-Sanij, A.A.; Xie, S.Q.; O'Connor, R.J. Analysis of Multimodal Sensor Systems for Identifying Basic Walking Activities. *Technologies* **2025**, *13*, 152. https://doi.org/10.3390/technologies13040152.
11. Kerdar, S.H.; Kirchhoff, B.M.; Adolph, L.; Bächler, L. A Study on Chatbot Development Using No-Code Platforms by People with Disabilities for Their Peers at a Sheltered Workshop. *Technologies* **2025**, *13*, 146. https://doi.org/10.3390/technologies13040146.
12. Marcaccini, G.; Seth, I.; Novo, J.; McClure, V.; Sacks, B.; Lim, K.; Ng, S.K.-H.; Cuomo, R.; Rozen, W.M. Leveraging Artificial Intelligence for Personalized Rehabilitation Programs for Head and Neck Surgery Patients. *Technologies* **2025**, *13*, 142. https://doi.org/10.3390/technologies13040142.
13. Urrea, C.; Garcia-Garcia, Y.; Kern, J.; Rodriguez-Guillen, R. Neuro-Visual Adaptive Control for Precision in Robot-Assisted Surgery. *Technologies* **2025**, *13*, 135. https://doi.org/10.3390/technologies13040135.
14. Lancioni, G.E.; Alberti, G.; Pezzuoli, F.; Abbinante, F.; Singh, N.N.; O'Reilly, M.F.; Sigafoos, J. Technology to Enable People with Intellectual Disabilities and Blindness to Collect Boxes with

Objects and Transport Them to Different Rooms of Their Daily Context: A Single-Case Research Series. *Technologies* **2025**, *13*, 131. https://doi.org/10.3390/technologies13040131.

15. Bishay, P.L.; Funes Alfaro, G.; Sherrill, I.; Reoyo, I.; McMahon, E.; Carter, C.; Valdez, C.; Riyaz, N.M.; Ali, S.; Lima, A.; et al. "The Foot Can Do It": Controlling the "Persistence" Prosthetic Arm Using the "Infinity-2" Foot Controller. *Technologies* **2025**, *13*, 98. https://doi.org/10.3390/technologies13030098.
16. Jayousi, S.; Cinelli, M.; Bigazzi, R.; Bianchi, S.; Scalvini, S.; Borghi, G.; Bernocchi, P.; Inchiostro, S.; Giovanazzi, A.; Mastellaro, M.; et al. Transforming Telemedicine: Strategic Lessons and Metrics from Italy's Telemechron Project (Telemechron Study). *Technologies* **2025**, *13*, 44. https://doi.org/10.3390/technologies13020044.
17. Mareş, S.; Deaconescu, A.; Deaconescu, T. Pneumatically Actuated Rehabilitation Equipment for the Sagittal and Frontal Plane Movements of the Neck Joint. *Technologies* **2025**, *13*, 39. https://doi.org/10.3390/technologies13010039.
18. Tenenbaum, G.; Ben-Zion, T.; Amichai-Hamburger, Y.; Galily, Y.; Lev, A. Smart Sport Watch Usage: The Dominant Role of Technology Readiness over Exercise Motivation and Sensation Seeking. *Technologies* **2025**, *13*, 24. https://doi.org/10.3390/technologies13010024.
19. Cruz-Flores, F.; Sánchez-Brito, A.L.; Campos Amezcua, R.; Barrera Sánchez, A.; Azcaray Rivera, H.R.; Martínez Mata, A.J.; Blanco Ortega, A. A Review of Assistive Devices in Synovial Joints: Records, Trends, and Classifications. *Technologies* **2025**, *13*, 292. https://doi.org/10.3390/technologies13070292.
20. Felsberg, D.T.; Pousti, R.; Howard, C.K.; Ross, S.E.; Raisbeck, L.D.; McGuirt, J.T.; Rhea, C.K. The Landscape of Virtual Reality Use in Mobility Rehabilitation from 2010–2023: A Scoping Review. *Technologies* **2025**, *13*, 167. https://doi.org/10.3390/technologies13050167.
21. Gherman, B.; Zima, I.; Vaida, C.; Tucan, P.; Pisla, A.; Birlescu, I.; Machado, J.; Pisla, D. Robotic Systems for Hand Rehabilitation—Past, Present and Future. *Technologies* **2025**, *13*, 37. https://doi.org/10.3390/technologies13010037.
22. Garofano, M.; Del Sorbo, R.; Calabrese, M.; Giordano, M.; Di Palo, M.P.; Bartolomeo, M.; Ragusa, C.M.; Ungaro, G.; Fimiani, G.; Di Spirito, F.; et al. Remote Rehabilitation and Virtual Reality Interventions Using Motion Sensors for Chronic Low Back Pain: A Systematic Review of Biomechanical, Pain, Quality of Life, and Adherence Outcomes. *Technologies* **2025**, *13*, 186. https://doi.org/10.3390/technologies13050186.
23. Pergantis, P.; Bamicha, V.; Doulou, A.; Christou, A.I.; Bardis, N.; Skianis, C.; Drigas, A. Assistive and Emerging Technologies to Detect and Reduce Neurophysiological Stress and Anxiety in Children and Adolescents with Autism and Sensory Processing Disorders: A Systematic Review. *Technologies* **2025**, *13*, 144. https://doi.org/10.3390/technologies13040144.
24. Camacho-Magriñán, P.; Sales-Lerida, D.; León-Jiménez, A.; Sanchez-Morillo, D. Indoor Environmental Monitoring and Chronic Respiratory Diseases: A Systematic Review. *Technologies* **2025**, *13*, 122. https://doi.org/10.3390/technologies13030122.

References

1. Available online: https://www.nichd.nih.gov/health/topics/rehabtech (accessed on 11 August 2025).
2. Agree, E.M. The potential for technology to enhance independence for those aging with a disability. *Disabil. Health J.* **2014**, *7* (Suppl. S1), S33–S39. [CrossRef] [PubMed] [PubMed Central]
3. Theng, L.B. (Ed.) *Assistive Technologies for Physical and Cognitive Disabilities*; Medical Information Science Reference/IGI Global: Hershey, PA, USA, 2015. [CrossRef]
4. Elsahar, Y.; Hu, S.; Bouazza-Marouf, K.; Kerr, D.; Mansor, A. Augmentative and Alternative Communication (AAC) Advances: A Review of Configurations for Individuals with a Speech Disability. *Sensors* **2019**, *19*, 1911. [CrossRef] [PubMed] [PubMed Central]
5. Available online: https://www.nidcd.nih.gov/health/assistive-devices-people-hearing-voice-speech-or-language-disorders (accessed on 11 August 2025).
6. Bonanno, M.; Saracino, B.; Ciancarelli, I.; Panza, G.; Manuli, A.; Morone, G.; Calabrò, R.S. Assistive Technologies for Individuals with a Disability from a Neurological Condition: A Narrative Review on the Multimodal Integration. *Healthcare* **2025**, *13*, 1580. [CrossRef] [PubMed]

7. Junaid, S.B.; Imam, A.A.; Balogun, A.O.; De Silva, L.C.; Surakat, Y.A.; Kumar, G.; Abdulkarim, M.; Shuaibu, A.N.; Garba, A.; Sahalu, Y.; et al. Recent Advancements in Emerging Technologies for Healthcare Management Systems: A Survey. *Healthcare* **2022**, *10*, 1940. [CrossRef] [PubMed] [PubMed Central]
8. Available online: https://iris.who.int/bitstream/handle/10665/354357/9789240049451-eng.pdf?sequence=1 (accessed on 11 August 2025).
9. Available online: https://www.who.int/standards/classifications/international-classification-of-functioning-disability-and-health (accessed on 11 August 2025).
10. Available online: https://www.who.int/tools/ata-toolkit/rata (accessed on 11 August 2025).
11. Special Issue: Assistive Technologies in Care and Rehabilitation: Research, Developments, and International Initiatives. Available online: https://www.mdpi.com/journal/technologies/special_issues/3JP949711D (accessed on 11 August 2025).

technologies

MDPI

Article

Neck Functional Status Assessment Using Virtual Reality Simulation of Daily Activities

José Angel Santos-Paz [1], Álvaro Sánchez-Picot [1], Elena Bocos-Corredor [2], Filippo Moggioli [2], Aitor Martin-Pintado-Zugasti [2], Rodrigo García-Carmona [1] and Abraham Otero [1,*]

1 Department of Information Technologies, Institute of Technology, Universidad San Pablo-CEU, CEU Universities, Campus Montepríncipe, 28660 Boadilla del Monte, Spain; jose.santospaz@ceu.es (J.A.S.-P.); alvaro.sanchezpicot@ceu.es (Á.S.-P.); r.garcia.carmona@gmail.com (R.G.-C.)

2 Department of Physiotherapy, School of Medicine, Universidad San Pablo-CEU, CEU Universities, Campus Montepríncipe, 28660 Boadilla del Monte, Spain; elena.bocoscorredor@ceu.es (E.B.-C.); filippo.moggioli@ceu.es (F.M.); martinpintado.a@gmail.com (A.M.-P.-Z.)

* Correspondence: aotero@ceu.es

Abstract: Neck pain is a significant global health concern and a leading cause of disability. Conventional clinical neck assessments often rely on maximal Cervical Range of Motion (CROM) measurements, which may not accurately reflect functional limitations experienced during activities of daily living (ADLs). This study introduces a novel approach to evaluate neck functional status by employing a virtual reality (VR) environment to simulate an apple-harvesting task. Three-dimensional head kinematics were continuously recorded in 60 participants (30 with clinically significant neck pain and 30 asymptomatic) as they performed the task. Spectral analysis of the data revealed that individuals with neck pain exhibited slower head rotation speed, particularly in the transverse and frontal planes, compared to the pain-free group, as evidenced by higher spectral power in the low-frequency band [0, 0.1] Hz and lower power in the [0.1, 0.5] Hz band. Furthermore, participants with neck pain required significantly more time to complete the apple-harvesting task. The VR system demonstrated high usability (SUS score = 84.21), and no adverse effects were reported. These findings suggest that VR-based assessment during simulated ADLs can provide valuable information about the functional impact of neck pain beyond traditional CROM measurements, potentially enabling remote evaluation and personalized telerehabilitation strategies.

Keywords: virtual reality; cervical range of motion; neck pain; functional neck assessment

1. Introduction

Global estimates suggest that approximately 1.71 billion individuals are affected by musculoskeletal disorders [1]. Musculoskeletal conditions account for a substantial proportion of years lived with disability (YLDs), particularly among adults of working age (20–54 years). As this age group represents the period of highest economic and social productivity, disability during these years can lead to significant losses in human capital. This burden is increasingly acknowledged in international policy frameworks due to its wide-ranging societal impact [2].

Women have a higher prevalence of musculoskeletal disorders than men across all age groups, with peak incidence between 40 and 44 years [3]. Regionally, the highest incidence and age-adjusted YLD rates were reported in North Africa and the Middle East, with Iran having the highest burden, while New Zealand had the lowest. Spain experienced the greatest decline in these rates between 1990 and 2021 [3]. Although a slight reduction in adjusted rates is projected, the absolute number of cases is expected to continue to rise due to population aging, with a projected 269 million people affected by 2050 [4].

Neck pain is one of the most common musculoskeletal disorders, representing a significant source of disability [1]. Neck pain presents a substantial public health burden, impacting an estimated 222 million individuals and contributing to 22 million years lived with disability (YLDs) [5]. The lifetime prevalence of neck pain is considerable, with 30% to 50% of the general population reporting experiencing this condition [6]. Suboptimal management of neck pain is a leading cause of disability within musculoskeletal disorders, ranking fourth and often leading to chronic pain syndromes that pose considerable clinical management challenges [7].

The increasing prevalence of musculoskeletal disorders, including neck pain, is compounded by population aging and the adoption of sedentary lifestyles [8]. These conditions constitute the foremost contributor to YLDs worldwide, accounting for approximately 149 million YLDs, or 17% of the global burden. Neck pain affects individuals across their lifespans, from young adulthood to advanced age, highlighting its extensive societal impact [1].

Clinical assessment of individuals presenting with neck pain commonly involves the evaluation of Cervical Range of Motion (CROM) to quantify the range of neck movement in various planes [9]. CROM is frequently employed as a baseline measurement prior to treatment planning, as well as for longitudinal monitoring of patient progress [10]. Individuals experiencing neck pain often have restricted CROM and may exhibit pain at the limits of motion [11]. Furthermore, these individuals may present compensatory trunk movements, either conscious or unconscious, in response to limited or painful neck movement [12].

CROM assessment quantifies the angular displacement of the neck within its planes of motion. Specifically, the sagittal plane, which bisects the body into left and right halves, encompasses flexion (anterior movement of the head, approximating the chin to the chest) and extension (posterior movement of the head, directing the gaze upwards). Angular measurement within this plane is commonly designated as pitch (see Figure 1). The transverse plane, dividing the body into superior and inferior segments, corresponds to rotational movement (axial rotation of the head to the left or right). Angular measurement within this plane is commonly designated as yaw (see Figure 1). Finally, the frontal plane, which partitions the body into anterior and posterior aspects, allows for lateral flexion (abduction of the head, approximating the ear to the shoulder). Angular measurement within this plane is commonly known as roll (see Figure 1).

Several instruments and methodologies are used to quantify cervical impairment. The goniometer remains a prevalent tool in clinical practice due to its portability, affordability, and ease of application [13]. This instrument facilitates the measurement of angular displacement within the sagittal (flexion–extension), transverse (rotation), and frontal (lateral flexion) planes. Despite the increasing availability of more advanced measurement systems, the goniometer continues to be widely used, especially in routine clinical assessments and in settings with limited access to high-cost equipment [14,15]. However, its inter-rater and intra-rater reliability has been reported to be moderate, with Intraclass Correlation Coefficient (ICC) values typically around 0.85 across movement directions [13,16].

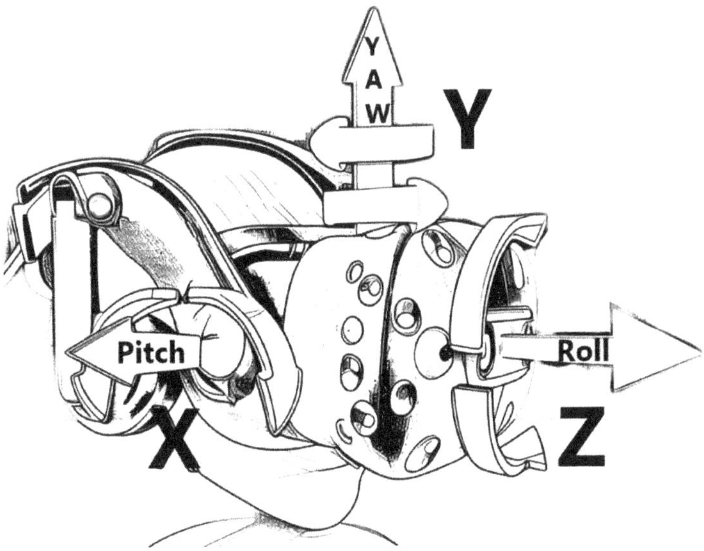

Figure 1. The assessment of Cervical Range of Motion (CROM) quantifies the angular displacement of the neck across its planes of movement. The Head-Mounted Display (HMD) supporting six degrees of freedom can capture movement along the X, Y, and Z axes, as well as rotation around each axis, commonly referred to as pitch (nodding), yaw (turning), and roll (tilting).

Alternative methodologies for CROM assessment include inclinometers, which operate by quantifying the angle of inclination relative to the vertical plane during cervical movements. These devices, available in both manual and digital configurations, provide a numerical representation of angular displacement across multiple planes [17,18]. Inertial measurement units (IMUs) have emerged as a promising technology for CROM assessment [19,20]. These compact, wireless sensors integrate accelerometers, gyroscopes, and magnetometers to track head kinematics and orientation in three-dimensional space. IMUs offer enhanced measurement reliability compared to goniometers and can be integrated into clinical protocols to quantify movement within the sagittal, transverse, and frontal planes. Furthermore, specialized CROM devices [17,21–24], incorporating integrated inclinometers and magnetometers, provide measurements of cervical motion across all planes.

Inertial sensors [19,20], electromagnetic tracking systems [25], and CROM devices [22] have demonstrated higher reproducibility and measurement precision. Inertial sensors have shown ICC values above 0.95 in most cases [20], while CROM devices present slightly more variable results, with reported ICCs ranging from 0.83 (for flexion–extension) to over 0.89 (for rotation and lateral flexion) [22]. These instruments offer greater reliability but also involve higher costs and operational complexity. Inclinometers [17] and electronic goniometers are also used in clinical and research settings, with digital versions generally offering improved performance. Reported ICCs for inclinometers range from 0.68 to 0.80 [17], while digital inclinometers tend to yield values above 0.85, showing better consistency [26]. Furthermore, photogrammetry techniques [27] and radiographic imaging [28] have been employed primarily in research environments due to their high cost, lack of portability, and need for complex setups. More recently, virtual reality (VR)-based systems have gained attention for their potential to combine immersive environments with accurate motion tracking [29–31]. These systems have shown high reliability in CROM assessment, with ICC values comparable to those of inertial systems (e.g., 0.94 for flexion–extension,

0.96 for rotation, and 0.91 for lateral flexion [31]), supporting their use in both clinical and experimental contexts.

The majority of prior investigations on the neck's functional status have primarily focused on evaluating the maximal cervical excursions exhibited by participants, representing the full active range of motion (ROM) [20,32–34]. While total ROM serves as a practical and straightforward metric for movement analysis, it offers a limited representation of functional capacity, as most activities of daily living (ADLs) do not necessitate maximal ROM [35]. For instance, previous research has questioned the clinical relevance of reductions in total ROM following cervical spine fusion with respect to ADLs and overall quality of life (QoL). The movement amplitudes required for ADLs are generally considered to be substantially lower than the full active ROM. Moreover, despite the utility of conventional methodologies in quantifying cervical movement, they frequently fail to capture clinically pertinent aspects such as movement speed, smoothness, trajectory, and compensatory trunk movements (consciously or unconsciously executed to alleviate pain or facilitate movement). Consequently, the diagnostic utility of CROM assessment as an isolated metric has been challenged, as some studies have provided limited evidence supporting its role in the diagnosis of specific cervical pathologies. This has fueled a growing interest in the development of alternative approaches that provide a more comprehensive representation of cervical spine function in real-world contexts [35–37].

CROM has been documented during various ADLs, including door manipulation, desk-based writing, and telephone usage. However, these findings were derived from a limited cohort of healthy university students utilizing multiple head-mounted inclinometers during experimental trials. The manual operation of these devices required the interruption of participant movements to allow the observer to take readings from the device indicators, thereby restricting data acquisition to static neck positions at the end of each activity [33]. In a more recent study, CROM was assessed during ADLs in 60 asymptomatic subjects aged 20 to 75 years. Using a noninvasive electrogoniometer and torsiometer, the full and functional Cervical ROM required to complete these simulated ADLs was measured. The results showed that, overall, ADLs require a relatively small percentage of total Cervical ROM. For example, when backing up a car, 32% of sagittal motion, 26% of lateral motion, and 92% of rotation were used. Activities related to personal hygiene, such as washing hands and hair, shaving, and applying makeup, involved significantly higher ROM compared to locomotor activities such as walking and ascending or descending stairs. These findings provide reference data that can allow clinicians to accurately assess the impact of the functional status of the neck on ADLs and to design therapies more focused on improving a patient's performance when performing ADLs and therefore a patient's quality of life [35].

A VR Head-Mounted Display (HMD) facilitates the continuous tracking of three-dimensional head position and rotation over time [38]. This tracking system provides six degrees of freedom (6DoF), encompassing both translational and rotational kinematics of the HMD (see Figure 1). The kinematic data, including three-dimensional position, orientation, and temporal timestamps, can be recorded continuously throughout the virtual reality experience. This methodology enables the uninterrupted measurement of CROM while participants engage in ADLs within a virtual environment (VE), thereby eliminating the need for movement interruption during data acquisition.

VR environments offer a unique advantage: they enable immersive and standardized assessment protocols that can be executed autonomously. In such systems, the VR experience guides users through specific cervical movements while simultaneously capturing motion data [31]. Through this motion data capture, it is possible to ensure that controlled repetitive movements of the neck joints during rehabilitation are performed properly, allowing recovery times to be shortened and improving the success of treatment [10].

These capabilities significantly enhance the potential of VR for telematic applications, including remote assessment, diagnosis, rehabilitation, and follow-up of cervical impairments. Recent studies have demonstrated the efficacy of VR-based interventions in improving Cervical Range of Motion, reducing pain, and enhancing functional outcomes in patients with chronic neck pain [39,40]. These findings underscore the viability of VR as a comprehensive tool in the telemanagement of cervical conditions.

Previous studies have demonstrated that VR setups are a reliable tool for measuring maximum CROM [31,41]. One of the advantages of VR technology is its relatively flat learning curve, allowing individuals with or without prior anatomical knowledge to use an HMD for cervical spine assessment. The objective of this observational cross-sectional study was to compare head kinematics between patients with chronic neck pain and asymptomatic participants during the performance of functional tasks in an immersive VR environment. To achieve this objective, we aimed to design a novel VR immersive experience to allow for the analysis of head kinematics during the performance of a whole-body functional task. Specifically, participants were required to retrieve virtual apples from simulated trees within a VE, utilizing natural head and neck movements to complete the task. The apple-harvesting task was chosen because it involves multiplanar movements, including whole-body movements in response to external stimuli for a duration that lasts a few minutes. This allows for a functional assessment that more closely resembles the ADLs a subject performs in their everyday life and aligns with previous recommendations for further research to examine neck kinematics for additional functional tasks [42].

Apples are located at various heights in the trees, and some may have fallen to the ground. The user is surrounded by trees; thus, she needs to search around for apples, pick them, and put them in a basket. We recorded the three-dimensional head kinematics of 60 participants (30 with clinically significant neck pain and 30 asymptomatic) during the apple retrieval task. Subsequently, we conducted a comparative analysis utilizing spectrograms generated from the head movement in its three motion planes to investigate whether participants with pain exhibited diminished movement speed compared to the pain-free cohort. The analysis shows that subjects without neck pain performed faster movements and required less time to complete the task compared to those with neck pain; these differences were statistically significant.

2. Materials and Methods

2.1. Participants

This was a descriptive, observational, cross-sectional study. It was conducted at CEU San Pablo University and received approval from the CEU San Pablo University Ethics Committee (approval code: 495/21/39). The study involved 60 participants, 30 individuals with neck pain and 30 asymptomatic individuals. They were recruited from the university's student and faculty population, as well as from patients at the university's polyclinic.

The inclusion criteria for the neck pain group required self-reported non-specific mechanical cervical pain of at least 3 months' duration and a pain intensity rating of 4 or higher on the 10-point numerical rating Visual Analogue Scale (VAS) [43] (see Section 2.4 for details). This cut-off value was selected to exclude patients with no pain or mild levels of pain, as usually pain intensity lower than 4/10 in VAS is considered mild [44,45]. Participants in the neck pain group were permitted to report concomitant headaches or upper cervical/shoulder discomfort. Exclusion criteria included a history of craniocervical surgery; bony deformities in the thoracic, cervical, or cranial region; vertigo/dizziness; and complex regional syndrome. Participants in the pain group had a mean neck pain intensity of 5.79 ± 1.38 on the VAS at the time of evaluation. The asymptomatic group consisted of participants reporting no cervical pain within the preceding three months and no history of neck pain treatment.

2.2. Experimental Setup

For this study, we utilized the HTC Vive Pro Eye™HMD (HTC Corporation, Taoyuan, Taiwan), a high-end VR system. The device features a dual OLED display with a combined resolution of 2880 × 1600 pixels (1440 × 1600 per eye). It offers a 110-degree field of view and a refresh rate of 90 Hz. The system includes SteamVR™ 2.0 tracking with two Lighthouse™ v2 base stations (Valve Corporation, Bellevue, WA, USA), which allow for precise 6DoF motion tracking, enabling accurate head movement recording.

The VR environment was powered by an HP OMEN™ laptop (HP Inc., Palo Alto, CA, USA) equipped with an Intel® Core™ i7-10750H processor, 16GB of RAM, and an 8GB NVIDIA® GeForce® RTX™ 2070 Super GPU. The system operated on Windows® 10 and ran the VR environment using SteamVR™. The experimental setup included a custom-developed VR application designed to simulate an apple-harvesting task described in the next section.

The Lighthouse™ v2 (Valve Corporation, USA) base stations provide precise positional and orientational tracking of the HMD. By detecting the temporal disparities in the illumination of photodiodes on the HMD and hand controllers via a sweeping laser array, these base stations provide the three-dimensional spatial data. This technology enhances the precision in capturing subtle and rapid user kinematics, thereby improving immersion through the accurate registration of virtual elements, such as picking apples in the apple-harvesting task within the VE. The configuration of the virtual scene is predicated solely on the initial physical position of the HMD, thereby ensuring a consistent and immersive representation of the simulated environment. An earlier study by the authors utilizing this same virtual reality equipment showed that, when used to assess maximum CROM in each plane, this setup had more reliability than a traditional goniometer [31].

2.3. Task Design

The Virtual Reality Toolkit (VRTK) is a collection of solutions to assist in the creation of VR applications [46]. As part of its demonstration capabilities, the VRTK includes a "Farmyard" example that showcases various locomotion systems, interaction paradigms, and control methodologies. This example features a range of activities set within a farmyard environment, such as a workshop scenario where users are required to place tools in their designated positions. It also incorporates diverse movement modalities and interactive objects, including a manipulable and fireable pistol, alongside several other items enabling user interaction.

The virtual reality application employed in this study is a modified version of VRTK v4 Beta's Farmyard example, specifically adapted to focus on the retrieval of apples from different trees. This version was developed using the Unity® 2018.4.33 engine.

At the beginning of the activity, the participant is positioned at the center of a virtual orchard consisting of three apple trees arranged in a triangular formation, one located anterior-right, one anterior-left, and one posterior. Each tree is located approximately 1.5 m from a central basket placed on the ground that is also placed near the participant, serving as the receptacle for the collected apples (see Figure 2d). A non-player character (NPC), represented as a farmer and positioned in front of the participant, provides visual instructions via floating text in Spanish (see Figure 2a). The NPC first welcomes the participant and explains the task, noting that some apples may also appear on the ground. Participants are instructed to collect the apples—using the grip button on either VR controller—and place them in the basket. Upon successful placement of an apple in the basket, another apple will spawn in a different location, and this process is repeated until a total of sixteen apples have been collected. Once all sixteen apples have been deposited, the NPC signals the completion of the task and expresses gratitude (see Figure 2a).

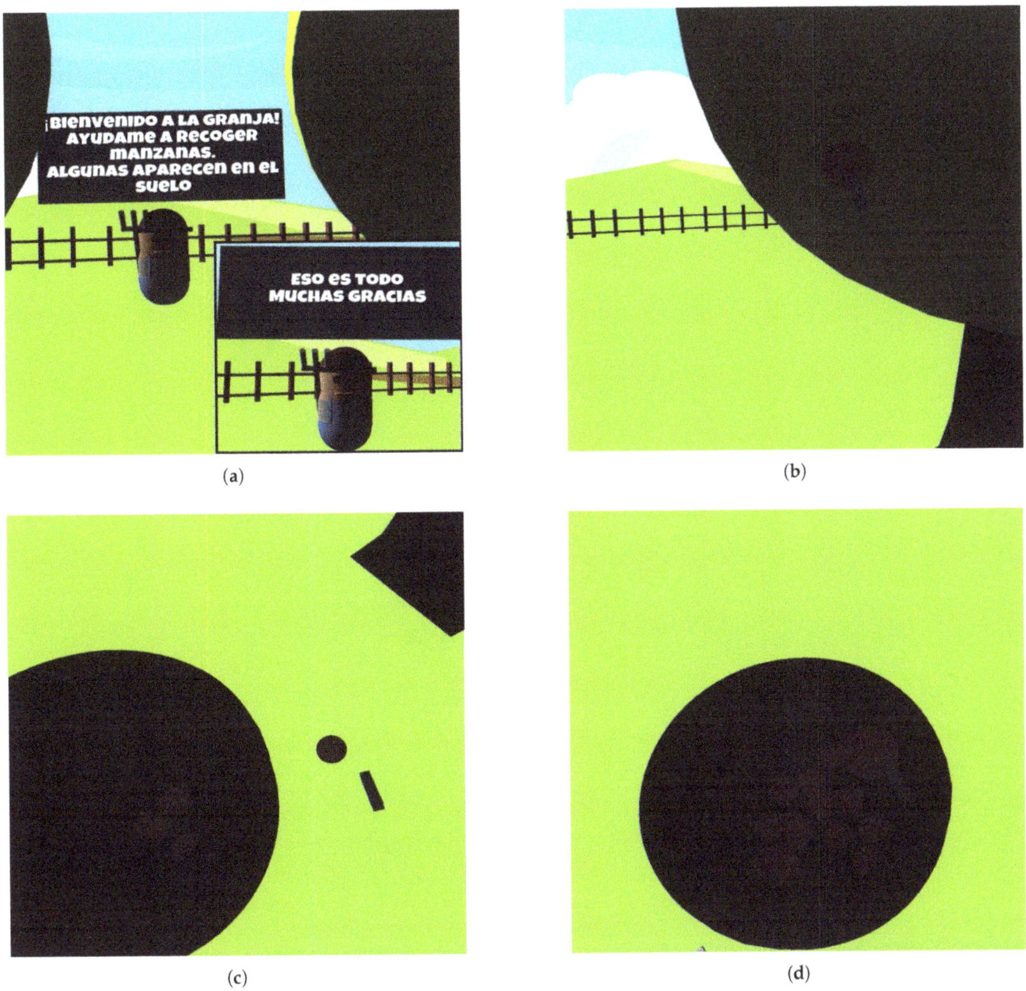

Figure 2. Images from the apple harvesting app used: (**a**) A farmer holding a sign that indicates the start and end of the task and provides instructions (In Spanish: "Welcome to the Farm! Help me collect apples. Some may appear on the ground." & "That's all, thank you very much.") for carrying out the task. (**b**) An apple that appears on a tree. (**c**) An apple that appears on the ground. (**d**) The basket where harvested apples are stored. Once an apple is placed in the basket, a new apple appears in one of the trees surrounding the user or on the ground.

The apple spawning sequence is predefined and identical for all participants to ensure experimental consistency. As part of an initial familiarization phase, the first four apples appear in each of the four possible locations: the first on the anterior-right tree (see Figure 2b), the second on the anterior-left tree, the third on the posterior tree, and the fourth on the ground (see Figure 2c). After this initial phase, the remaining twelve apples appear in varying order across the same four locations, ensuring that each tree and the ground hosts a total of four apples by the end of the task. Although the complete spawning sequence does not follow an obvious pattern (thus minimizing learning effects), all participants encounter the same distribution and order throughout the session. The positions of all apples are fixed and predefined in a comma-separated value (CSV) configuration file.

To ensure that all apples are within reach, the system calculates the user's initial head position using the HMD at the start of the session. Apple positions are then determined by applying fixed normalized vectors relative to this reference point. For arboreal apples, these vectors are anchored at the center of each tree's foliage, placing the apples visibly within the canopy and oriented toward the participant. Apples that spawn on the ground appear near the user's starting position. This approach ensures a standardized, visible, and accessible configuration for all users.

2.4. Data Collection and Measurement

Data collection was carried out in two different locations: in a lab at CEU San Pablo University and at its university polyclinic. This approach aimed to increase the sample size and ensure a more diverse participant pool. To standardize the setup across locations and minimize environmental variability, a 2 × 2 m area was marked on the floor at both sites. The VR base stations were placed in opposite corners of this area (front-left and back-right) to maximize motion capture coverage and ensure consistent tracking of head and neck movements across all participants (see Figure 3).

All participants provided their informed consent prior to the assessment. Subsequently, they completed a Visual Analogue Scale (VAS) questionnaire to assess pain levels [43]. VAS is a validated tool for assessing both acute and chronic pain. Participants indicate their pain intensity by placing a handwritten mark on a 10-centimeter line, which represents a continuum ranging from "no pain" to "worst pain imaginable". This method allows for a nuanced representation of pain levels, capturing the subjective experience of pain in a straightforward and effective manner. The information gathered from this questionnaire was used to classify participants into the appropriate study groups based on their reported neck pain at the time of measurement.

Before placing the HMD on the participant, a brief explanation of the task was provided. Participants were informed that they would be required to collect apples using the VR controllers and that the grip button on either hand should be used to grab each apple. No time constraints or speed-related goals were given, and participants were instructed to perform the task at their own pace and to move freely within the environment to reach the apples. The game mechanics appeared to be intuitive and engaging, allowing participants to complete the task without requiring additional instructions [47]. This ensured that movements performed during the task were as natural as possible, facilitating the assessment of functional Cervical ROM.

The HTC Vive Pro Eye™ continuously recorded head position and orientation during the task, capturing movements across the three CROM axes (see Figure 1). Headset and hand positions and rotations were tracked and saved at a sampling frequency of 50 Hz. The system uses Valve's SteamVR™ Lighthouse technology. The Lighthouse base stations emit structured infrared signals and sweeping laser beams, which are detected by photodiodes embedded on the surface of the HMD, controllers, and, when available, additional trackers. The timing differences in laser detection across photodiodes allow the system to calculate the position and orientation of the HMD and controllers in space, providing six degrees of freedom (three translational and three rotational). Additionally, the timestamps of when the apples are picked up and placed in the basket were also recorded for later analysis. To maintain consistency, the system was calibrated before each session, setting a neutral head position as the baseline reference. By allowing continuous motion recording throughout the task, this approach eliminated the need for manual readings or static postures [33], providing a more realistic and functional evaluation of cervical mobility.

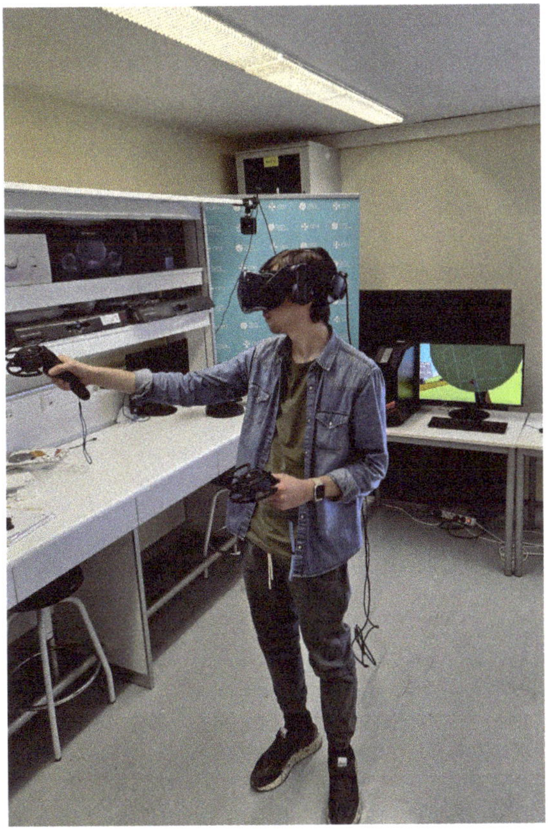

Figure 3. The image depicts a user performing the apple-harvesting task in the VE. The user is wearing an HMD and holding controllers within the designated measurement area, a 2 × 2 m open space. This area was physically marked at the measurement site. In the corner, one of the base stations can be seen, enabling precise tracking within the environment.

The recorded sessions, encompassing the entirety of each evaluation, were stored in 60 CSV files [48]. These are divided into two groups: "Group A" for asymptomatic participants and "Group B" for participants experiencing neck pain. Each file has a variable length, reflecting the differing durations of the session of each subject, and contains the following data elements: sample index, timestamp, device identifier (denoted as "H" for the Head-Mounted Display (HMD), "L" for the left controller, and "R" for the right controller), three-dimensional spatial coordinates in meters (designated as "X", "Y", "Z"), rotation quaternion components ("qX", "qY", "qZ", "qW"), and corresponding Euler angles for orientation ("x", "y", "z"). Furthermore, the instantiation and collection of virtual apples within the simulation were logged in this format: sample index, timestamp, and apple event (indicated as either "spawned" or "stored", along with a numerical identifier ranging from 0 to 15). All data processing was performed using MATLAB™ R2023b. A GitHub® repository containing the raw data from the 60 participants in the study, as well as the code to analyze the data, can be found at [48].

2.5. Spectral Analysis

The objective of spectral analysis is to quantify the number of slower, smoother movements and faster, more abrupt movements that each subject performs during the apple-harvesting task. Our hypothesis is that subjects with neck pain will perform slower movements than healthy subjects. To quantify the number of slow movements, spectral power will be calculated in the [0, 0.1] band, and for fast movements, spectral power will be calculated in the [0.1, 0.5] band. These two spectral power bands fall within the frequency ranges clearly associated with voluntary motor control [49]. Movements occurring outside the subjects' voluntary motor control will also be quantified by calculating the spectral power in the [0.5, 5] band [50]. All these calculations will be performed for each of the three planes of motion (frontal, transverse, and sagittal planes), as well as for the total three-dimensional movement. The detailed methodology for these calculations is explained below.

The data from the HMD and the apple positions were extracted from the CSV files. To prevent the time series of angles from containing fluctuations between $180°$ and $-180°$ degrees, which correspond to small movements around that position, a wrap angle function was applied such that $180°$ mapped to $180°$ and $-180°$ also mapped to $-180°$. Based on the angle of rotation in each plane, the magnitude of the three-dimensional head rotation was also computed for each subject.

For each recording, four spectrograms were computed: one for the movement in each plane and one for the total movement. A spectrogram depicts the frequency spectrum of a signal over time, with three axes: time, frequency, and magnitude (or power) at specific time-frequency points, calculated using the Short-Time Fourier Transform (STFT). Prior to spectrogram computation, the mean value was subtracted from each time series. To calculate the spectrogram, the signal was segmented into 512-sample sections (approximately 10 s in duration). A Hamming window function was applied to each of these segments. Subsequently, the Fast Fourier Transform (FFT) was calculated for each windowed section, thus obtaining the frequency content of that portion of the signal. This process was repeated throughout the entire signal, shifting the window by 128 samples at each step (approximately 2.5 s), which corresponds to a 384-sample overlap between consecutive segments. The result is a representation of how the signal's power spectral density varies in time and frequency. To obtain the spectral power in each band, the average of the absolute value of the spectrogram's spectral components falling within each band's ranges was calculated.

A custom function, "CustomPlotSpectrogram", was developed to visualize the results in a 2D top-down view, with color limits set between -10 and 90 decibels to facilitate magnitude comparisons across subjects [48]. By default, MATLAB™ adjusts the color scale used in spectrogram visualization based on the minimum and maximum power values present in that spectrogram. This prevents direct visual comparisons between two spectrograms. Our custom function fixes these limits to constant values for all spectrograms of all subjects, thus allowing the comparison of spectrograms from different subjects. The custom function also adds white vertical lines to mark the moments when apples were stored. As explained in the previous section, the log generated by the virtual reality application includes "apple stored" events, along with a timestamp indicating when each event occurred. This timestamp is used to draw the white vertical lines on the spectrogram's temporal axis to mark the moments when apples were stored. Figure 4 shows the spectrograms of a healthy subject and of a pain-affected subject. The axes units are time (seconds), frequency (Hz), and magnitude (dB/Hz).

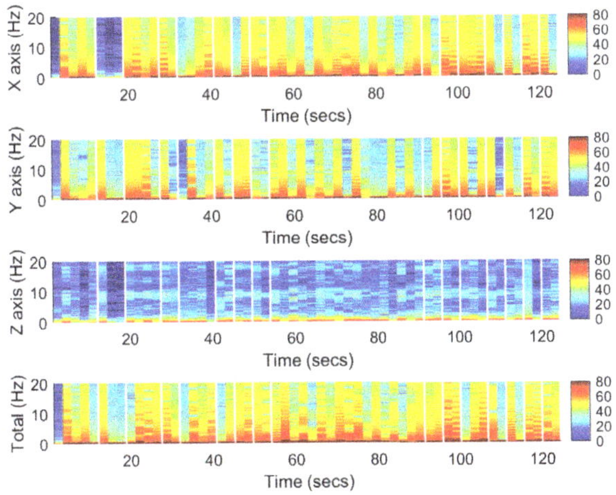

(**a**)

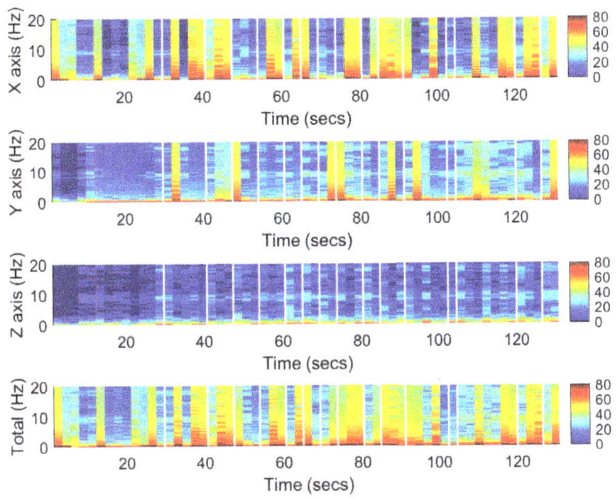

(**b**)

Figure 4. (**a**) The spectrogram of a healthy subject. (**b**) The spectrogram of a pain-affected subject. The vertical white lines correspond to the moments when apples are stored. The spectrograms show more power in the higher spectral components in the patients without neck pain.

2.6. Statistical Analysis

A statistical analysis was performed to characterize and quantify the variations in spectral power derived from the spectrogram data. From the spectrograms, the average spectral power for each subject was computed for three distinct frequency bands. The first band, spanning [0, 0.1] Hz, corresponds to relatively slow movements. The second band encompasses the range [0.1, 0.5] Hz, including rapid movements. These two frequency bands correspond to voluntary movements under the conscious control of the subject [49]. The third band extends from [0.5, 5] Hz and includes high-frequency movements outside the domain of voluntary postural control [50]. The initial 30 s of each spectrogram were excluded to mitigate the influence of quiescent periods, as these segments likely represent the participants' acclimation phase to the virtual reality environment and do not accurately reflect their natural movement kinematics. In Figure 4 it can be seen how at the beginning of the task, in all planes of movement and in the total movement, there is a greater prevalence of low frequencies (blue color) than for the rest of the task for both the subject with pain and the subject without pain.

To ascertain the presence of statistically significant differences in average spectral power between the two groups across the various frequency bands, a statistical analysis was conducted. First, the assumption of normality for the spectral power data within each group and for each frequency band was assessed using the Anderson–Darling test. This test was chosen for its sensitivity in detecting deviations from normality, particularly at the tails of the distribution. The null hypothesis for this test is that the data follow a normal distribution. If the Anderson–Darling test indicated that the data from both groups for a given frequency band were normally distributed, an independent-sample t-test was employed. Conversely, if the data in one or both groups for a given frequency band significantly deviated from a normal distribution, the non-parametric Mann–Whitney U test was utilized.

This methodology was applied to each of the three frequency bands for each of the four time series of head rotation (rotation in each of the three planes and total rotation). This involves the application of a total of 12 statistical tests. To mitigate the risk of spurious findings arising from multiple statistical comparisons, the False Discovery Rate (FDR) correction was applied to the resultant p-values obtained across all statistical tests [51]. This correction ranks the p-values in ascending order and then compares each p-value to a critical value that depends on its rank and the total number of tests. This method controls the expected proportion of significant results that are false positives, providing a set of FDR-adjusted p-values. This approach ensures greater validity and reliability of the findings, particularly in exploratory analyses involving numerous comparisons, as is the case of the analysis presented in this study.

The same procedure of normality testing and hypothesis evaluation was applied to the analysis of recording duration, to test for statistically significant differences in the time required by the subjects with and without pain to complete the apple-harvesting task.

2.7. System's Usability

To evaluate the usability of the VR experience, the Spanish version of the System Usability Scale (SUS) was employed [52]. This tool provides a straightforward method for users and researchers to evaluate usability, generating a single, easily interpretable score [53].

The SUS consists of ten alternating positive and negative statements, which participants rate from 1 ("Strongly Disagree") to 5 ("Strongly Agree"). The scores are calculated by adjusting the ratings for odd-numbered (positive) and even-numbered (negative) items, resulting in a total score ranging from 0 to 40. This total is then multiplied by 2.5 to create a scale from 0 to 100 [54]. A score between 68 and 84 indicates acceptable usability, while scores above 85 reflect excellent usability [52]. After completing the apple-harvesting task, participants anonymously filled out the SUS questionnaire to provide feedback on their VR experience.

3. Results

Table 1 shows the demographic characteristics of the participants in Groups A and B, with a total of 60 individuals included in the study. Group A consists of 14 women with an average age of (42 ± 14) years, a height of (166 ± 8) cm, and a weight of (65 ± 10) kg, alongside 16 men with a mean age of (29 ± 12) years, a height of (180 ± 6) cm, and a weight of (83 ± 19) kg. Group B comprises 21 women with a mean age of (31 ± 14) years, a height of (168 ± 8) cm, and a weight of (65 ± 12) kg, along with 9 men averaging (36 ± 15) years of age, (179 ± 8) cm in height, and (78 ± 14) kg in weight.

Table 1. Demographic characteristics of participants in Groups A and B.

Group	Gender	N	Age (Years)	Height (cm)	Weight (kg)
A	Women	14	41.57 ± 13.51	165.50 ± 7.79	64.57 ± 10.21
	Men	16	29.44 ± 12.25	180.38 ± 5.72	83.06 ± 19.28
	Total	30	35.10 ± 14.45	173.43 ± 10.21	74.43 ± 18.53
B	Women	21	30.67 ± 14.12	167.57 ± 8.19	64.76 ± 12.17
	Men	9	36.11 ± 14.51	178.89 ± 7.50	78.33 ± 14.13
	Total	30	32.30 ± 14.70	170.97 ± 9.69	68.83 ± 14.47
Total	Women	35	35.03 ± 15.09	166.74 ± 8.21	64.69 ± 11.59
	Men	25	31.84 ± 13.77	179.84 ± 6.59	81.36 ± 18.12
	Total	60	33.70 ± 14.52	172.20 ± 9.95	71.63 ± 16.72

Values are presented as mean ± standard deviation.

Table 2 shows the average spectral power for the 30 subjects without neck pain, for each of the three frequency bands, for each of the three planes of motion, and for the total movement. Table 3 shows the same information for the 30 subjects suffering from neck pain. The p-values of the statistical comparisons, after applying the FDR correction, can be found in Table 4.

The p-values presented in Table 4 indicate statistically significant differences in spectral power for the [0.1, 0.5] Hz band along the y-axis and the z-axis, as well as for total movement ($p = 0.0384$ in all the cases). These findings reveal that movements within this frequency range differ significantly between subjects with and without pain. No statistically significant differences were observed for any of the movement planes or for the total movement within the [0, 0.1] Hz and [0.5, 5] Hz frequency bands.

Table 2. Average spectral power and standard deviation for subjects without neck pain.

Frequency Bands	x-Axis	y-Axis	z-Axis	Total
[0, 0.1]	2.779 ± 0.858	9.348 ± 2.251	3.762 ± 1.165	5.274 ± 1.615
[0.1, 0.5]	5.793 ± 1.276	20.141 ± 2.611 *	7.898 ± 1.703 *	11.781 ± 1.579 *
[0.5, 5]	4.010 ± 0.803	24.463 ± 11.088	4.759 ± 0.951	8.309 ± 1.554

Values are presented as average spectral power (in 10^4 dB/Hz) ± standard deviation. * Indicates statistically significant differences.

Table 3. Average spectral power and standard deviation for subjects with neck pain.

Frequency Bands	x-Axis	y-Axis	z-Axis	Sum
[0, 0.1]	3.042 ± 0.795	10.476 ± 2.505	3.997 ± 1.303	5.201 ± 0.977
[0.1, 0.5]	5.473 ± 1.129	18.289 ± 2.672 *	6.777 ± 1.414 *	10.621 ± 1.676 *
[0.5, 5]	3.497 ± 1.093	23.866 ± 10.376	4.170 ± 1.380	7.438 ± 2.224

Values are presented as average spectral power (in 10^4 dB/Hz) ± standard deviation. * Indicates statistically significant differences.

The average time to accomplish the task for subjects with neck pain was (138.7 ± 43.4) seconds compared to (119.6 ± 23.8) seconds for those without pain. The Mann–Whitney U test indicated a statistically significant difference in task duration (p-value of 0.039) between the groups.

Table 4. Corrected p-values (using FDR) for each spectral band from the statistical tests assessing differences in average spectral power between subjects with neck pain and subjects without neck pain.

Frequency Bands (Hz)	x-Axis	y-Axis	z-Axis	Total
[0, 0.1]	0.2119	0.1438	0.5586	0.8883
[0.1, 0.5]	0.4100	0.0348	0.0348	0.0348
[0.5, 5]	0.1289	0.8883	0.1419	0.1438

The usability assessment using the SUS yielded an overall score of (84.21 ± 9.49), indicating a high level of user satisfaction with the virtual reality system used for the apple-harvesting task. This score falls between acceptable and excellent usability, suggesting that participants found the system intuitive and effective [52].

To study the possible influence of age on the usability of the virtual reality system, participants were divided into three age groups: young adults (18–25 years, n = 26), adults (26–45 years, n = 20), and individuals in later adulthood (46–65 years, n = 14). The normality assessment test indicated that the SUS score did not follow a normal distribution in all groups. Therefore, the non-parametric Kruskal–Wallis test was used to compare the medians of the SUS score between groups. The results indicated that there were no significant differences (p-value = 0.903). The means and standard deviations of the SUS scores were 84.1 ± 10.6 for the young group, 83.4 ± 9.7 for the adult group, and 85.5 ± 7.7 for the older group. These results indicate that the usability of the virtual reality experience is not affected by the user's age.

4. Discussion and Conclusions

The results of this study show that subjects with chronic neck pain exhibit consistently lower average spectral power in the [0.1, 0.5] Hz band for the y (transverse plane) and z (frontal plane) planes of motion and for the total movement when compared to asymptomatic controls (see Tables 2 and 3). These findings indicate that subjects without neck pain perform faster head movements in the frontal and transverse planes when performing a whole-body functional task. However, such a difference between groups was not observed for the sagittal plane. Tables 2 and 3 also show that the average spectral power in the [0, 0.1] Hz band is higher in subjects with neck pain for each of the three planes of motion compared to subjects without neck pain; however, these differences are not statistically significant (see Table 4). One interpretation of these data could be that subjects with neck pain, when rotating their heads to locate apples in the virtual trees, tend to do so more slowly than subjects without neck pain due to the pain they experience or the fear that the movement will induce pain.

The reduced head velocity seems to be aligned with previous evidence that has suggested that people with neck pain may have a slower head kinematics compared to asymptomatic individuals during functional movements [42]. However, there is little research analyzing functional tasks in individuals with neck pain that we could compare with our results. Moreover, to the best of our knowledge, there are no studies that share the same method of an immersive VR experience specifically designed for analyzing head kinematics during the performance of a complex whole-body functional task. Previous studies in the field have included analysis of neck or head motion during tasks such as walking [55], a typing task in sitting position [56], a VR game focused on isolated neck movements [57], or the task of transferring a weight with the upper limb [25].

The [0.5, 5] Hz frequency band captures very rapid movements outside the range of voluntary motor control. In this band, participants without neck pain again exhibit greater spectral power in the three planes of motion and in total movement, but these differences are not statistically significant (see Table 4). The meaning of this power band is difficult to interpret; however, a potential cause for these very rapid movements could be oscillations of the HMD due to a non-perfect fixation to the user's head. The HTC Vive Pro Eye™ is a relatively bulkier HMD, weighing 800 g with a somewhat uneven weight distribution, being significantly front-heavy. This can induce a high torque during the subject's rotational movements, potentially causing the HMD to continue rotating when the subject stops turning their neck in one direction [58]. The high torque caused by the weight and uneven weight distribution may lead to the HMD slipping relative to the subject's cranium, rotating more than the cranium, and subsequently returning to the original position due to the HMD's straps, causing vibrations and high-frequency movements. The fact that participants without neck pain exhibit faster movements (see Tables 2 and 3) would make this effect more pronounced in this group.

Subjects with neck pain required more time to collect the 16 apples in the virtual reality experience than subjects without neck pain (138.7 ± 43.4 s vs 119.6 ± 23.8 s), and this difference was statistically significant. This finding further suggests a greater slowness in the movements of subjects with neck pain and at the same time reflects a lower performance in the task of these subjects.

Regarding system usability, the SUS score obtained (84.21 ± 9.49) indicates that the experience is simple and intuitive. None of the subjects who used the experience reported adverse effects. This suggests that this virtual reality experience could be employed in the assessment of neck functional status without the need for assistance from a technician or a health professional. This could open doors to the use of the experience from a patient's home, allowing for remote assessment sessions as part of a virtual reality-based telerehabilitation program that integrates rehabilitation exercises and evaluation sessions for status monitoring and for adapting the rehabilitation exercises [59].

Currently, the evaluation of neck functional status is primarily based on the measurement of maximum ROM in the different planes. This assessment has little relation to the impact on a patient's ADLs [35–37], hence the interest in conducting assessments based on the quantification of metrics during the performance of ADLs, as proposed in this work. Although other studies have attempted to assess the neck during ADLs, these studies have used manual measurements that required the subject to stop at a point during task performance [33] or have employed electrogoniometers and torsiometers [35], which are more complex to use than a VR setup and require the use of physical objects and environments for patient assessment. The use of a VR experience allows for the simulation of these environments and objects, enabling activities (such as harvesting apples) that would not be feasible in a clinical setting or the patient's home. Furthermore, the use of VR provides an immersive and engaging environment that favors patient adherence to the treatment [60,61]. Although the current study included healthy individuals and participants with neck pain, the apple-harvesting task may be adapted for more impaired populations—such as frail older adults or individuals recovering from surgery—by modifying parameters like the location of the apples, required range of motion, or task duration. Future studies should explore the feasibility and usability of the system in these populations.

In this work, the spectral analysis has been proposed as a tool to assess kinematic differences between subjects with and without pain. This is based on the researchers' hypothesis that neck pain will influence movement smoothness, and thus acceleration, more than other metrics like velocity or range of motion. Nevertheless, it would be interesting to analyze in the future whether other types of metrics, different from spectral analysis, allow for a better functional assessment of the subjects.

The main limitation of the present study is the lack of quantification of compensatory movements performed with the trunk or the whole body [12]. It is possible that if compensatory movements had been captured and if the actual neck movement had been calculated by subtracting trunk rotation data from neck rotation data, there would have been more relevant differences in the spectral bands or more pronounced differences. In a future study, we intend to replicate the present study, employing a tracker on the subject's back to be able to analyze these compensatory movements. Furthermore, the differences in head kinematics between populations were analyzed through a cross-sectional study, so no inferences could be made in terms of causality. Future longitudinal research could provide more evidence on the possible causal direction of the relationship between head kinematics and the occurrence of the symptoms of neck pain.

Author Contributions: Conceptualization, R.G.-C., A.O. and A.M.-P.-Z.; methodology, R.G.-C., A.O. and A.M.-P.-Z.; software, Á.S.-P.; investigation, J.A.S.-P., E.B.-C. and F.M.; resources, R.G.-C. and A.O.; data curation, J.A.S.-P.; writing—original draft preparation, J.A.S.-P., R.G.-C. and A.O.; writing—review and editing, all the authors; supervision, R.G.-C. and A.O.; project administration, R.G.-C. and A.O.; funding acquisition, R.G.-C., A.O. and A.M.-P.-Z. All authors have read and agreed to the published version of the manuscript

Funding: This work was supported by the Spanish Ministry of Science, Innovation, and University under the grant European Regional Development Fund (ERDF), with project references IDI-20191120 and PID2021-127096OB-I00.

Institutional Review Board Statement: The study was conducted in accordance with the Declaration of Helsinki and approved by the Institutional Review Board (Ethics Committee) of the University San Pablo CEU (approval code: 495/21/39 on 22 March 2021).

Informed Consent Statement: Informed consent was obtained from all subjects involved in the study.

Data Availability Statement: The data and code supporting the results of this study are available at the following link: https://github.com/AbrahamOtero/FunctionalAssessmentOfTheNeck, accessed on 28 April 2025.

Conflicts of Interest: The authors declare no conflicts of interest.

Abbreviations

The following abbreviations are used in this manuscript:

6DoF	six degrees of freedom
ADLs	activities of daily living
CROM	Cervical Range of Motion
CSV	comma-separated value
ERDF	European Regional Development Fund
FDR	False Discovery Rate
FFT	Fast Fourier Transform
HMD	Head-Mounted Display
ICC	Intraclass Correlation Coefficient
IMUs	inertial measurement units
NPC	non-player character
QoL	quality of life
ROM	range of motion
STFT	Short-Time Fourier Transform
SUS	System Usability Scale
VAS	Visual Analogue Scale
VE	virtual environment
VR	virtual reality
VRTK	Virtual Reality ToolKit
YLDs	years lived with disability

References

1. World Health Organization. Musculoskeletal Conditions. 2022. Available online: https://www.who.int/news-room/fact-sheets/detail/musculoskeletal-conditions (accessed on 28 April 2025).
2. Disease, G.; Incidence, I.; Collaborators, P. Global, regional, and national incidence, prevalence, and years lived with disability for 354 diseases and injuries for 195 countries and territories, 1990–2017: A systematic analysis for the Global Burden of Disease Study 2017. *Lancet* **2018**, *392*, 1789–1858. Erratum in: *Lancet* **2019**, *393*, e44. [CrossRef]
3. Wu, H.; Li, Y.; Zou, C.; Guo, W.; Han, F.; Huang, G.; Sun, L. Global burden of neck pain and its gender and regional inequalities from 1990–2021: A comprehensive analysis from the Global Burden of Disease Study 2021. *BMC Musculoskelet. Disord.* **2025**, *26*, 94. [CrossRef] [PubMed]
4. GBD 2021 Neck Pain Collaborators. Global, regional, and national burden of neck pain, 1990–2020, and projections to 2050: A systematic analysis of the Global Burden of Disease Study 2021. *Lancet Rheumatol.* **2024**, *6*, e142–e155. [CrossRef] [PubMed]
5. Hoy, D.; March, L.; Woolf, A.; Blyth, F.; Brooks, P.; Smith, E.; Vos, T.; Barendregt, J.; Blore, J.; Murray, C.; et al. The global burden of neck pain: Estimates from the Global Burden of Disease 2010 study. *Ann. Rheum. Dis.* **2014**, *73*, 1309–1315. [CrossRef]
6. Hogg-Johnson, S.; van der Velde, G.; Carroll, L.J.; Holm, L.W.; Cassidy, J.D.; Guzman, J.; Côté, P.; Haldeman, S.; Ammendolia, C.; Carragee, E.; et al. The burden and determinants of neck pain in the general population: Results of the Bone and Joint Decade 2000–2010 Task Force on Neck Pain and Its Associated Disorders. *J. Manip. Physiol. Ther.* **2009**, *32*, S46–S60. [CrossRef]
7. Cohen, S.P. Epidemiology, diagnosis, and treatment of neck pain. *Mayo Clin. Proc.* **2015**, *90*, 284–299. [CrossRef]
8. Kazeminasab, S.; Nejadghaderi, S.A.; Amiri, P.; Pourfathi, H.; Araj-Khodaei, M.; Sullman, M.J.; Kolahi, A.A.; Safiri, S. Neck pain: Global epidemiology, trends and risk factors. *BMC Musculoskelet. Disord.* **2022**, *23*, 26. [CrossRef]
9. Sarig-Bahat, H.; Weiss, P.L.; Laufer, Y. Neck pain assessment in a virtual environment. *Spine* **2010**, *35*, E105–E112. [CrossRef]
10. Mareş, S.; Deaconescu, A.; Deaconescu, T. Pneumatically Actuated Rehabilitation Equipment for the Sagittal and Frontal Plane Movements of the Neck Joint. *Technologies* **2025**, *13*, 39. [CrossRef]
11. Stenneberg, M.S.; Rood, M.; de Bie, R.; Schmitt, M.A.; Cattrysse, E.; Scholten-Peeters, G.G. To what degree does active cervical range of motion differ between patients with neck pain, patients with whiplash, and those without neck pain? A systematic review and meta-analysis. *Arch. Phys. Med. Rehabil.* **2017**, *98*, 1407–1434. [CrossRef]
12. Van der Kruk, E.; Silverman, A.K.; Koizia, L.; Reilly, P.; Fertleman, M.; Bull, A.M.J. Age-related compensation: Neuromusculoskeletal capacity, reserve & movement objectives. *J. Biomech.* **2021**, *122*, 110385. [CrossRef]
13. Swinkels, R.A.; Swinkels-Meewisse, I.E. Normal values for cervical range of motion. *Spine* **2014**, *39*, 362–367. [CrossRef] [PubMed]

14. Reynolds, J.; Marsh, D.; Koller, H.; Zenenr, J.; Bannister, G. Cervical range of movement in relation to neck dimension. *Eur. Spine J.* **2009**, *18*, 863–868. [CrossRef]
15. Williams, M.A.; McCarthy, C.J.; Chorti, A.; Cooke, M.W.; Gates, S. A systematic review of reliability and validity studies of methods for measuring active and passive cervical range of motion. *J. Manip. Physiol. Ther.* **2010**, *33*, 138–155. [CrossRef]
16. Luedtke, K.; Schoettker-Königer, T.; Hall, T.; Enns, C.; Grassold, M.; Hasselhoff-Styhler, P.; Reimer, C. Concurrent validity and reliability of measuring range of motion during the cervical flexion rotation test with a novel digital goniometer. *BMC Musculoskelet. Disord.* **2020**, *21*, 535. [CrossRef]
17. Ghorbani, F.; Kamyab, M.; Azadinia, F. Smartphone applications as a suitable alternative to CROM device and inclinometers in assessing the cervical range of motion in patients with nonspecific neck pain. *J. Chiropr. Med.* **2020**, *19*, 38–48. [CrossRef]
18. Prushansky, T.; Deryi, O.; Jabarreen, B. Reproducibility and validity of digital inclinometry for measuring cervical range of motion in normal subjects. *Physiother. Res. Int.* **2010**, *15*, 42–48. [CrossRef]
19. Chalimourdas, A.; Dimitriadis, Z.; Kapreli, E.; Strimpakos, N. Test-re-test reliability and concurrent validity of cervical active range of motion in young asymptomatic adults using a new inertial measurement unit device. *Expert Rev. Med. Devices* **2021**, *18*, 1029–1037. [CrossRef]
20. Raya, R.; Garcia-Carmona, R.; Sanchez, C.; Urendes, E.; Ramirez, O.; Martin, A.; Otero, A. An inexpensive and easy to use cervical range of motion measurement solution using inertial sensors. *Sensors* **2018**, *18*, 2582. [CrossRef]
21. Feng, M.; Liang, L.; Sun, W.; Liu, G.W.; Yin, X.; Han, T.; Wei, X.; Zhu, L. Measurements of cervical range of motion using an optical motion capture system: Repeatability and validity. *Exp. Ther. Med.* **2019**, *18*, 4193–4202. [CrossRef]
22. Oliveira-Souza, A.I.S.; Carvalho, G.F.; Florêncio, L.L.; Fernández-de Las-Peñas, C.; Dach, F.; Bevilaqua-Grossi, D. Intrarater and interrater reliability of the flexion rotation test and cervical range of motion in people with migraine. *J. Manip. Physiol. Ther.* **2020**, *43*, 874–881. [CrossRef] [PubMed]
23. Wolan-Nieroda, A.; Guzik, A.; Mocur, P.; Druzbicki, M.; Maciejczak, A. Assessment of Interrater and Intrarater Reliability of Cervical Range of Motion (CROM) goniometer. *BioMed Res. Int.* **2020**, *2020*, 8908035. [CrossRef] [PubMed]
24. Lutke Schipholt, I.J.; Scholten-Peeters, G.G.M.; Logghe, S.; Koop, M.; Donders, S.; Stenneberg, M.S.; Coppieters, M.W. The CROM-VAS Test: A novel and reliable clinical test to assess immediate pain relief following treatment for movement-evoked neck pain. *Musculoskelet. Sci. Pract.* **2024**, *74*, 103191. [CrossRef] [PubMed]
25. Tsang, S.M.; Szeto, G.P.; Lee, R.Y. Altered spinal kinematics and muscle recruitment pattern of the cervical and thoracic spine in people with chronic neck pain during functional task. *J. Electromyogr. Kinesiol.* **2014**, *24*, 104–113. [CrossRef]
26. Law, E.Y.; Chiu, T.T. Measurement of cervical range of motion (CROM) by electronic CROM goniometer: A test of reliability and validity. *J. Back Musculoskelet. Rehabil.* **2013**, *26*, 141–148. [CrossRef]
27. Janjua, M.B.; Zhou, P.L.; Vasquez-Montes, D.; Moskovich, R. Photogrammetric analysis: An objective measure to assess the craniocervical range of motion after cervical laminoplasty surgeries. *J. Clin. Neurosci.* **2020**, *71*, 76–83. [CrossRef]
28. Rousseau, M.A.; Laporte, S.; Chavary-Bernier, E.; Lazennec, J.Y.; Skalli, W. Reproducibility of measuring the shape and three-dimensional position of cervical vertebrae in upright position using the EOS stereoradiography system. *Spine* **2007**, *32*, 2569–2572. [CrossRef]
29. Kiper, P.; Baba, A.; Alhelou, M.; Pregnolato, G.; Maistrello, L.; Agostini, M.; Turolla, A. Assessment of the cervical spine mobility by immersive and nonimmersive virtual reality. *J. Electromyogr. Kinesiol.* **2020**, *51*, 102397. [CrossRef]
30. Xu, X.; Chen, K.B.; Lin, J.H.; Radwin, R.G. The accuracy of the Oculus Rift virtual reality head-mounted display during cervical spine mobility measurement. *J. Biomech.* **2015**, *48*, 721–724. [CrossRef]
31. Santos-Paz, J.A.; Sánchez-Picot, Á.; Rojo, A.; Martín-Pintado-Zugasti, A.; Otero, A.; Garcia-Carmona, R. A novel virtual reality application for autonomous assessment of cervical range of motion: Development and reliability study. *PeerJ* **2022**, *10*, e14031. [CrossRef]
32. De Loose, V.; Van den Oord, M.; Burnotte, F.; Van Tiggelen, D.; Stevens, V.; Cagnie, B.; Danneels, L.; Witvrouw, E. Functional assessment of the cervical spine in F-16 pilots with and without neck pain. *Aviat. Space Environ. Med.* **2009**, *80*, 477–481. [CrossRef] [PubMed]
33. Bennett, S.E.; Schenk, R.J.; Simmons, E.D. Active Range of Motion Utilized in the Cervical Spine to Perform Daily Functional Tasks. *J. Spinal Disord. Tech.* **2002**, *15*, 307–311. [CrossRef] [PubMed]
34. Janczyk, R.; Janczyk, M.; Sibiński, M.; Drobniewski, M. Functional assessment and evaluation of health problems with the cervical spine among dental assistants and hygienists. *PostępPy Psychiatr. Neurol.* **2023**, *32*, 68–75. [CrossRef]
35. Bible, J.E.; Biswas, D.; Miller, C.P.; Whang, P.G.; Grauer, J.N. Normal functional range of motion of the cervical spine during 15 activities of daily living. *J. Spinal Disord. Tech.* **2010**, *23*, 15–21. [CrossRef]
36. Matamala-Gomez, M.; Slater, M.; Sanchez-Vives, M.V. Impact of virtual embodiment and exercises on functional ability and range of motion in orthopedic rehabilitation. *Sci. Rep.* **2022**, *12*, 5046. [CrossRef]

37. Flores-Cortes, M.; Guerra-Armas, J.; Pineda-Galan, C.; La Touche, R.; Luque-Suarez, A. Sensorimotor uncertainty of immersive virtual reality environments for people in pain: Scoping review. *Brain Sci.* **2023**, *13*, 1461. [CrossRef]
38. Lim, C.H.; Lee, S.C. The Effects of Degrees of Freedom and Field of View on Motion Sickness in a Virtual Reality Context. *Int. J. Hum.-Comput. Interact.* **2023**, *40*, 5884–5896. [CrossRef]
39. Guo, Q.; Zhang, L.; Han, L.; Gui, C.; Chen, G.; Ling, C.; Wang, W.; Gao, Q. Effects of Virtual Reality Therapy Combined With Conventional Rehabilitation on Pain, Kinematic Function, and Disability in Patients With Chronic Neck Pain: Randomized Controlled Trial. *JMIR Serious Games* **2024**, *12*, e42829. [CrossRef]
40. Nusser, M.; Kramer, M.; Knapp, S.; Krischak, G. Effects of virtual reality-based neck-specific sensorimotor training in patients with chronic neck pain compared with general sensorimotor training and a standard rehabilitation programme: A randomized controlled pilot trial. *J. Rehabil. Med.* **2021**, *53*, jrm00151. [CrossRef]
41. Trinidad-Fernández, M.; Bossavit, B.; Salgado-Fernández, J.; Abbate-Chica, S.; Fernández-Leiva, A.J.; Cuesta-Vargas, A.I. Head-Mounted Display for Clinical Evaluation of Neck Movement Validation with Meta Quest 2. *Sensors* **2023**, *23*, 3077. [CrossRef]
42. Moghaddas, D.; de Zoete, R.M.J.; Edwards, S.; Snodgrass, S.J. Differences in the kinematics of the cervical and thoracic spine during functional movement in individuals with or without chronic neck pain: A systematic review. *Physiotherapy* **2019**, *105*, 421–433. [CrossRef] [PubMed]
43. Delgado, D.A.; Lambert, B.S.; Boutris, N.; McCulloch, P.C.; Robbins, A.B.; Moreno, M.R.; Harris, J.D. Validation of Digital Visual Analog Scale Pain Scoring With a Traditional Paper-based Visual Analog Scale in Adults. *J. Am. Acad. Orthop. Surg. Glob. Res. Rev.* **2018**, *2*, e088. [CrossRef] [PubMed]
44. Boonstra, A.M.; Preuper, H.R.S.; Balk, G.A.; Stewart, R.E. Cut-off points for mild, moderate, and severe pain on the visual analogue scale for pain in patients with chronic musculoskeletal pain. *Pain* **2014**, *155*, 2545–2550. [CrossRef] [PubMed]
45. Serlin, R.C.; Mendoza, T.R.; Nakamura, Y.; Edwards, K.R.; Cleeland, C.S. When is cancer pain mild, moderate or severe? Grading pain severity by its interference with function. *Pain* **1995**, *61*, 277–284. [CrossRef]
46. Quan, W.; Liu, S.; Cao, M.; Zhao, J. A comprehensive review of virtual reality technology for cognitive rehabilitation in patients with neurological conditions. *Appl. Sci.* **2024**, *14*, 6285. [CrossRef]
47. Abbasi, M.; Váz, P.; Silva, J.; Martins, P. Enhancing Visual Perception in Immersive VR and AR Environments: AI-Driven Color and Clarity Adjustments Under Dynamic Lighting Conditions. *Technologies* **2024**, *12*, 216. [CrossRef]
48. Santos-Paz, J.A.; Sánchez-Picot, Á.; Bocos-Corredor, E.; Moggioli, F.; Martín-Pintado-Zugasti, A.; García-Carmona, R.; Otero, A. GitHub Repository Containing the Raw Data from the 60 Participants in the Study, as Well as the Code to Analyze It. 2025. Available online: https://github.com/AbrahamOtero/FunctionalAssessmentOfTheNeck (accessed on 28 April 2025).
49. Stensdotter, A.K.; Meisingset, I.; Pedersen, M.D.; Vasseljen, O.; Stavdahl, Ø. Frequency-dependent deficits in head steadiness in patients with nonspecific neck pain. *Physiol. Rep.* **2019**, *7*, e14013. [CrossRef]
50. Gresty, M.A.; Halmagyi, G.M. Abnormal head movements. *J. Neurol. Neurosurg. Psychiatry* **1979**, *42*, 705–714. [CrossRef]
51. Ni, Y.; Seffernick, A.E.; Onar-Thomas, A.; Pounds, S.B. Computing power and sample size for the false discovery rate in multiple applications. *Genes* **2024**, *15*, 344. [CrossRef]
52. Sevilla-Gonzalez, M.D.R.; Moreno Loaeza, L.; Lazaro-Carrera, L.S.; Bourguet Ramirez, B.; Vázquez, R.A.; Peralta-Pedrero, M.L.; Almeda-Valdes, P. Spanish version of the system usability scale for the assessment of electronic tools: Development and validation. *JMIR Hum. Factors* **2020**, *7*, e21161. [CrossRef]
53. Bangor, A.; Kortum, P.T.; Miller, J.T. An Empirical Evaluation of the System Usability Scale. *Int. J.-Hum.-Comput. Interact.* **2008**, *24*, 574–594. [CrossRef]
54. Brooke, J. SUS: A Quick and Dirty Usability Scale. In *Usability Evaluation in Industry*; Jordan, P.W., Thomas, B., McClelland, I.L., Weerdmeester, B., Eds.; Taylor & Francis: London, UK, 1996; pp. 189–194.
55. Falla, D.; Gizzi, L.; Parsa, H.; Dieterich, A.; Petzke, F. People with chronic neck pain walk with a stiffer spine. *J. Orthop. Sport. Phys. Ther.* **2017**, *47*, 268–277. [CrossRef] [PubMed]
56. Szeto, G.P.; Straker, L.M.; O'Sullivan, P.B. A comparison of symptomatic and asymptomatic office workers performing monotonous keyboard work—2: Neck and shoulder kinematics. *Man. Ther.* **2005**, *10*, 281–291. [CrossRef]
57. Bahat, H.S.; Weiss, P.L.; Laufer, Y. The effect of neck pain on cervical kinematics, as assessed in a virtual environment. *Arch. Phys. Med. Rehabil.* **2010**, *91*, 1884–1890. [CrossRef]
58. Astrologo, A.N.; Nano, S.; Klemm, E.M.; Shefelbine, S.J.; Dennerlein, J.T. Determining the effects of AR/VR HMD design parameters (mass and inertia) on cervical spine joint torques. *Appl. Ergon.* **2024**, *116*, 104183. [CrossRef]
59. Cerda, I.H.; Therond, A.; Moreau, S.; Studer, K.; Donjow, A.R.; Crowther, J.E.; Mazzolenis, M.E.; Lang, M.; Tolba, R.; Gilligan, C.; et al. Telehealth and Virtual Reality Technologies in Chronic Pain Management: A Narrative Review. *Curr. Pain Headache Rep.* **2024**, *28*, 83–94. [CrossRef]

60. Stasolla, F.; Passaro, A.; Curcio, E.; Di Gioia, M.; Zullo, A.; Dragone, M.; Martini, E. Combined deep and reinforcement learning with gaming to promote healthcare in neurodevelopmental disorders: A new hypothesis. *Front. Hum. Neurosci.* **2025**, *19*, 1557826. [CrossRef]
61. Alazba, A.; Al-Khalifa, H.; AlSobayel, H. RabbitRun: An immersive virtual reality game for promoting physical activities among people with low back pain. *Technologies* **2018**, *7*, 2. [CrossRef]

technologies

MDPI

Article

Touch to Speak: Real-Time Tactile Pronunciation Feedback for Individuals with Speech and Hearing Impairments

Anat Sharon [1], Roi Yozevitch [2,3] and Eldad Holdengreber [1,*]

[1] Department of Mechanical Engineering and Mechatronics, Ariel University, Ariel 40700, Israel; anat19970@gmail.com
[2] Department of Software and Computer Engineering, Ariel University, Ariel 40700, Israel; yozevitch@gmail.com
[3] Department of Electrical and Electronic Engineering, Ariel University, Ariel 40700, Israel
* Correspondence: eldadh@ariel.ac.il

Abstract: This study presents a wearable haptic feedback system designed to support speech training for individuals with speech and hearing impairments. The system provides real-time tactile cues based on detected phonemes, helping users correct their pronunciation independently. Unlike prior approaches focused on passive reception or therapist-led instruction, our method enables active, phoneme-level feedback using a multimodal interface combining audio input, visual reference, and spatially mapped vibrotactile output. We validated the system through three user studies measuring pronunciation accuracy, phoneme discrimination, and learning over time. The results show a significant improvement in word articulation accuracy and user engagement. These findings highlight the potential of real-time haptic pronunciation tools as accessible, scalable aids for speech rehabilitation and second-language learning.

Keywords: speech impairments; hearing impairments; haptic feedback; vibrotactile cues; speech therapy; pronunciation training; assistive technology

1. Introduction

Hearing and speech impairments pose significant challenges to millions of individuals worldwide, affecting their ability to communicate effectively and integrate into society. According to the World Health Organization (WHO), approximately 430 million people globally experience disabling hearing loss, with projections indicating that this number could rise to over 700 million by 2050 [1,2]. Additionally, speech impairments affect a substantial portion of the population, with an estimated 8% of children aged 3 to 17 in the United States having a communication disorder related to voice, speech, language, or swallowing [3]. These impairments can stem from various factors, including genetic conditions, injuries, diseases, and natural aging processes [4]. The impact on quality of life is significant, affecting education, employment, and social interactions [5,6]. Traditional interventions, such as speech therapy provided by Speech–Language Pathologists (SLPs), are crucial in improving communication abilities [7]. However, these methods often require significant human resources and time, limiting access and scalability [8].

To address these challenges, there is a growing need for innovative, automated solutions that can provide real-time feedback and assist in learning correct pronunciation without constant professional supervision [9,10]. Despite these promising developments, a notable gap remains in the domain of real-time, phoneme-level feedback for active speech production. Most existing systems are designed for passive perception (e.g., tactile word recognition or captioning), offer only partial phoneme coverage, or are tightly coupled with therapist-guided protocols. As such, there is a pressing need for solutions that support independent, scalable, and complete pronunciation training, particularly for users who cannot rely on auditory or visual feedback. Recent advancements in haptic feedback technologies have shown promising results in enhancing communication and interaction for individuals with sensory impairments [11,12]. Several haptic feedback devices have been developed to aid in communication and language acquisition [13,14]. For instance, the TActile Phonemic Sleeve (TAPS) translates phonemic elements of speech into tactile stimuli on the forearm, enabling users to learn and recognize English words through haptic feedback [15]. Other approaches, such as skin reading and vibrotactile information encoding, have demonstrated the potential to use tactile patterns to convey complex information [16,17]. Additionally, an intuitive cognition-based approach was introduced for generating speech through hand gestures, bridging the gap between physical movement and speech production [18]. Despite these advancements, significant gaps remain in existing solutions. Many current technologies provide either limited real-time assistance or focus on specific aspects of communication without offering comprehensive support. There is a need for integrated, user-responsive solutions to address the diverse and evolving needs of individuals with hearing and speech impairments. Recent studies highlight the value of cost-effective, real-time technologies—such as camera-based systems—for supporting motor rehabilitation in accessible, everyday settings [19].

Our Contribution

This research aims to develop a haptic feedback system to improve word pronunciation among people with speech and hearing impairments. By translating heard words into tactile information and comparing the tactile cues received from the device with the correct pronunciation, we seek to enable users to improve their pronunciation and speech production in a cognitively informed and effective manner. This approach can potentially enhance communication skills and ultimately improve the quality of life for individuals with hearing and speech impairments. By combining full phoneme coverage, spatially intuitive tactile encoding, and real-time closed-loop feedback, our system fills a critical gap in the assistive technology landscape. It is the first to support independent pronunciation learning through touch alone, without relying on speech therapists, vision, or hearing. This differentiates our work from previous approaches such as TAPS [20] or HAPOVER [4], which either lack production feedback, cover only a subset of phonemes, or focus on receptive learning tasks.

2. Related Work

2.1. Clinical Interventions: Speech–Language Pathologists

Speech–Language Pathologists (SLPs) are the cornerstone of therapeutic intervention, using structured exercises and real-time correction to guide patients toward improved articulation, fluency, and phonological awareness [21–24]. Clinical evidence supports their effectiveness in individualized care plans [21,22], but accessibility is constrained by cost, therapist availability, and geographic limitations, particularly for disadvantaged or remote populations [23]. Moreover, the reliance on face-to-face interaction limits scalability.

2.2. Real-Time Translation and Captioning Technologies

Technologies such as automatic speech recognition (ASR) and sign language translation have been developed to assist individuals with hearing disabilities by converting spoken language into readable or visual formats [25]. These tools are effective in enhancing communication comprehension, particularly in educational and public settings. However, they are one-directional: while they help users understand speech, they do not assist in producing or correcting speech, nor do they offer phoneme-specific feedback.

2.3. Haptic Feedback Systems for Language Support

Haptic feedback has emerged as a promising modality for sensory substitution, allowing tactile stimuli to carry linguistic information [26–30]. Recent frameworks for haptic language communication suggest that systems must go beyond basic vibration cues and consider perceptual, cognitive, and linguistic dimensions of tactile feedback. For instance, Reed et al. [14] conducted a comprehensive review of haptic language systems, classifying them by their encoding strategies (spatial, temporal, and intensity-based), user perceptual thresholds, and learning demands. They emphasized that effective tactile communication must align with linguistic salience and user learning curves, principles that directly informed our design, particularly the spatial mapping of distinct phonemes to vibration loci.

Several research efforts have explored its application in language learning:

- TActile Phonemic Sleeve (TAPS): A wearable system that encodes English phonemes into tactile patterns on the forearm. Tan et al. [20] demonstrated the acquisition of over 500 English words through repeated haptic exposure. However, TAPS is optimized for vocabulary comprehension, not for pronunciation output or real-time correction.
- HAPOVER System: Ilhan and Kaçanoğlu [4] introduced HAPOVER, a wearable pronunciation training device utilizing eight vibration motors to provide phoneme-level feedback. The system captures speech, extracts Mel-Frequency Cepstral Coefficients (MFCC), and compares them with reference templates using Dynamic Time Warping (DTW). If a mismatch is detected, it delivers corrective haptic signals to guide users toward accurate articulation. Their pilot study reported an 80.74% improvement in word pronunciation accuracy among second-language learners after training. Despite its promising results, HAPOVER uses a limited number of actuators and covers only a subset of phonemes, without a scalable design for full language production support.
- Skin Reading Interfaces: Luzhnica et al. [31] proposed encoding textual information using six-channel haptic displays. While innovative, the system focuses on passive reception and requires high cognitive training for interpretation.
- Vibrotactile Encoding Capacity: Novich and Eagleman [32] investigated how spatial and temporal patterns of vibration can encode complex information, estimating the throughput capacity of human skin. Their results highlight the potential—but also the limitations—of tactile systems for detailed language feedback.
- Tactile Vocoder with Envelope Expansion: Fletcher et al. [33,34] proposed an audio-to-tactile substitution approach using amplitude envelope expansion across multiple frequency bands. Their system demonstrated enhanced phoneme identification accuracy—especially for vowels and consonants—under noisy conditions, achieving an average improvement of 9.6%. The authors emphasized the clinical potential of such compact, low-power devices for real-time feedback. However, while promising for passive perception, this system does not provide active pronunciation correction or phoneme-level feedback tailored to speech production.
- Phoneme-Based Tactile Display: Jung et al. [35] developed a 4×6 tactile actuator array that maps 39 English phonemes to unique vibration patterns, allowing users to receive words and short messages via touch. In their study, participants achieved an average word recognition accuracy of 87% for trained four-phoneme words and 77% for novel words after 3–5 h of training. Additionally, a longitudinal experiment demonstrated

two-way tactile communication with 73% phoneme-level and 82% word-level accuracy, albeit at a limited transmission rate (approximately one message per minute). While this system effectively supports connected phoneme-level reception and real-world communication scenarios, it does not offer active feedback for pronunciation correction or real-time speech training.

- Phoneme-Based Tactile Display: Jung et al. [35] developed a 4 × 6 tactile actuator array that maps 39 English phonemes (their chosen inventory) to unique vibration patterns, allowing users to receive words and short messages via touch. In their study, participants achieved an average word recognition accuracy of 87% for trained four-phoneme words and 77% for novel words after 3–5 h of training. Additionally, a longitudinal experiment demonstrated two-way tactile communication with 73% phoneme-level and 82% word-level accuracy, albeit at a limited transmission rate (approximately one message per minute). While this system effectively supports connected phoneme-level reception and real-world communication scenarios, it does not offer active feedback for pronunciation correction or real-time speech training.

2.4. Limitations in Existing Approaches

Despite advancements, current systems tend to address only one dimension of the communication challenge. Table 1 provides a comparative summary of existing methods.

Table 1. Comparison of different approaches for speech communication systems.

Approach	Real-Time Feedback	Active Speech Production	Full Phoneme Coverage	Requires Therapist	Scalability
SLP (in-person) [21–24]	✓	✓	✓	✓	×
Real-Time Translation Tools [25,36,37]	✓	×	×	×	✓
TAPS [20]	×	×	Partial	×	Medium
HAPOVER [4]	✓	✓	Partial	×	Low–Medium
Tactile Vocoder [33,34]	✓	×	Partial (perceptual only)	×	Medium–High
Phoneme-Based Tactile Display [35]	×	×	✓	×	Medium
Our Proposed System	✓	✓	✓	×	✓

Most notably, no existing system fully supports real-time, closed-loop tactile feedback for speech correction. Systems like TAPS lack bidirectional feedback. Others focus on comprehension rather than production. Furthermore, few devices adapt to users dynamically or support comprehensive phoneme training based on International Phonetic Alphabet (IPA) standards.

2.5. Summary and Gap Analysis

Existing solutions for individuals with speech and hearing impairments include clinical therapy, translation systems, and haptic technologies. While SLPs [21–24] provide effective treatment, they are not scalable. Real-time translation tools [25] improve comprehension but do not support speech production.

Haptic systems—such as TAPS [20], HAPOVER [4], Fletcher's tactile vocoder [33,34], and Jung et al.'s phoneme display [35]—demonstrate the potential of tactile feedback for language learning. Some support passive recognition; others offer limited correction or communication. However, key limitations remain:

- Most systems lack real-time, corrective feedback.
- Phoneme coverage is often partial.
- Few are designed for active pronunciation training or broad scalability.

Our system addresses these gaps by providing:

- Real-time, closed-loop feedback;
- Full phoneme coverage;
- A scalable, therapist-free design aligned with cognitive and perceptual principles.

3. Method

This study examines whether users can learn to interpret phoneme-level haptic cues and pronounce words accurately in real time. We focus on two main questions: (1) Can participants reliably associate phonemes with specific tactile locations? (2) Does performance improve as phoneme set size increases?

We addressed these questions using a custom-built haptic system and a series of structured experiments, as detailed below.

3.1. System Overview

We developed a table-mounted device that delivers real-time vibrotactile cues corresponding to spoken output. The system integrates the following:

- Raspberry Pi 5 for speech processing and experiment control, running Python-based algorithms (ver 3.8).
- Arduino Uno to individually control up to 26 vibration motors.
- A microphone (speech input; not used during core haptic feedback phases).
- A speaker (optional auditory feedback; not used in the main experiments).
- A 3D-printed ergonomic hand rest for consistent contact and user comfort.

This configuration supports accurate haptic encoding of phonemes for speech learning and correction. The overall system architecture is shown in Figure 1.

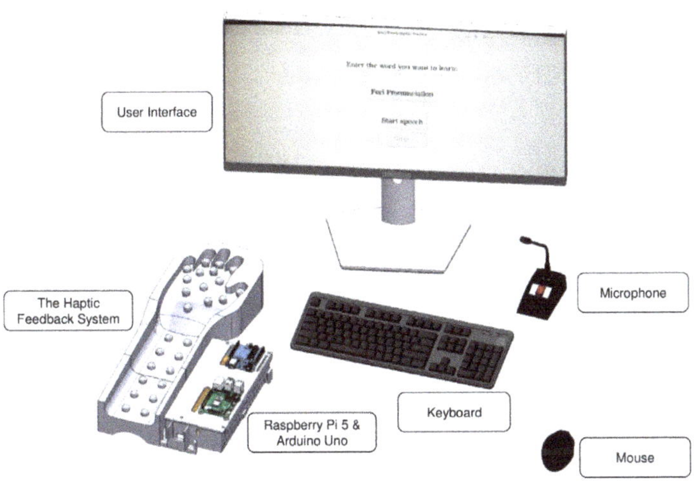

Figure 1. Block diagram of the haptic feedback system illustrating the information flow from speech input to vibrotactile output.

To assess system responsiveness, we measured the latency from word selection to the onset of the first haptic vibration. The average latency was $\approx$1.5 s, which was sufficient to maintain the perception of synchronicity for real-time pronunciation training tasks.

3.2. Phonemes and the International Phonetic Alphabet (IPA)

Spoken language consists of discrete sound units called *phonemes*, the smallest sounds that differentiate words within a language. For example, "pin" and "bin" differ by only one phoneme: /p/ versus /b/. English includes a distinct inventory of consonant and vowel phonemes, such as /t/, /s/, /m/, /i/, /æ/, and /o/.

To represent these sounds precisely, linguists use the International Phonetic Alphabet (IPA), a standardized set of symbols that directly encode pronunciation regardless of spelling. For instance, the word "sit" is written as /sɪt/ in IPA, making it clear how each letter should sound. IPA is widely used in linguistics, speech therapy, and language education for its clarity and universality.

In this study, all words and haptic patterns were selected and described using their IPA transcriptions. This ensured unambiguous communication of target sounds to both experimenters and participants, eliminating confusion from irregular spelling or pronunciation differences.

3.3. Haptic Feedback Selection

Multiple actuator types were evaluated; vibration motors were chosen for their

- Compactness and cost-effectiveness;
- Clear, discriminable tactile sensation;
- imple integration with microcontrollers.

Unlike prior protocols, each phoneme used in the experiment was mapped to a unique motor location. For each word, its phonemes were encoded as brief (250 ms) vibrations at corresponding spatial locations, with 50 ms pauses. Each vibration motor was a compact 10 mm diameter, 2 mm height coin-type actuator operating at 2.5–3.5 V. At 3 V, it delivered a rotational speed of $14,500$ RPM with a nominal current of 60 mA, ensuring clear and responsive tactile feedback suitable for wearable applications. Motors were run at a fixed frequency (approximately 130 Hz) and intensity, so spatial location alone cued phoneme identity. International Phonetic Alphabet (IPA) notation was used throughout to ensure clarity and avoid orthographic ambiguity. Words with ambiguous spelling or pronunciation were excluded.

3.4. Phoneme Conversion and Haptic Mapping Procedure

Each word used in the experiment was first converted into its International Phonetic Alphabet (IPA) transcription to ensure a precise, language-independent representation of pronunciation. This conversion was performed offline using automated tools, including the OpenAI API and the open-source `phonemizer` library [38]. The resulting phoneme sequences were manually verified for accuracy and consistency across all participants.

Importantly, no phoneme recognition or speech analysis was performed on participants' spoken responses. Instead, the IPA transcription served as a reliable foundation for generating the vibrotactile sequences, while pronunciation correctness was evaluated by a human operator during the experiment. Each unique phoneme from the IPA transcription was mapped to a specific vibration motor and spatial location on the haptic device. During each trial, the word's phonemes were delivered as a sequence of brief (approximately 250 ms) vibrations at the corresponding locations, separated by short pauses (about 50 ms). All motors operated at the same frequency and intensity, so the only distinguishing feature for each phoneme was its spatial position. Words with ambiguous spelling or multiple valid pronunciations were excluded to ensure clarity and reproducibility.

This systematic, automated mapping enabled this study to handle complex word lists while maintaining full experimental control over the haptic cues experienced by participants. Although English is variously analyzed as having 39–44 phonemes (depending on how diphthongs and rhotic vowels are treated), we adopted a 44-phoneme inventory in this work. Our device utilized 26 vibration motors. (An earlier prototype from our lab used the same actuator count for letter-level encoding; in the present work, we redesigned the mapping to operate at the phoneme level.) This motor count reflected practical constraints of the wearable form factor, power consumption, and user comfort rather than a one-to-one mapping to orthographic units.

To make the encoding intuitive, we followed three simple rules: vowels were placed on fingertip motors (higher tactile acuity), high-frequency phonemes were allocated to the most salient regions (e.g., palm, proximal digits), and low-frequency phonemes were assigned pragmatically—either grouped or encoded with two-motor combinations—without imposing further articulatory or spatial regularities. Accordingly, phonemes were mapped based on their relative frequency in English; for example, /ɪ/, /n/, and /t/ occur at 9.75%, 7.95%, and 7.59%, respectively [39], whereas the least frequent phonemes appear in less than 0.5% of words. This frequency-aware, rule-based scheme enabled scalable encoding of all required phonemes within the 26-motor constraint.

3.5. Mechanical Design and Assembly

Raspberry Pi controlled the experiment, converting each target word to an IPA phoneme sequence and relaying phoneme indices to Arduino, which activated the assigned motors in order. Motors were powered by a 9 V Li-ion battery for portability. The device was table-mounted; the user rested their hand for maximal contact with all vibration points. Mechanical parts were designed in SolidWorks V.2024 and 3D-printed with heat-resistant PLA+. Key features included

- Ergonomic hand fixture for comfortable, repeatable placement;
- Precise motor mounts to avoid vibratory overlap;
- Ventilation for electronics cooling.

Wiring was stabilized on perfboard. The assembled device is shown in Figure 2.

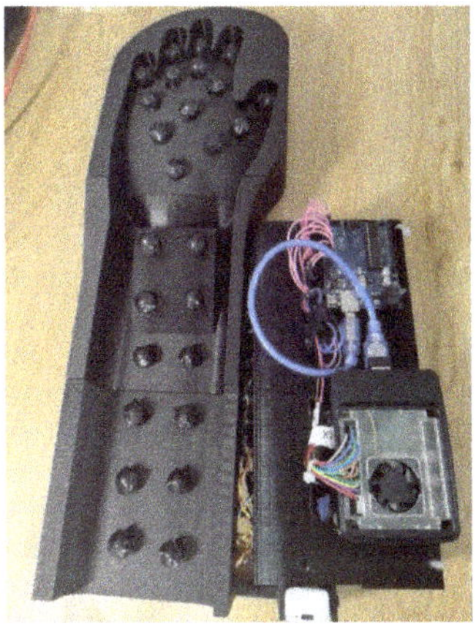

Figure 2. The assembled 3*D*-printed hand and forearm model was designed to deliver localized vibrotactile feedback across the fingers, palm, and lower forearm up to the wrist joint.

To clarify the user experience and operational flow, Figure 3 presents two complementary views of a participant interacting with the system during a pronunciation task. The setup included a visual display of target words, a calibrated microphone for speech input, and a tactile user interface that delivered immediate vibrotactile feedback. This physical arrangement supported the real-time feedback loop described above and enabled closed-loop pronunciation training.

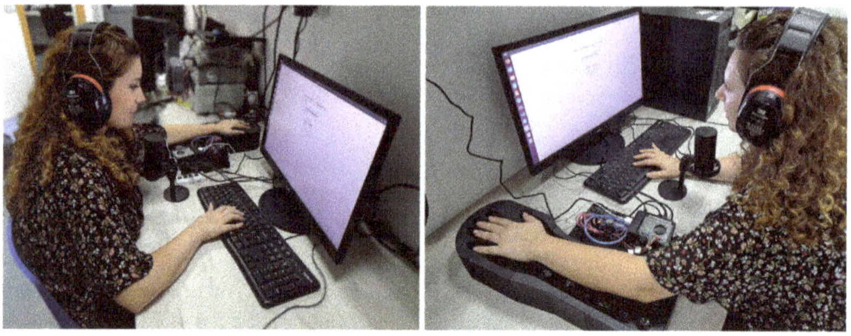

Figure 3. Dual-angle view of a participant using the system during a real-time pronunciation task. The user read a target word on the display, spoke into a calibrated microphone, and received immediate vibrotactile feedback via the tactile interface. The two perspectives highlight key components of the setup: the tactile unit, speech input, and visual guidance.

3.6. Experiment Protocol and Participants

In total, 20 adults (ages 22–49; 15 men, 5 women) participated. All were native Hebrew speakers and reported no formal training in phonetics/linguistics or speech therapy or prior experience with haptic phoneme-encoding systems. A brief pre-experiment questionnaire documented education level and prior exposure to phoneme instruction. All participants were undergraduate or graduate students or university staff members holding an academic degree. All gave informed consent and the protocol was IRB-approved. This initial study was conducted with participants without visual and hearing disabilities to evaluate the system's usability and decoding feasibility in a controlled environment prior to clinical testing.

Sessions were conducted in a quiet lab. Participants wore noise-canceling headphones playing white noise to eliminate auditory self-feedback (as can be seen in Figure 3). Each experimental phase (see Results for phoneme and word lists) included the following:

1. Familiarization: Participants learned the phoneme-to-motor mapping via isolated haptic cues.
2. Production Task: The experimenter delivered each word's phoneme sequence as haptic cues; participants pronounced the word aloud, relying solely on touch.
3. Correction: Incorrect attempts were met with a "not correct" prompt; repetition continued until success.
4. Timing: The researcher measured time from cue onset to successful pronunciation with a stopwatch.

No visual or software interface was used; all timing and feedback were manual.

The primary mode of feedback during the experiments was verbal confirmation from the experimenter. After each spoken response, the operator informed the participant whether their pronunciation was correct. No additional visual indicators (e.g., accuracy icons or success cues) were used. This setup ensured that participants relied solely on tactile input for pronunciation and auditory feedback only for correctness.

Pronunciation detection time (phase 4) was recorded and logged manually. One outlier—a participant whose phase 1 timing exceeded the group mean by more than two standard deviations—was removed from the dataset. Descriptive statistics (mean, SD) for the cleaned data appear in Section 4. The integration of a speech recognition engine, tactile encoding module, and visual interface enabled a closed-loop system for pronunciation correction. Together, these components formed the basis for real-time, user-guided articulation feedback. The following section presents the experimental validation of this system, including the evaluation protocol, key performance metrics, and participant outcomes.

In summary, the system integrates tactile encoding, controlled phoneme mapping, and live operator feedback to form a closed-loop platform for real-time pronunciation training. The design emphasizes simplicity, scalability, and cognitive alignment with the user's learning process. The following section presents the experimental validation of this approach, including performance metrics, learning curves, and participant outcomes.

4. Results

In this section, we report results from two experiments. **Experiment 1** (Word Recognition Task) tested initial learnability and decoding using a limited six-phoneme inventory and five words, with all 20 participants. **Experiment 2** (Learning Curves with Expanding Phoneme Sets) examined adaptation over time as the phoneme set and word list expanded across three sessions on separate days, with 10 participants (a subset of the original cohort). The procedural template (Familiarization, Production, Correction, Timing) was identical in both experiments; only the phoneme inventory, word sets, and number of participants differed.

4.1. Experiment 1—Word Recognition Task

The first experiment assessed the ability of participants to learn and recognize a set of five words, each constructed exclusively from a limited phoneme inventory (see Table 2). Twenty adult participants with no reported hearing or speech impairments took part in this phase. Each participant was sequentially trained to recognize the words *sit*, *pan*, *nap*, *pin*, and *satin*. For each word, the corresponding sequence of phoneme-coded haptic cues was delivered, and the participant had to correctly produce the spoken word.

Table 2. Phoneme inventory and word list for Phase 1, with IPA transcription.

Word	IPA Phonemes
Phonemes:	/p/, /æ/, /n/, /ɪ/, /s/, /t/
sit	/s/ /ɪ/ /t/
pan	/p/ /æ/ /n/
pin	/p/ /ɪ/ /n/
nap	/n/ /æ/ /p/
satin	/s/ /æ/ /t/ /ɪ/ /n/

Each word is listed alongside its IPA transcription to eliminate any ambiguity regarding pronunciation. The "Phonemes" row in the table highlights the complete inventory of phoneme sounds included in this phase; all selected words were composed solely from these six phonemes (/p/, /æ/, /n/, /ɪ/, /s/, /t/), which were mapped to specific spatial locations on the haptic device. This careful selection ensured that participants could focus exclusively on learning a limited, consistent set of haptic cues while minimizing confounding effects due to unfamiliar or ambiguous sounds. The inclusion of both monosyllabic (e.g., *sit, pan, pin, nap*) and a disyllabic word (*satin*) was designed to probe the effects of word length and phoneme sequence complexity on recognition and learning speed.

The average time (in seconds) required to successfully pronounce each word was as follows: 27.54 for *sit*, 39.70 for *pan*, 15.51 for *nap*, 19.14 for *pin*, and 51.94 for *satin*.

Figure 4 plots detection times for each Phase 1 word. The word *satin* stood out with the highest median and the widest spread, showing that the learning time was the longest and varied most across participants. By contrast, shorter words like *nap* and *pin* have lower, tighter boxes, meaning that they were detected faster and more consistently.

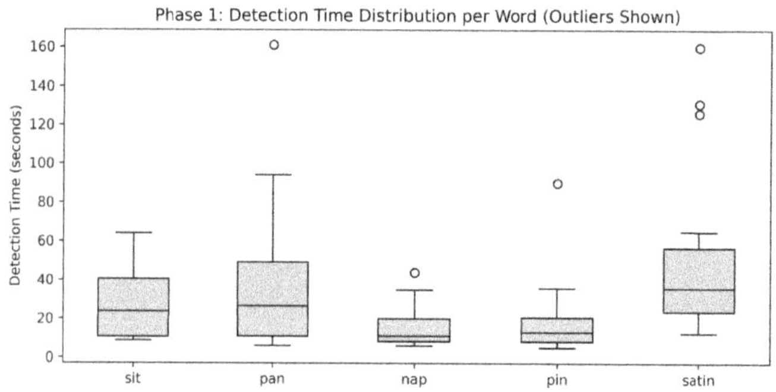

Figure 4. The box plot shows how long each Phase 1 word took to detect. The line in each box is the middle time, the box itself covers most of the scores, and dots are the rare extremes.

4.2. Experiment 2—Learning Curves with Expanding Phoneme Sets

The second experiment focused on how participants adapted to increasing complexity in the phoneme-to-haptic mapping task. This study involved 10 adult participants over three separate sessions, with each session (phase) conducted on a different day to allow for consolidation and to observe learning effects over time.

The first phase, described previously, used a foundational set of six phonemes and five corresponding words. In the subsequent phases, two additional phonemes were introduced at each stage, along with five new words constructed from the *expanded* phoneme inventory (including previous phonemes). The complete progression of phonemes and words for all phases is detailed in Table 3.

For each phase, the mean detection time for every participant was recorded, allowing us to calculate both the overall mean and standard deviation for each phase. This statistical summary provides insight into both the average performance and the consistency of recognition times as task complexity increased. By examining these values, one can also extract the learning curve across phases and observe how participants adapted to the expanding phoneme set. The summarized results for all phases are presented in Table 4.

The key finding from this experiment was that despite the increasing number of phonemes and the corresponding rise in word complexity, participants' average recognition time did not increase across phases. This suggests that once participants became familiar with the core principles of the haptic-phoneme mapping, they were able to generalize their skills to new, more complex word sets without any loss in speed.

These results underscore the intuitive and scalable nature of the haptic feedback system. Even as the task became more challenging, participants were able to maintain or even improve their performance, demonstrating effective learning and adaptation across sessions.

Table 3. Phoneme inventory and word list for each experimental phase, with IPA transcription.

Phase	Word	IPA Phonemes
Phase 1	**Phonemes:** /p/, /æ/, /n/, /ɪ/, /s/, /t/	
	sit	/s/ /ɪ/ /t/
	pan	/p/ /æ/ /n/
	pin	/p/ /ɪ/ /n/
	nap	/n/ /æ/ /p/
	satin	/s/ /æ/ /t/ /ɪ/ /n/
Phase 2	**New phonemes:** /m/, /k/ **All:** /p/, /æ/, /n/, /ɪ/, /s/, /t/, /m/, /k/	
	man	/m/ /æ/ /n/
	kit	/k/ /ɪ/ /t/
	mat	/m/ /æ/ /t/
	panic	/p/ /æ/ /n/ /ɪ/ /k/
	mantis	/m/ /æ/ /n/ /t/ /ɪ/ /s/
Phase 3	**New phonemes:** /d/, /l/ **All:** /p/, /æ/, /n/, /ɪ/, /s/, /t/, /m/, /k/, /d/, /l/	
	land	/l/ /æ/ /n/ /d/
	sand	/s/ /æ/ /n/ /d/
	sandal	/s/ /æ/ /n/ /d/ /ə/ /l/
	candle	/k/ /æ/ /n/ /d/ /ə/ /l/
	paddle	/p/ /æ/ /d/ /ə/ /l/

Table 4. Summary of pronunciation times (in seconds) by phase and gender.

Metric	Phase 1	Phase 2	Phase 3
Mean time (s), all	41.3	25.9	30.3
Fastest	11.4	12.4	10.6
Slowest	85.0	65.3	47.6

Key findings:

- Learning effect: Mean times dropped by 37% from Phase 1 to 2, indicating rapid adaptation. Phase 3 times increased slightly but remained 27% faster than initial performance.
- Outliers: One slow participant was excluded; the fastest individual achieved times below 12 s per word.

4.3. Qualitative Observations

Most participants reported that the phoneme–haptic code became intuitive after a short familiarization period as they quickly learned to associate specific spatial locations with particular speech sounds. In addition, the following was observed:

1. Native English advantage. Participants who were native in both Hebrew and English—or who had native-level proficiency in English—consistently achieved faster and more accurate detections. They were already accustomed to the mismatch between spelling and pronunciation; for example, they could segment *candle* as kændəl, whereas almost all native Hebrew speakers cannot distinguish *sheep* from *ship*.
2. Phoneme-load effect with learning curve. As predicted, tasks containing a larger inventory of phonemes posed a greater initial challenge; mean detection times fell across successive sessions, indicating a clear learning effect.

3. Gender parity. No statistically significant performance differences were observed between male and female participants ($p > 0.05$).
4. Zero-detection group. In addition to the 20 participants, four volunteers (two men and two women) failed to detect *even a single word*. None of these four were native English speakers, implying that some people—particularly those with little to no phonological experience in English—may find the task nearly impossible.
5. Usability impressions. Participants provided positive feedback regarding the usability of the system. Even those who did not successfully complete the tasks expressed appreciation for the intuitiveness of the tactile interface. Notably, it became evident that the hand's placement on the tactile platform played a crucial role in performance. Each participant naturally adjusted their hand to a position that felt most comfortable and effective for detecting the vibrations. This self-guided adjustment suggests that future designs may benefit from incorporating adaptable or user-customizable hand rests to enhance tactile perception and learning outcomes.

5. Conclusions and Future Work

The proposed haptic feedback system offers a novel approach to real-time pronunciation training through tactile cues. By mapping phonemes to spatial vibration patterns, users were able to interpret and articulate words without relying on hearing or vision. Across multiple sessions, participants showed consistent learning effects, with improved recognition speed and accuracy despite increasing task complexity.

Quantitative findings indicate a clear learning effect: mean completion times dropped by 37% from Phase 1 to Phase 2, with only a slight increase in Phase 3 despite added task complexity. Overall, performance in Phase 3 remained 27% faster than the initial phase, suggesting rapid adaptation to the phoneme-to-vibration mapping. These results demonstrate the feasibility and efficiency of real-time haptic pronunciation guidance, even under increasing cognitive and linguistic load.

While our system is designed for individuals with speech and hearing impairments, the current study was conducted with adults without visual and hearing disabilities to evaluate the core haptic encoding strategy in a controlled setting. This early-stage validation approach, common in assistive technology research, necessarily limits the generalizability of the results, a limitation we acknowledge.

Future trials with individuals from the target population, conducted in collaboration with speech therapists and educators, will assess the system's practical effectiveness, adaptability, and usability in therapeutic and educational contexts. We also plan to explore adaptations for reduced phoneme sets (e.g., Hebrew or early language acquisition) to better match the needs of different user groups. The tactile encoding can be reconfigured accordingly, allowing the system to support a wider range of languages and proficiency levels. For multilingual users, future versions could explore standardized tactile layouts across language phoneme sets, reducing the need to relearn mappings per language and improving cross-linguistic usability. This interdisciplinary direction will incorporate linguistic and physiological considerations into future system design.

Additional directions include enhancing the ergonomic design, increasing the resolution and perceptual clarity of the tactile signals, and integrating adaptive learning algorithms for personalized feedback. These steps aim to establish the system as a scalable, therapist-independent solution that improves pronunciation training and communication outcomes for individuals with speech and hearing impairments, as well as for second-language learners.

Author Contributions: Conceptualization, A.S. and E.H.; methodology, R.Y. and E.H.; software, A.S.; validation, E.H. and R.Y.; formal analysis, R.Y. and E.H.; investigation, A.S.; resources, E.H. and R.Y.; data curation, R.Y.; writing—original draft preparation, R.Y.; writing—review and editing, E.H. and R.Y.; visualization, A.S.; supervision, E.H.; project administration, E.H. All authors have read and agreed to the published version of the manuscript.

Funding: This research received no external funding.

Institutional Review Board Statement: Not applicable.

Informed Consent Statement: Informed consent was obtained from all subjects involved in the study.

Data Availability Statement: The raw data supporting the conclusions of this article will be made available by the authors on request.

Conflicts of Interest: The authors declare no conflicts of interest.

References

1. Kushalnagar, R. Deafness and hearing loss. In *Web Accessibility: A Foundation for Research*; Springer: Berlin/Heidelberg, Germany, 2019; pp. 35–47.
2. Graydon, K.; Waterworth, C.; Miller, H.; Gunasekera, H. Global burden of hearing impairment and ear disease. *J. Laryngol. Otol.* **2019**, *133*, 18–25. [CrossRef] [PubMed]
3. Guo, R. Advancing real-time close captioning: Blind source separation and transcription for hearing impairments. *Appl. Comput. Eng.* **2024**, *30*, 125–130. [CrossRef]
4. Ilhan, R.; Kaçanoğlu, K. HAPOVER: A Haptic Pronunciation Improver Device. *IEEJ Trans. Electr. Electron. Eng.* **2024**, *19*, 985–992. [CrossRef]
5. Greenwell, T.; Walsh, B. Evidence-based practice in speech-language pathology: Where are we now? *Am. J. Speech Lang. Pathol.* **2021**, *30*, 186–198. [CrossRef]
6. Tambyraja, S.R. Facilitating parental involvement in speech therapy for children with speech sound disorders: A survey of speech-language pathologists' practices, perspectives, and strategies. *Am. J. Speech Lang. Pathol.* **2020**, *29*, 1987–1996. [CrossRef]
7. CATy, M.È.; Kinsella, E.A.; DOyLE, P.C. Reflective practice in speech-language pathology: A scoping review. *Int. J. Speech Lang. Pathol.* **2015**, *17*, 411–420. [CrossRef]
8. Gomez-Risquet, M.; Cáceres-Matos, R.; Magni, E.; Luque-Moreno, C. Effects of Haptic Feedback Interventions in Post-Stroke Gait and Balance Disorders: A Systematic Review and Meta-Analysis. *J. Pers. Med.* **2024**, *14*, 974. [CrossRef]
9. Bogach, N.; Boitsova, E.; Chernonog, S.; Lamtev, A.; Lesnichaya, M.; Lezhenin, I.; Novopashenny, A.; Svechnikov, R.; Tsikach, D.; Vasiliev, K.; et al. Speech processing for language learning: A practical approach to computer-assisted pronunciation teaching. *Electronics* **2021**, *10*, 235. [CrossRef]
10. Pennington, M.C.; Rogerson-Revell, P.; Pennington, M.C.; Rogerson-Revell, P. Using technology for pronunciation teaching, learning, and assessment. In *English Pronunciation Teaching and Research: Contemporary Perspectives*; Palgrave Macmillan: London, UK, 2019; pp. 235–286.
11. Raghul, J.; Sreya, M.; Maithreye, S.; Durga Devi, K. Mobility Stick with Haptic Feedback for People with Vision Impairments. In Proceedings of the 2024 International Conference on Signal Processing, Computation, Electronics, Power and Telecommunication (IConSCEPT), Karaikal, India, 4–5 July 2024; pp. 1–6.
12. Kleinberg, D.; Yozevitch, R.; Abekasis, I.; Israel, Y.; Holdengreber, E. A haptic feedback system for spatial orientation in the visually impaired: A comprehensive approach. *IEEE Sens. Lett.* **2023**, *7*, 1–4. [CrossRef]
13. Emami, M.; Bayat, A.; Tafazolli, R.; Quddus, A. A survey on haptics: Communication, sensing and feedback. *IEEE Commun. Surv. Tutor.* **2024**, *27*, 2006–2050. [CrossRef]
14. Reed, C.M.; Tan, H.Z.; Jones, L.A. Haptic communication of language. *IEEE Trans. Haptics* **2023**, *16*, 134–153. [CrossRef]
15. Xia, J.; Pei, S.; Chen, Z.; Wang, L.; Hu, J.; Wang, J. Effects of Conventional Speech Therapy with Liuzijue Qigong, a Traditional Chinese Method of Breath Training, in 70 Patients with Post-Stroke Spastic Dysarthria. *Med. Sci. Monit. Int. Med. J. Exp. Clin. Res.* **2023**, *29*, e939623-1–e939623-10. [CrossRef] [PubMed]
16. de Groot, A.; Eijsvoogel, N.; van Well, G.; van Hout, R.; de Vries, E. Evidence-based decision-making in the treatment of speech, language, and communication disorders in Down syndrome; a scoping review. *J. Intellect. Disabil.* **2024**, 17446295241283659.
17. Martins, G.d.S.; Santos, I.R.D.d.; Brazorotto, J.S. Validation of an educational resource for speech therapists on the use of video feedback in training families of hearing-impaired children. *Audiol. Commun. Res.* **2024**, *29*, e2928. [CrossRef]

18. Holdengreber, E.; Yozevitch, R.; Khavkin, V. Intuitive cognition-based method for generating speech using hand gestures. *Sensors* **2021**, *21*, 5291. [CrossRef] [PubMed]
19. Yozevitch, R.; Frenkel-Toledo, S.; Elion, O.; Levy, L.; Ambaw, A.; Holdengreber, E. Cost-Effective and Efficient Solutions for the Assessment and Practice of Upper Extremity Motor Performance. *IEEE Sens. J.* **2023**, *23*, 23494–23499. [CrossRef]
20. Tan, H.Z.; Reed, C.M.; Jiao, Y.; Perez, Z.D.; Wilson, E.C.; Jung, J.; Martinez, J.S.; Severgnini, F.M. Acquisition of 500 English words through a TActile phonemic sleeve (TAPS). *IEEE Trans. Haptics* **2020**, *13*, 745–760. [CrossRef]
21. Weidner, K.; Lowman, J. Telepractice for adult speech-language pathology services: A systematic review. *Perspect. Asha Spec. Interest Groups* **2020**, *5*, 326–338. [CrossRef]
22. Powell, R.K. Unique contributors to the curriculum: From research to practice for speech-language pathologists in schools. *Lang. Speech Hear. Serv. Sch.* **2018**, *49*, 140–147. [CrossRef]
23. Thomas, S.; Schulz, J.; Ryder, N. Assessment and diagnosis of Developmental Language Disorder: The experiences of speech and language therapists. *Autism Dev. Lang. Impair.* **2019**, *4*, 2396941519842812. [CrossRef]
24. Raina, S. Schizophrenia: Communication disorders and role of the speech-language pathologist. *Am. J. Speech Lang. Pathol.* **2024**, *33*, 1099–1112. [CrossRef] [PubMed]
25. Otoom, M.; Alzubaidi, M.A. Ambient intelligence framework for real-time speech-to-sign translation. *Assist. Technol.* **2018**, *30*, 119–132. [CrossRef] [PubMed]
26. Shull, P.B.; Damian, D.D. Haptic wearables as sensory replacement, sensory augmentation and trainer—A review. *J. Neuroeng. Rehabil.* **2015**, *12*, 1–13. [CrossRef]
27. Giri, G.S.; Maddahi, Y.; Zareinia, K. An application-based review of haptics technology. *Robotics* **2021**, *10*, 29. [CrossRef]
28. Irigoyen, E.; Larrea, M.; Graña, M. A Narrative Review of Haptic Technologies and Their Value for Training, Rehabilitation, and the Education of Persons with Special Needs. *Sensors* **2024**, *24*, 6946. [CrossRef]
29. Levy, L.; Ambaw, A.; Ben-Itzchak, E.; Holdengreber, E. A real-time environmental translator for emotion recognition in autism spectrum disorder. *Sci. Rep.* **2024**, *14*, 31527. [CrossRef]
30. Levy, L.; Blum, Y.; Ambaw, A.; Yozevitch, R.; Holdengreber, E. Harnessing Haptic Technology for Real-Time Emotion Detection. *IEEE Sens. Lett.* **2025**, *9*, 5500804. [CrossRef]
31. Luzhnica, G.; Veas, E.; Pammer, V. Skin reading: Encoding text in a 6-channel haptic display. In Proceedings of the 2016 ACM International Symposium on Wearable Computers, Heidelberg, Germany, 12–16 September 2016; pp. 148–155.
32. Novich, S.D.; Eagleman, D.M. Using space and time to encode vibrotactile information: Toward an estimate of the skin's achievable throughput. *Exp. Brain Res.* **2015**, *233*, 2777–2788. [CrossRef]
33. Fletcher, M.D.; Akis, E.; Verschuur, C.A.; Perry, S.W. Improved tactile speech perception and noise robustness using audio-to-tactile sensory substitution with amplitude envelope expansion. *Sci. Rep.* **2024**, *14*, 15029. [CrossRef]
34. Fletcher, M.D.; Verschuur, C.A.; Perry, S.W. Improving speech perception for hearing-impaired listeners using audio-to-tactile sensory substitution with multiple frequency channels. *Sci. Rep.* **2023**, *13*, 13336. [CrossRef]
35. Jung, J.; Reed, C.M.; Martinez, J.S.; Tan, H.Z. Tactile Speech Communication: Reception of Words and Two-Way Messages through a Phoneme-Based Display. *Virtual Worlds* **2024**, *3*, 184–207. [CrossRef]
36. Anazia, E.K.; Eti, E.F.; Ovili, P.H.; Ogbimi, O.F. Speech-To-Text: A Secured Real-Time Language Translation Platform for Students. *FUDMA J. Sci.* **2024**, *8*, 329–338. [CrossRef]
37. Sanaullah, M.; Ahmad, B.; Kashif, M.; Safdar, T.; Hassan, M.; Hasan, M.H.; Aziz, N. A real-time automatic translation of text to sign language. *Comput. Mater. Contin.* **2022**, *70*, 2471–2488. [CrossRef]
38. Bernard, M.; Titeux, H. Phonemizer: Text to Phones Transcription for Multiple Languages in Python. *J. Open Source Softw.* **2021**, *6*, 3958. [CrossRef]
39. Hayden, R.E. The relative frequency of phonemes in General-American English. *Word* **1950**, *6*, 217–223. [CrossRef]

technologies

MDPI

Article

Non-Contact Platform for the Assessment of Physical Function in Older Adults: A Pilot Study

Ana Sobrino-Santos [1,2], Pedro Anuarbe [1,2], Carlos Fernandez-Viadero [2,3], Roberto García-García [4], José Miguel López-Higuera [1,2,5], Luis Rodríguez-Cobo [1,2,5,*,†] and Adolfo Cobo [1,2,5,†]

1 Photonics Engineering Group, Universidad de Cantabria, 39005 Santander, Spain
2 Instituto de Investigación Sanitaria Valdecilla (IDIVAL), 39011 Santander, Spain
3 Psychiatry Service, Marqués de Valdecilla University Hospital, 39011 Santander, Spain
4 Ambar Telecomunicaciones S.L., 39011 Santander, Spain
5 CIBER de Bioingeniería, Biomateriales y Nanomedicina, Instituto de Salud Carlos III, 28029 Madrid, Spain
* Correspondence: luis.rodriguez@unican.es
† These authors contributed equally to this work and share senior authorship.

Abstract: In the context of global population aging, identifying reliable, objective tools to assess physical function and postural stability in older adults is increasingly important to mitigate fall risk. This study presents a non-contact platform that uses a Microsoft Azure Kinect depth camera to evaluate functional performance related to lower-limb muscular capacity and static balance through self-selected depth squats and four progressively challenging stances (feet apart, feet together, semitandem, and tandem). By applying markerless motion capture algorithms, the system provides key biomechanical parameters such as center of mass displacement, knee angles, and sway trajectories. A comparison of older and younger individuals showed that the older group tended to perform shallower squats and exhibit greater mediolateral and anteroposterior sway, aligning with age-related declines in strength and postural control. Longitudinal tracking also illustrated how performance varied following a fall, indicating potential for ongoing risk assessment. Notably, in 30 s balance trials, the first 10 s often captured meaningful differences in stability, suggesting that short-duration stance tests can reliably detect early signs of imbalance. These findings highlight the feasibility of low-cost, user-friendly depth-camera technologies to complement traditional clinical measures and guide targeted fall-prevention strategies in older populations.

Keywords: functional assessment; depth cameras; squat; balance; falls; biomechanics

1. Introduction

Worldwide populations are aging at unprecedented rates. By 2030, it is estimated that one in six people globally will be 60 years or older, and the global count of individuals over 60 is expected to rise from 1.0 billion in 2020 to 1.4 billion [1]. By 2050, that number is projected to double to 2.1 billion [1]. Additionally, the population aged 80 and above will triple from 2020 to 2050, reaching 426 million [1]. This demographic shift creates a multitude of challenges in public health, particularly with increased risks of falls, frailty, and dependency.

Falls among older adults represent a major public health issue, with approximately 23.4% of those aged 65 and older experiencing at least one fall each year [2]. These incidents can lead to serious consequences, making falls a leading cause of injuries, hospitalizations, and even mortality in the elderly [3]. Beyond the immediate injuries, falls can precipitate long-term declines in function and independence, leading to sedentary behavior and a reduced quality of life for seniors [4]. Consequently, fall prevention is essential for enhancing healthy life expectancy and reducing healthcare system strain [5].

In this context, physical function assessments and biomechanical movement analysis are valuable tools for evaluating an older person's mobility and fall risk. Objective performance measures of gait and balance have well-documented clinical relevance—for example, slow walking speed or difficulty in chair-rise tests are associated with higher rates of future falls, disability, hospitalization, and even mortality [6]. Muscle weakness and impaired balance are well-established risk factors for falls [5]. Traditionally, functional assessments (such as static balance tests, gait analysis, or sit-to-stand tests) rely on time-based measurements or qualitative observation by professionals, which may limit the accuracy and objectivity of the evaluation.

Many widely used functional tests provide only coarse summary outcomes, such as the time to complete a Timed Up-and-Go (TUG) test [7], the number of repetitions in a chair stand test [8] or the composite score of the Short Physical Performance Battery (SPPB) [9], potentially overlooking subtle deficits in movement quality or motor control. Researchers have noted that objective sensor-based measures can be more sensitive than coarse clinical tests for detecting balance and gait impairments. For instance, an instrumented Timed Up-and-Go (iTUG) that uses wearable sensors can capture additional parameters beyond completion time, thereby identifying nuanced performance variables and improving fall-risk prediction. This evidence underscores the need for more objective, data-rich methods in geriatric care [10].

Markerless motion capture techniques offer a promising solution for objective, non-invasive, and high-resolution assessments in clinical and home settings. Various systems—including force platforms, wearable inertial sensors, and optical depth cameras—enable detailed quantification of biomechanical parameters, facilitating improved monitoring of functional status. Non-contact markerless systems use external cameras to track body kinematics without any sensors attached to the person. These vision-based devices capture three-dimensional movements of the body without requiring physical markers on the subject. Depth-sensing cameras in particular can directly measure distances to the body and construct a skeletal model in real time, providing rich motion data while being unobtrusive for the user.

Among depth cameras, the Microsoft Azure Kinect stands out as an evolution of the Kinect line, offering higher accuracy in 3D reconstruction, an improved working range, and an updated Software Development Kit (SDK). Several studies [11,12] have reported its effectiveness in quantifying gait, posture, and balance parameters, with relatively simple implementation and lower cost compared to traditional laboratory-based systems. This capability opens up opportunities to deploy objective mobility assessments in environments such as community clinics, nursing homes, or even patients' homes, which is particularly beneficial for monitoring at-risk older populations. Nevertheless, despite these technological advances, relatively few studies to date have focused on deploying markerless motion capture for comprehensive geriatric assessment. Recent reviews highlight that further research is still needed to establish the clinical usefulness of such markerless systems for quantifying functional performance in real-world older adult populations [13].

The present work proposes a non-contact functional evaluation platform based on a low-cost depth sensor (Azure Kinect), aimed at older adults. The system is designed to capture key biomechanical metrics during two simple physical function tests: self-selected depth squat exercise and static balance tests in four different stances. These test activities target indicators of lower-limb muscular capacity (e.g., squat depth) and balance—the domains most pertinent to mobility and fall risk in seniors—and the use of a marker-free sensor allows them to be evaluated objectively without the need for wearables or extensive setup.

The objectives are (1) to demonstrate the technical feasibility of using a non-contact depth sensor (Azure Kinect (Microsoft Corp., Redmond, WA, USA)) to measure relevant variables of physical function (balance and lower limb strength) in older adults, (2) to systematically compare these measurements with data from young healthy subjects, and (3) to explore the potential of this platform for early detection of physical decline. Through this approach, we aim to show that a markerless depth camera system can effectively provide accurate and actionable assessments of balance and lower-extremity function in older individuals.

2. Materials and Methods

2.1. System Design and Architecture

The proposed platform consists of a non-invasive evaluation system that integrates motion capture hardware and data processing software. The system is composed of the following: (i) an Azure Kinect depth sensor responsible for capturing the participant's movement in three dimensions and (ii) a software module for real-time visualization, data processing and biomechanical metric calculation. In Figure 1, a schematic of the overall architecture and data flow is shown.

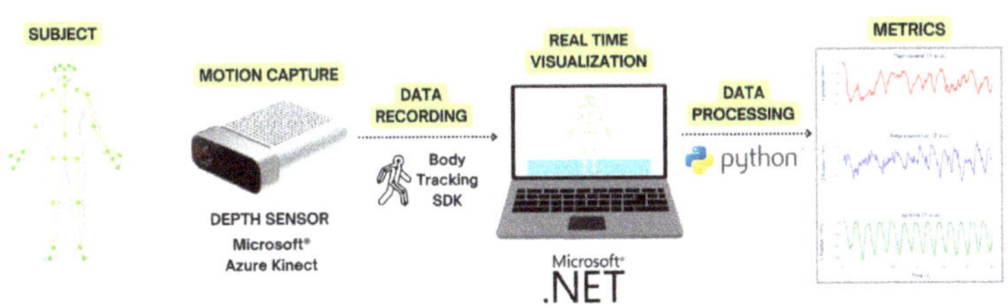

Figure 1. Overall architecture and data flow.

2.1.1. Azure Kinect

The Azure Kinect (Microsoft®) [14] is the system's central component. This next-generation device includes a 12-megapixel RGB camera, a 1-megapixel Time-of-Flight (ToF) depth sensor, an integrated inertial measurement unit (IMU), and an array of 7 microphones (Figure 2). The depth sensor emits an infrared pattern and measures the time-of-flight of the light to calculate distances, thus producing a depth map of the scene in real time. Unlike the previous Kinect v2 (Xbox One), Azure Kinect offers higher resolution and a wider field of view, improving spatial and temporal accuracy in human skeleton tracking. These characteristics make it suitable for capturing the key body movements relevant to functional evaluations.

To obtain the subject's posture, the platform uses Microsoft's body tracking SDK, which estimates the positions of a series of skeletal joints in each captured frame. Specifically, Azure Kinect returns 3D coordinates for 32 body joints—including the head, trunk, upper and lower extremities—at a frequency of up to 30 frames per second. This sampling rate (30 Hz) is sufficient for analyzing human movements in the selected tests since the main components of movement during balance and gait occur at low frequencies (generally below ~2–3 Hz) [15]. Biomechanical studies have shown, for instance, that rapid oscillations of postural sway rarely exceed 2 Hz, so the sensor's 30 Hz sampling covers the necessary dynamic range. In our study, however, we opted to record at 15 frames per second to reduce graphics-processing-unit (GPU) computational requirements; given that postural oscillations seldom exceed 2 Hz, this reduced rate is adequate to capture the necessary dynamics without demanding excessive processing power.

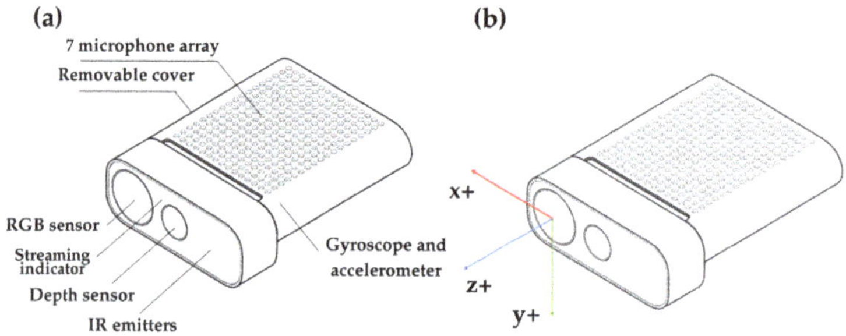

Figure 2. Azure Kinect (**a**) components and (**b**) 3D-coordinate system [14].

In its default configuration, the sensor's coordinate system is defined with the X axis running horizontally (with positive values toward the right of the camera), the Y axis oriented vertically (with positive values directed downward), and the Z axis representing depth (with positive values increasing away from the sensor), as shown in Figure 2. For the purposes of our biomechanical analyses, the raw Y values are later inverted so that upward movements are represented by positive values, thus facilitating the interpretation of vertical displacements during exercise.

The Azure Kinect was selected for this study due to its cost-effectiveness, ease of deployment, and enhanced tracking accuracy compared to earlier Kinect models.

2.1.2. Software Implementation

The software module of the platform was developed using a combination of languages: C# (v7.3) and Python (v3.12.4).

C# was used to interface with the Azure Kinect SDKs and perform, using the .NET framework, real-time data acquisition and preview of the tracked skeleton, allowing the clinician to verify that the subject is correctly positioned before data collection begins. Using the official Azure Kinect and Body Tracking SDKs, a simple desktop application was created in C# that initializes the camera, detects the subject, and begins recording the skeleton sequence when the evaluator indicates. This module not only allows the selection of the test type (squat or balance) to label the corresponding data but also continuously records the joint positions along with timestamps while the subject performs the exercise. Upon completion, the raw data are exported to CSV files, including joint identifiers, coordinates (position and orientation), timestamp, and a test label.

Python was used for data processing and metric calculation, thanks to its scientific ecosystem for efficient data manipulation (libraries like Numpy (v2.0), Pandas (v2.2.2) and SciPy (v1.14.1)) and visualization tools (libraries like Matplotlib (v3.9.1) and Plotly (v.5.24.1)). The software architecture follows a workflow in which the raw Kinect data (joint coordinates per frame) are stored and later processed by Python scripts that compute the biomechanical metrics.

In summary, the platform's design enables a rapid and objective evaluation: the older adult positions himself in front of the sensor and performs the designated exercises without needing markers or wearable devices; the system records the movement and, within seconds, calculates quantitative physical performance metrics. This ease of use and speed are essential for application in busy clinical settings.

2.2. Selected Exercises for Evaluation

Based on the experience provided by clinical personnel, two complementary functional tests were selected: (a) a dynamic lower-limb functional exercise (self-selected depth squats) and (b) static balance tests in progressively challenging stances (see Figures 3 and 4). The combination of these tests seeks to evaluate fundamental aspects of function in older adults: leg strength and postural stability.

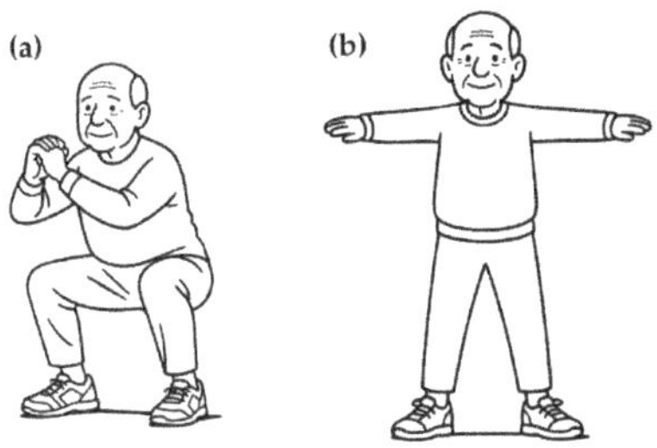

Figure 3. Illustration of the selected exercises: (**a**) self-selected depth squats and (**b**) static balance.

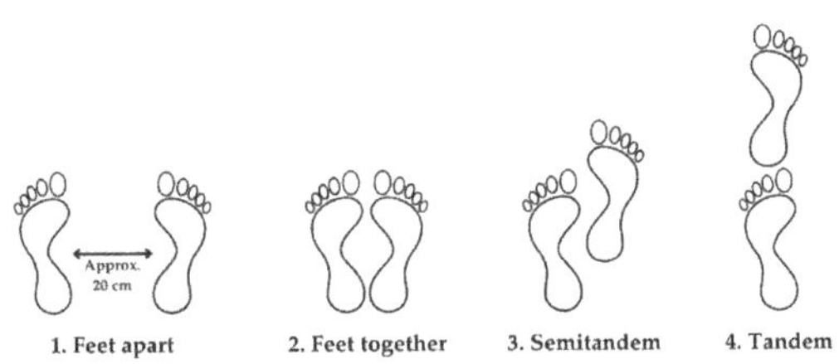

Figure 4. Overview of static balance stances.

2.2.1. Self-Selected Depth Squats

The first exercise consists of performing continuous self-selected depth squats for a duration of 30 s, according to the participant's capacity and comfort, without specifying a fixed depth; that is, each older adult descends as far as they feel safe and stable.

Squats are widely recognized as a fundamental movement for assessing lower-limb functional capacity related to strength rather than measuring muscle force directly. They involve coordinated activation of the quadriceps, hamstrings, and gluteal muscles, making them an effective proxy for evaluating the overall strength and mobility of the lower extremities.

In our study, we employ a self-selected depth squat, which allows evaluation of the effective range of motion and strength without forcing the participant into a posture that might be uncomfortable or risky for their joints. Unlike standardized squat protocols that may use a fixed target (e.g., sitting down on a chair), the self-selected approach respects individual variability in joint range and strength. This is particularly important for older adults, who often exhibit reduced flexibility and joint discomfort when forced to achieve a predetermined depth. By allowing a free-depth squat, our system captures the authentic functional performance of each participant, thereby providing a more accurate reflection of their lower-limb strength and mobility. Moreover, variations in squat depth can reveal asymmetries or compensatory strategies that might not be evident with a constrained movement.

2.2.2. Static Balance

The second part of the evaluation corresponds to static balance tests with progressively challenging stances. Four standing postures were selected—each with increasing difficulty—similar to those used in clinical balance assessments [9]. The selected stances, in order of increasing challenge, were as follows: (1) Feet apart (standing with feet shoulder-width apart, approximately 20 cm), (2) Feet together (both feet placed side-by-side), (3) Semitandem (one foot slightly ahead, with the heel of the front foot approximately halfway along the rear foot), and (4) Tandem (right foot directly in front of the left, heel-to-toe). These postures challenge the balance system progressively by reducing the base of support (see Figure 4).

The four selected stances allow multilevel evaluation of balance. The feet apart stance is very stable and almost all independent older adults can maintain it easily; it serves as a baseline reference for sway. When feet are together, the base is reduced, and slight increases in Center of Mass (CoM) oscillations are typically observed. The semitandem stance demands greater lateral balance and serves as an intermediate step; many older adults can hold it, though with more effort. Finally, the tandem stance is considerably challenging; failing to maintain 10 s in tandem is common in those with compromised balance. These stances are directly derived from validated clinical tests: for instance, the SPPB [9] measures the ability to maintain 10 s in these positions. However, our platform not only assesses whether a subject can maintain the posture for 10 s but also quantifies their movement during the task. Subtle differences in control can be captured; for example, two individuals might both maintain 10 s in tandem, but one does so almost motionless while the other sways noticeably; clinically they would receive the same score, but biomechanically their balance differs. The platform quantifies these differences using the metrics described in Section 2.3.

2.3. Metrics

2.3.1. Center of Mass (CoM)

The calculation of the overall CoM is central to the analysis of human movement and postural stability. In this study, we adopt an anthropometric model based on De Leva's modifications [16] to the classical segmental inertia parameters originally proposed by Zatsiorsky and Seluyanov [17]. According to this approach, the human body is divided into distinct segments—specifically, the trunk, thighs, shanks, and feet—with each segment assigned a specific percentage of the total body mass and a predetermined point of application representing its individual CoM (see Figure 5 and Table 1).

Table 1. Parameters for each unique segment.

Segment	Defining Joints	α (% of Length)	Relative Mass (kg) [1]
Trunk	PELVIS–NECK	55.14%	52.3
Thigh	HIP–KNEE	40.95%	17.0
Shank	KNEE–ANKLE	44.59%	5.2
Foot	ANKLE–FOOT	50%	1.65

[1] Renormalized masses to sum 100%.

For each segment i, the segmental CoM (CoM_i) is estimated by linear interpolation between the proximal and distal joint positions. For example, for the thigh, the CoM is calculated along the line joining the hip and knee, using a proportion α, that represents the percentage of the segment's length at which the CoM is located. Mathematically, if

$\vec{r}_{proximal}$ and $\vec{r}_{distal}$ are the position vectors of the proximal and distal joints, respectively, then the CoM for that segment is given by:

$$CoM_i = \vec{r}_{proximal} + \alpha \times \left(\vec{r}_{distal} - \vec{r}_{proximal}\right) \quad (1)$$

The overall body CoM is subsequently determined as the weighted average of all segmental centers of mass:

$$CoM_{total} = \frac{\sum_i (m_i \times CoM_i)}{\sum_i m_i} \quad (2)$$

where m_i denotes the mass fraction of segment i. In this study, we have deliberately excluded the head and arms from the CoM calculation to focus on the dynamics of the lower limbs and trunk. This decision is supported by previous research [18] showing that upper-body segments (arms and head) contribute additional variability in the mediolateral (ML) direction of CoM motion, which may obscure subtle differences in lower-limb performance during tasks such as squatting and static balance. The accurate estimation of the CoM is fundamental as it underpins subsequent analyses, including the detection of squat events and the assessment of postural sway.

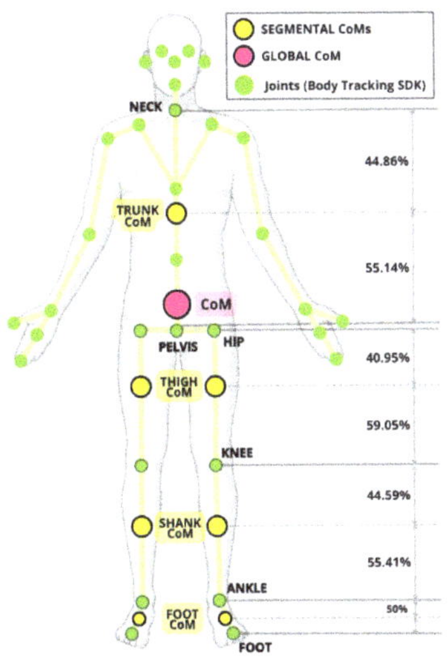

Figure 5. Segmental and Global CoMs based on De Leva's [16].

2.3.2. Joint Angles: Knee and Spine Alignment

Another set of metrics focuses on the key joint angles involved in the exercises: knee angle and a measure of spinal alignment. These parameters provide information on the subject's posture and technique during the movement, which is relevant for evaluating movement quality and potential compensations.

Knee angle is defined as the angle between the thigh and the shank. Using the coordinates of the hip, knee and ankle, the knee angle θ_{knee} is computed using the cosine law, via the dot product of the vectors representing the thigh ($\vec{v}_{thigh}$, hip to knee) and the shank ($\vec{v}_{shank}$, knee to ankle). That is:

$$\theta_{knee} = arcos\left(\frac{\vec{v}_{thigh} \cdot \vec{v}_{shank}}{\left\|\vec{v}_{thigh}\right\|\left\|\vec{v}_{shank}\right\|}\right) \tag{3}$$

This angle is approximately 180° when the leg is fully extended (standing upright) and decreases as the knee flexes (e.g., around 90° in a mid-depth squat). For each frame, the knee angle achieved in each leg is extracted and the minimum knee angle corresponds to the point of maximum flexion. This value serves as an indicator of squat depth complementary to the CoM descent: a lower minimum knee angle indicates greater flexion. For instance, if a subject only performs a shallow squat, their minimum knee angle might be around 140°, whereas a deeper squat might reach 100° or less.

Maintaining a straight back during squat is important to reduce injury risk and ensure that the load is borne by the legs. To quantify spinal posture, an index of back alignment was defined. The joints used are the pelvis, lumbar spine (spine_navel joint), thoracic spine (spine_chest joint), and neck. We then construct three sequential vectors:

- Vector 1 ($\vec{v}_1$): From the pelvis to the lumbar spine.
- Vector 2 ($\vec{v}_2$): From the lumbar spine to the thoracic spine.
- Vector 3 ($\vec{v}_3$): From the thoracic spine to the neck.

The angles between adjacent vectors are computed using the cosine law:

$$\theta_1 = arcos\left(\frac{\vec{v}_1 \cdot \vec{v}_2}{\left\|\vec{v}_1\right\|\left\|\vec{v}_2\right\|}\right) \theta_2 = arcos\left(\frac{\vec{v}_2 \cdot \vec{v}_3}{\left\|\vec{v}_2\right\|\left\|\vec{v}_3\right\|}\right) \tag{4}$$

If the spine were perfectly straight, these segments would be aligned and the angles would be close to 0°. To obtain a single index, the two angles are averaged and expressed as a deviation from perfect alignment, defined as:

$$Spine\ Alignment\ Index = 180^{\circ} - \frac{(\theta_1 + \theta_2)}{2} \tag{5}$$

Essentially, this value indicates how far the spine deviates from a straight line. A value near 0 would imply a very curved back (high $\theta_1 + \theta_2$), whereas higher values (e.g., 170°) indicate a straighter back. In our results, this index is reported in degrees; for example, an index of 175° suggests good alignment (almost straight spine, only 5° deviation on average per section), whereas 160° would indicate a notable forward bend during the squat. This calculation, while simplified (not distinguishing between lumbar or thoracic curvature), provides a quantitative measure of the subject's back posture during the exercise.

Together, the measures of knee angle and spinal alignment allow an assessment of the technique employed during the squat. This is important because, for example, a subject could achieve good depth (low CoM, knees around 100°) but at the expense of a heavily rounded back (low spine index), which is not ideal. Our metrics can detect such compensations. Similarly, if a subject has limited ankle or hip mobility, it may manifest as an abnormal posture that is reflected in these angles.

2.3.3. Symmetry Index

Movement symmetry is another important consideration, especially in bilateral exercises such as squats. Many older adults may exhibit differences in strength or mobility between their legs (for example, due to unilateral arthritis or past injuries), which could cause one leg to bear more load or have less flexion than the other during a squat. To quantify possible asymmetries, a Symmetry Index based on the knee angles was calculated.

The Symmetry Index (SI) is defined as the percentage difference between both legs relative to the mean value, using the common formula in biomechanics [19]:

$$\text{Symmetry Index} = \frac{\left|\theta_{\text{left}} - \theta_{\text{right}}\right|}{\frac{\theta_{\text{left}}+\theta_{\text{right}}}{2}} \times 100\% \tag{6}$$

where θ refers to the minimum knee angle reached during the squat for each side. This metric, widely used to quantify asymmetries in gait and movement, yields 0% if both sides are identical and increases as the difference grows. For example, if a subject flexes the left knee to 100° and the right to 110° at maximum depth, the SI would be $\frac{|100-110|}{(100+110)/2} \times 100 \approx 9.52\%$, indicating that one knee flexed about 9.5% less than the other.

2.3.4. Squat Detection and Squat Index

The system also performs automatic recognition of squat repetitions and extraction of the depth achieved in each. An algorithm was implemented to analyze the time series of the CoM to identify the movement cycles corresponding to each squat.

The vertical CoM signal (Y) (inverted for facilitating the interpretation) was chosen for detection because it exhibits a clear pattern: it decreases when lowering during a squat and increases when rising. In the CoM-Y signal, each complete squat appears as a valley (descent followed by ascent). SciPy's `find_peaks()` [20] function was used on the inverted signal (−CoM-Y). After an empirical tuning phase during the first two pilot sessions, the parameters were fixed for all subsequent recordings at prominence ≥ 20 mm, minimum inter-peak distance = 5 frames (≈0.33 s at 15 Hz), and a height threshold of −20 mm. These settings avoided counting minor sub-movements or brief pauses as separate repetitions and reliably isolated the instant of greatest descent for each squat.

The initial standing position is a critical reference for calculating squat depth. In our methodology, this position was determined by averaging the first three maximum peaks of the CoM-Y signal, based on the rationale that at the end of each squat the user returns to their initial standing posture, at least during the first squats. Averaging these maximum peaks, rather than simply taking the very first CoM-Y data points, mitigates the potential error that might occur if the recording starts while the subject is already performing the first squat. This approach ensures a more robust estimation of the baseline standing position. Once the initial standing position is established, the algorithm identifies the instants (t_i) corresponding to the deepest points during each squat. The squat depth is then calculated as the difference between the CoM-Y value at the initial standing position and the CoM-Y minimum at t_i.

Figure 6 illustrates an example of squat detection in the CoM-Y signal. The figure shows how the valleys correspond to individual squats, and it demonstrates the process of identifying both the initial standing position and the lowest points during each squat repetition.

To capture both the quantity and quality of the squatting performance, we introduce a Squat Index. This index is calculated as the product of the number of correctly detected squats and the mean squat depth. By combining these two aspects—repetition count and effective range of motion—the Squat Index provides a more comprehensive measure of squatting performance. We formulate this idea as:

$$\text{Squat Index} = N_{squats} \times \overline{d} \tag{7}$$

where N_{squats} is the number of correctly detected squats and $\overline{d}$ is their mean vertical depth in millimeters. Expressing the Squat Index in the original depth unit (mm) keeps it directly interpretable: one deep squat (e.g., 200 mm) has the same Squat Index as two half-depth squats (2 × 100 mm).

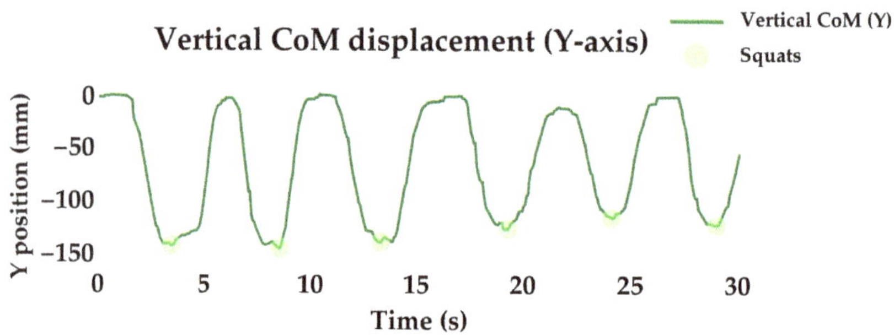

Figure 6. Example of squat detection in CoM Y-axis signal (participant ID6 (84 years, wheelchair)).

2.3.5. Balance Analysis

For the static balance tests, the derived metrics focused on quantifying the subject's postural sway during each stance. From the CoM trajectory (described in Section 2.3.1), several indicators were extracted:

- Maximum mediolateral (ML) and anteroposterior (AP) displacement: The maximum distance that the CoM deviated laterally (ML) and front-to-back (AP) from the center during the test. This provides an idea of the range of oscillation. For example, an ML max value of 20 mm means the greatest lateral deviation was 2 cm. Higher values suggest greater episodes of imbalance.
- Mean absolute deviation: The average absolute distance of the CoM from the center in both ML and AP directions. This reflects the sustained level of instability. For instance, if someone oscillates constantly by ±10 mm, the mean absolute deviation will be around 10 mm; if they hardly move from the center, it will be closer to 0.
- Elliptical confidence area (stabilographic area): The area of an ellipse that encompasses approximately 95% of the CoM trajectory was calculated. It was assumed that the distribution of CoM points is elliptical around the center. The standard deviations of the ML (σ_x) and AP (σ_z) positions were estimated. Then, applying a confidence factor (approximately 2.5), an ellipse with semi-axes $a = 2.5\sigma_x$ and $b = 2.5\sigma_z$ was constructed. The area of this ellipse is given by πab. This area (expressed in mm^2) serves as a measure to compare stability objectively: a smaller area implies the CoM remained within a small range, while a larger area indicates more dispersed oscillations. Each stance produces a different area. It is expected that more challenging stances will have larger areas (see Figure 7).

Given the differences in base of support, each metric is annotated with its corresponding stance. Direct comparisons are more meaningful between subjects in the same stance than across different stances.

It is important to note that for each balance posture, the initial position (i.e., the zero reference point) is determined by averaging the CoM position of the first 3 s of the test. This early phase estimation ensures that subsequent measurements of displacement and sway are relative to a stable and consistent starting position.

These objective measurements complement the simple observation of whether the subject can maintain the posture, providing a richer profile of their postural stability.

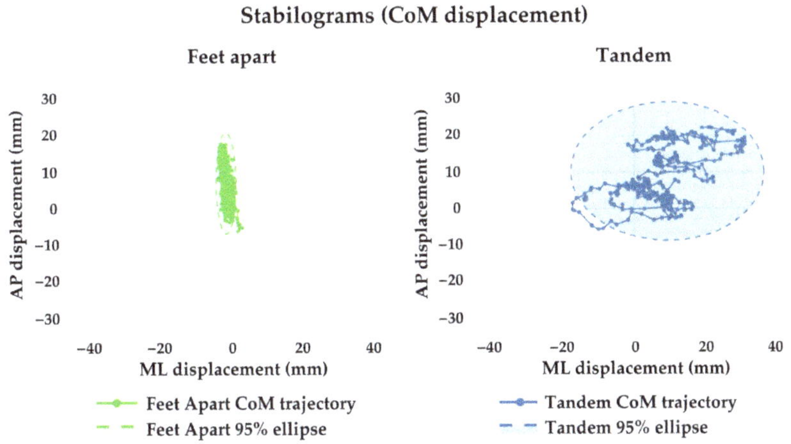

Figure 7. Example of stabilograms of Feet apart and Tandem balance stances.

2.4. Inclusion and Exclusion Criteria

Participants were included if they were aged 65 years or older, could stand independently for at least 30 s with or without assistive devices, and could understand simple verbal instructions. Participants were excluded if they had acute musculoskeletal injuries, severe cognitive impairment, or any condition that contraindicated participation in light physical activities.

All participants gave written informed consent.

2.5. Clinical Assessment

Scores for the Tinetti Performance-Oriented Mobility Assessment (POMA) [21,22] and the modified Barthel Index (mBI) [23,24] were extracted from each participant's most recent comprehensive evaluation performed $\leq$ months before Kinect testing by the nursing-home physiotherapy and nursing team. The 16-item POMA (9-item balance, 7-item gait), rated on a 0–2 scale, yields a maximum of 28 points; scores ≤ 24 indicate elevated fall-risk. The 10-item mBI (five-level rating; range 0–100) evaluates independence in basic activities of daily living (ADL). Internal consistency and sensitivity are superior to the original Barthel Index in older cohorts.

2.6. Statistical Analysis

The statistical plan was structured around the two primary research objectives. Objective 1 (technical feasibility in older adults) was addressed by summarizing, for the older group, knee-flexion, CoM-sway and squat-depth metrics and by testing whether their distributions met the expected biomechanical ranges reported in the literature (see H_{0a}). Objective 2 (systematic comparison with young adults) was tackled through between-group tests (H_{0b}) and within-subject repeated-measure tests to quantify stability of the metrics over time. The specific non-parametric procedures selected for each hypothesis are detailed below.

All statistical analyses were performed in Python 3.12 (Pandas 2.2, SciPy 1.14, Pingouin 0.5). Data normality was examined with the Shapiro–Wilk test. Because at least one variable per domain violated normality ($p < 0.05$) and the sample size was below thirty, non-parametric methods were selected.

- Between-group comparison (Older vs. Young): The independent Older vs. Young comparison was performed with the Mann–Whitney U test. Results are reported as the U statistic, the two-tailed p-value, and Cohen's d, calculated with the pooled standard deviation of the two groups to quantify the magnitude of the difference.
- Repeated-measures comparison: To examine changes across the three consecutive 10-s windows (0–10 s, 10–20 s, 20–30 s) within each participant, a Friedman test was applied. When the omnibus test reached significance, Bonferroni-adjusted Wilcoxon signed-rank tests identified the specific pairs that differed. The global effect size for the Friedman test is given as Kendall's W (0 indicating no agreement, 1 indicating complete agreement).
- Significance threshold: All tests were two-tailed with $\alpha = 0.05$.
- Type II error risk: Given the exploratory nature of this pilot ($n = 8$ older, $n = 8$ young), statistical power is limited; p-values close to 0.05 should therefore be interpreted cautiously. Effect-size estimates (Cohen's d and Kendall's W) are provided to aid interpretation until larger validation studies can be conducted.

Working hypotheses:

- H_{0a}: there is no difference between older and young adults in quantitative squat performance (minimum knee angle, CoM vertical displacement, Squat Index).
- H_{0b}: there is no difference between groups in postural-sway metrics (ML/AP displacements, 95% CoM-ellipse area) during static stances.

Rejection of either null hypothesis would support the technological feasibility of Azure Kinect to capture clinically relevant lower-limb and balance variables, thereby fulfilling Objectives 1–2.

2.7. Experimental Setup

The evaluations were conducted in a large room at the nursing home. The sensor (Azure Kinect) was mounted at a height of approximately 1 m and positioned 2–3 m away from the participant to ensure that the entire body was within the field of view. The room had neutral lighting and sufficient space.

Walking aids were removed from the base of support and placed behind the participant; all exercises were therefore executed unaided while a member of the study team provided standby supervision.

3. Results

3.1. Participant Characteristics

A preliminary evaluation was conducted with eight older adults (five women and three men) residing in a nursing home, with ages ranging from 71 to 94 years (median = 88.5 years; IQR = 80.8–92.0). Over a 7-week period, each participant was measured on nine occasions (two sessions per week during the first two weeks, followed by one session per week thereafter). These participants exhibited varying levels of physical fitness yet remained largely independent in their activities of daily living, as indicated by Modified Barthel Index scores close to 100 (median = 98; IQR = 95–100; range 90–100). Despite this functional independence, median Tinetti POMA was 26 (IQR = 24.5–28, range 23–28), indicating some gait-balance limitations; five of the eight volunteers used walking aids, and several reported at least one fall in the previous year. Detailed demographic and clinical data, including fall history, are presented in Table 2.

Table 2. Characteristics of older volunteers.

Age (Years)	Gender	Walking Aid	Tinetti	Barthel	Falls	
					Previous [1]	During [2]
87	Female	None	28	97	0	0
90	Female	Cane	23	98	0	0
92	Female	Cane	26	93	0	1
94	Female	Walker	26	90	5	1
71	Male	None	28	100	0	0
84	Male	Wheelchair	23	N/A	0	0
71	Male	None	28	100	4	0
92	Female	Walker	25	100	1	0

Summary statistics for the eight older participants: Age—median 88.5 (IQR 80.8–92; range 71–94); Tinetti—median 26 (IQR 24.5–28; range 23–28); Barthel—median 98 (IQR 95–100; 90–100). [1] Falls that occurred during the year prior to the start of the study. [2] Falls that occurred during the measurement sessions of the study.

It is worth noting that the participants' high Barthel and Tinetti scores indicate a relatively well-preserved functional status despite advanced age, although the presence of walking aids and previous falls suggests some degree of mobility impairment typical of older populations.

To provide a comparative benchmark, a sample of eight younger adults (three women and five men) aged 26 to 55 years was also recruited. None presented known musculoskeletal or balance disorders. Their baseline data can be found in Table 3. This younger cohort served as a control group, helping to determine whether the proposed platform could distinguish expected age-related differences in lower-limb strength (squatting tasks) and postural stability (static balance tests).

Table 3. Characteristics of younger volunteers.

Age (Years)	Gender
33	Male
34	Female
26	Female
26	Male
26	Female
26	Male
38	Male
55	Male

Informed consent was obtained prior to testing and it was verified that they could perform a partial squat and hold the semitandem position safely.

3.2. Comparison Between Older and Younger Adults

All participants completed the two main test protocols (self-selected depth squats and four progressively challenging static balance stances) while being tracked by the Azure Kinect sensor. A series of biomechanical metrics were extracted (Section 2.3), including the vertical displacement of the CoM during squats, knee angles, a spinal alignment index, symmetry indices for bilateral leg motion, and postural sway indicators during static balance.

To explore the platform's ability to differentiate between age groups, the metrics were compared following the analysis plan outlined in Section 2.6. Noteworthy findings are summarized below:

1. Squat Depth, Knee Flexion Angles and Squat Index:

The platform captured a clear tendency for older adults to exhibit less vertical displacement of the CoM during squats ($p < 0.001$), indicating more limited descent compared to the younger group. Correspondingly, their minimum knee angles (left and right) were significantly larger ($p < 0.001$), reflecting reduced knee flexion. For instance, the median minimum knee angle in the older group was about 110°, whereas the younger group reached about 60°. The calculated squat index, which combines both depth and repetition count, was also significantly lower in the older adults ($p < 0.001$). This underscores the reduced overall squatting performance potentially linked to age-related declines in lower-extremity strength and range of motion.

2. Spinal Alignment and Symmetry: No statistically significant differences were observed in the spinal alignment index ($p = 0.645$) or the symmetry index ($p = 0.505$) between the groups. This suggests that, although older adults descend less, their squat technique or distribution of load (left vs. right) may remain relatively balanced, and they do not exhibit marked asymmetries in knee flexion when performing the movement.
3. Static Balance Metrics: Static-balance metrics showed significant differences in several postural sway metrics between the older and younger adults. Specifically, older adults showed greater maximum ML displacement ($p = 0.01$), greater mean ML displacement ($p = 0.015$), greater maximum AP displacement ($p < 0.001$) and greater mean AP displacement ($p < 0.001$). The CoM trajectory ellipse area (a 95% confidence ellipse) was also significantly larger in older adults ($p < 0.001$).

Overall, these findings indicate that the proposed platform effectively differentiates older from younger adults in terms of squat depth and postural stability. Table 4 provides a detailed breakdown of the relevant U statistics and *p*-values, while Figure 8 illustrates some of these group-wise differences in squat and balance metrics.

Table 4. Comparison results of Biomechanical Metrics Between Older and Younger Adults using the Mann–Whitney U Test.

	Metric	Older Median	Younger Median	U Statistic	*p*-Value [1]	Cohen's d
Squats	Mean disp. in X-axis (mm)	2.44	−3.04	43	0.279	−0.02
	Mean disp. in Z-axis (mm)	−9.05	3.09	20	0.234	−0.42
	Mean disp. in Y-axis (mm)	−51.83	−142.27	64	<0.001	3.56
	Min. Knee Angle Left (°)	109.19	57. 93	64	<0.001	3.38
	Min. Knee Angle Right (°)	110.82	60. 97	64	<0.001	3.73
	Spinal Alignment	170.29	169.45	37	0.645	0.28
	Symmetry Index	3.38	2.68	39	0.505	0.20
	Number of squats	16.50	14.50	42	0.317	0.26
	Max. disp. in Y-axis (mm)	143.63	366.17	0	<0.001	−3.73
	Squat Index	1756.31	5401.51	1	<0.001	−3.12
Balance (10 s)	Max. ML Disp. (mm)	7.82	6.74	56	0.010	1.40
	Mean ML Disp. (mm)	3.37	2.48	55	0.015	1.40
	Max. AP Disp. (mm)	9.14	7.03	62	<0.001	2.16
	Mean AP Disp. (mm)	3.51	2.76	62	<0.001	2.23
	CoM Trajectory Ellipse Area (mm^2)	191.13	128.31	60	0.002	1.19

[1] *p*-values < 0.001 are reported as such for clarity.

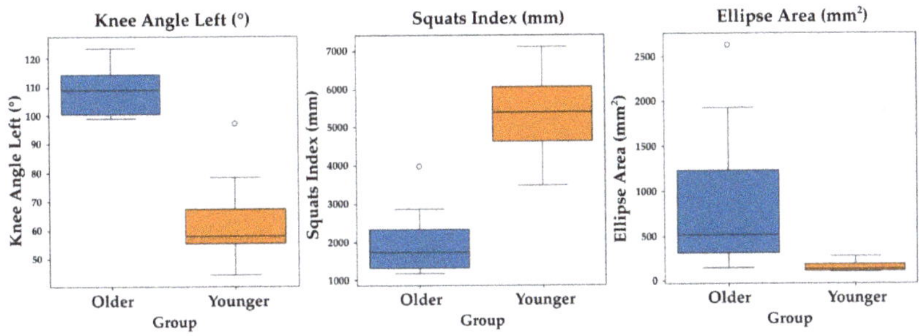

Figure 8. Comparison Results—box plots of knee angle range (degrees), squat index (dimensionless) and sway ellipse area (mm^2) in older (n = 8) and young (n = 8) participants.

3.3. 10-s vs. 30-s Balance Analysis

All participants were measured for 30 s in each balance posture (Feet Apart, Feet Together, Semitandem, and Tandem). During this period, the CoM) was continuously tracked. Figure 9 presents the group-averaged CoM displacement in ML and AP directions (±1 standard deviation) over the 30 s interval for each stance, combining all valid recordings.

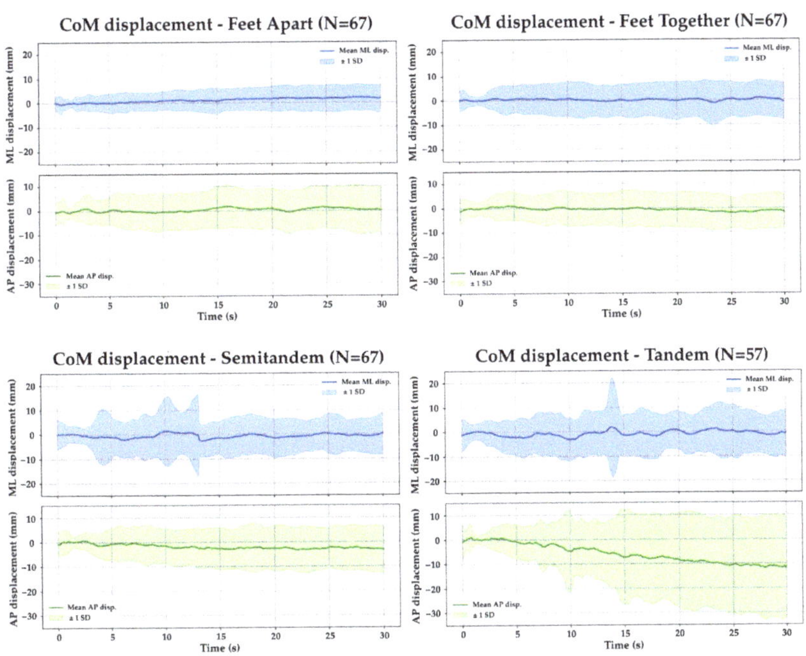

Figure 9. Group-Averaged CoM displacement in ML and AP directions during 30 s balance trials.Visual inspection suggests that the most pronounced fluctuations occur in the initial phase of each instance, with Tandem typically exhibiting wider variability due to its higher level of difficulty.

To formally assess whether the earliest portion of the trial (0–10 s) suffices to characterize each participant's sway, the 30 s were partitioned into three consecutive 10 s windows (0–10 s, 10–20 s, and 20–30 s) and a 95% confidence ellipse area was calculated in each window. Table 5 summarizes the results of a Friedman test for repeated measures. In every stance, Friedman revealed significant differences ($p < 0.05$) among the three intervals, indicating that at least one window diverges from the others.

Table 5. Friedman test and Wilcoxon pairwise (see Section 2.6) comparisons results for ellipse area across three consecutive 10-s windows.

Stance	χ^2 (p-Value)	Kendall's W	Window Pair	W-Stat	p-Corrected
Feet apart	6.75 (0.034)	0.578	0–10 vs. 10–20	1	0.047
			0–10 vs. 20–30	1	0.047
			10–20 vs. 20–30	12	1.000
Feet together	9.25 (0.010)	0.422	0–10 vs. 10–20	0	0.023
			0–10 vs. 20–30	5	0.234
			10–20 vs. 20–30	14	1.000
Semitandem	10.75 (0.005)	0.672	0–10 vs. 10–20	4	0.164
			0–10 vs. 20–30	0	0.023
			10–20 vs. 20–30	3	0.117
Tandem	8.857 (0.011)	0.633	0–10 vs. 10–20	7	0.891
			0–10 vs. 20–30	0	0.047
			10–20 vs. 20–30	9	1.000

Across all four static stances, the Friedman test revealed significant differences in the 95% CoM ellipse area among the three consecutive 10 s windows (feet apart $\chi^2(2) = 6.75$, $p = 0.034$; feet together $\chi^2(2) = 9.25$, $p = 0.010$; semitandem $\chi^2(2) = 10.75$, $p = 0.005$; tandem $\chi^2(2) = 8.86$, $p = 0.011$; Kendall's W ranging from 0.422 to 0.672; Table 5). Bonferroni-adjusted Wilcoxon pairwise tests (Table 5) showed that the 0–10 s window differed significantly from at least one later window in every stance (p-corrected ≤ 0.047), whereas the 10–20 s and 20–30 s windows seldom differed (p-corrected ≥ 0.117 in all 4 relevant comparisons; Table 5).

3.4. Longitudinal Case Examples

To illustrate the utility of our platform in detecting changes in postural control over time—and to provide a richer clinical context—two case examples are presented in Figure 10. For each participant (ID 1 and ID 4), the session-by-session number of squats, mean squat depth and mean CoM displacement metrics for Tandem stance are shown, alongside relevant clinical characteristics.

Participant ID 1 (Age: 87; No walking aid; Tinetti score = 28; Barthel Index = 97; No falls) exhibited relatively stable performance across nine sessions. The mean CoM displacement in both the ML and AP directions remained consistent over time, with only modest fluctuations in squat performance and tandem-stance sway. This stability aligns with the favorable clinical profile of ID 1, who, despite advanced age, demonstrates high functional scores and absence of falls.

In contrast, Participant ID 4 (Age: 94; Walking aid: Walker; Tinetti score = 26; Barthel Index = 90; 5 falls in the year prior to the study and 1 fall during the study) displayed marked variability. Notably, a fall occurred between Sessions 4 and 5 (indicated by a vertical dashed line in Figure 10). Following this event, the tandem-stance sway metrics (both ML and AP) fluctuated more noticeably, and squat performance also varied from session to session. These findings suggest that the fall—and the participant's more compromised clinical status—may have contributed to the increased instability and variability observed over time.

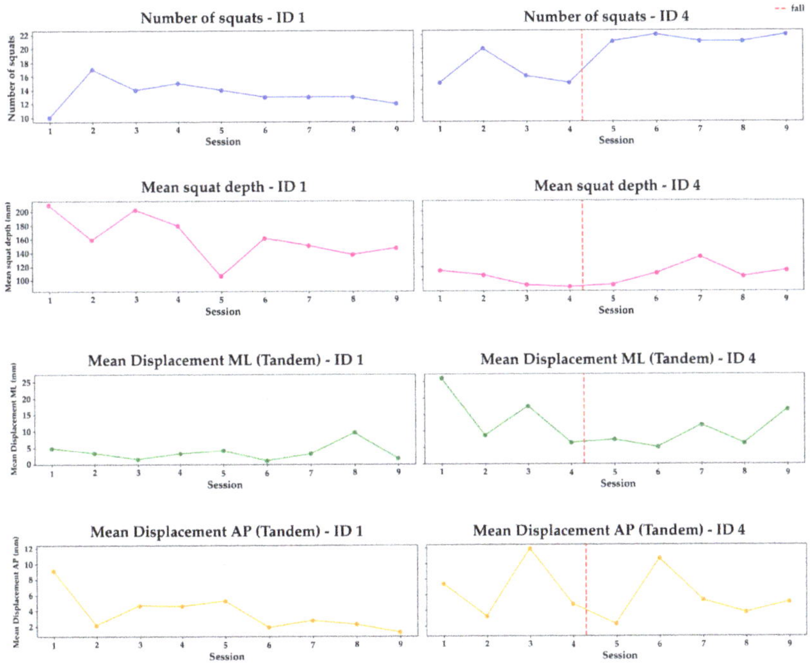

Figure 10. Longitudinal case examples: session-by-session changes in squat performance and tandem balance metrics. Colour coding: blue = number of squats; pink = mean squat depth; green = mean mediolateral (ML) displacement; orange = mean anteroposterior (AP) displacement. The vertical dashed red line marks the session in which a fall occurred.

By integrating these clinical characteristics, our analysis underscores the value of a longitudinal monitoring system that not only captures immediate postural adaptations (especially within the first 10 s) but also contextualizes them within the overall functional status of the individual. Such detailed insight can help clinicians tailor interventions more precisely, for instance, by identifying individuals (like ID 4) who may benefit from targeted balance training or fall-prevention strategies.

4. Discussion

In this study, we developed and tested a non-contact functional evaluation platform based on the Azure Kinect to assess lower-limb functional performance and balance in older adults through simple and clinically relevant tasks. Our approach leverages markerless motion capture to extract quantitative metrics—such as squat depth, knee angles and postural sway—which are essential for evaluating mobility and fall risk. Similar to recent advances in sensor-based frailty monitoring [25–27], our system aims to complement traditional clinical assessments by providing objective, high-resolution data during routine physical tasks. These findings fulfill Objective 1 by confirming technical feasibility, address Objective 2 through systematic older-versus-young comparisons (Section 3.2), and meet Objective 3 by revealing early phase sway (Section 3.3) and longitudinal variability (Figure 10) as indicators of incipient decline.

This study's goal regarding falls (Objective 3) was intentionally exploratory: our aim was only to verify that the Azure Kinect can in principle capture metrics linked to balance and lower-limb performance, not to derive fall predictors in a heterogeneous older sample. The presence of walking aids and previous falls in our cohort confirms a spectrum of impairment that the system can quantify, yet—given the small N—we purposely refrain from interpreting individual differences. A definitive evaluation of fall-risk metrics will require larger samples and subgroup analyses (e.g., older adults with vs. without a fall history or different frailty levels), which we have already planned for future work.

Our results indicate that the system reliably distinguishes between varying levels of functional performance. The squat test, quantified by the vertical displacement of the CoM, the number of squats and the minimum knee angles, consistently demonstrated that older adults perform shallower squats compared to younger individuals. This finding is consistent with previous reports that document reduced lower-extremity strength and joint mobility with advancing age [28]. By allowing participants to squat to a self-selected depth, we minimized discomfort yet still observed clear performance gaps relative to younger adults. We did not detect large asymmetries in knee flexion—suggesting that many older adults in this cohort maintained balanced bilateral usage, despite performing fewer and less complete squat cycles overall. These metrics complement traditional functional measures (e.g., the TUG, the 30 s chair stand or the SPPB) by providing additional parameters like knee angles or continuous motion trajectories, thereby enabling clinicians to detect subtler changes in mobility.

In the static balance tasks, the older group exhibited greater ML and AP sway, as evidenced by increased displacement metrics and larger 95% confidence ellipse areas. The greater sway observed in older adults is consistent with well-documented age-related declines in postural control [21–23]. These observations confirm that age-related sensorimotor degradation leads to diminished postural stability—a finding in line with prior investigations in geriatric populations [29–31]. While many standardized tests (e.g., Short Physical Performance Battery) rely on whether an individual can simply maintain a stance, our platform goes a step further by quantifying not just pass/fail but also the extent of sway in each stance. This additional resolution may be particularly valuable in identifying emerging balance problems at earlier stages.

Window-specific analysis showed that the 95% CoM ellipse-area was largest during the first 10 s of each stance and then plateaued; pairwise comparisons confirmed that 10–20 s seldom differed from 20–30 s, whereas 0–10 s differed from at least one later window in every stance. This pattern helps explain why brief 10-s balance tasks—such as the standing component of the Short Physical Performance Battery (SPPB) [9]—are able to expose postural instability so efficiently: they capture the most demanding adaptation phase, when individuals are still seeking equilibrium. Conversely, if the clinical aim is to characterize steady-state balance once the posture has stabilized, analyzing sway after the initial 10 s (for example, in the 10–20 s interval) appears sufficient; extending recordings to a full 30 s adds little additional information while lengthening test time.

Furthermore, our longitudinal observations highlight that repeated assessments can help track gradual or event-related changes in performance. One participant (ID 4) who had a walker and multiple fall incidents showed relatively large fluctuations in tandem-stance sway across sessions—particularly following an intervening fall. This variability contrasts with a more stable participant (ID 1), whose balance metrics remained consistent. Although our sample was small, this case-to-case difference underscores how a simple, markerless system could be used to monitor older adults over weeks or months, detecting fluctuations that traditional one-time evaluations might overlook. Previous research on wearable sensor-based monitoring has shown the value of repeated measures for anticipating and potentially preventing mobility-related incidents [25,26], and the present work suggests a similar strategy could be feasible with markerless devices. Each participant was tested at most once per day with rest between tasks, and no systematic practice or fatigue effect was evident (e.g., ID 1 remained stable across nine sessions). Larger longitudinal datasets will enable mixed-effects modelling that explicitly accounts for learning and fatigue.

However, several limitations must be acknowledged. First, our sample size was small (N = 8 per group), and the older cohort, while very aged, was relatively high-functioning (most had good baseline scores and few were recurrent fallers). Second, although prior studies have reported acceptable agreement between Kinect-based and laboratory-grade systems for measuring gait, joint angles, and balance [11,12,32], we did not perform a direct comparison with gold-standard motion capture or force plates. Future research with larger and more varied geriatric populations, including frailer individuals and those with a history of recurrent falls, as well as formal accuracy benchmarking, would help validate and extend these preliminary results.

Although the older adults in our sample exhibited the expected deficits relative to the young cohort—supporting the system's construct validity—this pilot study was not intended to establish new clinical indices or to delineate unique functional characteristics of older adults. Such finer-grained analyses will be pursued once a larger, clinically stratified dataset becomes available.

This platform, which requires minimal setup, operates with a non-contact design, and involves brief testing protocols, could be readily adopted in resource-limited settings such as community clinics or nursing homes, and it could enable early detection of mobility decline and promote targeted fall prevention strategies or strengthening interventions.

5. Conclusions

This pilot study demonstrates the feasibility of a simple, markerless Azure Kinect platform to capture quantitative squat and sway metrics in older adults without wearable sensors or specialized laboratories, and it reliably discriminated between eight older and eight younger participants by revealing shallower squat depth, larger minimum knee angles, and greater CoM sway in the older group. These results satisfy Objective 1, confirming that the system can acquire valid biomechanical data in older adults, and Objective 2, showing it can systematically differentiate them from young healthy controls. Crucially, the window-specific balance analysis—where the first ten seconds of each stance already exposed peak instability—and the session-to-session variability observed after a real fall illustrate the platform's capacity to flag subtle functional changes at an early stage, thereby fulfilling Objective 3 of exploring its potential for early detection of physical decline. Although validation in larger, clinically stratified cohorts and benchmarking against gold-standard instruments are still needed, the present findings point to a practical, non-contact solution that could enrich routine geriatric assessment with fine-grained biomechanical information and ultimately support targeted fall-prevention strategies.

Author Contributions: Conceptualization, A.S.-S., P.A., C.F.-V., R.G.-G., J.M.L.-H., L.R.-C. and A.C.; methodology, A.S.-S., C.F.-V. and L.R.-C.; software, A.S.-S. and P.A.; validation, A.S.-S. and P.A.; formal analysis, A.S.-S., P.A. and A.C.; investigation, A.S.-S. and C.F.-V.; resources, J.M.L.-H., L.R.-C. and A.C.; data curation, A.S.-S.; writing—original draft preparation, A.S.-S.; writing—review and editing, C.F.-V., R.G.-G., J.M.L.-H., L.R.-C. and A.C.; visualization, A.S.-S., P.A. and C.F.-V.; supervision, J.M.L.-H. and L.R.-C.; project administration, J.M.L.-H., L.R.-C. and A.C.; funding acquisition, R.G.-G., J.M.L.-H., L.R.-C. and A.C. All authors have read and agreed to the published version of the manuscript.

Funding: This work was supported by projects CPP2022-009714 funded by MICIU/AEI/10.13039/501100011033 and EU NextGenerationEU/PRTR; and PID2022-137269OB-C22 funded by MICIU/AEI/10.13039/501100011033 and FEDER, EU.

Institutional Review Board Statement: The study was conducted in accordance with the Declaration of Helsinki, and approved by the Committee on Ethics in Research with Medical Products of Cantabria (CEIm) (protocol code CPP2022-009714; approval date: 19 July 2024).

Informed Consent Statement: Informed consent was obtained from all subjects involved in the study.

Data Availability Statement: The datasets generated and/or analyzed during the current study are available from the corresponding author upon reasonable request.

Acknowledgments: The authors gratefully acknowledge the Nursing and Physiotherapy team at the San Cándido Foundation (Santander) for their collaboration and assistance during the data collection process. We also thank A. Perez Asensio and B. García García for their support during the measurements.

Conflicts of Interest: Author Roberto García-García is employed by the company Ambar Telecomunicaciones S.L. The remaining authors declare that the research was conducted in the absence of any commercial or financial relationships that could be construed as a potential conflict of interest.

Abbreviations

The following abbreviations are used in this manuscript:

AP	Anteroposterior
CoM	Center of Mass
CSV	Comma-Separated Values
GPU	Graphics Processing Unit
ML	Mediolateral
ToF	Time of Flight
TUG	Timed Up-and-Go
RGB	Red, Green, Blue
SDK	Software Development Kit
SI	Symmetry Index
SPPB	Short Physical Performance Battery

References

1. Ageing and Health. Available online: https://www.who.int/news-room/fact-sheets/detail/ageing-and-health (accessed on 3 March 2025).
2. Salari, N.; Darvishi, N.; Ahmadipanah, M.; Shohaimi, S.; Mohammadi, M. Global Prevalence of Falls in the Older Adults: A Comprehensive Systematic Review and Meta-Analysis. *J. Orthop. Surg. Res.* **2022**, *17*, 334. [CrossRef]
3. Nagano, H. Gait Biomechanics for Fall Prevention among Older Adults. *Appl. Sci.* **2022**, *12*, 6660. [CrossRef]
4. Marques, N.R.; Spinoso, D.H.; Cardoso, B.C.; Moreno, V.C.; Kuroda, M.H.; Navega, M.T. Is It Possible to Predict Falls in Older Adults Using Gait Kinematics? *Clin. Biomech.* **2018**, *59*, 15–18. [CrossRef] [PubMed]
5. Vaishya, R.; Vaish, A. Falls in Older Adults Are Serious. *JOIO* **2020**, *54*, 69–74. [CrossRef] [PubMed]
6. Patrizio, E.; Calvani, R.; Marzetti, E.; Cesari, M. Physical Functional Assessment in Older Adults. *J. Frailty Aging* **2021**, *10*, 141–149. [CrossRef] [PubMed]
7. Herman, T.; Giladi, N.; Hausdorff, J.M. Properties of the 'Timed Up and Go' Test: More than Meets the Eye. *Gerontology* **2010**, *57*, 203–210. [CrossRef]
8. Jones, C.J.; Rikli, R.E.; Beam, W.C. A 30-s Chair-Stand Test as a Measure of Lower Body Strength in Community-Residing Older Adults. *Res. Q. Exerc. Sport.* **1999**, *70*, 113–119. [CrossRef]
9. Guralnik, J.M.; Simonsick, E.M.; Ferrucci, L.; Glynn, R.J.; Berkman, L.F.; Blazer, D.G.; Scherr, P.A.; Wallace, R.B. A Short Physical Performance Battery Assessing Lower Extremity Function: Association With Self-Reported Disability and Prediction of Mortality and Nursing Home Admission. *J. Gerontol.* **1994**, *49*, M85–M94. [CrossRef]

10. Ortega-Bastidas, P.; Gómez, B.; Aqueveque, P.; Luarte-Martínez, S.; Cano-de-la-Cuerda, R. Instrumented Timed Up and Go Test (iTUG)—More Than Assessing Time to Predict Falls: A Systematic Review. *Sensors* **2023**, *23*, 3426. [CrossRef]
11. Clark, R.A.; Pua, Y.-H.; Fortin, K.; Ritchie, C.; Webster, K.E.; Denehy, L.; Bryant, A.L. Validity of the Microsoft Kinect for Assessment of Postural Control. *Gait Posture* **2012**, *36*, 372–377. [CrossRef]
12. Eltoukhy, M.A.; Kuenze, C.; Oh, J.; Signorile, J.F. Validation of Static and Dynamic Balance Assessment Using Microsoft Kinect for Young and Elderly Populations. *IEEE J. Biomed. Health Inform.* **2018**, *22*, 147–153. [CrossRef] [PubMed]
13. Jeyasingh-Jacob, J.; Crook-Rumsey, M.; Shah, H.; Joseph, T.; Abulikemu, S.; Daniels, S.; Sharp, D.J.; Haar, S. Markerless Motion Capture to Quantify Functional Performance in Neurodegeneration: Systematic Review. *JMIR Aging* **2024**, *7*, e52582. [CrossRef]
14. Azure Kinect DK: Desarrollo de Modelos de IA | Microsoft Azure. Available online: https://azure.microsoft.com/es-es/products/kinect-dk (accessed on 2 April 2025).
15. Winter, D.A. *Biomechanics and Motor Control of Human Movement*, 4th ed.; John Wiley & Sons, Inc.: Hoboken, NJ, USA, 2009.
16. de Leva, P. Adjustments to Zatsiorsky-Seluyanov's Segment Inertia Parameters. *J. Biomech.* **1996**, *29*, 1223–1230. [CrossRef]
17. Zatsiorsky, V.M.; Seluyanov, V.N.; Chungunova, L.G. Methods of Determining Mass-Inertial Characteristics of Human Body Segments. In *Contemporary Problems of Biomechanics*; CRC Press: Boca Raton, FL, USA, 1990; pp. 272–291.
18. Gill, N.; Preece, S.J.; Young, S.; Bramah, C. Are the Arms and Head Required to Accurately Estimate Centre of Mass Motion during Running? *Gait Posture* **2017**, *51*, 281–283. [CrossRef] [PubMed]
19. Błażkiewicz, M.; Wiszomirska, I.; Wit, A. Comparison of Four Methods of Calculating the Symmetry of Spatial-Temporal Parameters of Gait. *Acta Bioeng. Biomech.* **2014**, *16*, 29–35. [CrossRef]
20. Find_peaks—SciPy v1.15.2 Manual. Available online: https://docs.scipy.org/doc/scipy/reference/generated/scipy.signal.find_peaks.html (accessed on 1 April 2025).
21. Tinetti, M.E. Performance-Oriented Assessment of Mobility Problems in Elderly Patients. *J. Am. Geriatr. Soc.* **1986**, *34*, 119–126. [CrossRef]
22. Scura, D.; Munakomi, S. Tinetti Gait and Balance Test. In *StatPearls*; StatPearls Publishing: Treasure Island, FL, USA, 2025.
23. Mahoney, F.I.; Barthel, D.W. Functional Evaluation: The Barthel Index. *Md. State Med. J.* **1965**, *14*, 61–65. [PubMed]
24. Shah, S.; Vanclay, F.; Cooper, B. Improving the Sensitivity of the Barthel Index for Stroke Rehabilitation. *J. Clin. Epidemiol.* **1989**, *42*, 703–709. [CrossRef]
25. Park, C.; Sharafkhaneh, A.; Bryant, M.S.; Nguyen, C.; Torres, I.; Najafi, B. Toward Remote Assessment of Physical Frailty Using Sensor-Based Sit-to-Stand Test. *J. Surg. Res.* **2021**, *263*, 130–139. [CrossRef]
26. Arshad, M.Z.; Jamsrandorj, A.; Kim, J.; Mun, K.-R. Gait Events Prediction Using Hybrid CNN-RNN-Based Deep Learning Models through a Single Waist-Worn Wearable Sensor. *Sensors* **2022**, *22*, 8226. [CrossRef]
27. Friedrich, B.; Lau, S.; Elgert, L.; Bauer, J.M.; Hein, A. A Deep Learning Approach for TUG and SPPB Score Prediction of (Pre-) Frail Older Adults on Real-Life IMU Data. *Healthcare* **2021**, *9*, 149. [CrossRef]
28. Honda, K.; Sekiguchi, Y.; Shimazaki, S.; Suzuki, R.; Suzuki, T.; Kanetaka, H.; Izumi, S.-I. Effects of Aging on Whole-Body Center of Mass Movement and Lower Limb Joint Kinematics and Kinetics during Deep-Squat Movement. *J. Biomech.* **2022**, *134*, 110996. [CrossRef] [PubMed]
29. Prieto, T.E.; Myklebust, J.B.; Hoffmann, R.G.; Lovett, E.G.; Myklebust, B.M. Measures of Postural Steadiness: Differences between Healthy Young and Elderly Adults. *IEEE Trans. Biomed. Eng.* **1996**, *43*, 956–966. [CrossRef] [PubMed]
30. Seidler, R.D.; Bernard, J.A.; Burutolu, T.B.; Fling, B.W.; Gordon, M.T.; Gwin, J.T.; Kwak, Y.; Lipps, D.B. Motor Control and Aging: Links to Age-Related Brain Structural, Functional, and Biochemical Effects. *Neurosci. Biobehav. Rev.* **2010**, *34*, 721–733. [CrossRef] [PubMed]
31. Sturnieks, D.L.; St George, R.; Lord, S.R. Balance Disorders in the Elderly. *Neurophysiol. Clin. Clin. Neurophysiol.* **2008**, *38*, 467–478. [CrossRef]
32. Albert, J.A.; Owolabi, V.; Gebel, A.; Brahms, C.M.; Granacher, U.; Arnrich, B. Evaluation of the Pose Tracking Performance of the Azure Kinect and Kinect v2 for Gait Analysis in Comparison with a Gold Standard: A Pilot Study. *Sensors* **2020**, *20*, 5104. [CrossRef]

technologies

MDPI

Article

A Design-Based Research Approach to Streamline the Integration of High-Tech Assistive Technologies in Speech and Language Therapy

Anna Lekova [1,*], Paulina Tsvetkova [1,2], Anna Andreeva [1,3], Georgi Dimitrov [1,2], Tanio Tanev [1], Miglena Simonska [3], Tsvetelin Stefanov [1,2], Vaska Stancheva-Popkostadinova [3], Gergana Padareva [4], Katia Rasheva [2], Adelina Kremenska [1] and Detelina Vitanova [2]

[1] Institute of Robotics, Bulgarian Academy of Sciences, 1113 Sofia, Bulgaria; p.tsvetkova@ir.bas.bg (P.T.); anna_andreeva@swu.bg (A.A.); g.dimitrov@unibit.bg (G.D.); t.tanev@ir.bas.bg (T.T.); a.kostova012@gmail.com (A.K.)
[2] Faculty of Information Science, University of Library Studies and Information Technologies, 1784 Sofia, Bulgaria; k.rasheva@unibit.bg (K.R.); d.vitanova@unibit.bg (D.V.)
[3] Public Health, Health Care and Sport, South-West University, 2700 Blagoevgrad, Bulgaria; miglena_simonska@swu.bg (M.S.); v_stancheva@abv.bg (V.S.-P.)
[4] Faculty of Philology, South-West University, 2700 Blagoevgrad, Bulgaria; gerypadareva@swu.bg
* Correspondence: a.lekova@ir.bas.bg

Abstract: Currently, high-tech assistive technologies (ATs), particularly Socially Assistive Robots (SARs), virtual reality (VR) and conversational AI (ConvAI), are considered very useful in supporting professionals in Speech and Language Therapy (SLT) for children with communication disorders. However, despite a positive public perception, therapists face difficulties when integrating these technologies into practice due to technical challenges and a lack of user-friendly interfaces. To address this gap, a design-based research approach has been employed to streamline the integration of SARs, VR and ConvAI in SLT, and a new software platform called "ATLog" has been developed for designing interactive and playful learning scenarios with ATs. ATLog's main features include visual-based programming with graphical interface, enabling therapists to intuitively create personalized interactive scenarios without advanced programming skills. The platform follows a subprocess-oriented design, breaking down SAR skills and VR scenarios into microskills represented by pre-programmed graphical blocks, tailored to specific treatment domains, therapy goals, and language skill levels. The ATLog platform was evaluated by 27 SLT experts using the Technology Acceptance Model (TAM) and System Usability Scale (SUS) questionnaires, extended with additional questions specifically focused on ATLog structure and functionalities. According to the SUS results, most of the experts (74%) evaluated ATLog with grades over 70, indicating high acceptance of its usability. Over half (52%) of the experts rated the additional questions focused on ATLog's structure and functionalities in the A range (90–100), while 26% rated them in the B range (80–89), showing strong acceptance of the platform for creating and running personalized interactive scenarios with ATs. According to the TAM results, experts gave high grades for both perceived usefulness (44% in the A range) and perceived ease of use (63% in the A range).

Keywords: high-tech assistive technologies; socially assistive robots; virtual reality; conversational AI; software platform; visual programming; speech and language therapy; communication disorders; children; technology and usability assessment

1. Introduction

The present study follows a Design-Based Research (DBR) approach [1] to explore how high-tech assistive technologies (ATs), such as Socially Assistive Robots (SARs), virtual reality (VR) and conversational AI (ConvAI), can be easily integrated into and used in Speech and Language Therapy (SLT) for children and adults with communication disorders (CDs), as well as to identify the design principles that support the successful implementation of ATs in SLT. Scientific research shows that therapy with high-tech ATs improves the skills of children with CDs. According to Kouroupa [2], most interventions used humanoid (67%) robotic platforms; were predominantly based in clinics (37%), followed home, school, and laboratory (17%, respectively) environments; and targeted at improving social and communication skills (77%). In a 2023 survey of 53 speech and language therapists specializing in autism, approximately 92% reported being aware of VR; however, only 1.8% (1 therapist) had actually used it clinically [3]. The use of ATs shows low clinical adoption, likely due to the lack of a standardized methodology, high costs that make many technologies unaffordable, fast technological development, need for specialized training for therapists, and technical limitations related to the integration and programming of ATs. Additionally, there are increasing expectations for SAR autonomy and human-like speech recognition and response capabilities, allowing them to understand, generate and vocalize text. This highlights the significance of Natural Language Processing (NLP), Natural Language Generation (NLG) (a type of Generative AI), and cloud technologies as key assistive technologies in SLT. According to recent studies [4,5], the rapid progress of Large Language Models (LLMs) and Large Reasoning Models (LRMs), such as Generative Pre-trained Transformers (GPTs) with Chain-of-Thought (CoT) prompting for step-by-step decision making, will further enhance ConvAI and its relevance in SLT.

Despite the generally positive public perception of SARs, VR and ConvAI among therapists [6–15], one of the most significant challenges is how therapists individually integrate AT into their practice. Related difficulties include software programming, user-friendliness, and ease of setup and use. Santos et al. [15] highlighted these challenges in their discussion on interaction scenarios with ATs in future studies, emphasizing the need for user-friendly systems that minimize the requirement for technical skills among therapists. Additionally, there is a lack of ergonomic software platforms to effectively support SLT professionals in streamlining the design of interactive scenarios during intervention. User-friendly platforms often include visual programming features with pre-programmed graphical blocks, which is particularly helpful in educational and therapeutic settings [16].

Since there is a gap between the potential of ATs and their practical application in SLT, this study aims to contribute to the conceptualization of a design for integrating high-tech ATs and creating interactive, playful learning scenarios that support therapists in their practice. We report on a DBR study conducted over three years to develop and implement an ergonomic platform called ATLog, following the four phases of the DBR approach [1] and the logic of effective iteration outlined in [17]. According to [17], educational and therapeutic innovations are context-dependent and should be designed and implemented within real-world settings, requiring collaboration among researchers, practitioners, and stakeholders. In the frame of ATLog project [18], we systematically involved SLT professionals from the Logopedic Center at the South-West University in the iterative process of designing, developing, implementing and evaluating SLT interventions using ATs. This collaboration also focused on streamlining the design of interactive scenarios for playful learning with SARs, VR and ConvAI. Previous iterations have been reported in earlier work [19–23], detailing the building–testing cycles of the ATLog architecture, including the integration of various SARs, integration of AI cloud services for NLP/NLG into the

SARs' native software, and implementation of VR scenes for interactive speech and listening experiences. During these iterations, we optimized the client–server architecture to better integrate ATs and enhanced their communication protocols with pre-configured graphical blocks within a visual programming interface. These blocks were customized for specific treatment domains, therapy goals, and language skill levels, enabling dynamic combinations and adaptable scenarios tailored to the therapeutic needs of each child.

To ensure the effectiveness of the ATLog platform, it is essential to evaluate its acceptability and usability. According to the literature review, we performed a System Usability Scale (SUS) questionnaire [24], a highly effective instrument for evaluating the user experience of a novel platform. In addition, to examine the application's perceived usefulness and perceived ease of use, the Technology Acceptance Model (TAM) questionnaire was employed [25]. These questionnaires typically use a Likert scale to measure user opinions and are widely recognized instruments for analyzing and interpreting user behavior and the effectiveness of technological systems. The SUS and TAM questionnaires are often used together in such evaluations [26].

The research objectives of this study are as follows: (1) to design and (2) to evaluate an ergonomic platform to streamline the integration of high-tech ATs in SLT following the DBR approach. To achieve these objectives, the first phase in DBR involved consultations with SLT professionals to identify the challenges they face in integrating high-tech ATs, such as technical barriers, platform complexity and the need for an intuitive and flexible user interface tailored to therapeutic practice. A literature review was also conducted to examine existing technological solutions and systems relevant to CDs. In the second phase, iterative versions of the ATLog platform were developed. During the third phase, feedback on usability, logic flow and scenario effectiveness was collected from the pilot deployment in real SLT environments with children and therapists. The TAM and extended SUS questionnaires were employed to identify platform acceptance, usability issues and areas for improvement. Based on the data collection and analysis in this phase, the main design principle was identified during the fourth phase. This principle, along with a comprehensive framework for conceptualizing the design process and technical implementation guidelines for developers (provided in the **??** and Section B), are presented to support replication and further development.

The paper is organized as follows: Section 2 presents the related works. Section 3 describes the methodology of the study, materials and methods, and the validation approach. Section 4 presents the result implementation of the ATLog platform and the results from the TAM and SUS questionnaires, while Section 5 presents the Discussion. Then, conclusions, limitations and future directions follow.

2. Related Works

A literature review was conducted during the first phase of DBR to achieve the following: (1) explore the technical, ethical and cultural issues that hinder the acceptance and adoption of high-tech ATs by speech and language therapists, along with the methods used to validate technology acceptance and adoption; (2) analyze case studies demonstrating how high-tech ATs have been integrated into SLT; (3) review existing visual-based programming platforms that explore similar design solutions for intuitive and modular interfaces to diverse ATs.

2.1. Technical, Ethical and Cultural Issues That Hinder the Acceptance and Adoption of High-Tech ATs by Speech and Language Therapists

Despite the generally positive public perception of SARs, VR and ConvAI among therapists [6–15], one of the most significant technical challenges is the real integration of ATs into their practice, where flexibility, reliability and ease of use are critical. Concerns involve the need for an easy setup that does not require technical skills beyond a therapist's standard training or any software programming expertise. Further concerns include the absence of clear clinical guidelines, unfamiliarity with the technology, risk of system failures, and short training. Therapists' acceptance and use of ATs are strongly influenced by their confidence, the complexity of the ATs, technical limitations and the availability of support. Szabó et al. [7] point out that while speech and language therapists have access to a wide range of digital tools with potential therapeutic benefits, actual adoption depends heavily on several factors: the therapist's self-confidence in using digital tools, the time and effort required to learn them, insufficient technical infrastructure, and lack of peer or supervisory support. To address these barriers, user-friendly design and practical training, such as tutorials, troubleshooting guides and video lessons are essential. Santos et al. discussed in [15] the characteristics of interaction scenarios and the need for systems to be user-friendly for therapists, thus minimizing the requirements for technical skills. This supports the observations in [7], where therapists are seen as dual-role stakeholders—both as users of ATs and as facilitators who guide patients in accessing and using them effectively. Therefore, the experiences of both therapists and patients are essential to successful implementation. If therapists have negative initial experiences using ATs in therapy, they are more likely to discontinue their use. Additional concerns when integrating ConvAI include the accuracy of AI-generated outputs and the need for continuous monitoring to prevent the dissemination of incorrect information [27].

Concerns regarding the integration of SARs into SLT include the complexity of programming SARs for therapeutic purposes. This challenge lies not in simply making the robot operate, it requires robot behavior to align with complex therapeutic goals for enhancing communication and social skills, such as refining speech, improving listening, supporting turn-taking, and recognizing social cues. These are subtle, context-dependent abilities, and programming them is often time-consuming or exceeds the typical technical expertise of therapists, making a predefined, user-friendly interface essential.

Rupp et al. identified the key concerns and expectations of professionals in [10]:

- Technical expertise—therapists may lack the skills needed to program robots, raising concerns about their use in therapy;
- Software complexity—programming tools for SARs are often too complex or overly limited;
- Robot behavior—the robot must adapt to children's abilities, requiring customization based on individual needs;
- User-friendliness—the ease of setup and interface design are critical for adoption in clinical settings.

Conflicting perceptions arise among therapists when using SARs in real-world therapy sessions. The third research question in [9] explicitly asked: "*To what extent do therapists who have experienced SARs believe in their efficacy and intend to use them in their speech-language therapy practice to train children with language impairments?*", and the results revealed that therapists generally remained skeptical about the efficacy of SARs for improving the communication and social skills of children with language impairments. The study analyzed the usability, engagement and perceived benefits of SARs and virtual SARs (V-SARs) through questionnaires and group interviews. While therapists found both SARs and V-SARs easy to use, they noted that SAR setup was time-consuming and they remained careful about fully adopting such tools for improving communication and social interactions. Therapists observed that although both SARs and V-SARs effectively engaged children, SARs had more appeal and were seen as a companion, whereas V-SARs felt more like a training tool. Although therapists appreciated the engagement benefits of SARs, they were not ready to fully adopt them as primary therapeutic tools, expressing a preference for traditional, therapist-led approaches. Nonetheless, they did see value in SARs for supplementary roles in therapy, particularly in home environments.

Concerns regarding the integration of VR in SLT include the need for a stronger neuro-affirming evidence base supporting VR effectiveness, the absence of clear clinical guidelines, and a lack of adequate training for therapists to effectively integrate VR into their practice. Vaezipour et al. [28] examined speech and language therapists' acceptance of VR in communication rehabilitation by involving fifteen professionals in communication activities within an immersive VR kitchen environment. The study evaluated usability and motion sickness, and gathered qualitative feedback. While participants expressed positive attitudes toward VR's potential, the concerns raised in [28] are why the scores from the usability test were only average. Although the motion sickness was minimal, there were barriers such as unfamiliarity with the VR technology, insufficient training and technical complications, such as complex setup procedures, hardware limitations and risk of system failures.

Cost emerged as another significant concern, as the development of 3D applications, along with the acquisition, maintenance of VR equipment and required training, can be excessively expensive. Furthermore, many therapists remain uncertain about VR's actual clinical effectiveness, and this skepticism contributes to its limited adoption. Although public attitudes toward VR and AR are generally positive, as shown in [11], with both students and teachers highlighting educational benefits, these perceptions have not yet translated into widespread clinical use. The study in [3] found that despite VR being viewed as a promising tool for practical exercises, it has not been widely adopted in SLT. In fact, while 92% of speech–language therapists were aware of VR, only 1.8% had used it in therapy for autistic children. Further concerns were raised by Hashim et al. [29], who investigated stakeholder perspectives on applications with AR developed for children with CDs. Although the tool was seen as promising for supporting language learning among autistic children, stakeholders emphasized that substantial improvements would be needed to make vocabulary learning clinically useful. The review in [30] discusses the lack of tools to measure the outcomes of VR interventions in SLT aimed at improving communication skills.

Concerns regarding the integration of ConvAI in SLT practice are complex. One of the primary issues is the need for continuous monitoring to prevent the dissemination of inaccurate or inappropriate information [27]. Integrating generative AI tools (such as ChatGPT) into SLT also presents challenges, primarily due to the technical expertise required to refine these LLMs with existing therapeutic workflows and AT software. The integration of ConvAI into SARs is considered a key feature for enabling natural, human-like interactions with children. However, the complexity of implementing such integration remains a significant barrier. Robots such as Probo [31], QTrobot [32], FurhatAI [33], ARI [34], and Milo [35] have shown promising levels of acceptance due to their ConvAI capabilities. Advancements in LLMs and deep learning (DL) [36,37] are gradually improving user experiences and reducing skepticism toward ConvAI integration in SARs. Study [36] explores the enhancements of the Nao robot's language abilities using DL techniques, while [37] introduces FurChat—an embodied conversational agent powered by LLM and dialog management that enables open domain-specific conversations with facial expressions. Although these innovations demonstrate the growing potential of ConvAI, therapists often prefer generative AI (such as ChatGPT, DALL·E or Make-A-Video) for creating customized therapy materials rather than real-time interaction through ConvAI-enhanced SARs.

We examined the careful optimism among SLT professionals regarding AI adoption [12,13,38–40]. The identified concerns are as follow:

- Accessible training in AI basics—many therapists lack the background in AI or programming needed to effectively utilize or troubleshoot ConvAI systems. Continuous technical support and directions on how to use ChatGPT for speech therapy are essential to facilitate this transition [39].
- Time constraints—according to [12], 32.4% of professionals expressed interest in adopting new AI tools but mentioned limited time as a barrier. Some therapists (e.g., participants S27, S41) openly admitted that they tend to avoid using technology.
- Data privacy and compliance—therapists expressed concerns about compliance with privacy laws such as HIPAA and FERPA, especially when using AI tools for transcription or data processing (e.g., participant S10 in [12]).
- Rapid technological change—the speed at which AI technologies evolve makes it difficult for practitioners to stay up-to-date. One participant (S17) cited "keeping up with technology" as a top challenge.
- System compatibility and latency—the integration of AI systems into existing platforms can be technically demanding. Authors in [40] describe in detail the limitations of integrating ChatGPT into the Pepper robot. Compatibility issues (Pepper uses Python 2.7; ChatGPT APIs require Python 3.x) and dependency on stable internet connections often lead to latency, which disrupts smooth and real-time interaction.

Some speech and language therapists have raised additional concerns about inadequately programmed SARs or VR in interactive scenarios with children with special needs [2,41,42]. Poorly designed interactions can increase anxiety in children and reduce both therapist confidence and the overall acceptance of ATs. Successfully integrating SARs into existing healthcare or educational frameworks, therefore, demands considerable customization and ongoing efforts to ensure that these systems are aligned with the specific needs of both children and therapists. Key factors for successful adoption include adequate training for therapists, user-friendly and intuitive system design, adaptability to specific therapeutic goals, familiarity with the technology, and clear evidence of its clinical effectiveness. These elements are essential to foster trust; however, across the surveyed studies, there was a noticeable lack of simplified programming interfaces, seamless setup and operation, and adaptable features for designing interactive scenarios tailored to different therapeutic needs. Furthermore, to make the technology more accessible, software developers, engineers and therapists need to work together and to improve the usability of therapeutic robots.

How people view and accept ATs can differ depending on their culture [6,43,44]. The findings in [43] show that Chinese participants generally expressed positive feelings, viewing ConvAI agents more as sources of enjoyment and perceiving voice-based and physically embodied agents as warmer, more competent and emotionally engaging. In contrast, US participants saw ConvAI agents more functionally, with mixed or uncertain feelings. In Germany, cultural attitudes shifted notably during the COVID-19 pandemic, where the integration of ATs into SLT became not just an option, but a necessity [6]. Two online questionnaire-based studies are reported in [6], investigating the acceptance of technology among speech and language therapists in Germany. In the first study, external factors that inhibited or facilitated the adoption of video therapy and its potential future utilization were identified. In the second study, one of the research question is *"To what extent are speech and language therapists intending to use ICT in therapy in the future?"* and the modified model of the Unified Theory of Acceptance and Use of Technology (UTAUT) explained 58.8% of the variability in therapists' behavioral intention to use digital media. Both studies investigated facilitating and inhibiting factors for including video therapy in future speech and therapy services, and the results demonstrated an accelerated digital adoption in SLT services for telepractice.

Last but not least, integrating ATs into SLT raises important ethical and practical concerns. Although Severson et al. [45] identified social robots as among the most effective ATs in education and therapy for children, they emphasized that SARs must not give children the false impression of possessing emotions or consciousness. This raises concerns about emotional deception and unrealistic expectations, especially in vulnerable populations. There are also concerns about equity and accessibility—robots should be designed to serve all users fairly, avoiding over-personalization through machine learning that may reinforce biases or limit adaptability. Severson et al. further recommend that policymakers adopt evidence-based approaches to guide the certification and deployment of SARs in educational and clinical settings. Another concern is the ethical handling of child data, especially when used to train perceptual tools like speech or expression recognition systems. Ensuring data security, anonymization and regulatory compliance is critical. The survey in [46] reinforces these concerns, highlighting factors that affect therapists' adoption of ATs like SARs. These include trust, privacy, and ethical considerations, as well as cultural sensitivities and past experiences that may influence acceptance.

In exploring how to validate technology acceptance and adoption among therapists, we found that a range of qualitative methods were commonly used. To examine users' attitudes and concerns towards how constantly evolving hi-tech digital media technologies are used and accepted, the authors in [6] applied a modified model of UTAUT, while the authors in [7] used the original UTAUT model to assess the acceptance of apps and digital resources in SLT. The authors in [9] tested the usability and adoption of SARs among therapists via the Adoption of Technology (AoT), Quebec User Evaluation of Satisfaction with Assistive Technology (QUEST), and SUS questionnaire. In [28], the authors used the SUS, the NASA Task Load Index (NASA-TLX) for assessing subjective mental workload, and the Simulator Sickness Questionnaire (SSQ) to evaluate the acceptance, usefulness and usability of the SIM:Kitchen VR application for SLT. In [38], the authors applied the TAM2 model, which extends the original TAM, to assess the acceptance of chatbots as AI conversational partners in language learning, given their focus on specifically evaluating chatbots' role as an interactive agent. The TAM2 consists of 25 items from seven dimensions: perceived ease of use (PEU), perceived usefulness (PU), attitude (ATT), perceived behavior control (PBC), behavioral intention (BI), self-efficacy (SE), and personal innovativeness (PI). In the systematic review in [42], where the attitudes, acceptance, anxiety and trust toward social robots were analyzed, the measures employed by authors were the Almere Model of robot acceptance and UTAUT.

Based on the reviewed evaluation methods, we identified the SUS and TAM as the most suitable frameworks for assessing therapists' acceptance and adoption of the ATLog platform in Phase 3.

2.2. Findings from Case Studies Demonstrating How Hi-Tech ATs Have Been Integrated into SLT

While there are case studies that explore the integration of SARs or VR in SLT for children, to the best of our knowledge, no research papers have reported case studies involving the use of ConvAI, exploiting ChatGPT, Gemini, DeepSeek, etc., in SLT for children. As mentioned above, therapists have shown openness to the potential of generative AI for creating customized therapy materials, such as tailored stories, word lists, and sentences targeting specific speech or language goals, as well as educational resources like flashcards and interactive games. Du et al. [13] explores the potential adoption of ChatGPT as a promising tool in SLT for individuals with receptive and expressive language disorders. ChatGPT can help with vocabulary development through definitions and synonyms, generating stories for narrative skill practice, providing resources for literacy activities like reading and writing, assisting with bilingual therapy through translations, and offering information to enhance cultural competence during sessions. Therefore, we anticipate that the adoption of text-generative AI for conversations in SLT will increase in the near future also. Du et al. [13] advise therapists that, in addition to creating therapy materials, ChatGPT can simulate human-like interaction, allowing children to practice grammar and syntax, engage in social communication tasks such as turn-taking and topic maintenance, and learn by experience in a low-pressure conversational environment. Table 1 in [12] presents the speech and language therapists' perceptions of AI technologies. From 105 SLT practitioners, 79 are excited about AI's potential to improve communication outcomes and save time and 75 respondents see promise in its applications. S36 said, *"I would like to better understand AI and how it can support my work with students to improve their communication abilities"*. However, in response to RQ1: *"What aspects do they enjoy most about their job that should not be negatively impacted by AI?"*, most expressed frustration over the lack of time for preparation, planning and direct intervention with children and families.

Case studies exploring the integration of SARs in SLT are presented in Table 2 in the survey [47], which summarizes twelve empirical use cases for interactive scenarios with SARs [48–59]. Table 1 in the survey [46], which includes rows focused on children as end users, also presents examples of applications and experiments involving the use of social robots. Additional recent case studies can be found in [9,11,46,60]. Spitale et al. in [9] studied the use of SARs in SLT for children with language impairments. Over an 8-week period, 20 children and 6 speech-language therapists participated, with children randomly assigned to either a physical or virtual SAR condition. Key findings in [11] include the following: (1) significant improvements in linguistic skills in both SAR conditions; (2) greater engagement and speech occurrences observed in children interacting with the physical SAR. The study conducted by [60] demonstrated that humanoid educational robots can foster social and emotional skills. The study focuses on designing humanoid robots to engage students from both functional and affective perspectives and reports a pilot test involving 64 primary school students in Hong Kong, divided into control and experimental groups. The validity of the findings was ensured through a combination of questionnaires, observations, and language proficiency tests. The study employed motivational engagement theory to analyze the outcomes, which revealed that the experimental group, which interacted with humanoid robots, showed significant improvements in behavioral engagement (+13.24%), emotional engagement (+13.14%), cognitive engagement (+21.56%), and intrinsic motivation (+12.07%).

Two papers focused on case studies integrating VR in SLT for children and adolescents [61–65] examine the role of VR in enhancing speech and language skills, showcasing its interactivity, engagement and efficacy. A pilot randomized controlled trial (n = 32) comparing traditional speech therapy to VR-based therapy (using the VRRS system) in children with developmental language disorders showed greater gains in the VR group for language comprehension, naming, syntax and spontaneous speech [61]. The study by Macdonald [65] evaluated the impact of a single 30 min session of overexposure therapy on 29 adolescent students. The results showed a substantial decrease in public speaking anxiety and a notable increase in confidence and enjoyment of public speaking. We see its great potential for stuttering therapy, as well.

Pergantis in [66] presents 36 case studies involving different high-tech ATs, which are summarized in Table 2. These case studies provide detailed information on the type of study, participant characteristics (age, gender and diagnosis), intervention, type of technology, measurement tools, results, limitations, effect sizes, longitudinal effects and country. The studies emphasize the importance of user-centered design and therapist involvement to ensure effectiveness and promote adoption. They highlight the growing role of high-tech ATs, such as VR, serious games, and SARs, in supporting emotional regulation and communication development in children with ASD. Key findings from selected case studies in [66] relevant to CDs are as follows: (1) Virtual reality scenarios aimed at emotional regulation and social interaction demonstrated significant positive outcomes—a 14-week program involving children with ASD showed improvements in emotional expression and reduced stress responses, indicating VR's therapeutic potential for developing communication and coping strategies; (2) studies involving social robots such as KASPAR and PARO revealed encouraging results. KASPAR helped reduce anxiety-related behaviors in children with ASD, as indicated by physiological measures like heart rate variability. PARO, used with inpatient adolescents, also showed positive effects on mood and anxiety levels.

2.3. Existing Visual-Based Programming Platforms That Explore Similar Design Solutions for Intuitive and Modular at Interfaces

Many platforms propose interactive tools for designing and developing interactive scenarios with low-tech ATs in SLT for children and adolescents with CDs, such as Augmentative and Alternative Communication (AAC), customizable communication books with words and pictures, adaptive writing tools, interactive software for practicing skills, communication and social interaction, and mobile applications for smartphones and tablets. High-tech ATs are less commonly applied, although Tobii Dynavox [67] offers products and software specifically designed to support individuals with speech and language disorders, such as "TD Snap" and "Pathways" for visual scene displays. These tools enable therapists and caregivers to customize communication boards, symbols and workflows in order to meet a child's specific needs. However, the price is high and there is currently no dedicated visual-based programming platform.

Klavina et al. in [68] studied an additional type of high-tech AT with visual-based programing platform for VR, AI-empowered mobile applications and other AAC software to improve daily living skills and communications. Although the authors claimed that these tools offer engaging, user-friendly platforms that meet individual needs and improve learning, few were tailored to assist cross-disciplinary professionals with limited programming skills in integrating ATs and designing interactive scenarios for their interventions. Robotics platforms, like Ask Nao [69], Furhat Blockly [70], Vittascience Interface [71] and LEKA [72], focus on interaction and the development of interactive scenarios, but with a *high degree of universality*. Ask Nao, Vittascience and Furhat Blockly offer a simple drag-and-drop interface for building and controlling interactive behaviors for NAOv6 or Furhat without needing to write text code; however, they are not typically focused on a specific therapy, even though the blocks represent a variety of actions and interactions for creating dynamic and complex behaviors, along with the robot's capability to respond with empathy to the user's behavior. For instance, the Furhat visual platform facilitates speech and conversational interactions by design of facial expressions and lip synchronization, while also detecting user presence and recognizing user emotions. Ask Nao and LEKA's interfaces allow users to design and customize robot behaviors using graphical blocks, including gestures, speech, movements and sensory interactions. These tools are used for activities such as emotional engagement, sensory tasks and social skill development, but are not specifically tailored for SLT.

Open Access Virtual Reality Overexposure Therapy [73] is an open-access platform, compatible with various devices for VR public speaking, aimed at reducing public speaking anxiety. Platforms like ThingLink [74] enable users to create interactive VR scenarios for learning and training, offering opportunities for communication skill development through immersive and real-world simulations. However, despite their potential, limited accessibility remains a concern due to high costs and non-intuitive user interfaces, which can pose barriers for educators and therapists with limited technical expertise. The MagicItem tool for the dynamic behavior design of virtual objects with LLMs, presented in [75], explores how LLMs can shape the behavior of virtual objects in VR environments. By integrating LLMs with platform-specific scripting tools, therapists with minimal coding skills can easily define and control object behaviors, adding depth and interactivity to VR scenes. Similarly, therapy with VR [76] offers a set of customizable virtual reality scenarios designed to assist speech therapists in helping individuals enhance their vocal abilities, providing a versatile toolkit for therapeutic interventions in VR.

The platforms for integrating text-generative AI in SARs or VR usually exploit cloud services for enhancing the conversational capabilities of ATs. For example, the authors in [77] present a cloud-based platform designed to provide knowledge-based autonomous interactions for social robots and conversational agents, particularly beneficial for low-cost robots. LuxAI for QTrobot proposes a seamless integration of ChatGPT for language understanding and generation [78]. The Furhat conversational platform is also built on cloud services, utilizing NLP for understanding and NLG to generate responses.

2.4. Identified Issues and Areas for Improvement

During the first phase of DBR, we identified the following issues that need to be addressed:

- There is a need for an ergonomic platform that supports therapists in using various ATs. This platform should serve as a general hub, allowing therapists to seamlessly integrate ATs.
- The platform should offer a GUI that allows therapists to personalize the robot's receptive and expressive language, as well as interactions, to align with each child's therapeutic goals and developmental stage.
- The platform should provide secure data management, including storing and analyzing progress through quantitative performance metrics and session summaries.
- The platform should be tailored to SLT, which would save time for therapists in their intervention preparation. Visual programming platforms are generally universal in design and do not typically focus on specific therapies. They often lack pre-designed content, such as a content library with therapeutic interactive scenarios enhanced by ATs.
- There is a need for robot cooperation, which arises when a robot lacks certain functionalities, such as QR code reading or Automatic Speech Recognition (ASR). This calls for shared repositories and direct or message-based input/output channels to facilitate communication between robots and support such cooperation.
- There is a need for a remote mode in the platform for monitoring and controlling robots for children receiving therapy at home.
- There is a need for providing technical support for therapists, and training on how to integrate ATs through tutorials and video lessons. Therapists also need special training to use block-based GUIs, even though they are often intuitive.

To address the identified challenges, we initiated Phase 2 of the DBR process to design and develop ATLog—an innovative platform to facilitate the integration of ATs through a user-friendly visual programming editor, which uses graphical blocks tailored for SLT and allows therapists to configure and control various AT devices and resources without requiring advanced technical skills. Thus, the platform will enable customization by a modular combination of robot actions and VR scenes, broken down into micro-skills and micro-scenes, to suit the individual needs of each child. It will also include features like multi-robot cooperation, access to content repositories, secure communication protocols with authentication, built-in tools for quantitative assessment and a remote mode to support SLT from a distance.

3. Materials and Methods

3.1. Methodology

This section describes the research approach based on the four phases of the DBR process (Figure 1) using the Reeves model [1]. DBR focuses on applying research findings in practical, real-world settings with active stakeholder participation and continuous iterations. Iterations consist of repeated cycles of early and frequent building and testing, choosing flexible design versions that effectively support the goals and practices of professionals in each cycle. Thus, through the iterative process used to co-develop, test and refine the integration of SARs, VR and ConvAI into the novel ergonomic software platform ATLog, continuous improvements were achieved. Speech and language therapists actively contributed to streamlining the design of interactive scenarios for playful learning within the platform.

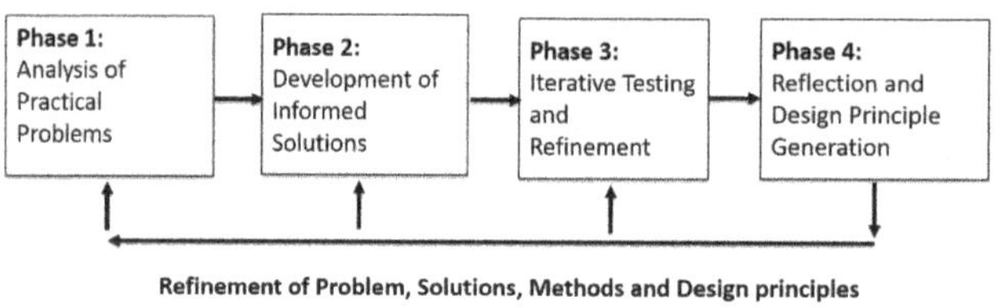

Figure 1. Four phases of the design-based research process using the Reeves DBR model, adapted from [1].

During Phase 1 of the DBR approach, we examined the objectives and therapeutic practices of therapists aiming to integrate high-tech ATs into SLT principles and methods. A literature review explored the technical, ethical and cultural barriers to adopting ATs and analyzed case studies of AT integration into SLT. The methodology of the design aligns with the theoretical foundations and principles of SLT: (1) Didactic—focusing on visibility and accessibility; (2) Ontogenetic—focusing on the systematic development of speech forms, functions and expressions. Other integrated principles include the Principle of Interactive Learning, the Principle of Student Activity, and the Principle of Personalized Learning. The methods integrated in the methodology are as follows: (1) the phonological awareness method, as a foundation for language and literacy development, focuses on identifying and manipulating language sounds, such as rhyming, blending, segmenting and changing individual phonemes within words; (2) the empirical method of knowledge acquisition, i.e., learning through practical interaction with the environment rather than theory; (3) embodiment learning, involving the body and physical actions in understanding; and (4) multisensory learning, which engages multiple senses to improve comprehension and knowledge retention. We also explored therapists' interest in using ConvAI with robots that lack built-in NLG abilities, like Nao, during SLT interventions. We analyzed the practical problems encountered and identified several technical challenges, including the need to improve speech recognition accuracy, generate context-aware human-like text, reduce response latency, implement multilingual TTS synthesis, and resolve communication issues between ATs that use different protocols.

During Phase 2, in the ongoing iteration of developing and testing the software architecture for integrating ConvAI in the Nao, Furhat and Emo robots, new technical solutions were implemented. The initially used Node-RED platform as central component had been replaced with 'Express server' in order to improve functionality and reduce system latency. This change took advantage of the lightweight client–server framework using Node.js for the backend, paired with a web server interface for the frontend. Using the 'spawn' module of Node.js, which allows the execution of Python or JavaScript files as child processes via server endpoints, streamlined the integration of ATs into the ATLog platform. This network solution ensures that only the child processes need updates when technology evolves, makes the maintenance easy. Furthermore, using a Node.js-based server instead of Node-RED reduced communication latency between ATs and the platform's web interface. At this stage, this time is neglected; however, the preliminary results from the quantitative analysis in [22] showed the need for further efforts to improve response times from the integrated cloud services and their communication reliability. The response API delay from Bulgarian ChatGPT currently averages around 3–4 s, and we started working on implementing response streaming to improve it.

During Phase 3, feedback on usability, logic flow and scenario effectiveness was collected from the pilot deployment in real SLT environments with children and therapists. The TAM and extended SUS questionnaires were employed to identify platform acceptance, usability issues and areas for improvement.

During Phase 4, based on the data collection and analysis, we identified areas for improvement and identified the main principle for conceptualizing the design process to guide future development and replication by other developers.

3.1.1. Developing and Accessing ATLog Therapy Solutions Using a Cyclical Approach

The methodology followed a cyclic process of design, testing and improvement for developing and evaluating platform interventions (solutions) in real-world therapy settings, with previous successful iterations reported in [19–23]. The solutions were compared and assessed to gather data for developing a new framework for conceptualizing the design processes. The iterations were conducted during experiments (which are still ongoing) at a Logopedic Center of South-West University in Blagoevgrad (Figure 2). The research procedure for the experiments was preregistered and approved by the Ethics Committee of the South-West University with protocol N 2410-1/29.10.2024.

Therapists actively contributed to the conceptualization and development of interactive scenarios with ATs, ensuring alignment with real SLT practices. At the beginning, they defined various scenarios for vocabulary acquisition and sentence construction with SARs, and scenes and interactions for language learning in the VR environment. Next, they prepared the robot replica to initiate and sustain conversations by programming predefined dialog structures and interactive prompts. These human-like interactions in language comprehension and speech production scenarios were continuously improved, resulting in a key innovation: fostering foundational vocabulary development through intensive but engaging verbal interaction with robots, making the process more enjoyable and encouraging sustained participation. Building on this foundation, the playful scenarios involve question-and-answer sessions, narration of fairy tales with subsequent analyses, and engaging spoken social communications with SARs or in VR. Through human-like conversations, children practice speaking and listening skills in a supportive, non-judgmental environment—in the secure world of robots and VR immersion. Additionally, children felt less anxious and self-conscious when interacting with a robot that misunderstood them or made jokes. This increased opportunities for practice, including outside of therapy sessions (e.g., at home), because ConvAI can be integrated easily into low-cost robots, such as the emotionally expressive robot Emo developed within the project.

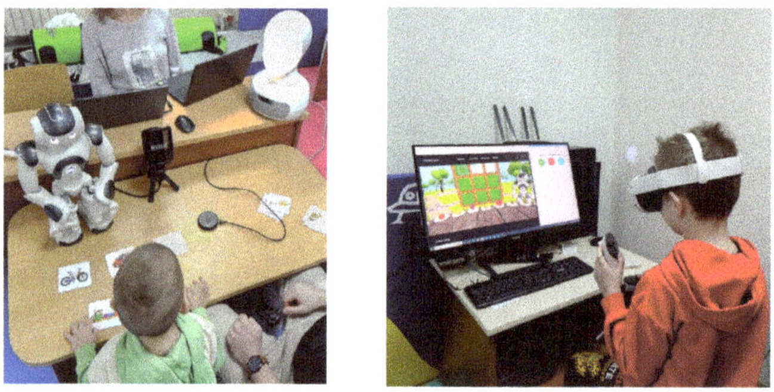

(a) (b)

Figure 2. Pilot experiments at the Logopedic Center of SWU: (**a**) Nao and Furhat cooperation during a playful scenario for 'Transport tools'; (**b**) VR Bingo 3 × 3 on topic 'fruits'.

3.1.2. Participants and Setup for the Qualitatively Assessment of ATLog

An online study was conducted to examine, via qualitative assessment, the potential of adopting ATLog platform in SLT practice. ATLog was evaluated by 27 experts using the TAM and SUS questionnaires, along with ten additional questions specifically focused on the ATLog structure and effectiveness. The selection criteria required experts to be practicing speech and language therapists, while excluding therapists in the ATLog project. Eligible candidates needed to have at least five years of professional experience, be actively engaged in clinical practice and work specifically with children and adolescents. The ATLog platform was demonstrated in front of 50 participants; however, only 27 SLT filled the surveys.

The experimental procedure for the SUS, extended with additional questions focused on ATLog functionality, was preregistered and approved by the Ethics Committee of IR-BAS under protocol N7/05.02.2025, while for the TAM—protocol N11/06.06.2025. There was a one-day face-to-face training session, consisting of a 4 h presentation and 4 h of platform demonstrations. At the beginning, each block for different ATs was explained, followed by the design and execution of example interactive scenarios. Two videos from the training were shared with the participants. Additionally, participants received a step-by-step tutorial consisting of four video lessons, covering explanations of blocks in different categories, as well as how to design and run an example scenario in ATLog. These videos are provided in the Supplementary Materials Videos S1–S4.

The average age of the participants was 37 years (SD = 8.37). All of them were female because this profession is practiced mainly by women in Bulgaria. The youngest SLT professional was 25 years and the oldest one was 56 years

3.1.3. Instruments for the Qualitatively Assessment of ATLog

The methodology included the System Usability Scale (SUS) and Technology Acceptance Model (TAM) during the Phase 3 of DBR. The reliability of questionnaires used in the study is presented in Table 1. The SUS evaluates three key dimensions of usability—effectiveness, efficiency and satisfaction. This questionnaire enables the assessment of a wide range of products and services, such as hardware, software, mobile devices, websites and applications. It has several advantages: (1) it is simple to administer, (2) it provides reliable results even with small sample sizes, and (3) it effectively distinguishes between usable and unusable systems. The questionnaire includes 10 items, each rated on 5-point Likert scale ranging from 'Strongly Agree' to 'Strongly Disagree'. They are focused on the usability of the platform, which content can be seen in Table 2. The remaining 10 questions (Table 3) are focused on ATLog structure, communication efficiency and the feasibility of designing interactive scenarios for SLT. The questionnaire evaluation confirmed therapists' acceptance of integrating ATs into SLT by effectively addressing user-friendliness and ensuring alignment with SLT practices. The responses were rated also via a 5-point Likert scale, ranging from 'Strongly Disagree' to 'Strongly Agree', consistent with the SUS questionnaire. Additionally, the survey finished with an open-ended question asking for any recommendations about the ATLog platform.

Table 1. Test results of the reliability of questionnaires used in the study.

Questionnaire	Cronbach's Alpha	N of Items	Description
SUS	0.798	10	Reliable
Design structure (communications and effectiveness in creating interactive scenarios in ATLog)	0.849	10	Reliable
PU subscale	0.906	6	Reliable
PEU subscale	0.922	6	Reliable

Table 2. SUS average scores for each statement.

No.	Question	Mean	SD	Interpretation
1	I think that I would like to use this system frequently.	4.1	0.8	Agree
2	I found the system is unnecessarily complex.	1.4	0.7	Disagree
3	I thought the system was easy to use.	4.3	0.8	Agree
4	I think that I would need the support of a technical person to be able to use this system.	2.4	1.2	Disagree
5	I found the various functions in this system were well integrated.	4.3	0.7	Agree
6	I thought there was too much inconsistency in this system.	1.4	0.8	Disagree
7	I would imagine that most people would learn how to use this system very quickly.	4.4	0.6	Agree
8	I found the system very cumbersome to use.	1.4	0.8	Disagree
9	I felt very confident using the system.	3.6	1.3	Agree
10	I need to learn a lot of things before I could get going with this system.	2.8	1.2	Disagree

The TAM is a widely used model for predicting and explaining user acceptance of technology before implementation. The TAM includes two key components: perceived usefulness (PU) and perceived ease of use (PEU). Both PU and PEU are assessed using six statements, the content of which can be seen in Table 4. Each statement is rated on a 7-point Likert scale, ranging from 'Strongly Disagree' to 'Strongly Agree'.

Table 3. ATLog Design Structure evaluation average scores for each statement.

No.	Question	Mean	SD	Interpretation
11	I would use ATLog if I had access to video tutorials and a methodological guide.	4.2	1.1	Agree
12	The platform is adequately structured for creating interactive scenarios with AT.	4.4	0.7	Agree
13	Creating scenarios in the Platform saves time.	4.3	0.8	Agree
14	The platform is suitable for managing SAR in real conditions.	4.3	0.8	Agree
15	The platform allows the child to take initiative (through QR code, text, voice).	4.8	0.4	Agree
16	The therapist has control over the AT in the platform during the intervention (stop button, voice command, and touch sensor).	4.9	0.4	Agree
17	The delay in responses from the text-generative AI is acceptable.	3.7	0.8	Agree
18	Each of the graphic blocks in the platform contains information about its therapeutic application.	4.6	0.6	Agree
19	The graphic blocks in the platform are informative enough for their use.	4.4	0.9	Agree
20	The platform supports the creation of personalized interactive scenarios with AT.	4.7	0.6	Agree

Table 4. TAM average scores for each statement.

	No.	Question	Mean	SD	Interpretation
PU	1	Using the ATLog platform would improve my performance at work.	6.1	0.7	Strongly agree
	2	Using the ATLog platform would increase my productivity.	6.1	0.7	Strongly agree
	3	Using the ATLog platform would increase my efficiency at work.	6.3	0.7	Strongly agree
	4	Using the ATLog platform would make my work easier.	6.4	0.7	Strongly agree
	5	Using the ATLog platform would be useful for my work.	6.4	0.7	A Strongly agree
	6	Using the ATLog platform in my work would allow me to complete my therapeutic tasks faster.	5.9	1.0	Strongly agree
PEU	7	Learning how to use the ATLog platform would be easy for me.	6.4	0.7	Strongly agree
	8	I could easily use the ATLog platform for therapy purposes.	6.4	0.8	Strongly agree
	9	The user interface to the ATLog platform is clear and understandable.	6.2	0.9	Strongly agree
	10	It would be easy for me to learn to work with the ATLog platform.	6.5	0.7	Strongly agree
	11	I think the ATLog platform is easy to use.	6.3	0.8	Strongly agree
	12	I think it will be easy for me to learn to use the ATLog platform.	6.4	0.7	Strongly agree

The SUS score for each participant was computed through a standardized approach [79,80]. Specifically, for odd-numbered statements, *1* was subtracted from the response, while for even-numbered statements, the response was subtracted from *5*. To normalize the scores and facilitate comparability across different evaluations, the individual scores were then multiplied by *2.5*. The same formula was applied to calculate the score for the second part of the questionnaire to enable a comparative analysis of the results of both. Since all statements in the second part were positively worded, the score for each respondent was derived by subtracting *1* from the response and subsequently multiplying by *2.5*. The average score from the study was used to assess the acceptability of the SUS test, with a *score of 70 applied as the passing threshold*, which was defined in [81]. Finally, the computed SUS scores, along with the scores from the second part of the questionnaire about the overall framework (Design Structure) and how the preprogrammed blocks are organized and communicate with ATs in creating interactive scenarios within the ATLog, were mapped to an absolute grading scale as proposed by [81]. In this scale, *A* corresponds to scores of *90–100*, *B* to *80–89*, *C* to *70–79*, *D* to *60–69*, and *F* to scores below *60*. As recommended by Lewis [82] to compare the results between the SUS and TAM questionnaires, we put PU and PEU on a 0–100-point scale and then averaged PU and PEU to obtain the overall TAM result, using the formula provided in [82]:

$$\mathrm{PU} = (\mathrm{AVERAGE}(\mathrm{Q1}, \mathrm{Q2}, \mathrm{Q3}, \mathrm{Q4}, \mathrm{Q5}, \mathrm{Q6}) - 1) \times (100/6) \quad (1)$$

$$\mathrm{PEU} = (\mathrm{AVERAGE}(\mathrm{Q7}, \mathrm{Q8}, \mathrm{Q9}, \mathrm{Q10}, \mathrm{Q11}, \mathrm{Q12}) - 1) \times (100/6) \quad (2)$$

The results from the questionnaires were analyzed using *IBM SPSS v26* to ensure the reliability of the results. Cronbach's alpha was employed to measure the internal consistency of the scales. Also, the nonparametric Spearman's rank-order correlation test was applied to evaluate the strength of the relationship between the parts of the questionnaires and to determine their correlation.

3.2. Materials

The hardware and software used in the ATLog platform are briefly presented below.

3.2.1. Hardware

Social Robots

- Nao [83]: A small humanoid robot for multimodal interaction through speech, body language, barcode reading and tactile sensors. Nao is one of the most widely used SARs in therapy for individuals with developmental, language and communication disorders [47]. For that reason, the ATLog platform contains more predefined Blockly blocks for Nao compared to other ATs.
- Furhat [84]: Currently the most advanced conversational social robot with an expressive face. Its human presence tracking, visual contact by eye-tracking camera, intuitive face-to-face interaction, and customizable diverse characters and voices contribute to real human-like interactions. The touchscreen interface, enhanced with images and text, further enriches communications.
- Emo, our second version (v2) of the emotionally expressive robot, v1 can be seen [85]: The robot has a 25 cm head that displays emotional states using emoticon-like facial features, with a dynamically changing mouth, eyes and eyebrows. Emo has six degrees of freedom to replicate human head movements. It can track a person in front of it to detect attendance, read QR codes and play audio files, and access cloud services for NLP and NLG. These capabilities make Emo suitable for emotional teaching and multi-robot cooperation in SLT.
- Double3 [86]: A robot for telepresence, designed to provide remote interaction with a dynamic presence. It is also considered as a social robot because it enables assistive interactions with both the therapists and other ATs during telepractice. Double3 has a high-definition camera, two-way audio and video capabilities, the ability to navigate physical spaces, and an interactive display to present text, images and videos. Double3 can scan remote QR codes, thus acting as a mediator in communications during telepractice.

VR Devices

- Headsets: Meta Quest 2, 3, 3S and Pro. Headsets run on the "Meta Quest OS" operating system, which is based on "Android" and can be used independently or connected to a computer via the "Meta Quest Link" program. The Meta Quest Pro headset was used during the experiments due to its eye-tracking.

- Camera for 360° Virtual Tours: XPhase Pro S2 with 25 sensors, each with 8 megapixels, providing a total resolution of 200 megapixels. It supports 360° tours, hot spots and side-by-side view, with 16-bit lossless format output.

Computing Devices

ATLog data processing, communications, storage and online display were conducted on a laptop (11th Gen Intel(R) Core(TM) i7-1165G7 @ 2.80 GHz, 8.00 GB RAM, MS Windows 11 Prof. 64-bit). The external touch monitor is Dell-P2424HT, 23.8", FHD, IPS, Anti-Glare, with built-in speakers.

3.2.2. Software

- Choregraphe [87]: a multi-platform desktop tool that allows users to create animations, behaviors and dialogs for the Nao robot. It has block-based visual interface for creating, customizing and uploading personalized behaviors, which are then uploaded to the robot for subsequent use through the ATLog frontend.
- NAOqi 2.8 [88]: NAOqi is the operating system for the Nao robot. Through its remote APIs, developers can interact with the robot from external IDEs over a network. These APIs allow users to access features such as speech recognition, motion control, vision processing and sensor data. Customized Python scripts in the ATLog backend enable these functionalities for subsequent use through the ATLog frontend.
- Furhat Kotlin SDK [89]: A software development kit designed for building interactive applications for the Furhat robot using Kotlin. This SDK is used to program the robot's real-time interactions, including speech, gestures, and dialog, as well as tablet-based interface to Furhat.
- Furhat Remote APIs [90]: The remote APIs enable developers to interact with the robot from external IDEs over a network. Using these APIs, the robot's movements, facial expressions and voice can be controlled remotely through the ATLog frontend.
- Double3 Developer SDK [91]: The D3 APIs, commands and events enable developers to use Double3 in developer mode. Thus, python scripts run directly in the Double3 operating system. The D3 software includes a built-in subscription/publishing system, allowing Double3 to send event messages or respond according to its programmed skills.
- EMO software: The control system of the robot is based on two Raspberry Pi 5 units and other Arduino-type microcontrollers. Running on Linux, it supports any compatible programming language.
- VR software for interactive scenarios in web environment: HTML, CSS and JavaScript for structuring the content, styling and layout. To enable virtual reality within the browser, webXR technology [92] is used to manage VR devices and handle controller inputs through an API that triggers events and interactions within the VR environment. Additionally, the THREE.js library, built on top of WebGL [93], accesses the underlying graphics hardware to render 3D content directly in the browser.
- 3DVista [94]: Software for 360° Virtual Tours enables the creation of interactive environments through integrated elements such as clickable hotspots, navigation arrows, and objects that are activated based on predefined therapeutic goals and outcomes. The virtual tours include components designed to support the development of spatial awareness, orientation and logical thinking. Specific interactive features for children

are included to facilitate navigation within environments and engage them through age-appropriate, game-based scenarios tailored to their individual needs.

- Cloud services for speech recognition and speech synthesis from MS Azure and Google and services for text generation from NLP Cloud [95], ChatGPT-4 of OpenAI [96], BgGPT of INSAIT [97].
- Express.js server [98]: A Node.js web application framework for developing the client–server model. Express.js is used to build the backend in ATLog, handling logic, communication and data processing.
- Visual programming interface, built on Google Blockly [99]: block-based programming interface allowing users to design graphical flows of blocks without programming skills.
- The internal memory, built on a Node.js object repository, stores and retrieves key-value pairs and acts as a temporary data storage for short-term operations.
- SQLite database [100]: persistent data storage for long-term data management to track and access the progress of the individual SLT interventions.

3.3. *ATLog Platform: Design and Features*

The platform architecture with network design solutions for the integration of SARs, VR devices and ConvAI in one platform is presented below. The integration of a block-based visual programming framework with Express server is presented, as well.

3.3.1. Platform Architecture

Figure 3 presents the architectural scheme of the ATLog platform, where a web-based interface facilitates the intuitive design of interactive scenarios, while Express server serves as the central backend component, managing communication with the frontend and among assistive technologies by processing incoming requests and responses. Express server processes incoming requests and responses through RESTful endpoints using standard HTTP methods and exchanges data in JSON format. However, it also includes some non-REST features, such as real-time streaming and command execution. The block-based graphical editor in the frontend removes the need for programming skills, enabling users to define a structured sequence of blocks (the scenario flow) that send requests to server endpoints in order to activate SAR skills, VR interactions, or NLP/NLG cloud services. Internal memory on the middleware enables data exchange among ATs, supporting cooperation between SARs, ConvAI and VR. For instance, text-generative AI (BgGPT) uses the physical presence of a Nao robot for QR code reading. The decoded text is saved in memory and later used for questioning BgGPT.

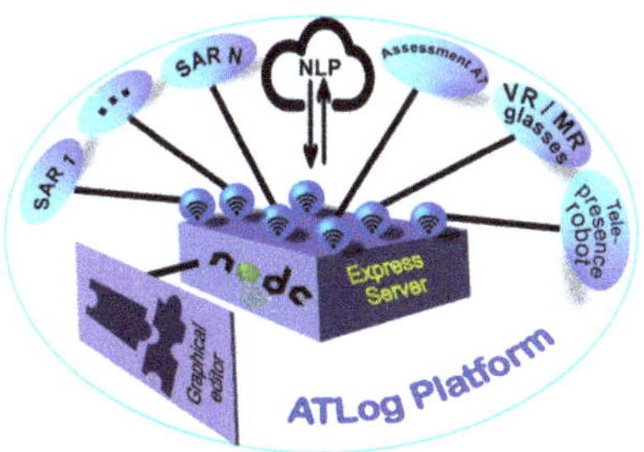

Figure 3. Architecture scheme of the ATLog platform.

3.3.2. Communication Protocols

- In Express server: standard HTTP protocols, along with child processes to access skills of SARs and VR scenarios. RESTful HTTP requests (GET, POST) are sent to cloud services for NLP and NLG. WebSocket protocol enables bidirectional communications in VR scenarios.
- In Blockly: HTTP GET and POST requests are used to send commands to Express server or external web resources.
- For file transfers: Files are securely transferred between the platform and the Nao robot via SCP (Secure Copy Protocol) over the LAN network, using SSH (Secure Shell) for encryption and authentication.
- For remote script execution on Nao and Furhat: TCP sockets are used for communication from the Express backend to NAOqi (on Nao) over IP, while for Furhat we use the Python SDK wrapper, which connects to the Furhat API via WebSocket.
- For remote script execution on Double3: python scripts are remotely executed using an SSH client via PuTTY. A developer mode and additional administrative rights are required to activate the camera and subscribe to events for Double3, such as reading QR codes (DRCamera.tags) using the command "camera.tagDetector.enable".
- For MQTT connections to Emo robot: Remote control and execution of scripts on the Emo robot by using the mqtt protocol within a PY 3.x virtual environment and paho-mqtt library. On the Raspberry Pi, a script runs as a communication bridge between the Raspberry Pi and the ATLog server.
- For database writing, the protocol is SQL, executed via the SQLite3 package for Node.js.

3.3.3. Network Solutions for the Integration of Block-Based Visual Programming with Express Server

Express server handles communication between Blockly graphical blocks and SARs or VR applications using HTTP, TCP, SSH, Websocket, SCP and SQL protocols, ensuring bidirectional and real-time responses. The server manages child processes and SSH connections in order to integrate the ATs in the platform. Dependencies that need to be installed comprise 'child_process' and 'ssh2' Node.js modules for process management and remote connections. The endpoints that use child processes execute server-side python- or JavaScripts for controlling robots and VR or calling NLP/NLG cloud services. This network solution ensures easy maintenance, since *only the scripts, which are used in the child processes, need updates when technology evolves*. Additionally, the ATLog interface uses HTTP requests to connect to external text-generative AI APIs, bypassing security limitations on unauthenticated devices like robots and VR glasses. The network solutions for integrating pre-programmed blocks with their corresponding endpoints in Express server are detailed in Section 4 and can be seen in Appendix **??**, Tables A1–A5.

- On the frontend (Blockly): ATLog sends HTTP GET and POST requests to the server to initiate the skills of ATs, retrieve data or send data to the internal ATLog repository. To ensure the correct execution of the next block in the scenario flow, specific handling of the backend response is mandatory for certain blocks.
- On the backend (Express server): ATLog uses standard TCP or HTTP protocols, along with child processes and several middleware, to access the skills of SARs and VR scenarios. It sends RESTful HTTP requests (GET, POST) to cloud services for NLP and NLG. Backend endpoints return responses to the frontend as needed.

- The VR endpoints on the backend run on a separate port, enabling bidirectional communication between the client and server using the socket.io library. Socket.io enhances the Websocket protocol by implementing organized communication spaces.
- VR streaming is provided through Meta's Meta Quest casting service [101], allowing the VR headset screen to be shared on an external monitor for observation by the therapist or other children.

3.3.4. Cooperation of ATs

Cooperation between Nao, Furhat, Emo and Double3 robots enhances the SLT session by enabling multimodal interactions, user presence detection, emotional responses and telepractice features, which are either lacking or less developed in individual robots. For example, the cooperation between Nao and Furhat alters the questioning approach, with Nao using QR codes for nonverbal children, while Furhat provides an advanced verbal recognition system. Furhat can further enhance Nao, Emo and Double3 robots by enabling them to subscribe to FurhatOS events and receive notifications when Furhat receives a new oral question from the child. Through calls to Furhat Remote API, these robots can also listen, speak and attend to children from external IDE. Emo can contribute by replicating child head movements and expressing its current emotions, making sessions more engaging and fun with natural, human-like mimicking. Emo can read QR codes in Bulgarian, a language not natively supported by Nao. Nao reads QR codes in English, requiring translation via cloud services, which inserts latency. Double3 can contribute to each robot through remote interactions with them during telepractice. According to our experimental test, when the child's face is displayed via video telepresence on the Double3 tablet in front of Furhat's camera, the child is detected from Furhat as active user and a unique ID is assigned, which remains fixed as long as the Double3 tablet stays in view of Furhat. This automatically initiates Furhat's transition from an 'idle' to an 'active' state, following the steps defined in the designed interactive scenario for the current telepractice.

3.4. Design Process of Interactive Scenario

To streamline the design of interactive scenarios, the ATLog frontend consists of preprogrammed graphical blocks that can be combined based on the existing ATs and logopedic materials. The platform employs a subprocess-oriented approach, breaking down SAR skills into microskills and VR interactive scenarios into smaller components, allowing the therapist to choose and combine microskills from different ATs. The blocks are assembled in a flow using a drag-and-drop interface.

A snapshot of the ATLog graphical interface is shown in Figure 4a. On the left, different colors represent various categories of ATs that are integrated into the platform. Nao's blocks are in green color, while the Furhat category is in dark blue. By the security block in the Furhat category (the red one in Figure 4a), all running ATs in the platform can be stopped. Thus, during the session, the Furhat robot listens for keywords like "stop" or "break" and terminates all spawned child processes, stops robot behaviors, closes open databases and shuts down Express server. Alternatively, the platform can be stopped using the *'Stop Code'* button (Figure 4a). The purple blocks are related to the ATLog internal repository, NLP/NLG cloud services, or logic blocks, one of which is the loop block 'repeat_execution' presented on the middle window in Figure 4b. It has an input parameter for the number of iterations and wraps any inner blocks inside *'for loop'* block to execute them multiple times. Thus, therapists determine how many times to repeat the execution of one or more blocks. Several instances of the ATLog block-based graphical interface can run separately, as shown in Figure 4b. This allows the therapist to partition the design of the scenario into parts, and by opening them in different tabs in a browser, they have the option to repeat some of the parts or to switch immediately to a certain part.

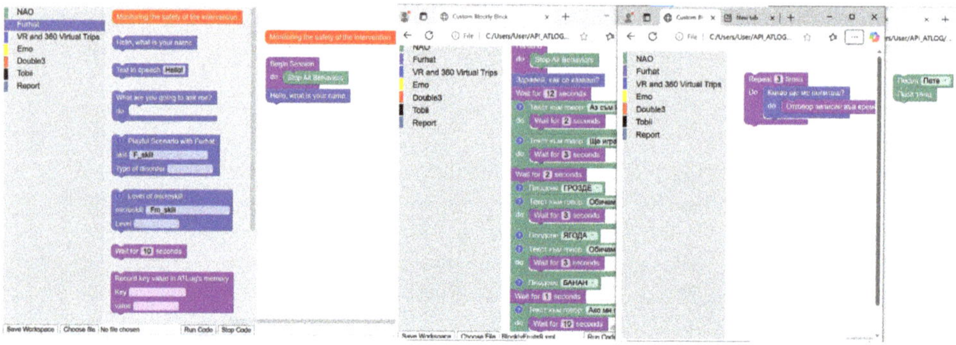

(**a**) (**b**)

Figure 4. (**a**) ATLog block-based graphical interface for visual programing with opened category for Nao robot; (**b**) three instances of ATLog block-based graphical interface running separately.

Each block has a pop-up window, accessible by pressing the question mark, which provides explanations of the therapy objectives, treatment domain, type of disorder and language skill level. Most of the blocks are hierarchical (structured with a drop-down menu) in order for therapists to select from predefined options. For example, a drop-down menu for the skill "Animals" presents choices corresponding to the hierarchical behavior '*WORDS_anim*' uploaded onto a Nao robot, which links to 9 sub-behaviors for different animals. Similar hierarchical blocks are: '*Ling 6-Sound Test*' (A, M, I, U, SH, S); '*Transports*'; '*Colors*'; '*Musical Instruments*'; '*Emotions*'; and '*Store*'. These blocks await a QR code on a double-sided flashcard illustrating the content, which should be shown to Nao. If the child selects the correct card, Nao responds with approval phrases and proceeds to the next block. If the child selects the wrong card, Nao waits for the correct one.

Nao can be asked a question by dragging '*TextQuestionBlock*'. The context and question must be specified in the block's fields. The default context is: "Say the information in a child-friendly way". For nonverbal children, an alternative option is to use '*QRquestionBlock*' by showing a QR code on a double-sided flashcard illustrating the question content. To cope with interactions not natively supported by Nao Bulgarian language, we use cloud-based TTS and ASR engines to convert text into audio, which is then dynamically uploaded to the robot's memory. By '*Text_to_speechBlock*', Nao plays the input text using an audio file, while by '*PlaytextBlock*', Nao plays the audio answer converted from Bulgarian ChatGPT (BgGPT). BgGPT provides a response in the backend and saves the answer in the ATLog repository. The '*FurhatQuestionBlock*' can be dragged to operate in parallel, allowing the child to continuously interact with Furhat during the session using prompts like 'Furhat, tell this?', which encourages active listening and speaking.

Figure 4a illustrates a block with 'do' input. Such blocks differ in how they handle responses and manage response data, with 'do' input blocks (doCode) allowing for additional actions to be triggered based on received responses. For example, the blocks for TTS and Q&A send requests to NLP/NLG cloud services and must wait for responses, using 'doCode' input blocks to handle text-to-speech synthesis.

Two types of temporary memory can be used: the one initialized when starting the ATLog and the other being the Nao robot's native memory. Blocks in green read or write in the Nao internal memory, while blocks in purple read or write in the memory of ATLog.

Each AT has in its category a *'RepositoryRead'* block, which retrieves a value from the ATLog repository using a specified key, and a *'RepositorySave'* block, which stores a value in the repository under a specified key. The persistent memory of the ATLog is a database and exists as a standalone category. Using the *'DB_save'* block, the therapist can save session observations and notes at the end of the therapy session. The information is anonymous, as each child is assigned a unique identity code. The records in the database can be exported in *csv* format.

ATLog frontend allows for the integration and execution of new skills through *"custom"* blocks. Anyone experienced in creating new behaviors in Choregraphe or programming via remote NAOqi can integrate new skills using two Nao custom blocks with input fields. The *'CustomBehavior'* block accepts the custom behavior name for behaviors designed in Choregraphe and uploaded to the NAO robot, while the *'CustomRemote'* block allows the execution of custom scripts remotely on NAOqi, enabling remote control of the NAO robot's capabilities. Similarly, for Furhat, new skills or microskills can be seamlessly integrated into the ATLog frontend using the *'CustomSkillBlock'*. It runs a custom skill prepared in Kotlin SDK and uploaded to Furhat robot.

More explanations for blocks in the different categories are provided in the Supplementary Materials Videos S1 and S2.

3.5. Ethics

The design and implementation of the ATLog platform raised ethical considerations for both developers and therapists, specifically regarding the assessment of risks linked with using AI systems. Although the European AI Act classifies conversational AI systems as having a low level of risk, ATLog adheres to its own Ethical Codex [102]. An ethical framework was established within the methodology to analyze potential risks associated with using text-generative AI, personal data and the protection of individuals' human rights. Throughout the development, ethical guidelines were followed to ensure data privacy and security through anonymization.

4. Implementation and Results

Following the proposed methodology in Section 3, this section provides the implementation of the ATLog platform. Technical details for developers on how AT devices and services interact within a client–server model can be seen in Appendix **??** (Tables A1–A5) and Appendix B (Table A6). This section also provides an example of how to design and execute an interactive scenario step-by-step using the platform. The final subsection presents the results of the ATLog platform usability assessment, including user-friendliness, functionality and technological acceptance as evaluated by the therapists.

4.1. Implementation of ATLog Platform

Figure 4 shows the implemented frontend, developed using the Blockly web-based visual programming framework. The frontend blocks control ATs by sending parameterized requests to the endpoints of a Node.js-based Express server, as detailed in Appendix **??**, Tables A1–A5. Table A6 in Appendix B provides an overview of Express server setup with the required dependencies, middleware and dynamic imports. The middleware section in Table A6 describes the processing of JSON and URL-encoded request bodies, along with specific configurations for serving static assets, including Three.js libraries for VR web-based integration and rendering 3D graphics in the browser using WebGL.

Server endpoints manage AT control by processing API requests from the frontend, executing pre-programmed scripts for certain ATs via child processes, or by using SSH connections and the MQTT protocol. Tables A1–A5 detail the relationships between block names; their functional descriptions; the required skill, microskill, or other files to be uploaded on the ATs; the input parameters; and the corresponding backend endpoints

Table A1 illustrates Nao blocks. When the user drags a Nao block in the Blockly workspace, it sends a request to the server endpoint, which executes either a behavior uploaded on Nao or 'child_process', which runs remote Nao API. Nao blocks activate specific endpoints (/nao1, /nao2, /nao3 or /naoUpload), forming a URL with input parameters. Such an example is http://serverIP:3000/*nao1?IP=${ipNao}&pyScript=${pyScript}*, where the *pyScript* parameter specifies the name of the PY 2.7 script to be executed on the Nao robot. Another example is http://serverIP:3000/*nao2?IP=${ipNao}&behname=${behname}*, where the *behname* parameter specifies the name of the uploaded behavior on the Nao robot to be executed. Some Nao blocks require the server endpoints to activate a virtual environment *(/venv)* to execute Python 3.x scripts, including those for NLP/NLG cloud services. The endpoint http://serverIP:3000/*nao3?IP=${ipNao}&filename=${filename}* specifies the script name to be executed. Some Nao blocks require input parameters such as port, Nao IP, password, file path on the server, file path on the robot and file name. One such endpoint is/*naoUpload*, which constructs a *pscp* command to upload the specified file from a local directory to the Nao robot via SSH.

Table A2 shows Furhat blocks that link endpoints using child_process to execute Python scripts that interface with Furhat remote APIs. The /*furhatRem* endpoint processes a GET request with the input parameters *${ipFurhat}*, *${pyScript}* and *${text}* (if TTS is required). The server captures the script output from 'stdout' and returns the response to Blockly, ensuring correct continuous block execution.

Table A3 summaries frontend blocks for Emo and Double3. The/*emo1* endpoint establishes a MQTT communication bridge to the Raspberry Pi 5 of Emo for remote control through a paho-mqtt library for message exchange. Different scripts run on the Emo robot, such as those for QR code scanning or playing audio, in response to block requests. The/*emo2* endpoint opens another type of MQTT session to the robot with different topics, such as 'audios', 'emotions', etc. The endpoint/*double3* opens an SSH session to the robot, requiring authentication, and runs shell commands and PY scripts in the remote robot environment, which interact with the Double3 Developer SDK, D3 API and events.

Table A4 summaries the general frontend blocks and their corresponding backend endpoints for functions not related to SARs and VR, such as '*RepeatBlock*', '*RepositoryReadBlock*', '*RepositorySaveBlock*', '*DB_saveBlock*', '*BG_GPT_Block*', '*QABlock*', and '*WaitBlock*'. A global repository, established for storing text in key–value pairs, is formatted in JSON (see established middleware in Table A6). It also transmits messages among robots and VR, enabling multi-robot cooperation scenarios where each robot's unique features are utilized. Since the Nao robot has a reliable and remote event subscription mechanism, all robots have a block in their category to declare events, raise events, subscribe to events and receive messages by callbacks, as well as to set and receive data to the internal Nao repository via the NAOqi framework. For instance, in order to ask for cooperation with the Nao robot, Furhat has to subscribe remotely to NAOqi Message Broker and QRevent in order to read the QR text that is in Nao memory. Robots can also be subscribed to Nao for audio playback cooperation through remote calls to NAOqi APIs or for TTS. This is useful when the robot does not have embedded TTS, such as Emo, or if TTS is not native for a specific language, such as Nao. Our solution is to use cloud service to obtain an audio file from the text and to play it on the robot, implemented by using gTTS (Google Text-to-Speech), a Python library, and a CLI tool that interfaces with Google Translate's text-to-speech API, generating spoken MP3 data and saving it to a file for playback on the robot. The synthesized audio file is uploaded to the robot using the PuTTY pscp network protocol. The Furhat robot comes with credentials for speaking voices like PollyVoice and Azure voices; however, the Bulgarian language is not supported with PollyVoice. We use personal Azure credentials; however, if they are unavailable, gTTS can also be used through Furhat's remote APIs, with the synthesized audio file uploaded to the web as Furhat plays files from a URL.

Table A5 summaries the VR frontend blocks. The *'Setup_VR_Session_Block'* sets up the WebSocket communication and assigns unique session IDs for both the therapist and the child. The *'Setup_VR_Scene_Block'* initializes a VR scene in Three.js, configuring the camera, VR controllers, renderer, and WebXR support and loading 3D models, while delivering static files such as frontend code, images, and styles from the "public" folder and dynamically generating HTML pages. The *'StartVRbutton_block'* activates the VR button in immersive mode within the browser. The *'360_Virtual_Tour'* block has a drop-down menu and fetches an interactive 360° virtual tour on a touchscreen, allowing children to explore familiar real-world settings (e.g., supermarket, house, museum) hosted on the ATLog project website. In the same way, the *'360_Virtual_Game'* block provides interactive 360° virtual games on a touchscreen, where children search for and identify objects from a preassigned list.

To streamline the design of blocks that must always be connected, a Blockly event function is utilized. This function is triggered automatically whenever the first block (block1) is moved or created in the Blockly workspace, providing information about the event type (e.g., MOVE or CREATE), the dragged block and its ID. The sequence is ensured by verifying that block1 has block2 connected as its previous block. If block2 is missing, the function automatically generates and links block2 for the correct sequence. An example of such a block is *'Song'*, connected in sequence with *'PoseDance'* (shown in the right window of Figure 4b).

4.2. Technical Challenges

- A virtual environment for different python versions must be activated through the 'venv' endpoint because the child processes for text translation, text generation or speech synthesis rely on PY 3.x or higher.
- We faced challenges with continuous block execution in Blockly. While child processes were still running, the run code in the JavaScript of the block had exited, causing the next block to start early. The solution was to use an *async* function with *await new Promise(resolve)*, which either waits for a server response indicating the child process has exited with code 0, or continuously checks the status of the child process by sending requests to a */monitor* endpoint. The second approach works better for blocks with more complex run code. When Nao blocks need to wait for Furhat child processes to finish, an *async* function continuously checks the status of the python process by sending requests to the */monitor/pyFurhat* endpoint. It waits for a response from the server, which indicates whether the Python process is still running or has been exited. Once the process is no longer running, the function exits the loop, and Nao blocks can start. Similarly, */monitor/pyNao1* and */monitor/pyNao2* endpoints allow for client-side functions to determine the child's status when Furhat blocks wait for Nao child processes to exit.
- Another challenge was that by default, Express sets a request body size limit of 100 KB when using the *express.json()* middleware. To handle larger payloads, such as saving responses from chatGPT in KEY=answer, the limit had to be increased to at least 500 KB by configuring the middleware to *express.json({limit: '500 kb'})*.

- We faced challenges with delay in the API response time of BgGPT. To address this, we experimented with response streaming using Server-Sent Events (SSEs) over an HTTP connection. We enhanced performance by delivering tokens in real time through an Express endpoint, which requests a streamed response from the BgGPT API and pipes the received chunks directly to the SARs TTS services.
- From the pilot experiment, where we tested interactive scenarios for stuttering using Furhat, we found that the embedded Furhat's speech recognition based on ML occasionally misinterpreted stuttered speech, sometimes recognizing it as fluent, while other times as '*NOMATCH*' (not fluent). The current solution relies on the SLT practitioners verbally instructing Furhat by saying "fluent" or "not fluent" to classify the stuttered speech correctly.
- We faced challenges with object selection and tracking the direction of the child's hand in VR Bingo (Figure 2b). In the previous DBR iteration, the objects (fruits) were placed on a round table (Figure 5a) and the children had difficulty changing the perspective in order to select the objects that were behind another one. The solution was to expand the round table along the X-axis in an ellipse and rearrange the objects to prevent overlap from the initial perspective (Figure 5b). Additionally, the invisible boxes representing the "hitbox" were initially too small and were adjusted to match the height of the objects (fruits), ensuring easier selection. The white ray used to track the direction of the child's hand was replaced with a longer and thicker red cylinder, significantly improving tracking accuracy.

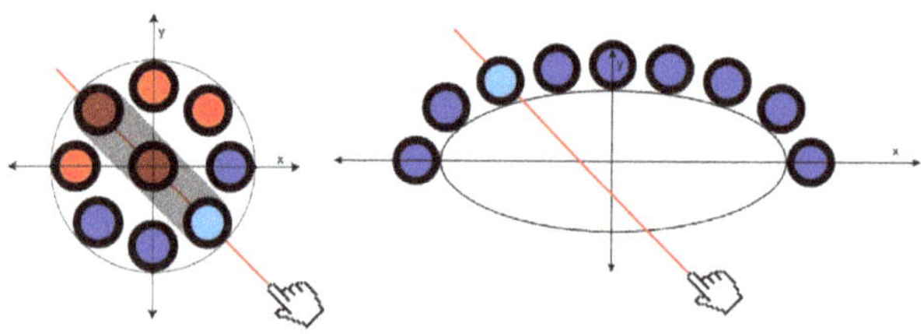

(**a**) (**b**)

Figure 5. Object selection challenges: (**a**) fruits placed on a round table; (**b**) fruits arranged in an ellipse layout. The red fruits (circles) are not reacable; blue means reacable objects.

4.3. Example Scenario, Development Steps and Runtime

Figure 6 presents an example scenario, written by an SLT practitioner, which needs to be designed using the ATLog frontend. Figure 7a illustrates the scenario flow of blocks. The block responsible for the first three rows (1–3) is the Furhat block for greeting the child, listening to its name and saving it in the internal repository. Then, Nao starts guiding the playful exercises by asking oral questions about looking, listening and showing the correct flashcard (rows 4–7). For speaking the text in row 4, the used block is the Nao 'TTS block'. The block automatically connected two blocks in the 'DO' input: (1) a narrating block and (2) a block specifying the required seconds for narrating, which are recorded in Nao's memory. A cloud-based speech recognition and TTS from Google engine were used, with a dedicated Nao block responsible for playing the converted response in audio format. This audio was dynamically uploaded to the robot's internal memory. The block responsible for rows 8–10 was '*Ask BgGPT with QR code*'. It waited for the child to show the QR code of the flashcard to the robot's eyes. BgGPT processed the request in the backend and saved the response in the repository. The default context was: 'Say in a child-friendly way". The block 'Ask BgGPT with QR code' automatically connected 'playtext_block,' which played the audio file containing the answer from BgGPT. For raw 12, the Furhat 'Ask BgGPT' block had to be dragged and placed in the 'repeat_execution' block with input parameters for three iterations (as shown in Figure 4b). For row 14, the Furhat 'microskill' block should be dragged, with 'stuttering' as the input parameter and 'phrase' as the selected level. During the interactions, a child can always ask "Furhat, tell this", prompting BgGPT to generate natural language responses, thus motivating the child to actively listen and speak.

Scenario #1 Theme: "Animals";
1. Furhat: "Hello! I'm Furhat. What's your name?";
2. Child: "My name is <name>";
3. Furhat: "Nice to meet you, <name>!";
4. Nao: "I'm Nao. Today we're going on an adventure! Are you ready?";
5. Child: "Yes!";
6. Nao: "We're going to play with different animals. Look, listen, and show me the picture of this animal (dog is selected)";
(Therapist positions two cards of a dog and a cat with QR code in front of the child.)
7. Child: Child shows the dog to Nao eyes.;
8. Nao: "Well done! If you show me any of these pictures, I'll tell you more."
9. Child: Shows the QR code of the cat to Nao eyes;
10. Nao: Reads QR, asks BgGPT and tells about the cat in a childish style;
11. Pause=10sec;
12. repeat (iteration times =3){
Furhat: "What more will you ask me?" Waits for a verbal question…
Child: Asks a question.;
Furhat: Furhat Action: Ask Q→Get response from BgGPT→Tell the answer: A
} until iteration==0 ↻
13. Pause=10sec;
14. Furhat: "Let's play something else! See animal picture on my tablet and tell what they eat?"; (microskill 'stuttering' with level 'phrase' are selected).
15. Nao: "Well done! You know the animals";

Figure 6. Example scenario #1 theme: "Animals".

Figure 7b illustrates the running behavior uploaded on Nao for 'WORDS_anim,' with the sub-behavior (microskill) 'dog', which was triggered by the 'Animals' block in the frontend. Videos S3 and S4 in the Supplementary Materials provide a detailed explanation specifically demonstrating the development steps and runtime of the scenario presented in Figure 6.

In addition to the example scenario presented in Figure 7, therapists using ATLog can design a wide range of interactive therapy activities that integrate speech, listening, visual cues, and AI-based dialog, as well as supporting phonological training, vocabulary development and social communication skills training in 2D or 3D VR environments. These activities include personalized interactions based on the child's name, object recognition tasks using QR codes, question–answer dialogs driven by NLP/NLG cloud services, and exercises such as "stuttering" or "phrase repetition". Activities can also trigger microskills within scenarios using various block types—such as sequential, parallel, and asynchronous blocks—that support diverse response-handling strategies. *'DoCode'* input blocks further allow the execution of specific actions based on received responses, such as playing the audio from ASR, narrating instructions, or prompting questions. The platform enables blocks repetition, setting time durations and combining multimodal inputs (e.g., visual, verbal and tactile).

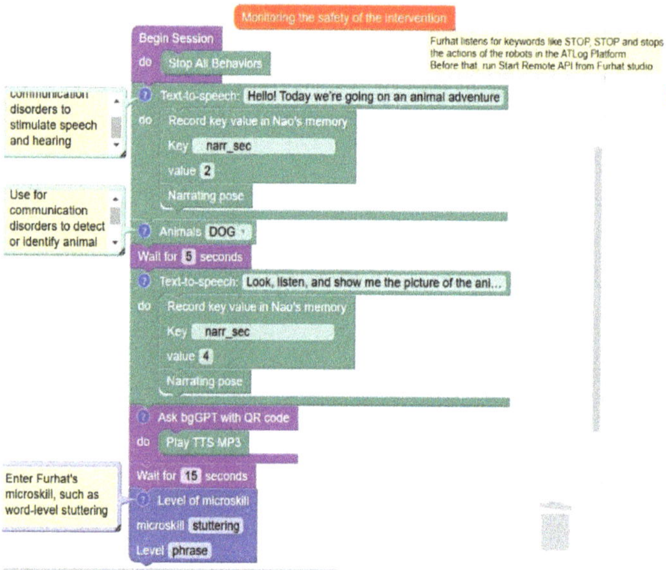

(**a**)

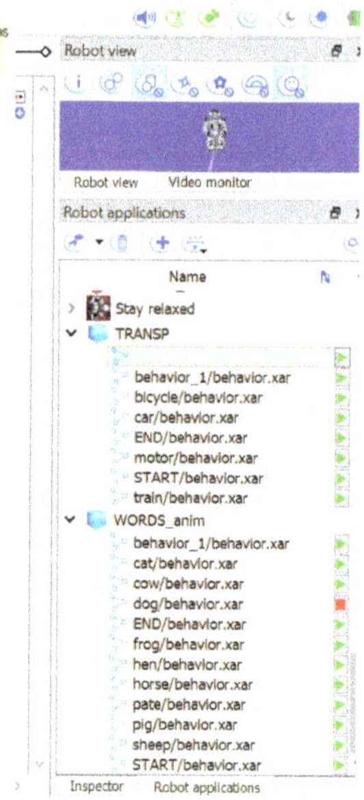

(**b**)

Figure 7. Scenario flow and activation (**a**) Developed in the ATLog frontend scenario #1. Skill block: "Animals", microskill 'DOG'. (**b**) Uploaded to robot Nao skill for 'WORDS_anim', the running 'dog' child behavior triggered by the corresponding Blockly block.

4.4. Results from the TAM and the SUS

The results from the online study, conducted to qualitatively assess the potential of using the ATLog platform by SLT professionals, along with an overview of the questionnaires, are presented in four figures and five tables.

The consistency and accuracy of all the questionnaires used were tested using Cronbach's Alpha. The researchers employed this method to determine the minimum reliability value of each construct, which is considered reliable if the Cronbach's Alpha value exceeds 0.60. The results in Table 1 show that the Cronbach's Alpha value of 0.798 confirms the validity of the SUS questionnaire. In terms of the Design Structure evaluation in the ATLog platform, the Cronbach's Alpha value is 0.849, indicating very strong reliability. The TAM questionnaire shows a very good consistency, with Cronbach's Alpha values of 0.906 and 0.922, respectively, for the PU and PEU subscales. These results reveal that all the questionnaires used for the study were consistent and trustworthy.

The mean score of the study was used to assess the acceptability of the SUS, with a score of 70 generally considered as the threshold for acceptable usability. The SUS survey data revealed an average score of 78, indicating that participants collectively perceive the ATLog platform as meeting acceptable usability standards. When interpreted using an adjective rating scale, this score corresponds to a "Good" level of usability. Furthermore, the results from the Design Structure evaluation within the ATLog platform yielded an average score of 86, indicating its features are acceptable.

The calculated SUS scores, along with the scores from the second part of the questionnaire, were assigned to an absolute grading scale as defined in [81]. In this scale, "A" corresponds to scores ranging from 90 to 100, "B"—to scores between 80 and 89, "C"—to scores between 70 and 79, "D"—to scores between 60 and 69, and "F"—to scores below 60.

The results for the SUS are illustrated in Figure 8. There were four SLT experts (15%) who evaluated the usability of the ATLog platform with a score between 52.5 and 57.5 (F). Eleven % of the participants gave Grade D. Most of the experts (74%) evaluated the usability of ATLog platform with scores over 70—Grades C (18.5%), B (25.9%) and A (29.6%).

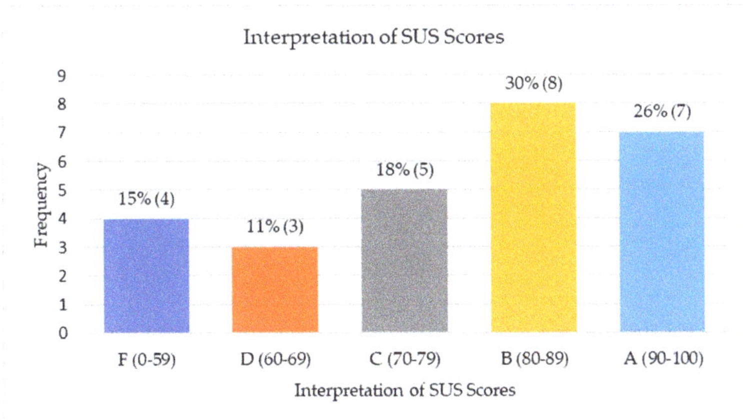

Figure 8. Absolute grading scale for the SUS scores.

The results for the Design Structure evaluation of the ATLog questionnaire are presented in Figure 9. There was only one expert who gave Grade F for the Design Structure evaluation of the ATLog platform; two experts rated it with Grade D and three gave it Grade C. Scores ranging from 80 to 89 were given by 25.9% of the therapists. Scores ranging from 90 to 100, corresponding to Grade A, accounted for 51.9%, indicating that the majority of experts gave the highest score for the platform.

As shown in Figure 10, the PU subscale scores of the TAM concerning the ATLog platform show different evaluations. A small proportion of professionals (11%; $n = 3$) rated the platform's usefulness as Grade D, while two (8%) assigned it Grade C. Ten professionals (37%) evaluated it more favorably as Grade B. The highest level of perceived usefulness—Grade A (scores between 90 and 100)—was reported by 44% of the therapists, indicating a strong positive assessment by nearly half of the respondents.

The findings related to the perceived ease of use subscale, as illustrated in Figure 11, reveal a generally positive evaluation of the ATLog platform. Three professionals (11%) assigned it Grade D, indicating lower ease of use, while two (8%) rated it as Grade C. Additionally, five experts (18%) provided it Grade B. The majority (63%) rated the platform within the 90–100 score range, corresponding to Grade A. This finding indicates a broad agreement among speech and language therapists concerning the ATLog platform's high level of perceived ease of use.

In the Likert scale assessment, a score above 3.00 is classified as positive (agree), while a score below 3.00 is considered negative (disagree). The SUS method adopts a balanced approach by incorporating five positive and five negative questions to assess both the strengths and weaknesses of a product, thereby minimizing response bias and enhancing the validity of the research findings. This methodological approach ensures a more objective and reliable evaluation of product usability by mitigating the risk of misinterpretation and inaccuracies in data analysis [80].

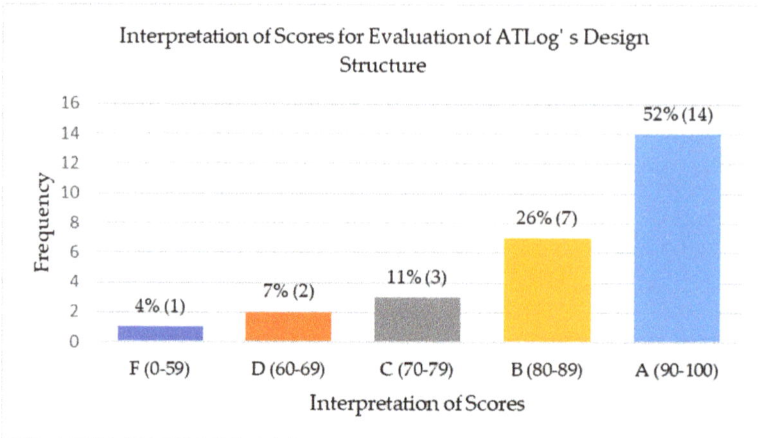

Figure 9. Absolute grading scale for the Design Structure evaluation of the ATLog platform scores.

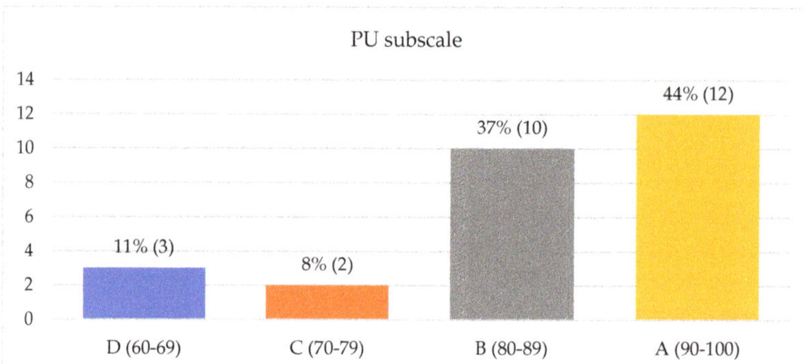

Figure 10. Absolute grading scale for the perceived usefulness subscale scores of the TAM.

The average scores of each statement of the SUS survey are presented in Table 2. Based on the results, all odd-numbered statements (1, 3, 5, 7, 9) received scores above 3 (from 3.6 to 4.4), indicating general agreement with these items. These positive responses indicate that the ATLog platform is perceived as easy to use, well-integrated, user-friendly, and efficient by the SLT practitioners. In contrast, all even-numbered statements (2, 4, 6, 8, 10) received scores below 3 (from 1.4 to 2.8), indicating disagreement among respondents. These responses suggest a low perceived level of complexity and a minimal need for technical support when using the platform. Also, the ATLog platform is regarded as easy to learn, consistent and user-friendly.

The results according to the average scores of each statement of the questionnaire about the Design Structure evaluation of ATLog platform are accessible in Table 3. All participants consistently agree with the positive aspects of the platform. The average scores were generally from 4.2 to 4.9, which suggests that professionals find the ATLog design user-friendly, well-organized and engaging. They particularly like features such as the child's ability to take initiative, the therapist's control over actions in the ATLog platform, and the personalization options for creating interactive scenarios. The platform is also seen as being adequately structured for managing scenarios and as informative and providing sufficient details for both therapeutic applications and interactions between the therapist, the ATs, and children and adolescents with CDs. These highly positive responses suggest that the design features of the ATLog platform are well-perceived and meet the needs of SLT practitioners, offering a high level of usability, individualization, control and functionality. While most responses were strongly positive, the statement for question 17 received a score of 3.7. As mentioned above [80], when the score is greater than 3, the statement is positive, indicating that professionals perceive the text-generative AI's reaction time to be acceptable. Although this remains in the positive range, it suggests a mild concern regarding response time. Therapists are generally accepting of the delay, but this result highlights an area for potential improvement, especially in contexts where real-time interaction is critical.

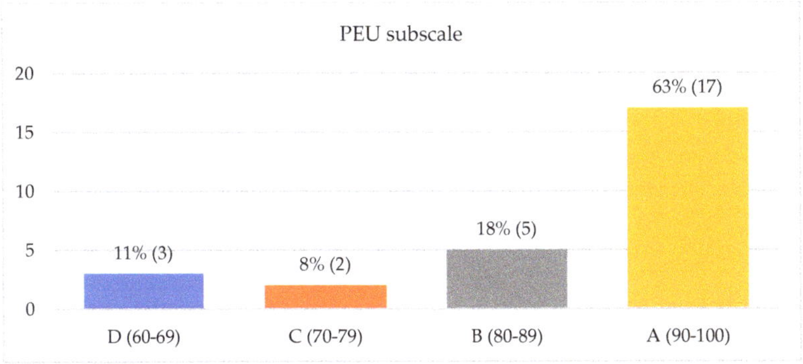

Figure 11. Absolute grading scale for the perceived ease of use subscale scores of the TAM.

The results for the mean scores of the TAM are presented in Table 4. All statements in the TAM questionnaire for both PU and PEU subscales received mean scores above 5.9, which indicates that the professionals mostly find the ATLog platform useful and easy to use. The statement "*Using the ATLog platform in my work would allow me to complete my therapeutic tasks faster*" was rated with the lowest score among all items (5.9), but it was still rated with "Strongly agree" and shows nuance in the SLT practitioners' opinions. The highest score (6.5) was about the statement "*It would be easy for me to learn to work with the ATLog platform*". Standard deviations ranged from 0.7 to 1.0, indicating consistent responses and a strong positive perception of the ATLog platform's usefulness and ease of use.

A correlation analysis was conducted to explore the relationships between the SUS, the Design Structure evaluation of the ATLog platform, and the TAM (represented by PU and PEU subscales). A summary of the results about Spearman's rho correlation analysis is presented in Table 5. The findings show a Spearman's rho correlation coefficient of 0.450, which indicates a moderate positive correlation between the two questionnaires, the SUS and Design Structure evaluation of the ATLog platform. This suggests that as values in the SUS increase, values in the Design Structure evaluation of the ATLog survey tend to increase as well. The p-value of 0.018 is less than 0.05, meaning that the correlation is statistically significant ($p < 0.05$). This indicates that professionals who perceived the platform as well-structured were more likely to report higher system usability. However, the Design Structure evaluation of the ATLog platform did not significantly correlate with PU ($r = 0.095$) or PEU ($r = -0.022$), suggesting limited direct impact on them. The SUS exhibited weak, non-significant positive correlations with both PU ($r = 0.262$) and PEU ($r = 0.243$), implying that while perceptions of usefulness and ease of use may contribute to usability perceptions, the relationships were not statistically robust in this dataset.

Table 5. Correlation analysis for the questionnaires (Spearman's rho).

Correlations	SUS	Design Structure of ATLog Platform	PU	PEU
SUS	1			
Design Structure of ATLog platform	0.450 *	1		
PU	0.262	0.095	1	
PEU	0.243	−0.022	0.879 **	1

*. Correlation is significant at the 0.05 level (2-tailed); **. Correlation is significant at the 0.01 level (2-tailed).

A strong and statistically significant correlation was found between PEU and PU ($r = 0.879$, $p < 0.01$), supporting the TAM hypothesis that ease of use strongly influences the perceived usefulness of the presented ATLog platform.

5. Discussion

By reducing technical barriers and aligning design with therapeutic needs, we aim to foster innovative practices among SLT practitioners and increase their engagement with high-tech ATs through a user-friendly visual programming interface and a seamless integration of ATs. ATLog utilizes RESTful APIs to ensure standardized and secure communication with ATs, making the system accessible without requiring advanced technical expertise. The platform is built to be flexible, allowing therapists easily customize it to fit each child's therapy needs. By decomposing complex SAR and VR functionalities into therapy-specific microskills, represented by pre-configured graphical blocks, therapists can intuitively design personalized therapy scenarios aligned with targeted goals and the language level of each child, without engaging in software coding.

The technical details provided for developers enable easy replication and extension of the ATLog platform design.

5.1. Technological Innovation of ATLog Platform

ATLog offers customizable resources tailored to specific therapeutic goals, treatment domains and language skill levels. The platform is designed with a subprocess-oriented approach, where SAR skills and VR scenarios are broken down into microskills represented as pre-programmed graphical blocks. The interoperability and scalability of ATLog's open-access framework and expandable design provide opportunities for integration with additional ATs, extending its functionality. The integrated mobile telepresence robots will facilitate remote speech therapy interventions.

5.2. Human–Computer Interaction (HCI)

Through ATLog's frontend, speech therapists can independently select and combine ATs based on their needs. The platform's visual programming interface allows therapists to assemble predefined blocks for robotic behaviors, 3D scenes, interactive elements and cloud-based text generation in multiple languages. HCI using ATLog, with integrated NLP and NLG in SARs/VRs, enhances human-like natural language interactions and helps encourage intensive listening and speaking in children.

5.3. Social and Economic Impact

The proposed approach of integrating high-tech ATs in ATLog allows for the seamless integration of other ATs, appropriate to different language skill levels and communication needs. ATLog enhances accessibility by enabling therapists to design structured and personalized SLT scenarios with ATs. The design is intuitive and empowers those without advanced technical and programming expertise or a large budget. Through dynamic combinations of pre-programed blocks for specific AT devices and resources, ATLog facilitates the design of individualized therapy interventions tailored to each child's needs. Since ATLog is an open-access, universal software platform, it minimizes the need for costly custom solutions, making ATs more affordable. Additionally, it will support professionals working with children with CDs across different settings, such as resource centers, schools and healthcare institutions.

5.4. User Behavior Analysis

5.4.1. SUS Q1–10

The SUS helps assess usability by measuring how easy and efficient SLT practitioners find the ATLog platform. The results in Table 1 show that the SUS questionnaire has a Cronbach's Alpha of 0.798, indicating strong reliability. This score demonstrates that the questionnaire is highly consistent in measuring the usability of the ATLog platform. When comparing this value with other studies that apply the SUS, we find that reliability scores range from 0.83 to 0.97 [79]. Our score (0.798) is slightly lower but still within the strong range, which aligns well with typical values found in the literature.

An SUS average score of 70 is considered the threshold for acceptable usability [81]. In our study, the ATLog platform received an average SUS score of 78, indicating that the participants perceived it as having good usability. When mapped onto the adjective rating scale [81], this score corresponds to a "Good" usability level, reflecting the professionals' positive experience with the platform. When comparing this result to other studies, the ATLog platform outperforms the average SUS score for Internet platforms. According to research in [79], where the authors analyzed 77 surveys in the Internet platforms category, the mean SUS score was 66.25 (SD = 12.42). This score is below the 70 point usability acceptability threshold, indicating that many Internet platforms may present usability challenges or require improvements to meet user expectations. Furthermore, the score for the Design Structure evaluation of ATLog platform was 86, categorizing it as "Excellent". This suggests that while the overall platform usability is well-received, the specific actions and functionalities therapists engage with are perceived as even more intuitive and efficient.

Figure 8 reveals that while most participants rated ATLog positively, some variation in individual ratings was observed. Specifically, 74.07% of professionals rated the SUS at 70 or higher, with grades of C (18.5%), B (25.9%), or A (29.6%). This indicates that the majority of users found the platform's usability to be acceptable, good, or excellent. Eleven percent gave a grade of D, indicating an SUS score between 60 and 69, suggesting the need for improvement, while 15% of professionals rated usability in the range [52.5–57.5], corresponding to "F". Most professionals rated the ATLog Design Structure evaluation positively, with 89% giving an SUS grade of A, B, or C, indicating high intuitiveness and efficiency. Only 11% gave a D or F score, suggesting some usability challenges to be explored.

To analyze the average scores for each statement in the two parts of the questionnaire, the SUS and Design Structure evaluation of the ATLog platform, we followed the approach used in [103]: statements with scores above 3.00 were classified as positive (agree), while those below 3.00 were considered negative (disagree). Scores very close to 3.00 were challenging to classify as distinctly positive or negative, as they lie near the neutral point of the Likert scale. An example of a borderline assessment is Q10 in Table 2. A score of 2.8 was the average for Q10. This indicates a slight tendency toward disagreement but not a definitive or strong view. This means that SLT practitioners do not strongly agree with the notion that they need to learn a lot before using the ATLog Platform, but they may still feel that some learning is required. This result suggests that professionals believe they do not need to learn a great amount of information before using the ATLog platform. While the score is closer to the neutral point, it still indicates that therapists feel the system is somewhat accessible or easy to understand without requiring extensive learning. However, the score of 2.8 implies that some may feel the need for some basic knowledge before using the ATLog platform effectively. If we compare the outliner Q10 average score with the one for Q7 (4.4), which is the opposite statement (positive), there is a big difference. It shows that the participants believe that the ATLog platform is easy for most people to learn quickly. The difference between the Q7 value and 3 is greater than the difference between the Q10 value and the neutral 3, where 1.4 (Q7) > 0.2 (Q10), with the difference between the two values being 1.2. The difference between the two values highlights a clear contrast in the therapists' perceptions. The score for Q7 shows strong agreement that the ATLog Platform is easy to learn. This result supports the conclusion that the ATLog has a user-friendly design, requiring minimal introduction of information for new users. However, the presence of some slight hesitation in Q10 suggests that offering additional resources, such as videos or training materials, could further enhance user confidence and ensure a smoother learning process for all professionals.

5.4.2. Q11–20

The second part of the questionnaire provided a more detailed analysis of user behavior, focusing on how therapists interact with the ATLog platform and their perception of its functionality and user-friendliness. In comparison, the reliability test results are even stronger, with a Cronbach's Alpha value of 0.849. This is an indication of excellent consistency and reliability. This score places the reliability of the ATLog survey in the very high range. The strong reliability scores in both sections of the questionnaire used in the current study (SUS and Design Structure evaluation in the survey) are well suited for measuring usability and the experience of SLT practitioners. However, it is important to note that even higher reliability could be achieved. It would be valuable to study a larger and more diverse group of professionals working with children and adolescents with CD and using the platform to assist technology-based interventions. These advancements could help enhance the results.

Research by Bangor et al. established a correlation between the participants' age and their scores on the SUS survey [81]. Contrary to the established relationship, our study did not observe such an association. These findings are supported by the results obtained in a systematic review of 30 scientific studies evaluating the usability of educational technology, where [103] found that there was no statistically significant correlation between the age of the respondents and the SUS scores. Future studies could explore this relationship further by including a larger number of SLT practitioners.

Regarding the open-ended question, the feedback from the experts highlights the ATLog platform's' potential and usefulness. A total of 41% of participants did not provide any comments in this section. Four participants described the platform as interesting and beneficial, especially for professionals and children with CDs. Additionally, 22% of the responses emphasized the need for broader promotion and awareness among more professionals. Interest in training sessions was expressed by 11% of participants. One participant raised concerns about delays in robot responses affecting the session flow. Another one suggested simplifying scenario creation to involve only one robot. This can be achieved in the ATLog frontend when only one SAR category is utilized.

5.4.3. TAM Q1–12

The results from the TAM assessment demonstrate that speech and language therapists perceive the ATLog platform as both highly useful and easy to use (Table 4). This aligns with the TAM's core premise that perceived usefulness and ease of use are critical for successful technology adoption in professional contexts. A particularly strong result was seen for the item *"It would be easy for me to learn to work with the ATLog platform"*, which received the highest mean score (M = 6.5), reflecting high user confidence in learning and using the system. This finding suggests that ATLog is intuitive, user-friendly, and easy to use and learn, allowing therapists to start using it quickly with minimal training.

While overall acceptance was high, some nuances emerged. The statement *"Using the ATLog platform in my work would allow me to complete my therapeutic tasks faster"* received the lowest mean score (M = 5.9; SD = 1.0), which, although still positive, suggests some hesitation about the platform's impact on time efficiency. This may reflect limited real-world experience with the platform or uncertainty about integrating its diverse features—such as combining ATs or uploading custom data—into everyday practice. The slightly higher standard deviation also points to varied individual perceptions regarding time savings, underscoring the need for hands-on training or the demonstration of practical efficiencies.

TAM subscales revealed particularly high reliability, with Cronbach's Alpha values of 0.906 for PU and 0.922 for PEU. These results not only exceed the conventional threshold of 0.70 for acceptable reliability [104] but fall within the range considered excellent, indicating that the TAM constructs were measured with a high degree of internal coherence. These results confirm that the measurement tools used in this study were both statistically reliable and psychometrically valid, enabling confident interpretation of the observed relationships between design structure, usability, and user acceptance. The high reliability of the measures strengthens the overall validity of the study's conclusions and confirms the appropriateness of using these standardized tools in the evaluation of user experience within digital platforms like ATLog.

The distribution of responses further reveals interesting patterns, as shown in Figures 10 and 11. For PU, 81% of participants gave higher ratings (Grades B or A), with 44% awarding the top rating (A). This suggests a strong overall validation of the ATLog platform's ability to support therapeutic tasks, despite some variability. For PEU, responses were even more favorable and consistent—63% of SLT practitioners rated the platform in the top range (90–100, Grade A), and only 11% offered lower ratings (Grade D), indicating few concerns about usability.

In summary, the evaluation of ATLog via the TAM provides robust evidence of its high perceived usefulness and ease of use among speech and language therapists. While the platform is generally seen as supportive and accessible, future implementations should emphasize hands-on training and efficiency in practice to address any remaining uncertainties and promote sustained adoption in therapeutic settings.

5.4.4. Correlation Analysis Between the SUS, the Design Structure Evaluation of the ATLog Platform, and the TAM

The Design Structure evaluation of the ATLog platform demonstrated a moderate and statistically significant correlation with the SUS, as shown in Table 5. This finding suggests that a well-organized and intuitively structured interface plays a critical role in enhancing users' overall usability perceptions. However, the Design Structure evaluation did not significantly correlate with PU or PEU, indicating that while structural clarity improves usability perceptions, it may not directly influence users' judgments of a system's utility or simplicity.

Interestingly, both PU and PEU showed weak and non-significant correlations with SUS, suggesting that while these subscales are central to the TAM, they may not directly contribute to how usable a system is perceived to be when measured by the SUS. This might reflect how the SUS primarily captures users' overall satisfaction with the ATLog platform's functionality and interface, whereas PU and PEU are more related to anticipated performance outcomes and cognitive effort, respectively.

The most robust finding was the very strong and highly significant correlation between PEU and PU ($r = 0.879$, $p < 0.01$). This is consistent with the original TAM framework [25], which suggests that systems perceived as easy to use are more likely to be seen as useful. This reinforces the idea that ease of interaction is a major driver of perceived effectiveness, especially in digital platforms like ATLog.

Together, these findings suggest a partial validation of the TAM in the context of usability and system design. While ease of use remains a critical determinant of perceived usefulness, system usability (as measured by the SUS) is more directly affected by the quality of the ATLog platform's Design Structure evaluation than by perceived usefulness or ease of use alone.

6. Conclusions

Following the four-phase Design-Based Research process proposed by Reeves, we identified and addressed the practical challenges faced by speech and language therapists in accepting and adopting high-tech ATs, such as Socially Assistive Robots, VR and conversational AI. Through iterative development, in collaboration with and based on feedback from therapists, we designed and refined ATLog—a visual programming platform that enables the integration of ATs and the intuitive creation of personalized, interactive and playful learning scenarios. As a result, the *Design-Based Principle* identified is as follows: *"Streamlining the integration of high-tech ATs (SARs, VR, ConvAI) in SLT can be achieved through an ergonomic software platform, such as ATLog. It lowers technical barriers through visual programming tools, such as a Google Blockly-based frontend, and a lightweight Express server that acts as the backend hub, managing all communications between the frontend and the ATs. The platform enables scenario personalization and supports the modular design of therapy activities through predefined graphical blocks aligned with specific therapeutic goals and skill levels".*

To foster innovative thinking in therapists, the resulting design principle highlights the need to lower technical barriers through therapy-centered modularity and customizable tools. By breaking down complex AT functionalities into modular microskills aligned with specific therapy goals and language levels, ATLog empowers therapists to streamline the integration of ATs within SLT practice and to design and run interactive, playful scenarios without requiring advanced technical skills.

The identified principle is validated by the results of the TAM and SUS surveys, which suggest that the platform is well-designed, intuitive and effective. Most of the SLT practitioners (74%) evaluated the SUS of the ATLog platform with scores over 70, indicating high acceptance of its usability and functionality, assigning grades C (18.5%), B (25.9%) and A (29.6%). Over half (52%) of the experts rated the additional questions focused on ATLog's structure and functionalities in the A range (90–100), while 26% rated them in the B range (80–89), showing strong acceptance of the platform for creating and running personalized interactive scenarios with ATs. According to the TAM results, experts gave high grades for both perceived usefulness (44% in the A range) and perceived ease of use (63% in the A range). However, based on the open questions, there are still areas for improvement, particularly in enhancing integration and compatibility with other ATs, refining the user interface, and expanding educational resources with more step-by-step guides and interactive tutorials for beginners. The comparative strength of the ease-of-use ratings over perceived usefulness may indicate that while the platform is user-friendly, its practical value in clinical contexts might still be under evaluation or may be context-dependent.

6.1. Limitations

Despite promising outcomes, this study has several limitations that may affect the generalizability of the findings. The iterative evaluations were conducted within a limited range of SLT contexts and therapy types, and broader validation is needed to assess the platform's long-term impact and adoption. While ATLog simplifies technical complexity, its effectiveness in improving therapy outcomes requires further empirical investigation through large-scale, longitudinal studies involving children with CDs. Additionally, the questionnaires used in the study were performed only by stakeholders who participate in the training session, which limited the diversity of perspectives captured. Finally, the research was conducted within a national context, primarily focusing on Bulgaria, which may restrict the transferability of the results to other regions due to cultural, economic and systemic differences in how ATs are adopted globally.

6.2. Future Directions

While the current study focused on therapists' perspectives on designing structured playful scenarios in the physical, digital and virtual world using the ATLog platform, future research will evaluate the platform's impact on therapy outcomes by assessing how ATLog supports skill development in children and adolescents with CDs. A six-month experimental study involving 20 children and adolescents is currently ongoing in real-world therapy settings. By the end of the year, we aim to evaluate the intervention's effectiveness in enhancing skill acquisition through increased engagement and motivation by ATs, as well as to generate new insights for refining the design of the ATLog platform. Future development will also include the integration of other ATs, such as Oculus VR glasses, further refinement of the Emo robot for emotional learning, automatic phonological and linguistic assessment of disordered speech, and ATLog telepractice capabilities.

Supplementary Materials: The following supporting information can be downloaded at: https://www.mdpi.com/article/10.3390/technologies13070306/s1, Video S1: ATLog_lesson1, Video S2: ATLog_lesson2, Video S3: ATLog_lesson3, Video S4: ATLog_lesson4.

Author Contributions: Conceptualization, A.L., G.D., T.T. and A.A.; methodology, A.L., P.T., A.A., M.S., V.S.-P. and G.P.; software, A.L., A.K., K.R., G.D., T.T., D.V., T.S. and P.T.; validation, A.L., G.D., T.S., P.T., K.R., A.K. and D.V.; formal analysis, M.S., A.A., V.S.-P. and G.P.; data curation, A.A. and P.T.; writing—original draft preparation, A.L., P.T., A.A. and T.S.; writing—review and editing, V.S.-P., G.D., D.V., T.T., A.A. and K.R.; visualization, A.L., T.T., T.S., A.A. and P.T.; project administration, A.L., G.D. and M.S. All authors have read and agreed to the published version of the manuscript.

Funding: The research findings are supported by the Bulgarian National Scientific Research Fund, Project No KP-06-H67/1.

Institutional Review Board Statement: The ethical procedures inherent to these surveys were approved by the ethical committee of the Institute of Robotics Bulgarian Academy of Sciences (ECSR; Decision No. 7/21.07.2023, par. 4 of the Scientific Council of IR-BAS). This procedure was formalized in the protocols No. 7/05.02.2025 and No. 11/06.06.2025, issued by the Ethics Committee for Scientific Research, regarding a request submitted by Anna Lekova.

Informed Consent Statement: Written informed consent was obtained from all subjects involved in this survey.

Data Availability Statement: We provide data supporting the reported results at https://osf.io/3z65m/ (last access on 11 July 2025).

Acknowledgments: We acknowledge the technical support by the European Regional Development Fund under the Operational Program "Scientific Research, Innovation and Digitization for Smart Transformation 2021–2027", Project CoC "Smart Mechatronics, Eco- and Energy Saving Systems and Technologies", BG16RFPR002-1.014-0005.

Conflicts of Interest: The authors declare no conflicts of interest related to this study.

Abbreviations

The following abbreviations are used in this article:

AAC	Alternative and Augmented Communication
ATs	Assistive Technologies
CDs	Communication Disorders
ConvAI	Conversational AI
DBR	Design-Based Research
GPT	Generative Pre-trained Transformer
IDE	Integrated Development Environment
LLMs	Large Language Models
LRMs	Large Reasoning Models
NLG	Natural Language Generation
NLP	Natural Language Processing
PEU	Perceived Ease of Use
PU	Perceived Usefulness
PY	Python
Q&A	AI questions and answers
RQ	Research Question
SARs	Socially Assistive Robots
SCP	Secure Copy Protocol
SLT	Speech and Language Therapy
SUS	System Usability Scale
TAM	Technology Acceptance Model
VR	Virtual Reality

Appendix A

Table A1. Nao robot frontend blocks with corresponding backend endpoints.

Frontend Block Name	Description	Microskill/File Uploaded on the Robot	Input Parameters	Backend Endpoint	Fetching Endpoint(s) with Parameters
StartBlock	Initializes the session. ***Connected endpoints in doCode of the block***: *StopAll_BehaviorsBlock* and *AutonomousModeBlock*.	No	N/A	N/A	N/A
Autonomous ModeBlock	Enables or disables autonomous behavior on Nao robot.	No	ipNao, STATE (FieldCheckbox: TRUE, FALSE)	/nao1	http://serverIP:3000/nao1?IP=${ipNao}&state=${STATE}&pyScript=auton
StopAll_BehaviorsBlock	Stops ongoing behaviors on Nao robot.	No	ipNao	/nao1	http://serverIP:3000/nao1?IP=${ipNao}&pyScript=stopBehav2
VolumeBlock	By entering an integer from 0 to 100, the Nao robot's volume level can be adjusted.	No	ipNao, VOLUME	/nao1	http://serverIP:3000/nao1?IP=${ipNao}&volume=${VOLUME}&pyScript=volume
HelloBlock	Nao animation—greeting while in a seated position.	Yes	ipNao	/nao2	http://ipServer:3000/${endpoint}?IP=${ipNao}&BN=User/hello-6f0483/behavior_1
Read_qr_code Block	Initiates QR code reading in front of Nao's eyes. Reads from Nao's memory. Saves in ATLog repository with a key = QR. ***Connected endpoints in doCode of the block:*** *NaoMemoryRead* and *RepositorySaveBlock*.	Yes	ipNao KEY	/nao2	http://serverIP:3000/${endpoint}?IP=${ipNao}&BN=User/qr-19f134/behavior_1 ***Connected endpoints:*** *http://serverIP:3000/monitor/pyNao2*
LingSounds Block	Nao says the Ling sound, defined by the input parameter, and waits to recognize the QR code shown to it.	Yes	ipNao, LING_SOUND: A, I, U, M, S, Sh	/nao2	http://serverIP:3000/${endpoint}?IP=${ipNao}&BN=ling-2b453a/${LING_SOUND}
TransportationBlock	Nao says the name and play sounds for a transportation tool and waits to recognize the QR code shown to it.	Yes	ipNao, TRANSPORT: Bicycle, Car, Train, Motor, Airplane, etc.	/nao2	http://serverIP:3000/${endpoint}?IP=${ipNao}&BN=transports-c868b7/${TRANSPORT}
AnimalsBlock	Nao says the animal's name, plays its sound, and waits to recognize the QR code shown to it.	Yes	ipNao, ANIMAL: Cat, Dog, Cow, Sheep, Frog, Horse, Monkey, Pate, Pig, etc.	/nao2	http://serverIP:3000/${endpoint}?IP=${ipNao}&BN=animals-486c82/${ANIMAL}
FruitsBlock	Nao says the fruit's name and waits to recognize the QR code shown to it.	Yes	ipNao, FRUIT: strawberry, bannana, apple, etc.	/nao2	http://serverIP:3000/${endpoint}?IP=${ipNao}&BN= fruits-f0887f/${FRUIT}
Vegetable Block	Nao says the vegetables's name and waits to recognize the QR code shown to it.	Yes	ipNao, VEGETABLE: cucumber, cabbage,	/nao2	http://serverIP:3000/${endpoint}?IP=${ipNao}&BN=vegetables-7e6223/${VEGETABLE}

Table A1. *Cont.*

Frontend Block Name	Description	Microskill/File Uploaded on the Robot	Input Parameters	Backend Endpoint	Fetching Endpoint(s) with Parameters
ShapesBlock	Nao says the shape's name and waits to recognize the QR code shown to it.	Yes	ipNao, SHAPE: Triangle, Rectangle, Circle, Square, Star, Moon, etc.	/nao2	http://serverIP:3000/${endpoint}?IP=${ipNao}&BN=shapes-cc46c2/${SHAPE}
ColorsBlock	Nao says the color's name and waits to recognize the QR code shown to it.	Yes	ipNao, COLOR: Green, Orange, Red, Blue, Pink, White, Yellow, etc.	/nao2	http://serverIP:3000/${endpoint}?IP=${ipNao}&BN=colors-dd3988/${COLOR}
MusicalInstr Block	Nao plays music with animation for an instrument (defined by the input parameter).	Yes	ipNao, INSTRUMENT: Trumpet, Guitar, Maracas, Piano, Drums, Violin, etc.	/nao2	http://serverIP:3000/${endpoint}?IP=${ipNao}&BN=instruments-78257e/${INSTRUMENT}
EmotionsBlock	Nao performs an animation for the emotion defined by the input parameter.	Yes	ipNao, EMOTION: sad, happy, scared, tired, neutral	/nao2	http://serverIP:3000/${endpoint}?IP=${ipNao}&BN=emotions-f6ef56/${EMOTION}
FairytaleBlock	Nao narrates a fairy tale, defined by the input parameter, and its mp3 is uploaded on Nao folder: home/nao/fairs/. ***Connected in sequence blocks:*** NarratingBlock.	Yes	ipNao, FAIRY_TALE_NAME: MuriBird, CatMum, 3cats, smallCat, 3catsMum, etc.	/nao2	http://serverIP:3000/${endpoint}?IP=${ipNao}&BN=story-afb24d/${ FAIRY_TALE_NAME }
StoryBlock	Nao tells a story with sequential in time scenes by three or more flashcards (the story is defined by input parameter).	Yes	ipNao, STORY_NAME: tomato, cake, sleep, cat, etc.	/nao2	http://serverIP:3000/${endpoint}?IP=${ipNao}&BN=[story_nina-97b2d5,story_emi-e0be5f,story_cat-7f9f13, story_mimisleep-afcea3]
SongBlock	Nao sings a song (defined by the input parameter), and its mp3 is uploaded on Nao folder: home/nao/songs/. ***Connected in sequence blocks:*** DanceBlock.	Yes	ipNao, SONG_NAME: song1, song2, song3, song4, song5, etc.	/nao1	http://serverIP:3000/${endpoint}?IP=${ipNao}&filepath=${filepath}&filename=${SONG_NAME}&pyScript=play_mp3
MarketPlay Block	Nao simulates market-related interactions with the child using 3D objects embedded with barcodes (real or toys), such as toothbrush, cash desk, payment card, etc.	Yes	ipNao, MarketItem: Juice, Salad, Bathroom, Teeth, etc.	/nao2	http://serverIP:3000/${endpoint}?IP=${ipNao}&BN=market-6f6441/${MarketItem}
TouchSensor Block	Nao detects a touch on its tactile sensors and plays the corresponding mp3 for the touched body_part, uploaded on the robot in folder home/nao/body/.	Yes	ipNao, SENSOR: Head_Front, RArm, Larm, LFoot/Bumper RFoot/Bumper	/nao1	http://serverIP:3000/${endpoint}?IP=${ipNao}&touch=${SENSOR}&pyScript =touchBodyPart
Head_tactile_ sensorBlock	Activates the tactile sensor on Nao head to stop any currently running microskill. ***Connected in sequence block:*** *StopAll_behaviours.*	No	ipNao, SENSOR Head_Front, Head_Middle Head_Rear	/nao1	http://serverIP:3000/${endpoint}?IP=${ipNao}&bodyPart&{SENSOR}&pyScript =touchHead
NaoMemory ReadBlock	Reads a value from Nao's memory key.	No	ipNao, KEY	/nao1	http://serverIP:3000/${endpoint}?IP=${ipNao}&key=${KEY}&pyScript=ALmemory_get
NaoMemory SaveBlock	Writes a {key: value} to Nao's memory.	No	ipNao, KEY, VALUE	/nao1	http://serverIP:3000/${endpoint}?IP=${ipNao}&key=${KEY}&value=${VALUE}& pyScript=ALmemory_set
DeclareEvent Block	Declares an event name in Nao's memory.	No	ipNao, EVENT	/nao1	http://serverIP:3000/${endpoint}?IP=${ipNao}&name=${ EVENT }&pyScript=ALmemory_decl
RaiseEvent Block	Raises a declared event in Nao's memory.	No	ipNao, EVENT	/nao1	http://serverIP:3000/${endpoint}?IP=${ipNao}&name=${ EVENT }&pyScript=ALmemory_raise

Table A1. *Cont.*

Frontend Block Name	Description	Microskill/File Uploaded on the Robot	Input Parameters	Backend Endpoint	Fetching Endpoint(s) with Parameters
PlayAudio Block	Plays audio files uploaded to the robot in Nao folder home/nao/audio/.	Yes	ipNao, path, file_name	/nao1	http://serverIP:3000/nao1?IP=${robot_ip}&filepath=${path}&filename=${file_name}&pyScript=play_mp3
UploadFile Block	Uploads a file on Nao robot in folder:/home/nao/tts/with name: tts.mp3.	No	ipNao, passwordNao, file_path, file_name	/naoUpload	http://serverIP:3000/naoUpload?IP=${ipNao}&password=${passwordNao}${file_path}${file_name}
Text_to_speechBlock	Nao plays the input text as audio file. Text is converted to speech by GoogleTTS or MSAzureTTS. The generated tts.mp3 file is uploaded to NAO folder:/home/nao/tts/.	No	ipNao, passwordNao text filename: tts.mp3, filepath on Nao:/home/nao/tts/	/nao3	http://serverIP:3000/${endpoint}?IP=${ipNao}&filepath=${path}&filename=${file_name}?TEXT=${text} ***Connected endpoints:*** *http://serverIP:3000/venv;http://serverIP:3000/monitor/pyNao1* http://serverIP:3000/naoUpload?*IP=${ipNao}*&password=${passwordNao}${file_path}${file_name} *http://serverIP:3000/nao1?IP=${robot_ip}&filepath=${path}&filename=${file_name}&pyScript=play_mp3*
PlaytextBlock	Nao plays the current answer in the ATLog repository as audio file. Answer is converted to tts.mp3 and uploaded to Nao directory/home/nao/tts/.	No	ipNao, passwordNao file_name, file_path, KEY=answer	/nao3	http://serverIP:3000/${endpoint}?IP=${ipNao}&filepath=${path}&filename=${file_name}?TEXT=${answer}} ***Connected endpoints:*** http://serverIP:3000/repository/answer *http://serverIP:3000/venv;http://serverIP:3000/monitor/pyNao1* http://serverIP:3000/naoUpload?*IP=${ipNao}*&password=${passwordNao}${file_path}${file_name} *http://serverIP:3000/nao1?IP=${robot_ip}&filepath=${path}&filename=${file_name}&pyScript=play_mp3*
QRquestion Block	Nao waits for a QR code to be shown, decodes it to generate a text-based question, sends the question to bgGPT, and stores the received answer in the repository. It then plays the answer as an audio file. ***Connected endpoints in doCode of the block: PlaytextBlock.***	No	ipNao, Question, Context, KEY =answer, VALUE	/nao1 /nao2 /nao3 /bgGPT /repository */monitor/pyNao1* */monitor/pyNao2*	***Connected endpoints:*** *http://serverIP:3000/nao2?*IP=${ipNao}&*BN=qr-19f134* *http://serverIP:3000/monitor/pyNao2* *http://serverIP:3000/nao1?IP=*${ipNao}*&key=QR&pyScript=ALmemory_get2* *http://serverIP:3000/venv; ttp://serverIP:3000/monitor/pyNao1* http://serverIP:3000/bgGPT?question=${question}&context=${context} *http://serverIP:3000/repository?key=${KEY}&value=${VALUE*
TextQuestion Block	Retrieves the questions and context entered in the input fields, sends them to bgGPT, stores the generated answer in the repository, and Nao plays the current response. ***Connected endpoints in doCode of the block:* PlaytextBlock.**	No	ipNao, Question, Context, KEY: answer, VALUE	/nao1 /nao3 /bgGPT /repository	***Connected endpoints:*** *http://serverIP:3000/venv* http://serverIP:3000/bgGPT?question=${question}&context=${context} *http://serverIP:3000/monitor/pyNao1* *http://serverIP:3000/repository?key=${KEY}&value=${VALUE*
Narrating Block	Nao animation—for narrating pose. **Connected in sequence blocks**: *NaoMemorySave* with {key= narr_sec, value= VALUE}.	Yes	ipNao VALUE (Seconds for narrating)	/nao2	http://serverIP:3000/${endpoint}?IP=${ipNao}&BN=User/slow_narrating-0de14c/behavior_1
Thinking Block	Nao animation—thinking pose in a seated position.	Yes	ipNao	/nao2	http://serverIP:3000/${endpoint}?IP=${ipNao&BN=User/thinking-b54157/behavior_1
Narrating_sit Block	Nao animation—pose for storytelling in a seated position.	Yes	ipNao	/nao2	http://serverIP:3000/${endpoint}?IP=${ipNao}&BN=User/narr_sit-a1f157/behavior_1
Dance Block	Nao animation—performing dance movements.	Yes	ipNao	/nao2	http://serverIP:3000/${endpoint}?IP=${ipNao}&BN=User/dancing-e1h145/behavior_1
CustomBehavior Block	Runs a custom skill prepared in Choregraphe and uploaded to Nao.	Yes	ipNao, BEHAVIOR_NAME (Unique Behavior ID on Nao)	/nao2	http://serverIP:3000/${endpoint}?IP=${ipNao}&?id=${BEHAVIOR_NAME}
CustomRemote Block	Runs a custom python script by remote NAOqi.	No	ipNao, PY_SCRIPT (Unique py script name)	/nao1	http://serverIP:3000/${endpoint}?IP=${ipNao}&${endpoint}id=${PY_SCRIPT}

Table A2. Furhat robot frontend blocks with corresponding backend endpoints.

Frontend Block Name	Description	Microskill/File Uploaded on the Robot	Input Parameters	Backend Endpoint	Fetching Endpoint(s) with Parameters
Monitoring SafetyBlock	Furhat listens for keywords like 'STOP', and stops the actions of the integrated ATs in the current session.	No	ipFurhat	/furhatRem	http://serverIP:3000/furhatRem?IP=${ipFurhat}&scriptName=fur_stop.py ***Connected endpoints:*** *http://serverIP:3000/venv* *http://serverIP:3000/furhat?IP=${ipFurhat}&?id=RemoteAPI* *http://serverIP:3000/stop-server*
CustomSkill Block	Runs a custom skill prepared in KotlinSSDK and uploaded to Furhat.	Yes	ipFurhat, SKILL_NAME	/furhat	http://serverIP:3000/${endpoint}?IP=${ipFurhat}&?id=${SKILL_NAME}
FurhatTTS Block	Specifies the text to vocalize (TTS).	No	ipFurhat, Text to Vocalize	/furhatRem	http://serverIP:3000/${endpoint}?IP=${ipFurhat}&scriptName=fur_tts.py&text=${text} ***Connected endpoints:*** *http://serverIP:3000/venv* *http://serverIP:3000/${endpoint}?IP=${ipFurhat}&?id=RemoteAPI*
FurhatAsk NameBlock	Asks the user their name and saves the response in the internal repository.	No	ipFurhat, KEY: name	/furhatRem	http://serverIP:3000/${endpoint}?IP=${ipFurhat}&scriptName=fur_name.py **Connected endpoints:** http://serverIP:3000/venv; http://serverIP:3000/monitor/pyFurhat http://serverIP:3000/${endpoint}?IP=${ipFurhat}&?id=RemoteAPI http://serverIP:3000/repository?key=${KEY}
FurhatSpeak AnswerBlock	Furhat speaks the answer stored in the internal repository.	No	ipFurhat, KEY: answer	/furhatRem	http://serverIP:3000/${endpoint}?IP=${ipFurhat}&scriptName=furhat_rem_textFur.py' **Connected endpoints:** http://serverIP:3000/venv http://serverIP:3000/${endpoint}?IP=${ipFurhat}&?id=RemoteAPI http://serverIP:3000/repository?key=${KEY}
FurhatQuestionBlock	Listens to a question, **fetches the question to bgGPT** and stores the answer in the repository. ***Connected endpoints in doCode of the block:*** ***FurhatSpeakAnswerBlock.***	No	ipFurhat, Question, Context, KEY: answer, VALUE	/furhatRem	http://serverIP:3000/${endpoint}?IP=${ipFurhat}&scriptName=furhat_rem_question.py' ***Connected endpoints:*** *http://serverIP:3000/venv;* http://serverIP:3000/monitor/pyFurhat *http://serverIP:3000/${endpoint}?IP=${ipFurhat}&?id=RemoteAPI* http://serverIP:3000/bgGPT?question=${question}&context=${context} *http://serverIP:3000/repository?key=${KEY}&value=${VALUE}*
FurhatRepeat Block	Listens to a spoken phrase with attempts to repeat it, unless it returns a 'NOMATCH' response.	No	ipFurhat, text_intent	/furhatRem	http://serverIP:3000/${endpoint}?IP=${ipFurhat}&scriptName=fur_understand.py ***Connected endpoints:*** *http://serverIP:3000/venv* *http://serverIP:3000/${endpoint}?IP=${ipFurhat}&scriptName=fur_tts.py&text=${text}*

Table A3. Frontend blocks for robots EMO and Double3 with corresponding backend endpoints.

Frontend Block Name	Description	Microskill/File Uploaded on the Robot	Input Parameters	Backend Endpoint	Fetching Endpoint(s) with Parameters
Start_EMO_mqqt_ session1	Establishes MQTT session1 (via Python paho-mqtt bridge).	remote_paho_ mqtt.py	ipEmo, Port, Username, Password (PUP)	/emo1	http://serverIP:3000//${endpoint}?IP=${ipEmo}&PUP=${PUP} ***Connected endpoints:*** *http://serverIP:3000/venv*
Start_EMO_mqtt_ session2	Establishes an MQTT session2 (via MQTT net library).	Yes	ipEmo, Port, Username, (PU), TOPIC, file_name	/emo2	http://serverIP:3000//${endpoint}?IP=${ipEmo}&PU=${PU}&topic=${TOPIC}&file=${file_name}
ReadQRcode	Initiates QR code reading in front of EMO. Saves in ATLog repository with a key = QR. ***Connected in sequence blocks:*** *RepositorySaveBlock.*	Yes	ipEmo, Port, Username, Password (PUP), KEY	/emo1	http://serverIP:3000/${endpoint}?IP=${ipEmo}&PUP=${PUP}&script=*qr_reader_atlog.py* ***Connected endpoints:*** *http://serverIP:3000/venv*
UploadFile Block	Uploads a file after serialization to Emo robot with topic = 'upload'.		ipEmo, Port, Username, (PU), TOPIC, data	/emoUpload	http://serverIP:3000/${endpoint}?*IP=${ipEmo}*&PU=${PU}&topic=${TOPIC}&serialization=${data}***Connected endpoints:*** *http://serverIP:3000/emo2*
EmoPlay AudioBlock	Emo plays audio file uploaded on Emo folder/home/emo/audio/ topic = 'audios'.	Yes	ipEmo, Port, Username, (PU), TOPIC, filename filename	/emoPlay	http://serverIP:3000/${endpoint}?IP=${ipEmo}&PU=${PU}&topic=${TOPIC}&filename=${name} ***Connected endpoints:*** *http://serverIP:3000/emo2*
EmoChat TextBlock	Emo plays the current answer from BgGPT in the internal repository as audio file. Answer is converted in tts.mp3 and uploaded to Emo folder/home/emo/tts/ topic is 'answer'.	Yes	ipEmo, Port, Username, (PU), TOPIC, filename filename/home/emo/tts/, KEY	/emoChat	http://serverIP:3000/${endpoint}?IP=${ipEmo}&PU=${PU}&topic=${TOPIC}&filename=${file_name}?TEXT=${answer}) ***Connected endpoints:*** http://serverIP:3000/repository/answer *http://serverIP:3000/venv* *http://serverIP:3000/emoUpload; http://serverIP:3000/emoPlay*
EmoQRquestionBlock	Waiting for a QR code, decode it to prepare a question, **fetch the question to bgGPT** and stores the answer in the repository. Emo plays the current answer. ***Connected endpoints in doCode of the block:*** ***EmoPlayAudioBlock***	No	ipEmo, Question, Context, KEY: answer, VALUE	/qrEmo	http://serverIP:3000/${endpoint}?IP=${ipEmo}&PUP=${PUP} ***Connected endpoints:*** *http://serverIP:3000/emo1* *http://serverIP:3000/venv* *http://serverIP:3000/emo1?IP=${ipEmo}&pyScript=qr_reader_atlog.py* http://serverIP:3000/bgGPT?question=${question}&context=${context} *http://serverIP:3000/repository?key=${KEY}&value=${VALUE}* *http://serverIP:3000/emo2/emoUpload* *http://serverIP:3000/emo2/emoPlay*
Start_D3_session	Opens an SSH session to a Double3 (D3) robot and runs PY scripts that interact with the Double3 Developer SDK and D3 API.	Yes	ipD3, Port, Username, Password (PUP), script_name	/double3	http://serverIP:3000/double3?IP=${ipD3}&PUP=${PUP}&script=alive.py
D3QRBlock	Opens an SSH session to D3 and runs PY script that reads QR codes via D3 robot.	Yes	ipD3, Port, Username, Password (PUP), script_name	/double3	http://serverIP:3000/double3?IP=${ipD3}&PUP=${PUP}&script=readQR.py
D3 ControlBlock	Opens an SSH session to a D3 and run PY script with parameters.	Yes	ipD3, Port, Username, Password (PUP), script_name, PARAM	/double3	http://serverIP:3000/double3?IP=${ipD3}&PUP=${PUP}&script=${script_name}&param=${PARAM}

Table A4. General frontend blocks with corresponding backend endpoints.

Frontend Block Name	Description	Microskill/File Uploaded on the Robot	Input Parameters	Backend Endpoint	Fetching Endpoint(s) with Parameters
Stop Code (button)	Sends a request to shut down the server by terminating the all active child processes and closes the database connections	No	No	/stop-server	http://serverIP:3000/stop-server
Repository ReadBlock	Reads a value in ATLog's repository with a specified key	N/A	KEY	/repository	http://serverIP:3000//${endpoint}?&key=${ KEY}
Repository SaveBlock	Saves a value in ATLog's repository with the specified key	N/A	KEY, VALUE	/repository2	http://serverIP:3000//${endpoint}?&key=${ KEY}&value=${VALUE}
DB_save Block	Saves session observations or assessments in ATLog's database	No	postData: ID, VALUE (childID, observations, date and time recorded automatically)	/save-child-notes	http://serverIP:3000/${endpoint} with JSON: { method: 'POST', headers: { 'Content-Type': 'application/json; charset=utf-8' }, body: JSON.stringify(${JSON.stringify(postData)}) }
BG_GPT Block	Sends questions and context entered in the input fields to the BgGPT APIs (Bulgarian ChatGPT)	No	QUESTION, CONTEXT	/bgGPT	http://serverIP:3000/bgGPT?question=${QUESTION}&context=${CONTEXT}
QABlock	Sends questions and context to NLPcloud	No	QUESTION, CONTEXT	/QA	http://serverIP:3000/QA?question=${QUESTION}&context=${CONTEXT}
WaitBlock	Makes the robot wait for a specified number of seconds	No	SECONDS	N/A	**Blockly local run** await new Promise(resolve => setTimeout(resolve, ${ SECONDS }));
RepeatBlock	Wraps (one or more) blocks in a loop to execute it multiple times based on a variable number of iterations. *In doCode of the block*: any block(s)	No	ITERATIONS		**Blockly local run** loop to repeat execution ${ITERATIONS} times ***Connected endpoints*** = some_of ([*http://serverIP:3000/monitor/pyNao1,* *http://serverIP:3000/monitor/pyNao2,* *http://serverIP:3000/monitor/pyFurhat]}*

Table A5. VR frontend blocks with corresponding backend endpoints.

Frontend Block Name	Description	Microskill/File Uploaded on the Server	Input Parameters	Backend Endpoint	Fetching Endpoint(s) with Parameters
Setup_VR_Session_Block	Sets up Express server, WebSocket communication, assigns unique session IDs for the therapists and the child.	Socket.io, JavaScript ES6 Modules	VRsceneID	/startVR	http://serverIP:3005/${VRsceneID}/startVR
Setup_VR_Scene_Block	Initializes a VR scene in Three.js with camera, VR controllers, renderer, WebXR support and 3D model loading. Delivers static files (frontend code, images, styles) from the "public" folder. Dynamically generates HTML pages.	JavaScript ES6 Modules	sessionID, BINGO SIZE: 3x3,4x4,5x5, SCENARIO: animals, fruits, vegetables, transports.	/sessions:id/setup	http://serverIP:3005/sessions/${sessionID}/setup with JSON:{method: 'POST', headers: { 'Content-Type': 'application/json; }, body: JSON.stringify (${JSON.stringify({ "bingoSize": BINGO_SIZE, "scenario": SCENARIO })}) }
StartVRbutton_Block	Starts VR button in the immersive mode of the browser.	Socket.io, Three.js, WebXR, JavaScript ES6 Modules	N/A	/startVRbutton	http://serverIP:3005/startVRbutton

Table A5. *Cont.*

Frontend Block Name	Description	Microskill/File Uploaded on the Server	Input Parameters	Backend Endpoint	Fetching Endpoint(s) with Parameters
360_Virtual_Tour	An interactive 360° virtual tour on a touchscreen where children explore common places, as well as educational spaces. The tours are hosted on the ATLog project website.	N/A	SPACE: house, hypermarket, museum	N/A	Blockly local runtime for fetch request https://atlog.ir.bas.bg/images/tours/${SPACE}/index.htm
360_Virtual_Game	An interactive 360° virtual game on a touchscreen, where children search for and identify objects from a preassigned list. The games are hosted on the ATLog project website.	N/A	SCENARIO: animals, fruits, vegetables, transports	N/A	Blockly local runtime for fetch request https://atlog.ir.bas.bg/images/tours/${SCENARIO}/index.htm

Appendix B

Table A6. Express server setup.

Dependencies that Need to be Installed by Npm	Dynamic Imports Used for:
const express = require('express');	Express framework to create a web server.
const app = express();	Creating an instance of the Express application.
const {spawn } = require('child_process');	Running child processes (e.g., executing PY scripts).
const {Client } = require('ssh2');	SSH2 client module to establish SSH connections.
const {exec } = require('child_process');	Exec to run shell commands asynchronously.
const fetch = require('node-fetch');	Node-fetch for making HTTP requests.
const repository = {};	Initializing an empty object to store key-value pairs.
const Database = require('better-sqlite3');	SQLite database interactions (better-sqlite3).
const fs = require('fs');	File System (fs) module to handle file operations.
const path = require('path');	Path module to manipulate file paths.
const http = require('http');	HTTP module to create an HTTP server for VR session.
const socketIo = require('socket.io');	Socket.IO library for real-time communication in VR.
const server = http.createServer(app);	Create an HTTP server using the Express app.
const io = socketIo(server);	Initialize Socket.IO by passing the HTTP server.
const os = require('os');	OS module to interact with the operating system.
Middleware (built into Express)	**Establishing a middleware to:**
app.use(express.json());	Parse JSON request bodies.
app.use(express.urlencoded({extended: true }));	Parse URL-encoded request bodies.
app.use((req, res, next) => {res.setHeader('Content-Type', 'application/json; charset=utf-8'); next(); });	Set the response header to JSON format with UTF-8 encoding.
app.use(express.static('public'));	Deliver static files from the public directory.
app.use(morgan('dev'));	Log HTTP requests in "dev" format.
const corsOptions = {	
origin: function (origin, callback) {...};	Handle requests only for LAN devices, based on the request's origin or IP address.
app.use(cors(corsOptions));	
app.use(express.static(__dirname + '/public'));	Listen for HTTP requests with a path starting with/public. Deliver static files (e.g., HTML, CSS, JS).
app.use(express.urlencoded({ extended: true }));	Parse URL-encoded request bodies (e.g., form data).
paths = ["/geometries", "/textures", "/sounds", "/styles"];	
paths.forEach((path) => {	Deliver static files from directories corresponding to the paths:/geometries;/textures;/sounds;/styles.
app.use(path, express.static(__dirname + path));});	
app.use('/build/',express.static(path.join(__dirname, 'node_modules/three/build')));	Deliver Three.js build files from the build directory under the "/build" route.
app.use('/jsm/',express.static(path.join(__dirname, 'node_modules/three/examples/jsm')));	Deliver Three.js modules from the "jsm" directory under the "/jsm" route.

References

1. Reeves, T. Design Research from a Technology Perspective. In *Educational Design Research*; Routledge: London, UK, 2006; pp. 64–78.
2. Kouroupa, A.; Laws, K.R.; Irvine, K.; Mengoni, S.E.; Baird, A.; Sharma, S. The Use of Social Robots with Children and Young People on the Autism Spectrum: A Systematic Review and Meta-Analysis. *PLoS ONE* **2022**, *17*, e0269800. [CrossRef]
3. Mills, J.; Duffy, O. Speech and Language Therapists' Perspectives of Virtual Reality as a Clinical Tool for Autism: Cross-Sectional Survey. *JMIR Rehabil. Assist. Technol.* **2025**, *12*, e63235. [CrossRef]
4. Peng, L.; Nuchged, B.; Gao, Y. Spoken Language Intelligence of Large Language Models for Language Learning. *arXiv* **2025**, arXiv:2308.14536.
5. Austin, J.; Benas, K.; Caicedo, S.; Imiolek, E.; Piekutowski, A.; Ghanim, I. Perceptions of Artificial Intelligence and ChatGPT by Speech-Language Pathologists and Students. *Am. J. Speech-Lang. Pathol.* **2025**, *34*, 174–200. [CrossRef] [PubMed]
6. Leinweber, J.; Alber, B.; Barthel, M.; Whillier, A.S.; Wittmar, S.; Borgetto, B.; Starke, A. Technology Use in Speech and Language Therapy: Digital Participation Succeeds through Acceptance and Use of Technology. *Front. Commun.* **2023**, *8*, 1176827. [CrossRef]
7. Szabó, B.; Dirks, S.; Scherger, A.-L. Apps and Digital Resources in Speech and Language Therapy—Which Factors Influence Therapists' Acceptance? In *Universal Access in Human–Computer Interaction. Novel Design Approaches and Technologies. HCII 2022*; Antona, M., Stephanidis, C., Eds.; Springer: Cham, Switzerland, 2022; Volume 13308, pp. 379–391. [CrossRef]
8. Hastall, M.R.; Dockweiler, C.; Mühlhaus, J. Achieving End User Acceptance: Building Blocks for an Evidence-Based User-Centered Framework for Health Technology Development and Assessment. In *Universal Access in Human–Computer Interaction. Human and Technological Environments*; Antona, M., Stephanidis, C., Eds.; Springer: Cham, Switzerland, 2017; pp. 13–25. [CrossRef]
9. Spitale, M.; Silleresi, S.; Garzotto, F.; Mataric, M. Using Socially Assistive Robots in Speech-Language Therapy for Children with Language Impairments. *Int. J. Soc. Robot.* **2023**, *15*, 1525–1542. [CrossRef]
10. Rupp, R.; Wirz, M. Implementation of Robots into Rehabilitation Programs: Meeting the Requirements and Expectations of Professional and End Users. In *Neurorehabilitation Technology*, 2nd ed.; Reinkensmeyer, D.J., Juneal-Crespo, L., Dietz, V., Eds.; Springer: Cham, Switzerland, 2022; pp. 263–288.
11. Lampropoulos, G.; Keramopoulos, E.; Diamantaras, K.; Evangelidis, G. Augmented Reality and Virtual Reality in Education: Public Perspectives, Sentiments, Attitudes, and Discourses. *Educ. Sci.* **2022**, *12*, 798. [CrossRef]
12. Suh, H.; Dangol, A.; Meadan, H.; Miller, C.A.; Kientz, J.A. Opportunities and Challenges for AI-Based Support for Speech-Language Pathologists. In Proceedings of the 3rd Annual Symposium on Human—Computer Interaction for Work (CHIWORK 2024), New York, NY, USA, 9–11 June 2024; pp. 1–14. [CrossRef]
13. Du, Y.; Juefei-Xu, F. Generative AI for Therapy? Opportunities and Barriers for ChatGPT in Speech-Language Therapy. *Unpubl. Work 2023.* Available online: https://openreview.net/forum?id=cRZSr6Tpr1S (accessed on 20 June 2025).
14. Fu, B.; Hadid, A.; Damer, N. Generative AI in the Context of Assistive Technologies: Trends, Limitations and Future Directions. *Image Vis. Comput.* **2025**, *154*, 105347. [CrossRef]
15. Santos, L.; Annunziata, S.; Geminiani, A.; Ivani, A.; Giubergia, A.; Garofalo, D.; Caglio, A.; Brazzoli, E.; Lipari, R.; Carrozza, M.C.; et al. Applications of Robotics for Autism Spectrum Disorder: A Scoping Review. *Rev. J. Autism Dev. Disord.* **2023**. [CrossRef]
16. Sáez-López, J.M.; del Olmo-Muñoz, J.; González-Calero, J.A.; Cózar-Gutiérrez, R. Exploring the Effect of Training in Visual Block Programming for Preservice Teachers. *Multimodal Technol. Interact.* **2020**, *4*, 65. [CrossRef]
17. Rees Lewis, D.; Carlson, S.; Riesbeck, C.; Lu, K.; Gerber, E.; Easterday, M. The Logic of Effective Iteration in Design-Based Research. In Proceedings of the 14th International Conference of the Learning Sciences: The Interdisciplinarity of the Learning Sciences (ICLS 2020), Nashville, TN, USA, 19–23 June 2020; Gresalfi, M., Horn, I.S., Eds.; International Society of the Learning Sciences: Bloomington, IN, USA; Volume 2, pp. 1149–1156.
18. ATLog Project. Available online: https://atlog.ir.bas.bg/en (accessed on 20 June 2025).
19. Lekova, A.; Tsvetkova, P.; Andreeva, A.; Simonska, M.; Kremenska, A. System Software Architecture for Advancing Human-Robot Interaction by Cloud Services and Multi-Robot Cooperation. *Int. J. Inf. Technol. Secur.* **2024**, *16*, 65–76. [CrossRef]
20. Andreeva, A.; Lekova, A.; Tsvetkova, P.; Simonska, M. Expanding the Capabilities of Robot NAO to Enable Human-Like Communication with Children with Speech and Language Disorders. In Proceedings of the 25th International Conference on Computer Systems and Technologies (CompSysTech 2024), Sofia, Bulgaria, 28–29 June 2024; pp. 63–68. [CrossRef]
21. Lekova, A.; Tsvetkova, P.; Andreeva, A. System Software Architecture for Enhancing Human-Robot Interaction by Conversational AI. In Proceedings of the 2023 International Conference on Information Technologies (InfoTech), Varna, Bulgaria, 19–20 October 2023; pp. 1–6. [CrossRef]

22. Lekova, A.; Vitanova, D. Design-Based Research for Streamlining the Integration of Text-Generative AI into Socially-Assistive Robots. In Proceedings of the 2024 International Conference "ROBOTICS & MECHATRONICS", Sofia, Bulgaria, 29–30 October 2024.
23. Kolev, M.; Trenchev, I.; Traykov, M.; Mavreski, R.; Ivanov, I. The Impact of Virtual and Augmented Reality on the Development of Motor Skills and Coordination in Children with Special Educational Needs. In *Lecture Notes of the Institute for Computer Sciences, Social Informatics and Telecommunications Engineering: Computer Science and Education in Computer Science*; Springer Nature Switzerland: Cham, Switzerland, 2023; Volume 514, pp. 171–181. [CrossRef]
24. Brooke, J. SUS—A Quick and Dirty Usability Scale. In *Usability Evaluation in Industry*; CRC Press: Boca Raton, FL, USA, 1996; pp. 189–194.
25. Davis, F. Perceived usefulness, perceived ease of use, and user acceptance of information technology. *MIS Q.* **1989**, *13*, 319–340. [CrossRef]
26. Cheah, W.; Jusoh, N.; Aung, M.; Ab Ghani, A.; Rebuan, H.M.A. Mobile technology in medicine: Development and validation of an adapted system usability scale (SUS) questionnaire and modified technology acceptance model (TAM) to evaluate user experience and acceptability of a mobile application in MRI safety screening. *Indian J. Radiol. Imaging* **2023**, *33*, 36–45. [CrossRef] [PubMed]
27. Hariri, W. Unlocking the Potential of ChatGPT: A Comprehensive Exploration of Its Applications, Advantages, Limitations, and Future Directions in Natural Language Processing. *arXiv* **2023**, arXiv:2304.02017.
28. Vaezipour, A.; Aldridge, D.; Koenig, S.; Theodoros, D.; Russell, T. "It's Really Exciting to Think Where It Could Go": A Mixed-Method Investigation of Clinician Acceptance, Barriers and Enablers of Virtual Reality Technology in Communication Rehabilitation. *Disabil. Rehabil.* **2022**, *44*, 3946–3958. [CrossRef]
29. Hashim, H.U.; Md Yunus, M.; Norman, H. Augmented Reality Mobile Application for Children with Autism: Stakeholders' Acceptance and Thoughts. *Arab World Engl. J.* **2021**, *12*, 130–146. [CrossRef]
30. Rasheva-Yordanova, K.; Kostadinova, I.; Georgieva-Tsaneva, G.; Andreeva, A.; Tsvetkova, P.; Lekova, A.; Stancheva-Popkostandinova, V.; Dimitrov, G. A Comprehensive Review and Analysis of Virtual Reality Scenarios in Speech and Language Therapy. *TEM J.* **2025**, *14*, 1895–1907. [CrossRef]
31. Vanderborght, B.; Simut, R.; Saldien, J.; Pop, C.; Rusu, A.S.; Pintea, S.; Lefeber, D.; David, D.O. Using the Social Robot Probo as a Social Story Telling Agent for Children with ASD. *Interact. Stud.* **2012**, *13*, 348–372. [CrossRef]
32. LuxAI. QTrobot for Schools & Therapy Centers. Available online: https://luxai.com/robot-for-teaching-children-with-autism-at-home/ (accessed on 20 June 2025).
33. Furhat Robotics. Furhat AI. Available online: https://www.furhatrobotics.com/furhat-ai (accessed on 20 June 2025).
34. PAL Robotics. ARI. Available online: https://pal-robotics.com/robot/ari/ (accessed on 20 June 2025).
35. RoboKind Milo Robot. Available online: https://www.robokind.com/?hsCtaTracking=2433ccbc-0af8-4ade-ae0b-4642cb0ecba4%7Cb0814dc8-76e1-447d-aba7-101e89845fb7 (accessed on 20 June 2025).
36. She, T.; Ren, F. Enhance the Language Ability of Humanoid Robot NAO through Deep Learning to Interact with Autistic Children. *Electronics* **2021**, *10*, 2393. [CrossRef]
37. Cherakara, N.; Varghese, F.; Shabana, S.; Nelson, N.; Karukayil, A.; Kulothungan, R.; Farhan, M.; Nesset, B.; Moujahid, M.; Dinkar, T.; et al. FurChat: An Embodied Conversational Agent Using LLMs, Combining Open and Closed-Domain Dialogue with Facial Expressions. In Proceedings of the 24th Annual Meeting of the Special Interest Group on Discourse and Dialogue (SIGDIAL 2023), Prague, Czech Republic, 11–13 September 2023; pp. 588–592. [CrossRef]
38. Belda-Medina, J.; Calvo-Ferrer, J.R. Using Chatbots as AI Conversational Partners in Language Learning. *Appl. Sci.* **2022**, *12*, 8427. [CrossRef]
39. ChatGPT Prompting for SLPs. Available online: https://eatspeakthink.com/chatgpt-for-speech-therapy-2025/ (accessed on 20 June 2025).
40. Bertacchini, F.; Demarco, F.; Scuro, C.; Pantano, P.; Bilotta, E. A Social Robot Connected with ChatGPT to Improve Cognitive Functioning in ASD Subjects. *Front. Psychol.* **2023**, *14*, 1232177. [CrossRef] [PubMed]
41. Salhi, I.; Qbadou, M.; Gouraguine, S.; Mansouri, K.; Lytridis, C.; Kaburlasos, V. Towards Robot-Assisted Therapy for Children with Autism—The Ontological Knowledge Models and Reinforcement Learning-Based Algorithms. *Front. Robot. AI* **2022**, *9*, 713964. [CrossRef] [PubMed]
42. Naneva, S.; Sarda Gou, M.; Webb, T.L.; Prescott, T.J. A Systematic Review of Attitudes, Anxiety, Acceptance, and Trust Towards Social Robots. *Int. J. Soc. Robot.* **2020**, *12*, 1179–1201. [CrossRef]
43. Liu, Z.; Li, H.; Chen, A.; Zhang, R.; Lee, Y.C. Understanding Public Perceptions of AI Conversational Agents. In Proceedings of the 2024 CHI Conference on Human Factors in Computing Systems (CHI 2024), Honolulu, HI, USA, 11–16 May 2024; pp. 1–17. [CrossRef]

44. Gerlich, M. Perceptions and Acceptance of Artificial Intelligence: A Multi-Dimensional Study. *Soc. Sci.* **2023**, *12*, 502. [CrossRef]
45. Severson, R.; Peter, J.; Kanda, T.; Kaufman, J.; Scassellati, B. Social Robots and Children's Development: Promises and Implications. In *Handbook of Children and Screens*; Christakis, D.A., Hale, L., Eds.; Springer: Cham, Switzerland, 2024; pp. 627–633. [CrossRef]
46. Youssef, K.; Said, S.; Alkork, S.; Beyrouthy, T. A Survey on Recent Advances in Social Robotics. *Robotics* **2022**, *11*, 75. [CrossRef]
47. Georgieva-Tsaneva, G.; Andreeva, A.; Tsvetkova, P.; Lekova, A.; Simonska, M.; Stancheva-Popkostadinova, V.; Dimitrov, G.; Rasheva-Yordanova, K.; Kostadinova, I. Exploring the Potential of Social Robots for Speech and Language Therapy: A Review and Analysis of Interactive Scenarios. *Machines* **2023**, *11*, 693. [CrossRef]
48. Estévez, D.; Terrón-López, M.-J.; Velasco-Quintana, P.J.; Rodríguez-Jiménez, R.-M.; Álvarez-Manzano, V. A Case Study of a Robot-Assisted Speech Therapy for Children with Language Disorders. *Sustainability* **2021**, *13*, 2771. [CrossRef]
49. Ioannou, A.; Andreva, A. Play and Learn with an Intelligent Robot: Enhancing the Therapy of Hearing-Impaired Children. In *Human–Computer Interaction—INTERACT 2019*; Lamas, D., Loizides, F., Nacke, L., Petrie, H., Winckler, M., Zaphiris, P., Eds.; Lecture Notes in Computer Science; Springer: Cham, Switzerland, 2019; Volume 11747, pp. 436–452. [CrossRef]
50. Lee, H.; Hyun, E. The Intelligent Robot Contents for Children with Speech-Language Disorder. *J. Educ. Technol. Soc.* **2015**, *18*, 100–113.
51. Lekova, A.; Andreeva, A.; Simonska, M.; Tanev, T.; Kostova, S. A System for Speech and Language Therapy with a Potential to Work in the IoT. In Proceedings of the 2022 International Conference on Computer Systems and Technologies (CompSysTech 2022), Ruse, Bulgaria, 16–17 June 2022; pp. 119–124. [CrossRef]
52. QTrobot for Special Needs Education. Available online: https://luxai.com/assistive-tech-robot-for-special-needs-education/ (accessed on 20 June 2025).
53. Vukliš, D.; Krasnik, R.; Mikov, A.; Zvekić Svorcan, J.; Janković, T.; Kovačević, M. Parental Attitudes Towards the Use of Humanoid Robots in Pediatric (Re)Habilitation. *Med. Pregl.* **2019**, *72*, 302–306. [CrossRef]
54. Szymona, B.; Maciejewski, M.; Karpiński, R.; Jonak, K.; Radzikowska-Büchner, E.; Niderla, K.; Prokopiak, A. Robot-Assisted Autism Therapy (RAAT): Criteria and Types of Experiments Using Anthropomorphic and Zoomorphic Robots. *Sensors* **2021**, *21*, 3720. [CrossRef]
55. Nicolae, G.; Vlădeanu, C.; Saru, L.-M.; Burileanu, C.; Grozăvescu, R.; Crăciun, G.; Drugă, S.; Hatiș, M. Programming the NAO Humanoid Robot for Behavioral Therapy in Romania. *Rom. J. Child Adolesc. Psychiatry* **2019**, *7*, 23–30.
56. Gupta, G.; Chandra, S.; Dautenhahn, K.; Loucks, T. Stuttering Treatment Approaches from the Past Two Decades: Comprehensive Survey and Review. *J. Stud. Res.* **2022**, *11*. [CrossRef]
57. Chandra, S.; Gupta, G.; Loucks, T.; Dautenhahn, K. Opportunities for Social Robots in the Stuttering Clinic: A Review and Proposed Scenarios. *Paladyn J. Behav. Robot.* **2022**, *13*, 23–44. [CrossRef]
58. Bonarini, A.; Clasadonte, F.; Garzotto, F.; Gelsomini, M.; Romero, M.E. Playful Interaction with Teo, a Mobile Robot for Children with Neurodevelopmental Disorders. In Proceedings of the 7th International Conference on Software Development and Technologies for Enhancing Accessibility and Fighting Info-exclusion (DSAI 2016), Vila Real, Portugal, 1–3 December 2016; pp. 223–231. [CrossRef]
59. Kose, H.; Yorganci, R. Tale of a Robot: Humanoid Robot Assisted Sign Language Tutoring. In Proceedings of the 11th IEEE-RAS International Conference on Humanoid Robots, Bled, Slovenia, 26–28 October 2011; pp. 105–111. [CrossRef]
60. Fung, K.Y.; Lee, L.H.; Sin, K.F.; Song, S.; Qu, H. Humanoid Robot-Empowered Language Learning Based on Self-Determination Theory. *Educ. Inf. Technol.* **2024**, *29*, 18927–18957. [CrossRef]
61. Cappadona, I.; Ielo, A.; La Fauci, M.; Tresoldi, M.; Settimo, C.; De Cola, M.C.; Muratore, R.; De Domenico, C.; Di Cara, M.; Corallo, F.; et al. Feasibility and Effectiveness of Speech Intervention Implemented with a Virtual Reality System in Children with Developmental Language Disorders: A Pilot Randomized Control Trial. *Children* **2023**, *10*, 1336. [CrossRef]
62. Purpura, G.; Di Giusto, V.; Zorzi, C.F.; Figliano, G.; Randazzo, M.; Volpicelli, V.; Blonda, R.; Brazzoli, E.; Reina, T.; Rezzonico, S.; et al. Use of Virtual Reality in School-Aged Children with Developmental Coordination Disorder: A Novel Approach. *Sensors* **2024**, *24*, 5578. [CrossRef]
63. Maresca, G.; Corallo, F.; De Cola, M.C.; Formica, C.; Giliberto, S.; Rao, G.; Crupi, M.F.; Quartarone, A.; Pidalà, A. Effectiveness of the Use of Virtual Reality Rehabilitation in Children with Dyslexia: Follow-Up after One Year. *Brain Sci.* **2024**, *14*, 655. [CrossRef] [PubMed]
64. Mangani, G.; Barzacchi, V.; Bombonato, C.; Barsotti, J.; Beani, E.; Menici, V.; Ragoni, C.; Sgandurra, G.; Del Lucchese, B. Feasibility of a Virtual Reality System in Speech Therapy: From Assessment to Tele-Rehabilitation in Children with Cerebral Palsy. *Children* **2024**, *11*, 1327. [CrossRef] [PubMed]
65. Macdonald, C. Improving Virtual Reality Exposure Therapy with Open Access and Overexposure: A Single 30-Minute Session of Overexposure Therapy Reduces Public Speaking Anxiety. *Front. Virtual Real.* **2024**, *5*, 1506938. [CrossRef]

66. Pergantis, P.; Bamicha, V.; Doulou, A.; Christou, A.I.; Bardis, N.; Skianis, C.; Drigas, A. Assistive and Emerging Technologies to Detect and Reduce Neurophysiological Stress and Anxiety in Children and Adolescents with Autism and Sensory Processing Disorders: A Systematic Review. *Technologies* **2025**, *13*, 144. [CrossRef]
67. Tobii Dynavox Global: Assistive Technology for Communication. Available online: https://www.tobiidynavox.com/ (accessed on 20 June 2025).
68. Klavina, A.; Pérez-Fuster, P.; Daems, J.; Lyhne, C.N.; Dervishi, E.; Pajalic, Z.; Øderud, T.; Fuglerud, K.S.; Markovska-Simoska, S.; Przybyla, T.; et al. The Use of Assistive Technology to Promote Practical Skills in Persons with Autism Spectrum Disorder and Intellectual Disabilities: A Systematic Review. *Digit. Health* **2024**, *10*, 20552076241281260. [CrossRef]
69. Ask NAO. Available online: https://www.asknao-tablet.com/en/home/ (accessed on 20 June 2025).
70. Furhat Blockly. Available online: https://docs.furhat.io/blockly/ (accessed on 20 June 2025).
71. Vittascience Interface for NAO v6. Available online: https://en.vittascience.com/nao/?mode=mixed&console=bottom&toolbox=vittascience (accessed on 20 June 2025).
72. LEKA. Available online: https://leka.io (accessed on 20 June 2025).
73. Platform for VR Public Speaking. Available online: https://www.virtualrealitypublicspeaking.com/platform (accessed on 20 June 2025).
74. ThingLink. Available online: https://www.thinglink.com/ (accessed on 20 June 2025).
75. Kurai, R.; Hiraki, T.; Hiroi, Y.; Hirao, Y.; Perusquía-Hernández, M.; Uchiyama, H.; Kiyokawa, K. MagicItem: Dynamic Behavior Design of Virtual Objects with Large Language Models in a Commercial Metaverse Platform. *IEEE Access* **2025**, *13*, 19132–19143. [CrossRef]
76. Therapy withVR. Available online: https://therapy.withvr.app/ (accessed on 20 June 2025).
77. Grassi, L.; Recchiuto, C.T.; Sgorbissa, A. Sustainable Cloud Services for Verbal Interaction with Embodied Agents. *Intell. Serv. Robot.* **2023**, *16*, 599–618. [CrossRef]
78. LuxAI. Complete Guide to Build a Conversational Social Robot QTrobot with ChatGPT. Available online: https://luxai.com/blog/complete-guide-to-build-conversational-social-robot-qtrobot-chatgpt/ (accessed on 20 June 2025).
79. Lewis, J.R. The system usability scale: Past, present, and future. *Int. J. Hum. Comput. Interact.* **2018**, *34*, 577–590. [CrossRef]
80. Mulia, A.P.; Piri, P.R.; Tho, C. Usability analysis of text generation by ChatGPT OpenAI using system usability scale method. *Procedia Comput. Sci.* **2023**, *227*, 381–388. [CrossRef]
81. Bangor, A.; Kortum, P.T.; Miller, J.T. An empirical evaluation of the system usability scale. *Int. J. Hum. Comput. Interact.* **2008**, *24*, 574–594. [CrossRef]
82. Lewis, J.R. Comparison of Four TAM Item Formats: Effect of Response Option Labels and Order. *J. Usability Stud.* **2019**, *14*, 224–236.
83. Aldebaran. NAO Robot. Available online: https://aldebaran.com/en/nao6/ (accessed on 20 June 2025).
84. Furhat Robotics. The Furhat Robot. Available online: https://www.furhatrobotics.com/furhat-robot (accessed on 20 June 2025).
85. Tanev, T.K.; Lekova, A. Implementation of Actors' Emotional Talent into Social Robots Through Capture of Human Head's Motion and Basic Expression. *Int. J. Soc. Robot.* **2022**, *14*, 1749–1766. [CrossRef]
86. Double Robotics. Double3 Robot for Telepresence. Available online: https://www.doublerobotics.com/double3.html (accessed on 20 June 2025).
87. Aldebaran. Choregraphe Software Overview. Available online: http://doc.aldebaran.com/2-8/software/choregraphe/choregraphe_overview.html (accessed on 20 June 2025).
88. Aldebaran. NAOqi API and SDK 2.8. Available online: http://doc.aldebaran.com/2-8/news/2.8/naoqi_api_rn2.8.html?highlight=naoqi (accessed on 20 June 2025).
89. Furhat Robotics. Furhat SDK Documentation. Available online: https://docs.furhat.io/getting_started/ (accessed on 20 June 2025).
90. Furhat Robotics. Furhat Remote API. Available online: https://docs.furhat.io/remote-api/ (accessed on 20 June 2025).
91. Double Robotics. Double3 Developer SDK. Available online: https://github.com/doublerobotics/d3-sdk (accessed on 20 June 2025).
92. W3C. WebXR Device API. Available online: https://www.w3.org/TR/webxr/ (accessed on 20 June 2025).
93. Dirksen, J. *Learning Three.js—The JavaScript 3D Library for WebGL*, 2nd ed.; Packt Publishing: Birmingham, UK, 2015; ISBN 978-1-78439-221-5.
94. 3DVista Virtual Tour Software. Available online: https://www.3dvista.com/en/ (accessed on 20 June 2025).
95. NLP Cloud API Platform. Available online: https://nlpcloud.com/ (accessed on 20 June 2025).
96. OpenAI. ChatGPT-4 Research Overview. Available online: https://openai.com/index/gpt-4-research/ (accessed on 20 June 2025).
97. INSAIT. BgGPT Language Model. Available online: https://bggpt.ai/ (accessed on 20 June 2025).
98. Express.js. Node.js Web Application Framework. Available online: https://expressjs.com/ (accessed on 20 June 2025).
99. Google Developers. Blockly for Developers. Available online: https://developers.google.com/blockly (accessed on 20 June 2025).

100. Node.js. SQLite Module Documentation. Available online: https://nodejs.org/api/sqlite.html (accessed on 20 June 2025).
101. Meta. Casting from Meta Quest 3 to Computer. Available online: https://www.oculus.com/casting/ (accessed on 20 June 2025).
102. ATLog Ethical Codex. Available online: https://atlog.ir.bas.bg/en/results/ethical-codex (accessed on 20 June 2025).
103. Vlachogianni, P.; Tselios, N. Perceived Usability Evaluation of Educational Technology Using the Post-Study System Usability Questionnaire (PSSUQ): A Systematic Review. *Sustainability* **2023**, *15*, 12954. [CrossRef]
104. Lah, U.; Lewis, J.R.; Šumak, B. Perceived usability and the modified technology acceptance model. *Int. J. Hum. Comput. Interact.* **2020**, *36*, 1216–1230. [CrossRef]

technologies

MDPI

Article

Vision-Based Activity Recognition for Unobtrusive Monitoring of the Elderly in Care Settings

Rahmat Ullah [1,*], Ikram Asghar [2], Saeed Akbar [3], Gareth Evans [4], Justus Vermaak [5], Abdulaziz Alblwi [6] and Amna Bamaqa [6]

[1] School of Computer Science and Electronic Engineering, University of Essex, Colchester CO4 3SQ, UK
[2] Department of Computing & Games, Teesside University, Middlesbrough TS1 3BX, UK; i.asghar@tees.ac.uk
[3] Department of Physical & Numerical Sciences, Qurtuba University of Science & Information Technology, Peshawar 25150, Pakistan; saedakbr@qurtuba.edu.pk
[4] Centre of Excellence in Mobile and Emerging Technologies, University of South Wales, Pontypridd CF37 4BD, UK; gareth.evans@southwales.ac.uk
[5] Skystrm Limited, Barry CF62 5BE, UK; justus@henleycarecentre.com
[6] Department of Computer Science, Applied College, Taibah University, P.O. Box 344, Madinah 41477, Saudi Arabia; ablwi@taibahu.edu.sa (A.A.); abamaqa@taibahu.edu.sa (A.B.)
* Correspondence: rahmat.ullah@essex.ac.uk

Abstract: As the global population ages, robust technological solutions are increasingly necessary to support and enhance elderly autonomy in-home or care settings. This paper presents a novel computer vision-based activity monitoring system that uses cameras and infrared sensors to detect and analyze daily activities of elderly individuals in care environments. The system integrates a frame differencing algorithm with adjustable sensitivity parameters and an anomaly detection model tailored to identify deviations from individual behavior patterns without relying on large volumes of labeled data. The system was validated through real-world deployments across multiple care home rooms, demonstrating significant improvements in emergency response times and ensuring resident privacy through anonymized frame differencing views. Upon detecting anomalies in daily routines, the system promptly alerts caregivers and family members, facilitating immediate intervention. The experimental results confirm the system's capability for unobtrusive, continuous monitoring, laying a strong foundation for scalable remote elderly care services and enhancing the safety and independence of vulnerable older individuals.

Keywords: activity recognition; action recognition; daily living activity recognition; elderly care; fall detection; remote monitoring

1. Introduction

According to recent statistics from the World Health Organization, the global population is aging rapidly. By the end of this decade, one in every six people worldwide will be over the age of 60. This demographic shift is anticipated to grow, with projections suggesting that there will be over 2 billion people aged 60 and above by the year 2050. Historically, trends of aging populations were predominantly observed in developed and high-income countries. However, current projections indicate that aging will also become a significant phenomenon in low and middle-income countries. By 2050, nearly 80% of the elderly population will reside in these regions [1]. It is crucial to investigate and implement care-based and health monitoring technologies in the living environments of the ageing population, such as care homes and independent homes, to ensure timely care is provided when needed [2].

The aging population presents a complex mix of challenges and opportunities. As life expectancy increases, individuals have more opportunities to engage in new learning experiences, embark on different career paths later in life, and contribute their knowledge and skills to society. However, the full participation of elderly individuals in these opportunities heavily depends on their health. Many older adults face a range of medical issues, including sensory impairments, mobility restrictions, and chronic conditions such as diabetes and dementia, which can significantly impact their quality of life [3].

Monitoring the daily activities of elderly individuals is crucial for assessing their health status. These activities, encompassing daily routines, physical movements, eating habits, sleeping patterns, and more, serve as vital indicators of their overall health [4]. By carefully observing and tracking these activities, caregivers, family members, and healthcare providers can detect any deviations from normal patterns, providing early warning signs of potential health issues. Moreover, monitoring physical activity can pinpoint changes in mobility and balance, potentially flagging early signs of conditions that could lead to falls or other serious health complications [5].

In today's rapidly advancing technological landscape, integrating artificial intelligence (AI) and computer vision into healthcare monitoring systems can significantly enhance the efficiency and effectiveness of care. These technologies offer the revolutionary potential to improve the management of healthcare facilities, particularly those catering to vulnerable groups such as the elderly or those with chronic health conditions [6]. Traditional monitoring methods often struggle to detect emergencies or significant health changes in real time, highlighting the need for more innovative solutions to these challenges. The COVID-19 pandemic, for instance, has exposed high mortality rates among older adults in care facilities, largely due to inadequate monitoring and care, underscoring the importance of robust remote monitoring systems that can ensure continuous care and timely interventions [7].

Research into wearable sensors for monitoring human activity provides a complex perspective, emphasizing the benefits and limitations of such technology, especially for the elderly. While wearable sensors can offer detailed insights into an individual's health and activity levels, they may not always be reliable for elderly users who might forget to wear them or find them uncomfortable. This can lead to significant gaps in data collection and reduce the effectiveness of monitoring based solely on these devices [8,9]. Furthermore, due to unique environmental challenges, traditional deep learning techniques are often inadequate for accurately identifying activities within specific indoor settings, such as care homes. These models rely on large volumes of labeled data to identify and classify activities indicative of health risks.

Indoor Human Activity Recognition requires models that are specifically tailored to the typical activities of the environment. Therefore, a one-size-fits-all model is not appropriate for specialized settings, as noted in a review by Bhola et al. [8]. Anomaly detection models are a great alternative to traditional machine learning techniques for human activity detection. These models can effectively operate with unlabeled data.

This paper proposes a vision-based monitoring system designed to enable effective remote monitoring in elderly care settings. The key contributions of our work are as follows:

- A novel computer vision system is developed that integrates cameras and infrared sensors to monitor daily activities of elderly individuals without requiring wearable devices.
- We implement lightweight anomaly detection algorithms capable of identifying deviations from normal behavior patterns without relying on large volumes of labeled

data. This makes the system highly suitable for real-world care home environments where critical events are rare and collecting large volumes of labeled anomaly data is not impractical.
- The system is evaluated through deployments in real elderly care settings, demonstrating significant improvements in emergency response times and overall resident safety.
- The system maintains resident privacy by employing frame differencing techniques that anonymize video outputs while retaining critical movement information for accurate activity recognition.

In contrast to many deep learning-based approaches requiring substantial computational resources, extensive labeled datasets, and complex maintenance, the proposed lightweight system leverages simple frame differencing and anomaly detection techniques. This design ensures real-time performance, minimizes installation and operational costs, preserves resident privacy, and offers high scalability for elderly care environments. Our system demonstrates that in safety-critical applications like remote elderly monitoring, purposeful algorithmic simplicity can translate into greater practicality, reliability, and faster emergency responses than overly complex models.

2. Related Work

Recent computer vision and machine learning studies demonstrate significant advancements across various applications, from aerial surveillance to autonomous vehicle navigation and human-computer interaction. A comprehensive review of the current landscape in video-based human activity recognition systems, examining the essential components such as object segmentation, feature extraction, activity detection, and classification, is conducted in [10]. The survey spans three primary application areas: surveillance, entertainment, and healthcare. While noting the significant advancements in the field, the paper also identifies persistent challenges and technical hurdles that impede practical, real-world implementation. A comprehensive scoping and in-depth examination of audio and video-based human activity recognition systems within healthcare settings is presented in [11]. The review provides a critical evaluation of the performance, robustness, and scalability of these systems, as well as their privacy and security implications. Despite their potential, there are still challenges in implementing such systems into clinical practice due to privacy concerns and the complexity of real-world implementation.

2.1. Vision-Based Human Activity Recognition Systems

A Diminutive Multi-Dimensional Locality Coding Convolutional Neural Network (DMLC-CNN) is proposed for human activity recognition from UAV-captured videos [12]. The model introduces a novel feature extraction and encoding process suitable for complex and dynamic backgrounds in aerial surveillance, resulting in superior accuracy compared to traditional methods. Similarly, deep learning techniques recognize in-bed movements from video streams in a clinical setting in [13]. The paper proposed a 3D MoCap combined with skeleton-based action recognition as a promising technique for improving the accuracy of clinical in-bed monitoring systems. However, the effectiveness of the proposed methods heavily relies on the availability of high-quality, labeled datasets for training and validation, which are scarce in clinical contexts.

A system was designed to provide real-time feedback to stroke patients performing daily activities necessary for independent living. It used overhead cameras and histogram-based recognition methods to monitor the position and movement of the patient's hands and the objects they manipulate [14]. The key events are recognized and interpreted in the context of a model of the coffee-making task. A computer vision-based human activity recognition system for assisted living systems was proposed in [15]. The proposed system addresses some of the limitations of traditional sensor-based systems by using a numerical dataset derived from key-joint angles, distances, and slopes. This approach, using data from 20,000 images to detect five human postures, sitting, standing, walking, lying, and falling enabled efficient training and high-accuracy detection. A video sensor-based HAR system for elderly care was proposed in [16]. The proposed system used depth imaging sensors to generate human skeletons and joint information for precise activity recognition. This approach outperforms traditional RGB sensor-based systems by providing richer data necessary for detailed analysis of elderly activities within smart environments. An AI-driven privacy-preserving monitoring system for elderly care was proposed in [17]. Their system employs the YOLOv8 model to detect individuals in real-time and replaces them with anonymized 2D avatars, ensuring privacy protection. However, the proposed system's performance can be less effective under varying environmental conditions like lighting and obstacles, which can hinder sensor accuracy and activity recognition. Moreover, it requires high computational resources for complex algorithms, raising concerns about its feasibility in real-time applications.

2.2. *Wearable Sensor-Based Human Activity Recognition Systems*

Wearable technology is attracting considerable interest for its ability to track and improve physical activity in older adults [18]. An extensive review of the advancements in smart home technologies specifically tailored for elderly healthcare is presented in [19]. Their work underscores the integration of e-health and assisted living technologies within the Internet of Things (IoT) framework. The authors discuss critical components such as sensors, actuators, and communication networks that are instrumental in monitoring and assisting the elderly. A study was conducted by [20], which showed that wearable devices, along with mobile-based intermittent coaching, can significantly boost physical activity and health outcomes, especially in pre-frail older adults. Similarly, Smirnova et al. found that accelerometers, commonly used in wearable technology, provide reliable measurements of physical activity and are better predictors of five-year mortality in older adults than traditional methods [21]. A similar study identified wearable devices as crucial facilitators of physical activity, especially for older adults with cardiovascular diseases or associated risks [22].

A comprehensive review is conducted on the use of wearable sensors in human activity recognition (HAR), mainly through deep learning approaches [23]. The paper highlights the wide range of applications for wearable technologies, from fitness and lifestyle enhancement to critical roles in healthcare and rehabilitation. An ensemble measurement-based deep learning model is proposed in [24], which utilizes four Convolutional Neural Networks (CNN) and Long Short-Term Memory (LSTM)-based models for smartphone sensor-based Human HAR problems. The model was tested on three publicly available datasets and demonstrated commendable performance in activity prediction with reasonable accuracy. However, the lack of advanced processing techniques for time-series sensor data potentially impacts its performance effectiveness.

2.3. *Fall Detection Systems and Low-Light Activity Recognition*

Recent advancements in human activity monitoring have also emphasized the significance of fall detection, particularly for the elderly, using different machine and deep learning models. For instance, a modified NASNet model incorporating Local Binary Patterns (LBP) features distinguishes itself by achieving an impressive accuracy, precision, recall, and F1 score of 99% [25]. A similar study developed a vision-based fall detection system capable of operating under low-light conditions. Their method involves enhancing images and tracking objects using a dual illumination estimation algorithm and then utilizing YOLOv7 + Deep SORT/w DUAL for fall detection [26]. A framework for Human Activity Recognition in low-light conditions using a dual stream network that combines Convolutional Neural Networks and Transformers is proposed in [27]. This cloud-assisted IoT framework enhances video frame quality at the edge and utilizes an optimized network architecture for efficient and accurate activity recognition in low-lighting scenarios.

However, despite these positive findings, research remains inconclusive regarding the absolute validity and reliability of these devices for evaluating physical activity and health-related outcomes in older adults, highlighting the need for further research and adaptation to suit this age group better [28] In conclusion. In comparison, substantial evidence supports the effectiveness of wearable devices in monitoring and enhancing physical activity among older adults. There is a simultaneous recognition of the necessity for continued research, particularly in terms of device adaptability and reliability in this age group.

3. Materials and Methods

This study used a co-design approach. The research process started with multiple requirements workshops between the research team, care industry experts, and end users to understand the care industry's needs. The research aimed to develop a system that provides a way to demonstrate the possibilities of applying computer vision techniques within the care industry. Based on the nature of this study, the prototyping approach was best suited for the system development. The data to test the system's performance was collected through a pilot study, which records a person's movements in a predefined scenario. The data were captured with the help of cameras and infrared sensors, which monitor an individual's movements. The pilot study data marked a first step in determining the suitability and efficiency of the developed system.

3.1. Proposed Method

A series of computer vision algorithms and data handling methods are used. These algorithms are pivotal for the real-time monitoring and activity analysis of elderly residents in care environments. By using these techniques, the system provides detailed insights into daily activities and quickly identifies any deviations that may indicate potential health or safety concerns. Using raw image data requires extensive data cleaning and pre-processing techniques. This process required lots of experimentation to ensure optimal results while providing the user with enough flexibility and control. An illustrative diagram of this process can be seen in Figure 1, which outlines the sequence from frame capture to motion detection.

Frame differencing was used to detect the movement in data obtained using camera and infrared sensors. In this method, the captured video frames are converted into grayscale. The absolute difference between consecutive frames is calculated to highlight areas where motion has occurred. This difference image undergoes a binary thresholding process, simplifying the image to binary values representing motion and no-motion areas. This step is crucial for isolating relevant motion data from background noise.

Once motion is detected through frame differencing, the system uses a moving average filter to assess the continuity and significance of detected movements. This helps distinguish between incidental movements, such as a curtain fluttering, and significant activities like walking or falling. Logging an activity as 'true motion' is made based on the consistency and duration of detected movement across several frames. The Algorithm 1 gives pseudocode for the Frame Differencing Algorithm. The algorithm processes each frame to identify significant movements by comparing differences, applying a binary threshold, and analyzing contours for robust motion detection.

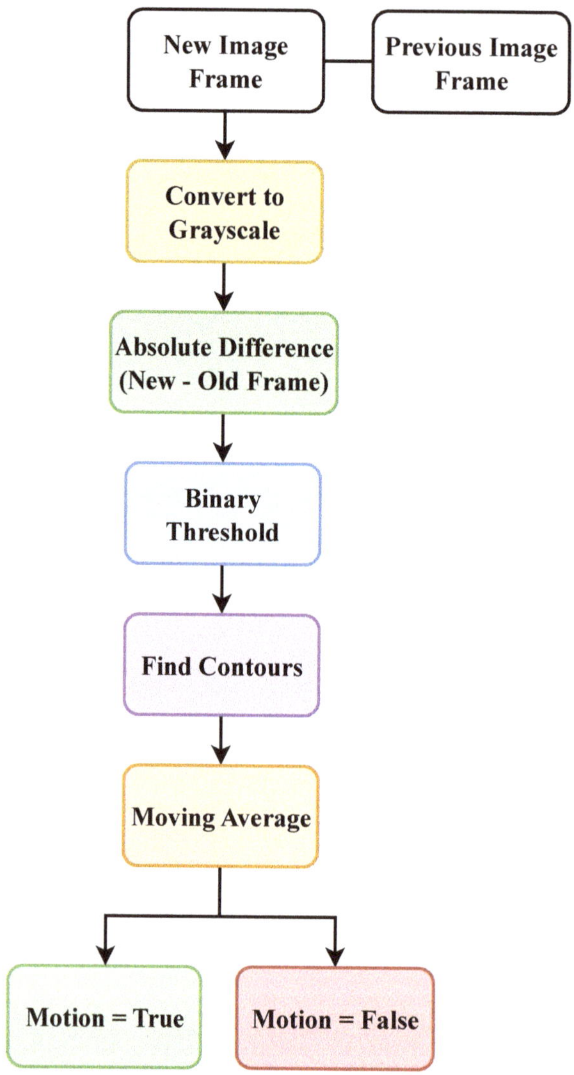

Figure 1. Workflow of the frame differencing algorithm. The process starts with converting video frames to grayscale and then computing the absolute difference between consecutive frames. The resulting difference image is then held in a binary format, isolating significant movement areas.

Several key parameters and techniques are utilized to optimize the detection and analysis of motion. These parameters include the detection threshold, binary threshold, and window length, each contributing uniquely to the system's efficacy.

Thresholding in computer vision is used to segment images, effectively separating the foreground from the background [29]. The detection threshold is crucial for determining the existence of motion based on the number of contours identified in processed images. This parameter was adjusted from 1 to 125, where 1 indicates a higher sensitivity to motion, capturing finer movements. Conversely, a higher threshold value makes the system less sensitive and useful in environments where incidental movements are common. This flexibility allows the system to be finely tuned in real time to suit different operational conditions, ensuring that motion detection is accurate and relevant to the specific care setting.

Algorithm 1: Frame Differencing Algorithm used in motion detection

```
Result: Detect motion in video frames and mark frames containing significant
        motion
Initialize: previous_frame ← NULL;
foreach frame in video stream do
    Convert frame to grayscale;
    if previous_frame is not NULL then
        absolute_difference ← ComputeAbsoluteDifference(frame, previous_frame);
        binary_image ← ApplyBinaryThreshold(absolute_difference);
        contours ← FindContours(binary_image);
        if contours exist then
            motion_average ← CalculateMovingAverage(contours);
            if motion_average indicates significant motion then
                Mark frame as containing motion;
                Store or process frame as required;
            end
        end
    end
    previous_frame ← frame;
end
```

Binary thresholding is applied following frame differencing to distinguish between static and dynamic elements within the frame. The binary image results in pixels set to '1' (white) where differences are detected and '0' (black) elsewhere. Adjusting the binary threshold impacts the sensitivity of motion detection; for example, a lower threshold captures slight differences between frames, enhancing sensitivity, while a higher threshold requires more significant differences for detection, reducing sensitivity. This parameter is pivotal for adjusting the system's response to varying activity levels and environmental conditions.

The window length parameter addresses the temporal aspect of motion detection. By considering multiple frames at once, the system can more reliably determine whether the detected motion is consistent and significant rather than transient or background noise. The algorithm maintains an array of motion values where each new frame's motion result (either '0' or '1') is added, and the oldest value is removed. If the sum of this array exceeds a predefined limit (e.g., five in a ten-frame window), the system confirms the presence of sustained motion. This approach minimizes false positives and enhances the reliability of the system in dynamically changing environments. This pseudocode in Algorithm 2 represents the moving average algorithm used for motion detection.

The proposed algorithm adopts a sliding window approach to aggregate and analyze motion values from consecutive video frames. Denote v_t as the binary motion value at time t, where v_t is 0 (no motion) or 1 (motion detected). These values are stored in an array A, with a predefined window length W, typically set to $W = 10$. Each new frame updates A by appending v_t and removing the oldest value, effectively shifting the array by one position.

Algorithm 2: Moving Average Algorithm for Motion Detection

```
Data: motionWindow, windowLength, motionData
Result: averageMotion indicating the motion status
for each new frame do
    motionWindow[currentIndex] ← Cast motionData to integer;
    if currentIndex ≥ windowLength then
        Reset currentIndex to 0;
        Reset motionSum to 0;
    end
    for i ← 0 to windowLength-1 do
        motionSum ← motionSum + motionWindow[i];
    end
    if motionSum ≥ (windowLength/2) then
        averageMotion ← 1;
    else
        averageMotion ← 0;
    end
end
```

The mathematical representation of the update mechanism for array A at time t is expressed as:

$$A_t = v_{t-W+1}, v_{t-W+2}, \ldots, v_t \tag{1}$$

The decision-making process involves calculating the sum S_t of the elements within A_t. If $S_t > 5$, the algorithm concludes that sustained motion is present within the window, indicating a reliable detection of actual motion:

$$S_t = \sum_{i=t-W+1}^{t} v_i \tag{2}$$

For example, after processing 10 frames, if the majority of frames within A indicate motion (e.g., $[1,1,1,1,1,1,0,0,0,0]$), then $S_t = 6$ and the algorithm signals motion detection by setting "averageMotion" to 1, suggesting true motion. Conversely, if fewer than half the frames show motion, such as in $[1,0,0,0,1,1,0,0,0,0]$ with $S_t = 3$, "averageMotion" is set to 0, indicating no significant motion is detected. This distinction is crucial for minimizing false positives from transient or incidental movements.

The algorithm's effectiveness and accuracy are further refined through empirical testing of various binary threshold settings to identify the optimal configuration that accurately reflects true motion in specific environments. This tailored optimization is vital for adapting the system to meet the unique requirements and safety protocols necessary for monitoring scenarios, such as in care homes for the elderly, ensuring both security and comfort.

3.2. Anomaly Detection

Anomaly detection is a technique used to identify deviations from expected patterns, similar to outlier detection in machine learning. This method finds extensive applications in various sectors, such as intrusion detection in network systems, fraud detection in financial sectors, identification of health anomalies in medicine, and more [30]. Even though it is widely used, its integration into smart home technologies is still in its nascent stage. Anomaly detection addresses the challenges associated with the need for labeled data, as it effectively processes unbalanced or singular-class datasets. In this work, the anomaly detection model is designed to identify deviations from typical behavior patterns considered normal for each resident. This model is simpler than deep neural networks, making it easier to train and requiring less data. The main concept behind this model is to establish a normal activity profile for each resident based on their routine daily activities. This profile acts as a baseline for identifying any anomalous behavior.

To implement the anomaly detection, daily activity data were collected for each resident to develop a comprehensive profile of their normal behavior. This involved monitoring various activities throughout the day and capturing patterns of movement and interaction within the care environment. Once this profile is established, the anomaly detection model continuously monitors the incoming data against the established norms. When the system detects activities that deviate significantly from the normal profile, it flags these as anomalies. This real-time detection allows for immediate responses, where the system can generate alerts for caregivers or family members, prompting timely intervention.

This method is particularly effective in environments where individuals have consistent daily routines, making it easier to spot deviations that could indicate potential health issues or emergencies. The implementation of this anomaly detection model not only enhances the safety and well-being of the elderly residents by providing immediate alerts but also contributes to a more personalized approach to care as the system adjusts and learns from each individual's behavioral patterns.

4. Results and Analysis

4.1. Data Used in Experiments

To validate the proposed system, we conducted a pilot study in a simulated elderly care environment using volunteer participants. A total of four volunteers were recruited to perform daily activities and occasional anomaly events across four separate monitored rooms. Each room was equipped with cameras and infrared sensors integrated with our vision-based monitoring system. The volunteers were asked to perform a set of typical activities of daily living (ADL), including sitting, standing, walking, lying down, and moving between rooms, as well as to simulate abnormal scenarios such as prolonged inactivity, sudden falls, and absence from expected zones.

Across the sessions, over 150 h of continuous monitoring footage were recorded and analyzed. Data were collected over multiple sessions to ensure variability in lighting, room conditions, and participant behavior. No personal identifiable information was recorded, as privacy protection was a fundamental design aspect of our system. The monitoring relied solely on anonymized frame differencing outputs, where individuals were represented as motion contours rather than identifiable images.

This dataset allowed us to evaluate the system's ability to: (1) accurately detect motion and non-motion events; (2) identify deviations from normal activity patterns using anomaly detection algorithms; and (3) measure system robustness under different environmental conditions, such as lighting changes or background movements.

Although no formal numerical metrics were computed at this stage, qualitative validation was performed by manually cross-verifying system-generated activity logs against video footage, confirming that detected motion events and room transitions matched expected real-world behaviors.

4.2. System Workflow and Monitoring Process

The basic functionality of the proposed system system is depicted in the flow diagram as shown in Figure 2. The diagram shows a step-by-step process for monitoring, collecting data, and updating activity logs. As shown in the flow diagram, when monitoring begins, a new frame is received and processed for each room (Room 1 to Room 4). For each room, the system checks the frame for motion (frame differencing) and determines whether there is motion (True or False). This information is added to a rolling window if motion is detected, which likely represents an ongoing log or buffer. Subsequently, the activity log is updated, and the user interface (UI) is updated to reflect the new data.

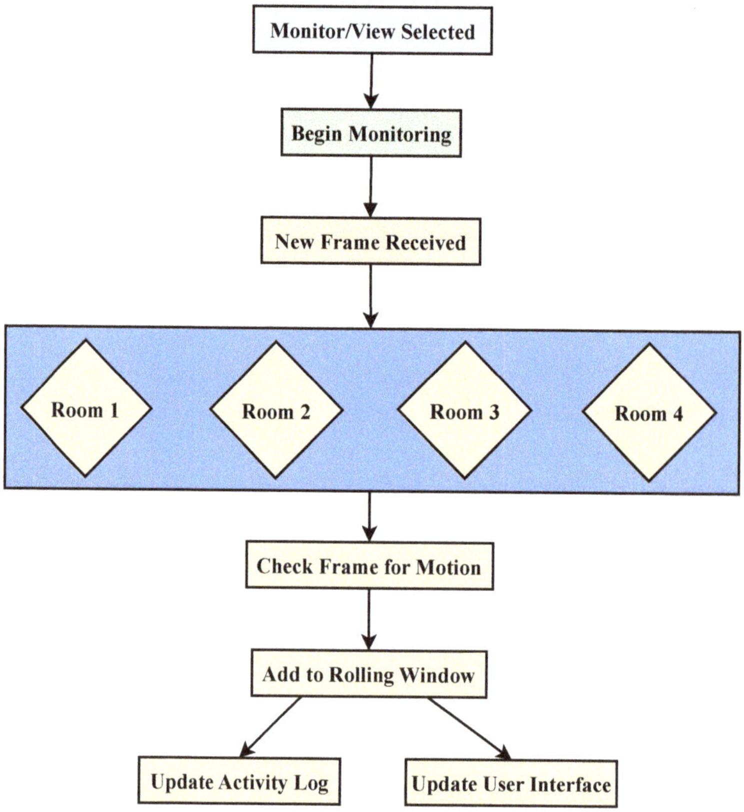

Figure 2. Schematic representation of the system's operational flow, illustrating the process from user-initiated monitoring to motion detection and data logging across multiple rooms.

In a care setting, it is crucial to have monitoring systems that can adapt to different environments and meet the specific needs of the care providers. To enhance its adaptability to various care settings, the system incorporates several adjustable parameters that allow fine-tuning of its operations. One such parameter is the activity update rate, which controls the temporal resolution of activity logging. A lower value means that activity is logged more frequently, capturing more detail about short-duration movements. A higher value would reduce the system's responsiveness but could be beneficial in reducing data storage requirements or minimizing the noise from insignificant movements.

Another critical adjustable feature is the detection threshold. The detection threshold is a crucial parameter for tuning the system's motion detection algorithm. A lower threshold makes the system highly responsive to even slight movements, which could be essential in scenarios where the safety of individuals is a priority. In contrast, a higher threshold reduces sensitivity, which might be suitable in environments where minor movements are not critical to detect or where there is a need to filter out false positives caused by incidental movements.

The detection threshold is used to facilitate frame differencing, where the image is divided into binary classes: pixels with unchanged frame values are set to 0 (black), indicating no motion, and pixels with different frame values are set to 1 (white), indicating motion. This binary segmentation is crucial as it distinctly highlights areas of movement. This parameter can also be used to tweak the motion detection sensitivity (1 being sensitive, 125 being less sensitive). This can be tuned in real-time while the application is running. The image shown in Figure 3 demonstrates frame differencing using a binary threshold value of 3. A lower threshold value is far more sensitive to detecting a difference between the frames, making overall motion detection more sensitive.

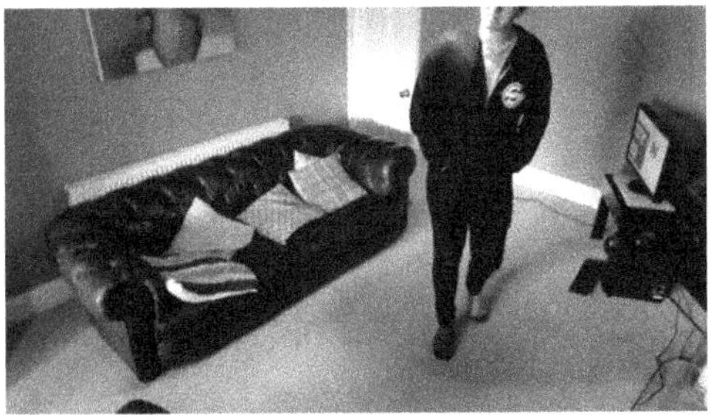

(**a**)

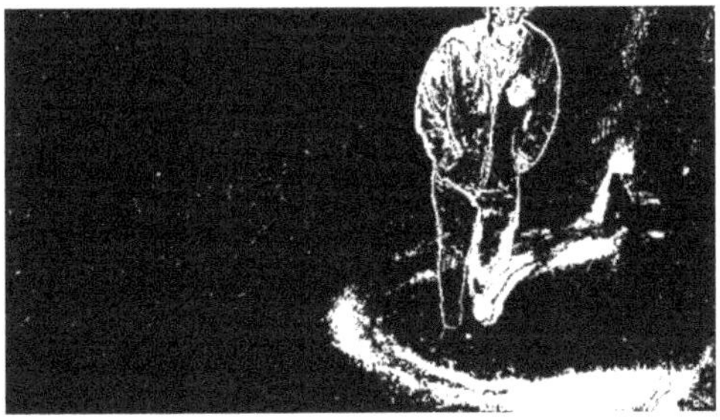

(**b**)

Figure 3. Illustration of the effect of detection threshold settings on motion detection outputs. (**a**) The original room environment. (**b**) Enhanced focus on relevant movements.

For our experiment, a binary threshold value of 16 was used. This value was determined to provide optimal performance for reliable motion detection in the demonstrated environment. It is important to note that this threshold value is not universally applicable; it will need to be adjusted and fine-tuned based on the specific requirements and conditions of each scenario to ensure the system functions effectively.

Lastly, the window length parameter adjusts the breadth of frame consideration. Increasing the window length parameter enhances the algorithm's robustness against false positives by considering a broader set of frames, thus allowing for a more reliable motion assessment. However, this parameter introduces a trade-off between the system's sensitivity and immunity to sporadic non-relevant movements. The array-based implementation facilitates a dynamic motion analysis across consecutive frames, providing a buffer that smooths out anomalies and ensures that detected motion is not an isolated incident but a consistent activity. These parameters collectively ensure that the system can be customized effectively, making it a versatile and reliable tool for enhancing the safety and monitoring capabilities within a smart care home.

4.3. Data Analysis

This subsection describes the data analysis modules of the system. The system provides a MonitorView module that is the heart of the application, encompassing advanced computer vision and motion detection capabilities. Users must first select a residence from the Residence page with a double-click action to access it. Upon selection, the user is directed to the MonitorView interface. Before initiating the monitoring process, the user must configure the system by visiting the settings page to select the appropriate video files intended for the motion detection test. Once the files are chosen, the user can start the motion detection scenario by clicking the green play button within the MonitorView, enabling the system to begin analyzing and detecting motion within the video feed.

In the proposed system, the data collection and analysis capabilities are demonstrated through the 'Motion Active' room display within the 'Overview' tab, as depicted in Figure 4. This interface provides an immediate and thorough understanding of an occupant's activities. It employs a donut chart for a lucid representation of time spent in various rooms, offering a quick visual interpretation of the occupant's spatial movements. The activity log, an integral part of this tab, catalogs detailed room activities alongside precise timestamps. This log is essential for granular analysis in the AnalysisView, where data stored in JSON format can be meticulously examined.

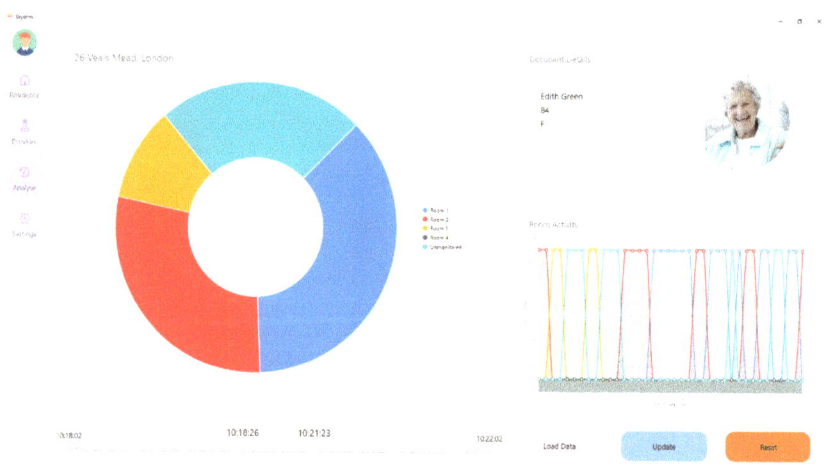

Figure 4. Data analysis of stored JSON file. The diagram shows the activities of one occupant/patient in different rooms.

Additionally, the system can monitor multiple rooms simultaneously via the 'Rooms' tab, as shown in Figure 5. Each active room is marked with a distinct green circle, enabling users to quickly identify areas of current activity. The real-time update functionality of these indicators is paramount for ensuring timely and accurate monitoring. This multi-room surveillance feature enhances the system's utility by providing a comprehensive view of the entire monitored space, which is crucial for complete situational awareness and prompt response to any irregular activities or emergencies.

In deploying and evaluating the proposed system, considerable attention was given to the privacy and anonymity of the real-time data collected from cameras within care homes. The system's user interface is designed with a selector switch that enables the toggling between the raw camera feed and the frame differencing video output, as shown in Figure 6.

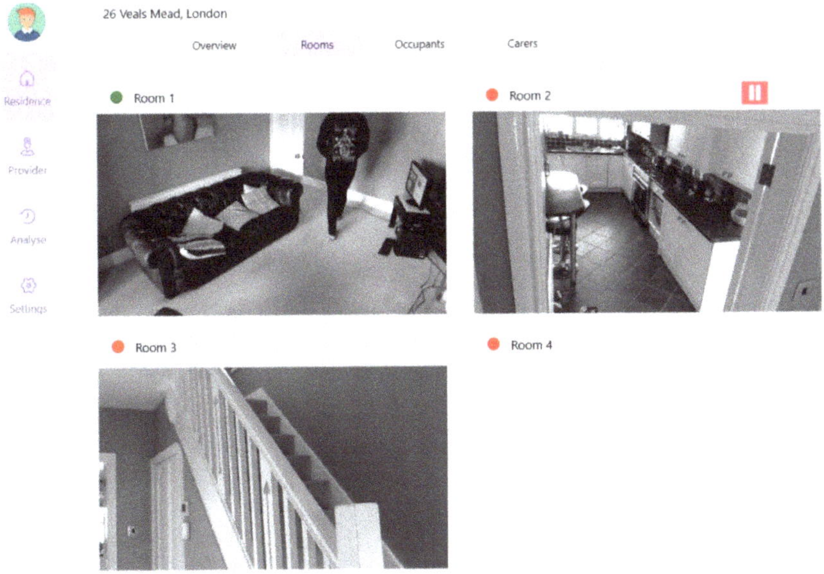

Figure 5. Simultaneous activity monitoring in differing rooms.

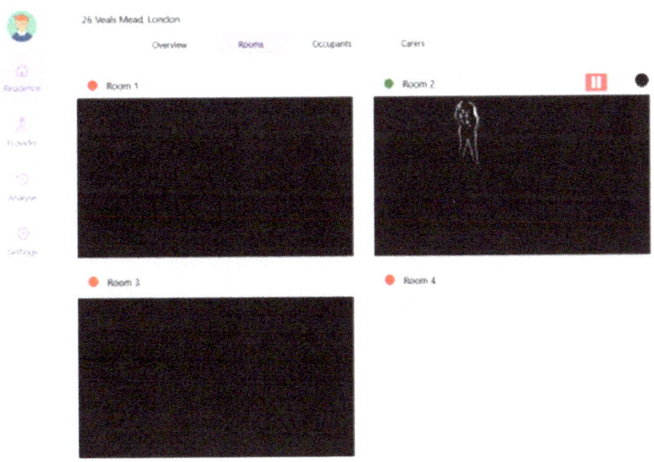

Figure 6. Toggling between the raw camera feed and the frame differencing video.

This feature played a crucial role during the testing phase, allowing us to validate the system's performance without compromising resident privacy. More importantly, this functionality lays the groundwork for future operational use, where any demonstration or review of the recorded footage can be conducted in a manner that maintains the anonymity of individuals. The frame differencing view abstracts the individuals into non-identifiable moving shapes, ensuring that the system can be used in real-world settings without infringing on personal privacy. This approach to data handling not only meets ethical standards but also aligns with legal privacy requirements, underscoring the system's applicability in sensitive environments where the dignity and rights of individuals are paramount.

A vital aspect of the developed system's utility is its sophisticated data visualization capabilities, which are essential in presenting complex data streams in an accessible manner. The system employs a sophisticated user interface for data analysis and visualization, designed to handle, display, and analyze the data collected during monitoring. Users can load data into the system, which then updates the UI to reflect the information in an interactive format. Features like adjustable sliders allow users to navigate through timestamps, facilitating detailed examination of specific events or periods. The AnalysisView system can reset and clear the UI, providing a fresh start for new data analysis without residual data from previous sessions. The Workflow of the Analysis View is depicted in Figure 7.

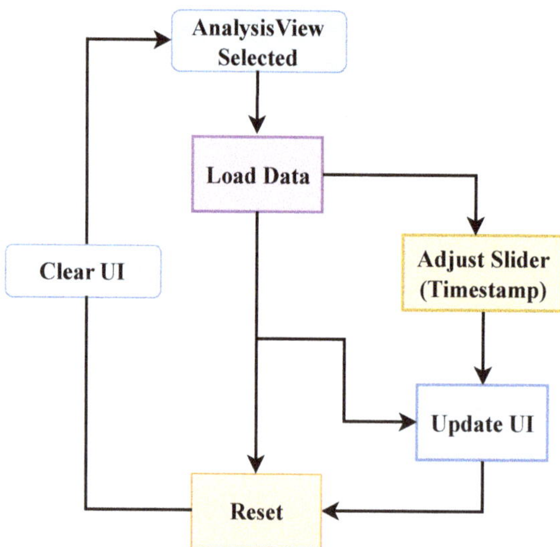

Figure 7. Data Handling and Visualization Workflow. The process begins with loading data into the system, which triggers updates to the user interface to reflect new information.

AnalysisView also supports extensive data handling capabilities. Data collected during monitoring sessions is stored in JSON format, containing detailed logs of activities along with associated metadata like timestamps and sensor readings. This format supports efficient data manipulation and retrieval, which is essential for analyzing long-term trends and immediate concerns in elderly care.

The combination of these algorithms and the AnalysisView interface equips caregivers and health professionals with the tools needed to monitor the well-being of elderly residents effectively, ensuring timely intervention and improved care outcomes. The detailed data flow through the AnalysisView interface and the precise steps involved in motion detection through frame differencing is crucial for understanding how the proposed system enhances elderly care through technology.

One of the primary visualization tools employed is the donut chart, which has proven highly effective for this application. This graphical representation offers an immediate overview of the distribution of an occupant's activities, identifying the rooms frequented over a user-defined period as shown in Figure 8a. Such a visual summary is invaluable for building activity profiles for occupants, particularly those living alone. By observing the proportion of time spent in various areas, caregivers can quickly discern normal patterns and, crucially, pinpoint any anomalies that may suggest changes in behavior or potential emergencies.

Additionally, the system uses line graphs to present motion data over time, offering a dynamic and temporal view of resident activities. Each entry in the graph signifies a motion event, categorized as either 'true' (1) or 'false' (0), allowing for a clear depiction of activity levels and movements throughout the care home. A particularly insightful feature of the line graph is its ability to trace the transitions between different rooms, adding a layer of context to the activity data as shown in Figure 8b. This not only aids in the immediate understanding of daily routines but also serves as a reliable record against which any deviations can be measured.

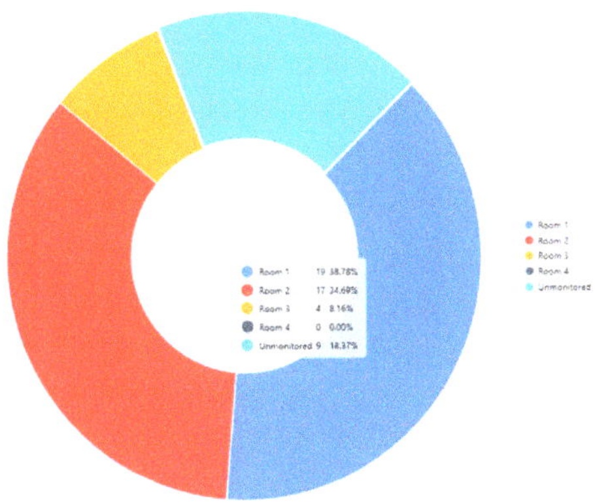

(**a**)

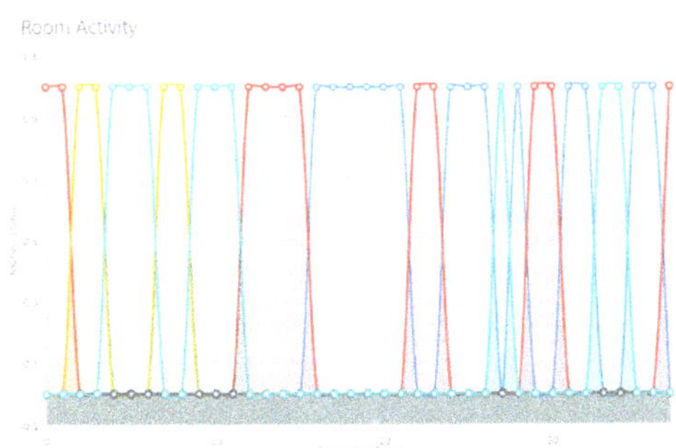

(**b**)

Figure 8. Data visualizations. (**a**) A donut chart representing the most frequently visited rooms within the last n period, where n is a user-defined parameter. (**b**) A line graph displaying a distinct record of the occupant's activity for the specified period.

During the testing phase, using pre-recorded scenarios, the line graphs were instrumental in validating the system's logs against expected outcomes. The exact match between the logged data and the footage's manual observations confirmed the motion detection's precision. The congruence between the visualized data and the actual events confirms the accuracy of the system's motion detection capabilities and its potential as a foundation for further development.

These visualization techniques simplify the interpretation of complex data for caregivers and underpin the system's potential for advanced applications, such as predictive analytics and deeper behavior analysis. By employing such intuitive data visualizations, the system ensures that critical information is conveyed effectively, supporting timely decision-making and enhancing the overall care experience within elderly care homes.

4.4. Comparative Analysis with Existing Methodologies

In the context of existing methodologies for elderly monitoring, many systems utilize complex machine learning models or deep neural networks that often require substantial computational resources and large volumes of labeled training data [11,13,17]. By contrast, the proposed system employs a lightweight frame differencing-based approach combined with anomaly detection, providing reliable motion detection without the need for extensive data preprocessing or model training.

While formal quantitative comparisons based on detection rates or false positive rates were not computed at this stage, internal qualitative validation demonstrated the system's capability to detect motion and room transitions accurately. Compared to vision-based systems such as depth-sensor approaches [16] and privacy-preserving avatar systems [17], our solution achieves a balance between real-time performance, user privacy, and operational simplicity, making it particularly suitable for deployment in resource-constrained elderly care environments. Future work will involve conducting formal benchmarking studies against other state-of-the-art solutions using standardized datasets and metrics.

5. Discussion

Camera-based Human Activity Recognition uses video or images captured by cameras to identify and categorize human activities. Unlike wearable or ambient sensors, which often lack detailed information, camera sensors can provide comprehensive data [31]. They can determine a person's location, environment, facial expressions, poses, gestures, and even mood. The implementation of the vision-based system in elderly care settings represents a critical evolution in monitoring technologies. It blends computer vision with anomaly detection to enhance residents' safety and independence [32]. These systems underscore the potential of integrating sophisticated monitoring solutions into traditional care practices to improve the monitoring of elderly activities.

Preliminary findings from the system's deployment show that it can identify daily activities and detect deviations from established behavioral patterns. These features are essential for anticipating potential emergencies and enhancing the overall management of elderly care. Importantly, the use of simple anomaly detection models instead of complex deep learning-based approaches is a deliberate design choice. In elderly care environments, lightweight algorithms provide critical advantages: they reduce computational demands, minimize system maintenance complexity, improve interpretability for caregivers, and allow real-time operation without sacrificing accuracy. Using simple anomaly detection models in place of more complex machine learning or neural network-based algorithms ensures that the system remains efficient and user-friendly, reducing computational requirements while maintaining a high level of accuracy.

This purposeful simplicity also supports privacy preservation, as it eliminates the need to store or process large volumes of sensitive video data, relying instead on anonymized motion-based outputs. Furthermore, by avoiding deep learning models that require extensive labeled datasets and continuous retraining, the proposed system achieves greater robustness and scalability for practical deployment across multiple care settings.

A critical aspect of the system's functionality is the adjustability of parameters such as the activity update rate, detection threshold, and window length. These parameters are essential as they allow the system to be finely tuned to suit the specific environmental conditions and care needs. For example, adjusting the activity update rate can help manage the volume of data logged, enhancing the focus on significant movements rather than minor or irrelevant ones. Similarly, the detection threshold is vital for tailoring the system's sensitivity, enabling it to detect subtle movements critical in high-risk situations or to avoid false alarms in less dynamic environments.

Furthermore, the binary threshold and window length adjustments play a significant role in activity recognition accuracy. They ensure that only meaningful activities are recorded and analyzed, reducing the likelihood of false positives and enhancing the system's reliability. Such adaptability improves the system's performance and applicability across various care settings, demonstrating a versatile approach to elderly care. Despite these advancements, the proposed system may face challenges in implementing new technologies in sensitive environments. Variations in individual behaviors and the dynamic nature of care settings can sometimes affect the accuracy of the readings, leading to potential false positives or missed detections. These issues highlight the need for ongoing refinements and algorithm adjustments based on continuous feedback and accumulated data.

Limitations

While the proposed system demonstrates practical applicability and strong performance in simulated care environments, several limitations exist. First, the current validation is based on qualitative analysis using pre-recorded scenarios, and no formal numerical evaluation (e.g., detection accuracy, false positive rate) has yet been conducted using annotated ground truth datasets. Second, the system has not been directly compared against other existing motion detection or fall detection frameworks due to the prototype nature of the work and limited access to standardized datasets. Third, while the algorithm is lightweight and well-suited for privacy-conscious environments, more complex behaviors may not be accurately captured without the integration of advanced learning techniques. Future work will focus on real-world deployment, quantitative benchmarking, and evaluation against state-of-the-art systems.

6. Conclusions and Future Work

This study presents an unobtrusive monitoring system for elderly people in care settings. The system uses advanced computer vision techniques and anomaly detection algorithms to monitor elderly people in care settings. The system tracks daily activities and intelligently analyzes patterns to identify deviations from normal routines. The system logs these events, which can be visualized later for further analysis. The real-time notifications allow immediate intervention when potential health risks are detected, significantly reducing response times and potentially preventing emergencies. The system's effectiveness in a real-world setting has set the stage for further advancements in the field. Future work will focus on refining the accuracy of the algorithms to decrease the likelihood of false positives and increase the system's reliability. Integration with additional sensor data, such as wearable devices or environmental sensors, could provide valuable context for activity recognition and anomaly detection. Furthermore, exploring advanced machine learning techniques, including deep learning and reinforcement learning, may unlock new insights and predictive capabilities within the system.

Author Contributions: Conceptualization, R.U., I.A. and J.V.; methodology, G.E.; software, G.E.; validation, R.U., I.A., J.V. and G.E.; formal analysis, J.V.; investigation R.U., I.A., S.A., A.A. and A.B., resources, J.V.; data curation, G.E. and J.V.; writing—original draft preparation, R.U., I.A. and S.A.; writing—review and editing, R.U., I.A., S.A., A.A. and A.B.; visualization, R.U., I.A. and S.A.; supervision, J.V.; project administration, J.V. All authors have read and agreed to the published version of the manuscript.

Funding: The European Regional Development Fund (ERDF) and the Welsh Government funded this project. The expert knowledge sharing by CEMET and Skystrm colleagues is also acknowledged.

Institutional Review Board Statement: Ethical review and approval were waived for this study due to the fully anonymized nature of the dataset and the absence of sensitive personal information. All participants provided informed consent for their anonymized data to be used in research, in accordance with our organization's data privacy policies.

Informed Consent Statement: Informed consent was obtained from all subjects involved in the study.

Data Availability Statement: The data presented in this study are available on request from the corresponding author due to privacy concerns.

Conflicts of Interest: Author Justus Vermaak was employed by the company Skystrm Limited. The remaining authors declare that the research was conducted in the absence of any commercial or financial relationships that could be construed as a potential conflict of interest.

References

1. Tan, M.P. Healthcare for older people in lower and middle income countries. *Age Ageing* **2022**, *51*, afac016. [CrossRef] [PubMed]
2. Saied, I.; Alzaabi, A.; Arslan, T. Unobtrusive Sensors for Synchronous Monitoring of Different Breathing Parameters in Care Environments. *Sensors* **2024**, *24*, 2233. [CrossRef] [PubMed]
3. Maresova, P.; Krejcar, O.; Maskuriy, R.; Bakar, N.A.A.; Selamat, A.; Truhlarova, Z.; Horak, J.; Joukl, M.; Vítkova, L. Challenges and opportunity in mobility among older adults–key determinant identification. *BMC Geriatr.* **2023**, *23*, 447. [CrossRef]
4. Awotunde, J.B.; Ayoade, O.B.; Ajamu, G.J.; AbdulRaheem, M.; Oladipo, I.D. Internet of things and cloud activity monitoring systems for elderly healthcare. In *Internet of Things for Human-Centered Design: Application to Elderly Healthcare*; Springer: Singapore, 2022; pp. 181–207.
5. Hussain, A.; Khan, S.U.; Rida, I.; Khan, N.; Baik, S.W. Human centric attention with deep multiscale feature fusion framework for activity recognition in Internet of Medical Things. *Inf. Fusion* **2024**, *106*, 102211. [CrossRef]
6. Eyiokur, F.I.; Kantarcı, A.; Erakın, M.E.; Damer, N.; Ofli, F.; Imran, M.; Križaj, J.; Salah, A.A.; Waibel, A.; Štruc, V.; et al. A survey on computer vision based human analysis in the COVID-19 era. *Image Vis. Comput.* **2023**, *130*, 104610. [CrossRef]
7. Asghar, I.; Ullah, R.; Griffiths, M.G.; Evans, G.; Vermaak, J. Skystrm: An Activity Monitoring System to Support Elderly Independence Through Smart Care Homes. In Proceedings of the 2023 6th Conference on Cloud and Internet of Things (CIoT), Lisbon, Portugal, 20–22 March 2023; pp. 119–126.
8. Bhola, G.; Vishwakarma, D.K. A review of vision-based indoor HAR: State-of-the-art, challenges, and future prospects. *Multimed. Tools Appl.* **2024**, *83*, 1965–2005. [CrossRef]
9. Ullah, R.; Arslan, T. PySpark-based optimization of microwave image reconstruction algorithm for head imaging big data on high-performance computing and Google cloud platform. *Appl. Sci.* **2020**, *10*, 3382. [CrossRef]
10. Ke, S.R.; Thuc, H.L.U.; Lee, Y.J.; Hwang, J.N.; Yoo, J.H.; Choi, K.H. A review on video-based human activity recognition. *Computers* **2013**, *2*, 88–131. [CrossRef]
11. Cristina, S.; Despotovic, V.; Pérez-Rodríguez, R.; Aleksic, S. Audio-and Video-based Human Activity Recognition Systems in Healthcare. *IEEE Access* **2024**, *12*, 8230–8245. [CrossRef]
12. Sinha, K.P.; Kumar, P. Human activity recognition from UAV videos using a novel DMLC-CNN model. *Image Vis. Comput.* **2023**, *134*, 104674. [CrossRef]
13. Karácsony, T.; Jeni, L.A.; De la Torre, F.; Cunha, J.P.S. Deep learning methods for single camera based clinical in-bed movement action recognition. *Image Vis. Comput.* **2024**, *143*, 104928. [CrossRef]

14. Ghali, A.; Cunningham, A.S.; Pridmore, T.P. Object and event recognition for stroke rehabilitation. In Proceedings of the Visual Communications and Image Processing 2003, Lugano, Switzerland, 8–11 July 2003; Volume 5150, pp. 980–989.
15. Gaikwad, S.; Bhatlawande, S.; Shilaskar, S.; Solanke, A. A computer vision-approach for activity recognition and residential monitoring of elderly people. *Med. Nov. Technol. Devices* **2023**, *20*, 100272. [CrossRef]
16. Jalal, A.; Kamal, S.; Kim, D. A depth video sensor-based life-logging human activity recognition system for elderly care in smart indoor environments. *Sensors* **2014**, *14*, 11735–11759. [CrossRef]
17. Wang, C.Y.; Lin, F.S. AI-driven privacy in elderly care: Developing a comprehensive solution for camera-based monitoring of older adults. *Appl. Sci.* **2024**, *14*, 4150. [CrossRef]
18. Gillani, N.; Arslan, T. Intelligent sensing technologies for the diagnosis, monitoring and therapy of alzheimer's disease: A systematic review. *Sensors* **2021**, *21*, 4249. [CrossRef]
19. Majumder, S.; Aghayi, E.; Noferesti, M.; Memarzadeh-Tehran, H.; Mondal, T.; Pang, Z.; Deen, M.J. Smart homes for elderly healthcare—Recent advances and research challenges. *Sensors* **2017**, *17*, 2496. [CrossRef]
20. Jang, I.Y.; Kim, H.R.; Lee, E.; Jung, H.W.; Park, H.; Cheon, S.H.; Lee, Y.S.; Park, Y.R. Impact of a wearable device-based walking programs in rural older adults on physical activity and health outcomes: Cohort study. *JMIR MHealth UHealth* **2018**, *6*, e11335. [CrossRef] [PubMed]
21. Smirnova, E.; Leroux, A.; Cao, Q.; Tabacu, L.; Zipunnikov, V.; Crainiceanu, C.; Urbanek, J.K. The predictive performance of objective measures of physical activity derived from accelerometry data for 5-year all-cause mortality in older adults: National Health and Nutritional Examination Survey 2003–2006. *J. Gerontol. Ser. A* **2020**, *75*, 1779–1785. [CrossRef] [PubMed]
22. Jiang, Y.; Zeng, K.; Yang, R. Wearable device use in older adults associated with physical activity guideline recommendations: Empirical research quantitative. *J. Clin. Nurs.* **2023**, *32*, 6374–6383. [CrossRef]
23. Zhang, S.; Li, Y.; Zhang, S.; Shahabi, F.; Xia, S.; Deng, Y.; Alshurafa, N. Deep learning in human activity recognition with wearable sensors: A review on advances. *Sensors* **2022**, *22*, 1476. [CrossRef]
24. Bhattacharya, D.; Sharma, D.; Kim, W.; Ijaz, M.F.; Singh, P.K. Ensem-HAR: An ensemble deep learning model for smartphone sensor-based human activity recognition for measurement of elderly health monitoring. *Biosensors* **2022**, *12*, 393. [CrossRef] [PubMed]
25. Umer, M.; Alarfaj, A.A.; Alabdulqader, E.A.; Alsubai, S.; Cascone, L.; Narducci, F. Enhancing fall prediction in the elderly people using LBP features and transfer learning model. *Image Vis. Comput.* **2024**, *145*, 104992. [CrossRef]
26. Zi, X.; Chaturvedi, K.; Braytee, A.; Li, J.; Prasad, M. Detecting human falls in poor lighting: Object detection and tracking approach for indoor safety. *Electronics* **2023**, *12*, 1259. [CrossRef]
27. Hussain, A.; Khan, S.U.; Khan, N.; Rida, I.; Alharbi, M.; Baik, S.W. Low-light aware framework for human activity recognition via optimized dual stream parallel network. *Alex. Eng. J.* **2023**, *74*, 569–583. [CrossRef]
28. Teixeira, E.; Fonseca, H.; Diniz-Sousa, F.; Veras, L.; Boppre, G.; Oliveira, J.; Pinto, D.; Alves, A.J.; Barbosa, A.; Mendes, R.; et al. Wearable devices for physical activity and healthcare monitoring in elderly people: A critical review. *Geriatrics* **2021**, *6*, 38. [CrossRef]
29. Yu, Y.; Wang, J.; Li, N. Foreground and background separated image style transfer with a single text condition. *Image Vis. Comput.* **2024**, *143*, 104956. [CrossRef]
30. Galvão, Y.M.; Castro, L.; Ferreira, J.; Neto, F.B.d.L.; Fagundes, R.A.d.A.; Fernandes, B.J. Anomaly Detection in Smart Houses for Healthcare: Recent Advances, and Future Perspectives. *SN Comput. Sci.* **2024**, *5*, 136. [CrossRef]
31. Kolkar, R.; Geetha, V. Issues and challenges in various sensor-based modalities in human activity recognition system. In *Applications of Advanced Computing in Systems: Proceedings of International Conference on Advances in Systems, Control and Computing*; Springer: Singapore, 2021; pp. 171–179.
32. Zhang, Y.; Liang, W.; Yuan, X.; Zhang, S.; Yang, G.; Zeng, Z. Deep Learning Based Abnormal Behavior Detection for Elderly Healthcare Using Consumer Network Cameras. *IEEE Trans. Consum. Electron.* **2023**, *70*, 2414–2422. [CrossRef]

technologies

MDPI

Article

The Impact of Real-World Interaction on the Perception of a Humanoid Social Robot in Care for Institutionalised Older Adults

Slawomir Tobis [1,*], Joanna Piasek-Skupna [2], Aleksandra Suwalska [3] and Katarzyna Wieczorowska-Tobis [4,5]

[1] Department of Occupational Therapy, Poznan University of Medical Sciences, 60-781 Poznan, Poland
[2] Institute of Robotics and Machine Intelligence, Poznan University of Technology, 60-965 Poznan, Poland; joanna.piasek-skupna@put.poznan.pl
[3] Department of Mental Health, Chair of Psychiatry, Poznan University of Medical Sciences, 60-572 Poznan, Poland; asuwalska@ump.edu.pl
[4] Chair and Department of Palliative Medicine, Poznan University of Medical Sciences, 61-245 Poznan, Poland; kwt@tobis.pl
[5] Department of Human Nutrition and Dietetics, Poznan University of Life Sciences, 60-624 Poznan, Poland
* Correspondence: stobis@ump.edu.pl

Abstract: (1) Background: For the residents of long-term care (LTC) units, a humanoid social robot (HSR) may be not only a caregiver but also a companion. The aim of our study was to analyse changes in its perception following a real-world interaction; (2) Methods: One hundred LTC residents were assessed twice with the Godspeed Questionnaire Series (GQS): after viewing a photograph of HSR TIAGo only and after interacting with it in a practical manner. The perception parameters were evaluated on a scale of 1–5 in five series: I-*Anthropomorphism*, II-*Animation*, III-*Likeability*, IV-*Perceived intelligence*, and V-*Perceived safety*. (3) Results: In the post-interaction assessment of the TIAGo robot, no lower scores were observed relative to the first (photo-based) scoring. Positive changes were observed in III ($p < 0.001$), I ($p < 0.01$), II ($p < 0.05$), and IV ($p < 0.05$). In multivariable analysis, high levels of loneliness constituted a correlate for improvement after interaction in I ($p < 0.05$); computer skills—in III ($p < 0.01$), and GDS score corresponding to depression—in IV ($p < 0.01$). (4) Conclusions: Our study reveals a positive change in older people's perception of an HSR after interacting with it. Interaction is thus an indispensable element in the development process. Developers and implementers should pay particular attention to the robot's smart functions, movements, and responsiveness.

Keywords: humanoid robot; social robot; robot perception; robot acceptance; correlates; long-term care

1. Introduction

For various reasons, many people face the necessity of relocating to a care institution at some point [1]. In most instances, this procedure cannot be described as easy to accept. Upon moving in, older individuals begin the process of establishing their homes within the new environment. Four factors associated with this transition have been identified as particularly crucial: continuity, the preservation of personal identity, a sense of belonging, and the ability to remain active and engaged in work [2]. Meeting these needs can prove complex, as the institutional structure of long-term care (LTC) settings has been shown to influence the functioning of older individuals and their decision-making processes [3]. The restriction of autonomy perpetuates the stereotype of LTC residents as passive [4]. Their perceived lack of control often leads to a sense of powerlessness [5], which is especially evident among those with dementia [6], many of whom report experiencing a poor quality of life [7]. These challenges underscore the inherent issues within LTC units that require attention. Furthermore, the growing populations of older adults and the simultaneous decline in the number of younger individuals in contemporary societies—not limited to developed countries—contribute to an expanding care gap (a growing insufficiency in the availability of both formal and informal caregivers). LTC systems worldwide, especially in the aftermath of the COVID-19 pandemic, are struggling with inadequate staffing levels [8]. Consequently, it is imperative to explore and implement novel solutions that, among other goals, can contribute to optimising the time budgets of LTC employees. While staff members regard non-pharmacological interventions as vital for enhancing resident care, there has been relatively little discourse on the implementation of innovative interventions or technologies, highlighting the need to raise awareness in this area [9]. This calls for novel approaches to efficient and ethical LTC. The application of new technologies [10], including social robots [11], in care for older adults presents a promising solution, particularly when these technologies are perceived as reasonable, appropriate, and easy to use by prospective users [12].

The barriers, facilitators, and intentions associated with the use of humanoid social robots (HSRs) in care have been extensively studied, including by our team [13–19] (e.g., consistently worse attitudes of formal caregivers than those of older adults). A systematic review conducted by Papadopoulos et al. [20] found that many of the enablers (enjoyment, personalisation, and familiarisation), as well as barriers (limited capabilities and negative preconceptions), are related to the perception of the robot. Among the conclusions drawn, key insights touch on the acceptance of proposed solutions. We have demonstrated that assessing potential users' needs and requirements and providing opportunities for tangible interaction with the robot is essential, as this interaction influences factors related to acceptance [21]. We have also highlighted that the perception of the robot is of central importance when considering its various potential roles and functions [22]. Therefore, the aim of this study was to analyse changes in the perception of an HSR resulting from the opportunity to experience its operation, investigate the correlates of these changes, and discuss their implications for the implementation of robotic solutions in LTC. The first research question was thus: does interaction with an HSR influence the perception of its usefulness, acceptability, and implementation potential in LTC facilities? The second research question was: what are the correlates of change of perception of the robot? Based on these questions, we formulated six hypotheses.

In contrast to the Pepper robot, which features articulated arms and a skirt-shaped base [23], our TIAGo robot did not possess a human-like body or extremities. Consequently, we hypothesise that this absence of anthropomorphic features will negatively influence anthropomorphism-related parameters (H1). Animacy is typically characterised by an agent's capacity to act autonomously, as opposed to being passively controlled [24]. This distinction may account for the lower animacy ratings observed for static robots such as Furhat in comparison to mobile robots like Pepper or NAO [25]. Therefore, as the TIAGo robot is capable of autonomous activity, we expect that interaction with TIAGo will result in an increased animacy score (H2). The robot's appearance is recognised as an important factor of its likeability [26]; however, older adults may prefer its functionality over appearance [27]. Accordingly, we anticipate that direct interaction with the TIAGo robot will similarly enhance likeability ratings among older adults in our study, particularly due to the hands-on availability of its various functions (H3). Perceived intelligence in robots is contingent upon their demonstrated competence. Given the technological constraints of the TIAGo platform, we postulate that perceived intelligence will remain unchanged following interaction with the robot (H4). Finally, perceived safety is influenced by the robot's physical size; larger robots may be viewed as less safe [25]. Therefore, we hypothesise that the substantial size of the TIAGo robot will not positively affect perceived safety following interaction (H5). Furthermore, as we showed previously that attitudes toward the robot were not correlated with sociodemographic factors, self-assessment scores or selected items of the Comprehensive Geriatric Assessment [28], we expect that there will be no universal correlates of the perception of the robot (H6).

2. Materials and Methods

2.1. Research Methodology

The study model allowed for a comparison of perceptions of the HSR TIAGo (PAL Robotics, Spain) after viewing a photograph and following direct interaction. Ethical approval for this study was granted by the Bioethics Committee of Poznan University of Medical Sciences under Protocol No. 711/18.

2.2. Study Group

This study involved older individuals (aged 60 years and above) from six LTC homes in the Greater Poland region. Initially, informational sessions were held to explain the aims of the project. All residents who expressed interest were screened for functional capacity, which included assessments of basic activities of daily living (ADL) using the Barthel Index (BI) [29], cognitive functions using the Mini-Mental State Examination (MMSE) [30], and mood using the Geriatric Depression Scale (GDS) [31]. Additionally, participants completed a questionnaire containing demographic data (age, gender assigned at birth, education) and declarative self-assessment items rated on a 1–5 scale. These items included the following:

- Computer skills (1—no skills, 5—excellent skills);
- Ease of use of technology (1—extreme difficulty/lack of ability, 5—no issues with new technologies);
- Health status (1—the worst possible, 5—the best health condition);
- Physical fitness (1—the worst possible, 5—the highest possible independence);
- Loneliness (1—no loneliness, 5—extreme loneliness).

2.3. Ethical Considerations

For ethical reasons, all interested individuals participated in the subsequent stages of the meeting; however, the analysis of results included only those participants who scored at least 15 points on the MMSE, which is considered to indicate the ability to engage in logical communication, understand questions, and provide appropriate responses [32,33]. The subjects were also verbally asked whether they would like to express any ethical reservations about this study.

2.4. The TIAGo Robot

We used a customised version of the TIAGo robot that incorporated several sensors (an RGB-D camera, a thermal camera, RFID equipment, a laser scanner, various environment sensors, and radar distance sensors), a microphone, a loudspeaker, and a tablet for communication with the user, mounted on the robot's chest section. The robot was wirelessly coupled with a remote computer and connected to the Internet. It was able to navigate in a semi-autonomous manner or follow the user based on the thermal sensor. The options available during the interaction included reminders, safety measures, dietary recommendations, physical exercises, cognitive games, video connectivity (e.g., for contacting friends), and the provision of news and weather. Presentation of environmental values based on local and networked sensors (temperature, humidity, air pressure, air quality, etc.) was also accessible.

2.5. Procedure

After participants viewed a photograph of the TIAGo, they expressed their opinions on its perception for the first time. They were then given the opportunity to interact with the robot in person for as long as they deemed necessary (Figure 1). A detailed description of the presentation can be found in a previous publication [20]. The interaction lasted from approximately 90 to 150 min (the duration was determined by the number of participating subjects and their interest in operating the robot). The final stage of the meeting involved a re-assessment of the participants' perceptions of the robot, taking into account their interaction experience.

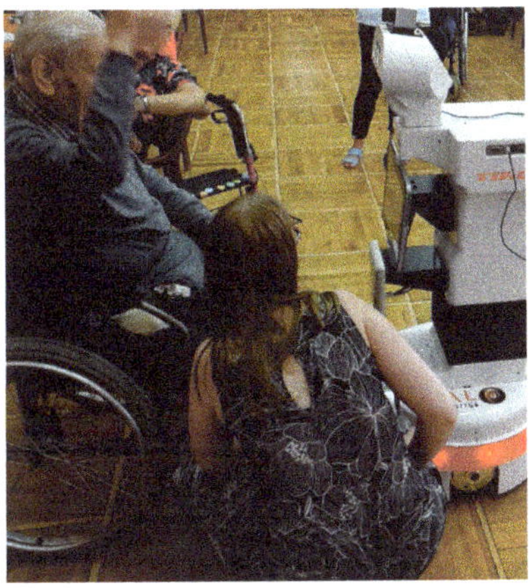

Figure 1. The interaction of long-term care home residents with HSR TIAGo.

The Godspeed Questionnaire Series (GQS) was employed to assess robot perceptions. The Polish-language version of the questionnaire was validated in a separate study [22]. The GQS consists of five series of terms related to the robot: 1—*Anthropomorphism*, 2—*Animacy*, 3—*Likeability*, 4—*Perceived intelligence*, and 5—*Perceived safety*. Each item is rated using five-point semantic differentials with opposing terms. Respondents are asked to rate each category on a scale from 1–5 (e.g., *Dead* (1) vs. *Alive* (5) from the *Animacy* series).

In this study, we also analysed factors that could potentially influence perception, including the following:

- Demographic data (age, gender, education);
- Self-assessment (subjective) items;
- Objective data on functional capacity (cognitive functions, presence of depressive symptoms, and ADL performance).

2.6. Statistical Analysis

Statistical analysis was conducted using STATISTICA 13.3 software (StatSoft, Poland). The results were presented as means, standard deviations, and medians due to the non-normal distribution of some variables, verified using the Shapiro–Wilk test.

The perceptions of the robot, as assessed after viewing the photograph and after interaction (paired data), were compared using the Wilcoxon test. Differences for individual parameters were analysed using the χ^2 test, considering the following:

- Demographic data: age (60–79 years vs. 80+), gender (F vs. M), and education (less than secondary vs. at least secondary);
- Self-assessment items: scores below the central value vs. scores equal to or greater than the central value (i.e., 1–2 vs. 3–5, except for loneliness, where 4–5 vs. 1–3 was used, as 5 represents the most negative score);
- Objective data on functional capacity:
    - Cognitive function assessment via the MMSE scale: participants with at least 24 points (indicating no more than mild cognitive impairment) vs. those with a lower score;
    - Depression symptom assessment via the GDS scale: participants scoring up to 5 points vs. those with a higher score;
    - ADL performance on the Barthel scale: participants with scores below 80 vs. those scoring at least 80.

A multiple regression model (logistic regression) was employed to assess simultaneous interdependence between variables, yielding the odds ratio (OR) and the confidence interval (CI) with a 95% confidence limit. All variables found to be significant in the univariable analysis were included in the multiple linear regression analysis. A p-value of <0.05 was considered statistically significant, while p-values between 0.05 and 0.10 were interpreted as indicative of non-significant trends.

3. Results

This study involved 100 older adults (aged 60 years or more), with a mean age of 76.6 $\pm$ 8.9 years (median 75.5 years; the oldest participant was 94 years old). Of these, 47 respondents were aged 75 years or older. There were 53 women among the participants. The largest group (41 participants) had completed secondary education, while only nine held a university degree.

The mean declared computer skills score was 1.6 $\pm$ 1.3 (median 1.0), with 79 participants reporting no skills and only eight indicating excellent skills. The mean score for ease of use of technology was considerably higher at 3.0 $\pm$ 1.6 (median 3.0), as only 31 participants reported a lack of abilities, while 25 indicated no problems with technology.

The mean value of the respondents' self-assessment of health was 3.0 $\pm$ 1.1 (median 3.0), with 13 participants giving the lowest and eight people—the highest rating. The mean score for physical fitness was 3.2 $\pm$ 1.2 (median 3.0), with the lowest and highest ratings provided by nine and 15 participants, respectively. Regarding declared loneliness, the mean score was 2.6 $\pm$ 1.6 (median 2.5), with 18 subjects indicating extreme loneliness and 41 reporting no loneliness.

The mean BI score was 77.0 $\pm$ 23.4 (median 85.0). No participant scored between 0 and 20 points (indicating total dependency), and 21 subjects achieved the maximum score of 100 points, indicating no limitations in independence. The mean score on the MMSE was 23.3 $\pm$ 4.1 (median 23.5). Fifty participants scored below 24, suggesting advanced cognitive impairment, with 21 scoring between 15 and 19 points. Thirty-one subjects scored within the normal range (27–30 points). The mean GDS score was 3.9 $\pm$ 2.9 (median 3.0), with 75 participants scoring within the range indicating no depressive symptoms (1–5 points). The remaining participants had higher scores, with three individuals presenting symptoms of severe depression (GDS score of 11 points or above).

3.1. The Impact of Interaction with the TIAGo Robot on GQS Results

No perception scores were lower on any parameter or GQS series in the post-interaction assessments compared to those based on the robot's photograph. Mean perception scores for all series were higher after the interaction, except for the *Perceived Safety* series (mean ± SD; median: 3.7 ± 0.9; 3.7 vs. 3.9 ± 0.9; 4.0)—see Figure 2.

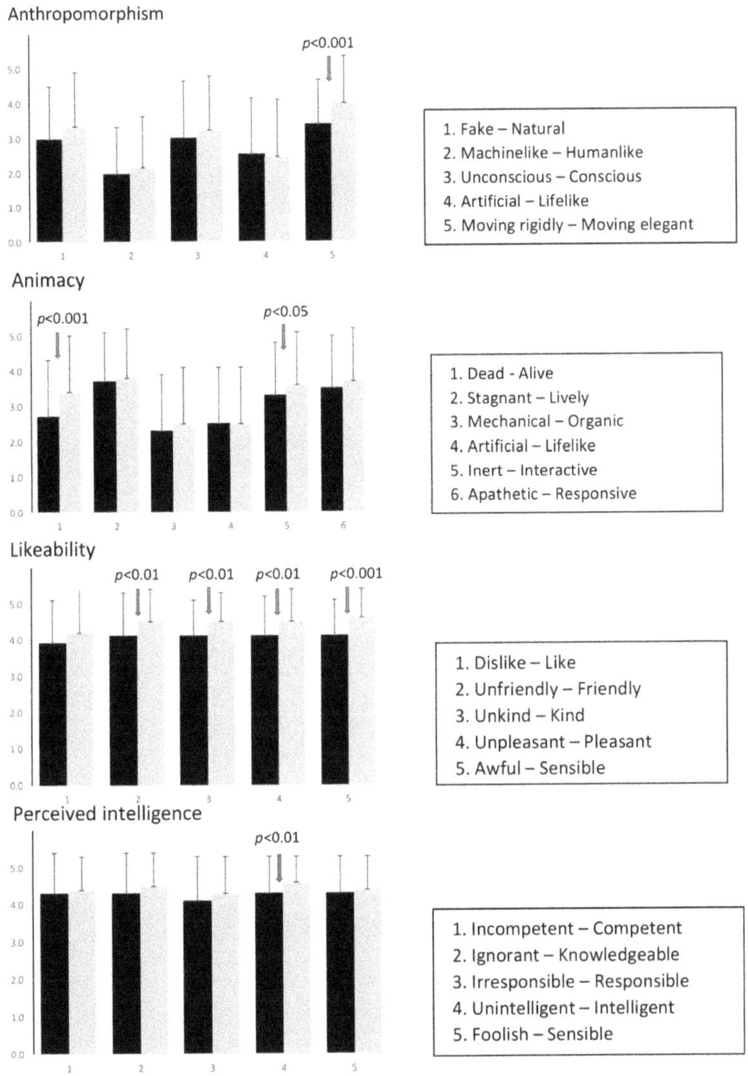

Figure 2. The impact of interaction with the TIAGo robot on the perception of the robot by older people in the GQS assessment (black bars indicate results before, and grey bars indicate after interaction).

The most substantial changes were observed in the *Likeability* series (4.1 ± 0.9; 4.2 vs. 4.4 ± 0.8; 4.8; $p < 0.001$). These changes were related to changes in ratings for all components of the parameters in this series, with the exception of the *Dislike–Like* item, for which an insignificant trend was observed (3.9 ± 1.2; 4 vs. 4.2 ± 1.3; 5; $p = 0.058$). Specifically, significant increases were noted in the following parameters: *Unfriendly–*

Friendly (4.1 ± 1.2; 4.5 vs. 4.5 ± 0.9; 5.0; $p < 0.01$), *Unkind–Kind* (4.1 ± 1.0; 4.6 vs. 4.5 ± 0.8; 5.0; $p < 0.01$), *Unpleasant–Pleasant* (4.1 ± 1.1; 5.0 vs. 4.5 ± 0.9; 5.0; $p < 0.01$), and *Awful–Nice* (4.1 ± 1.0; 4.0 vs. 4.6 ± 0.8; 5.0; $p < 0.001$).

In the *Anthropomorphism* series (2.8 ± 1.0; 2.8 vs. 3.0 ± 1.0; 3.0; $p < 0.01$), the higher perception was primarily linked to a change in the perception of the robot's movement parameter (*Moving rigidly* vs. *Moving elegantly*: 3.4 ± 1.3; 3.0 vs. 4.0 ± 1.4; 5.0; $p < 0.0001$) as no significant changes were noted for other parameters (*Machinelike–Humanlike*: 2.0 ± 1.4; 1.0 vs. 2.2 ± 1.5; 1.0, *Unconscious–Conscious:* 3.0 ± 1.6; 3.0 vs. 3.2 ± 1.5; 3.0, *Artificial–Lifelike*: 2.5 ± 1.6; 3.0 vs. 2.5 ± 1.5; 3.0). For the *Fake–Natural* item, an insignificant trend was noted (3.0 ± 1.5; 3.0 vs. 3.3 ± 1.0; 3.0; $p = 0.0896$).

Significantly higher perception scores were also recorded for the *Animacy* series (3.0 ± 0.9; 2.8 vs. 3.3 ± 1.0; 3.3; $p < 0.01$), primarily driven by a change in the *Dead–Alive* item (2.7 ± 1.6; 3 vs. 3.3 ± 1.6; 4; $p < 0.001$), and the *Inert–Interactive* parameter (3.3 ± 1.6; 3 vs. 3.6 ± 1.5; 4; $p < 0.05$). No changes were observed for the remaining parameters.

The mean score of the *Perceived Intelligence* series was also higher (4.2 ± 0.9; 4.6 vs. 4.4 ± 0.7; 4.8; $p < 0.05$), primarily due to an increase in the *Unintelligent–Intelligent* item (4.3 ± 1.0; 5 vs. 4.6 ± 0.7; 5; $p < 0.01$). For other items, no significant changes were noted.

3.2. Correlates of Change in Perception of the TIAGo Robot After Interacting with It

The frequency of higher perception of the TIAGo robot following interaction, compared to perception based on the photograph, with a distinction between the analysed parameters, is presented in Table 1.

Table 1. The characteristics of study subjects whose perception improved after interaction with HSR TIAGo.

Parameter		Anthropo Morphism	Animacy	Likeability	Perceived Intelligence	Perceived Safety
Age (years)	60–74 (n = 43)	28 (65.1%)	25 (58.1%)	28 (65.1%)	22 (51.2%)	21 (48.8%)
	≥75 (n = 57)	30 (52.6%)	34 (59.6%)	24 (42.1%) $p = 0.0272$	20 (35.1%)	22 (38.6%)
Gender	Females (n = 53)	31 (58.5%)	29 (54.7%)	21 (39.6%)	17 (32.0%)	27 (50.9%)
	Males (n = 47)	27 (57.4%)	30 (63.8%)	31 (65.9%) $p = 0.0099$	25 (53.2%) $p = 0.0428$	14 (29.8%) $p = 0.0419$
Education	Below secondary (n = 44)	28 (63.6%)	29 (65.9%)	24 (54,5%)	22 (50.0%)	17 (38.6%)
	At least secondary (n = 56)	30 (53.6%)	30 (53.6%)	28 (50.0%)	20 (35.7%)	26 (46.4%)
Ease of use of technology	1–2 (n = 40)	27 (67.5%)	24 (60.0%)	22 (55.5%)	15 (37.5%)	18 (45.0%)
	3–5 (n = 60)	31 (51.7%)	35 (58.3%)	30 (50.0%)	27 (45.0%)	25 (41.7%)
Computer skills	1–2 (n = 81)	46 (56.8%)	46 (56.8%)	36 (44.4%)	30 (37.0%)	33 (40.7%)
	3–5 (n = 19)	12 (63.2%)	13 (68.4%)	16 (84.2%) $p = 0.0020$	12 (63.2%) $p = 0.0435$	10 (52.6%)
BI	≤80 (n = 48)	28 (58.3%)	32 (66.7%)	24 (50.0%)	20 (41.7%)	24 (50.0%)
	>80 (n = 52)	30 (57.7%)	27 (51.9%)	28 (53.8%)	22 (42.3%)	19 (36.5%)
MMSE	≤23 (n = 50)	33 (66.0%)	32 (64.0%)	25 (50.0%)	20 (40.0%)	22 (44.0%)
	>23 (n = 50)	25 (50.0%)	27 (54.0%)	27 (54.0%)	22 (44.0%)	21 (42.0%)
GDS	<6 (n = 75)	40 (53.3%)	42 (56.0%)	39 (52.0%)	31 (41.3%)	25 (33.3%)
	≥6 (n = 25)	18 (72.0%)	17 (68.0%)	13 (52.0%)	11 (44.0%)	18 (72.0%) $p = 0.0010$

Table 1. *Cont.*

Parameter		Anthropo Morphism	Animacy	Likeability	Perceived Intelligence	Perceived Safety
Physical fitness	1–2 (n = 26)	16 (61.5%)	17 (65.4%)	11 (42.3%)	9 (34.6%)	10 (38.5%)
	3–5 (n = 74)	26 (35.1%) $p = 0.0226$	42 (56.8%)	41 (55.4%)	33 (44.6%)	46 (62.2%) $p = 0.0418$
Health status	1–2 (n = 18)	18 (64.3%)	18 (64.3%)	14 (50.0%)	15 (53.6%)	17 (60.7%)
	3–5 (n = 72)	40 (55.6%)	41 (56.9%)	38 (52.8%)	27 (37.5%)	26 (36.1%) $p = 0.0419$
Loneliness *	1–3 (n = 68)	33 (48.5%)	40 (58.8%)	37 (54.4%)	29 (42.6%)	25 (36.8%)
	4–5 (n = 30)	23 (76.7%) $p = 0.0142$	17 (56.7%)	13 (43.3%)	12 (40.0%)	16 (53.3%) $p = 0.0817$

* Two participants provided no values.

In the multivariable analysis, which assessed all variables being significant in the univariable analysis, we found that the odds ratios for a better perception of the robot after interaction were higher for the *Anthropomorphism* series: individuals who declared high levels of loneliness had an odds ratio of 3.34 (95% confidence interval: 1.26–8.87; $p < 0.05$). For the *Likeability* series, subjects with declared computer literacy had an OR of 6.74 (95% CI: 1.74–26.09; $p < 0.01$). For the *Perceived safety* series, participants with a GDS score indicative of depression had an OR of 4.75 (95% CI: 1.63–13.87; $p < 0.01$).

No correlates were identified for the remaining series. The results of the multi-parameter analysis are presented in detail in Table 2.

Table 2. Multivariable analysis of correlates of improvement after interaction with HSR TIAGo.

	Series I: Anthropomorphism			
		OR	**95% CI**	***p***
Physical fitness	1–2 vs. 3–5	1.665	0.618–4.487	0.314
Loneliness	4–5 vs. 1–3	3.340	1.258–8.872	**0.016**
	Series III: Likeability			
		OR	**95% CI**	***p***
Age (years)	60–74 vs. at least 75	2.126	0.860–5.257	0.102
Gender	Males vs. females	2.332	0.953–5.706	0.064
Computer skills	3–5 vs. 1–2	6.735	1.738–26.093	**0.006**
	Series IV: Perceived intelligence			
		OR	**95% CI**	***p***
Gender	Males vs. females	2.283	0.997–5.228	0.051
Computer skills	3–5 vs. 1–2	2.719	0.945–7.821	0.064
	Series V: Perceived safety			
		OR	**95% CI**	***p***
Gender	Males vs. females	0.421	0.168–1.055	0.065
Physical fitness	3–5 vs. 1–2	0.763	0.238–2.441	0.648
Health status	3–5 vs. 1–2	0.511	0.164–1.597	0.248
Loneliness	4–5 vs. 1–3	1.381	0.524–3.642	0.514
GDS	6 and above vs. less than 6	4.753	1.628–13.871	**0.004**

4. Discussion

Based on the literature and our previous studies, attitudes toward the use of HSRs in care settings are deeply intertwined with various aspects of their perception [22,28,34]; we thus pose the question of whether a real-world interaction influences the perception of the robot. Understanding how LTC residents perceive a robot is essential for the successful implementation of robotic solutions [35], which could ultimately reduce staff workload. Staffing in LTC institutions is a critical issue, affecting not only the overall quality of life for residents but also their mental health, as demonstrated by Chappell et al. [36].

Our study is one of the first to analyse the impact of institutionalised subjects' real-world interaction with an HSR on their perception of the robot. While numerous studies on robot perception have been published, few incorporate actual interaction with the technology, particularly in the context of its use in care. D'Onofrio et al. assessed post-exposure perceptions of a robot's usefulness and found positive feedback, regardless of the participants' familiarity with new technologies [37], similar to our findings. Beer et al. applied a 2.5-h exposure to a robot and observed an improvement in perceived ease of use [38]—a parameter generally related to perception (this aspect of technology acceptance has been recently strengthened in an analysis using a Large Language Model [39]). Moreover, Ke et al. noted an improvement in LTC residents with dementia after 32 weeks of interaction with a robot [40], which complements the results we obtained. Our study assessed the change in perception of the HSR TIAGo between viewing it in a photograph and interacting with it in full contact. We previously demonstrated that a tangible interaction with an HSR changes attitudes towards the robot, with perception being a key factor [21]. This current study also examined potential correlates of the robot's perception, including demographic data, self-assessment information, and selected items of the Comprehensive Geriatric Assessment.

Our results show a generally positive change in older people's perceptions of an HSR. The greatest difference, congruently with our H3, was observed in the *Likeability* series, with almost all items being rated higher after the interaction. It is consistent with the study by Robinson et al. using the Pepper HSR [41]. This observation is significant because the *Likeability* series captures elements related to the human–robot relationship, such as friendliness and kindness. Reciprocal responses are known to play an important role in shaping these relationships [42].

The *Anthropomorphism* series also showed improvement (matching our H1), primarily due to the movement parameter (e.g., *Moving rigidly–Moving elegantly*). Notably, Schulz et al. analysed the characteristics of the Fetch robot and found that participants preferred to engage in interaction with the robot rather than watch it move [43]. The robot's movement quality seems important for its perception; however, the uncanny valley effect (UVE) should also be considered in this context. Tu et al. demonstrated differences in UVE perception between younger and middle-aged adults and older individuals, suggesting that the robot's motor functions should be designed with the target group in mind [44].

Scores for the *Animacy* series improved significantly, primarily due to the *Dead–Alive* and *Inert–Interactive* items, consistent with our H2. This suggests that future robot users may place a high value on how quickly the robot reacts and prefer more dynamic behaviour.

The *Perceived intelligence* series was also rated higher post-interaction (confirming our H4), with the *Unintelligent–Intelligent* item driving this change. Hence, prospective users seem to expect robots to exhibit intelligence, and interaction with the TIAGo reinforced the perception of an HSR as such. Similar results were obtained by Sturgeon et al. using the relatively small NAO HSR (presented in a video sequence), though no change was observed in our study for the *Perceived safety* series, reflecting our H5. This finding warrants further investigation because comfort, experience, familiarity, predictability, sense of control, transparency, and trust are key factors influencing perceived safety in human–robot interaction [45].

In the multivariable analysis, no common correlates for change in all series were found, as suggested in our H6. Loneliness was observed to correlate with changes in *Anthropomorphism* scores. Single-assessment studies by Chen et al. [46], Li and Sung [47], and Dang and Liu, particularly for Western cultures [48], have also noted a relationship between loneliness and anthropomorphism, which suggests that special attention should be paid to human-like features when designing robotic interventions for people experiencing loneliness. This is a critical consideration, given that older adults transitioning to LTC facilities are often lonely. For changes in the *Likeability* series, computer skills were found to be a correlate, a finding not previously demonstrated. Hence, computer literacy appears to play a positive role in moderating the acceptance of HSRs in care. Gender yielded an insignificant trend here. The literature data related to the impact of gender on the acceptance of robots are inconsistent: from no [49] to substantial influence [50]. Our univariable analysis indicated that males scored *Likeability* and *Perceived intelligence* better, whereas females scored *Perceived safety better.* For *Perceived safety*, a GDS score indicating depression was a correlate (a trend also observed in a pilot study by Harrington et al. [51]). This finding is important because safety features are a priority for prospective HSR users in care [52]. GDS, commonly used as a screening tool for mood and depression, could serve as an indicator of the significance of safety functions in robot design. In univariate analysis, physical fitness and loneliness were also significant factors influencing changes in *Perceived safety*. While our participants consistently interacted in close proximity to the machine, Rugabotti et al. observed that spatial aspects may also affect the perceived safety of the robot [53]. All this suggests that the perception of safety in an HSR is a multifaceted phenomenon, as highlighted in previous studies [53,54], and should be carefully examined during the pre-implementation phase of robotic interventions. Indicated factors may shape user expectations and acceptance, ultimately affecting the success of robotic integration not only in long-term care settings. From a clinical perspective, the findings underscore the importance of tailoring robotic solutions to their older users. Integrating robots that are perceived as responsive, friendly, and intuitive may contribute to improved mood, greater social stimulation, and potentially reduce caregiver burden.

The results of this study support the hypothesis that interaction with the robot led to a positive change in its perception. Participants demonstrated significantly improved evaluations across multiple dimensions, particularly in terms of likeability. These observations indicate that real-world interaction plays a critical role in shaping user attitudes towards robotic solutions, reinforcing the value of experiential exposure in promoting acceptance and trust in assistive technologies.

Limitations

The cross-sectional nature of this study means that the results suggest important relationships but cannot establish causality. Furthermore, the first interaction with a robot may be influenced by the novelty effect; however, participants had sufficient time to operate the robot as they saw fit. Despite these limitations, the study group can be considered relatively large for this type of analysis.

5. Conclusions

Real-world interaction with an HSR results in both qualitative and quantitative changes in its perception. To obtain reliable results, studies on HSR perception and acceptance should incorporate actual interaction with the robot. Developers and staff responsible for implementing these systems should pay particular attention to the robot's smart functions, movements, and responsiveness. It is essential to thoroughly understand the target group's characteristics before designing the robot, particularly in terms of loneliness, mood (including symptoms of depression), and computer literacy. Our findings may also benefit the LTC management and staff when preparing interventions using HSRs. Their deployment should be accompanied by staff training and user education to maximise therapeutic potential and ensure effective interaction between users and robotic systems.

Author Contributions: Conceptualisation, S.T.; methodology, S.T. and K.W.-T.; formal analysis, S.T. and A.S.; investigation, S.T. and J.P.-S.; data curation, S.T.; writing—original draft preparation, S.T.; writing—review and editing, K.W.-T., J.P.-S. and A.S.; visualisation, S.T.; supervision, K.W.-T. All authors have read and agreed to the published version of the manuscript.

Funding: This research received no external funding.

Institutional Review Board Statement: This study was conducted in accordance with the Declaration of Helsinki and approved by the Bioethics Committee of Poznan University of Medical Sciences under Protocol No. 711/18, approval date: 14 June 2018.

Informed Consent Statement: Informed consent was obtained from all subjects involved in this study.

Data Availability Statement: Dataset available on request from the corresponding author.

Acknowledgments: The authors would like to thank PAL Robotics, Spain, for customising the TIAGo robot and making it available for this study.

Conflicts of Interest: The authors declare no conflicts of interest.

Abbreviations

The following abbreviations are used in this manuscript:

LTC	long-term care
HSR	humanoid social robot
ADL	activities of daily living
BI	Barthel Index
MMSE	Mini-Mental State Examination
GDS	Geriatric Depression Scale
GQS	Godspeed Questionnaire Series
OR	odds ratio
CI	confidence interval

References

1. Young, Y. Factors associated with permanent transition from independent living to nursing home in a continuing care retirement community. *J. Am. Med. Dir. Assoc.* **2009**, *10*, 491–497. [CrossRef] [PubMed]
2. Cooney, A. 'Finding home': A grounded theory on how older people 'find home' in long-term care settings. *Int. J. Older People Nurs.* **2012**, *7*, 188–199. [CrossRef] [PubMed]
3. Vaismoradi, M.; Wang, I.L.; Turunen, H.; Bondas, T. Older people's experiences of care in nursing homes: A meta-synthesis. *Int. Nurs. Rev.* **2016**, *63*, 111–121. [CrossRef] [PubMed]
4. Theurer, K.; Mortenson, W.B.; Stone, R.; Suto, M.; Timonen, V.; Rozanova, J. The need for a social revolution in residential care. *J. Aging Stud.* **2015**, *35*, 201–210. [CrossRef]
5. Behuniak, S.M. Toward a political model of dementia: Power as compassionate care. *J. Aging Stud.* **2010**, *24*, 231–240. [CrossRef]
6. Alzheimer's Society. *Alzheimer's Society Low Expectations: Attitudes on Choice, Care and Community for People with Dementia in Care Homes*; Alzheimer's Society: London, UK, 2017.

7. Toot, S.; Swinson, T.; Devine, M.; Challis, D.; Orrell, M. Causes of nursing home placement for older people with dementia: A systematic review and meta-analysis. *Int. Psychogeriatr.* **2017**, *29*, 195–208. [CrossRef]
8. Predali, D. COVID-19: A worldwide hecatomb in long-term care facilities. In *Handbook on COVID-19 Pandemic and Older Persons: Narratives and Issues from India and Beyond*; Shankardass, M.K., Ed.; Springer Nature: Singapore, 2023; pp. 21–54.
9. Travers, J.L.; Wittenberg, G.F.; Gifford, D.R.; Reddy, A.; McLaughlin, M.M.; Baier, R.R. Providers' perspectives on high-quality dementia care in long-term care. *J. Am. Med. Dir. Assoc.* **2022**, *23*, 2030.e1–2030.e8. [CrossRef]
10. Wilson, M.G.; Gauvin, F.P.; DeMaio, P.; Alam, S.; Drakos, A.; Soueidan, S.; Costa, A.; Reid, R.; Simeonov, D.; Sixsmith, A.; et al. Enhancing the use of technology in the long-term care sector in canada: Insights from citizen panels and a national stakeholder dialogue. *Healthc. Manag. Forum* **2022**, *35*, 310–317. [CrossRef]
11. Getson, C.; Nejat, G. The adoption of socially assistive robots for long-term care: During COVID-19 and in a post-pandemic society. *Healthc. Manag. Forum* **2022**, *35*, 301–309. [CrossRef]
12. Felding, S.A.; Koh, W.Q.; Teupen, S.; Budak, K.B.; Laporte Uribe, F.; Roes, M. A scoping review using the almere model to understand factors facilitating and hindering the acceptance of social robots in nursing homes. *Int. J. Soc. Robot.* **2023**, *15*, 1115–1153. [CrossRef]
13. Lukasik, S.; Tobis, S.; Kropinska, S.; Suwalska, A. Role of assistive robots in the care of older people: Survey study among medical and nursing students. *J. Med. Internet Res.* **2020**, *22*, e18003. [CrossRef] [PubMed]
14. Łukasik, S.; Tobis, S.; Suwalska, J.; Łojko, D.; Napierała, M.; Proch, M.; Neumann-Podczaska, A.; Suwalska, A. The role of socially assistive robots in the care of older people: To assist in cognitive training, to remind or to accompany? *Sustainability* **2021**, *13*, 10394. [CrossRef]
15. Sawik, B.; Tobis, S.; Baum, E.; Suwalska, A.; Kropinska, S.; Stachnik, K.; Perez-Bernabeu, E.; Cildoz, M.; Agustin, A.; Wieczorowska-Tobis, K. Robots for elderly care: Review, multi-criteria optimization model and qualitative case study. *Healthcare* **2023**, *11*, 1286. [CrossRef] [PubMed]
16. Tobis, S.; Cylkowska-Nowak, M.; Wieczorowska-Tobis, K.; Pawlaczyk, M.; Suwalska, A. Occupational therapy students' perceptions of the role of robots in the care for older people living in the community. *Occup. Ther. Int.* **2017**, *2017*, 9592405. [CrossRef]
17. Tobis, S.; Piasek-Skupna, J.; Neumann-Podczaska, A.; Suwalska, A.; Wieczorowska-Tobis, K. The effects of stakeholder perceptions on the use of humanoid robots in care for older adults: Postinteraction cross-sectional study. *J. Med. Internet Res.* **2023**, *25*, e46617. [CrossRef]
18. Tobis, S. Education and training in gerontechnology. In *Gerontechnology. A Clinical Perspective*; Pilotto, A., Maetzler, W., Eds.; Springer International Publishing: Cham, Switzerland, 2023; pp. 163–173.
19. Piasek, J.; Wieczorowska-Tobis, K. Acceptance and long-term use of a social robot by elderly users in a domestic environment. In Proceedings of the 2018 11th International Conference on Human System Interaction (HSI), Gdansk, Poland, 4–6 July 2018; pp. 478–482.
20. Papadopoulos, I.; Koulouglioti, C.; Lazzarino, R.; Ali, S. Enablers and barriers to the implementation of socially assistive humanoid robots in health and social care: A systematic review. *BMJ Open* **2020**, *10*, e033096. [CrossRef]
21. Tobis, S.; Piasek, J.; Cylkowska-Nowak, M.; Suwalska, A. Robots in eldercare: How does a real-world interaction with the machine influence the perceptions of older people? *Sensors* **2022**, *22*, 1717. [CrossRef]
22. Tobis, S.; Piasek-Skupna, J.; Suwalska, A. The godspeed questionnaire series in the assessment of the social robot tiago by older individuals. *Sensors* **2023**, *23*, 7251. [CrossRef]
23. Pandey, A.K.; Gelin, R. A mass-produced sociable humanoid robot: Pepper: The first machine of its kind. *IEEE Robot. Autom. Mag.* **2018**, *25*, 40–48. [CrossRef]
24. Bartneck, C.; Kulić, D.; Croft, E.; Zoghbi, S. Measurement instruments for the anthropomorphism, animacy, likeability, perceived intelligence, and perceived safety of robots. *Int. J. Soc. Robot.* **2008**, *1*, 71–81. [CrossRef]
25. Thunberg, S.; Arnelid, M.; Ziemke, T. Older adults' perception of the furhat robot. In Proceedings of the 10th International Conference on Human-Agent Interaction, Christchurch, New Zealand, 5–8 December 2022; Association for Computing Machinery: Christchurch, New Zealand, 2022; pp. 4–12.
26. Haring, K.S.; Watanabe, K.; Velonaki, M.; Tossell, C.C.; Finomore, V. Ffab—The form function attribution bias in human–robot interaction. *IEEE Trans. Cogn. Dev. Syst.* **2018**, *10*, 843–851. [CrossRef]
27. Robinson, F.; Nejat, G. An analysis of design recommendations for socially assistive robot helpers for effective human-robot interactions in senior care. *J. Rehabil. Assist. Technol. Eng.* **2022**, *9*, 20556683221101389. [CrossRef] [PubMed]
28. Tobis, S.; Piasek-Skupna, J.; Neumann-Podczaska, A.; Religioni, U.; Suwalska, A. Determinants of attitude to a humanoid social robot in care for older adults: A post-interaction study. *Med. Sci. Monit.* **2023**, *29*, e941205. [CrossRef] [PubMed]
29. Mahoney, F.I.; Barthel, D.W. Functional evaluation: The barthel index. *Md. State Med. journal* **1965**, *14*, 61–65.

30. Folstein, M.F.; Folstein, S.E.; McHugh, P.R. "Mini-mental state": A practical method for grading the cognitive state of patients for the clinician. *J. Psychiatr. Res.* **1975**, *12*, 189–198. [CrossRef]
31. Marc, L.G.; Raue, P.J.; Bruce, M.L. Screening performance of the 15-item geriatric depression scale in a diverse elderly home care population. *Am. J. Geriatr. Psychiatry* **2008**, *16*, 914–921. [CrossRef]
32. Chopra, M.P.; Sullivan, J.R.; Feldman, Z.; Landes, R.D.; Beck, C. Self-, collateral- and clinician assessment of depression in persons with cognitive impairment. *Aging Ment. Health* **2008**, *12*, 675–683. [CrossRef]
33. Henneges, C.; Reed, C.; Chen, Y.F.; Dell'Agnello, G.; Lebrec, J. Describing the sequence of cognitive decline in alzheimer's disease patients: Results from an observational study. *J. Alzheimers Dis.* **2016**, *52*, 1065–1080. [CrossRef]
34. David, D.; Thérouanne, P.; Milhabet, I. The acceptability of social robots: A scoping review of the recent literature. *Comput. Hum. Behav.* **2022**, *137*, 107419. [CrossRef]
35. Vandemeulebroucke, T.; Dzi, K.; Gastmans, C. Older adults' experiences with and perceptions of the use of socially assistive robots in aged care: A systematic review of quantitative evidence. *Arch. Gerontol. Geriatr.* **2021**, *95*, 104399. [CrossRef]
36. Chappell, V.; Kirkham, J.; Seitz, D.P. Association between long-term care facility staffing levels and antipsychotic use in us long-term care facilities. *J. Am. Med. Dir. Assoc.* **2022**, *23*, 1787–1792.e1. [CrossRef] [PubMed]
37. D'Onofrio, G.; Fiorini, L.; Hoshino, H.; Matsumori, A.; Okabe, Y.; Tsukamoto, M.; Limosani, R.; Vitanza, A.; Greco, F.; Greco, A.; et al. Assistive robots for socialization in elderly people: Results pertaining to the needs of the users. *Aging Clin. Exp. Res.* **2019**, *31*, 1313–1329. [CrossRef] [PubMed]
38. Beer, J.M.; Prakash, A.; Smarr, C.A.; Chen, T.L.; Hawkins, K.; Nguyen, H.; Deyle, T.; Mitzner, T.L.; Kemp, C.C.; Rogers, W.A. Older users' acceptance of an assistive robot: Attitudinal changes following brief exposure. *Gerontechnology* **2017**, *16*, 21–36. [CrossRef] [PubMed]
39. Kim, S.D. Application and challenges of the technology acceptance model in elderly healthcare: Insights from chatgpt. *Technologies* **2024**, *12*, 68. [CrossRef]
40. Ke, C.; Lou, V.W.; Tan, K.C.; Wai, M.Y.; Chan, L.L. Changes in technology acceptance among older people with dementia: The role of social robot engagement. *Int. J. Med. Inform.* **2020**, *141*, 104241. [CrossRef]
41. Robinson, N.L.; Hicks, T.N.; Suddrey, G.; Kavanagh, D.J. The robot self-efficacy scale: Robot self-efficacy, likability and willingness to interact increases after a robot-delivered tutorial. In Proceedings of the 2020 29th IEEE International Conference on Robot and Human Interactive Communication (RO-MAN), Naples, Italy, 31 August–4 September 2020; pp. 272–277.
42. Sandoval, E.B.; Brandstatter, J.; Yalcin, U.; Bartneck, C. Robot likeability and reciprocity in human robot interaction: Using ultimatum game to determinate reciprocal likeable robot strategies. *Int. J. Soc. Robot.* **2021**, *13*, 851–862. [CrossRef]
43. Schulz, T.; Holthaus, P.; Amirabdollahian, F.; Koay, K.L.; Torresen, J.; Herstad, J. Differences of human perceptions of a robot moving using linear or slow in, slow out velocity profiles when performing a cleaning task. In Proceedings of the 2019 28th IEEE International Conference on Robot and Human Interactive Communication (RO-MAN), New Delhi, India, 14–18 October 2019; pp. 1–8.
44. Tu, Y.C.; Chien, S.E.; Yeh, S.L. Age-related differences in the uncanny valley effect. *Gerontology* **2020**, *66*, 382–392. [CrossRef]
45. Akalin, N.; Kristoffersson, A.; Loutfi, A. Do you feel safe with your robot? Factors influencing perceived safety in human-robot interaction based on subjective and objective measures. *Int. J. Hum. Comput. Stud.* **2022**, *158*, 102744. [CrossRef]
46. Chen, S.C.; Moyle, W.; Jones, C.; Petsky, H. A social robot intervention on depression, loneliness, and quality of life for taiwanese older adults in long-term care. *Int. Psychogeriatr.* **2020**, *32*, 981–991. [CrossRef]
47. Li, X.; Sung, Y. Anthropomorphism brings us closer: The mediating role of psychological distance in user–ai assistant interactions. *Comput. Hum. Behav.* **2021**, *118*, 106680. [CrossRef]
48. Dang, J.; Liu, L. Do lonely people seek robot companionship? A comparative examination of the loneliness–robot anthropomorphism link in the united states and China. *Comput. Hum. Behav.* **2023**, *141*, 107637. [CrossRef]
49. Sorensen, L.; Sagen Johannesen, D.T.; Melkas, H.; Johnsen, H.M. User acceptance of a home robotic assistant for individuals with physical disabilities: Explorative qualitative study. *JMIR Rehabil. Assist. Technol.* **2025**, *12*, e63641. [CrossRef]
50. Abel, M.; Buccino, G.; Binkofski, F. Perception of robotic actions and the influence of gender. *Front. Psychol.* **2024**, *15*, 1295279. [CrossRef] [PubMed]
51. Harrington, E.E.; Bishop, A.J.; Do, H.M.; Sheng, W. Perceptions of socially assistive robots: A pilot study exploring older adults' concerns. *Curr. Psychol.* **2021**, *42*, 2145–2156. [CrossRef]
52. Tobis, S.; Neumann-Podczaska, A.; Kropinska, S.; Suwalska, A. Unraq—A questionnaire for the use of a social robot in care for older persons. A multi-stakeholder study and psychometric properties. *Int. J. Environ. Res. Public Health* **2021**, *18*, 6157. [CrossRef]

53. Rubagotti, M.; Tusseyeva, I.; Baltabayeva, S.; Summers, D.; Sandygulova, A. Perceived safety in physical human–robot interaction—A survey. *Robot. Auton. Syst.* **2022**, *151*, 104047. [CrossRef]
54. Akalin, N.; Kristoffersson, A.; Loutfi, A. Evaluating the sense of safety and security in human–robot interaction with older people. In *Social Robots: Technological, Societal and Ethical Aspects of Human-Robot Interaction*; Korn, O., Ed.; Springer International Publishing: Cham, Switzerland, 2019; pp. 237–264.

technologies

MDPI

Article

A Socially Assistive Robot as Orchestrator of an AAL Environment for Seniors †

Carlos E. Sanchez-Torres, Ernesto A. Lozano, Irvin H. López-Nava *, J. Antonio Garcia-Macias and Jesus Favela *

Department of Computer Scicence, CICESE, Ensenada 22870, Mexico; hello@sanchezcarlosjr.com (C.E.S.-T.); ernilozpa@gmail.com (E.A.L.); jagm@cicese.mx (J.A.G.-M.)

* Correspondence: hussein@cicese.mx (I.H.L.-N.); favela@cicese.mx (J.F.); Tel.: +52-646-175-0500 (I.H.L.-N & J.F.)

† This paper is an extended version of our paper published in the 15th International Conference on Ubiquitous Computing & Ambient Intelligence (UCAmI 2023), Riviera Maya, México, 28–30 November 2023; "An Open Framework for Nonverbal Communication in Human-Robot Interaction", https://doi.org/10.1007/978-3-031-48642-5_3.

Abstract: Social robots in Ambient Assisted Living (AAL) environments offer a promising alternative for enhancing senior care by providing companionship and functional support. These robots can serve as intuitive interfaces to complex smart home systems, allowing seniors and caregivers to easily control their environment and access various assistance services through natural interactions. By combining the emotional engagement capabilities of social robots with the comprehensive monitoring and support features of AAL, this integrated approach can potentially improve the quality of life and independence of elderly individuals while alleviating the burden on human caregivers. This paper explores the integration of social robotics with ambient assisted living (AAL) technologies to enhance elderly care. We propose a novel framework where a social robot is the central orchestrator of an AAL environment, coordinating various smart devices and systems to provide comprehensive support for seniors. Our approach leverages the social robot's ability to engage in natural interactions while managing the complex network of environmental and wearable sensors and actuators. In this paper, we focus on the technical aspects of our framework. A computational P2P notebook is used to customize the environment and run reactive services. Machine learning models can be included for real-time recognition of gestures, poses, and moods to support non-verbal communication. We describe scenarios to illustrate the utility and functionality of the framework and how the robot is used to orchestrate the AAL environment to contribute to the well-being and independence of elderly individuals. We also address the technical challenges and future directions for this integrated approach to elderly care.

Keywords: ambient assisted living; service orchestration; computational notebook; human–robot interaction; social robots; nonverbal communication

1. Introduction

Ambient Assisted Living (AAL) environments are smart living spaces designed to enhance the quality of life and independence of elderly or disabled individuals through seamlessly integrated technology. These environments combine sensors, actuators, and intelligent systems to monitor residents' health and activities, provide timely assistance, and ensure safety without being intrusive. By adapting to users' needs and preferences,

AAL environments aim to support aging in place, reduce the burden on caregivers, and promote overall well-being through a combination of proactive and reactive technological interventions [1].

Socially Assistive Robots (SARs) are increasingly considered a component of an AAL. As social robots, they are physical agents designed to communicate with humans while also providing healthcare and caregiving support, such as assisting with activities of daily living, providing companionship, and monitoring health [2].

Given their verbal and nonverbal communication abilities and physical presence, SARs can serve as interactive and intuitive interfaces to the network of sensors and devices present in an AAL environment. By acting as a central hub, these robots can interpret data from various AAL systems, communicate information to users naturally and engagingly, and execute commands to control smart home features, bridging the gap between advanced technology and human-friendly interaction in assisted living spaces.

We present a framework for an adaptable AAL environment that leverages a social robot as a user-friendly interface to smart home services and a computational notebook for customizing the environment by incorporating additional sensors and services. Unlike a basic hub, this framework supports service orchestration, allowing the AAL environment to manage and adapt to complex, dynamic scenarios. It builds on a platform designed to recognize both verbal and nonverbal communication, enabling the social robot to respond appropriately [3], and uses the Eva robot, which has been successfully used to guide interventions with older adults with dementia [4,5].

This work is organized as follows. Section 2 discusses the need for service orchestration in AAL environments. In Section 3 we present the architecture of the framework proposed, including its main components. Section 4 illustrates how the framework composes various services to implement different AAL scenarios. In Section 5 we discuss the novelty of the approach, comparing with service orchestration and the use of social robots in AAL, and present some of the ethical and privacy considerations on the use of the platform. Finally, Section 7 concludes this work and discusses possible future work.

2. Orchestration of Ambient Assisted Living Services

AAL environments include many networked sensors, computers, and services aimed at supporting elderly or disabled individuals. Its hardware components usually include motion and pressure sensors, wearable devices, lighting systems, voice assistants, and health monitoring devices. These components support a variety of services such as medication reminders, video conferencing, fall detection, and home automation. As social robots become popular, they are increasingly becoming part of AALs.

As an AAL environment expands with new components and services, it creates opportunities for innovative integrated functionalities. However, this growth also increases the complexity of system management and coordination. For example, integrating a user's smartwatch with sleep detection capabilities could enable the system to postpone medication reminders until the user wakes up, demonstrating how new components can enhance existing services in sophisticated ways.

Voice assistants can function as hubs in smart environments, interfacing with users through voice commands and communicating with various sensors and services. Common examples include turning lights on or notifying users about visitors at the door. These assistants seamlessly integrate multiple smart home functionalities, providing a centralized and intuitive control point for the user.

While software hubs excel at managing connections and data flow, they are limited in handling complex multi-step processes that require sophisticated decision making. Software orchestration [6], on the other hand, is designed to manage these intricate workflows, coordinating actions across various systems and adapting to changing conditions.

Recent years have seen an increased interest and research in robotic assistants that can perform tasks focused on social integration, affective bonding, and cognitive training [7]. While verbal communication remains the primary mode of interaction between SARs and humans, non-verbal communication can be particularly effective in AAL environments to trigger services based on the user´s presence, emotional state, or physical behaviors. For instance, facial expression analysis could detect signs of discomfort, prompting an appropriate response; motion sensors detecting an elder standing up in the middle of the night could automatically activate soft lighting for safety; and body posture tracking might trigger fall prevention services. This multimodal approach creates a more intuitive and seamless interaction with the AAL environment.

Social robots can take a variety of shapes and can have different affordances to enact and recognize nonverbal communication cues, showcasing various types of nonverbal human–robot interactions. Some well-known examples include NAO (https://en.wikipedia.org/wiki/Nao_(robot)), accessed on 27 March 2025, which can track faces, make eye contact, imitate human gestures, and respond to touch. It can also exhibit emotions through its LED lights and body movements. The Cozmo (https://www.digitaldreamlabs.com/products/cozmo-robot, accessed on 27 March 2025) robot uses its expressive digital eyes, body language, and sounds to communicate with users, allowing it to exhibit excitement, frustration, and curiosity. Another example is Jibo (https://robotsguide.com/robots/jibo, accessed on 27 March 2025), which uses facial recognition and expressive animations to establish emotional connections with users by exhibiting nonverbal cues like nodding, blinking, and expressing curiosity through head movements. While most of these efforts have focused on sensors within the robot, in an AAL environment, the sensing capabilities can be distributed throughout the living space, allowing for more comprehensive and unobtrusive monitoring of the user's nonverbal cues.

Environmental and wearable sensors, such as cameras, motion detectors, and smartwatches, can work in tandem with the robot's sensors to create a more complete picture of the user's state and behavior. For example, a smartwatch can detect gait patterns and potential fall risks, while ambient microphones can pick up patterns in voice tone that might indicate emotional states. Integrating robot and environmental sensing enables a more context-aware and responsive system capable of interpreting subtle nonverbal cues that a robot alone might miss.

Moreover, this expanded sensing network allows the social robot to act as an intelligent interface to the broader AAL system, translating environmental data into appropriate social responses and actions. This synergy between the robot and the environment enhances the capability for nonverbal communication and creates a more seamless and natural assisted living experience for the user.

2.1. Nonverbal Interactions in HRI

Human–robot interaction can incorporate various forms of nonverbal communication in an AAL environment. These interactions utilize a broad spectrum of communication modalities and cues that go beyond spoken language [8]. The following are some categories of nonverbal interactions in AAL scenarios:

1. Visual cues: Analyze a person's facial expressions, such as smiles, frowns, raised eyebrows, or narrowed eyes, to infer emotions like happiness, sadness, surprise, or anger; this also includes eye gaze tracking and whether a person is making or avoiding direct eye contact. All these might be signs of interest or discomfort.

2. Paralanguage: Tones of voice, such as volume and speed, can indicate mood, exertion, or health status. Detecting non-speech vocalizations such as sighs or groans might indicate stress or pain.
3. Gestures: Hand movements or arm motions to communicate with humans. Gestures can include pointing to objects, waving, making other meaningful movements to indicate actions and directions, or engaging in collaborative tasks.
4. Body Language and Posture: By observing a person's posture and overall body movements, a robot can interpret cues like open or closed body position, leaning in or away, hand movements, gait analysis or crossed arms, providing insights into the person's level of comfort, engagement, or risk.
5. Proxemics: Understanding the distance between the robot and the person using sensors, such as the camera, allowing the robot to assess the person's comfort level with proximity and adjust its behavior accordingly.
6. Time-based cues or chronemics: Patterns of user activities, including time to respond to robot interactions, day–night activities, and chrononutrition.

These types of nonverbal interactions are crucial in making human–robot interactions more natural, intuitive, and socially engaging.

2.2. Design Scenarios

We describe three scenarios of human–robot interaction in the AAL environment that were developed to identify the design requirements for the proposed framework. These scenarios highlight three main roles social robots can play in ALL: companionship and emotional support, communication facilitation, and health monitoring. They are derived from design sessions with caregivers [9] and proven applications of social robots in elder care [10].

2.2.1. Scenario 1: Guiding an Exercise Routine

Elsa is an older adult who performs her exercise routine each morning. The robot activates the physiological sensor in Elsa's smartwatch to continuously measure her heart rate when she starts her exercise routine. One morning, while exercising, Elsa's heart rate increases beyond a predefined threshold, which is considered dangerous or inappropriate for her health. Thus, the social robot will issue a verbal warning to advise her to stop or decrease the intensity of the exercise to avoid health risks.

2.2.2. Scenario 2: Gaze and Proxemics to Initiate an Interaction

Eva is a social robot used to assist Roberto, a patient who lives alone at home and exhibits signs of dementia. He often feels disoriented and lonely. When feeling like talking to someone, he approaches Eva to get its attention and initiate an interaction. As he approaches her, the robot can analyze and calculate how far Roberto is from it using an integrated camera. If the distance between them is greater than three meters, Eva will begin to move her head to track him. As Roberto approaches while looking at the robot, the robot will change its behavior to be more interactive and affective. When Eva notices that Roberto keeps looking at it for more than two seconds, the robot will initiate an interaction: "Hi Roberto, how have you been today?", and the conversation will continue, incorporating elements of cognitive stimulation therapy until Roberto decides to terminate the interaction.

2.2.3. Scenario 3: Sleep Disturbances

Ana usually sleeps soundly, but tonight, after three hours of rest, she becomes restless. Eva cannot determine a probable cause by analyzing diurnal sleep patterns, environmental temperature, noise, or Ana's food and water intake that day. At 2 a.m., Eva detects that Ana is awake based on her smartwatch's heart rate and accelerometer data. Eva attempts to comfort and encourage Ana to go back to sleep by performing a mindfulness activity. However, Ana stands up and tells Eva that she must use the bathroom. Responding to Ana's movements, detected by motion sensors, Eva activates soft lighting at the base of Ana's bed to guide her safely to the bathroom. Ana goes to the toilet twice that night, which is unusual for her. Unable to identify a clear cause for this behavior, Eva informs a caregiver to check for a possible urinary tract infection. Meanwhile, Eva reminds Ana the next day not to drink too much water before bedtime and adjusts the room temperature to an optimal level for sleep.

3. Architecture of the AAL Orchestration Framework

We present the proposed AAL orchestration architecture, focusing on its features rather than implementation details, from a domain perspective. In this context, the architecture's competence refers to the domain it operates in (e.g., nonverbal scenarios, behaviors, and tasks). In contrast, its performance depends on implementation factors such as technology choices, algorithms, and design practices.

Our architectural framework is a flow-based programming engine that orchestrates microservices through streams. Inspired by [11], our proposal emphasizes distributed and data-driven strategies. These are characteristics that form the basis for our proposed framework and that we could not find in already existing platforms. For example ROS [12], the most widely used platform, consists of a set of software libraries and tools to build robot applications; as flow-based features are not present, third-party proposals (such as [13,14]) have recently appeared.

An AAL environment relies on distributed algorithms running across multiple interconnected nodes without strict centralized control, and online algorithms (including stream and dynamic algorithms), which process input incrementally rather than all at once, resembling nonmonotonic logic. In addition, reactive programming provides operational semantics that respond to external events and seamlessly manage time-dependent data flows, such as asynchronous environmental signals.

The proposed engine architecture is event-driven and utilizes a combination of publish/subscribe models through various communication protocols with different fault-tolerance mechanisms, along with a computational notebook that enables users to create reactive microservices. In this context, an event is defined as an immutable object, denoted as the evaluation of the signal, $s(t_0)$, or the change in the state of the system, originating from a subsystem. In discrete time increments, this object yields a stream, the signal $s(t)$. A producer generates an event that multiple consumers can process.

The messaging system operates in one of three ways: (i) producers send direct messages without intermediaries, (ii) messages are routed through a message broker, or (iii) events are logged for later processing. In this work, we refer to both producers and consumers as microservices—independently deployable and loosely coupled, unlike monolithic software.

Once the consumer receives a stream, several processing approaches can be applied:

- Data synchronizers store or present data in a storage system.
- Tasks trigger events that influence the environment.
- Pipeline stages aggregate events from input streams, producing one or more output streams that pass through various transformations before reaching a task or data synchronizer via pipe-and-filter operations.

Thus, a service forms a graph of dependencies among microservices, connected by different protocols, working together to achieve a specific competence.

What can be done with the stream once it is in the hands of the consumer? How can the consumer process it and when can we achieve a specific competence? Those are classified as data synchronizers, tasks, and pipeline stages. Data synchronizers are tasked with storing or presenting data on a storage system. Tasks push events that affect the environment. Pipeline stages receive events from multiple input streams to produce one or more output streams that go through different stages until they reach a task or data synchronizers applying pipe-and-filter operations. Therefore, a service is a graph of dependencies within microservices joined by different protocols designed to achieve a specific competence.

In contrast to other alternatives, the process decision mechanism introduces a perspective of fault tolerance in microservices. At the worker level, we implement a "let it crash" policy with a supervisor.

Figure 1 illustrates the data flow within an example of a service, where the nodes symbolize microservices and the edges represent communication protocols. A real-time conversation, which is a specific competence, with a social robot involves understanding communication to either wake up or put the system to sleep. Instead of using a hot-word to wake up the assistant, the rest of the system remains largely inoperative until sufficient evidence is obtained to make a decision. In addition, a conversation involves the user managing sessions, where the social robot can recall the voice, face, and other characteristics of the user to interact in the best way customized for that user. When EvaNotebook, a component designed to build microservices on the fly, wakes up the system based on available information, it customizes the Large Language Model (LLM) to respond based on a specific scenario by injecting a system prompt and restoring previous sessions. The Rhasspy is then used to vocalize the robot's response and listen to the user's intention. Whisper transforms speech into text and sends it back to EvaNotebook. Therefore, we form a feedback loop where different consumers emit events that we must inject into the LLM and react accordingly. In the background, the system records data for later analysis.

The remainder of this section focuses on the physical and logical components needed to build AAL services, including the social robot, wearable and environmental sensors, an MQTT Broker, and EvaNotebook.

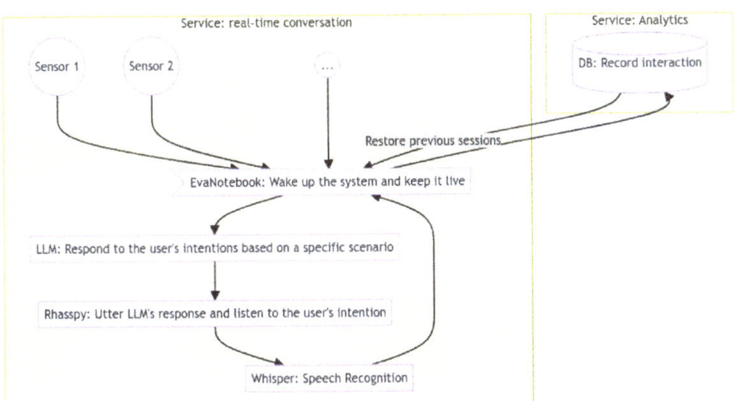

Figure 1. A typical topological data flow in our event-driven architecture.

3.1. The Eva Social Robot

EVA is an open-hardware robotic platform (https://eva-social-robot.github.io/, accessed on 27 March 2025) characterized by its modular design and low cost. It incorporates several sensors and supports verbal and nonverbal communication. The platform was initially developed as a social assistant robot to interact with and assist people with dementia [4]. EVA has been used in other scenarios, such as helping children with emotional regulation [15].

3.2. EvaNotebook

EvaNotebook (https://notebook.sanchezcarlosjr.com, accessed on 27 March 2025) is a computational notebook designed to operate within a browser environment without needing a client–server architecture. Its design lends itself to developing prototypes, experimental processes, and system scenarios, mainly emphasizing multilingual programming for event-driven architectures. It achieves this with the assistance of a decentralized database and incorporates various application protocols, including WebRTC, WebSockets, and MQTT, providing a higher level of abstraction. Our notebook extends the Jupyter Notebook v4.5 JSON schema, introducing a block-based application framework incorporating dynamic dependencies and configurations through an advanced plugin architecture delineated in the metadata. Each code block within our system operates based on an actor model with a supervision tree model similar to Elang. In the actor model, a code block can send a limited number of messages, spawning a finite number of new actors and defining its behavior for processing incoming text messages. In this approach, each worker is executed on different nodes, adopting a DAG (Directed Acyclic Graph) execution model instead of a linear model. This method is advantageous because it is often more practical to move the code to where the data and other critical dependencies reside rather than relocating the data itself.

3.3. MQTT Broker

We have adopted a pub-sub architecture with loosely coupled components, allowing us to scale and adapt services more quickly than a centralized architecture. This approach enables us to externalize the processing and view the social robot and the rest of the environment as both subscribers and emitters of events. As a communication protocol to distribute these events, we use MQTT, the current standard protocol for IoT, a lightweight messaging protocol designed for efficient communication in constrained environments. The platform deploys an instance of Eclipse Mosquitto (https://mosquitto.org/, accessed on 27 March 2025), an open-source message broker that implements the MQTT protocol on a local network to guarantee low latency and ensure responsiveness.

3.4. Sensors

Several sensors integrated into social robots like Eva, in the user and/or the environment, are used to gather data. These sensors provide valuable insights into human emotions, physical cues, and environmental context by capturing and analyzing data. Eva can leverage this information to deliver personalized and adaptive interactions, fostering various benefits for individuals. Some of the advantages that this offers to multiple interactions are:

- Emotional understanding. Eva can perceive a person's emotional state and respond accordingly by analyzing physiological signals and facial expressions.
- Contextual adaptation. Environmental sensors, including microphones and cameras, allow EVA to sense and respond to the environment around it.

- Supportive and assistive capabilities. The framework processes data to offer support to individuals. For instance, if Eva detects an increase in heart rate or signs of stress through wearable sensors, it can trigger relaxation techniques, breathing exercises, or soothing music to alleviate anxiety.
- Data sharing and integration. Eva's ability to deliver information captured by these sensors via MQTT to other devices or algorithms opens up further analysis and integration opportunities.

3.5. Voice Assistant

For verbal interaction with the user, the framework uses Rhasspy (https://rhasspy.readthedocs.io/en/latest/, accessed on 27 March 2025), an open-source toolkit for creating personalized voice assistants with a strong focus on user privacy. It enables developers to build custom voice interfaces for controlling devices and services through MQTT. A standout feature of Rhasspy is its commitment to data protection. By default, the system is designed to function completely offline, ensuring that all voice processing occurs within the user's local network. This approach eliminates the need to transmit voice data to external servers, thereby safeguarding user privacy [16].

3.6. Data Analysis Models

The framework can use pre-trained gestures and emotions in posture recognition modules to infer relevant activities, behaviors, and nonverbal cues. Several EvaNotebooks have been developed to recognize gaze direction, proximity, object recognition, posture, etc. These can be adapted or customized to the problem and run synchronously with other tasks.

4. Implementing Assistive Services

In this section, we illustrate how the services described in the scenarios presented in Section 2.2 are implemented using the orchestration paradigm supported by the framework.

4.1. Scenario 1: Guiding an Exercise Routine

Figure 2 shows a sequence diagram to explain the interaction of Scenario 1, described in Section 2.2.1. The social robot Eva initiates the interaction by indicating to the elder the exercise routine to be performed. The robot initiates a service in EvaNotebook to be notified when the user's heart rate deviates from established parameters. When this happens, the microservice in EvaNotebook will warn the user so that he adjusts the routine, advises the user to take a break, and/or triggers a notification to a third party of the situation.

This scenario requires access to data from sensors that are not integrated into the robot but worn by the subject. The components of the proposed framework operate together to accomplish the task.

1. Adding a sensor. The device with the physiological sensor is added to the environment by registering with the broker, and a JSON specification is used to indicate the frequency of the data sent to the broker. The user wears a sensor that monitors their heart rate during the exercise routine, such as a smartwatch with an optical ECG or a chest strap monitor with ECG electrodes. Both types of monitoring devices can be connected via Bluetooth. Sensors requiring synchronous communication, such as video, can be connected directly to the consumer.
2. Data collection. A service coded in a notebook for processing ECG data registers to the broker when executed. By using the Pulsoid API, the data can be transferred to the EvaNotebook for processing.

3. Data processing. A script in EvaNotebook is used to analyze the incoming data, which can be plotted in real-time for visualization purposes. If the heart rate parameters are out of range, a message can be enabled with Rhasspy. The EvaNotebook can also connect to the SendGrid API, which provides the necessary tools for sending notifications via email and text. This functionality is designed to send alert notifications to a caregiver or an individual associated with the user.

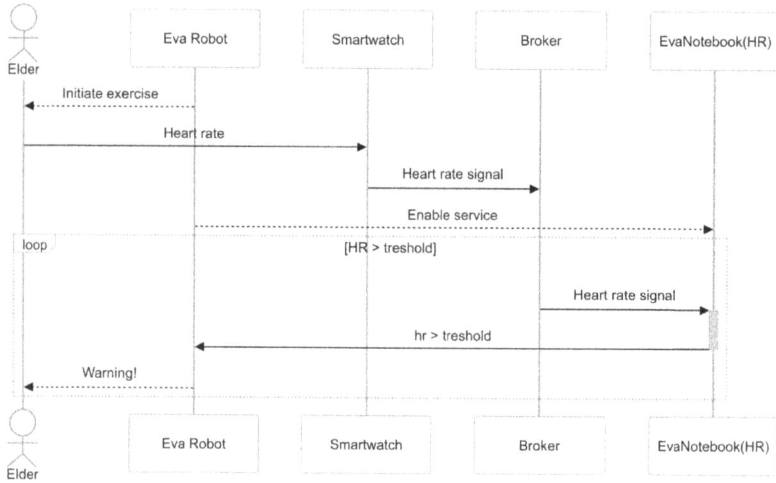

Figure 2. Eva guides the exercise routine of the user, monitoring his heart rate.

4.2. Scenario 2: Gaze and Proxemics to Initiate an Interaction

In this scenario, the social robot Eva initiates an interaction when it detects the presence of an individual at a certain distance. It uses the camera and a facial recognition algorithm to infer gaze direction and proximity.

This is implemented in an EvaNotebook that extends the "WakeFace" microservice proposed in [17] as an alternative to the wakeword method to initiate an interaction. The extension consists of using proximity in addition to gaze direction to adapt the interaction according to the following criteria:

1. Distance greater than three meters: When Eva detects a person walking at a distance of more than three meters, the robot activates its visual tracking function. Eva turns its neck and directs its gaze toward the person as long as the person keeps moving. The robot adjusts its neck's speed and range of motion to follow the person's movement smoothly and naturally. However, Eva does not initiate verbal interaction or ask questions at this distance.
2. Distance less than three meters: When the person comes within approximately three meters of Eva, the robot emits a soft auditory signal to capture the person's attention and then initiates a verbal interaction. For example, it might say, "Hello! How are you today?" or "Welcome! Can I help you with something?"
3. The service of a real-time conversation: Once Eva has initiated the conversation, it waits for the user's response. If the person responds positively or shows interest, Eva continues the dialogue smoothly and naturally, enacting conversation-based therapy using an LLM with a prompt tailored to the individual and relevant context [18].

The code below is an extract from the WakeFace microservice written in EvaNotebook, specifically in a WebWorker of JavaScript. It illustrates how the microservice subscribes to relevant MQTT events. The obtained camera data is then sent to the ML modules responsible for assessing gaze direction and proximity (MediaPipe). The code uses a pipe-and-filter architecture to handle asynchronous events, allowing for streaming processing via operators. The code listens to the camera stream, ignoring frames where no face is detected. When a face is detected, it tests if the user is facing the camera and within 3 m; if so, it runs the wakeup script to greet the user and initiate a conversation. The use of a pipe-and-filter approach facilitates adding complexity to the service, for instance, by using a model to infer the mood of the user and modify the greeting script accordingly. If the facial emotion recognition model is available, this would imply adding a line of code to the script. Additionally, this service is in itself a notebook that can be used as a component by more sophisticated services.

Listing 1. WakeFace microservice that runs on Evanotebook.

```
begin
  // import mediapipe
  zip(
   listen('Mqtt', 'camera stream').pipe(
     map(frame => mediapipe.faceDetector.detect(frame).detections[0]),
     // Ignore frames when no face detected.
     filter(landmarks => landmarks !== undefined),
     // Check if the user is facing the robot
     map(landmarks => testIfUserLooksAtCamera(landmarks))
   ),
    listen('Mqtt', 'camera stream').pipe(
     map(frame => mediapipe.faceLandmarks.detect(frame).detections[0]),
     filter(landmarks => landmarks !== undefined),
     map(landmarks => testIfUserIsADistanceLessThan3Meters(landmarks))
    )
  ).pipe(
      filter(
     // Run wakeup script if user close and facing the robot
       ([userLooksAtCamera, userIsAdistanceLessThan3Meters]) =>
            userLooksAtCamera && userIsAdistanceLessThan3Meters),
      tap(_ => mqtt.publish('wakeup'))
  )
end
```

Mediapipe is used to detect face landmarks. Afterward, the code estimates whether the person is looking at Eva. Different approaches to achieve this include solving PnP, Procrustes Analysis, SVD, or defining an ROI. On the other hand, we calculate the user's distance to the camera using, for instance, the pinhole camera model. Then, we combine both streams to determine whether to wake up the system.

Once the conversation starts, EvaNotebook prompts ChatGPT using its API. The prompt describes the scenario, such as reminiscence therapy or cognitive stimulation. Then, it indicates general recommendations for talking with people with dementia, such as using short sentences and avoiding criticizing and correcting. Then, the user's profile and preferences are provided, and finally, a sample conversation.

4.3. Scenario 3: Sleep Disturbance

The scenario on sleep disturbance mentioned above can help highlight several of the technical advantages offered by EvaNotebook and the orchestration framework:

1. Reactive Programming. EvaNote offers transparent layers of inter-communication tools in a distributed, heterogeneous computing environment, inspired by Marimo, ViNE, and the principles of Functional Reactive Programming [19,20]. EvaNote

presents a reactive programming environment that guarantees transparency for developers in distributed settings. When a code block is executed, EvaNote promptly reacts by automatically triggering the execution of subsequent cells that rely on the variables defined in the initial block. This functionality streamlines the workflow, eliminating the tedious and error-prone process of manually re-executing dependent cells. When a cell is removed, EvaNote proactively purges its variables from the program's memory using a Garbage Collector, thereby avoiding any hidden states that could lead to unpredictable results. In this scenario, when a condition is met (person wakes up), the AAL environment reacts by triggering an appropriate response for a given context (time = 2 a.m.) to encourage Ana to get back to sleep or contact a caregiver.

2. Service Coordination. A notebook includes code blocks that define one or more services and are deployed independently of other services leveraging a mobile agent strategy, allowing them to self-replicate and use metadata to determine their execution context autonomously—be it within a computing cluster, as a standalone microservice, or on a blockchain framework. Each code block in EvaNotebook operates based on either an actor model or a shared memory paradigm. The execution environment is server-agnostic. The process decision mechanism introduces a different perspective for the notebook, adopting a DAG (Directed Acyclic Graph) execution model instead of a linear model. In this approach, each block is executed on different nodes. This method is advantageous because it is often more practical to move the code to where the data and other critical dependencies reside rather than relocating the data itself. In the sleep scenario, the service that monitors night behaviors depends on the sleep data and other relevant data that could cause abnormal behavior (gender, frequency of visits to the bathroom, water intake, room temperature).
3. Data Storage. As a Distributed File System, EvaNotebook uses "EvaFS," a specialized metadata layer designed to function as file system middleware by positioning itself atop existing storage infrastructures. EvaFS enhances the functionality of underlying storage systems by managing metadata, thereby facilitating more sophisticated data operations and interactions without directly handling data storage. The metadata produced by a sensor or a service, such as HR or accelerometer raw data, is described in JSON.
4. End-user Programming. End-user development enables users, particularly those without formal programming skills, to create, modify, or enhance software without necessitating code recompilation [21]. This approach integrates the low-code paradigm with techniques like programming by example and visual programming. EvaNotebook supports end-user programming via a flexible architecture powered by the virtualization of WebComponents, which allows the dynamic modification of the playbook executor across various nodes. The user can modify a service if, for instance, a new device is added to the environment, such as indicating that the new under-bed lights should be turned on when the older adult stands up from bed at night.
5. Collaboration. EvaNotebook supports seamless real-time collaboration through a transparent mechanism replicating the working environment. Its security infrastructure is underpinned by an Identity and Access Management (IAM) system, coupled with a secure storage solution known as Vault, which ensures secure user authentication and safeguards sensitive data. In the scenario above, a caregiver can access some or all of the notebooks in the AAL environment to monitor variables or edit a service directly. For instance, it could edit a sleep service to set the thermostat to 18 degrees Celsius when the user goes to bed.

5. Ethics and Privacy Considerations

Introducing social robots in elderly care scenarios requires careful consideration regarding privacy and ethical issues. Integrating AI in assistive robots introduces concerns regarding collecting, storing, and utilizing user data; SARs often use cameras, microphones, and sensors to interact with users, which can lead to constant monitoring and a loss of personal privacy. As described in Section 3.5, we handle locally the transmission and processing of data related to voice interactions with the robot without external servers or communication links; this includes using MQTT over SSL to enable secure communications. Although we have taken measures to protect data transmission, it is still necessary to implement secure data storage measures (including encryption and access controls) to protect stored data from unauthorized access or breaches. Other measures we intend to incorporate into future system versions include techniques to anonymize or de-identify data whenever possible, thus safeguarding user identities.

Evaluation of the system with actual users will require obtaining explicit consent from users for data collection and usage, providing them with the ability to access, modify, or delete their data; this should include establishing clear data retention policies, specifying the duration of data storage and procedures for secure deletion. If actual (elderly) users are not capable of giving informed consent (for example, in cases of dementia or other cognitive impairments), it may be necessary to involve family members or legal guardians. Informed consent is a process that we have duly followed in all interventions (e.g., [4,5,9]) where we have used the same SAR system.

It is also essential to remember that the primary ethical consideration is to guarantee the safety and well-being of the elderly interacting with the robot. Therefore, measures should be taken to protect them from physical, emotional, and psychological harm. In case of error or malfunction (e.g., if a robot fails to alert for a fall), it is critical to establish clear accountability guidelines in order to define the responsibilities of system developers, caregivers, and care institutions.

6. Discussion

A thorough examination of the literature does not yield many instances where social robots act as services orchestrators in AAL settings. We can find frameworks that apply service orchestration to robot application development [22].

Within the healthcare sector, hospOS is a platform for orchestrating service robots in hospitals, aimed at alleviating the shortage of healthcare workers [23]. Similarly to our approach, the design of hospOS is informed by scenarios or case studies. However, their approach is on the autonomous navigation of the service robot triggered by a workflow request made by the staff on a web application rather than the end user communicating directly with the robot, as required in an AAL environment.

The need to orchestrate services has been recognized in the context of ambient assisted living. An experimental ambient orchestration system was built on top of the universAAL middleware [24] to address the challenge of interoperability of various commercial devices [24]. The underlying technology is based on web services. This approach is similar to the one we propose in the sense that it supports the interconnection of diverse devices that are registered as nodes in the universAAL middleware. However, the emphasis is on inter-device interaction, rather than the role of the user, which in our proposal relies on human–robot interaction.

Similarly, in [25], the authors propose an ontology that supports the creation and orchestration of services in an AAL environment. The approach also focuses on the problem of the technical integration of diverse devices, rather than their seamless interaction with the user.

The MPOWER project focuses on modeling user needs to support the orchestration of AAL services [26]. It describes two pilot scenarios that prioritize service automation and care provider interaction with the system, rather than requiring the elderly to initiate orchestration as we propose.

The use of SARs has shown potential for emotional connection, as in the case of CuDDler [27], where a participant with visual agnosia formed a strong emotional bond with the robot through tactile interaction, linking it to memories of her dog, thus highlighting the variability of responses and the potential therapeutic benefit for select individuals.

On the other hand, the role of social robots is increasingly being explored as part of AAL systems [28]. This includes predicting user activities to provide proactive assistance [29], monitoring air quality and triggering alerts [30], monitoring and providing social and cognitive stimulation to older adults [31], and assisting in performing household tasks [32]. While users interact directly with these robots, the services provided are usually independent of each other and predefined in advance, and do not require the adaptive orchestration of devices and services.

The proposed approach facilitates the development of social robots that have demonstrated utility in older adult care, but might require tailoring to the individual or context of use. These applications include guiding exercise routines [10], leading therapy sessions for individuals with dementia [4], and providing mealtime assistance to those with dementia [5].

The proposed orchestration architecture seeks to bridge the gap between programming effort and service complexity in social robots for elderly care. While graphical programming languages offer an intuitive, end-user-friendly approach [33], they often lack the flexibility and expressiveness needed to handle intricate, real-world scenarios. Conversely, XML-based or other text-heavy programming methods provide the necessary control for complex tasks [34], but are too cumbersome for non-technical users. This architecture strikes a balance by combining high-level abstractions, in the form of notebooks that implement atomic services, that simplify service creation with underlying modular components capable of managing sophisticated interactions. By doing so, it empowers caregivers and other end-users to design and customize robot behaviors without requiring advanced programming skills, while still accommodating the nuanced demands of elderly care environments. The result is a scalable, adaptable framework that democratizes robot programming without sacrificing functionality.

Although the scenarios used to demonstrate the orchestration platform have not been validated with actual users, we have previously conducted interventions using the Eva robot to guide therapy sessions for individuals with dementia [4] and supporting older adults with eating disorders [5]. Additionally, other applications, such as employing a social robot as an exercise coach for older adults, have been successfully implemented [10]. Therefore, our focus is on enabling the deployment of such services using a socially assistive robot (SAR), rather than on assessing user adoption or the clinical efficacy of the interventions themselves.

Our proposed approach centers on human–robot interaction, creating an intelligent interface that enables end-users to seamlessly orchestrate devices and services toward both explicit and implicit goals—a novel approach not previously documented in existing research literature.

7. Conclusions and Future Work

This paper presented a novel framework for integrating social robotics with Ambient Assisted Living technologies to improve elderly care. The proposed approach leverages the unique capabilities of social robots as central orchestrators in AAL environments, combining their emotional engagement abilities with comprehensive monitoring and support features. By using a social robot as an intuitive interface to complex smart home systems, developers can create a more accessible and user-friendly environment for seniors and their caregivers.

Implementing a computational P2P notebook for environment customization, reactive services, and machine learning models for non-verbal communication recognition enhances the system's adaptability and responsiveness to individual needs. The human–robot interaction scenarios presented illustrate this framework's practical applications and benefits in real-world settings.

Two key components of the framework are a broker server that distributes messages from sensors, actuators, and analysis modules, and the P2P computational network used to quickly develop and test prototypes that can become components of more complex scenarios. We illustrate the use of the framework with multimodal scenarios that use various sensors and inference models.

Future work includes exploring different perspectives on failure tolerance, as relying solely on a single worker's perspective is insufficient. Implementing Collaborative Filtering or Graph Machine Learning with Consensus algorithms is an effective strategy to enhance fault tolerance and decision making.

The current paradigm of end-user programming involves writing or editing scripts in a notebook, which might be too complex for most users. We plan to add an automatic programming feature supported by an LLM using prompt-tuning and the Retrieval Augmented Generation paradigm. The documentation of new services, including examples of their use, will be added as an external context. Thus, the user could create a new notebook using instructions in natural language such as, "Ask me if I took my medication when I go to bed if I have not already done that."

As the global population ages, innovative solutions like the one proposed become increasingly crucial. By combining the strengths of social robotics and AAL technologies, we can create more effective, efficient, and compassionate care environments for our elderly population. This integrated approach not only has the potential to revolutionize elderly care but also to set new standards for human–robot interaction in assistive contexts.

Author Contributions: Conceptualization, I.H.L.-N. and J.F.; methodology, C.E.S.-T., I.H.L.-N. and J.F.; software, C.E.S.-T. and E.A.L.; validation, E.A.L., C.E.S.-T. and J.A.G.-M.; writing—original draft preparation, J.F., C.E.S.-T.; writing—review and editing, I.H.L.-N. and J.A.G.-M. All authors have read and agreed to the published version of the manuscript.

Funding: This research was funded by the Mexican Ministry of Science, Humanities, Technology and Innovation (SECIHTI) thru scholarships provided to the first two authors.

Data Availability Statement: Data are contained within the article.

Conflicts of Interest: The authors declare no conflict of interest.

References

1. Blackman, S.; Matlo, C.; Bobrovitskiy, C.; Waldoch, A.; Fang, M.L.; Jackson, P.; Mihailidis, A.; Nygård, L.; Astell, A.; Sixsmith, A. Ambient assisted living technologies for aging well: A scoping review. *J. Intell. Syst.* **2016**, *25*, 55–69. [CrossRef]

2. Abdi, J.; Al-Hindawi, A.; Ng, T.; Vizcaychipi, M.P. Scoping review on the use of socially assistive robot technology in elderly care. *BMJ Open* **2018**, *8*, e018815. [CrossRef]
3. Lozano, E.A.; Sánchez-Torres, C.E.; López-Nava, I.H.; Favela, J. An Open Framework for Nonverbal Communication in Human-Robot Interaction. In Proceedings of the 15th International Conference on Ubiquitous Computing & Ambient Intelligence (UCAmI 2023), Lima, Peru, 22–24 November 2023; Bravo, J., Urzáiz, G., Eds.; Springer: Cham, Switzerland, 2023; pp. 21–32.
4. Cruz-Sandoval, D.; Morales-Tellez, A.; Sandoval, E.B.; Favela, J. A Social Robot as Therapy Facilitator in Interventions to Deal with Dementia-Related Behavioral Symptoms. In Proceedings of the 2020 ACM/IEEE International Conference on Human-Robot Interaction, New York, NY, USA, 23–26 March 2020; HRI '20; pp. 161–169. [CrossRef]
5. Astorga, M.; Cruz-Sandoval, D.; Favela, J. A Social Robot to Assist in Addressing Disruptive Eating Behaviors by People with Dementia. *Robotics* **2023**, *12*, 29. [CrossRef]
6. Thomas, E. *Service-Oriented Architecture: Concepts, Technology and Design*; Prentice Hall: Upper Saddle River, NJ, USA, 2005.
7. Robinson, H.; MacDonald, B.; Broadbent, E. The role of healthcare robots for older people at home: A review. *Int. J. Soc. Robot.* **2014**, *6*, 575–591. [CrossRef]
8. Urakami, J.; Seaborn, K. Nonverbal cues in human–robot interaction: A communication studies perspective. *ACM Trans. Hum.-Robot Interact.* **2023**, *12*, 1–21. [CrossRef]
9. Cruz-Sandoval, D.; Tentori, M.; Favela, J. A Framework to Design Engaging Interactions in Socially Assistive Robots to Mitigate Dementia-Related Symptoms. *J. Hum.-Robot Interact.* **2024**, *14*, 3700889. [CrossRef]
10. Cauli, N.; Reforgiato Recupero, D. Dr.VCoach: Employment of advanced deep learning and human–robot interaction for virtual coaching. *Intel. Serv. Robot.* **2025**, *35*, 123–135. [CrossRef]
11. Pineda, L.A.; Rodríguez, A.; Fuentes, G.; Rascon, C.; Meza, I.V. Concept and functional structure of a service robot. *Int. J. Adv. Robot. Syst.* **2015**, *12*, 6. [CrossRef]
12. Quigley, M.; Gerkey, B.; Smart, W.D. *Programming Robots with ROS: A Practical Introduction to the Robot Operating System*; O'Reilly Media, Inc.: Sebastopol, CA, USA, 2015.
13. Wang, S.H.; Tu, C.H.; Huang, C.C.; Juang, J.C. Execution Flow Aware Profiling for ROS-based Autonomous Vehicle Software. In Proceedings of the Workshop Proceedings of the 51st International Conference on Parallel Processing, Chicago, IL, USA, 15–18 August 2022; pp. 1–7.
14. Lumpp, F.; Panato, M.; Bombieri, N.; Fummi, F. A design flow based on docker and kubernetes for ros-based robotic software applications. *ACM Trans. Embed. Comput. Syst.* **2024**, *23*, 1–24. [CrossRef]
15. Rocha, M.; Valentim, P.; Barreto, F.; Mitjans, A.; Cruz-Sandoval, D.; Favela, J.; Muchaluat-Saade, D. Towards Enhancing the Multimodal Interaction of a Social Robot to Assist Children with Autism in Emotion Regulation. In *Pervasive Computing Technologies for Healthcare*; Lewy, H., Barkan, R., Eds.; Springer: Cham, Sitzerland, 2022; pp. 398–415.
16. Filipe, L.; Peres, R.S.; Tavares, R.M. Voice-activated smart home controller using machine learning. *IEEE Access* **2021**, *9*, 66852–66863. [CrossRef]
17. Villa, L.; Hervás, R.; Cruz-Sandoval, D.; Favela, J. Design and evaluation of proactive behavior in conversational assistants: Approach with the eva companion robot. In *International Conference on Ubiquitous Computing and Ambient Intelligence*; Springer: Berlin/Heidelberg, Germany, 2022; pp. 234–245.
18. Favela, J.; Cruz-Sandoval, D.; Parra, M.O. Conversational Agents for Dementia using Large Language Models. In Proceedings of the 2023 Mexican International Conference on Computer Science (ENC), Guanajuato, Mexico, 11–13 September 2023; pp. 1–7.
19. Perez, I.; Dedden, F. The Essence of Reactivity. In Proceedings of the 16th ACM SIGPLAN International Haskell Symposium, Berlin, Germany, 21–22 August 2023; pp. 18–31.
20. Kleppmann, M.; Wiggins, A.; Van Hardenberg, P.; McGranaghan, M. Local-first software: You own your data, in spite of the cloud. In Proceedings of the 2019 ACM SIGPLAN International Symposium on New Ideas, New Paradigms, and Reflections on Programming and Software, Portland, OR, USA, 21–23 October 2019; pp. 154–178.
21. Barricelli, B.R.; Cassano, F.; Fogli, D.; Piccinno, A. End-user development, end-user programming and end-user software engineering: A systematic mapping study. *J. Syst. Softw.* **2019**, *149*, 101–137. [CrossRef]
22. Qi, L.; Zhang, X.; Chen, H.; Bian, N.; Ma, T.; Yin, J. A Novel Distributed Orchestration Engine for Time-Sensitive Robotic Service Orchestration Based on Cloud-Edge Collaboration. *IEEE Trans. Ind. Inform.* **2025**, 45, 215–229. [CrossRef]
23. Schmidt, S.; Sommer, D.; Greiler, T.; Wahl, F. hospOS: A Platform for Service Robot Orchestration in Hospitals. In Proceedings of the ICT4AWE, Vienna, Austria, 9–11 April 2024; pp. 221–228.
24. Brestovac, G.; Marin, D.; Oroz, T.; Vidović, A.; Bozóki, S.; Grguric, A.; Mošmondor, M.; Galinac Grbac, T. Ambient orchestration in assisted environment. *Eng. Rev.* **2014**, *34*, 119–129.
25. Grguric, A.; Huljenic, D.; Mosmondor, M. AAL ontology: From design to validation. In Proceedings of the 2015 IEEE International Conference on Communication Workshop (ICCW), London, UK, 8–12 June 2015; pp. 234–239. [CrossRef]

26. Stav, E.; Walderhaug, S.; Mikalsen, M.; Hanke, S.; Benc, I. Development and evaluation of SOA-based AAL services in real-life environments: A case study and lessons learned. *Int. J. Med. Inform.* **2013**, *82*, e269–e293. [CrossRef]
27. Moyle, W.; Jones, C.; Sung, B.; Bramble, M.; O'Dwyer, S.; Blumenstein, M.; Estivill-Castro, V. What effect does an animal robot called CuDDler have on the engagement and emotional response of older people with dementia? A pilot feasibility study. *Int. J. Soc. Robot.* **2016**, *8*, 145–156. [CrossRef]
28. Cruces, A.; Jerez, A.; Bandera, J.P.; Bandera, A. Socially Assistive Robots in Smart Environments to Attend Elderly People—A Survey. *Appl. Sci.* **2024**, *14*, 5287. [CrossRef]
29. de Carolis, B.; Ferilli, S.; Macchiarulo, N. Ambient Assisted Living and Social Robots: Towards Learning Relations between User's Daily Routines and Mood. In Proceedings of the Adjunct Proceedings of the 30th ACM Conference on User Modeling, Adaptation and Personalization, New York, NY, USA, 3–7 July 2022; UMAP '22 Adjunct; pp. 123–129. [CrossRef]
30. Marques, G.; Pires, I.M.; Miranda, N.; Pitarma, R. Air Quality Monitoring Using Assistive Robots for Ambient Assisted Living and Enhanced Living Environments through Internet of Things. *Electronics* **2019**, *8*, 1375. [CrossRef]
31. Luperto, M.; Monroy, J.; Moreno, F.A.; Lunardini, F.; Renoux, J.; Krpic, A.; Galindo, C.; Ferrante, S.; Basilico, N.; Gonzalez-Jimenez, J.; et al. Seeking at-home long-term autonomy of assistive mobile robots through the integration with an IoT-based monitoring system. *Robot. Auton. Syst.* **2023**, *161*, 104346. [CrossRef]
32. A Multirobot System in an Assisted Home Environment to Support the Elderly in Their Daily Lives. *Sensors* **2022**, *22*, 7983. [CrossRef]
33. Öztürk, Ö. A Methodology for end user programming of ROS-based service robots using jigsaw metaphor and ontologies. *Intel. Serv. Robot.* **2024**, *17*, 745–757. [CrossRef]
34. Rocha, M.; Favela, J.; Muchaluat-Saade, D. Design and Evaluation of an XML-Based Language for Programming Socially Assistive Robots. *Int. J. Soc. Robot.* **2025**, *28*, 245–258. [CrossRef]

technologies

MDPI

Article

Analysis of Multimodal Sensor Systems for Identifying Basic Walking Activities

John C. Mitchell [1,*], Abbas A. Dehghani-Sanij [1], Sheng Q. Xie [2] and Rory J. O'Connor [3,4]

1 School of Mechanical Engineering, University of Leeds, Leeds LS2 9JT, UK; a.dehghani@leeds.ac.uk
2 School of Electronic and Electrical Engineering, University of Leeds, Leeds LS2 9JT, UK; s.q.xie@leeds.ac.uk
3 Academic Department of Rehabilitation Medicine, University of Leeds, Leeds LS1 3EX, UK; medrjo@leeds.ac.uk
4 NIHR Devices for Dignity, Sheffield Teaching Hospitals NHS Trust, Sheffield S10 2JF, UK
* Correspondence: l15j3cm@leeds.ac.uk

Abstract: Falls are a major health issue in societies globally and the second leading cause of unintentional death worldwide. To address this issue, many studies aim to remotely monitor gait to prevent falls. However, these activity data collected in studies must be labelled with the appropriate environmental context through Human Activity Recognition (HAR). Multimodal HAR datasets often achieve high accuracies at the cost of cumbersome sensor systems, creating a need for these datasets to be analysed to identify the sensor types and locations that enable high-accuracy HAR. This paper analyses four datasets, USC-HAD, HuGaDB, Camargo et al.'s dataset, and CSL-SHARE, to find optimal models, methods, and sensors across multiple datasets. Regarding window size, optimal windows are found to be dependent on the sensor modality of a dataset but mostly occur in the 2–5 s range. Support Vector Machines (SVMs) and Artificial Neural Networks (ANNs) are found to be the highest-performing models overall. ANNs are further used to create models trained on the features from individual sensors of each dataset. From this analysis, Inertial Measurement Units (IMUs) and three-axis goniometers are shown to be individually capable of high classification accuracy, with Electromyography (EMG) sensors exhibiting inconsistent and reduced accuracies. Finally, it is shown that the thigh is the optimal location for IMU sensors, with accuracy decreasing as IMUs are placed further down away from the thigh.

Keywords: artificial neural networks; classification algorithms; decision trees; human activity recognition; K-nearest neighbors; machine learning; random forests; sensor systems; support vector machines; wearable sensors

1. Introduction

Falling is a significant health issue in society. The World Health Organisation (WHO) estimates that each year 37.3 million falls require medical attention, while 684,000 falls are fatal [1], making falls the second leading cause of unintentional death worldwide. Among people who fall, certain groups are at a higher risk due to cognitive or physical impairments, which can be attributed to factors including age [1,2], recent surgery [3], or conditions such as Parkinson's disease [4], dementia [5], stroke [6], multiple sclerosis [7], and amputation [8].

Many technological developments in recent years have led to an increased capability for monitoring gait in people at a high risk of falling, such as the widespread adoption of smartphones and smartwatches containing sensors, the Internet of Things (IoT) and body sensor networks, and improvements in wearable sensors. With these advances, many studies aim to automate the process of gait analysis by collecting real-time data from wearable sensors during tasks such as level-ground walking, navigating ramps, or ascending and descending stairs [9]. The data from these sensors can be analysed to aid healthcare professionals in diagnosing conditions affecting gait [10], performing gait analysis [11], or for use in detecting fall events so that the severity of future falls can be reduced [9,12,13].

However, to enable remote, real-time gait analysis, the context from which the data are extracted must be provided to the specialist who is reviewing the data. Typically, this context is obtained through the process of Human Activity Recognition (HAR), where classification methods are used to determine walking activity in real time from the collected data [9,14]. As many of these classification methods are supervised [9,14–17], a training dataset is required to build models capable of identifying activities with high accuracy. Past studies have created such datasets with a wide array of sensors, pre-processing techniques, classification methods, and validation methods, resulting in difficulty determining the most important factors that contribute towards obtaining high accuracy when designing novel sensor systems [9,14,18].

In the literature, Human Activity Recognition (HAR) studies can be separated into two categories that focus on convenience, typically making use of a smartphone or smartwatch [9,19], or accuracy by implementing a multimodal sensor system which can be cumbersome to wear [9,20,21]. In addition to the potential for accuracy, multimodal systems typically collect more appropriate quantities of data for remote gait analysis by allowing the system to collect data from multiple areas of interest through a body sensor network [22].

Existing studies on finding the optimal sliding window parameters for HAR have demonstrated a range of results in different contexts. Banos et al. [23] studied the effect of window size on classification performance for a single dataset featuring accelerometers placed on each thigh, shank, upper arm, and forearm and the back [24]. This work highlights the need for a balance between high accuracy and rapid decision times and finds that larger window sizes do not correlate to increased classification performance, with the optimal window sizes occurring below 2 s using Decision Trees (DTs), K-Nearest Neighbors (KNN), naïve Bayes, and a nearest-centroid classifier. Similarly, Niazi et al. [25] analysed the co-dependency of window size and sample rate to determine what parameters enable the highest classification accuracy using Random Forests (RFs) and a single hip-worn accelerometer. This study found that window sizes of 2–10 s were optimal, contrasting the results of Banos et al. [23]. Both of these studies highlight that future work is needed to consider additional technologies and sensor types. Li et al. [26] discuss the difficulty of determining an optimal window size for a given application, instead choosing to use different window sizes for each activity based on the temporal properties of that activity, which increases classification performance. Finally, Dehghani et al. [27] considered the effects of using overlapping sliding windows against non-overlapping sliding windows with both subject-dependent and subject-independent cross-validation on HAR performance using data collected using inertial sensors with DTs, KNN, naïve Bayes, and a nearest-centroid classifier. This study found that performance across all classifiers was reduced when using subject-independent cross-validation and that, under this condition, the use of overlapping sliding windows did not improve the performance of the models when compared to non-overalpping windows [27].

Regarding sensor placement, Duan et al. [28] placed seven accelerometers on the upper arm, wrists, thighs, and chest to determine how sensor location affected classification accuracy. This study found that sensors placed on the subjects' dominant side, the right side in all cases for this study, exhibited increased performance, with the right wrist being the highest-performing sensor type when used alone. Furthermore, this study evaluated the use of RF models along with deep learning techniques such as convolutional neural networks, transformers, and long short-term memory models with the latter. Kulchyk et al. [29] analysed the performance of sensors positioned on the sternum, left thigh, right ankle, and right shoulder using a convolutional neural network for both subject-dependent and subject-independent cross-validation. This study found the right ankle to be the optimal sensor location, with multiple pairs of sensors including the ankle sensor resulting in 100% classification accuracy [29]. Finally, Khan et al. [30] placed five sensor nodes consisting of accelerometers and gyroscopes on each forearm, the waist, and each ankle and performed HAR using simple logistic regression, naïve Bayes, and sequential minimal optimisation classifiers. The study found that individual sensor performance was dependent on activity type, with sensors on the chest and thigh being optimal for stationary tasks, whilst sensors on the thigh, lower back, and ankle performed better at movement tasks [30]. Many studies that consider sensor placement for HAR consider only accelerometers or Inertial Measurement Units (IMUs) [28–32], leaving much room for sensor position analysis using additional technologies which can capture motion data.

Overall, these studies highlight a gap in the literature for multi-dataset studies which aim to identify trends in both optimal window size and optimal sensor placement across multiple datasets and with additional motion-related technologies and sensors. As stated by Banos et al. [23], these types of studies form a guideline for future researchers faced with determining sensor locations and sliding window parameters in the future and contribute towards a knowledge database of the interactions between analytical parameters and sensors in HAR using different classifiers so that researchers and system designers can avoid performing lengthy brute-force searches across high-dimensional search spaces for individual applications of HAR.

The contributions of this study, therefore, are to identify these optimal analytical methods, sensor placements, and sensor types which will contribute towards existing knowledge of HAR classification co-dependencies such as window size, sensor type, and sensor location. This novel approach using a normalised cross-comparison of different datasets by controlling variables such as the number of participants, activity types, the sample rate, and window size for the sliding window technique creates a robust analysis that can identify trends with increased generalisability when compared with the current state-of-the-art. Therefore, the results of this study will offer reliable insights into the performance capabilities of individual sensor types and how these differ based on their locations on the body. The results of this analysis will help future researchers effectively design more lightweight sensor systems which decrease the computational burden of HAR while maintaining high levels of accuracy, comfort, and convenience.

2. Materials and Methods

Four datasets were selected for this study which feature a wide variety of sensor systems, an appropriate number of participants for sufficient model generalisation, and walking activities comparable between datasets. A description of each dataset along with the reasons it was chosen for this analysis follows.

2.1. Dataset 1: USC-HAD

The USC-HAD dataset [33] was published in 2012 and features 14 participants with a mean (standard deviation; std) age, height, and weight of 30.1 (std: 7.2) years, 170 (std: 6.8) cm, and 64.6 (std: 12.1) kg, respectively. Each subject was equipped with a single 'MotionNode' IMU containing a 3-axis accelerometer, gyroscope, and magnetometer, totalling 9 data channels. The IMU was mounted to the participants' anterior right hip in a pouch designed for mobile phones. Data were recorded using a laptop which was held under the arm, pressed to the waist by the subject and connected to the IMU via a cable.

The USC-HAD dataset features 12 activities which were performed at the participants' own pace [33]. These activities were walking forwards, left, and right, walking upstairs and downstairs, running, jumping, sitting, standing, sleeping, and going up and down in a lift.

USC-HAD was chosen because this dataset has been widely explored in the literature since its publication [15,16,34]. Therefore, this dataset acts as a control for the newer datasets to validate the chosen methods and models.

2.2. Dataset 2: HuGaDB

The HuGaDB dataset [35] was published in 2017 and features 18 participants with a mean age, height, and weight of 23.67 (std: 3.69) years, 179.06 (std: 9.85) cm, and 73.44 (std: 16.67) kg, respectively. The sensor system worn by each participant consisted of IMU sensors placed at the thigh, shank, and foot and an Electromyography (EMG) sensor placed on the vastus lateralis, each of which were sampled at around 60 Hz. This setup was mirrored on each leg, for a total of six IMUs and two EMG sensors.

Participants were asked to perform the following 12 activities at a usual pace: walking, running, navigating stairs, sitting (stationary), sitting down, and standing up, standing (stationary), cycling, going up and down in a lift, and sitting in a car [35].

2.3. Dataset 3: Camargo et al.

Camargo et al. [36] created an open-source dataset for the study of lower-limb biomechanics in 2021, featuring 22 healthy participants with a mean age, height, and weight of 21 (std: 3.4) years, 170 (std: 7.0) cm, and 68.3 (std: 10.83) kg, respectively. Subjects were equipped with 11 EMG sensors, 3 goniometers, and 4 six-axis IMUs on their right side only. Sensor locations and sample rates can be found in Table 1.

Table 1. The sensor type, position, and sample rate of each sensor in the Camargo et al. dataset.

Sensor	Position	Sample Rate
Goniometer	Hip Knee Trunk	1000 Hz
Inertial Measurement Unit	Trunk Thigh Shank Foot	200 Hz
Electromyography Sensor	Gastrocnemius Medialis Tibialis Anterior Soleus Vastus Medialis Vastus Lateralis Rectus Femoris Biceps femoris Semitendinosus Gracilis Gluteus Medius Right External Oblique	1000 Hz

Whilst participants only performed six basic activities, the transition states were also labelled, raising the activity count to 19 [36]. With the 'idle' class removed as no activities were performed, 18 walking activities remained, consisting of six core activities and the transitions between them. These core activities were ramp ascent, ramp descent, stair ascent, stair descent, stand, turning, and walking.

2.4. Dataset 4: CSL-SHARE

CSL-SHARE is a dataset published in 2021 for the purpose of exploring activity recognition for common sport-related movements [37]. The sensor system is a multimodal, knee-mounted system featuring 2 6-axis IMUs placed on the thigh and shank, 4 EMG sensors placed on the vastus medialis, tibialis anterior, biceps femoris, and gastrocnemius, a goniometer placed on the lateral knee, and an airborne microphone. Like the Camargo et al. dataset, these sensors were placed on the right leg only. The CSL-SHARE dataset features 22 activities and was upscaled to 1000Hz due to differing sample rates for the various sensors [37].

2.5. Summary of Datasets

The datasets chosen for this study cover a variety of environments, activities, and sensor configurations. Analysis of the datasets with the same Machine Learning (ML) models and pre-processing methods will provide insight into how sensor configuration and type affect classification accuracy in HAR. A comparison of these datasets can be found in Table 2.

Table 2. A summary of the properties of each dataset in this analysis.

Dataset Features	USC-HAD	Camargo et al.	HuGaDB	CSL-SHARE
Participants	14	22	18	20
Mean Age (Years)	30.1	21	23.67	30.5
Mean Height (cm)	170	170	179.06	N/A
Mean Weight (kg)	64.6	68.3	73.44	N/A
IMU Sensors	1	4	6	2
EMG Sensors	0	11	2	4
Goniometers	0	3	0	1
Acoustic Sensors	0	0	0	1
Activities	12	18	12	22
Sample Rate	100 Hz	200 Hz/1000 Hz	60 Hz	100 Hz/1000 Hz

2.6. Dataset Preprocessing

2.6.1. Normalisation Between Datasets

As this study focuses on the sensor types in the HAR datasets, steps were taken to remove the variations between datasets. Of the variables in Table 2, participant numbers, activity types, and sample rates were normalised. To achieve this, the number of participants in each dataset was limited to the minimum number available across all datasets, which was 14, with additional participants being excluded from the datasets where appropriate to maintain a fair comparison between the datasets. For example, in CSL-SHARE, participants 2, 11, and 16 contained different data due to varying protocol versions, device communication issues, and a participant stopping early due to knee pain. As such, these participants were removed, before cropping the number of participants down to 14. Of the activities included in the chosen datasets, only walking, standing, stair ascent, and stair descent were common across all datasets and are activities of interest with respect to fall-related research [38,39]. Therefore, the additional activities were removed from each dataset. Finally, 100 Hz was chosen as the common sample rate, resulting in the sample rate for the Camargo et al. and CSL-SHARE datasets being subsampled to 100 Hz, whilst HuGaDB was interpolated up to 300 Hz with 5th-order polynomial interpolation, before being subsampled to 100 Hz.

2.6.2. Filtering

Before data could be presented to the Machine Learning models, a series of preprocessing steps had to be performed to prepare the data for use by the Machine Learning models. This process began with a 4th-order low-pass Butterworth filter with a cut-off frequency of 7 Hz before windowing and feature extraction occurred. This cut-off frequency was chosen through testing and laid around the 10 Hz mark, which is typical for analyses using inertial sensors [19].

2.7. Feature Extraction

As is typical when performing classification with time-series data, semi-overlapping sliding windows are used to extract statistical features such that a single sample represents a larger time window of raw data. The size of these windows and the amount of overlap varies between studies, with lower window sizes being preferable for real-time classification, whilst larger window sizes consider more of the gait cycle per sample which may result in higher classification accuracies. For this study, a search was performed to identify trends in accuracy from a 1 s to 10 s window size, with a 75% window overlap for each window size. This overlap was chosen to combine co-dependent sliding window parameters and reduce computation times.

For each window of the time-series data, a wide array of statistical features were extracted to enable the ML models to make accurate predictions. There is little consensus on which features are necessary for accurate HAR, with many studies considering a mean of 15 features [15,40–46]. This analysis included 22 features from each sensor, including commonly chosen features from existing research [15,42–45,47]. Most of these features were extracted from the raw data in the time domain, with Fourier transforms being used to obtain additional features from the frequency domain. Feature selection methods were then used to eliminate noisy features before classification. This combination of increased feature numbers with appropriate feature selection techniques to accommodate this ensured that relevant data from each sensor were present to allow a sensor-focussed analysis. The list of included features is as follows:

- Maximum value.
- Minimum value.
- Mean.
- Median.
- Standard deviation.
- Mean absolute deviation.
- Median absolute deviation.
- Number of zero crossings.
- Root mean square.
- Maximum gradient.
- Kurtosis.
- Skewness.
- Variance.
- Interquartile range.
- Entropy.

- Energy.
- Maximum frequency amplitude.
- Mean frequency amplitude.
- Maximum power spectral density.
- Mean power spectral density.
- Frequency kurtosis.
- Frequency skewness.

After feature extraction, the data were split into train and test data by leaving out the data from a single subject. Scikit-Learn's 'MinMaxScaler' function was then fit to the train set and applied separately to the train and test sets to scale each feature between 0 and 1. Principal Component Analysis (PCA) was performed to reduce the number of features. As with the scaler, the PCA was fit to the train set and applied separately to the train and test sets. The number of selected principal components varied for each dataset due to the different features which were dependent on the sensors but was controlled by choosing the minimum amount required to retain 95% of the variance of the full feature set. Finally, another round of scaling was performed to prepare the data for the Machine Learning algorithms.

2.8. Cross-Validation and Test Data

Two methods of cross-validation and testing are prevalent in the literature for gait- and fall-related studies: subject-dependent analysis using Train-Test Split (TTS) cross-validation and subject-independent analysis using Leave-One-Subject-Out (LOSO) cross-validation [27,48]. TTS cross-validation uses a set percentage of the total data from all subjects as test and validation data, whilst LOSO leaves out the data from a specific subject. Each of these methods of cross-validation offers differing advantages and disadvantages, with TTS creating models with higher accuracies at the cost of poor generalisation, whilst LOSO typically creates models with lower accuracies that perform better with data from new subjects. For this study, both TTS and LOSO cross-validations are used to make the results applicable to both types of devices and to be more comparable with existing and future studies.

2.9. Models

For classification, the KNN, Support Vector Machine (SVM), DT, RF, and Artificial Neural Network (ANN) models, an ensemble voting classifier, and an ensemble stacking classifier were chosen due to their prevalence in the literature. Ensemble models were constructed from each of the individual models (KNN, SVM, DT, RF, and ANN), with either a voting or a logistic regression classifier fusing the decisions. This inclusion of a variety of ML models reduced variations in classifier performance that could be introduced due to the various properties of each model, such as how prone they are to overfitting and how dataset size affects their classification performance.

Hyperparameter tuning was performed using 25 iterations of the Scikit-Optimize Bayesian hyperparameter search. All models were trained on a computer with 32 GB of RAM, a 12th Generation Intel i9-12900K processor, and a 12 GB Nvidia RTX 3060 GPU using the Scikit-Learn library for Python version 3.9.18.

2.10. Performance Metrics and Evaluation

To assess the performance of each model, this study considered both macro-average accuracy and the F1-score. While macro-average accuracy provides a straightforward overview of a model by reporting the mean classification accuracy across all classes, it can be misleading in the presence of large class imbalances, as it does not account for differences in class distribution. To address this, the macro-average F1-score was also reported, which provides a more balanced measure of performance across classes. For each dataset, walking was the primary class, with around 10× more walking data than stair ascent and stair descent data. Standing data varied between datasets but were typically around 2–3× more numerous than data in the stair ascent and stair descent classes.

3. Results

To determine the optimal window size for sliding window feature extraction, each model was trained using the PCA-reduced feature set for each window size, ranging from 1 to 10 s. We selected 10 s as the maximum time due to issues with class distributions and the number of samples in each class at larger window sizes. This process was repeated three times for each model to reduce the impact of random initialisations, which can lead to models becoming stuck in local minima during training. The results for subject-dependent cross-validation can be seen in Figures 1–4, whilst the results for subject-independent cross-validation can be found in Figures 5–8. A full list of performance metrics for each dataset and window size can be found in Appendix A.

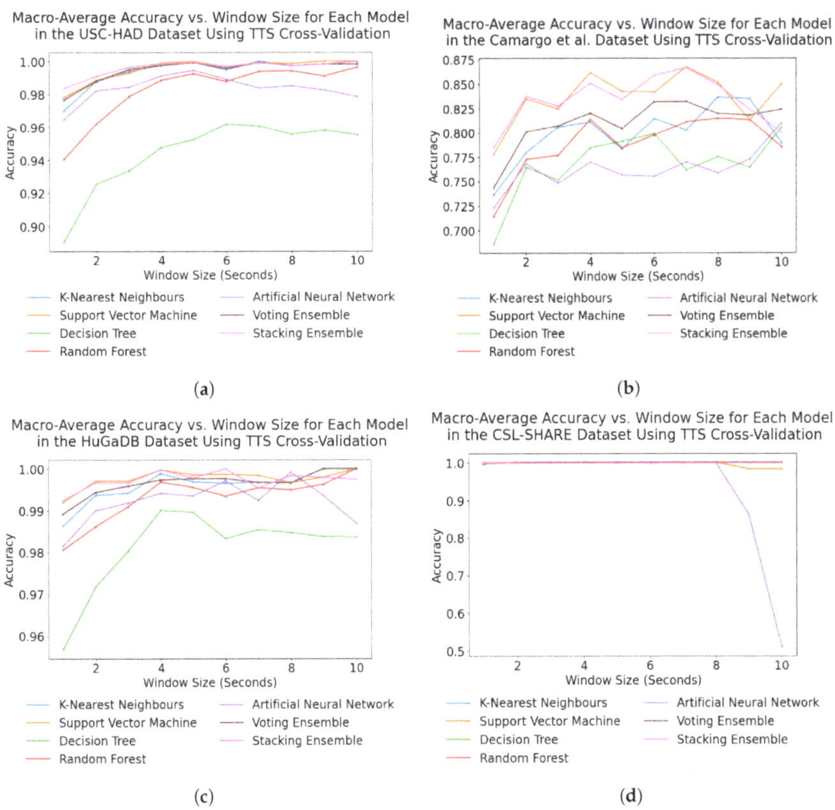

Figure 1. Trend graphs showing the mean accuracy across all models and window sizes for the four datasets in this analysis when using TTS cross-validation. (**a**) USC-HAD. (**b**) Camargo et al. (**c**) HuGaDB. (**d**) CSL-SHARE.

3.1. Subject-Dependent Cross-Validation

3.1.1. Determining Optimal Window Sizes

Figures 1 and 2 show the mean performance of each model over the three repeat trials for each window size. The trend lines present in these figures demonstrate an increase in both accuracy and the F1-score with window size for subject-dependent cross-validation using TTS across all models and all datasets. The exceptions to this trend suggest that overfitting may have occurred as the number of samples decreased, with some models decreasing in performance with 9 and 10 s window sizes, where the number of data from each class was at a minimum. This issue was most prevalent with the ANNs among the smaller datasets, whilst the Camargo et al. dataset was the only one in which the ANN performance metrics did not drop at higher window size values. Although performance generally trended upwards with window size, all datasets except for CSL-SHARE, which exhibited 100% accuracy and a 100% F1-score for most models at all window sizes, plateaued at around 4–5 s. Furthermore, CSL-SHARE appeared to exhibit reduced performance at higher window sizes for both the ANN and SVM, likely due to a lack of data.

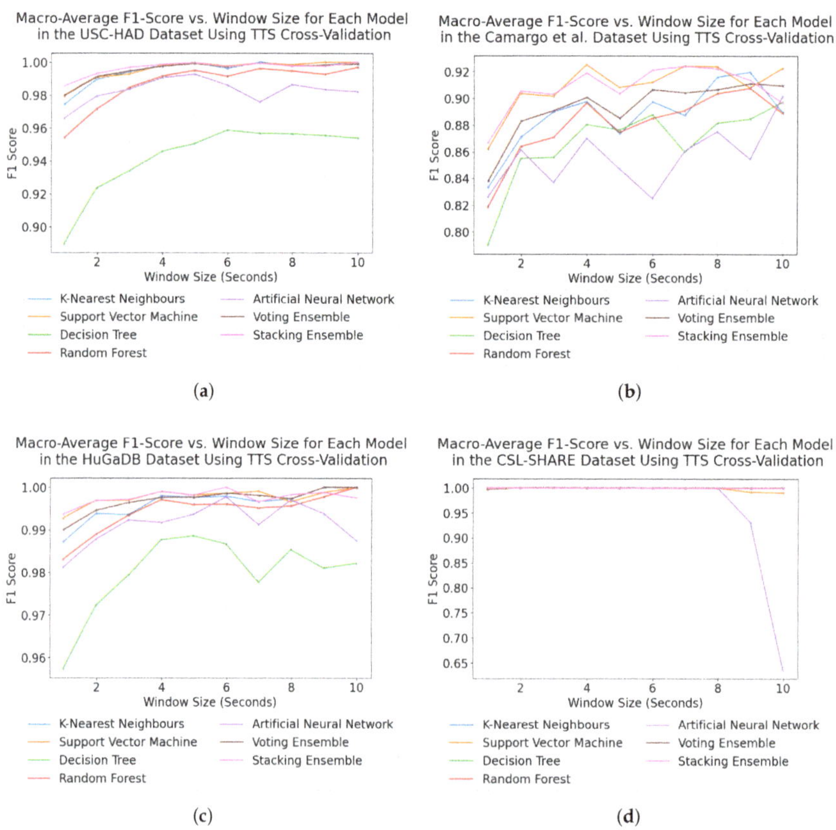

Figure 2. Trend graphs showing the mean F1-score across all models and window sizes for the four datasets in this analysis when using TTS cross-validation. (**a**) USC-HAD. (**b**) Camargo et al. (**c**) HuGaDB. (**d**) CSL-SHARE.

Figures 3 and 4 show the average highest-performing model among all window sizes, along with the average accuracy and F1-score at each window size across all models. These figures highlight the SVM and the stacking ensemble classifier as the most capable models across all window sizes and that the best model performances occurred at window sizes of 4–8 s.

Regarding the individual (non-ensemble) highest-performing model, all models performed fairly similarly between datasets, with the SVM being the only model that performed significantly higher than others with average accuracies of 99.6%, 83.7%, 99.8%, and 100% and average F1-scores of 99.7%, 90.9%, 99.8%, and 100% on each of the USC-HAD, Camargo et al., HuGaDB, and CSL-SHARE datasets, respectively. However, these results also suggest there may be an issue with the Camargo et al. dataset, as the average accuracies for all models and window sizes were far more reduced for this dataset when compared with the others. An overview of the highest-performing individual models can be found in Table 3.

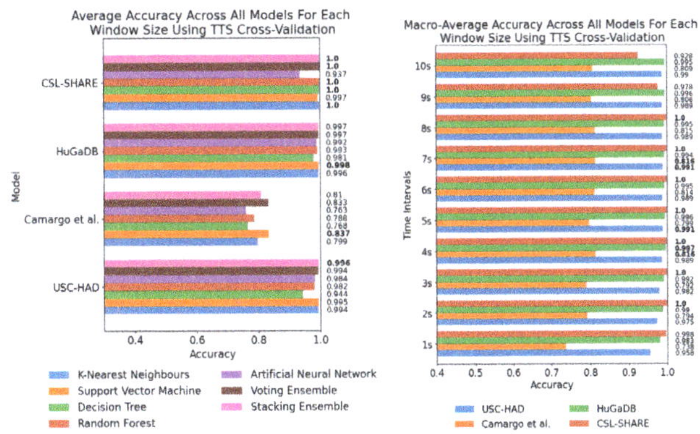

(a) (b)

Figure 3. Model and window size effect on classification accuracy across all four datasets using TTS cross-validation. The highest-performing model for each dataset and window size is marked in bold. (**a**) Average accuracy for each model across all window sizes for each dataset. (**b**) Average accuracy across all models at each window size from 1 to 10 s for each dataset.

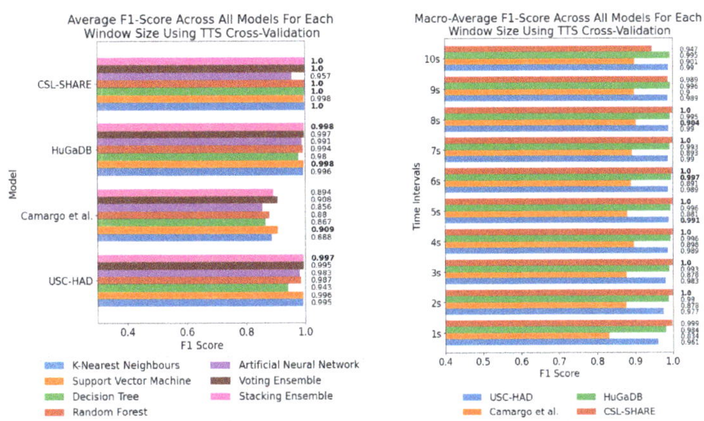

(a) (b)

Figure 4. Model and window size effect on F1-score across all four datasets using TTS cross-validation. The highest-performing model for each dataset and window size is marked in bold. (**a**) Average F1-score for each model across all window sizes for each dataset. (**b**) Average F1-score across all models at each window size from 1 to 10 s for each dataset.

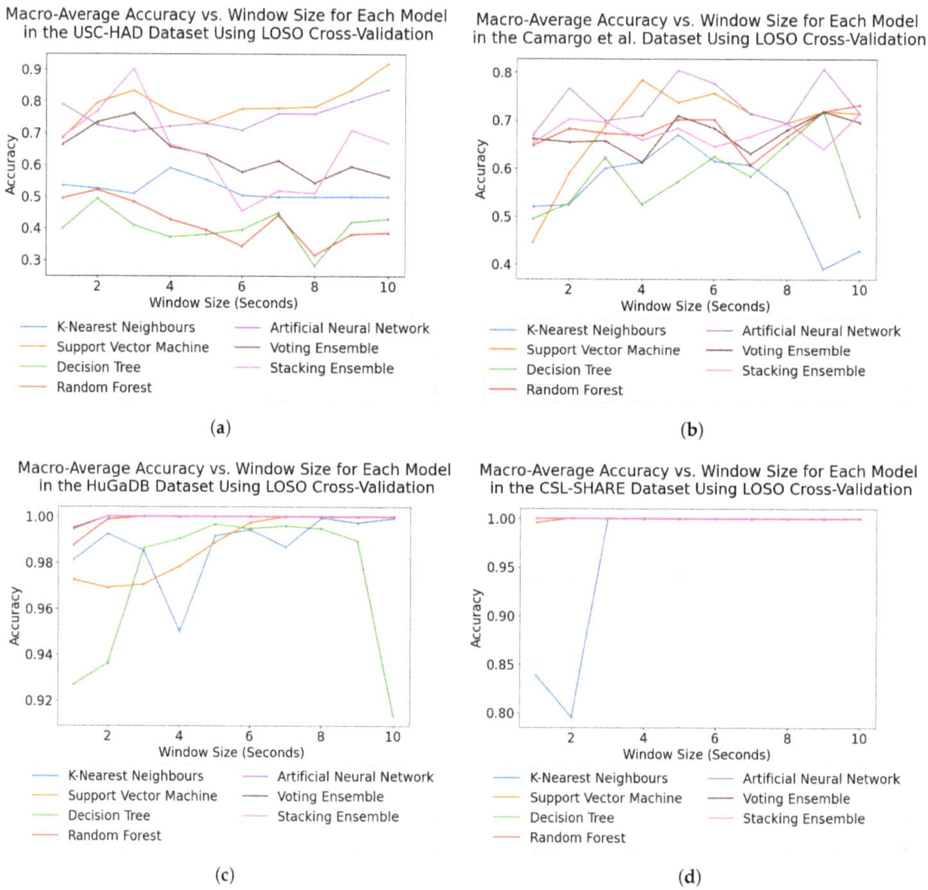

Figure 5. Trend graphs showing the mean accuracy across all models and window sizes for the four datasets in this analysis when using LOSO cross-validation. (**a**) USC-HAD. (**b**) Camargo et al. (**c**) HuGaDB. (**d**) CSL-SHARE.

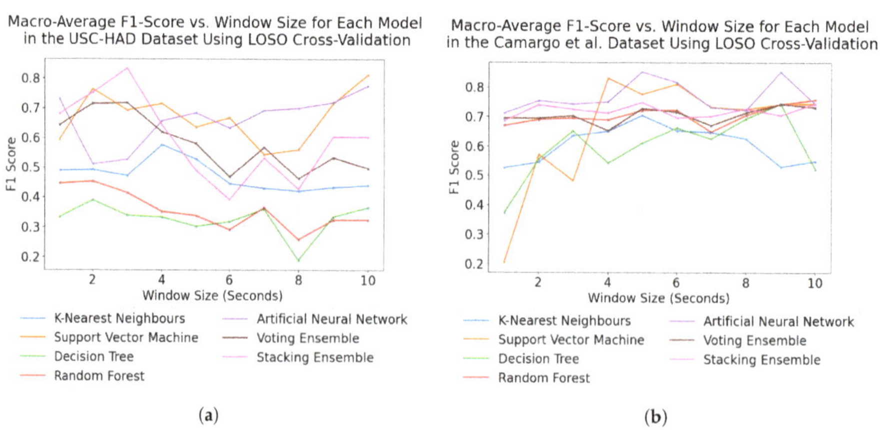

Figure 6. *Cont.*

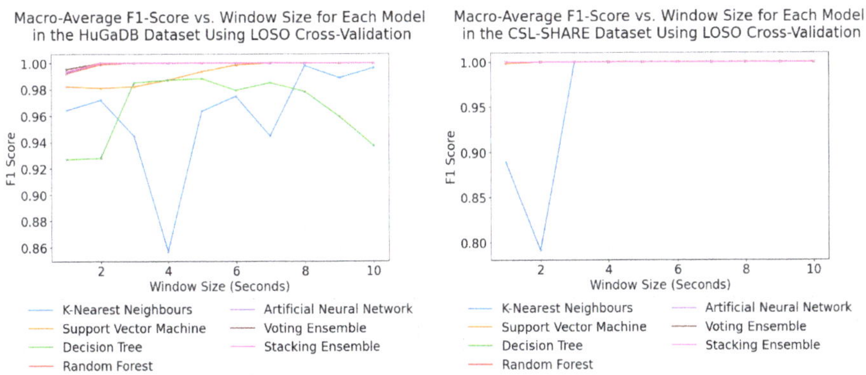

(c) (d)

Figure 6. Trend graphs showing the mean F1-score across all models and window sizes for the four datasets in this analysis when using LOSO cross-validation. (**a**) USC-HAD. (**b**) Camargo et al. (**c**) HuGaDB. (**d**) CSL-SHARE.

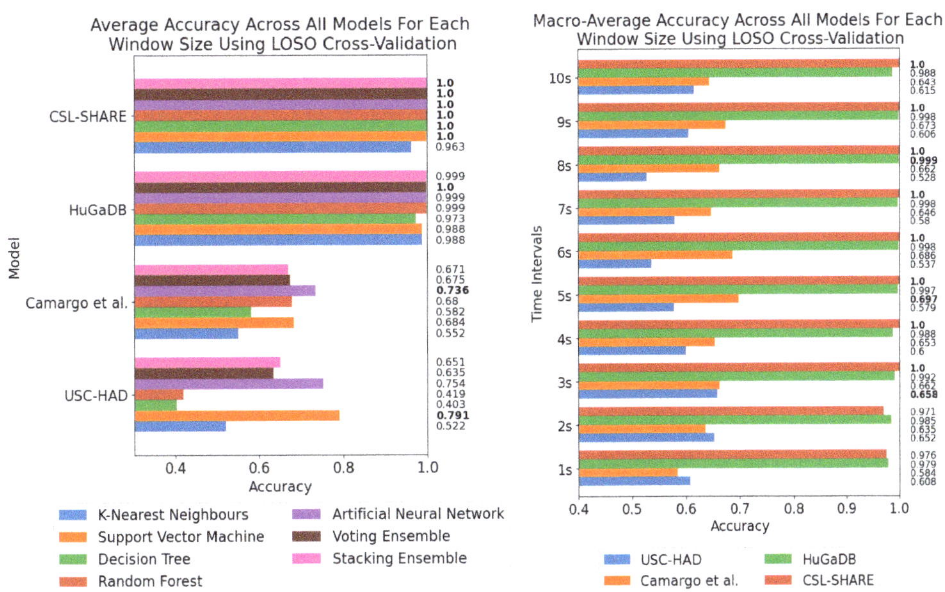

(a) (b)

Figure 7. Model and window size effect on classification accuracy across all four datasets using LOSO cross-validation. The highest-performing model for each dataset and window size is marked in bold. (**a**) Average accuracy for each model across all window sizes for each dataset. (**b**) Average accuracy across all models at each window size from 1 to 10 s for each dataset.

3.1.2. Individual Sensor Analysis

The optimal window sizes for each dataset were used to determine the sensor importance for achieving high accuracies among the four core activities. As USC-HAD contained just a single sensor, it was excluded from this analysis. Due to its high performance across all datasets, and due to the SVM failing to converge on these reduced datasets, an ANN was trained to classify between the four activities using data from individual sensors.

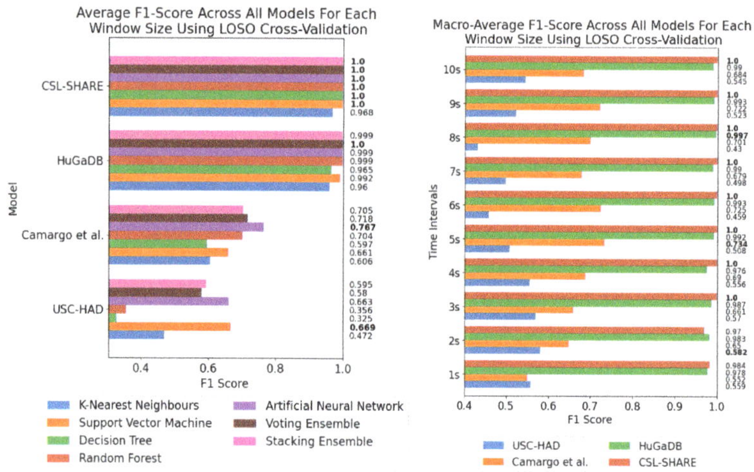

(a) (b)

Figure 8. Model and window size effect on F1-score across all four datasets using LOSO cross-validation. The highest-performing model for each dataset and window size is marked in bold. (**a**) Average F1-score for each model across all window sizes for each dataset. (**b**) Average F1-score across all models at each window size from 1 to 10 s for each dataset.

Tables 4–6 show the precision, recall, F1-score, and accuracy of the ANN trained from features extracted from each sensor in the Camargo et al., HuGaDB, and CSL-SHARE datasets, respectively. These tables highlight IMUs as the most effective individual sensors, exhibiting accuracies of 87.4–100% and F1-scores of 74.4–100% across all datasets. Goniometers also appear as high-performing sensors, with the three-axis goniometers at the hip and ankle in the Camargo et al. dataset exhibiting performance metrics marginally lower than those of the IMUs, with accuracies of 86.8% and 87.4% and F1-scores of 74.2% and 70.8%, respectively. Following the three-axis goniometers, both the Camargo et al. and CSL-SHARE datasets feature two-axis goniometers at the knee, which enabled accuracies of 74.2% and 99.6%, respectively. However, with an F1-score of just 44.5% for the Camargo et al. knee goniometer, this may suggest that two-axis goniometers lacked the data dimensionality for high-accuracy HAR. Finally, the EMG sensors exhibited the lowest performance metrics across all datasets. Among the EMG sensors, placement heavily affected classification accuracy, with the vastus lateralis and biceps femoris performing extremely poorly, whilst the tibialis anterior, soleus, gastrocnemius, and vastus medialis generally outperformed EMG sensors placed on other muscles. However, even the highest-performing EMG sensors in each dataset exhibit F1-scores significantly lower than those of the IMUs.

3.2. Subject-Independent Cross-Validation

3.2.1. Determining Optimal Window Sizes

Figure 5 shows the performance trends of each model at each window size for the four datasets in this study using LOSO cross-validation. The maximum accuracy for USC-HAD occurred at a 10 s window size with the SVM exhibiting an accuracy of 91.9% and an F1-score of 81.2%, whilst the Camargo et al. dataset achieved a maximum accuracy of 80.8% and an F1-score of 85.2% at 9 s using the ANN. Both the CSL-SHARE and HuGaDB datasets achieved a 100% classification accuracy and an F1-score with multiple model types at 1 and 2 s, respectively, which was maintained up to a window size of 10 s. The DT, RF, and KNN models performed erratically across all datasets and window sizes, which caused the stacking and voting ensemble methods to underperform when compared to the ANN and SVM.

Table 3. Maximum accuracy, precision, recall, and F1-Score for each dataset, non-ensemble model, and method of cross-validation.

Dataset	Model	Window Size (s)	Acc (%)	Prec (%)	Rec (%)	F1-Score (%)
USC-HAD TTS	SVM	5	99.90	99.73	99.90	99.81
USC-HAD LOSO	SVM	10	91.89	79.29	91.89	81.17
Camargo et al. TTS	SVM	4	86.15	92.56	92.52	92.51
Camargo et al. LOSO	ANN	5	80.41	86.66	86.06	85.19
HuGaDB TTS	SVM	4	99.97	99.82	99.97	99.90
HuGaDB LOSO	ANN	2	100	100	100	100
CSL-SHARE TTS	ALL	2	100	100	100	100
CSL-SHARE LOSO	ALL	3	100	100	100	100

Table 4. Subject-dependent performance metrics of each individual sensor in the Camargo et al. dataset.

Sensor	Precision	Recall	F1-Score	Accuracy
Trunk IMU	0.801	0.798	0.799	0.897
Thigh IMU	0.753	0.751	0.744	0.874
Shank IMU	0.778	0.769	0.772	0.881
Foot IMU	0.814	0.787	0.774	0.894
Gastrocnemius Medialis EMG	0.716	0.630	0.621	0.758
Tibialis Anterior EMG	0.636	0.547	0.523	0.755
Soleus EMG	0.676	0.620	0.629	0.774
Vastus Medialis EMG	0.459	0.493	0.470	0.652
Vastus Lateralis EMG	0.158	0.256	0.169	0.458
Rectus Femoris EMG	0.185	0.252	0.212	0.374
Biceps Femoris EMG	0.296	0.348	0.302	0.561
Semitendinosus EMG	0.216	0.296	0.242	0.423
Gracilis EMG	0.763	0.460	0.456	0.652
Gluteus Medius EMG	0.348	0.357	0.316	0.577
Right External Oblique EMG	0.372	0.372	0.336	0.594
Ankle Goniometer	0.741	0.747	0.708	0.874
Knee Goniometer	0.410	0.500	0.445	0.742
Hip Goniometer	0.753	0.744	0.742	0.868

Figure 7 shows the mean accuracies across all time windows and models. From Figure 7a, the SVMs and ANNs appear as the classifiers with the highest classification accuracy where there is a statistically significant difference between classifier performances, with the SVMs achieving 79.1%, 68.4%, 98.8%, and 99.9% accuracies and F1-scores of 66.9%, 66.1%, 99.2%, and 100%, whilst the ANNs achieved 75.4%, 73.6%, 99.9%, and 100% accuracies and F1-scores of 66.3%, 76.7%, 99.9% and 100% on each of the USC-HAD, Camargo et al., HuGaDB, and CSL-SHARE datasets, respectively. As such, the ANN and SVM can clearly be identified as the highest-performing model types across all datasets, as seen in Table 3. Concerning window size, each dataset presented a different window size at which the maximum mean accuracy occurred. For USC-HAD, the highest mean accuracy and F1-score across all models occurred at 2–3 s window sizes, whilst for the Camargo et al. dataset, these occurred at 5 s, both of which were similar to the time at which model accuracy plateaued using subject-dependent cross-validation. Both HuGaDB and CSL-SHARE achieved accuracies of 100% with several models, but due to the lower accuracies with other models, their highest mean performances occurred at 8 s for HuGaDB and any value from 3 to 10 s for CSL-SHARE.

Table 5. Subject-dependent performance metrics of each individual sensor in the HuGaDB dataset.

Sensor	Precision	Recall	F1-Score	Accuracy
Right Thigh IMU	0.990	0.994	0.992	0.995
Left Thigh IMU	0.993	0.996	0.995	0.997
Right Shank IMU	0.995	0.997	0.996	0.998
Left Shank IMU	0.989	0.990	0.989	0.993
Right Foot IMU	0.973	0.979	0.976	0.987
Left Foot IMU	0.978	0.984	0.981	0.991
Right Vastus Lateralis EMG	0.669	0.509	0.506	0.775
Left Vastus Lateralis EMG	0.597	0.478	0.457	0.783

Table 6. Subject-dependent performance metrics of each individual sensor in the CSL-SHARE dataset.

Sensor	Precision	Recall	F1-Score	Accuracy
Vastus Medialis EMG	0.691	0.699	0.695	0.661
Tibialis Anterior EMG	0.659	0.648	0.644	0.592
Biceps Femoris EMG	0.430	0.383	0.391	0.367
Gastrocnemius EMG	0.582	0.550	0.534	0.475
Airborne Microphone	0.550	0.536	0.534	0.454
Thigh IMU	1.000	1.000	1.000	1.000
Shank IMU	1.000	1.000	1.000	1.000
Knee Goniometer	0.997	0.996	0.997	0.996

3.2.2. Individual Sensor Analysis

As with the subject-dependent individual sensor analysis, the ANN was trained on the features extracted from each individual sensor. Tables 7–9 show the performance metrics for each sensor used in the Camargo et al., HuGaDB, and CSL-SHARE datasets, respectively. Like with the subject-dependent analysis, the IMUs achieved the highest accuracies across two of the three datasets, whilst the EMG sensors exhibited consistently poor performances. In this scenario, performance metrics were generally reduced, with only the EMG sensors placed on the gastrocnemius medialis and gluteus medius for the Camargo et al. dataset and the vastus medialis for the CSL-SHARE dataset achieving accuracies and F1-scores above 50%. The three-axis goniometers on the hip from the Camargo et al. dataset exhibited higher performance metrics than the IMUs in this case, with the ankle goniometer outperforming all but the foot IMU, whilst the two-axis goniometers positioned on the knee in the Camargo et al. and CSL-SHARE datasets exhibited much lower performance metrics.

Overall, the trends among these sensors were largely the same as with the subject-dependent analysis, with the main difference being the high performance of the three-axis goniometers, along with an overall reduction in accuracy for the two-axis goniometers and EMG sensors, further highlighting the volatility of performance when using these sensors.

Table 7. Subject-independent performance metrics of each individual sensor in the Camargo et al. dataset.

Sensor	Precision	Recall	F1-Score	Accuracy
Trunk IMU	0.781	0.787	0.754	0.787
Thigh IMU	0.299	0.547	0.386	0.547
Shank IMU	0.680	0.720	0.679	0.720
Foot IMU	0.795	0.800	0.788	0.800
Gastrocnemius Medialis EMG	0.513	0.600	0.532	0.600
Tibialis Anterior EMG	0.272	0.227	0.226	0.227
Soleus EMG	0.599	0.347	0.381	0.347
Vastus Medialis EMG	0.110	0.173	0.120	0.173
Vastus Lateralis EMG	0.453	0.307	0.361	0.307
Rectus Femoris EMG	0.072	0.147	0.085	0.147
Biceps Femoris EMG	0.475	0.400	0.409	0.400
Semitendinosus EMG	0.404	0.307	0.307	0.307
Gracilis EMG	0.080	0.173	0.110	0.173
Gluteus Medius EMG	0.548	0.667	0.556	0.667
Right External Oblique EMG	0.419	0.187	0.157	0.187
Ankle Goniometer	0.738	0.800	0.759	0.800
Knee Goniometer	0.285	0.267	0.229	0.267
Hip Goniometer	0.927	0.880	0.859	0.880

Table 8. Subject-independent performance metrics of each individual sensor in the HuGaDB dataset.

Sensor	Precision	Recall	F1-Score	Accuracy
Right Thigh IMU	1.000	1.000	1.000	1.000
Left Thigh IMU	0.970	0.966	0.966	0.984
Right Shank IMU	1.000	1.000	1.000	1.000
Left Shank IMU	0.976	0.997	0.986	0.992
Right Foot IMU	0.953	0.960	0.952	0.982
Left Foot IMU	0.874	0.824	0.779	0.923
Right Vastus Lateralis EMG	0.211	0.290	0.229	0.478
Left Vastus Lateralis EMG	0.428	0.330	0.330	0.726

Table 9. Subject-independent performance metrics of each individual sensor in the CSL-SHARE dataset.

Sensor	Precision	Recall	F1-Score	Accuracy
Vastus Medialis EMG	0.846	0.634	0.624	0.757
Tibialis Anterior EMG	0.475	0.375	0.332	0.456
Biceps Femoris EMG	0.366	0.361	0.270	0.417
Gastrocnemius EMG	0.300	0.458	0.354	0.573
Airborne Microphone	0.525	0.517	0.475	0.427
Thigh IMU	0.992	0.993	0.992	0.990
Shank IMU	0.935	0.931	0.924	0.903
Knee Goniometer	0.884	0.767	0.706	0.738

4. Discussions

The results of the window size analysis did not exhibit a consistent peak or plateau, with accuracies appearing volatile across the four datasets for each window size and trend lines displaying misaligned peaks. Furthermore, the averaging of accuracies across all models at each window size showed no clear single optimal window size across the four datasets and methods of cross-validation.

It must be noted that the performance metrics of the Camargo et al. dataset did not align with the other multimodal datasets in terms of overall classification accuracy. These systems all made use of the same six-axis IMU positioned on the thigh, yet the Camargo et al. dataset achieved significantly reduced accuracies when trained on only this sensor when compared to HuGaDB and CSL-SHARE. Given the large number of controlled variables in this study, this indicates a difference in experimental procedure or activity data distribution, which negatively affects the results of the Camargo et al. dataset. Figure 9a shows the confusion matrix for an SVM trained on the Camargo et al. dataset, which shows that the misclassifications are between the stair ascend and stair descend classes. This is also shown not to be caused by sample weighting, as Figure 9b,c show the confusion matrices for the HuGaDB and CSL-SHARE datasets, respectively, which feature more extreme sample weightings than the Camargo et al. dataset whilst achieving 100% accuracy.

Figure 9 highlights SVMs as the most effective individual models for HAR using subject-dependent cross-validation, with ANNs proving more effective when using subject-independent cross-validation. This is likely due to the tendency for ANNs to overfit, which was further pronounced by the use of a TTS in creating test data for subject-dependent cross-validation, whereas SVMs typically perform well in these scenarios due to the maximisation of the margin when creating a decision boundary.

For subject-dependent cross-validation, peak accuracies occurred at smaller window sizes, ranging from 2–5 s. The trend lines in Figures 1 and 5 also exhibit rises in accuracy for some models as they approach a 10-s window size, indicating that, if the dataset contains enough samples in each class for this to be viable, larger window sizes offer richer features which lead to higher classification accuracies. For subject-independent cross-validation, the highest-performing model accuracies occurred at 2, 3, 5, and 10 s for the HuGaDB, CSL-SHARE, Camargo et al., and USC-HAD datasets, respectively. Apart from USC-HAD, this further highlights the range of 2–5 s as an effective range of window sizes in achieving high classification accuracy for the core activities of HAR.

Aside from the Camargo et al. dataset, the multimodal datasets achieved much higher classification accuracies when using the same models and window sizes, which allowed high accuracies to be obtained with much smaller window sizes. This has significant implications when considering the delay time, portability, and convenience of systems, as increasing the number of sensors can enable high-accuracy HAR using very computationally inexpensive methods such as DT. These computationally low-cost methods can also allow designers of real-time HAR systems to incorporate low-power computational devices with reduced size profiles and battery consumption, therefore increasing the comfort and convenience of the devices. Additionally, the fact that high accuracies can be obtained in multimodal systems with low window sizes means that much faster response times can be achieved for real-time HAR systems, as some models trained on the CSL-SHARE dataset achieved 100% accuracy using just 1 s windows with a 0.25 s fixed delay time caused by the step size. Whilst it was shown that accuracy at each window size was dependent on the sensor types used in each dataset, further work is needed to identify how model performance varies with window size for each individual sensor type. This will enable the building of a knowledge database to help future researchers choose a window size given a sensor system without the need for lengthy, brute-force approaches to finding the most appropriate window size, combination of sensors, and choice of model for each novel dataset produced in this field.

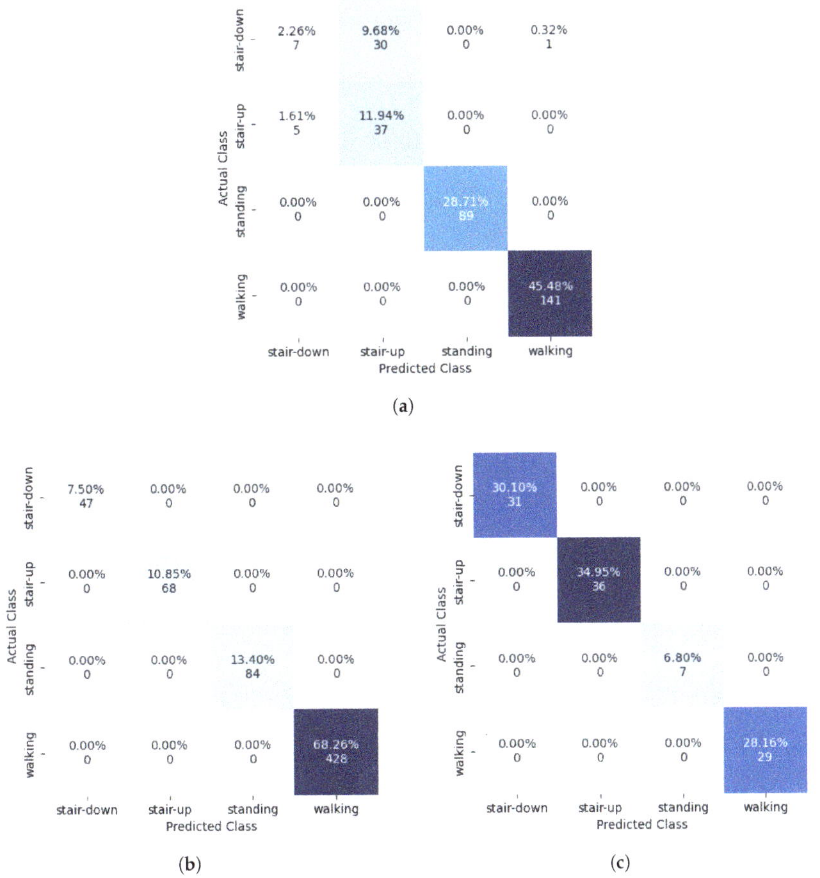

Figure 9. Confusion matrices of an SVM trained on data from a single EMG sensor using LOSO cross-validation. (**a**) Camargo et al. Vastus Lateralis. (**b**) HuGaDB Vastus Lateralis. (**c**) CSL-SHARE Vastus Medialis EMG.

Regarding individual sensor types, the IMUs and three-axis goniometers generally exhibited the highest accuracies, followed by the two-axis goniometers and finally the EMG sensors. Among IMU locations, accuracy varied among the different locations, with no clear ranking between all datasets. Only the Camargo et al. and CSL-SHARE datasets featured goniometers, with the three-axis goniometers at the thigh and ankle in the Camargo et al. dataset showing large performance improvements over the two-axis goniometers located on the knee in both the Camargo et al. and CSL-SHARE datasets. Goniometers are low-power devices with fewer data dimensions than IMUs which can be incorporated into smart clothing devices to improve comfort and convenience. Given the competitive performance of goniometers in this study, three-axis goniometers should be considered in future datasets and HAR systems. On the other hand, EMG sensor performance was volatile between locations and datasets, which may be due to differences in filtering methods, varying placements on muscles, or changes in experimental procedures. As such, it is not currently possible to compare the locations of these sensors, particularly with so few datasets for reference. More datasets are required to accurately rank the locations of these sensors so that the impact of differences in experimental setup can be minimised.

Regarding the sample rates of each dataset, no correlation was present between the native sample rates of each dataset and the final classification accuracy, with the HuGaDB dataset exhibiting far higher accuracies than USC-HAD and the Camargo et al. dataset, despite having the lowest native sample rate of 60 Hz. As such, whilst sample rate is expected to have an effect at even lower values, 60 Hz can be considered a sufficient sample rate for high-accuracy HAR.

These results align with the findings of Banos et al. [23], who found that increased window size does not necessarily increase activity classification performance across many datasets. However, our study also offers insight into the reason for this assumption, with subject-dependent cross-validation demonstrating this pattern until accuracy and F1-score began to reduce at larger window size values due to insufficient sample sizes. Crucially, this work considers both subject-dependent and subject-independent methods of cross-validation, which highlights how the choice of cross-validation method impacts the selection of an optimal window size, which was not considered in the study [23]. Niazi et al. [25] considered the effect of window size and sample rate on classification accuracy using an RF classifier, where it was reported that window sizes could appear optimal between 2–10 s using subject-dependent cross-validation. Our results support these findings and demonstrate that this also applies to additional classical Machine Learning models such as the ANN, SVM, KNN, and DT. Duan et al. [28] considered the optimal placement of sensors using deep learning techniques for a single dataset, finding that sensors placed on the right leg exhibited increased performance. Our results align with the findings of this study, with the HuGaDB dataset demonstrating that, when subject-independent cross-validation was used, the performance metrics of the right leg were higher than those of the left. Finally, Khan et al. [30] report that sensor performance is dependent on the activities being performed in the dataset. By removing the variation between datasets, our study controlled for this factor, resulting in a reliable ranking of sensor locations that achieved high performances and offer future researchers the information necessary to build effective HAR systems.

Finally, this study featured several limitations due to the computational cost of performing this analysis. The first of these limitations was the lack of investigation into the effects of window step size, which was set to 25% of the total window size. This could have been set to a fixed time value for all window sizes or have been individually analysed to explore the co-dependent effects of step size and window size. Furthermore, the availability of datasets which feature a sufficiently large number of participants and sensors, along with the core activities included in this study, was limited, resulting in the inclusion of just four datasets.

5. Conclusions and Future Work

This study is the first of its kind in providing a bias-reduced, normalised, cross-dataset analysis to determine and rank the highest-performing sensor types for Human Activity Recognition. First, ANNs were found to be the highest-performing models across multiple multimodal HAR datasets, closely followed by SVMs, with the optimal window size being in the range of 2–5 s when using the semi-non-overlapping sliding window approach to feature engineering with a 75% overlap. Where datasets were large enough to reduce the impact of class imbalance, or models were sufficiently powerful to generalise with smaller sample numbers, accuracies were also shown to trend upwards with larger window sizes of 9–10 s. Regarding the contributions of individual sensor types to classification accuracy, IMUs placed on the thigh and three-axis goniometers on the thigh and ankle were the overall largest contributors to high-accuracy HAR, whilst EMG sensors were found to exhibit volatile accuracies which was likely due to the difficulty in ensuring that the sensors were in the same place and calibrated equally for different subjects. It remains appropriate for researchers to collect large HAR datasets and to investigate alternative methods of HAR using multimodal sensor systems and smart clothing to investigate how the size and inconvenience of these systems can be minimised whilst maintaining high accuracy using low-computational-complexity classification methods.

This study was limited by the scarcity of open multimodal gait datasets with large numbers of sensors and common activities. As a result, future work in this area should consider more datasets, activities (including fall-related activities), and sensor types to investigate how classifier performance in HAR is affected by these properties. Additionally, elements such as step size, the proportion of data for each activity, and time-series features should be investigated for their contribution towards achieving efficient and convenient high-accuracy HAR. Finally, the time and space complexity of these algorithms should be considered under the various window sizes to evaluate the feasibility of deploying these optimised models in real-world HAR applications.

Author Contributions: Conceptualisation, J.C.M., A.A.D.-S., S.Q.X., R.J.O.; methodology, J.C.M.; software, J.C.M.; validation, J.C.M.; formal analysis, J.C.M.; investigation, J.C.M.; resources, J.C.M.; data curation, J.C.M.; writing—original draft preparation, J.C.M.; writing—review and editing, A.A.D.-S., S.Q.X., R.J.O.; visualisation, J.C.M.; supervision, A.A.D.-S., S.Q.X., R.J.O.; project administration, A.A.D.-S., S.Q.X., R.J.O.; funding acquisition, A.A.D.-S. All authors have read and agreed to the published version of the manuscript.

Funding: This research was funded by the United Kingdom Research and Innovation (UKRI)—Engineering and Physical Sciences Research Council (EPSRC) (grant number EP/T517860/1).

Institutional Review Board Statement: Not applicable.

Informed Consent Statement: Not applicable.

Data Availability Statement: Data are contained within the article and available upon request by contacting the authors.

Conflicts of Interest: The authors declare no conflicts of interest.

Abbreviations

The following abbreviations are used in this manuscript:

ANN	Artificial Neural Network
DT	Decision Tree
EMG	Electromyography
HAR	Human Activity Recognition
IMU	Inertial Measurement Unit
IoT	Internet of Things
KNN	K-Nearest Neighbors
LOSO	Leave-One-Subject-Out
ML	Machine Learning
PCA	Principal Component Analysis
RF	Random Forest
SVM	Support Vector Machine
TTS	Train–Test Split

Appendix A

Figures A1 and A2 along with Tables A1–A8 show the performance metrics of each dataset and method of cross-validation, including the mean, standard deviation, and 95% confidence intervals.

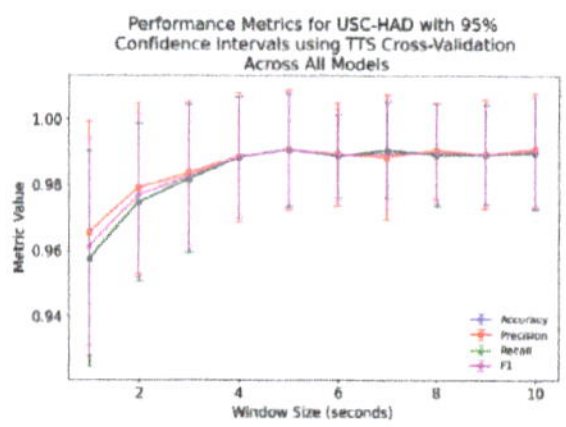

(a)

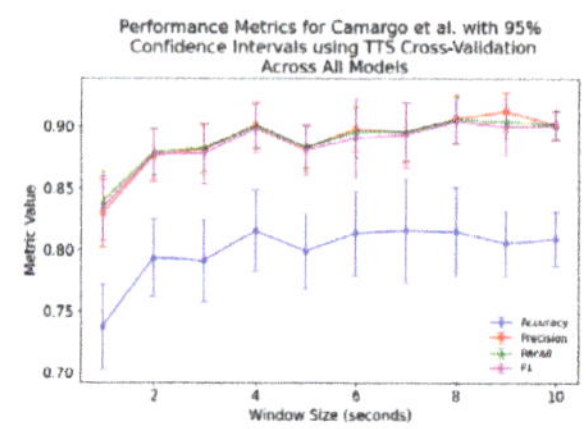

(b)

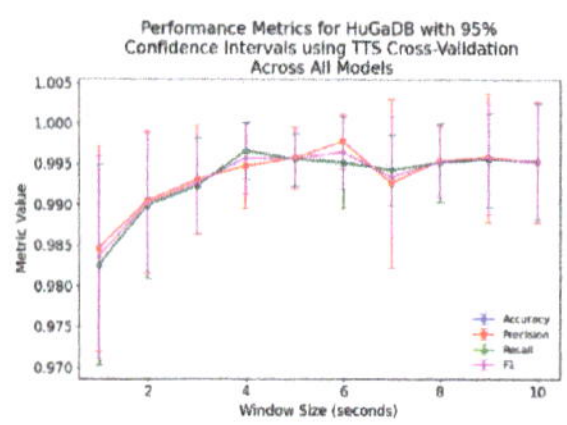

(c)

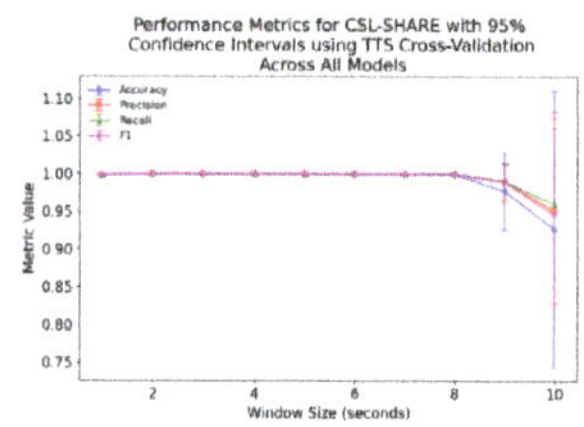

(d)

Figure A1. Trend graphs showing the macro-averaged performance metrics across all models and window sizes for the four datasets in this analysis when using TTS cross-validation. (**a**) USC-HAD. (**b**) Camargo et al. (**c**) HuGaDB. (**d**) CSL-SHARE.

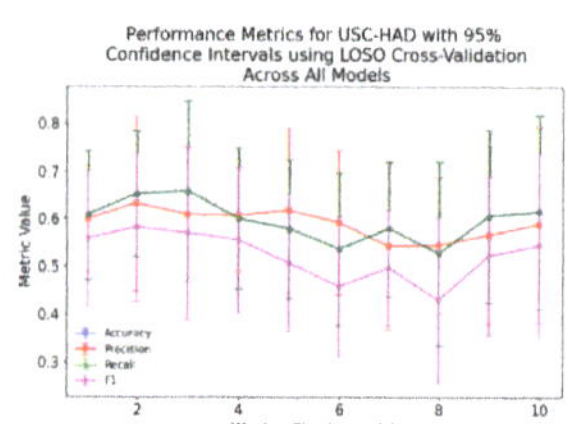

(a)

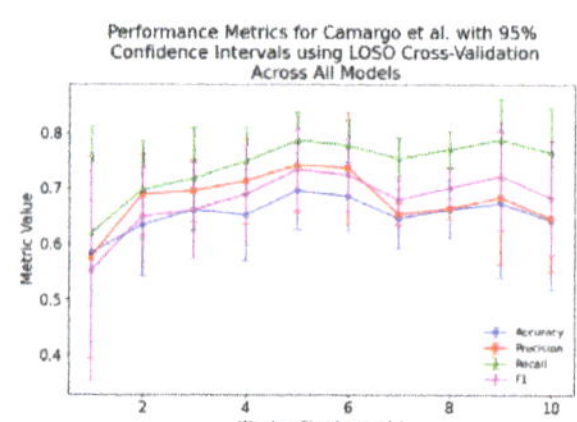

(b)

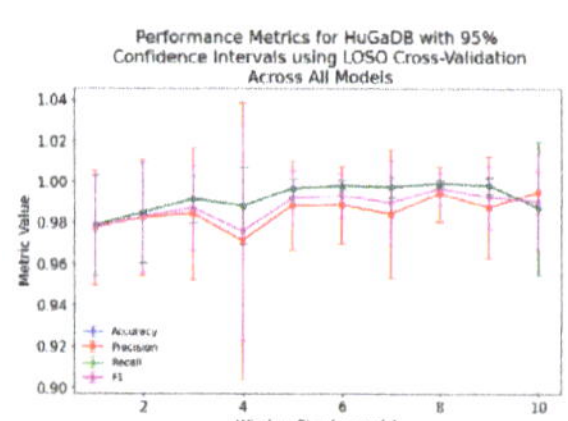

(c)

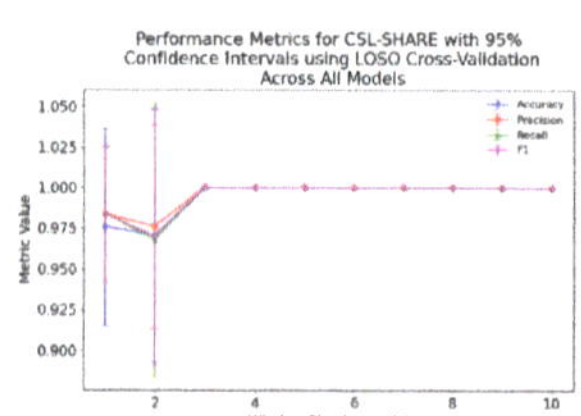

(d)

Figure A2. Trend graphs showing the macro-averaged performance metrics across all models and window sizes for the four datasets in this analysis when using TTS cross-validation. (**a**) USC-HAD. (**b**) Camargo et al. (**c**) HuGaDB. (**d**) CSL-SHARE.

Table A1. Performance metrics for the USC HAD dataset using TTS cross-validation with 95% confidence intervals.

Window (s)	Metric	Mean	Std	CI Low	CI High
1	Accuracy	0.9577	0.0328	0.9273	0.9881
	Precision	0.9654	0.0341	0.9339	0.9970
	Recall	0.9577	0.0328	0.9273	0.9881
	F1-score	0.9613	0.0332	0.9306	0.9920
2	Accuracy	0.9749	0.0240	0.9527	0.9971
	Precision	0.9791	0.0262	0.9549	1.0034
	Recall	0.9749	0.0240	0.9527	0.9971
	F1-score	0.9769	0.0248	0.9540	0.9999
3	Accuracy	0.9820	0.0224	0.9613	1.0027
	Precision	0.9838	0.0221	0.9633	1.0043
	Recall	0.9820	0.0224	0.9613	1.0027
	F1-score	0.9829	0.0222	0.9624	1.0034
4	Accuracy	0.9885	0.0185	0.9714	1.0057
	Precision	0.9886	0.0197	0.9704	1.0068
	Recall	0.9885	0.0185	0.9714	1.0057
	F1-score	0.9886	0.0191	0.9709	1.0062
5	Accuracy	0.9910	0.0172	0.9750	1.0069
	Precision	0.9908	0.0186	0.9736	1.0080
	Recall	0.9910	0.0172	0.9750	1.0069
	F1-score	0.9909	0.0179	0.9743	1.0074
6	Accuracy	0.9889	0.0126	0.9773	1.0005
	Precision	0.9895	0.0158	0.9750	1.0041
	Recall	0.9889	0.0126	0.9773	1.0005
	F1-score	0.9892	0.0140	0.9762	1.0022
7	Accuracy	0.9907	0.0146	0.9772	1.0042
	Precision	0.9886	0.0191	0.9710	1.0063
	Recall	0.9907	0.0146	0.9772	1.0042
	F1-score	0.9896	0.0168	0.9740	1.0051
8	Accuracy	0.9893	0.0155	0.9749	1.0036
	Precision	0.9906	0.0147	0.9771	1.0042
	Recall	0.9893	0.0155	0.9749	1.0036
	F1-score	0.9899	0.0152	0.9758	1.0040
9	Accuracy	0.9894	0.0152	0.9754	1.0035
	Precision	0.9895	0.0166	0.9741	1.0049
	Recall	0.9894	0.0152	0.9754	1.0035
	F1-score	0.9894	0.0159	0.9747	1.0041
10	Accuracy	0.9898	0.0170	0.9741	1.0055
	Precision	0.9909	0.0174	0.9749	1.0070
	Recall	0.9898	0.0170	0.9741	1.0055
	F1-score	0.9903	0.0172	0.9744	1.0062

Table A2. Performance metrics for the USC HAD dataset using LOSO cross-validation with 95% confidence intervals.

Window (s)	Metric	Mean	Std	CI Low	CI High
1	Accuracy	0.6083	0.1353	0.4831	0.7334
	Precision	0.5992	0.1117	0.4959	0.7025
	Recall	0.6083	0.1353	0.4831	0.7334
	F1-score	0.5589	0.1424	0.4272	0.6907
2	Accuracy	0.6521	0.1317	0.5303	0.7739
	Precision	0.6319	0.1831	0.4626	0.8012
	Recall	0.6521	0.1317	0.5303	0.7739
	F1-score	0.5817	0.1563	0.4372	0.7262
3	Accuracy	0.6579	0.1900	0.4821	0.8336
	Precision	0.6092	0.1416	0.4783	0.7402
	Recall	0.6579	0.1900	0.4821	0.8336
	F1-score	0.5705	0.1804	0.4036	0.7373
4	Accuracy	0.6004	0.1481	0.4635	0.7374
	Precision	0.6065	0.1163	0.4990	0.7141
	Recall	0.6004	0.1481	0.4635	0.7374
	F1-score	0.5561	0.1524	0.4152	0.6970
5	Accuracy	0.5795	0.1451	0.4453	0.7137
	Precision	0.6181	0.1726	0.4584	0.7777
	Recall	0.5795	0.1451	0.4453	0.7137
	F1-score	0.5079	0.1443	0.3745	0.6414
6	Accuracy	0.5372	0.1601	0.3891	0.6852
	Precision	0.5928	0.1511	0.4530	0.7326
	Recall	0.5372	0.1601	0.3891	0.6852
	F1-score	0.4586	0.1453	0.3241	0.5930
7	Accuracy	0.5799	0.1415	0.4490	0.7108
	Precision	0.5434	0.1746	0.3819	0.7049
	Recall	0.5799	0.1415	0.4490	0.7108
	F1-score	0.4982	0.1205	0.3868	0.6096
8	Accuracy	0.5279	0.1938	0.3486	0.7071
	Precision	0.5455	0.1416	0.4145	0.6764
	Recall	0.5279	0.1938	0.3486	0.7071
	F1-score	0.4304	0.1727	0.2706	0.5901
9	Accuracy	0.6061	0.1817	0.4380	0.7741
	Precision	0.5663	0.1864	0.3939	0.7387
	Recall	0.6061	0.1817	0.4380	0.7741
	F1-score	0.5227	0.1661	0.3691	0.6764
10	Accuracy	0.6150	0.2031	0.4271	0.8028
	Precision	0.5895	0.2052	0.3997	0.7793
	Recall	0.6150	0.2031	0.4271	0.8028
	F1-score	0.5448	0.1925	0.3668	0.7228

Table A3. Performance metrics for the CSL-SHARE dataset using TTS cross-validation with 95% confidence intervals.

Window (s)	Metric	Mean	Std	CI Low	CI High
1	Accuracy	0.9984	0.0015	0.9970	0.9998
	Precision	0.9988	0.0012	0.9977	0.9999
	Recall	0.9988	0.0012	0.9977	0.9999
	F1-score	0.9988	0.0012	0.9977	0.9999
2	Accuracy	1.0000	0.0000	N/A	N/A
	Precision	1.0000	0.0000	N/A	N/A
	Recall	1.0000	0.0000	N/A	N/A
	F1-score	1.0000	0.0000	N/A	N/A
3	Accuracy	1.0000	0.0000	N/A	N/A
	Precision	1.0000	0.0000	N/A	N/A
	Recall	1.0000	0.0000	N/A	N/A
	F1-score	1.0000	0.0000	N/A	N/A
4	Accuracy	1.0000	0.0000	N/A	N/A
	Precision	1.0000	0.0000	N/A	N/A
	Recall	1.0000	0.0000	N/A	N/A
	F1-score	1.0000	0.0000	N/A	N/A
5	Accuracy	1.0000	0.0000	N/A	N/A
	Precision	1.0000	0.0000	N/A	N/A
	Recall	1.0000	0.0000	N/A	N/A
	F1-score	1.0000	0.0000	N/A	N/A
6	Accuracy	1.0000	0.0000	N/A	N/A
	Precision	1.0000	0.0000	N/A	N/A
	Recall	1.0000	0.0000	N/A	N/A
	F1-score	1.0000	0.0000	N/A	N/A
7	Accuracy	1.0000	0.0000	N/A	N/A
	Precision	1.0000	0.0000	N/A	N/A
	Recall	1.0000	0.0000	N/A	N/A
	F1-score	1.0000	0.0000	N/A	N/A
8	Accuracy	1.0000	0.0000	N/A	N/A
	Precision	1.0000	0.0000	N/A	N/A
	Recall	1.0000	0.0000	N/A	N/A
	F1-score	1.0000	0.0000	N/A	N/A
9	Accuracy	0.9778	0.0514	0.9302	1.0254
	Precision	0.9904	0.0222	0.9698	1.0109
	Recall	0.9896	0.0241	0.9674	1.0119
	F1-score	0.9891	0.0255	0.9655	1.0127
10	Accuracy	0.9277	0.1839	0.7576	1.0977
	Precision	0.9523	0.1223	0.8391	1.0654
	Recall	0.9607	0.1000	0.8682	1.0532
	F1-score	0.9469	0.1366	0.8206	1.0732

Table A4. Performance metrics for the CSL-SHARE dataset using LOSO cross-validation with 95% confidence intervals.

Window (s)	Metric	Mean	Std	CI Low	CI High
1	Accuracy	0.9762	0.0609	0.9199	1.0325
	Precision	0.9837	0.0421	0.9448	1.0227
	Recall	0.9841	0.0412	0.9460	1.0222
	F1-score	0.9838	0.0419	0.9451	1.0225
2	Accuracy	0.9708	0.0773	0.8993	1.0423
	Precision	0.9762	0.0629	0.9181	1.0344
	Recall	0.9683	0.0840	0.8906	1.0459
	F1-score	0.9701	0.0790	0.8971	1.0432
3	Accuracy	1.0000	0.0000	N/A	N/A
	Precision	1.0000	0.0000	N/A	N/A
	Recall	1.0000	0.0000	N/A	N/A
	F1-score	1.0000	0.0000	N/A	N/A
4	Accuracy	1.0000	0.0000	N/A	N/A
	Precision	1.0000	0.0000	N/A	N/A
	Recall	1.0000	0.0000	N/A	N/A
	F1-score	1.0000	0.0000	N/A	N/A
5	Accuracy	1.0000	0.0000	N/A	N/A
	Precision	1.0000	0.0000	N/A	N/A
	Recall	1.0000	0.0000	N/A	N/A
	F1-score	1.0000	0.0000	N/A	N/A
6	Accuracy	1.0000	0.0000	N/A	N/A
	Precision	1.0000	0.0000	N/A	N/A
	Recall	1.0000	0.0000	N/A	N/A
	F1-score	1.0000	0.0000	N/A	N/A
7	Accuracy	1.0000	0.0000	N/A	N/A
	Precision	1.0000	0.0000	N/A	N/A
	Recall	1.0000	0.0000	N/A	N/A
	F1-score	1.0000	0.0000	N/A	N/A
8	Accuracy	1.0000	0.0000	N/A	N/A
	Precision	1.0000	0.0000	N/A	N/A
	Recall	1.0000	0.0000	N/A	N/A
	F1-score	1.0000	0.0000	N/A	N/A
9	Accuracy	1.0000	0.0000	N/A	N/A
	Precision	1.0000	0.0000	N/A	N/A
	Recall	1.0000	0.0000	N/A	N/A
	F1-score	1.0000	0.0000	N/A	N/A
10	Accuracy	1.0000	0.0000	N/A	N/A
	Precision	1.0000	0.0000	N/A	N/A
	Recall	1.0000	0.0000	N/A	N/A
	F1-score	1.0000	0.0000	N/A	N/A

Table A5. Performance metrics for the Camargo et al. dataset using TTS cross-validation with 95% confidence intervals.

Window (s)	Metric	Mean	Std	CI Low	CI High
1	Accuracy	0.7379	0.0347	0.7058	0.7701
	Precision	0.8294	0.0274	0.8041	0.8547
	Recall	0.8394	0.0250	0.8163	0.8625
	F1-score	0.8336	0.0262	0.8093	0.8579
2	Accuracy	0.7939	0.0311	0.7651	0.8227
	Precision	0.8764	0.0212	0.8568	0.8960
	Recall	0.8796	0.0190	0.8621	0.8972
	F1-score	0.8776	0.0203	0.8589	0.8964
3	Accuracy	0.7916	0.0331	0.7610	0.8223
	Precision	0.8819	0.0199	0.8634	0.9003
	Recall	0.8830	0.0186	0.8658	0.9003
	F1-score	0.8784	0.0249	0.8554	0.9013
4	Accuracy	0.8158	0.0329	0.7854	0.8462
	Precision	0.9012	0.0185	0.8840	0.9183
	Recall	0.9002	0.0179	0.8837	0.9168
	F1-score	0.8985	0.0194	0.8805	0.9164
5	Accuracy	0.7994	0.0303	0.7714	0.8274
	Precision	0.8827	0.0188	0.8653	0.9001
	Recall	0.8836	0.0169	0.8679	0.8992
	F1-score	0.8813	0.0205	0.8623	0.9002
6	Accuracy	0.8140	0.0343	0.7823	0.8458
	Precision	0.8981	0.0180	0.8815	0.9148
	Recall	0.8959	0.0205	0.8769	0.9149
	F1-score	0.8908	0.0317	0.8615	0.9201
7	Accuracy	0.8159	0.0424	0.7767	0.8552
	Precision	0.8952	0.0238	0.8732	0.9172
	Recall	0.8958	0.0236	0.8740	0.9176
	F1-score	0.8932	0.0265	0.8687	0.9177
8	Accuracy	0.8151	0.0359	0.7819	0.8484
	Precision	0.9066	0.0200	0.8881	0.9251
	Recall	0.9057	0.0194	0.8877	0.9237
	F1-score	0.9042	0.0191	0.8866	0.9219
9	Accuracy	0.8058	0.0266	0.7811	0.8304
	Precision	0.9125	0.0159	0.8978	0.9272
	Recall	0.9046	0.0137	0.8919	0.9173
	F1-score	0.9001	0.0228	0.8790	0.9211
10	Accuracy	0.8093	0.0223	0.7887	0.8300
	Precision	0.9018	0.0113	0.8913	0.9123
	Recall	0.9014	0.0116	0.8906	0.9121
	F1-score	0.9010	0.0118	0.8901	0.9120

Table A6. Performance metrics for the Camargo et al. dataset using LOSO cross-validation with 95% confidence intervals.

Window (s)	Metric	Mean	Std	CI Low	CI High
1	Accuracy	0.5844	0.0941	0.4973	0.6714
	Precision	0.5760	0.1825	0.4072	0.7448
	Recall	0.6194	0.1948	0.4392	0.7996
	F1-score	0.5517	0.1966	0.3699	0.7336
2	Accuracy	0.6351	0.0917	0.5503	0.7199
	Precision	0.6892	0.0738	0.6210	0.7575
	Recall	0.6983	0.0883	0.6167	0.7800
	F1-score	0.6495	0.0901	0.5662	0.7328
3	Accuracy	0.6623	0.0382	0.6270	0.6976
	Precision	0.6961	0.0564	0.6440	0.7482
	Recall	0.7183	0.0935	0.6318	0.8047
	F1-score	0.6613	0.0882	0.5798	0.7429
4	Accuracy	0.6531	0.0817	0.5775	0.7287
	Precision	0.7135	0.0765	0.6428	0.7842
	Recall	0.7507	0.0598	0.6954	0.8059
	F1-score	0.6896	0.0900	0.6063	0.7728
5	Accuracy	0.6970	0.0703	0.6320	0.7620
	Precision	0.7428	0.0871	0.6623	0.8234
	Recall	0.7879	0.0502	0.7414	0.8343
	F1-score	0.7339	0.0735	0.6660	0.8019
6	Accuracy	0.6865	0.0630	0.6282	0.7448
	Precision	0.7385	0.1009	0.6452	0.8318
	Recall	0.7794	0.0447	0.7380	0.8208
	F1-score	0.7249	0.0657	0.6641	0.7857
7	Accuracy	0.6463	0.0531	0.5971	0.6954
	Precision	0.6538	0.0197	0.6356	0.6720
	Recall	0.7547	0.0395	0.7182	0.7913
	F1-score	0.6793	0.0430	0.6396	0.7191
8	Accuracy	0.6622	0.0513	0.6148	0.7096
	Precision	0.6638	0.0183	0.6469	0.6808
	Recall	0.7717	0.0334	0.7409	0.8026
	F1-score	0.7010	0.0360	0.6678	0.7343
9	Accuracy	0.6735	0.1338	0.5497	0.7972
	Precision	0.6843	0.1205	0.5729	0.7958
	Recall	0.7890	0.0740	0.7206	0.8575
	F1-score	0.7225	0.0965	0.6332	0.8117
10	Accuracy	0.6429	0.1241	0.5280	0.7577
	Precision	0.6465	0.0943	0.5593	0.7337
	Recall	0.7657	0.0818	0.6901	0.8413
	F1-score	0.6843	0.1025	0.5895	0.7791

Table A7. Performance metrics for the HuGaDB dataset using TTS cross-validation with 95% confidence intervals.

Window (s)	Metric	Mean	Std	CI Low	CI High
1	Accuracy	0.9826	0.0123	0.9712	0.9940
	Precision	0.9846	0.0126	0.9729	0.9963
	Recall	0.9826	0.0123	0.9712	0.9940
	F1-score	0.9836	0.0124	0.9721	0.9951
2	Accuracy	0.9899	0.0089	0.9817	0.9982
	Precision	0.9904	0.0086	0.9825	0.9984
	Recall	0.9899	0.0089	0.9817	0.9982
	F1-score	0.9902	0.0087	0.9822	0.9982
3	Accuracy	0.9924	0.0058	0.9870	0.9978
	Precision	0.9931	0.0067	0.9869	0.9993
	Recall	0.9924	0.0058	0.9870	0.9978
	F1-score	0.9927	0.0062	0.9870	0.9984
4	Accuracy	0.9966	0.0035	0.9934	0.9999
	Precision	0.9948	0.0052	0.9900	0.9996
	Recall	0.9966	0.0035	0.9934	0.9999
	F1-score	0.9957	0.0043	0.9917	0.9997
5	Accuracy	0.9956	0.0032	0.9927	0.9985
	Precision	0.9958	0.0038	0.9922	0.9993
	Recall	0.9956	0.0032	0.9927	0.9985
	F1-score	0.9957	0.0035	0.9924	0.9989
6	Accuracy	0.9952	0.0056	0.9900	1.0004
	Precision	0.9978	0.0034	0.9947	1.0010
	Recall	0.9952	0.0056	0.9900	1.0004
	F1-score	0.9965	0.0045	0.9924	1.0007
7	Accuracy	0.9943	0.0043	0.9903	0.9983
	Precision	0.9927	0.0104	0.9831	1.0023
	Recall	0.9943	0.0043	0.9903	0.9983
	F1-score	0.9935	0.0074	0.9866	1.0003
8	Accuracy	0.9953	0.0049	0.9908	0.9998
	Precision	0.9955	0.0043	0.9915	0.9995
	Recall	0.9953	0.0049	0.9908	0.9998
	F1-score	0.9954	0.0045	0.9912	0.9995
9	Accuracy	0.9956	0.0057	0.9903	1.0009
	Precision	0.9959	0.0080	0.9886	1.0033
	Recall	0.9956	0.0057	0.9903	1.0009
	F1-score	0.9958	0.0068	0.9895	1.0020
10	Accuracy	0.9954	0.0071	0.9889	1.0020
	Precision	0.9954	0.0075	0.9884	1.0023
	Recall	0.9954	0.0071	0.9889	1.0020
	F1-score	0.9953	0.0073	0.9885	1.0021

Table A8. Performance metrics for the HuGaDB dataset using LOSO cross-validation with 95% confidence intervals.

Window (s)	Metric	Mean	Std	CI Low	CI High
1	Accuracy	0.9789	0.0244	0.9564	1.0015
	Precision	0.9777	0.0279	0.9519	1.0035
	Recall	0.9789	0.0244	0.9564	1.0015
	F1-score	0.9781	0.0251	0.9549	1.0013
2	Accuracy	0.9852	0.0244	0.9627	1.0077
	Precision	0.9827	0.0284	0.9564	1.0090
	Recall	0.9852	0.0244	0.9627	1.0077
	F1-score	0.9828	0.0267	0.9581	1.0075
3	Accuracy	0.9917	0.0115	0.9811	1.0024
	Precision	0.9846	0.0322	0.9548	1.0144
	Recall	0.9917	0.0115	0.9811	1.0024
	F1-score	0.9874	0.0204	0.9685	1.0063
4	Accuracy	0.9884	0.0188	0.9711	1.0058
	Precision	0.9714	0.0674	0.9090	1.0337
	Recall	0.9884	0.0188	0.9711	1.0058
	F1-score	0.9758	0.0529	0.9269	1.0247
5	Accuracy	0.9967	0.0047	0.9924	1.0011
	Precision	0.9886	0.0217	0.9685	1.0087
	Recall	0.9967	0.0047	0.9924	1.0011
	F1-score	0.9921	0.0135	0.9796	1.0046
6	Accuracy	0.9981	0.0026	0.9956	1.0005
	Precision	0.9889	0.0189	0.9715	1.0064
	Recall	0.9981	0.0026	0.9956	1.0005
	F1-score	0.9932	0.0112	0.9829	1.0035
7	Accuracy	0.9975	0.0050	0.9929	1.0021
	Precision	0.9845	0.0313	0.9556	1.0135
	Recall	0.9975	0.0050	0.9929	1.0021
	F1-score	0.9899	0.0208	0.9707	1.0091
8	Accuracy	0.9992	0.0020	0.9974	1.0010
	Precision	0.9942	0.0137	0.9815	1.0069
	Recall	0.9992	0.0020	0.9974	1.0010
	F1-score	0.9966	0.0081	0.9891	1.0041
9	Accuracy	0.9981	0.0039	0.9945	1.0018
	Precision	0.9878	0.0248	0.9649	1.0107
	Recall	0.9981	0.0039	0.9945	1.0018
	F1-score	0.9926	0.0153	0.9784	1.0067
10	Accuracy	0.9875	0.0327	0.9573	1.0177
	Precision	0.9951	0.0104	0.9855	1.0047
	Recall	0.9875	0.0327	0.9573	1.0177
	F1-score	0.9905	0.0235	0.9687	1.0123

References

1. World Health Organization (WHO). *Falls*; WHO: Geneva, Switzerland, 2021.
2. Pfortmueller, C.A.; Lindner, G.; Exadaktylos, A.K. Reducing fall risk in the elderly: Risk factors and fall prevention, a systematic review. *Minerva Med.* **2014**, *105*, 275–281. [PubMed]
3. Lo, C.W.T.; Tsang, W.W.N.; Yan, C.H.; Lord, S.R.; Hill, K.D.; Wong, A.Y.L. Risk factors for falls in patients with total hip arthroplasty and total knee arthroplasty: A systematic review and meta-analysis. *Osteoarthr. Cartil.* **2019**, *27*, 979–993. [CrossRef] [PubMed]

4. Fasano, A.; Canning, C.G.; Hausdorff, J.M.; Lord, S.; Rochester, L. Falls in Parkinson's disease: A complex and evolving picture. *Mov. Disord.* **2017**, *32*, 1524–1536. [CrossRef] [PubMed]
5. Härlein, J.; Dassen, T.; Halfens, R.J.G.; Heinze, C. Fall risk factors in older people with dementia or cognitive impairment: A systematic review. *J. Adv. Nurs.* **2009**, *65*, 922–933. [CrossRef]
6. Batchelor, F.A.; Mackintosh, S.F.; Said, C.M.; Hill, K.D. Falls after stroke. *Int. J. Stroke* **2012**, *7*, 482–490. [CrossRef]
7. Gunn, H.J.; Newell, P.; Haas, B.; Marsden, J.F.; Freeman, J.A. Identification of risk factors for falls in multiple sclerosis: A systematic review and meta-analysis. *Phys. Ther.* **2013**, *93*, 504–513. [CrossRef]
8. Hunter, S.W.; Batchelor, F.; Hill, K.D.; Hill, A.M.; Mackintosh, S.; Payne, M. Risk factors for falls in people with a lower limb amputation: A systematic review. *PM R* **2017**, *9*, 170–180.e1. [CrossRef]
9. Wang, Y.; Cang, S.; Yu, H. A survey on wearable sensor modality centred human activity recognition in health care. *Expert Syst. Appl.* **2019**, *137*, 167–190. [CrossRef]
10. Zhao, H.; Wang, R.; Qi, D.; Xie, J.; Cao, J.; Liao, W.H. Wearable gait monitoring for diagnosis of neurodegenerative diseases. *Measurement* **2022**, *202*, 111839. [CrossRef]
11. Chen, S.; Lach, J.; Lo, B.; Yang, G.Z. Toward pervasive gait analysis with wearable sensors: A systematic review. *IEEE J. Biomed. Health Inform.* **2016**, *20*, 1521–1537. [CrossRef]
12. Hu, X.; Qu, X. Pre-impact fall detection. *Biomed. Eng. Online* **2016**, *15*, 61. [CrossRef] [PubMed]
13. Tamura, T.; Yoshimura, T.; Sekine, M.; Uchida, M.; Tanaka, O. A wearable airbag to prevent fall injuries. *IEEE Trans. Inf. Technol. Biomed.* **2009**, *13*, 910–914. [CrossRef] [PubMed]
14. De-La-Hoz-Franco, E.; Ariza-Colpas, P.; Quero, J.M.; Espinilla, M. Sensor-Based Datasets for Human Activity Recognition—A Systematic Review of Literature. *IEEE Access* **2018**, *6*, 59192–59210. [CrossRef]
15. Nguyen, H.D.; Tran, K.P.; Zeng, X.; Koehl, L.; Tartare, G. Wearable Sensor Data Based Human Activity Recognition using Machine Learning: A new approach. *arXiv* **2019**, arXiv:1905.03809. [CrossRef]
16. Murad, A.; Pyun, J.Y. Deep Recurrent Neural Networks for Human Activity Recognition. *Sensors* **2017**, *17*, 2556. [CrossRef]
17. Jiang, W.; Yin, Z. Human Activity Recognition Using Wearable Sensors by Deep Convolutional Neural Networks. In Proceedings of the 23rd ACM International Conference on Multimedia (MM '15), Brisbane, Australia, 26–30 October 2015; pp. 1307–1310. [CrossRef]
18. Das Antar, A.; Ahmed, M.; Ahad, M.A.R. Challenges in Sensor-based Human Activity Recognition and a Comparative Analysis of Benchmark Datasets: A Review. In Proceedings of the 2019 Joint 8th International Conference on Informatics, Electronics & Vision (ICIEV) and 2019 3rd International Conference on Imaging, Vision & Pattern Recognition (icIVPR), Spokane, WA, USA, 30 May–2 June 2019; pp. 134–139. [CrossRef]
19. Straczkiewicz, M.; James, P.; Onnela, J.P. A systematic review of smartphone-based human activity recognition methods for health research. *NPJ Digit. Med.* **2021**, *4*, 148. [CrossRef]
20. Chung, S.; Lim, J.; Noh, K.J.; Kim, G.; Jeong, H. Sensor Data Acquisition and Multimodal Sensor Fusion for Human Activity Recognition Using Deep Learning. *Sensors* **2019**, *19*, 1716. [CrossRef]
21. Diraco, G.; Rescio, G.; Siciliano, P.; Leone, A. Review on human action recognition in smart living: Sensing Technology, Multimodality, Real-time Processing, Interoperability, and resource-Constrained Processing. *Sensors* **2023**, *23*, 5281. [CrossRef]
22. Majumder, S.; Mondal, T.; Deen, M.J. Wearable sensors for remote health monitoring. *Sensors* **2017**, *17*, 130. [CrossRef]
23. Banos, O.; Galvez, J.M.; Damas, M.; Pomares, H.; Rojas, I. Window Size Impact in Human Activity Recognition. *Sensors* **2014**, *14*, 6474–6499. [CrossRef]
24. Baños, O.; Damas, M.; Pomares, H.; Rojas, I.; Tóth, M.A.; Amft, O. A benchmark dataset to evaluate sensor displacement in activity recognition. In Proceedings of the 2012 ACM Conference on Ubiquitous Computing (UbiComp '12), Pittsburgh, PA, USA, 5–8 September 2012; pp. 1026–1035. [CrossRef]
25. Niazi, A.H.; Yazdansepas, D.; Gay, J.L.; Maier, F.W.; Ramaswamy, L.; Rasheed, K.; Buman, M.P. Statistical Analysis of Window Sizes and Sampling Rates in Human Activity Recognition. In Proceedings of the HEALTHINF, Porto, Portugal, 21–23 February 2017; pp. 319–325.
26. Li, H.; Abowd, G.D.; Plötz, T. On specialized window lengths and detector based human activity recognition. In Proceedings of the 2018 ACM International Symposium on Wearable Computers (ISWC '18), Singapore, 8–12 October 2018; pp. 68–71. [CrossRef]
27. Dehghani, A.; Sarbishei, O.; Glatard, T.; Shihab, E. A Quantitative Comparison of Overlapping and Non-Overlapping Sliding Windows for Human Activity Recognition Using Inertial Sensors. *Sensors* **2019**, *19*, 5026. [CrossRef]
28. Duan, Y.; Fujinami, K. Effect of Combinations of Sensor Positions on Wearable-sensor-based Human Activity Recognition. *Sens. Mater.* **2023**, *35*, 2175–2193. [CrossRef]

29. Kulchyk, J.; Etemad, A. Activity Recognition with Wearable Accelerometers using Deep Convolutional Neural Network and the Effect of Sensor Placement. In Proceedings of the 2019 IEEE SENSORS, Montreal, QC, Canada. 27–30 October 2019; pp. 1–4. [CrossRef]
30. Khan, M.U.S.; Abbas, A.; Ali, M.; Jawad, M.; Khan, S.U.; Li, K.; Zomaya, A.Y. On the Correlation of Sensor Location and Human Activity Recognition in Body Area Networks (BANs). *IEEE Syst. J.* **2018**, *12*, 82–91. [CrossRef]
31. Maurer, U.; Smailagic, A.; Siewiorek, D.; Deisher, M. Activity recognition and monitoring using multiple sensors on different body positions. In Proceedings of the International Workshop on Wearable and Implantable Body Sensor Networks (BSN'06), Cambridge, MA, USA, 3–5 April 2006; pp. 4–116. [CrossRef]
32. Orha, I.; Oniga, S. Study regarding the optimal sensors placement on the body for human activity recognition. In Proceedings of the 2014 IEEE 20th International Symposium for Design and Technology in Electronic Packaging (SIITME), Bucharest, Romania, 23–26 October 2014; pp. 203–206. [CrossRef]
33. Zhang, M.; Sawchuk, A.A. USC-HAD: A daily activity dataset for ubiquitous activity recognition using wearable sensors. In Proceedings of the 2012 ACM Conference on Ubiquitous Computing (UbiComp '12), Pittsburgh, PA, USA, 5–8 September 2012; pp. 1036–1043. [CrossRef]
34. Han, C.; Zhang, L.; Tang, Y.; Huang, W.; Min, F.; He, J. Human activity recognition using wearable sensors by heterogeneous convolutional neural networks. *Expert Syst. Appl.* **2022**, *198*, 116764. [CrossRef]
35. Chereshnev, R.; Kertesz-Farkas, A. HuGaDB: Human Gait Database for Activity Recognition from Wearable Inertial Sensor Networks. *arXiv* **2017**, arXiv:1705.08506. Available online: http://arxiv.org/abs/1705.08506 (accessed on 16 September 2023).
36. Camargo, J.; Ramanathan, A.; Flanagan, W.; Young, A. A comprehensive, open-source dataset of lower limb biomechanics in multiple conditions of stairs, ramps, and level-ground ambulation and transitions. *J. Biomech.* **2021**, *119*, 110320. [CrossRef]
37. Liu, H.; Hartmann, Y.; Schultz, T. CSL-SHARE: A Multimodal Wearable Sensor-Based Human Activity Dataset. *Front. Comput. Sci.* **2021**, *3*, 90. [CrossRef]
38. Gay, J.L.; Cherof, S.A.; LaFlamme, C.C.; O'Connor, P.J. Psychological Aspects of Stair Use: A Systematic Review. *Am. J. Lifestyle Med.* **2019**, *16*, 109–121. [CrossRef]
39. Bridenbaugh, S.A.; Kressig, R.W. Laboratory Review: The Role of Gait Analysis in Seniors' Mobility and Fall Prevention. *Gerontology* **2010**, *57*, 256–264. [CrossRef]
40. Zhang, M.; Sawchuk, A. A Feature Selection-Based Framework for Human Activity Recognition Using Wearable Multimodal Sensors. In Proceedings of the 6th International ICST Conference on Body Area Networks (BodyNets '11), Beijing, China, 7–8 November 2011; ACM: New York, NY, USA, 2011. [CrossRef]
41. Li, F.; Shirahama, K.; Nisar, M.; Köping, L.; Grzegorzek, M. Comparison of Feature Learning Methods for Human Activity Recognition Using Wearable Sensors. *Sensors* **2018**, *18*, 679. [CrossRef]
42. Zurbuchen, N.; Bruegger, P.; Wilde, A. A comparison of machine learning algorithms for fall detection using wearable sensors. In Proceedings of the 2020 International Conference on Artificial Intelligence in Information and Communication (ICAIIC), Fukuoka, Japan, 19–21 February 2020.
43. Zia, U.; Khalil, W.; Khan, S.; Ahmad, I.; Khan, M.N. Towards human activity recognition for ubiquitous health care using data from awaist-mounted smartphone. *Turk. J. Electr. Eng. Comput. Sci.* **2020**, *28*, 646–663. [CrossRef]
44. Zhang, H.; Chen, Z.; Zanotto, D.; Guo, Y. Robot-Assisted and Wearable Sensor-Mediated Autonomous Gait Analysis. In Proceedings of the 2020 IEEE International Conference on Robotics and Automation (ICRA), Paris, France, 31 May–31 August 2020. [CrossRef]
45. Reches, T.; Dagan, M.; Herman, T.; Gazit, E.; Gouskova, N.; Giladi, N.; Manor, B.; Hausdorff, J. Using Wearable Sensors and Machine Learning to Automatically Detect Freezing of Gait during a FOG-Provoking Test. *Sensors* **2020**, *20*, 4474. [CrossRef] [PubMed]
46. Chen, Z.; Zhang, L.; Cao, Z.; Guo, J. Distilling the Knowledge From Handcrafted Features for Human Activity Recognition. *IEEE Trans. Ind. Inform.* **2018**, *14*, 4334–4342. [CrossRef]
47. Hassan, M.M.; Uddin, M.Z.; Mohamed, A.; Almogren, A. A robust human activity recognition system using smartphone sensors and deep learning. *Future Gener. Comput. Syst.* **2018**, *81*, 307–313. [CrossRef]
48. Ferrari, A.; Micucci, D.; Mobilio, M.; Napoletano, P. On the Personalization of Classification Models for Human Activity Recognition. *IEEE Access* **2020**, *8*, 32066–32079. [CrossRef]

technologies

MDPI

Article

Understanding Technology Perception in Autism with Separate Analyses for Anxiety and Depression Using Quantum Circuit Simulation Approach †

Gema Benedicto-Rodríguez [1,2,*], Vanessa Zorrilla-Muñoz [2,3,*], Nicolas Garcia-Aracil [2], Eduardo Fernandez [2,4] and José Manuel Ferrández [1]

1 Department of Electronics and Computer Technology, Universidad Politécnica de Cartagena, 30202 Murcia, Spain; jm.ferrandez@uptc.es
2 Bioengineering Institute, Miguel Hernández University of Elche, 03202 Elche, Spain; nicolas.garcia@umh.es (N.G.-A.); e.fernandez@umh.es (E.F.)
3 Bioengineering Institute of Gender Studies, University Carlos III of Madrid, 28903 Madrid, Spain
4 Networking Research Centre of Bioengineering, Biomaterials and Nanomedicine (CIBER-BBN), 03202 Elche, Spain
* Correspondence: gema.benedicto@edu.upct.es (G.B.-R.); vzorrilla@umh.es (V.Z.-M.)

† This paper is an extended version of our paper published in the Third International Conference on Innovations in Computing Research (ICR'24), Athens, Greece, 12–14 August 2024; "Technological Influence on the Measurement of Quality of Life in Persons with Autism Spectrum Disorder", doi:10.1007/978-3-031-65522-7_60.

Abstract: Background: This work explores the current use of technologies and the perception of their impact on people diagnosed with Autism Spectrum Disorder (ASD) and other comorbidities—Chronic Anxiety (CA) and Chronic Depression (CD). Autistic people often experience anxiety and/or depression. These mental health issues are exacerbated by social stigma, affecting their quality of life (QoL) and well-being. Aims: The study aims to analyze how emerging technologies can reduce communication difficulties, as well as stress, anxiety, and depression, and thus improve QoL for individuals with ASD and comorbidities like CA and CD. Methods: This study analyzes data from the secondary questionnaire 'Encuesta de Discapacidad, Autonomía Personal y situaciones de Dependencia (EDAD)' developed in 2020–2021 by the 'Instituto Nacional de Estadística (INE)' for people with ASD (n = 241), ASD and CA (n = 61), and ASD and CD (n = 29). The analysis includes Pearson correlation tests to examine the relationship between various factors affecting QoL. Results: The results highlight differences in difficulties affecting the QoL of ASD persons. Pearson correlation analysis showed significant negative correlations in communication and learning for ASD patients, with similar patterns in the separate analyses of CA and CD. More significant variables were found in the 'Learning' and 'Communication' indices for ASD, while CA and CD represented more significant variables in 'Mobility' index. Conclusions: This work suggests that technological interventions, such as the integration of advanced technologies, could enhance emotional regulation and social skills in individuals with ASD. In this sense, the quantum computing approach could help in the emerging technologies impact evaluation, analyzing devices adapted to the user to optimize their QoL and well-being.

Keywords: technologies quality of life; autism; anxiety; depression; quantum computing algorithm

1. Introduction

The WHO (2023) estimates that one in every hundred people under 18 years of age suffers from Autism Spectrum Disorder (ASD) [1].

For these reasons, the early detection of ASD is essential. However, currently, there is no biological test that allows its diagnosis. As a consequence, the evaluation is mainly based on the use of validated scales [2], which in turn necessitate clinical evaluation, and this directly impacts the functional capabilities and quality of life (QoL) of the person who suffers this disease.

QoL, both for individuals with ASD and neurotypicals, is understood as a multidimensional concept that refers to people's perception of their existence within the values and environment in which they are situated, related to their goals, expectations, concerns, and norms [1]. From both medical and physiotherapeutic perspectives, managing ASD involves addressing not only the cognitive and behavioral symptoms, but also the physical challenges that can significantly affect daily life [3]. Physiotherapy, tailored to the specific needs of individuals with ASD, can improve motor function, sensory processing, and propioception, which are often compromised. These physical improvements can lead to enhanced self-efficacy and independence, potentially reducing anxiety and depression symptoms by fostering a better sense of control over one's environment [4,5]. Medical interventions, on the other hand, focus on pharmacological and non-pharmacological treatments for co-occurring mental health issues, aiming to stabilize mood and behavior in a way that complements physical therapy efforts [6], thereby contributing to an overall better quality of life.

Moreover, familiar caregivers for ASD patients often experience a reduction in QoL, especially in parents of children with ASD, who face significant physical, social, and emotional stress [7].

1.1. Co-Occurrence of Anxiety and Depression in ASD

People with ASD can live with various mental disorders (MDS), and vice versa. For example, the symptoms of anxiety may be present in autistic people (this is not the case in all cases of autism) and the characteristics of autism may manifest in people with an anxiety disorder. The prevalence of anxiety in individuals with ASD varies widely, with estimates ranging from 11% to 84%, depending on the sample and methodology used [8]. However, a higher percentage of anxiety was found in young people with ASD (63%), where 17% showed traditional anxiety disorders and only 15% showed atypical symptoms of TA related to ASD. The current prevalence of ASD and anxiety remains a contentious issue, as highlighted Sánchez et al. [9]. The symptoms of anxiety observed in people with autism form an independent entity from ASD [8].

1.2. Perception of Technology in ASD, Anxiety, and Depression

The perceptions that people with autism, anxiety and depression have of technologies play an important role in the design of therapies and their effectiveness. According to previous studies, people with autism can experience technology in a variety of ways, ranging from as a potential source of stress and sensory overload, to offering devices that are tailored to each individual's specific needs [10]. As for anxiety, the perception of technology is ambiguous, as technologies can offer a positive sense of control and predictability, but constant exposure can produce emotional overload [11].

However, in depression, a positive perception arises as technology offers a form of avoidance or distraction from emotional symptoms, which can always vary depending on the nature of the symptoms [12]. However, some research has shown that cognitive behavioral therapy apps are effective for treating depression, as long as users maintain a positive attitude toward technologies [12].

The moment technologies adapt to people's needs, people begin to perceive them as useful and non-invasive. In this way, they manage to have a significant impact on their quality of life (QoL), and therefore, the perception of technology becomes fundamental for the development of effective therapeutic tools. Otherwise, technologies can be perceived as counterproductive [13]. This user-centered approach can contribute to the creation of technological solutions that enhance emotional well-being, social inclusion and personal development [14].

1.3. Challenges of Co-Morbidity: Anxiety and Depression in ASD

In this context, it is also common for adolescents with both anxiety and autism to experience high levels of social anxiety or depressive symptoms compared to neurotypical adolescents [11,15]. People with both conditions often face serious challenges in managing intolerance and uncertainty, and in carrying out daily activities, which undoubtedly affects their QoL. Anxiety can have a negative impact on the QoL of individuals with ASD, as well as other types of mental conditions, among which depression stands out [16–19]. According to the WHO [1], it is estimated that 5% of adults suffer from depression, but it also affects minors [18] and the young, being found in around 2.8% of children under 13 years of age and 5.6% of those aged 13–18 years [20]. That is, its incidence increases from early adolescence and may persist into adulthood [21]. Furthermore, the risk of depression increases with age [1,22].

According to a study by Hudson, Hall and Harkness [23], the combined prevalence rate of depression and ASD ranges from 12 to 14%, and is higher in adolescent and child populations [24]. Hollocks et al. [25] found that the combined prevalence rates of both diseases varied between 23 and 37% over a lifetime, suggesting that individuals with ASD may be at a higher risk of developing depressive disorders than individuals without ASD [23,24,26]. Although it is evident that the prevalence of depressive disorders is higher in youth, it is highly variable depending on the type of study conducted and the cultural, temporal, contextual, and environmental factors considered [27].

Among the social causes of depression, there is a focus on cognitive processes due to failures in an individual's information processing system. Another argument cites the social images and strategies that the individual and surrounding community use to cope with depression (adaptation strategies, social support, self-esteem, and self-image) [28,29].

Childhood depression can be related to severe deficiencies in various areas of life, including social, family, personal, and educational aspects, which manifest over time as an emotional response [20]. The comorbidity of anxiety and depression significantly complicates daily life for individuals with ASD, impacting stress management, social interactions, and access to support services, which affect QoL [30,31].

1.4. Technological Intervention for Emotional Regulation

These factors underscore the importance of a comprehensive approach in managing individuals with ASD who also have anxiety and depression.

Consequently, developing intervention strategies that address both ASD characteristics and additional conditions to enhance QoL and promote healthy, satisfying personal development is crucial. Moreover, addressing emotional regulation through technology promises to enhance QoL and help manage stress, including complications such as anxiety or depression in individuals with ASD.

In line with this context, a recent suggestion has been made of the significant therapeutic benefits of using socially disruptive technologies to delve into emotional regulation in individuals with ASD [32], as well as patients with mental illnesses such as anxiety and/or depression [33]. It is foreseeable that new technologies could help improve QoL in individuals affected by disability by reducing communication gaps and managing stressful situations [34].

This is linked to how people perceive technology in relation to the difficulties they face on a daily basis, which is the focus of this study. The results suggest that interventions should focus on a deeper understanding of how people with ASD, anxiety, and depression perceive technology, with the aim of improving the design, development, and advancement of therapeutic technologies that are practical, accessible to all people, and, above all, effective.

1.5. The Role of Quantum Computing in Collaborative AI

In this regard, generative algorithms could represent an approach to generate useful tools that explore the correlations between ASD, anxiety, and depression. For example, collaborative artificial intelligence (CAI) techniques have demonstrated the ability to handle correlations and complex patterns in diverse datasets that traditional computational methods may find challenging due to their increasing exponential complexity. CAI enables the combination of knowledge and capabilities from multiple agents or models to analyze large and complex datasets more effectively. For instance, CAI has demonstrated positive results in Quantitative Modeling in Drug Discovery [35] and Employ Service Coproduction [36]. Moreover, the agent-based model produces a more comprehensive analysis by leveraging distributed expertise and perspectives. Additionally, databases with limited data can be enhanced using CAI to augment and refine the existing information through synthetic data generation or advanced data imputation techniques. For this reason, exploring the application of algorithms in quantum computing (QC) could be particularly interesting. QC offers potential advantages in handling complex correlations and patterns within diverse datasets, which traditional computing methods may struggle with due to their exponential growth in complexity. Moreover, QC could potentially enhance the analysis of dependencies between variables, particularly in domains regarding QoL and others relevant to Autism Spectrum Disorder (ASD) and other comorbidities (Chronic Anxiety (CA) and Chronic Depression (CD)). By leveraging QA, it may be possible to uncover deeper insights into the interplay of these variables, thereby informing more targeted interventions and therapies aimed at improving quality of life and managing stress in individuals affected by these conditions. In this context, the objective of this study is to investigate the prevalence and impact of anxiety and depression in persons affected by Autism Spectrum Disorder (ASD) and to develop a comprehensive, technology-enhanced intervention strategy that addresses these comorbid conditions to improve their QoL. This study [37] aims to explore the role of perceived technology and its observed impact on persons with Autism Spectrum Disorder (ASD), and separately, Chronic Anxiety (CA) and Chronic Depression (CD), concerning aspects related to their daily challenges.

2. Materials and Methods

2.1. Objective of the Study

To carry out the objectives of this study, separate analyses will be conducted for each condition to identify distinct patterns, and evaluate how technology can positively influence the QoL in these groups.

2.2. Data Collection

To accomplish this, data are collected from the 'Encuesta de Discapacidad, Autonomía Personal y situaciones de Dependencia (EDAD)' of the 'Instituto Nacional de Estadística (INE)' [38]. This large-scale survey targets individuals residing in family households in Spain, collected during 2020. The survey is based on the statistic that 4.38 million people (94.9 per thousand inhabitants) had some form of disability in Spain during the year 2020 [38]. The questionnaire underwent validation by the National Institute of Statistics (INE) before implementation. This study received approval from the Ethics Committee of the Miguel Hernández University of Elche (code AUT.IB.EFJ.240202).

The EDAD survey provides a robust dataset, but certain limitations and potential biases should be acknowledged. The survey's focus on individuals in family households may exclude those living in institutional settings, such as care facilities, potentially under-representing the full scope of disability prevalence in Spain. Additionally, self-reported data, which form the basis of the questionnaire, may be subject to recall bias or varying interpretations of disability among respondents. The data, collected solely in 2020, may also reflect specific socio-economic or health-related conditions unique to that year, such as the impact of the COVID-19 pandemic, which could limit their generalizability to other time periods. These factors should be considered when interpreting the study's findings.

A two-stage stratified sampling approach was employed using a multi-channel methodology, including computer-assisted web interviewing (CAWI), computer-assisted telephone interview (CATI), and paper questionnaires sent via ordinary mail. Upon locating individuals with disabilities, data from individual questionnaires were collected through computer-assisted personal interviews (CAPI). Ultimately, 11,650 participants were included, comprising 4790 males (41.12%) and 6890 females (58.88%).

The prevalence rate for Autism Spectrum Disorder (ASD) was 2.07%, while Chronic Anxiety (CA) 17.77% and Chronic Depression (CD) were seen in 18.70% of the total 11,650 surveyed individuals. Notably, within the group of individuals with CD, 0.25% also suffered from CA, and 12.40% had ASD (Table 1).

Table 1. Diagnosed conditions and associated comorbidities in the case of Autism Spectrum Disorder (ASD), Chronic Anxiety (CA) and Chronic Depression (CD) (n = 11,650).

People Diagnosed with...	Med. Age ± SD	Total	Freq. Total (%)	Total ASD	Freq. ASD (%)
Autism Spectrum Disorder (ASD)	36.34 ± 2.71	241	2.07		
Chronic Anxiety (CA)	63.06 ± 0.37	2070	17.77	61	0.52
Chronic Depression (CD)	43.56 ± 6.16	2179	18.70	29	0.25

2.3. Measuring Instruments

The secondary questionnaire applied aspects related to quality of life (QoL) based on the index of the WHOQOL-100 scale used by the World Health Organization (WHO) [1], which has previously been validated in ASD patients [31,39–41]. This multidimensional construct [42] focuses on physical, emotional, and social well-being, which includes physical health perception, physiological state, level of independence, social relationships, and relationships with the environment, as shown in Table 2.

Each question in the survey used a Likert scale ranging from 1 to 4 points. The question addressing the perception of technology and its impact on quality of life was: 'In your opinion, has the use of new technologies improved aspects of your daily life?'. This question served as the cornerstone for measuring technology perception among individuals with Autism Spectrum Disorder (ASD) who are also affected by co-occurring conditions such as Chronic Anxiety (CA) and Chronic Depression (CD), providing critical insights into how technological advancements influence their daily experiences.

Table 2. Index, description of variables and number of variables that make up the index.

Domains	Description of Variables	Number of Variables that Make up the Index
Communication	Some variables are related to the definition of communication [43], including the following: Difficulties in speaking in an understandable way or saying meaningful sentences; speaking comprehensively or saying meaningful sentences when using the assistive device; understanding the meaning of what others say to you; understanding the meaning of what others say to you when you receive help	11
Learning	Some variables are related with the definition of learning [44]. Included are those variables that determine the level of difficulty in paying attention with the gaze or maintaining attention with the ear; learning how to do simple things; learning to do simple things when you receive personal help or assistance; carrying out simple tasks	7
Mobility	Some variables are related with the definition of mobility [45]. Difficulty is measured in variables such as changing posture; changing posture when receiving personal help or assistance; keeping the body in the same position; keeping the body in the same position when receiving personal help or assistance; walking or moving around your home; walking or moving around your home when you receive personal help or assistance.	16
Self-care	Some variables are related with the definition of self-care [46]. These include variables that measure the level of difficulty when washing and drying different parts of the body; washing and drying different parts of the body when receiving personal help or assistance; performing basic body care; performing basic care of the body when receiving personal help or assistance	14
Domestic life or social support	Some variables are related with the definition of cosmetic life or social support [47]. These include variables that measure difficulties in managing the household budget, planning expenses, or organizing purchases; managing the household budget, planning expenses, or organizing shopping when you receive personal help or assistance; preparing meals; preparing meals when you receive personal help or assistance; taking care of other household chores	6

Table 2. *Cont.*

Domains	Description of Variables	Number of Variables that Make up the Index
Interpersonal relationships	Some variables are related with the definition of interpersonal relationships [48]. These inlcude those that measure aspects related to the display of affection; respect or feelings, relationships with strangers, creating and maintaining relationships with friends and neighbors, acquaintances, and colleagues; starting a family or maintaining family relationships; creating and maintaining romantic or sexual relationships.	5

2.4. Statistical Methods

Statistical analysis of the mean indices was performed with all variables of the specified domains 'Communication', 'Learning', 'Mobility', 'Self-care' 'Domestic Life or Social Support' and 'Interpersonal Relationships' and the dependent variable "Do you believe that the use of new technologies has improved aspects of your daily life?', using STATA/MP 17.0 software. Mean index and standard error analyses are presented for the ASD variables.

This questionnaire employed a Likert scale, which presents challenges for parametric tests due to its ordinal nature. The Likert scale categorizes responses into ordered categories without assuming equal intervals between them, making it non-continuous and less suitable for traditional parametric analyses. Therefore, an ANOVA analysis was conducted to explore potential differences among groups based on Likert-scale responses related to the dependent variable. In addition to ANOVA, several non-parametric tests were performed, such as Spearman's correlation and the Kruskal–Wallis test.

Non-parametric tests offer a robust alternative when the assumptions for parametric tests are violated, such as the non-normality or heterogeneity of variances. By incorporating both parametric and non-parametric analyses, a comprehensive understanding of the data can be achieved, ensuring the robustness and reliability in the findings.

These tests were used to examine the relationship between each independent variable and the dependent variable 'Do you believe that the use of new technologies has improved aspects of your daily life?'. For the Spearman test, a p-value < 0.05 indicates a statistically significant correlation. For Kruskall–Wallis, if the p-value is ≥ 0.05, there is not enough evidence to support significant differences between the medians of the compared categories.

2.5. Reliability and Internal Consistency Analysis

Given the questionnaire nature of the study, an analysis of internal consistency using Cronbach's alpha was conducted across the various domains encompassing the independent variables and the dependent variable. The test of average interitem correlation was conducted to assess the internal consistency within each domain of the questionnaire. For Cronbach's alpha, a minimum value of 0.70 is typically considered acceptable for research purposes, indicating sufficient reliability. The average interitem correlation should ideally fall between 0.15 and 0.50, suggesting moderate to strong interrelatedness among the variables within each domain. This analysis provides insights into how closely related the items within each domain are, ensuring that the questionnaire measures the intended constructs reliably.

2.6. Factor Analysis

For the ASD and CA groups, and the ASD and CD groups, a factor analysis will be conducted to evaluate two aspects—uniqueness and the Kaiser–Meyer–Olkin (KMO) measure—as well as the factor structure using Varimax rotation. Varimax rotation will be used as an orthogonal technique to simplify the interpretation of the factors by maximizing high factor loadings on some factors and minimizing low loadings on others. This will facilitate the identification of variables that are strongly associated with each factor, making the resulting model more interpretable and useful for data analysis. Uniqueness measures the proportion of each variable's variability that is not explained by the extracted factors. Low uniqueness values below 0.5 indicate that a variable is well represented by the factors, which reinforces the validity of the factor model. Values above 0.6 suggest that the sample is adequate, while values below 0.5 indicate that the data are not ideal for this analysis.

2.7. Quantum Algorithms

Based on the results, an appropriate quantum algorithm will be used to analyze the relationships between the independent variable of technology 'Do you believe that the use of new technologies has improved aspects of your daily life?' and the specific domains wherein dependent variables have obtained significance according to the *p*-value Pearson correlation.

The proposed algorithm will use the Hamiltonian operator, which is particularly suitable for modeling complex interactions between variables. Hamiltonians are fundamental in quantum simulation, allowing for the simulation of the temporal evolution of a quantum system. This capability is particularly valuable for studying how correlations between variables change over time or under different conditions [49,50].

By using quantum simulation techniques, one can obtain an exact description of the interactions, surpassing the limitations of classical methods.

This adaptability allows for the efficient handling of both small and large systems, making Hamiltonians a scalable solution for quantum data analysis [51].

3. Results

For each domain, the analysis includes statistical evaluations using both parametric and non-parametric methods. Non-parametric tests do not assume a normal distribution of data, which is advantageous when dealing with diverse and heterogeneous datasets like those found in studies of ASD and related developmental conditions.

3.1. Parametric and Non-Parametric Statistical Analysis

Table 3 concerns the statistical analysis of the data. In the domain of Communication, there are pronounced differences in several areas. For instance, the item "…speak in an understandable way or make sentences that make sense" has an ANOVA value of 9.60 and $p < 0.05$, indicating substantial variability in how different groups can effectively articulate their thoughts. This suggests that some groups may face challenges in clear verbal expression, impacting their overall communication effectiveness. Similarly, the item "…understand the meaning of what others say" has an ANOVA value of 6.13 with $p < 0.05$, showing differences in comprehension abilities. For example, individuals who can better understand spoken language might have a more effective interaction with others compared to those who struggle with comprehension.

Table 3. Statistical analysis for parametric (Barltlett's test, Shapiro–Wilk, skewness–kurtosis and ANOVA) and non-parametric tests (Spearman (rho) and Kruskal–Wallis (Chi-squared with ties).

						Shaphiro–Wilk and Skewness–Kurtosis tests					
Domain	**Difficulty Level for…**	**Mean**	±	**S.D.**	**Bartlett's Test Chi2(2) ***	**Pr (Skewness) ***	**Pr (Kurtosis) ***	**Adj Chi2(2) ***	**ANOVA (F) ***	**Spearman (rho) ***	**Kruskal–Wallis (Chi Squared with Ties)**
	…speak in an understandable way or say sentences that make sense	1.959184	±	0.0709385	0.6257 *	0.8103 *	0.0009	9.60	3.63 *	0.6242	6.806
	…speak in an understandable way or say meaningful sentences when using the assistive device	2.606061	±	0.1439394	2.4316 *	0.6348 *	0.7915 *	0.30 *	0.58	−0.0904	2.568
	…understand the meaning of what others say	1.815534	±	0.0658057	0.7495 *	0.3253	0.0189	6.13	1.69	0.0000	4.080
	…understand the meaning of what others say to you when you receive help	2.481481	±	0.0897718	0.9155 *	0.4246	0.4305 *	1.29 *	2.06	−0.1286	7.303
	…understand and express themselves through written language	2.245.614	±	0.0677463	4.1487 *	0.0704	0.0000	16.31	2.49	0.3952	9953 *
COMMUNICATION	…understand and express themselves through gestures, symbols, drawings or sounds	1.922078	±	0.0842445	2.9057 *	0.6355 *	0.0000	14.27	6.69 *	−0.2020	9755 *
	…hold a dialogue and exchange ideas with one or more people	2.117117	±	0.0649308	2.5252 *	0.4960	0.0035	8.07	2.47	0.3984	5.238
	…use the telephone (landline or mobile) or other communication devices or techniques	2.2	±	0.0758348	0.8640 *	0.1182	0.0000	35.46	1.50	0.3582	7.824
	…use the telephone or other communication devices or techniques when receiving help	2.612903	±	0.1111329	1.2219	0.7389 *	0.1064 *	2.84 *	1.01	0.3984	7.783
	…use remote written communication systems	2.42268	±	0.0715487	0.9242 *	0.0019	0.1429 *	3.29 *	2.68	0.4166	3.741
	…use remote written communication systems when receiving help	2.653846	±	0.1313712	2.7316	0.4364	0.1133 *	1.68 *	2.09	0.1444	5.878

Table 3. *Cont.*

						Shaphiro–Wilk and Skewness–Kurtosis tests					
Domain	Difficulty Level for...	Mean	±	S.D.	Bartlett's Test Chi2(2) *	Pr (Skewness) *	Pr (Kurtosis) *	Adj Chi2(2) *	ANOVA (F) *	Spearman (rho) *	Kruskal–Wallis (Chi Squared with Ties)
LEARNING	...pay attention with your eyes or keep your attention with your ears	1.791667	±	0.0626825	4.5721	0.5265	0.2657 *	22.65	5.01 *	−0.1306	10.570 *
	...learn to do simple things	2.044944	±	0.0797566	0.4567	0.7632 *	0.0000	0.27 *	5.18 *	−0.0833	9.213
	...learn to do simple things when receiving personal help or assistance	2.5	±	0.0904326	2.5418	0.7078 *	0.7153 *	13.85	1.17	−0.0388	9.250
	...carry out simple tasks	2.017241	±	0.0998831	3.5982	0.9225 *	0.0000	5.64 *	5.01 *	−0.2899	9.271
	...carry out simple tasks when receiving personal help or assistance	2.5	±	0.140698	0.5132	0.6868 *	0.0163	6.91	0.47	0.0596	3.678
	...carry out complex tasks	2.293103	±	0.0692834	1.6118	0.0194	0.0000	4.26 *	4.94 *	−0.2145	12.600 *
	...carry out complex tasks when receiving personal help or assistance	2.621053	±	0.1005906	3.9635	0.7766 *	0.0000	9.60	2.23	−0.2332	7.793
MOBILITY	...change position	2.038462	±	0.141212	0.6533	0.8930 *	0.1679 *	8.06	0.80	.	4.832
	...change posture when receiving personal help or assistance	2.590909	±	0.2246603	0.6855	0.7807 *	0.1128 *	31.22	0.87	.	1.755
	...keep the body in the same position	2.034483	±	0.1263621	3.2550	0.9187 *	0.3872 *	.	1.78	.	6.666
	...keep the body in the same position when receiving help or personal assistance	2.565217	±	0.1867772	2.4995	0.6384 *	0.6510 *	2.80 *	0.60	.	5.328
	...walk or move around your home	2.130435	±	0.1578555	1.8263	0.6167 *	0.0826 *	3.20 *	0.20	.	4.201
	...walk or move around in your home when you receive help or personal assistance	2.6	±	0.210263	1.6960	0.5093 *	0.6103 *	4.62 *	0.43	.	3.899
	...walk or move outside your home	2.541667	±	0.0891167	0.0137	0.0060	0.7536 *	6.58	1.96	.	3.318
	...walk or move outside your home when you receive help or personal assistance	2.414634	±	0.1560785	1.2133	0.6326 *	0.0482	18.79	1.99	.	1.915
	...move using means of transport as a passenger	2.538462	±	0.1007571	0.4217	0.0008	0.6935 *	18.40	0.36	.	1.254

Table 3. *Cont.*

Domain	Difficulty Level for…	Mean	±	S.D.	Bartlett's Test Chi2(2) *	Pr (Skewness) *	Pr (Kurtosis) *	Adj Chi2(2) *	ANOVA (F) *	Spearman (rho) *	Kruskal–Wallis (Chi Squared with Ties)
						Shaphiro–Wilk and Skewness–Kurtosis tests					
	…move using means of transport as a passenger when receiving personal help or assistance	2.511628	±	0.1608811	7.4477	0.5180	0.0029	10.43	1.22	.	0.832
	…driving vehicles without adaptations	2.862069	±	0.0957745	.	0.0000	0.0000	10.00	0.00	.	1.685
	…driving vehicles when receiving personal help or assistance	3.666667	±	0.3333333	.	.	.	27.99	.	.	.
	…manipulate and move objects, using hands and arms	2.054054	±	0.115898	1.1332	0.8358 *	0.1097 *	7.94	0.85	.	5.230
	…manipulate and move objects, using hands and arms when receiving personal help or assistance	2.862069	±	0.1770318	9.6770	0.5613 *	0.1084 *	59.60	0.60	.	2.312
	…manipulate small objects with hands and fingers	2.212121	±	0.1287879	14.4606	0.3499	0.0544 *	11.56	2.76	.	11.236 *
	…manipulate small objects with hands and fingers when receiving personal help or assistance	2.884615	±	0.1866871	13.5468	0.8958 *	0.0071	73.47	1.73		4.566
SELF-CARE	…wash and dry the different parts of the body	2.239437	±	0.0929395	1.1548	0.1091	0.0000	4.83 *	0.17	−0.0425	1.778
	…wash and dry the different parts of the body when receiving help or personal assistance	2.666667	±	0.1300316	1.1743	0.5711 *	0.0000	11.97	0.48	−0.0065	2.645
	…perform basic body care	2.544118	±	0.0796001	0.6105	0.0005	0.6149 *	44.75	3.33 *	0.2487	2.931
	…perform basic body care when receiving personal help or assistance	2.878788	±	0.1304737	0.2709	0.1082	0.0023	7.18	4.04 *	0.1744	2.008
	…go to the toilet and relieve yourself or take care of your intimate hygiene	2.157895	±	0.1085028	0.0259	0.3216	0.0000	12.45	3.03	−0.1146	5.903

Table 3. *Cont.*

Domain	Difficulty Level for…	Mean	±	S.D.	Bartlett's Test Chi2(2) *	Shapiro–Wilk and Skewness–Kurtosis tests Pr (Skewness) *	Pr (Kurtosis) *	Adj Chi2(2) *	ANOVA (F) *	Spearman (rho) *	Kruskal–Wallis (Chi Squared with Ties)
	…go to the toilet and relieve yourself or take care of your intimate hygiene when you receive help or personal assistance	2.849057	±	0.1410005	4.4321	0.2696 *	0.0051	25.49	1.37	−0.2387	7.649
	…dress or undress	2.103448	±	0.1118768	2.4061	0.5013 *	0.0000	21.37	0.86	0.0427	2.838
	…dressing or undressing when receiving personal help or assistance	2.535714	±	0.141798	1.5484	0.9943 *	0.0002	19.09	0.87	−0.1461	4.665
	…eat and drink	1.977778	±	0.1329118	0.2832	0.8941 *	0.0000	8.26	2.80	−0.2343	5.132
	…eat and drink when receiving personal help or assistance	2.302326	±	0.1579733	1.3172	0.2263 *	0.0653 *	10.97	2.25	−0.2100	4.365
	…comply with medical prescriptions	0.1579733	±	0.0859398	0.7047	0.0001	0.9239 *	6.65	1.05	0.2560	4.795
	…fulfill medical prescriptions when receiving personal help or assistance	2.726027	±	0.1382929	2.0651	0.3132 *	0.0000	9.22	0.99	0.0374	6.149
	…avoid dangerous situations	2.41791	±	0.0854637	5.5222	0.0099	0.2554 *	7.18	1.03	−0.0526	7.126
	…avoid dangerous situations when receiving personal help or assistance	2.967213	±	0.1440386	1.5263	0.0571	0.0006	12.45	0.36	−0.0823	2.638
DOMESTIC LIFE	…manage the household budget, plan expenses or organize purchases	2.681319	±	0.0622711	3.9341	0.0000	0.0108	25.49	2.20	−0.1464	7.544
	…manage the household budget, plan expenses or organize purchases when you receive personal help or assistance	3.567164	±	0.0979756	1.6465	0.0000	0.0128	21.37	0.42	−0.0330	8.239
	…prepare meals	2.630435	±	0.0631953	4.8575	0.0000	0.0853 *	19.09	2.83	−0.2279	7.243
	…prepare meals when receiving personal help or assistance	3.131579	±	0.1144661	5.5536	0.0081	0.1230 *	8.26	1.83	−0.0186	7.257
	…take care of other chores around the house	2.494382	±	0.0734451	4.3456	0.0003	0.7782 *	10.97	1.44	−0.0997	4.225

Table 3. *Cont.*

Domain	Difficulty Level for…	Mean	±	S.D.	Bartlett's Test Chi2(2) *	Pr (Skewness) *	Pr (Kurtosis) *	Adj Chi2(2) *	ANOVA (F) *	Spearman (rho) *	Kruskal–Wallis (Chi Squared with Ties)
						Shaphiro–Wilk and Skewness–Kurtosis tests					
	…take care of other chores around the house when you receive personal help or assistance	3.04	±	0.1114038	8.7014	0.0249 *	0.1397 *	6.65	2.16	−0.1224	3.370
INDIVIDUAL RELATION-SHIPS	…show affection, respect or feelings	1.891304	±	0.0732439	2.2537	0.5269 *	0.0014	9.22	1.87	−0.1925	8.445
	…associating with unknown people	2.131148	±	0.059295	0.9925	0.5114 *	0.0355	4.87 *	3.77 *	−0.1927	7.782
	…create and maintain relationships with friends, neighbors, acquaintances, subordinates, superiors or colleagues	2	±	0.0636778	0.9231	1.000	0.0000	22.70	2.22	−0.1633	6.626
	…form a family or maintain family relationships	2.5	±	0.0832816	2.6687	0.0009	0.9094 *	9.46	1.91	−0.0392	6.463
	…create and maintain sentimental, partner or sexual relationships	2.546667	±	0.0742369	0.3646	0.0004	0.6230 *	10.87	0.32	−0.0574	2.151
	Do you believe that the use of new technologies has improved aspects of your daily life?	2.647059	±	0.0743089		0.0002	0.6863 *	12.27			

Note: For Bartlett's test (chi2(2)), if * $p > 0.05$, the data refused the assumption of equal variances. In the Shapiro–Wilk test and skewness–kurtosis tests, if Pr (skewness) and Pr (kurtosis) are greater than 0.05 and/or Adj. chi2(2) probability, that is * $p > 0.05$, it suggests that the data may plausibly follow a normal distribution. For ANOVA, * $p < 0.05$. For Spearman test, * $p < 0.05$ suggests the correlation is statistically significant. For the Kruskal–Wallis test, if * $p < 0.05$, there is enough evidence to claim that there are significant differences between the medians of the compared categories.

The item "...use the telephone (landline or mobile) or other communication devices" exhibits an exceptionally high ANOVA value of 35.46 with $p < 0.05$, highlighting significant differences in the ability to use communication devices. This variance could be due to factors such as familiarity with technology or the presence of physical or cognitive barriers that affect device usage. For instance, individuals with more advanced communication skills might use phones and other devices more efficiently, whereas others might face challenges due to less familiarity or physical limitations.

In the Learning domain, significant differences are seen in the ability to perform both simple and complex tasks. For instance, the item "...carry out simple tasks" has an ANOVA value of 5.01 with $p < 0.05$, indicating notable variability in performing basic tasks. This may reflect differences in cognitive processing or support received, whereby some individuals can manage simple tasks independently, while others might require assistance.

The item "...carry out complex tasks" shows an ANOVA value of 4.94 with $p < 0.05$, revealing differences in handling more intricate tasks. This could include activities requiring higher levels of problem-solving or multi-step processes. The Kruskal–Wallis test confirms this with a value of 12.600 and $p < 0.05$, indicating significant differences in the median abilities of groups. For example, individuals who can effectively manage complex tasks might have developed better cognitive strategies or received more comprehensive support compared to those who find such tasks challenging.

In the Mobility domain, significant differences are apparent in various physical activities. For example, the item "...change position" has an ANOVA value of 8.06 with $p < 0.05$, indicating variability in how groups manage physical repositioning. This difference could be influenced by physical strength, coordination, or the presence of assistive devices.

The item "...manipulate small objects with hands and fingers" demonstrates significant differences with a Kruskal–Wallis value of 11.236 and $p < 0.05$, highlighting variations in fine motor skills. For example, individuals with dexterity issues may struggle with tasks requiring precise hand movements, affecting their ability to perform everyday activities like buttoning a shirt or handling small tools.

The item "...walk or move around inside the home" has an ANOVA value of 1.82 with $p < 0.05$, reflecting differences in the ability to navigate indoor environments. These differences could be related to physical strength, balance, or the layout of the living space. Variability in mobility can impact an individual's independence and their ability to perform routine tasks within their home.

In the Self-Care domain, significant differences are observed in personal hygiene and daily care tasks. For example, the item "...perform basic body care" shows an ANOVA value of 3.33 with $p < 0.05$, indicating variability in managing personal hygiene tasks. This may include activities such as bathing or grooming, where some individuals may require more support due to physical or cognitive limitations.

The item "...eat and drink" demonstrates significant differences, with a Kruskal–Wallis value of 5.132 and $p < 0.05$, reflecting variability in the ability to perform eating and drinking activities. This could be influenced by factors such as fine motor skills, oral motor function, or access to appropriate utensils and food. Individuals facing difficulties in this area might need assistance with mealtimes, impacting their nutritional intake and overall well-being.

In the Domestic Life domain, significant differences are observed in managing household responsibilities. For instance, the item "...manage the household budget" has an ANOVA value of 2.20 with $p < 0.05$, indicating variability in financial management skills. Some individuals may handle budgeting tasks with ease, while others might struggle, possibly due to differences in financial literacy or support systems.

The item "...prepare meals" shows a Kruskal–Wallis value of 7.243 with $p < 0.05$, suggesting differences in meal preparation abilities. This could reflect varying levels of culinary skills or access to resources like cooking facilities and ingredients. Individuals who are more skilled in meal preparation might be able to cook diverse and nutritious meals, whereas others might face challenges that limit their dietary options.

The item "...go to the toilet and relieve yourself or take care of your intimate hygiene" also shows variability, with an ANOVA value of 3.03 and $p < 0.05$, indicating differences in managing personal hygiene related to toileting. This task may present challenges for individuals with mobility issues or cognitive impairments, affecting their ability to maintain personal hygiene independently.

In the Individual Relationships domain, most items did not show statistically significant differences. For example, the items "...show affection, respect or feelings" (with ANOVA values around 1.87 and $p > 0.05$) and "...create and maintain relationships with friends, neighbors, acquaintances, subordinates, superiors, or colleagues" (with ANOVA values around 2.22 and $p > 0.05$) did not reveal significant variability. These results suggest that skills related to forming and maintaining relationships are relatively consistent across different groups, indicating that such interpersonal abilities might be less influenced by the factors that affect other domains.

In the context of the provided data, several variables exhibited skewness or kurtosis that deviated from normality, as indicated by the Shapiro–Wilk test and the skewness–kurtosis results.

3.2. Pearson Correlation Analysis for ASD, ASD and CA and, and ASC and CD

Individuals with ASD alone have a negative correlation of −0.2994 ($p < 0.05$), indicating moderate difficulty. This difficulty is exacerbated in those with ASD + CA, who exhibit a stronger negative correlation of −0.5765 ($p < 0.05$), pointing to a more significant challenge in learning simple tasks.

This difficulty is more pronounced in individuals with ASD + CA, who have a strong negative correlation of −0.6375 ($p < 0.05$), reflecting significant challenges with fine motor tasks.

However, individuals with ASD + CA show a weaker positive correlation of 0.0424, while those with ASD + CD have a negative correlation of −0.1291, indicating more pronounced difficulties.

This difficulty is more pronounced for individuals with ASD + CA (−0.4367) and ASD + CD (−0.5433), indicating that meal preparation becomes increasingly challenging with additional conditions.

For example, individuals with ASD alone show a slight negative correlation of −0.1795 for 'associating with unknown people', suggesting some difficulty, but less severe compared to other domains. This variability suggests that the impact on individual relationships may be more influenced by personal experiences than by the presence of specific additional conditions (Table 4).

Table 4. Pearson Correlation results for ASD, ASD with CA, ASD with CD and the dependent variable 'Do you believe that the use of new technologies has improved aspects of your daily life?'.

Domain	Difficulty Level for…	ASD (n = 241)	ASD with CA (n = 61)	ASD with CD (n = 29)
COMMUNICATION	…speak in an understandable way or say sentences that make sense	−0.2053 *	−0.4067	−0.4143
	…speak in an understandable way or say meaningful sentences when using the assistive device	−0.1318	0.7559	.
	…understand the meaning of what others say	−0.1804	−0.4446 *	−0.7354 *
	…understand the meaning of what others say to you when you receive help	−0.2365 *	−0.1869	−0.4437
	…understand and express themselves through written language	−0.1887 *	−0.2460	−0.2768
	…understand and express themselves through gestures, symbols, drawings or sounds	−0.3095 *	−0.5649 *	−0.4299
	…hold a dialogue and exchange ideas with one or more people	−0.0496	−0.3928	−0.5486
	…use the telephone (landline or mobile) or other communication devices or techniques	−0.1081	−0.2764	−0.5993
	…use the telephone or other communication devices or techniques when receiving help	−0.2147	−0.0000	−0.5000
	…use remote written communication systems	−0.0472	−0.0475	−0.6198
	…use remote written communication systems when receiving help	−0.2489	0.2000	−0.4677
LEARNING	…pay attention with your eyes or keep your attention with your ears	−0.3116 *	−0.1667	−0.6142
	…learn to do simple things	−0.2994 *	−0.5765 *	−0.7385
	…learn to do simple things when receiving personal help or assistance	−0.2106	−0.0578	.
	…carry out simple tasks	−0.3779 *	−0.3850	.
	…carry out simple tasks when receiving personal help or assistance	−0.1201	0.3665	.
	…carry out complex tasks	−0.2828 *	−0.2718	−0.3543
	…carry out complex tasks when receiving personal help or assistance	−0.2351 *	0.1414	0.0184

Table 4. *Cont.*

Domain	Difficulty Level for...	ASD (n = 241)	ASD with CA (n = 61)	ASD with CD (n = 29)
MOBILITY	...change position	−0.2028	−0.1887	−0.2342
	...change posture when receiving personal help or assistance	−0.2284	−0.0463	−0.1766
	...keep the body in the same position	−0.3374	−0.3915	−0.3263
	...keep the body in the same position when receiving help or personal assistance	−0.2033	0.1942	0.0913
	...walk or move around your home	−0.0637	0.1295	−0.0425
	...walk or move around in your home when you receive help or personal assistance	−0.2490	−0.2340	−0.4678
	...walk or move outside your home	−0.1833	−0.1970	−0.4468
	...walk or move outside your home when you receive help or personal assistance	−0.1430	−0.2428	−0.0778
	...move using means of transport as a passenger	−0.0988	0.3502	0.7660 *
	...move using means of transport as a passenger when receiving personal help or assistance	−0.0996	0.2810	0.6847
	...driving vehicles without adaptations	0.0091	.	.
	...driving vehicles when receiving personal help or assistance	.	.	.
	...manipulate and move objects, using hands and arms	−0.0613	0.0400	0.3208
	...manipulate and move objects, using hands and arms when receiving personal help or assistance	−0.2310	−0.2037	−0.4082
	...manipulate small objects with hands and fingers	−0.3429	−0.6375 *	−0.1715
	...manipulate small objects with hands and fingers when receiving personal help or assistance	−0.3015	−0.3338	−0.1741
SELF-CARE	...wash and dry the different parts of the body	−0.0506	0.0970	0.0000
	...wash and dry the different parts of the body when receiving help or personal assistance	−0.0418	−0.0251	0.0000
	...perform basic body care	0.0874	0.0424	−0.1291
	...perform basic body care when receiving personal help or assistance	−0.0639	−0.0807	−0.1768
	...go to the toilet and relieve yourself or take care of your intimate hygiene	−0.2954 *	−0.1874	−0.6625
	...go to the toilet and relieve yourself or take care of your intimate hygiene when you receive help or personal assistance	−0.2593	−0.1423	−0.3151

Table 4. *Cont.*

Domain	Difficulty Level for…	ASD (n = 241)	ASD with CA (n = 61)	ASD with CD (n = 29)
	…dress or undress	−0.1740	0.1755	0.0000
	…dressing or undressing when receiving personal help or assistance	−0.1621	0.0987	0.1291
	…eat and drink	−0.3267 *	−0.4105	−0.5571
	…eat and drink when receiving personal help or assistance	−0.2102	−0.7172 *	−0.9191 *
	…comply with medical prescriptions	−0.0128	−0.2002	−0.5130
	…fulfill medical prescriptions when receiving personal help or assistance	−0.1544	−0.1881	−0.6198
	…avoid dangerous situations	−0.1513	−0.1015	−0.6355
	…avoid dangerous situations when receiving personal help or assistance	−0.1316	−0.0248	−0.3151
DOMESTIC LIFE	…manage the household budget, plan expenses or organize purchases	−0.1831	−0.2202	−0.4348
	…manage the household budget, plan expenses or organize purchases when you receive personal help or assistance	0.0886	0.0696	−0.2140
	…prepare meals	−0.2307 *	−0.4367 *	−0.5433
	…prepare meals when receiving personal help or assistance	−0.0543	−0.0896	−0.2895
	…take care of other chores around the house	−0.1795	−0.3359	−0.5333
	…take care of other chores around the house when you receive personal help or assistance	−0.1544	−0.0791	−0.3481
INDIVIDUAL RELATIONSHIPS	…show affection, respect or feelings	−0.0918	0.0262	−0.1959
	…associating with unknown people	−0.1795 *	−0.0167	0.0669
	…create and maintain relationships with friends, neighbors, acquaintances, subordinates, superiors or colleagues	−0.1587	−0.1518	0.0176
	…form a family or maintain family relationships	−0.1094	0.2160	0.1066
	…create and maintain sentimental, partner or sexual relationships	−0.0675	0.1259	0.0449

* $p < 0.05$.

3.3. Reliability and Consistency Analysis

The Cronbach's alpha values are consistently above 0.8, such as 0.8326 and 0.8417 (Table 5), reflecting good internal consistency.

3.4. Quantum Associative Memory Algorithm

To explicitly incorporate the role of quantum simulation in analyzing the relationships between technology use, Autism Spectrum Disorder (ASD), and related conditions like anxiety and depression, this study employs quantum simulation techniques to model complex interactions among variables. Specifically, we focus on the independent variable 'Do you believe that the use of new technologies has improved aspects of your daily life?' and its correlations with dependent variables tied to functional domains in ASD (e.g., difficulties in communication and task performance), identified through significant Pearson's correlations ($p < 0.05$). Quantum simulation enhances this analysis by representing each variable as a qubit within a quantum system, leveraging the Hamiltonian operator to capture intricate interactions and energy states that classical methods may oversimplify. Unlike traditional approaches, quantum simulation exploits superposition and entanglement to explore nonlinear relationships and temporal dynamics, offering a more nuanced understanding of how technology influences these domains in ASD and co-occurring conditions. For instance, the Quantum Associative Memory (QAM) algorithm is applied to associate technology use with multiple dependent variables simultaneously, revealing patterns that might be computationally infeasible with classical techniques. This approach not only provides a precise mathematical framework, but also scales efficiently to larger datasets, facilitating deeper insights into the interplay of autism, mental health, and technological impact.

In summary, the QAM algorithm would facilitate the exploration and understanding of how technology influences specific domains differently across ASD and CA, leveraging the significant correlations identified in Table 1 and the mean index analyses conducted.

The dependent variables are selected by the significant Pearson's correlation for the cases of ASD in CA/CD, which are the following:

A1. Difficulties in understanding and expressing themselves through written language;
A2. Difficulties in learning how to do simple things when receiving personal help or assistance;
A3. Difficulties in carrying out complex tasks when receiving personal help or assistance.

In addition, there is the dependent variable 'A4. Do you believe that the use of new technologies has improved aspects of your daily life?'

To represent these variables in a quantum model, we assigned one qubit to each independent variable and one to the dependent variable. The coefficients αi and βi represent the influences of the independent variables on the dependent variable and the self-interactions of the dependent variable, respectively. The proposed model is a Hamiltonian in QAM, and it is expressed by

$$H = \sum_{i=1}^{3} i\alpha i Ai + \beta i Bi + \sum i\ \delta i Ai Bi \quad (1)$$

where the following pertains:

αi are the coefficients of the independent variables A1, A2, and A3;

β is the coefficient of the dependent variable A4;

δi are the interaction coefficients between each independent variable Ai and the dependent variable B.

Table 5. Average inter-item correlation and Cronbach's α for ASD, ASD and CA and ASD and CD.

Domain	Difficulty Level for...	ALL VARIABLES (n = 241)		SELECTED VARIABLES ASD + CA (n = 61)				SELECTED VARIABLES ASD + CD (n = 29)	
		Average Interitem Correlation	Cronbach's α	Average Interitem Correlation	Cronbach's α	Uniqueness	KMO	Average Interitem Correlation	Cronbach's α
COMMUNICATION	...speak in an understandable way or say sentences that make sense	0.3114	0.8326	−0.0285	0.1051			−0.1626	
	...speak in an understandable way or say meaningful sentences when using the assistive device	0.3258	0.8417						
	...understand the meaning of what others say	0.3288	0.8435						
	...understand the meaning of what others say to you when you receive help	0.3124	0.8333	−0.0104				−0.1587	
	...understand and express themselves through written language	0.3028	0.8269	−0.2226 *	0.5339	0.0827 *	0.4773	0.0888	0.2804
	...understand and express themselves through gestures, symbols, drawings or sounds	0.3213	0.8389	−0.0003				−0.0380	0.1910
	...hold a dialogue and exchange ideas with one or more people	0.2905	0.8183						
	...use the telephone (landline or mobile) or other communication devices or techniques	0.2997	0.8248						
	...use the telephone or other communication devices or techniques when receiving help	0.3098	0.8316						
	...use remote written communication systems	0.3198	0.8380						
	...use remote written communication systems when receiving help	0.3153	0.8351						
	Do you believe that the use of new technologies has improved aspects of your daily life?	0.4597	0.9035	−0.0590				0.0557	0.1910
		0.3243	0.8521	0.0328	0.1451			−0.0505	

Table 5. *Cont.*

Domain	Difficulty Level for…	ALL VARIABLES (n = 241) Average Interitem Correlation	ALL VARIABLES (n = 241) Cronbach's α	SELECTED VARIABLES ASD + CA (n = 61) Average Interitem Correlation	SELECTED VARIABLES ASD + CA (n = 61) Cronbach's α	SELECTED VARIABLES ASD + CA (n = 61) Uniqueness	SELECTED VARIABLES ASD + CA (n = 61) KMO	SELECTED VARIABLES ASD + CD (n = 29) Average Interitem Correlation	SELECTED VARIABLES ASD + CD (n = 29) Cronbach's α
LEARNING	…pay attention with your eyes or keep your attention with your ears	0.4079	0.8283	0.3401 **	0.7204	0.5882	0.3679	0.4839 **	0.7895
	…learn to do simple things	0.3883	0.8163	0.2250	0.5921			0.3057	0.6378
	…learn to do simple things when receiving personal help or assistance	0.4107	0.8299	0.3294 **	0.7107	0.2864 *	0.3047		
	…carry out simple tasks	0.3825	0.8126						
	…carry out simple tasks when receiving personal help or assistance	0.4087	0.8287						
	…carry out complex tasks	0.3961	0.8211	0.2498 *	0.6247			0.3161 **	0.6496
	…carry out complex tasks when receiving personal help or assistance	0.4064	0.8273	0.3585 **	0.7364	0.1763 *	0.6243 *	0.5467 **	0.8283
	Do you believe that the use of new technologies has improved aspects of your daily life?	0.4719	0.8622	0.4138	0.7792			0.4630	0.7752
		0.4083	0.8466	0.3173	0.7361			0.4173	0.7817
SELF-CARE	…wash and dry the different parts of the body	0.4127	0.9077						
	…wash and dry the different parts of the body when receiving help or personal assistance	0.4011	0.9036						
	…perform basic body care	0.4226	0.9111						
	…perform basic body care when receiving personal help or assistance	0.3975	0.9023						
	…go to the toilet and relieve yourself or take care of your intimate hygiene	0.4021	0.9040	0.4105 **	0.5921			0.5571 **	0.7155
	…go to the toilet and relieve yourself or take care of your intimate hygiene when you receive help or personal assistance	0.3960	0.9018						

Table 5. *Cont.*

Domain		ALL VARIABLES (n = 241)		SELECTED VARIABLES ASD + CA (n = 61)				SELECTED VARIABLES ASD + CD (n = 29)	
	Difficulty Level for…	Average Interitem Correlation	Cronbach's α	Average Interitem Correlation	Cronbach's α	Uniqueness	KMO	Average Interitem Correlation	Cronbach's α
	…dress or undress	0.4031	0.9044						
	…dressing or undressing when receiving personal help or assistance	0.3922	0.9003						
	…eat and drink	0.4101	0.9068	0.1874 *	0.3157			0.6625 **	0.7970
	…eat and drink when receiving personal help or assistance	0.4055	0.9052						
	…comply with medical prescriptions	0.4229	0.9112						
	…fulfill medical prescriptions when receiving personal help or assistance	0.4036	0.9045						
	…avoid dangerous situations	0.4043	0.9048						
	…avoid dangerous situations when receiving personal help or assistance	0.4033	0.9044						
	Do you believe that the use of new technologies has improved aspects of your daily life?	0.4605	0.9228	0.5926	0.7442			0.4472	0.6180
		0.4090	0.9121	0.3619	0.6299			0.5663	0.7596
DOMESTIC LIFE	…manage the household budget, plan expenses or organize purchases	0.4512	0.8315						
	…manage the household budget, plan expenses or organize purchases when you receive personal help or assistance	0.4760	0.8450						
	…prepare meals	0.4488	0.8301	0.4367 **	0.6079			0.5433 **	0.7040
	…prepare meals when receiving personal help or assistance	0.4453	0.8281						
	…take care of other chores around the house	0.4169	0.8110						

Table 5. *Cont.*

Domain	Difficulty Level for...	ALL VARIABLES (n = 241)		SELECTED VARIABLES ASD + CA (n = 61)				SELECTED VARIABLES ASD + CD (n = 29)	
		Average Interitem Correlation	Cronbach's α	Average Interitem Correlation	Cronbach's α	Uniqueness	KMO	Average Interitem Correlation	Cronbach's α
	...take care of other chores around the house when you receive personal help or assistance	0.4295	0.8187						
	Do you believe that the use of new technologies has improved aspects of your daily life?	0.6258	0.9094						
		0.4697	0.8611						
INDIVIDUAL RELATIONSHIPS	...show affection, respect or feelings	0.3252	0.7067						
	...associating with unknown people	0.3226	0.7043	0.0167	0.0328			0.0699	0.1254
	...create and maintain relationships with friends, neighbors, acquaintances, subordinates, superiors or colleagues	0.3130	0.6950						
	...form a family or maintain family relationships	0.3232	0.7048						
	...create and maintain sentimental, partner or sexual relationships	0.3199	0.7016						
	Do you believe that the use of new technologies has improved aspects of your daily life?	0.5111	0.8394						
		0.3482	0.7622						
	Note: * Cronbach's alpha > 0.7. * Average iteritem correlation with moderate interrelatedness: 0.15 to 0.3. ** Strong 0.3–0.5. Uniqueness * with values <0.5 indicates the variable is well represented by the factors. KMO * for values >0.6 indicates the sample is adequate for the analysis.				I_17	0.2072	0.5593		
						Overall KMO	0.4838		

The quantum circuit graph using logic gates is represented in Figure 1, where the following pertains:

1. Hadamard gates (H) initialize qubits in a superposition;
2. CNOT gates (with a point) represent the interactions between the independent and dependent variables;
3. Measurement gates (M) measure the final state of the qubits.

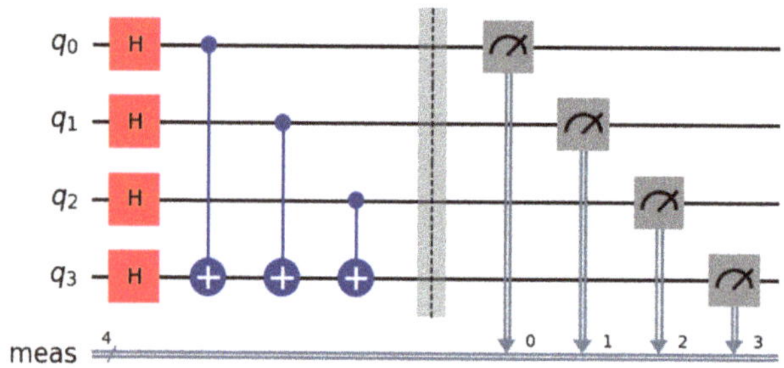

Figure 1. Quantum circuit representation with superposition (four Hadamard gates) and entanglement (three CNOT gates), and measurement at the end.

The quantum circuit begins with the application of Hadamard gates to each qubit, thereby creating an initial state of superposition. Subsequently, CNOT gates are used to entangle the qubits corresponding to the independent variables Ai with the qubit of the dependent variable B. Finally, a measurement is performed on the B qubit to obtain results that reflect the quantum correlations between the variables, as predicted by the defined Hamiltonian.

This quantum simulation not only provides a visual and mathematical representation of the interactions between the variables of interest, but also allows the exploration of quantum phenomena such as superposition and entanglement, which can reveal nonlinear and complex relationships between the study variables. Measurement results offer a unique quantum perspective on how independent variables impact the dependent variable within the theoretical framework of quantum mechanics applied to modeling complex systems.

Algebraically, this quantum circuit starts with the 16-dimensional state vector for $|0000\rangle$, represented as $|\psi0\rangle = (100\ldots.0)$, and applies the tensor product of four Hadamard matrices, $H4 = H{\otimes}H{\otimes}H{\otimes}H$, where $H = \frac{1}{\sqrt{2}}\ (1\ 1\ 1 - 1\ )$, to create a uniform superposition across all possible four-qubit states, resulting in $|\psi1\rangle = H4|\psi0\rangle = \frac{1}{4}\ (111\ldots1)$.

Each qubit's transformation by the Hadamard gate yields an equal distribution of amplitudes. Following this, three CNOT gates are applied, each represented by a 16×16 permutation matrix where qubits 0, 1, and 2 control qubit 3, leading to entanglement; the final state is given by $|\psi2\rangle = \mathrm{CNOT2,3{\cdot}CNOT1,3{\cdot}CNOT0,3}{\cdot}|\psi1\rangle$, where each CNOT matrix permutes specific rows based on the control–target relationship. The final state vector after these operations reflects a complex superposition and entanglement pattern, which requires much computation to describe explicitly due to the intricacy of the entanglement involved.

This quantum circuit, implemented using Qiskit, consists of four qubits initialized in the $|0\rangle$ state. First, Hadamard gates (H) are applied to each qubit, creating an equal superposition of all possible 4-bit states, ranging from $|0000\rangle$ to $|1111\rangle$. Subsequently, three controlled-NOT (CNOT) gates are applied, where qubits 0, 1, and 2 act as control qubits, and qubit 3 serves as the target qubit. These CNOT gates entangle the state of qubit

3 with the states of the first three qubits, resulting in a highly entangled quantum state. The circuit is then visualized using using the Phyton library Matplotlib ("mpl") to display its structure graphically.

```
# Create a quantum circuit with 4 qubits
qc = QuantumCircuit(4)
# Apply Hadamard gates to each qubit
qc.h(0)
qc.h(1)
qc.h(2)
qc.h(3)
# Apply CNOT gates with qubits 0, 1, and 2 as controls and qubit 3 as the target
qc.cx(0, 3)
qc.cx(1, 3)
qc.cx(2, 3)
# Add measurement to all qubits
qc.measure_all()
# Draw the circuit
qc.draw("mpl")
```

The representation of this circuit is included in Figure 1.

The analysis of the quantum circuit results shows a relatively uniform distribution of correlations across the 16 possible states, with counts ranging between 49 and 78 (see Figure 2). This suggests that the correlations between the variables A1, A2 and A3 (representing difficulties in various areas) and the dependent variable A4 (reflecting the perceived improvement through technology use) are fairly balanced. However, the state 1110, with 78 counts, stands out as the most dominant, indicating a stronger correlation in this case. This state reflects a significant interaction between the variables, where the difficulties in A1, A2, and A3 are associated with a perception of improvement in A4. This suggests that in this particular pattern of interactions, the influence of the difficulties on the perception of technology is more pronounced. On the other hand, the state 0111, with 49 counts, shows the fewest measurements, indicating a weaker or less significant correlation compared to other states. However, the presence of several intermediate states with counts ranging between 60 and 70 reflects a balanced distribution of probabilities, suggesting that the relationships between the variables are generally consistent, although there is no single dominant state. This variability is typical in quantum systems, where the behavior of the variables does not follow a predictable linear structure. This pattern of distribution can be attributed to the quantum entanglement between the qubits. The CNOT gates applied between the qubits corresponding to the independent variables (A1, A2, A3) and the dependent variable (A4) create a non-classical correlation between these qubits, allowing the probabilities of the states to be distributed in a complex and entangled manner. Entanglement means that the state of each qubit cannot be described independently, but is intrinsically linked to the state of the other qubits. This phenomenon is key to explaining the uniformity in the counts, while also accounting for the dominance of certain states like 1110, which reflect stronger interactions between the variables. In summary, while the counts are relatively uniform across the range of states, quantum entanglement generates complex relationships between the variables, favoring certain states with higher correlation, such as state 1110, which represents the most significant interactions between the variables in the model.

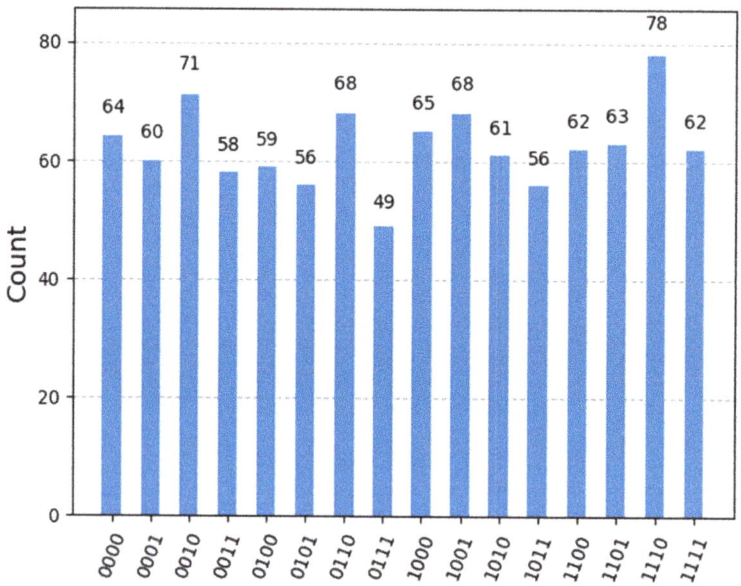

Figure 2. Quantum state measurement histogram for 16 states (X) and counts (Y).

4. Discussion

The analysis results provide a detailed insight into how individuals with ASD and associated conditions (such as concomitant developmental conditions, CD, or additional conditions, AC) perform in various domains of daily life. Both parametric and non-parametric statistical methods are employed to assess differences and relationships in areas such as communication, learning, mobility, self-care, domestic life, and individual relationships. The findings underscore the importance of combining parametric and non-parametric methods to accurately capture variability and strengthen the study's conclusions. Furthermore, this approach reinforces the need for the development of a differentiated approach for carrying out technological or combined interventions, adapting to the specific needs of each diagnostic group.

The results suggest that the domains in which people find the most challenges are Communication and Learning, finding a significant correlation between communication skills and the ability to learn and perform simple tasks with the dependent variable, that is, the positive impact of new technologies. However, the Mobility and Personal Care domains are also correlated, but show a different pattern from the previous two domains, indicating differences in each subdomain in relation to technology.

In the domain of Communication, significant differences are observed in key skills, such as the ability to speak intelligibly and understand what others say. ANOVA values and tests like Kruskal–Wallis show variability between groups, suggesting that persons face greater challenges in verbal expression and the use of communication devices, which may be related to their level of familiarity with technology or cognitive and physical barriers.

Regarding Learning, differences are evident in the ability to perform simple and complex tasks. The analysis shows that individuals with ASD and additional conditions (AC or CD) face greater difficulties, which may be due to differences in cognitive processing or the type of support received. For example, the ability to perform complex tasks is more affected in individuals with ASD and CD, reflecting potential challenges in advanced cognitive strategies.

The analysis of the Mobility domain reveals significant differences in physical activities, such as changing positions or manipulating small objects. Non-parametric tests, such as the Kruskal–Wallis test, highlight variability in fine motor skills, where some groups show considerable difficulties, possibly due to dexterity or coordination issues.

In Self-Care, significant differences are evident in tasks related to personal hygiene and feeding. For example, some individuals with ASD require more support to perform basic body care or to eat and drink, impacting their independence and overall well-being.

In the domain of Domestic Life, skills related to managing household responsibilities, such as preparing meals or managing a budget, also show significant variability. Persons with ASD and additional conditions may face greater difficulties in these areas, which could be due to a lack of culinary or financial management skills.

In the domain of Individual Relationships, it is observed that the skills required to show affection or maintain relationships do not show such pronounced differences between groups, suggesting that these abilities may be less influenced by the conditions affecting other domains. Among the different factors presented by this population with ASD are sensory overload [52], low flexibility in routines, and difficulties in interpreting and managing different social situations, all of which are related to the high prevalence of anxiety in this study. The same is true for high levels of depression, which seems to be linked to the accumulation of negative experiences that lead to the desire for social isolation and future alexithymia [53]. Both disorders have a considerable impact on the quality of life of people with ASD, aggravating their difficulties in mobility, independence, and interpersonal relationships.

Additionally, the reliability and internal consistency analysis shows that domains like Self-Care and Domestic Life exhibit high internal consistency across different groups, with Cronbach's alpha values above 0.8, indicating strong measurement reliability. However, the Individual Relationships domain presents more variability, particularly in subgroups with comorbid conditions like ASD + CA, where lower correlation coefficients and Cronbach's alpha values suggest reduced reliability.

This may be due to the differences in the symptom profiles and needs that are addressed in the three disorders, which are reflected in the indices that make up QoL. In the case of ASD, they have difficulties in the perception of emotions and cognitive deficits, which can affect the development of communication skills and social interaction. For this reason, they present challenges for communication, and the main motivation of some studies is the analysis of the communication process in ASD [54,55].

This is why variability is found in the structure of the indices, with ASD affecting socialization and learning skills more, while AC and CD may present a greater impact on mobility or other areas. In major depressive disorder, among the symptoms that patients present are the absence of facial expression and few body movements, as well as changes in speech [56].

From other perspectives, the results of this paper indicate that Autism Spectrum Disorder (ASD) tends to be chronic and debilitating, affecting the quality of life (QoL) and necessitating timely intervention. Technology could be useful in the domains of learning and communication for people with ASD, although the results are different in the case of mobility and self-care. However, similar patterns are found in AC and CD, that is, both can affect specific areas of quality of life but do so in a different ways, varying between people.

Although this study highlights the importance of combining statistical methods to assess variability across different domains of daily life, the rapid evolution of technologies may alter the dynamics observed and analyzed. As new tools and approaches are introduced, new correlations and patterns in the data that have not yet been identified may emerge. For example, integrating advanced artificial intelligence and machine learning techniques in data analysis could reveal new insights into how technologies impact various domains of daily functioning in individuals with ASD and associated conditions. These technological advances could provide a more detailed and precise understanding, helping to tailor interventions more effectively and personally to people's needs.

4.1. Future Patterns in New and Emerging Technologies to Treat ASD and Concomitant Developmental Conditions Such as Anxiety and Depression

The QAM algorithm applied theoretically in this work could be very useful in avoiding the dysfunctionality of questionnaires and facilitating a more precise and efficient assessment of psychological and behavioral characteristics, improving the quality and reliability of the data collected. The QAM algorithm allows for the association of multiple input variables (such as technology use and various domains) with output variables on their correlations. It can effectively handle the diverse and scattered nature of the variables observed, providing insights into how technology impacts different domains across conditions like ASD, CA, and CD. In this study, the QAM algorithm facilitates the exploration and understanding of how technology influences specific domains differently across ASD, CA, and CD, leveraging significant correlations identified and mean index analyses. By emphasizing variables consistently identified as significant across both CA and CD groups, this study aims to enhance the robustness of its findings and interpretations. Moreover, the study introduces the Quantum Associative Memory (QAM) algorithm to model the impacts of independent variables, such as difficulties in communication and task management, on perceptions of how technology influences daily life. This quantum approach allows for the exploration of complex, nonlinear relationships between variables, offering insights that traditional statistical methods might overlook, thereby broadening the understanding of how technology affects different domains across ASD, CA, and CD conditions, which could be combined with different therapies and technologies. For example, PsicAP therapy has shown efficacy in treating anxiety, depression, and somatization, highlighting the importance of emotional regulation and digital interventions [57], which could be combined with emerging technologies such QAM or existing technologies such social robots.

Apart from QAM, the determination of which strategies are the most suitable for each individual needs to comply with standardized criteria. For example, emotion is a criterion that is useful to consider from different perspectives, and with the help of technological devices. The second criterion is the application of non-invasive techniques, which includes bracelets, mobile applications, skin or temperature sensors, facial recognition technology, virtual reality or augmented reality devices, voice analysis technology, physical activity tracking devices (movement patterns and activity), and electrodermal sensors (GSR) [58].

Moreover, social robots are among the devices that are involved in emotion recognition. These machines were created in the 1990s, and have the ability to communicate with people through language; they can perform certain behaviors and adapt to social norms in different contexts such as hospitals, educational centers, work, and even in the home environment. To do this, social robots are capable of understanding a wide variety of human actions and responding to them with a human-like appearance, as well as showing certain traits that make up a personable personality and appearance, being able to engage in conversations with a high level of complexity, and achieving a certain level of confidence. with the person through the empathy that a social robot can produce [59].

An example of a social robot used to meet emotional criteria is Asimo, developed in 2000, which has the ability to identify faces and voices and converse in several languages, and even has the ability to manipulate objects using tactile sensors in its hands [60].

Another example is the iCub humanoid robot developed in Italy, which is part of the RobotCub project and has been created for research on human cognition and artificial intelligence. It can crawl, express emotions through the face, and learn and solve different activities and challenges in order to avoid moving obstacles [61].

The NAO humanoid robot, developed in France, has evolved into five different versions. It has abilities such as movement and adaptation to the surrounding environment, and maintains balance due to the degrees of freedom that characterize it. It can listen and chat with humans, in addition to detecting objects that are around it, with access to the internet.

It was followed later by the Pepper robot. This intelligent social robot was initially created by Aldebaran Robotics and later incorporated by Softbank Robotics, and is known as the first humanoid robot, designed to live among humans. Pepper communicates in a natural and friendly manner with all the people around him, with movements similar to those of humans. Its voice is pleasant, and it can recognize not only faces but also different voices and movements, responding to them in different contexts. It adapts its behavior to the interlocutor, although its size draws attention as compared to NAO, as Pepper is taller and larger, in addition to supporting a tablet with which to maintain a more visual and close interaction. However, the main uses of this robot are in shops and gastronomic establishments, or in education studies, via a Japanese app that provides online classes through the robot's screen [62]. In line with technology that can strengthen our emotional intelligence, Pepper is implemented and equipped with skills for social interaction, allowing it to open new lines of research into autism. Other humanoid robots, such Keepon, promise to be very collaborative and effective, helping to improve social relationships, but also ground greater analyses and expressions of feelings [63]. Other positive examples applied in the context of autism include animal-like robots (zoomorphic), such as the AIBO dog or Kasha, which have been used in autism studies to treat verbal engagement and social communication, with positive results [64].

Recently, the Kaspar robot has been used to promote cooperative play, reduce isolation, and improve body awareness and the sense of self in children with ASD. Kaspar is equipped with touch sensors that allow children to observe how their actions affect the robot's movement, encouraging turn-taking interactions, a rare behavior in children with ASD. However, Kaspar has limitations in its behavioral reaction capacity, as it cannot perform actions such as walking, grasping objects, or making fine hand gestures [64].

In comparison, the QTrobot is smaller than the Pepper robot; this is a great advantage due to its similarity with the physical dimensions of a child, and its voice is friendlier, dedicated to teaching new communicative, emotional and social skills in children diagnosed with autism or in special education settings [65]. Also considered are the robotic toys used in the study of Autism Spectrum Disorder (ASD), a set of mini-humanoid robots that look like dolls that are part of a project called Robota. The Robota studies have two main objectives: to test the reactions of children with autism to the human characteristics of a robot, and to assess their ability to distinguish between their actions and those of others. The results indicate children's initial preference for interacting with a simple robot rather than a human or a more humanoid robot. Some children are able to communicate with the robot without the therapist present, but the robot is usually used as a mediator between the therapist and the children [66].

The current uses of disruptive technologies such as social robots have sparked widespread debate over their alleged dangers, inadequate therapeutic applicability, and social acceptance. However, there is no consensus regarding the emotional alignment offered by the use of such robots. From another perspective, technology could affect how interventions are carried out for such diseases from a holistic view, based on the positive results on QoL derived via therapies addressing anxiety interventions under the auspices of social skills. However, in the medium term, if these symptoms do not progress appropriately, other psychological disorders may develop.

In this way, they can offer advances in areas such as diagnosis and the personalization of treatment, as well as modeling and simulation, helping us to understand in a deeper way the underlying mechanisms of developmental disorders. In addition, this can involve the optimization of technology-based therapies, such as social robots and virtual reality applications that improve adherence to therapy, and offer new solutions for data security and privacy (as they protect sensitive information) and, in many cases, the protection of minors.

Additionally, future studies must consider not only the potential benefits of these technologies, but also their ethical implications, such as data privacy and the impacts on human interactions. Concerns about the use of these tools must be addressed comprehensively to ensure that the rights and dignity of the individuals using them are respected. As new technologies are developed and adopted, it is crucial for researchers and professionals in the field to collaborate in establishing ethical standards and best practices that balance innovation with the protection of individuals and their well-being.

4.2. Limitations of the Study

In social psychology studies, structural equation modeling is used to relate the scores of different tests, usually administered in groups or via online questionnaires. However, participants in these studies may not be fully engaged, affecting the accuracy of their responses. The absence of the researcher during questionnaire administration can also lead to inaccurate responses. Recent models in personality and social psychology, despite being complex, often do not consider the tendency of participants to provide socially desirable answers.

Additionally, some researchers assume high reliability between scales with similar items without proper evaluation. The quality of tests varies, and it is crucial for researchers to assess their validity before using them. The inability to distinguish between reliable and low-validity tests can result in the prolonged and dogmatic use of these tools without an adequate empirical basis [67].

This study, like other psychological questionnaires, questions the meaning of 'measurement' in psychological testing. While numbers are produced during scoring, their validity as true measurements of behavior is debatable. Philosophers argue that psychological test numbers differ from physical measurements, and may be inappropriate for statistical analyses. Psychological traits may not be truly quantifiable, highlighting the inadequacy of conventional statistical methods for addressing this complexity [67].

A brief review of prior studies on the relationship between mental health, technology perception, and quality of life in ASD, anxiety, and depression shows that raising an autistic child significantly impacts parental quality of life. It causes emotional, social, physical, and economic stress, with autism traits leading to greater parental stress than other disabilities. This stress results in poorer quality of life, less social support, dissatisfaction in relationships, feelings of isolation, and career sacrifices to care for autistic individuals [68,69].

Added to this, the next limitation of this study is the presence of social conception and the influence of individual perceptions. In this regard, the importance of supporting caregivers in emotional and social aspects must be highlighted, giving them the social recognition they deserve, because when we face many daily difficulties, they can generate anxiety, becoming something overwhelming that causes negative effects on the person's QoL, as well as on their cognitive domain, and therefore, on their relationships with the environment, being considered maladaptive. For example, factors associated with ASD, such as the presentation of psychiatric comorbidities, the family environment, income level, or even parental roles, affect the levels of anxiety of both autistic people and their family or friends ç [70]. One of the aspects that most influences the quality of life of parents with children with autism is the low support they receive from society to be able to take care of their children. This can affect the severity of the autistic traits. Although anxiety is not always negative, it can represent an advantage in adapting to our environment if accompanied by appropriate coping strategies [68]. Therefore, it should not be underestimated that certain domains analyzed in ASD, CA, and CD did not show significant correlations. However, this does not necessarily mean that this accurately reflects the true situation. Various factors could contribute to this lack of correlation, including the complexity of measuring outcomes in these conditions, the diversity of symptoms and presentations within each disorder, or the limitations of the assessment tools used. Moreover, the nature of correlation in psychological and developmental disorders is intricate and multifaceted. It often involves dynamic interactions between biological, environmental, and individual factors, which may not always manifest in straightforward statistical relationships.

5. Conclusions

This study has provided valuable insights into the impact of technology on the quality of life (QoL) of individuals with Autism Spectrum Disorder (ASD), Chronic Anxiety (CA), and Chronic Depression (CD). The findings show that the perceptions these individuals have of technology (especially user-centered technologies) play a significant role in their perceived improvements in well-being.

The perception of technology by people with ASD, anxiety, and/or depression can provide information about the level of difficulty they perceive and their quality of life (QoL). This suggests that person-centered technologies can improve both cognitive abilities (such as memory and joint attention) and physical functions in people with autism, improve anxiety management, alleviate depression, and support people with dementia.

Personalized apps and devices have proven effective in enhancing different functions for participants. For individuals with ASD, such interventions led mainly to cognitive and communicative benefits—with memory and joint attention being two critical areas. Improvements in these functions help the individuals with ASD in being able to participate better in social interactions, as well as other daily activities. On the other hand, participants with ASD and CD reported improvements primarily in the mobility and self-care domains. This finding indicates that individuals with these disorders derive greater benefits from being able to carry out daily activities with more independence and less anxiety.

Personalizing technologies may be the best way to ensure that therapeutic benefits are maximized for particular groups. Quantum computing algorithms have, indeed, found use in applications analyzing large data volumes; basically, they can accommodate complex pattern recognition where traditional methods fail. This has enabled the discovery of some deeper relationships and correlations among the key variables (ASD, AC, and DC) that could help in designing more appropriate technological interventions specifically tailored to individual users' needs. These algorithms have allowed a much keener and finer examination of the challenges and requirements of people with ASD as well as anxiety and depression, which can subsequently enhance existing technological interventions.

In summary, the lack of human resources in mental health provided by the state, with fewer professionals in psychiatry and psychology, represents one of the daily barriers that influence affected people and their environment, which could be alleviated through technological advances. This offers adequate tools to improve mental health, thus improving the quality of life of many people with autism, anxiety and depression, and their caregivers.

Suggestions for Future Developments

This study offers valuable information, but there are several potential fields of study for future research and technological developments. It is suggested to explore areas such as virtual reality, augmented reality and wearable devices to improve emotional regulation and cognitive functions in people with ASD, anxiety and depression.

In addition, the use of artificial intelligence (through machine learning and other techniques) could tailor, and therefore further personalize, interventions to users. It is key to consider the scalability of these technologies in different population and cultural contexts, and to develop interventions tailored to them. The impacts of caregiver involvement in technology interventions to improve emotional and social support should also be investigated. Finally, applying quantum computing together with artificial intelligence to other disorders could bring about significant advances in the field of mental health.

Author Contributions: G.B.-R. preparation, preparation, method, exploitation of data, bibliography, review. V.Z.-M. preparation, exploitation of data, methods and results, review. N.G.-A. review, approval, and search for funding. E.F. review, approval, search for funding. J.M.F. review, approval, search for funding. All authors have read and agreed to the published version of the manuscript.

Funding: This project received funding from the grant PID2020-115220RB-C22 funded by MCIN/AEI/10.13039/501100011033 and, as appropriate, from 'ERDF A way of making Europe', the "European Union" or the 'European Union NextGenerationEU/PRTR'; grant RTI2018-098969-B-100 from the Spanish 'Ministry of Science, Innovation and Universities', grant PROMETEO/2019/119 from the Valencian Community (Comunitat Valenciana) in Spain, and INNTA1/2022/23 Project 'Innovation Agent for the Bioengineering Institute, Miguel Hernandez University' (2022–2024), co-financed by Valencian Community EU-FEDER Program, 2021–2027 and the Accessible Technologies Award from Indra and Fundación Universia.

Institutional Review Board Statement: This study was carried out with the ethical approval of the Miguel Hernández University, with the code AUT.IB.EFJ.240202. All stages of the research were carried out in accordance with established ethical standards. Secondary data from the National Institute of Statistics (INE) of Spain are used. The INE obtains informed consent and guarantees the confidentiality of participants' data through the established CATI (computer-assisted telephone interview) and CAWI (computer-assisted web interview) methods. To analyze the secondary data, we received ethical approval from the Miguel Hernández University, ensuring compliance with all ethical regulations relevant to our specific use of the data, with the code AUT.IB.EFJ.240202.

Informed Consent Statement: Informed consent was obtained from all subjects involved in the study.

Data Availability Statement: The data from the "Survey of Disability, Personal Autonomy and Dependency Situations (2020)", developed by the National Institute of Statistics (INE), are available at https://www.ine.es/dyngs/INEbase/en/operacion.htm?c=Estadistica_C&cid=1254736176782&idp=1254735573175. Accessed on 15 June 2024. The methodology employed for the questionnaire encompassed various aspects related to QoL based on the WHO dimensions of the WHOQOL-100 scale, available at https://www.who.int/tools/whoqol/whoqol-100.

Conflicts of Interest: The authors declare no conflicts of interest.

References

1. WHOQOL-Measuring Quality of Life | The World Health Organization. Available online: https://www.who.int/tools/whoqol (accessed on 6 December 2023).
2. Martínez, V.T.P.; Montero, O.A.A. Necesidades de aprendizaje de los especialistas de Medicina General Integral sobre los trastornos del espectro autista. *Rev. Cuba. Med. Gen. Integral.* **2013**, *29*, 267–280.
3. Oreskovic, N.M.; Neumeyer, A.M.; Duggan, M.P.; Kuhlthau, K.A. Assessment of Walking Routes as a Possible Approach for Promoting Physical Activity in Children with Autism Spectrum Disorder: Brief Report. *Dev. Neurorehabilit.* **2020**, *23*, 59–63. [CrossRef] [PubMed]
4. Ferreira, J.P.; Toscano, C.V.A.; Rodrigues, A.M.; Furtado, G.E.; Barros, M.G.; Wanderley, R.S.; Carvalho, H.M. Effects of a Physical Exercise Program (PEP-Aut) on Autistic Children's Stereotyped Behavior, Metabolic and Physical Activity Profiles, Physical Fitness, and Health-Related Quality of Life: A Study Protocol. *Front. Public Health* **2018**, *6*, 47. [CrossRef]
5. Huang, J.; Du, C.; Liu, J.; Tan, G. Meta-Analysis on Intervention Effects of Physical Activities on Children and Adolescents with Autism. *Int. J. Environ. Res. Public. Health* **2020**, *17*, 1950. [CrossRef]
6. Majhi, S.; Kumar, S.; Singh, L. A Review on Autism Spectrum Disorder: Pathogenesis, Biomarkers, Pharmacological and Non-Pharmacological Interventions. *CNS Neurol. Disord. Drug Targets* **2023**, *22*, 659–677. [CrossRef]
7. Susniene, D.; Jurkauskas, A. The Concepts of Quality of Life and Happiness–Correlation and Differences. *Eng. Econ.* **2009**, *63*. Available online: https://inzeko.ktu.lt/index.php/EE/article/view/11648 (accessed on 6 December 2023).
8. Sakip, S.R.M.; Zukri, A.Z.M.; Rahim, P.R.M.A. Assessing the Relationship Between Environmental, Psychological, Physical and Social Towards the Quality of Life. *Int. J. Sustain. Constr. Eng. Technol.* **2023**, *14*, 256–265. [CrossRef]
9. Happiness or Quality of Life? Or Both? | Journal of Education Culture and Society. Available online: https://jecs.pl/index.php/jecs/article/view/1408 (accessed on 16 December 2024).
10. Beneytez, C. Síntomas de ansiedad en los trastornos del espectro del autismo desde un enfoque transdiagnóstico. Universidad Complutense de Madrid. 2019. Available online: https://dialnet.unirioja.es/servlet/tesis?codigo=223238 (accessed on 16 December 2024).
11. Kerns, C.M.; Kendall, P.C. Autism and anxiety: Overlap, similarities, and differences. In *Handbook of Autism and Anxiety*; en Autism and Child Psychopathology Series; Springer International Publishing/Springer Nature: Cham, Switzerland, 2014; pp. 75–89. [CrossRef]
12. Sánchez-Cueva, M.S.; Marín, F.A.; Alonso-Esteban, Y. Ansiedad y trastornos del espectro del autismo: Notas para la intervención psicoeducativa. *Siglo. Cero.* **2022**, *53*, 4930. [CrossRef]
13. White, S.W.; Oswald, D.; Ollendick, T.; Scahill, L. Anxiety in children and adolescents with autism spectrum disorders. *Clin. Psychol. Rev.* **2009**, *29*, 216–229. [CrossRef]
14. Jenkinson, R.; Milne, E.; Thompson, A. The relationship between intolerance of uncertainty and anxiety in autism: A systematic literature review and meta-analysis. *Autism Int. J. Res. Pract.* **2020**, *24*, 1933–1944. [CrossRef]
15. Ghaziuddin, M.; Ghaziuddin, N.; Greden, J. Depression in persons with autism: Implications for research and clinical care. *J. Autism Dev. Disord.* **2002**, *32*, 299–306. [CrossRef]
16. Hofvander, B.; Delorme, R.; Chaste, P.; Nydén, A.; Wentz, E.; Ståhlberg, O.; Herbrecht, E.; Stopin, A.; Anckarsäter, H.; Gillberg, C.; et al. Psychiatric and psychosocial problems in adults with normal-intelligence autism spectrum disorders. *BMC Psychiatry* **2009**, *9*, 35. [CrossRef] [PubMed]
17. Lever, A.G.; Geurts, H.M. Psychiatric Co-occurring Symptoms and Disorders in Young, Middle-Aged, and Older Adults with Autism Spectrum Disorder. *J. Autism Dev. Disord.* **2016**, *46*, 1916–1930. [CrossRef] [PubMed]
18. van Heijst, B.F.; Deserno, M.K.; Rhebergen, D.; Geurts, H.M. Autism and depression are connected: A report of two complimentary network studies. *Autism* **2020**, *24*, 680–692. [CrossRef] [PubMed]
19. Hopkins, K.; Crosland, P.; Elliott, N.; Bewley, S.; On behalf of the Clinical Guidelines Update Committee B. Diagnosis and management of depression in children and young people: Summary of updated NICE guidance. *BMJ* **2015**, *350*, h824. [CrossRef]
20. Kelvin, R. Depression in children and young people. *Paediatr. Child Health* **2016**, *26*, 540–547. [CrossRef]
21. Zenebe, Y.; Akele, B.; W/Selassie, M.; Necho, M. Prevalence and determinants of depression among old age: A systematic review and meta-analysis. *Ann. Gen. Psychiatry* **2021**, *20*, 55. [CrossRef]
22. Hudson, C.C.; Hall, L.; Harkness, K.L. Prevalence of Depressive Disorders in Individuals with Autism Spectrum Disorder: A Meta-Analysis. *J. Abnorm. Child Psychol.* **2019**, *47*, 165–175. [CrossRef]
23. Menezes, M.; Harkins, C.; Robinson, M.F.; Mazurek, M.O. Treatment of Depression in Individuals with Autism Spectrum Disorder: A Systematic Review. *Res. Autism Spectr. Disord.* **2020**, *78*, 101639. [CrossRef]

24. Hollocks, M.J.; Lerh, J.W.; Magiati, I.; Meiser-Stedman, R.; Brugha, T.S. Anxiety and depression in adults with autism spectrum disorder: A systematic review and meta-analysis. *Psychol. Med.* **2019**, *49*, 559–572. [CrossRef]
25. Earls, F. The epidemiology of depression in children and adolescents. *Pediatr. Ann.* **1984**, *13*, 23–31.
26. Fernández, F.C.; Martínez, Á.M.; Martín, A.B.B.; Pérez-Fuentes, M.D.C.; Jurado, M.D.M.M.; Linares, J.J.G. Prevalencia de la depresión en España: Análisis de los últimos 15 años. *Eur. J. Investig. Health Psychol. Educ.* **2015**, *5*, 267. [CrossRef]
27. Pardo, G.; Sandoval, A.; Umbarila, D. ADOLESCENCIA Y DEPRESIÓN. *Rev. Colomb. Psicol.* **2004**, *13*, 13–28.
28. Nabeshima, T.; Kim, H.-C. Involvement of Genetic and Environmental Factors in the Onset of Depression. *Exp. Neurobiol.* **2013**, *22*, 235–243. [CrossRef] [PubMed]
29. Álvaro-Estramiana, J.L.; Garrido-Luque, A.; Schweiger-Gallo, I. Causas sociales de la depresión. Una revisión crítica del modelo atributivo de la depresión. *Rev. Int. Sociol.* **2010**, *68*, 333–348. [CrossRef]
30. Moscoso, D.R.B.; Narvaez, L.C.V.; Ortiz, L.F.A.; Ramos, R.A.; Gonzalez, E.M.V. Ansiedad y depresión en adolescentes. *Rev. Bol. Redipe* **2021**, *10*. [CrossRef]
31. Theoharides, T.C.; Kavalioti, M.; Tsilioni, I. Mast Cells, Stress, Fear and Autism Spectrum Disorder. *Int. J. Mol. Sci.* **2019**, *20*, 3611. [CrossRef]
32. Espada, J.P.; Orgilés, M.; Méndez, X.; Morales, A. Problemas relacionados con la regulación emocional: Depresión y problemas de ansiedad. *Libro Blanco Salud Ment. Infanto-Juv.* **2021**, *1*, 18–31.
33. Charlton, R.A.; McQuaid, G.A.; Wallace, G.L. Social support and links to quality of life among middle-aged and older autistic adults. *Autism Int. J. Res. Pract.* **2023**, *27*, 92–104. [CrossRef]
34. MacKenzie, K.T.; Theodat, A.; Beck, K.B.; Conner, C.M.; Mazefsky, C.A.; Eack, S.M. Correlates of Quality of Life in Autistic Individuals. *Res. Autism Spectr. Disord.* **2024**, *115*, 102401. [CrossRef]
35. Kouroupa, A.; Laws, K.R.; Irvine, K.; Mengoni, S.E.; Baird, A.; Sharma, S. The use of social robots with children and young people on the autism spectrum: A systematic review and meta-analysis. *PLoS ONE* **2022**, *17*, e0269800. [CrossRef] [PubMed]
36. Health Quality Ontario. Internet-Delivered Cognitive Behavioural Therapy for Major Depression and Anxiety Disorders: A Health Technology Assessment. *Ont. Health Technol. Assess. Ser.* **2019**, *19*, 1–199.
37. Jamwal, R.; Jarman, H.K.; Roseingrave, E.; Douglas, J.; Winkler, D. Smart home and communication technology for people with disability: A scoping review. *Disabil. Rehabil. Assist. Technol.* **2022**, *17*, 624–644. [CrossRef] [PubMed]
38. Fellinghauer, B.; Reinhardt, J.D.; Stucki, G.; Bickenbach, J. Explaining the disability paradox: A cross-sectional analysis of the Swiss general population. *BMC Public Health* **2012**, *12*, 655. [CrossRef]
39. Niero, M. Disability paradox: I disabili e la felicità. *SALUTE E Soc* **2005**, 32–46. Available online: https://www.francoangeli.it/riviste/articolo@Model.IDArticolo (accessed on 6 December 2023).
40. Cruceanu, G.L.; Clemente-Belmonte, S.; Herrero-Sanz, R.; Ayala, A.; Zorrilla-Muñoz, V.; Agulló-Tomás, M.S.; Martínez-Miguelez, C.; Fernández-Mayoralas, G. Evaluation of Older People Digital Images: Representations from a Land, Gender and Anti-ageist Perspective. *Land* **2023**, *12*, 18. [CrossRef]
41. Van Dooren, M.; De Croon, R.; Swillen, A.; Verbert, K. Bridging the Communication Gap Between People With Cognitive Impairments and Their Caregivers Using mHealth Apps: User-Centered Design and Evaluation Study With People With 22q11 Deletion Syndrome. *JMIR Hum. Factors* **2023**, *10*, e44290. [CrossRef] [PubMed]
42. Zannat, N.; Mahmud, M. Exploring mindmend: An innovative mental health support app for autistic adolescents and their caregivers. *J. Digit. Syst. Dev.* **2024**, *2*, 1–16. [CrossRef]
43. Terranova, N.; Renard, D.; Shahin, M.H.; Menon, S.; Cao, Y.; Hop, C.E.C.A.; Hayes, S.; Madrasi, K.; Stodtmann, S.; Tensfeldt, T.; et al. Artificial Intelligence for Quantitative Modeling in Drug Discovery and Development: An Innovation and Quality Consortium Perspective on Use Cases and Best Practices. *Clin. Pharmacol. Ther.* **2024**, *115*, 658–672. [CrossRef]
44. Blaurock, M.; Büttgen, M.; Schepers, J. Designing Collaborative Intelligence Systems for Employee-AI Service Co-Production. *J. Serv. Res.* **2024**, 10946705241238751. [CrossRef]
45. Benedicto-Rodriguez, G.; Zorrilla-Muñoz, V.; Fernandez, E.; Ferrandez, J.M. Technological Influence on the Measurement of Quality of Life in Persons with Autism Spectrum Disorder. In Proceedings of the Third International Conference on Innovations in Computing Research (ICR'24), Athens, Greece, 12–14 August 2024; Daimi, K., Al Sadoon, A., Eds.; Springer Nature: Cham, Switzerland, 2024; pp. 691–698. [CrossRef]
46. Hong, J.; Bishop-Fitzpatrick, L.; Smith, L.E.; Greenberg, J.S.; Mailick, M.R. Factors Associated with Subjective Quality of Life of Adults with Autism Spectrum Disorder: Self-Report Versus Maternal Reports. *J. Autism Dev. Disord.* **2016**, *46*, 1368–1378. [CrossRef] [PubMed]
47. Jariwala, K.; Khanna, R.; West-Strum, D.; Bentley, J.P.; Banahan, B.F.I.; Holmes, E.R.; Barnard, M. Psychometric properties of the world health organization's quality of life-bref instrument (WHOQOL-BREF) among adults with autism. *Value Health* **2014**, *17*, A194. [CrossRef]

48. Mason, D.; Rodgers, J.; Garland, D.; Wilson, C.; Parr, J.; McConachie, H. Measuring quality of life in autistic adults: The reliability and validity of the Brief Version of the World Health Organization Quality of Life scal. *AMRC Open Res.* **2022**, *4*, 3. [CrossRef]
49. Mouelhi, Y.; Jouve, E.; Castelli, C.; Gentile, S. How is the minimal clinically important difference established in health-related quality of life instruments? Review of anchors and methods. *Health Qual. Life Outcomes* **2020**, *18*, 136. [CrossRef]
50. Klefbeck, K. Educational Approaches to Improve Communication Skills of Learners with Autism Spectrum Disorder and Comorbid Intellectual Disability: An Integrative Systematic Review. *Scand. J. Educ. Res.* **2023**, *67*, 51–68. [CrossRef]
51. De Houwer, J.; Barnes-Holmes, D.; Moors, A. What is learning? On the nature and merits of a functional definition of learning. *Psychon. Bull. Rev.* **2013**, *20*, 631–642. [CrossRef]
52. Metz, D.H. Mobility of older people and their quality of life. *Transp. Policy* **2000**, *7*, 149–152. [CrossRef]
53. Jordan, M. The power of connection: Self-care strategies of social wellbeing. *J. Interprof. Educ. Pract.* **2023**, *31*, 100586. [CrossRef]
54. Savari, K.; Naseri, M.; Savari, Y. Evaluating the Role of Perceived Stress, Social Support, and Resilience in Predicting the Quality of Life among the Parents of Disabled Children. *Int. J. Disabil. Dev. Educ.* **2023**, *70*, 644–658. [CrossRef]
55. Dainton, M.; Conville, R.L.; Rogers, L.E. The Meaning of "Relationship" in Interpersonal Communication. *J. Marriage Fam.* **1999**, *61*, 546. [CrossRef]
56. Bogolyubov, N.N. *A Method for Studying Model Hamiltonians: A Minimax Principle for Problems in Statistical Physics*; Elsevier: Amsterdam, The Netherlands, 2013.
57. Chabane, L.; Lazarescu, A.; Verley, G. Effective Hamiltonians and Lagrangians for Conditioned Markov Processes at Large Volume. *J. Stat. Phys.* **2022**, *187*, 6. [CrossRef]
58. Cervera-Lierta, A.; Kottmann, J.S.; Aspuru-Guzik, A. Meta-Variational Quantum Eigensolver: Learning Energy Profiles of Parameterized Hamiltonians for Quantum Simulation. *PRX Quantum* **2021**, *2*, 020329. [CrossRef]
59. Wilde, F.; Kshetrimayum, A.; Roth, I.; Hangleiter, D.; Sweke, R.; Eisert, J. Scalably learning quantum many-body Hamiltonians from dynamical data. *arXiv* **2022**, arXiv:2209.14328. [CrossRef]
60. Altman, E.; Brown, K.R.; Carleo, G.; Carr, L.D.; Demler, E.; Chin, C.; DeMarco, B.; Economou, S.E.; Eriksson, M.A. Quantum Simulators: Architectures and Opportunities. *PRX Quantum* **2021**, *2*, 017003. [CrossRef]
61. O'Neill, M.; Jones, R.S. Sensory-perceptual abnormalities in autism: A case for more research? *J. Autism Dev. Disord.* **1997**, *27*, 283–293. [CrossRef]
62. Kinnaird, E.; Stewart, C.; Tchanturia, K. Investigating alexithymia in autism: A systematic review and meta-analysis. *Eur. Psychiatry J. Assoc. Eur. Psychiatr.* **2019**, *55*, 80–89. [CrossRef]
63. Alberdi-Fernández, A. Habilidades Comunicativas en Trastornos del Espectro Autista. Bachelor's Thesis, Universidad Internacional de la Rioja, Logroño, Spain, 2015. Available online: https://reunir.unir.net/handle/123456789/3219 (accessed on 16 December 2024).
64. Guerrero, L.C.; Padilla, E.M. Habilidades sociales y comunicativas a través del arte en jóvenes con trastorno del espectro autista (TEA). *Estud. Pedagógicos Valdivia* **2017**, *43*, 47–64. [CrossRef]
65. Coryell, W. Trastornos Depresivos-Trastornos Psiquiátricos. Manual MSD Versión Para Profesionales. Available online: https://www.msdmanuals.com/es/professional/trastornos-psiqui%C3%A1tricos/trastornos-del-estado-de-%C3%A1nimo/trastornos-depresivos (accessed on 16 December 2024).
66. González-Blanch, C.; Umaran-Alfageme, O.; Cordero-Andrés, P.; Muñoz-Navarro, R.; Ruiz-Rodríguez, P.; Medrano, L.A.; Ruiz-Torres, M.; Collado, E.D.; Cano-Vindel, A. Grupo de Investigación PsicAP. Tratamiento psicológico de los trastornos emocionales en Atención Primaria: El manual de tratamiento transdiagnóstico del estudio PsicAP. *Ansiedad Estrés* **2018**, *24*, 1–11. [CrossRef]
67. Hernandez, J.; Riobo, I.; Rozga, A.; Abowd, G.D.; Picard, R.W. Using electrodermal activity to recognize ease of engagement in children during social interactions. *MIT Web Domain*. 2014. Available online: https://dspace.mit.edu/handle/1721.1/107809 (accessed on 16 December 2024).
68. Fong, T.; Nourbakhsh, I.; Dautenhahn, K. A survey of socially interactive robots. *Robot. Auton. Syst.* **2023**, *42*, 143–166. [CrossRef]
69. Shigemi, S. ASIMO and Humanoid Robot Research at Honda. In *Humanoid Robotics: A Reference*; Goswami, A., Vadakkepat, P., Eds.; Springer: Dordrecht, The Netherlands, 2019; pp. 55–90. [CrossRef]
70. O'Reilly, Z.; Navare, U.P.; Marchesi, S.; Wykowska, A. Does Embodiment and Interaction Affect the Adoption of the Intentional Stance Towards a Humanoid Robot? In *Social Robotics: 14th International Conference, ICSR 2022, Florence, Italy, December 13–16, 2022, Proceedings, Part I*; Springer: Berlin/Heidelberg, Germany, 2023; pp. 357–366. [CrossRef]

technologies

MDPI

Article

Leveraging Artificial Intelligence for Personalized Rehabilitation Programs for Head and Neck Surgery Patients

Gianluca Marcaccini [1,2], Ishith Seth [1,3,4,*], Jennifer Novo [5], Vicki McClure [1], Brett Sacks [1], Kaiyang Lim [1], Sally Kiu-Huen Ng [4], Roberto Cuomo [2] and Warren M. Rozen [1,3]

1 Department of Plastic and Reconstructive Surgery, Peninsula Health, Frankston, VIC 3199, Australia
2 Department of Plastic and Reconstructive Surgery, University of Siena, 53100 Siena, Italy
3 Faculty of Medicine and Surgery, Central Clinical School, Monash University, Clayton, VIC 3004, Australia
4 Department of Plastic and Reconstructive Surgery, Austin Health, Heidelberg, VIC 3084, Australia
5 Faculty of Medicine and Surgery, The University of Notre Dame, Sydney, NSW 2008, Australia
* Correspondence: iseth@phcn.vic.gov.au

Abstract: Background: Artificial intelligence (AI) and large language models (LLMs) are increasingly used in healthcare, with applications in clinical decision-making and workflow optimization. In head and neck surgery, postoperative rehabilitation is a complex, multidisciplinary process requiring personalized care. This study evaluates the feasibility of using LLMs to generate tailored rehabilitation programs for patients undergoing major head and neck surgical procedures. Methods: Ten hypothetical head and neck surgical clinical scenarios were developed, representing oncologic resections with complex reconstructions. Four LLMs, ChatGPT-4o, DeepSeek V3, Gemini 2, and Copilot, were prompted with identical queries to generate rehabilitation plans. Three senior clinicians independently assessed their quality, accuracy, and clinical relevance using a five-point Likert scale. Readability and quality metrics, including the DISCERN score, Flesch Reading Ease, Flesch–Kincaid Grade Level, and Coleman–Liau Index, were applied. Results: ChatGPT-4o achieved the highest clinical relevance (Likert mean of 4.90 ± 0.32), followed by DeepSeek V3 (4.00 ± 0.82) and Gemini 2 (3.90 ± 0.74), while Copilot underperformed (2.70 ± 0.82). Gemini 2 produced the most readable content. A statistical analysis confirmed significant differences across the models ($p < 0.001$). Conclusions: LLMs can generate rehabilitation programs with varying quality and readability. ChatGPT-4o produced the most clinically relevant plans, while Gemini 2 generated more readable content. AI-generated rehabilitation plans may complement existing protocols, but further clinical validation is necessary to assess their impact on patient outcomes.

Keywords: artificial intelligence; large language models; head and neck surgery; postoperative care; ChatGPT; DeepSeek

1. Introduction

Artificial intelligence (AI) is increasingly transforming healthcare, with applications ranging from diagnostic assistance to perioperative management and rehabilitation planning. Recent studies have demonstrated the ability of AI-driven models to improve decision-making in surgical and postoperative care, particularly through large language models (LLMs) and natural language processing (NLP) techniques [1,2]. For instance, AI has been successfully applied in thoracic surgery to enhance diagnostic precision and predict postoperative complications, underscoring its expanding role in surgical specialties.

Given the growing body of evidence supporting AI's integration into clinical workflows, this study aims to assess the feasibility of using LLMs for generating personalized rehabilitation programs for patients undergoing major head and neck surgery [1–3]. Among AI-driven tools, large language models (LLMs), such as ChatGPT, DeepSeek, Gemini 2, and Copilot, have gained significant attention for their ability to generate medical information and answer clinical questions based on extensive datasets [4,5].

LLMs in medicine are trained on large repositories of medical literature, clinical guidelines, and anonymized patient case information, allowing them to synthesize complex information and generate sophisticated and structured responses that align with evidence-based practices [4,5]. While LLMs are already being used to streamline administrative tasks and automate clinical documentation, there is growing interest in their potential beyond these functions, particularly in developing tailored patient rehabilitation programs for patients recovering from complex surgeries [6].

Head and neck surgery (HNS) often involves oncological patients who require extensive surgical intervention and complex reconstructions, particularly in cases of squamous cell carcinoma (SCC), basal cell carcinoma (BCC), and other aggressive cutaneous or mucosal malignancies. These procedures range from simple local excisions to complex reconstructions involving microvascular free flaps, mandibulectomies, and radical neck dissections. While these surgeries are often lifesaving, they are also associated with significant morbidity, frequently resulting in functional impairments that affect speech, swallowing, mastication, airway patency, and facial nerve function [7]. The severity of these postoperative complications depends on patient factors, the extent of tissue resection, and the need for adjuvant radiotherapy or chemotherapy treatment, which can further impact function and prolong recovery [8]. Microvascular free flap reconstructions, while providing vascularized soft tissue and bony support, are not without risk, with higher complication rates in previously irradiated fields [8,9]. Additionally, surgical site infections, wound dehiscence, hematomas, and percutaneous fistulae are known postoperative challenges following extensive resections, often requiring prolonged wound management and staged interventions [7,10].

Given this, rehabilitation following HNS must be highly individualized and often requires a multidisciplinary approach with input from surgeons, speech therapists, dietitians, physiotherapists, and psychologists to optimize functional and aesthetic outcomes [11]. Current rehabilitation protocols for HNS patients are primarily guided by standard clinical pathways and expert consensus [9,10]. However, these approaches may not fully account for patient-specific variables, such as age, comorbidities, tumor location, and the extent of resection. This is an area where AI and LLMs could offer a novel solution by utilizing large sets of data to predict patient rehabilitation trajectories, recommend structured postoperative care instructions, and provide real-time clinical support to surgeons, ultimately enhancing patient outcomes.

This study aims to assess the feasibility of using LLMs to generate personalized rehabilitation programs for patients undergoing HNS by comparing the recommendations of multiple LLMs against expert-reviewed standards. By doing so, this study seeks to determine whether AI-generated rehabilitation programs can complement traditional approaches and improve postoperative outcomes. Additionally, this study will assess the readability and quality of LLM-generated responses using validated tools, such as the DISCERN score and Flesch Reading Ease Score, to provide insights into their applicability in patient education and clinical decision-making.

2. Materials and Methods

This experimental study was designed to assess the capacity of LLMs to generate personalized rehabilitation programs for patients undergoing head and neck surgery. Given that the study utilized hypothetical clinical scenarios rather than real patient data, formal ethical approval was not required. However, all research activities adhered to the ethical principles of the Declaration of Helsinki.

Ten hypothetical clinical scenarios were developed to encompass a range of head and neck surgical procedures. These scenarios were designed by three senior clinicians with expertise in head and neck surgery, ensuring clinical relevance and representativeness. Each scenario was based on real-world cases commonly encountered in surgical practice, incorporating key variables such as patient demographics, comorbidities, tumor location, extent of resection, and reconstructive techniques. The scenarios were iteratively refined through expert review to ensure they reflected a broad spectrum of complexity and post-operative rehabilitation needs. To standardize AI model evaluation, a consistent prompt structure was used for all scenarios, focusing on the recommended rehabilitation program and necessary supportive care measures.

The following prompt was added post-hypothetical scenario: "What rehabilitation program and services are recommended for this patient to optimize their postoperative recovery, considering their specific clinical condition, surgical procedure, and potential risk factors?". These scenarios were formulated by senior clinicians with expertise in head and neck surgery, ensuring their relevance and clinical validity.

2.1. Generation of Rehabilitation Programs

Four state-of-the-art LLMs, ChatGPT-4o, DeepSeek V3, Gemini 2, and Copilot, were selected based on their relevance and accessibility for medical applications. The choice of these models aimed to ensure a balanced comparison between well-established AI tools and emerging alternatives, allowing for a comprehensive evaluation of their suitability in generating rehabilitation programs. ChatGPT-4o was included due to its demonstrated accuracy in medical contexts and its strong performance in previous studies assessing AI-generated clinical recommendations [1–5]. DeepSeek V3 was selected as an emerging model designed for complex reasoning, offering a distinct approach to AI-generated text with an emphasis on scientific and technical content. Gemini 2, developed by Google, was incorporated for its strong capabilities in language understanding and its optimization for producing highly readable outputs, which could be beneficial in patient-centered rehabilitation programs. Copilot, integrated within Microsoft's ecosystem, was chosen to evaluate how general-purpose AI models perform in specialized medical tasks. By including these four LLMs, this study aims to capture a broad spectrum of AI capabilities, from established models optimized for clinical reasoning to newer competitors designed for diverse applications. To ensure consistency in evaluation, all models were prompted simultaneously on 10 February 2025, using identical clinical scenarios.

2.2. Evaluation of LLM-Generated Rehabilitation Programs

Three senior clinicians (WMR, SN, and RC), with over 40 years of cumulative experience, independently assessed the rehabilitation programs suggested by the LLMs for accuracy, clinical relevance, and appropriateness. The clinicians were selected based on their expertise in head and neck surgery and postoperative rehabilitation, each with over ten years of experience in tertiary academic centers. Their selection aimed to ensure a high level of clinical judgment and familiarity with current rehabilitation protocols. To minimize bias, evaluations were conducted independently, and the inter-rater agreement was analyzed to assess consistency in their assessments. Similar studies evaluating AI-generated medical recommendations have also relied on small expert panels for initial validation [9]. Future research may benefit from expanding the number of reviewers to enhance generalizability and account for inter-rater variability. The assessments were conducted using a five-point Likert scale (1 = Poor, 5 = Excellent) to measure the quality of the responses quantitatively.

To further assess the readability, clarity, and reliability of the generated rehabilitation plans, standardized text analysis metrics were applied, including the following:

- DISCERN Score—evaluating the reliability and quality of health information.
- Flesch Reading Ease Score—measuring the ease of comprehension.
- Flesch–Kincaid Grade Level—indicating the educational level required to understand the text.
- Coleman–Liau Index—assessing the complexity of the generated text.

2.3. Data Analysis

The Likert scale ratings assigned by the two senior clinicians were analyzed for inter-rater reliability using Cohen's kappa coefficient to assess consistency in evaluation. A descriptive statistical analysis was performed to compare the mean scores of each LLM, identifying trends in accuracy and clinical utility. A comparative study of the readability and quality assessment metrics was also conducted, examining model variations and their suitability for patient and clinician use.

3. Results

Quantitative Analysis

To evaluate the performance of four AI models (ChatGPT-4o, DeepSeek V3, Gemini 2, and Copilot) on surgical case responses, we conducted both descriptive and inferential analyses across several metrics. Descriptive statistics revealed that ChatGPT-4o achieved the highest performance in subjective evaluation, with a Likert scale mean of 4.90 $\pm$ 0.32, followed by DeepSeek V3 (4.00 $\pm$ 0.82) and Gemini 2 (3.90 $\pm$ 0.74), while Copilot's responses scored markedly lower, with a mean of 2.70 $\pm$ 0.82. In terms of the DISCERN score, which assesses the quality and reliability of the provided information, ChatGPT-4o, DeepSeek V3, and Gemini 2 produced comparable results (ranging from 46.90 $\pm$ 2.60 to 47.20 $\pm$ 2.53), whereas Copilot consistently scored 40.00.

The readability metrics further differentiated the models. The Flesch Reading Ease Score was notably higher for Gemini 2 (12.25 $\pm$ 7.22), suggesting that its texts are more straightforward to comprehend. At the same time, the Flesch–Kincaid Grade Level for Gemini 2 (16.60 $\pm$ 1.40) was lower than the other models, indicating reduced complexity. The Coleman–Liau Index, which also reflects text complexity, showed less pronounced differences among the models, with mean values ranging from 18.23 $\pm$ 0.79 for Copilot to 19.68 $\pm$ 1.32 for ChatGPT-4o.

A one-way variance analysis (ANOVA) was performed for each metric to determine whether these differences were statistically significant. The analysis revealed significant differences among the models for the Likert scale ($F(3, 36) = 16.50$, p value < 0.001), the DISCERN score ($F(3, 36) = 24.63$, p value < 0.001), the Flesch Reading Ease ($F(3, 36) = 4.35$, p value ≈ 0.01), and the Flesch–Kincaid Grade Level ($F(3, 36) = 11.82$, p value < 0.001). In contrast, the result for the Coleman–Liau Index was marginally non-significant ($F(3, 36) = 2.84$, p value ≈ 0.06). These findings indicate that the observed differences in performance and text quality across the AI models are unlikely due to chance, supporting the validity of the differences noted in the descriptive analysis and justifying further post hoc testing to precisely identify which pairs of models differ significantly in performance (Table 1).

Table 1. Mean and median values of AI output across various evaluation metrics.

AI Model	N	Likert Mean	Likert SD	DISCERN Mean	DISCERN SD	Flesch Reading Ease Mean	Flesch Reading Ease SD	Flesch–Kincaid Grade Level Mean	Flesch–Kincaid Grade Level SD	Coleman–Liau Index Mean	Coleman–Liau Index SD
ChatGPT-4o	10	4.90	0.32	46.90	2.60	5.02	8.09	18.44	1.42	19.68	1.32
DeepSeek V3	10	4.00	0.82	46.90	2.60	3.05	4.78	20.15	1.53	19.29	1.39
Gemini 2	10	3.90	0.74	47.20	2.53	12.25	7.22	16.60	1.40	18.50	1.46
Copilot	10	2.70	0.82	40.00	0.00	4.99	3.29	19.23	1.18	18.23	0.79

Statistical analyses were performed using Python (version 3.9) and its associated libraries, including SciPy and Statsmodels. We calculated descriptive statistics means and standard deviations for each metric and conducted a one-way analysis of variance to evaluate differences among the AI models. Prior to testing, we assessed assumptions of normality and homogeneity of variances, and all *p* values were computed with a significance level set at 0.05. To ensure the accuracy of our analysis, we performed an independent verification of the results using ChatGPT as a supplementary tool, confirming the validity of our findings (Table 2).

Table 2. One-way ANOVA analysis between four AI models across various evaluation metrics.

Metric	F-Value	Degrees of Freedom Between	Degrees of Freedom Within	*p* Value	Test
Likert Scale	16.50	3	36	<0.001	One-way ANOVA
DISCERN Score	24.63	3	36	<0.001	One-way ANOVA
Flesch Reading Ease	4.35	3	36	~0.01	One-way ANOVA
Flesch–Kincaid Grade Level	11.82	3	36	<0.001	One-way ANOVA
Coleman–Liau Index	2.84	3	36	~0.06	One-way ANOVA

Supplementary Table S1 shows responses from large language models to the following clinical scenario prompt: "What rehabilitation program and services are recommended for this patient to optimize their postoperative recovery, considering their specific clinical condition, surgical procedure, and potential risk factors?"

4. Discussion

This study explores the potential role of large language models (LLMs) in generating rehabilitation programs for patients undergoing head and neck surgery. While AI has been increasingly applied in clinical decision support and administrative tasks, its use in postoperative rehabilitation planning remains an emerging area. By comparing multiple LLMs (ChatGPT-4o, DeepSeek V3, Gemini 2, and Copilot) using standardized clinical scenarios and expert evaluation, this study provides insights into the strengths and limitations of AI-generated rehabilitation recommendations. The dual assessment of clinical relevance and readability offers a structured approach to understanding how these models perform in generating patient-centered rehabilitation plans. These findings contribute to the ongoing discussion on integrating AI into multidisciplinary care, highlighting potential applications and areas for further refinement. The integration of AI-generated rehabilitation plans into clinical practice could enhance multidisciplinary decision-making by providing structured, evidence-based recommendations tailored to individual patient needs. In particular, these tools could be valuable in settings with limited access to specialized rehabilitation providers, where AI models may help bridge the gap in expertise. Moreover, by standardizing rehabilitation protocols, AI has the potential to reduce variability in care while promoting adherence to best practices. However, for these technologies to be effectively implemented, further research is needed to assess their adaptability to real-world clinical scenarios, their ability to account for patient-specific factors, and their integration into electronic health record (EHR) systems to streamline their use in daily practice.

The key findings reveal that ChatGPT-4o achieved the highest subjective performance, as evidenced by a Likert scale mean of 4.90 $\pm$ 0.32. At the same time, DeepSeek V3 and Gemini 2 recorded moderate scores (4.00 $\pm$ 0.82 and 3.90 $\pm$ 0.74, respectively), and Copilot performed significantly lower with a mean of 2.70 $\pm$ 0.82. In parallel, the DISCERN score, a measure of the quality and reliability of clinical information, was similar for ChatGPT-4o, DeepSeek V3, and Gemini 2 (ranging from 46.90 $\pm$ 2.60 to 47.20 $\pm$ 2.53), whereas Copilot consistently scored 40.0. Readability metrics further differentiated the models: Gemini 2 produced outputs with a notably higher Flesch Reading Ease (12.25 $\pm$ 7.22) and a lower Flesch–Kincaid Grade Level (16.60 $\pm$ 1.40), suggesting its texts are easier to understand. Meanwhile, the Coleman–Liau Index demonstrated smaller variations among the models, ranging from 18.23 $\pm$ 0.79 for Copilot to 19.68 $\pm$ 1.32 for ChatGPT-4o. A one-way analysis of variance confirmed that these differences were statistically significant for the Likert scale ($F(3, 36) = 16.50$, p value < 0.001), DISCERN score ($F(3, 36) = 24.63$, p value < 0.001), Flesch Reading Ease ($F(3, 36) = 4.35$, p value ≈ 0.01), and Flesch–Kincaid Grade Level ($F(3, 36) = 11.82$, p value < 0.001), while the Coleman–Liau Index result was marginally non-significant ($F(3, 36) = 2.84$, p value ≈ 0.06). Therefore, ChatGPT-4o's superior performance, coupled with the enhanced readability of Gemini 2, underscores the nuanced strengths of current AI technologies.

Regarding the subjective evaluation, the superior Likert score of ChatGPT-4o suggests that its outputs are perceived as highly acceptable and coherent by clinical experts. This observation is consistent with the emerging literature that emphasizes the growing capability of large language models to solve complex clinical problems intelligently and even outperform traditional clinical decision-making in certain scenarios. The high rating may reflect ChatGPT-4o's advanced natural language processing abilities, which enable it to generate nuanced and contextually appropriate recommendations [12–15]. While this study involved a limited number of evaluators, all were senior specialists in head and neck surgery, ensuring a high level of clinical expertise. Expanding the panel of reviewers in future studies could help refine the assessment by incorporating a broader range of clinical perspectives. However, given the structured evaluation criteria used, the key performance trends observed across different LLMs are likely to remain consistent.

In contrast, the moderate Likert scores for DeepSeek V3 and Gemini 2 indicate that while these models are competent, they might not capture the same level of subtlety or contextual integration as ChatGPT-4o. However, Copilot's significantly lower rating likely stems from its design as a general-purpose AI rather than a model optimized for medical applications. Unlike ChatGPT-4o and Gemini 2, which are trained using extensive medical literature, Copilot's responses were more generic and lacked clinical depth. Additionally, its outputs were often less structured and detailed, making them less useful for rehabilitation planning. These findings highlight the importance of using AI models specifically trained for medical contexts to ensure clinically relevant recommendations. Such discrepancies highlight the importance of selecting the appropriate AI model based on specific clinical applications and demonstrate that not all AI algorithms are equally effective, a point corroborated by previous research [16].

The analysis of the DISCERN scores further supports these interpretations. The comparable scores for ChatGPT-4o, DeepSeek V3, and Gemini 2 suggest that these models can produce reliable and evidence-based information essential for formulating safe rehabilitation protocols. In contrast, Copilot's consistently lower score may indicate deficiencies in its content generation process, raising concerns about its reliability for clinical decision support. These findings align with the broader trend of exploring AI's potential in perioperative care while emphasizing the need for rigorous quality control.

Readability is a critical factor in the practical application of rehabilitation protocols. Gemini 2's higher Flesch Reading Ease Score and lower Flesch–Kincaid Grade Level imply that its outputs are more accessible, which could facilitate better understanding among clinicians and patients. However, while readability metrics such as DISCERN, Flesch Reading Ease, Flesch–Kincaid Grade Level, and Coleman–Liau Index provide objective measures of text complexity, they also have inherent limitations when applied to medical texts. These indices primarily evaluate structural aspects of language, such as sentence length and word difficulty, but do not assess whether the content is clinically accurate, contextually appropriate, or effectively communicates complex medical concepts. For example, a text with a high readability score may be oversimplified and omit essential clinical details, while a more complex text with a lower score may contain crucial information needed for precise rehabilitation planning. Furthermore, these metrics were originally developed for general educational materials rather than specialized medical content, making their direct applicability to AI-generated rehabilitation programs somewhat limited. Therefore, while readability scores provide useful insights into the accessibility of AI-generated content, they should be interpreted alongside qualitative expert assessments to ensure that rehabilitation plans are both comprehensible and clinically sound.

Using standardized readability measures in our study allows for a valid comparison with the existing literature and reinforces that clarity is paramount in clinical documentation. Although the Coleman–Liau Index did not reveal stark differences among the models, its relatively stable values suggest that while basic text complexity may be similar, other aspects of readability, such as sentence structure and vocabulary, play a more pivotal role in ensuring effective communication.

The statistical significance established through the one-way analysis of variance lends robust support to these findings. The highly significant p values (all below 0.01, except for the borderline result of the Coleman–Liau Index) confirm that the observed differences in performance, quality, and readability among the models are not due to random variation. This reinforces the validity of our conclusions and suggests that each model's distinct strengths and weaknesses are inherent to its design and training data.

It is vital for all who use LLMs to understand that their output is not static. The same prompt entered today will likely not return the same result if entered a year later. These results have broader implications within the context of AI integration in clinical practice. The ability of large language models to generate structured rehabilitation protocols aligns with previous research on AI-assisted clinical decision-making. While prior studies have explored the role of LLMs in generating medical guidelines and decision support tools [12,13], their application in postoperative rehabilitation planning remains less examined. This study builds upon the existing research by evaluating AI-generated rehabilitation recommendations specifically in head and neck surgery, an area where patient-specific variability often limits standardized protocols. However, as with other AI applications in healthcare, the integration of LLMs in rehabilitation requires further validation to ensure their clinical reliability and adaptability [16–18]. For instance, while AI algorithms have shown superiority in specific decision-making tasks, translating this potential into a reliable clinical tool requires adherence to principles such as TURBO (Testable, Usable, Reliable, Beneficial, Operable) to ensure consistent performance [15].

Furthermore, the dynamic nature of AI outputs, wherein the same input may yield different results over time due to continuous updates in training data, necessitates that these tools be used under strict clinical supervision [18]. This study, like others in the field, acknowledges that while AI can provide valuable insights and augment clinical practice, its output must be validated through prospective studies, randomized controlled trials, and longitudinal research. Additionally, integrating AI with established technologies such as Virtual Surgical Planning, a cornerstone in head and neck surgery, could further refine patient-specific rehabilitation strategies and optimize surgical outcomes.

This study has several limitations that should be considered when interpreting the findings. Firstly, the rehabilitation programs generated by LLMs were evaluated using hypothetical clinical scenarios rather than real patient data, which may limit the direct applicability of the results to clinical practice. Secondly, the number of expert reviewers was limited to three senior clinicians, which, although providing a high level of expertise, may not fully capture the diversity of clinical perspectives. Furthermore, clinician assessments are inherently subjective and may be influenced by individual biases, prior experiences, or expectations, introducing potential variability in the evaluation of LLM outputs. Expanding the panel and incorporating blinded or standardized assessment protocols in future studies could help mitigate these biases and enhance reliability. Thirdly, while readability metrics were used to assess text complexity, they do not fully capture the nuances of patient comprehension or the effectiveness of AI-generated recommendations in real-world rehabilitation settings. Finally, as LLMs continue to evolve, their outputs are subject to ongoing updates, meaning that future versions of these models may yield different results. Prospective studies involving real patient cases and longitudinal follow-up are necessary to validate the clinical utility of AI-generated rehabilitation programs.

This comprehensive analysis demonstrates significant differences in the performance, quality, and readability of rehabilitation protocols generated by various AI models [17–19]. The superior performance of ChatGPT-4o, coupled with the enhanced readability of Gemini 2, underscores the nuanced strengths of current AI technologies while highlighting areas needing improvement [20]. These findings contribute to the evolving landscape of AI in perioperative care by providing critical insights that can inform future research and clinical practice [21]. Moving forward, multidisciplinary collaborations and rigorous clinical validations must guide the integration of AI into healthcare, ensuring that these advanced tools ultimately translate into improved patient outcomes and safer, more effective clinical interventions [22].

5. Conclusions

This study demonstrates that large language models can generate clinically relevant rehabilitation programs for patients undergoing head and neck surgery, with significant variation in quality and readability among models. ChatGPT-4o outperformed others in clinical relevance, as assessed by expert reviewers, while Gemini 2 produced more readable responses. Copilot consistently scored lower across all metrics, highlighting variability in AI-generated outputs. While LLMs show promise in supporting postoperative care, their outputs require rigorous validation before clinical implementation. The findings underscore the need for multidisciplinary oversight and ongoing refinement of AI tools to ensure their reliability in patient rehabilitation. Future research should focus on real-world clinical trials to assess the impact of AI-driven rehabilitation programs on patient outcomes. Integrating AI with existing multidisciplinary approaches could enhance personalized rehabilitation strategies, ultimately improving the functional recovery and quality of life for head and neck surgery patients.

Supplementary Materials: The following supporting information can be downloaded at https://www.mdpi.com/article/10.3390/technologies13040142/s1, Supplementary Figure S1: Representative image. Supplementary Table S1: Responses from large language models to the clinical scenario prompt: "What rehabilitation program and services are recommended for this patient to optimize their postoperative recovery, considering their specific clinical condition, surgical procedure, and potential risk factors?".

Author Contributions: Conceptualization, I.S., G.M., J.N., and V.M.; methodology, I.S., G.M., and J.N.; software, G.M.; validation, S.K.-H.N., R.C., and W.M.R.; formal analysis, I.S., G.M., J.N., V.M., and B.S.; investigation, I.S.; resources, G.M.; data curation, G.M.; writing—original draft preparation, I.S., G.M., J.N., K.L., V.M., and B.S.; writing—review and editing, all authors; visualization, B.S. and G.M.; supervision, R.C., S.K.-H.N., and W.M.R. All authors have read and agreed to the published version of the manuscript.

Funding: This research received no external funding.

Institutional Review Board Statement: Not applicable.

Informed Consent Statement: Not applicable, as this study did not involve human participants.

Data Availability Statement: The authors confirm that the data supporting this study's findings are available within the article.

Conflicts of Interest: The authors declare no conflicts of interest.

Abbreviations

The following abbreviations are used in this manuscript:

AI	Artificial intelligence
HNS	Head and neck surgery
LLMs	Large language models
SCC	Squamous cell carcinoma
BCC	Basal cell carcinoma
ANOVA	One-way analysis of variance

References

1. DiDonna, N.; Shetty, P.N.; Khan, K.; Damitz, L. Unveiling the Potential of AI in Plastic Surgery Education: A Comparative Study of Leading AI Platforms' Performance on In-training Examinations. *Plast. Reconstr. Surg. Glob. Open* **2024**, *12*, e5929. [CrossRef]
2. Aleem, M.U.; Khan, J.A.; Younes, A.; Sabbah, B.N.; Saleh, W.; Migliore, M. Enhancing Thoracic Surgery with AI: A Review of Current Practices and Emerging Trends. *Curr. Oncol.* **2024**, *31*, 6232–6244. [CrossRef] [PubMed]
3. Bajwa, J.; Munir, U.; Nori, A.; Williams, B. Artificial intelligence in healthcare: Transforming the practice of medicine. *Future Healthc. J.* **2021**, *8*, e188–e194. [CrossRef] [PubMed]
4. Busch, F.; Hoffmann, L.; Rueger, C.; van Dijk, E.H.; Kader, R.; Ortiz-Prado, E.; Makowski, M.R.; Saba, L.; Hadamitzky, M.; Kather, J.N. Current applications and challenges in large language models for patient care: A systematic review. *Commun. Med.* **2025**, *5*, 26.
5. Clusmann, J.; Kolbinger, F.R.; Muti, H.S.; Carrero, Z.I.; Eckardt, J.-N.; Laleh, N.G.; Löffler, C.M.L.; Schwarzkopf, S.-C.; Unger, M.; Veldhuizen, G.P.; et al. The future landscape of large language models in medicine. *Commun. Med.* **2023**, *3*, 141. [CrossRef]
6. Sumner, J.; Lim, H.W.; Chong, L.S.; Bundele, A.; Mukhopadhyay, A.; Kayambu, G. Artificial intelligence in physical rehabilitation: A systematic review. *Artif. Intell. Med.* **2023**, *146*, 102693. [CrossRef]

7. Bhattacharyya, N.; Fried, M.P. Benchmarks for mortality, morbidity, and length of stay for head and neck surgical procedures. *Arch. Otolaryngol. Head Neck Surg.* **2001**, *127*, 127–132. [CrossRef] [PubMed]
8. Tan, B.K.; Por, Y.C.; Chen, H.C. Complications of head and neck reconstruction and their treatment. *Semin. Plast. Surg.* **2010**, *24*, 288–298. [CrossRef]
9. Walia, A.; Lee, J.J.; Jackson, R.S.; Hardi, A.C.; Bollig, C.A.; Graboyes, E.M.; Zenga, J.; Puram, S.V.; Pipkorn, P. Management of flap failure after head and neck reconstruction: A systematic review and meta-analysis. *Otolaryngol. Head Neck Surg.* **2022**, *167*, 224–235. [CrossRef]
10. Genden, E.M.; Rinaldo, A.; Suárez, C.; Wei, W.I.; Bradley, P.J.; Ferlito, A. Complications of free flap transfers for head and neck reconstruction following cancer resection. *Oral Oncol.* **2004**, *40*, 979–984. [CrossRef]
11. Seth, I.; Marcaccini, G.; Lim, K.; Castrechini, M.; Cuomo, R.; Ng, S.K.-H.; Ross, R.J.; Rozen, W.M. Management of Dupuytren's Disease: A Multi-Centric Comparative Analysis Between Experienced Hand Surgeons Versus Artificial Intelligence. *Diagnostics* **2025**, *15*, 587. [CrossRef] [PubMed]
12. List, M.A.; Knackstedt, M.; Liu, L.; Kasabali, A.; Mansour, J.; Pang, J.; Asarkar, A.A.; Nathan, C.A. Enhanced recovery after surgery, current, and future considerations in head and neck cancer. *Laryngoscope Investig. Otolaryngol.* **2023**, *8*, 1240–1256. [CrossRef]
13. Prasad, A.; Chorath, K.; Barrette, L.X.; Go, B.; Deng, J.; Moreira, A.; Rajasekaran, K. Implementation of an enhanced recovery after surgery protocol for head and neck cancer patients: Considerations and best practices. *World J. Otorhinolaryngol. Head Neck Surg.* **2022**, *8*, 91–95. [CrossRef] [PubMed]
14. Loftus, T.J.; Tighe, P.J.; Filiberto, A.C.; Efron, P.A.; Brakenridge, S.C.; Mohr, A.M.; Rashidi, P.; Upchurch, G.R.; Bihorac, A. Artificial intelligence and surgical decision-making. *JAMA Surg.* **2020**, *155*, 148–158. [CrossRef] [PubMed]
15. Palenzuela, D.L.; Mullen, J.T.; Phitayakorn, R. AI versus MD: Evaluating the surgical decision-making accuracy of ChatGPT-4. *Surgery* **2024**, *176*, 241–245. [CrossRef]
16. Hashimoto, D.A.; Rosman, G.; Rus, D.; Meireles, O.R. Artificial intelligence in surgery: Promises and perils. *Ann. Surg.* **2018**, *268*, 70–76. [CrossRef]
17. Seth, I.; Lim, B.; Phan, R.; Xie, Y.; Kenney, P.S.; Bukret, W.E.; Thomsen, J.B.; Cuomo, R.; Ross, R.J.; Ng, S.K.; et al. Perforator selection with computed tomography angiography for unilateral breast reconstruction: A clinical multicentre analysis. *Medicina* **2024**, *60*, 1500. [CrossRef]
18. Abi-Rafeh, J.; Xu, H.H.; Kazan, R.; Tevlin, R.; Furnas, H. Large language models and artificial intelligence: A primer for plastic surgeons on the demonstrated and potential applications, promises, and limitations of ChatGPT. *Aesthetic Surg. J.* **2024**, *44*, 329–343. [CrossRef]
19. Roberts, R.H.; Ali, S.R.; Dobbs, T.D.; Whitaker, I.S. Can large language models generate outpatient clinic letters at first consultation that incorporate complication profiles from UK and USA aesthetic plastic surgery associations? In *Aesthetic Surgery Journal Open Forum*; Oxford University Press: Oxford, UK, 2024; Volume 6, p. ojad109. [CrossRef]
20. Mohapatra, D.P.; Thiruvoth, F.M.; Tripathy, S.; Rajan, S.; Vathulya, M.; Lakshmi, P.; Singh, V.K.; Haq, A.U. Leveraging Large Language Models (LLM) for the plastic surgery resident training: Do they have a role? *Indian J. Plast. Surg.* **2023**, *56*, 413–420. [CrossRef]
21. Kwon, D.Y.; Wang, A.; Mejia, M.R.; Saturno, M.P.; Oleru, O.; Seyidova, N.; Taub, P.J. Adherence of a Large Language Model to Clinical Guidelines for Craniofacial Plastic and Reconstructive Surgeries. *Ann. Plast. Surg.* **2024**, *92*, 261–262. [CrossRef]
22. Seth, I.; Xie, Y.; Rodwell, A.; Gracias, D.; Bulloch, G.; Hunter-Smith, D.J.; Rozen, W.M. Exploring the role of a large language model on carpal tunnel syndrome management: An observation study of ChatGPT. *J. Hand Surg.* **2023**, *48*, 1025–1033. [CrossRef] [PubMed]

technologies

MDPI

Article

Technology to Enable People with Intellectual Disabilities and Blindness to Collect Boxes with Objects and Transport Them to Different Rooms of Their Daily Context: A Single-Case Research Series

Giulio E. Lancioni [1,*], Gloria Alberti [1], Francesco Pezzuoli [2], Fabiana Abbinante [1], Nirbhay N. Singh [3], Mark F. O'Reilly [4] and Jeff Sigafoos [5]

1 Lega F. D'Oro Research Center, 60027 Osimo, Italy; alberti.g@legadelfilodoro.it (G.A.); abbinante.f@legadelfilodoro.it (F.A.)
2 Department of Architecture and Design, University of Camerino and LiMiX Srl, 63100 Ascoli Piceno, Italy; francesco.pezzuoli@unicam.it
3 College of Medicine, Augusta University, Augusta, GA 30912, USA; nirbz52@gmail.com
4 Department of Special Education, University of Texas at Austin, TX 78712, USA; markoreilly@austin.utexas.edu
5 School of Education, Victoria University of Wellington, Wellington 6140, New Zealand; jeff.sigafoos@vuw.ac.nz
* Correspondence: giulio.lancioni@uniba.it

Abstract: (1) Background: People with intellectual disabilities and blindness tend to be withdrawn and sedentary. This study was carried out to assess a new technology system to enable seven of these people to collect boxes containing different sets of objects from a storage room and transport them to the appropriate destination rooms. (2) Methods: The technology system used for the study involved tags with radio frequency identification codes, a tag reader, a smartphone, and mini speakers. At the start of a session, the participants were called by the system to take a box from the storage room. Once they collected a box, the system identified the tags attached to the box, called the participants to the room where the box was to be transported and delivered, and provided them with preferred music stimulation. The same process was followed for each of the other boxes available in the session. (3) Results: During baseline sessions without the system, the mean frequency of boxes handled correctly (collected, transported, and put away without research assistants' guidance) was zero or virtually zero. During the intervention sessions with the system, the participants' mean frequency of boxes handled correctly increased to between about 10 and 15 per session. (4) Conclusions: These findings suggest that the new technology system might be helpful for people like the participants of this study.

Keywords: technology; tags; tag reader; blindness; intellectual disability; verbal instructions; encouragements; orientation cues

1. Introduction

1.1. Background

People with severe intellectual disabilities and visual impairment are often withdrawn and sedentary and lag behind in their developmental process [1–4]. In essence, this (marginality and passivity) condition may be connected to their problems in critical areas, such as activity engagement, orientation and mobility, communication, and motivation [5–10]. For example, activity engagement requires appropriate object use and motivation to perform the actions (object use responses) involved in the activity [11,12]. Yet, many of these people may have a limited ability to discriminate and handle objects and no specific interest in using those objects for completing a specific activity/task [11–15]. Orientation and mobility may be prerequisites to gather objects for the activities and to practice basic physical exercise essential for wellbeing [10,12–14]. Yet, many of these people tend to have difficulties orienting and moving even in small indoor areas and, thus, tend to remain sedentary rather than exploring their context [12,16–19].

The complexity of this situation and the need to alleviate the negative consequences associated with it have prompted the development of a variety of intervention programs aimed at promoting people's general progress and wellbeing [5,6,12,18]. In particular, efforts were made to develop programs assisted by technology that would provide the types of support necessary for the participants to advance in specific areas of their rehabilitation process [18–21]. For example, programs were developed in which technology was adopted to enable the participants to use simple motor actions to make clear requests that would lead to satisfactory (reinforcing) consequences from the environment (consequences that would foster the participants' motivation to repeat their requests) [22–24]. Programs were developed to enable the participants to carry out basic physical exercise independent of staff or caregivers' direct supervision [25–28]. Those programs typically involved the use of technology devices to monitor the participants' exercise responses and possibly (a) provide the participants with encouragements to emit those responses and (b) follow those responses with brief stimulation events that were expected to motivate the participants to maintain/strengthen the responses.

1.2. Related Work

Programs were also developed to enable participants to orient within a work room and carry out simple activities within such a room. For example, Lancioni et al. [29] designed a program that involved a smartphone with an Android system, which was fitted with Amazon Alexa, MacroDroid, and Philips Hue applications, as well as indoor motion sensors and mini speakers. The technology was to help seven participants to collect objects from three different areas of the room and bring those objects to a central desk located in the same room through the provision of spatial cues, verbal instructions, and positive stimulation. At the start of a session, the participants were called to one of the three areas of the room from which they had to take objects. The calls served as encouragements as well as spatial cues that would help the participants to orient to that area and reach it and were emitted by the mini speaker available in that area. As they reached that area (i.e., were detected by the motion sensor available there), they received praise and the instruction to take an object. The instruction was then followed by the activation of the mini speaker available at the central desk, which called the participants to the desk. As they reached the desk (i.e., were detected by the motion sensor available there), the speaker on that desk delivered praise, the instruction to put away the object transported, and 15 s of preferred stimulation.

At the end of the stimulation, the mini speaker of the next area to be reached started calling the participants. The process was repeated for each of the other objects to be collected and transported, and a session lasted until all the objects available (i.e., 18 in total) had been transported to the central desk or a 30 min period had elapsed, whichever came first. The results showed that the participants were able to transport and put away between 13 and 18 objects per session during the intervention sessions. Their mean frequency was zero or near zero before the intervention.

Lancioni et al. [30] designed a program that involved the use of a barcode reader, a series of barcodes, a smartphone fitted with a special application, and a mini speaker or headphones. The technology served to enable seven participants to find different room entrances distributed along the two sides of a corridor and deliver objects at those rooms. Each session included seven different trials. At each trial, the participants were to walk to a specific room and enter the room with the object they had to deliver, and then they would receive 20 s of preferred stimulation. A trial started with the research assistants guiding the participants to a specific position of the corridor, providing them with an object that they were to transport to one of the rooms, and typing the number of the destination room into the smartphone. The room entrances were marked with barcodes reproduced on sheets of paper. Those barcodes could be decoded by a small barcode reader that the participants wore at their ankle or waist. Based on the barcodes decoded, the smartphone provided the participants with different verbal messages, which were delivered via the mini speaker or the headphones the participants had. The message would invite the participants to walk forward (when the barcode detected indicated that the entrance did not correspond to the destination where the object was to be delivered) or stop and enter the room (when the barcode detected indicated that the entrance was that of the destination room). The results showed that the mean frequency of trials correctly completed (with the participants entering the right room) per session varied from about six to nearly seven during the intervention with the technology, while it was between zero and two before the intervention.

1.3. Objectives

The aim of the present study was to extend the scope of Lancioni et al.'s intervention programs [29,30], which are summarized above in several ways. First, this study aimed to enable participants to collect boxes containing different sets of objects from a storage room and transport them to five different destination rooms, thus expanding the activity context used by Lancioni et al. [29]. Second, the boxes were to be transported to the pertinent destination rooms, that is, to the rooms that were connected to the objects the boxes contained. For example, a box containing soap and grooming items was to be transported to a washroom, whereas a box with food and drink items was to be transported to the room used as a snack area. This new activity arrangement (supplying different rooms with different/appropriate types of material) was thought to have practical and vocational relevance [2,8,21]). Third, the technology system used during the study, which included tags with radio frequency identification codes, a tag reader, a smartphone, and mini speakers, was set to guide the participants to the different pertinent rooms automatically throughout the entire activity session (i.e., without any need for research assistants' inputs, such as those scheduled by Lancioni et al. [30]). These three new aspects were thought to make the intervention program set up in the present study more relevant from a rehabilitation standpoint and more functional and convenient from a technological standpoint than previous programs. The study included seven participants with intellectual disabilities and blindness and relied on a single-case research methodology.

2. Materials and Methods

2.1. Participants

Table 1 lists the seven participants by using their pseudonyms and reports their chronological ages and their age equivalents for daily living skills (personal subdomain), which were computed via the second edition of the Vineland Adaptive Behavior Scales [31,32]. Their chronological age ranged from 25 to 45 years. Their Vineland age equivalents ranged from 2 years and 8 months to 4 years. All the participants were diagnosed with congenital encephalopathy associated with intellectual disability and blindness. The seventh participant (Edgar) also presented with ambulation difficulties. Specifically, he walked when he had some form of physical support. For example, he could walk and transport objects by using a shopping cart (see below). No Intelligence Quotient scores were available for the participants, but the psychological services of the rehabilitation and care contexts that they attended considered their intellectual disability level to fall within the moderate-to-severe range (Eloise) or the severe range (all the others).

Table 1. Participants' chronological ages and Vineland age equivalents for daily living skills (personal sub-domain).

Participants (Pseudonyms)	Chronological Age (Years)	Vineland Age Equivalents [1] (Years, Months)
Dean	45	2, 8
Ryan	43	3, 2
Ruth	26	3, 1
Eloise	38	4, 0
Graham	25	3, 0
George	45	2, 10
Edgar	41	2, 8

[1] The age equivalents are based on the Italian standardization of the Vineland scales [31].

The participants represented a convenience sample, in that they were recruited from rehabilitation and care centers belonging to a single organization [33]. Their recruitment, however, was carried out based on a number of conditions, which had been verified through preliminary observations and interviews. First, they were adults who needed to increase their levels of mobility and occupational engagement (the functional use of objects). Second, they had difficulties orienting and traveling in indoor contexts and were totally dependent when in outdoor contexts. Third, they were able to orient to sound cues (i.e., voices or other types of sounds) and could reach the sound source and the destination it represented within relatively small indoor contexts. Fourth, they could respond to simple verbal instructions concerning the use of objects such as "take" and "put away" the object. Fifth, they were interested in various forms of environmental stimulation (e.g., music and songs), so such stimulation was considered important to motivate their activity engagement (e.g., collecting and transporting boxes with objects). Sixth, staff personnel considered the use of technology support to promote mobility and occupational engagement a valuable objective and thus endorsed the study.

2.2. Ethical Considerations

The participants' regular staff viewed the study as a positive opportunity for the participants. In fact, the study was deemed to offer the participants the chance to increase their mobility and occupational engagement, as well as their access to preferred stimulation. This access was expected to motivate their involvement and make it enjoyable for them. Given their condition, they could not provide a clear/reliable response as to their interest in the study or read and sign a consent form for it. In view of that, the participants' legal representatives read and signed the consent form on their behalf. This study complied with the 1964 Helsinki Declaration and its later amendments and was approved by an institutional Ethics Committee.

2.3. Setting, Responses, Sessions, Instruction Cues, Research Assistants, and Stimuli

The setting was an area of the centers that the participants attended, which involved a corridor with room entrances on both sides. In total, six rooms were included: one serving as storage room and the others as destination rooms (see Figure 1). The storage room contained a desk with 15 different boxes of 25 × 19 × 17 cm. Each box contained specific objects (e.g., toilet, food, or cleaning items). Each of the destination rooms had a large carton (placed on a chair) right after its entrance. A response consisted of taking one of the boxes from the storage room, transporting the box to the pertinent destination room, and depositing the box in the carton displayed in that room. For example, boxes containing grooming items were to be transported to a washroom and deposited in the carton available there, while boxes containing leisure items were to be transported to a room used as leisure area and deposited in the carton of that room (see the Introduction). A session lasted until the participants had transported all the 15 boxes available on the desk of the storage room, a 20 min period had elapsed, or several instances of research assistants' guidance had occurred (see the Baseline for the First Six Participants Section). The participants typically had one session per day, 3 to 6 days a week.

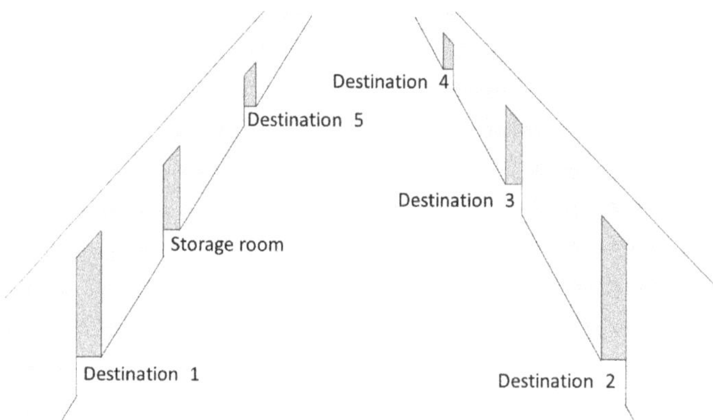

Figure 1. Schematic representation of the setting with entrances to the storage room and the five destination rooms.

The instruction cues consisted of single words or combinations of two or three words presented by the technology system during the intervention sessions. Specifically, the cues included expressions such as the following: (a) "Come here" and "Take a box", which were presented from the desk with the boxes at intervals of about 5–7 s every time the participants were to go to such desk and collect a box; (b) "NAME plus walk", or "Over here", which was presented from the room where the box that the participants had collected was to be transported; and (c) "Box down" or "Box in carton", which was presented when the participants were to deposit the transported box into the carton.

Four research assistants (two women and two men) were employed to implement the sessions and record the data. They held a university degree in psychology and were familiar with different data recording procedures and the technology systems/solutions employed with people with different types of disabilities.

The stimuli provided to the participants in connection with their depositing a box in a carton included music and song segments combined with verbal approval. The music and song stimuli were selected through a stimulus preference screening procedure. The procedure involved the presentation of two or three 10 s clips of each song or music piece included in the preference evaluation for a minimum of 10 non-consecutive times distributed over different evaluation periods. Stimuli were selected for use during the intervention phase of the study if the research assistants involved in the screening agreed that they had elicited the participants' positive reactions (e.g., alerting and smiling) in at least 50% of their presentations.

2.4. Technology System for the First Six Participants

The technology system used for the first six participants (i.e., Dean, Ryan, Ruth, Eloise, Graham, and George) included (a) tags with radio frequency identification codes suitable for NFC; (b) a tag reader; (c) an Android smartphone with a light sensor, which was equipped with the Talking Hands application [34] and the MacroDroid application; and (d) six mini speakers. The smartphone was fixed at the participants' waist. The mini speakers were displayed in the storage room and the five destination rooms (one speaker per room).

The tags (5.4 × 8.5 × 0.1 cm; NFC MIFARE RFID, 1 K 13.56 MHz) were fixed onto the sides of the boxes that the participants were to transport and deposit in the cartons available in the destination rooms. All the tags attached to a specific box had the same code, which could be easily identified by the tag reader.

The tag reader consisted of two watch-like devices linked to one another. During the intervention (i.e., when the technology system was used), one of the devices (4.5 × 4.5 × 0.9 cm) was strapped to the palm of the participants' right hand (see Figure 2) and contained an NFC module which was designed to identify the tags attached to the different boxes with objects. The other device (6.5 × 4 × 1.5 cm) was strapped to the participants' right wrist and contained an electronic circuit that was designed to send the smartphone Bluetooth signals about the tags identified.

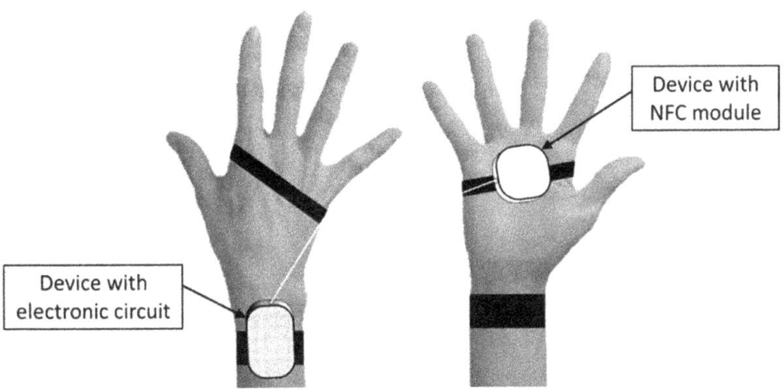

Figure 2. A schematic representation of the tag reader's watch-like devices and how the participants wore them.

At the start of each session, the participants were called to take a box by the mini speaker of the storage room (see Figure 3). When the participants collected a box, their tag reader identified the box's tags and sent a Bluetooth signal to the smartphone. The smartphone decoded the Bluetooth signal through the Talking Hands application. Decoding a Bluetooth signal (recognizing the tags' code for the box being collected) led to the activation of the MacroDroid application, which (a) triggered the mini speaker of the room to which the box was to be transported and (b) ensured that the mini speaker presented the participants with the instructions to reach that room. The instructions (i.e., verbal encouragements to reach the room that were repeated every 5–7 s; see Section 2.3 also provided orientation and spatial guidance for the participants traveling to the room.

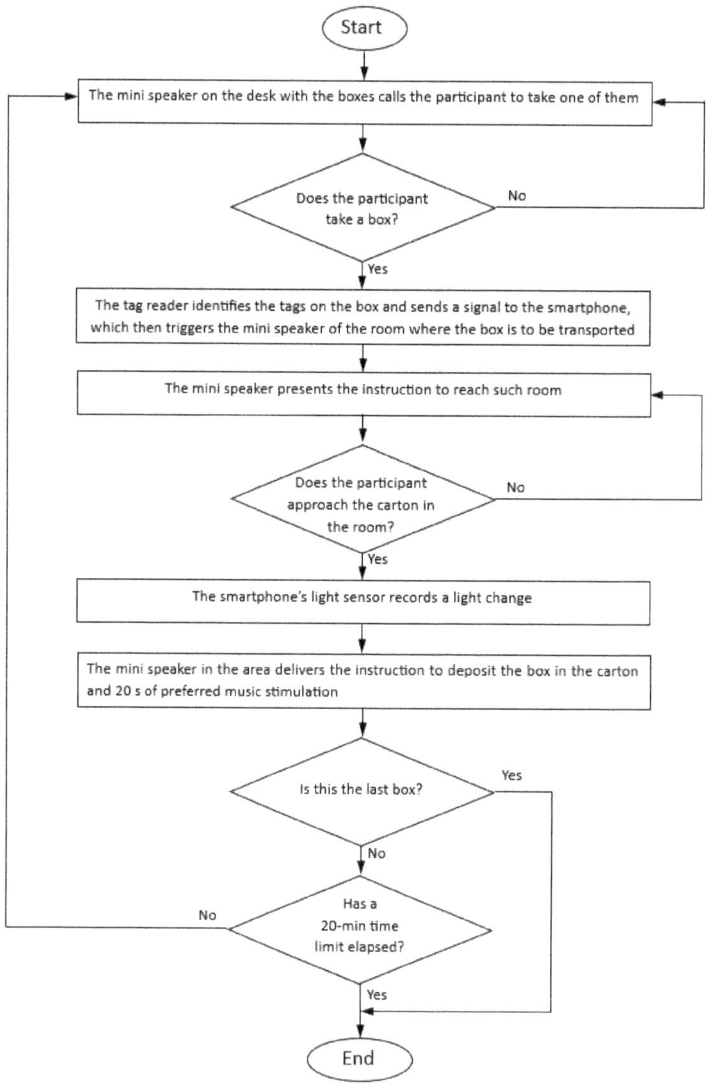

Figure 3. Flowchart summarizing the functioning of the technology system.

Once the participants entered the room and approached the carton where the box was to be deposited, the smartphone's light sensor detected a light change (i.e., a reduction in light intensity caused by the smartphone's proximity to the carton; see Figure 4). Based on this change, the MacroDroid caused the mini speaker available in the area to deliver (a) the instruction to deposit the box in the carton and (b) (3–4 s thereafter) 20 s of preferred music stimulation. Once the stimulation was over, the MacroDroid triggered the mini speaker of the storage room to present the instructions to reach the desk and take a box (see Section 2.3). The box was then to be transported to the pertinent destination room following the procedure described above. The same procedure was applied to each box to be collected, transported, and deposited during the session.

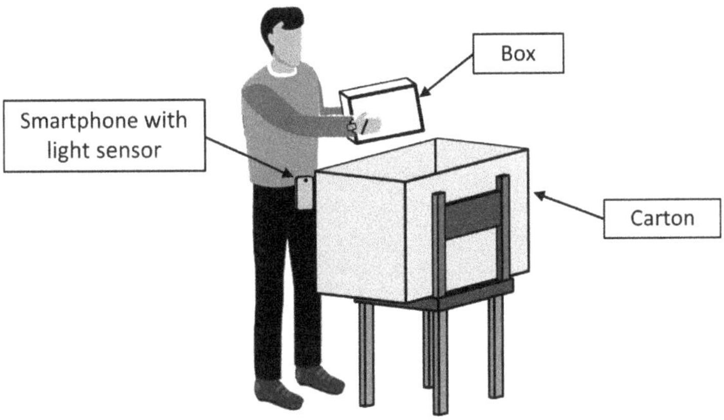

Figure 4. Schematic representation of the smartphone's position at the participants' waist and its proximity to the carton when the participants approached it to deposit a box (i.e., the proximity caused the smartphone's light sensor to detect a reduction in light intensity).

2.5. Technology System for the Seventh Participant

The technology system used for the seventh participant (i.e., Edgar) included the same components as the system used for the first six participants. Yet, the position and functioning of some of those components differed as Edgar walked with the support of a shopping cart and used the cart for transporting the boxes (see the Participants Section). The cart was adapted so that (a) only a small sector of it (i.e., the one close to the handle) was open and accessible for placing the boxes (see Figure 5) and (b) the tag reader and the smartphone were fixed at the bottom of that sector (see Figure 5).

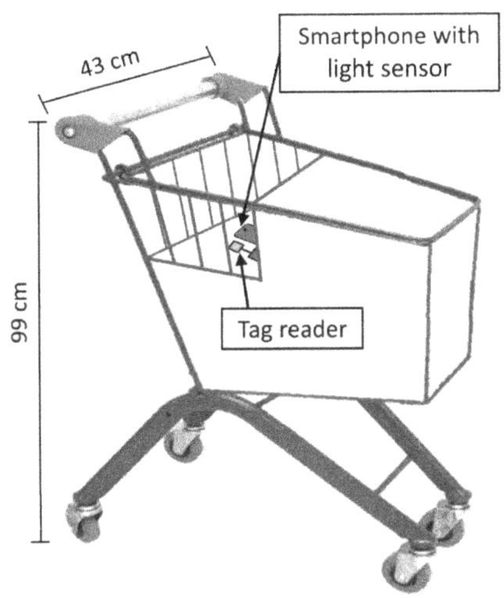

Figure 5. Schematic representation of the shopping cart used for Edgar with measures of its height and handle wideness. Only a small sector of the cart (i.e., the one close to the handle) was open and accessible. All the rest, which is white in the figure, was closed. The smartphone and tag reader were fixed at the bottom of the open sector.

As soon as Edgar placed a box in the cart, the tag reader would identify the tags attached to the box and send a signal to the smartphone. The smartphone decoded the signal and activated (via the MacroDroid) the mini speaker of the destination room where the box was to be transported and deposited. The mini speaker presented encouragement (orientation) messages, as it had done for the other participants. Once in the room, he was to take the box from the cart, causing a change for the smartphone's light sensor. This change led the MacroDroid to trigger the emission of the instruction to put the box in the carton. About 5 s after this instruction, a 20 s presentation of preferred music started. The end of the music led to the instructions to reach the storage room and take a box. The same process was followed for the other boxes to be used during the session.

2.6. Data Recording

Data recording concerned (a) the number of boxes correctly handled (i.e., collected, transported, and placed in the carton of the right destination room, independently of any research assistants' guidance), (b) the research assistants' guidance instances, and (c) the length of the sessions. The measures were recorded by the research assistants implementing the sessions. Inter-rater agreement was assessed in more than 23% of the sessions of the single participants, with a reliability observer watching those sessions and scoring the measures. The percentage of agreement (computed by dividing the number of sessions in which both the research assistants and the reliability observer had the same scores for the boxes being correctly handled and for the research assistants' guidance, with differences of less than 1.5 min for the session lengths, by the total number of sessions carried out with the reliability observer and then multiplying by 100%) was above 93% for all the participants.

2.7. Experimental Conditions and Data Analysis

The first six participants (Dean, Ryan, Ruth, Eloise, Graham, and George) were exposed to the study according to a non-concurrent multiple baseline design across participants [35]. During the initial phase of the study, they received baseline sessions in which the technology system was not in use. The number of baseline sessions differed across them, as required by the design. The baseline phase was followed by an intervention phase, during which the technology system was available (see below). For the seventh participant (Edgar), the study was carried out according to an ABAB design [35], in which A represented baseline conditions (without the system), and B represented intervention conditions (with the system).

The research assistants were in charge of the baseline and intervention sessions of all the participants. To ensure that the sessions were implemented accurately (i.e., to ensure a high level of procedural fidelity [36]), the research assistants were provided with (a) three or four preliminary practice sessions to familiarize them with the baseline and intervention conditions and (b) feedback on whether or not they had been procedurally accurate after regular sessions. Feedback was provided by a study supervisor who had access to videos of the sessions.

The participants' frequency of boxes correctly handled during the baseline and intervention sessions was summarized in graphic form. The difference between the baseline and the intervention frequency levels was assessed through the Percentage of Nonoverlapping Data (PND) method [37]. This method, which is a practical tool for the evaluation of single-case research data, allowed us to verify for each participant the percentage of intervention sessions in which the frequency of boxes correctly handled was higher than the highest baseline value.

2.7.1. Baseline for the First Six Participants

The baseline phase included 5 to 10 sessions during which the system was not available. Familiar objects were attached to the boxes to be transported and to the doorframes of the rooms to which those boxes were to be transported. For example, a toothpaste tube would be attached to the boxes that were to be transported to the washroom as well as to the doorframe of that room. At the start of a session, the participants were guided to touch the objects on the doorframes. Then, they were instructed to (a) take a box, (b) touch the object attached to the box (e.g., a cup), and (c) find (enter) the room with the cup.

If the participants transported the box to the correct room destination and deposited that in the carton available there, the research assistants provided verbal praise, guided the participants to the desk with the boxes, and instructed them to take a box. If the participants failed to make any progress toward the destination for 30–60 s or entered a wrong destination room, the research assistants provided verbal and physical guidance to help them find the correct room and deposit the box in the carton available there. Depositing the box in the carton led to verbal praise even when the response was carried out with the research assistants' guidance. The session lasted until the participants had transported all the 15 boxes available, a 20 min time period had elapsed, or research assistants' guidance had occurred on four consecutive boxes, whichever came first.

2.7.2. Intervention for the First Six Participants

The intervention included 59 to 78 sessions, with differences in the number of sessions being largely due to the participants' availability. The technology system was in use and worked as described in the Technology System Section and summarized in Figure 3. The research assistants provided guidance only if the participants failed to make progress for over 60 s. The intervention sessions were preceded by four to seven familiarization (practice) sessions, during which the research assistants' guidance was available to help the participants respond to the system instructions without hesitation or breaks and experience the system praise and music.

2.7.3. Baseline for the Seventh Participant

Each of the two baseline (A) phases available for Edgar included six sessions. The conditions were as those described for the first six participants, except that he was to place the boxes in the cart and walk with the cart to the destinations.

2.7.4. Intervention for the Seventh Participant

The two intervention (B) phases available included 29 and 51 sessions, respectively. During those sessions, Edgar was provided with the technology system that worked as described in the technology system section concerning him. The first intervention phase was preceded by eight familiarization (practice) sessions, which were similar to those described for the first six participants.

3. Results

The six graphs of Figure 6 report the baseline and intervention data for the first six participants. Each data point represents the mean frequency of boxes correctly handled per session over a block of two sessions. Blocks of three sessions (at the end of the baseline or intervention phases) are marked with an arrow. The graphs do not report the introduction (practice) sessions preceding the start of the intervention phase. Figure 7 reports the baseline and intervention data for Edgar, which are plotted as in Figure 6.

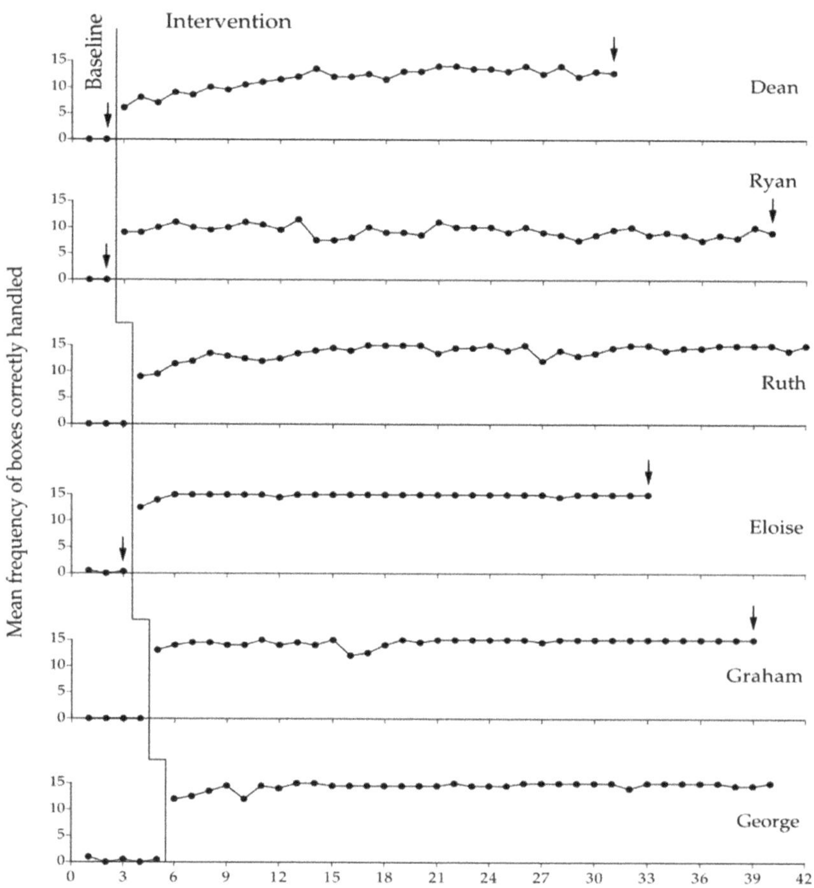

Figure 6. The figure reports the baseline and intervention data for the first six participants. Each data point represents the mean frequency of boxes correctly handled per session over a block of two sessions. Blocks of three sessions are marked with an arrow.

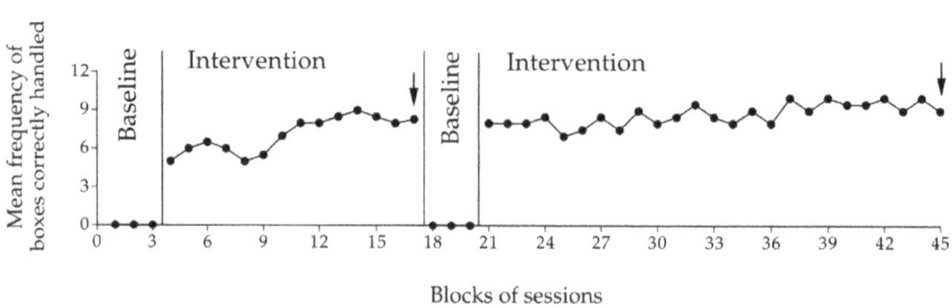

Figure 7. The figure reports the baseline and intervention data for Edgar, which are plotted as in Figure 6.

Figure 6 shows that only two of the first six participants, namely Eloise and George, managed to handle some of the boxes correctly (i.e., totals of 2 and 4, respectively) during the baseline sessions. Given the participants' difficulties, research assistants' guidance was regularly required, and all the participants' baseline sessions were interrupted following four consecutive instances of research assistants' guidance. The length of those sessions was below 10 min.

During the intervention phase, all the participants showed a clear performance improvement. Eloise, Graham, and George were able to correctly handle nearly all the boxes available in the sessions (i.e., their mean frequency of boxes correctly handled per session was about or above 14.5). Their mean session length was about 16.5, close to 20, and 18 min, respectively. Ruth's mean frequency of boxes correctly handled per session was about 13.5. In some sessions, she managed to handle all 15 boxes correctly within the 20 min allowed. In most of the sessions, however, she would handle between 12 and 14 boxes. Ryan and Dean's mean frequency of boxes correctly handled per session was about 9 and 12, respectively. Their sessions always ended after the 20 min time limit had elapsed. Research assistants' guidance was virtually absent or very sporadic for all six participants. In fact, the discrepancies in their data reflected their differences in performance speed and dexterity more than their level of independence, which was high for all of them. The PND method showed indices of 1 for all the participants, given that their frequency of boxes correctly handled during the intervention sessions was always higher than their baseline best performance.

Edgar did not manage to handle any box correctly during the baseline phases (see Figure 7), and the sessions were interrupted after four consecutive instances of research assistants' guidance. During the first intervention phase, his mean frequency of boxes handled correctly was about 7 per session. During the second intervention phase, the mean frequency was about 8.5 per session. The sessions were always ended after the 20 min limit had elapsed. Research assistants' guidance occurred on a few occasions during the initial sessions of the first intervention phase and then became highly sporadic and virtually absent. His relatively low frequency of boxes handled correctly was largely due to the fact that he was rather slow in taking and putting away boxes and also in his walking with the shopping cart. The PND index for him was 1 as it was for the previous participants.

4. Discussion

The results show that the seven participants succeeded in correctly collecting, transporting, and depositing boxes with objects within an activity context that included six different rooms (i.e., a storage room and five destination rooms). These data expand upon previous evidence in this area, in that the participants managed to carry out their activity engagement (a) using a relatively large and articulated activity context, (b) delivering the material (boxes) by transporting it to the pertinent destination rooms [20,29,30], and (c) relying on a technology system that did not require research assistants' input throughout the sessions [30]. In light of the new evidence/findings, several considerations may be in order.

First, enabling people to transport boxes with different objects to the pertinent destination rooms might be seen as an important achievement that could have practical and vocational implications. In fact, one might envisage the use of activities such as supplying different rooms with different/appropriate types of material as viable within domestic and vocational (supported employment) contexts [38–40]. The possibility of being successfully involved in those forms of activity independently of staff could thus represent a new perspective for people's futures with expectedly positive consequences for their developmental and social progress and for their quality of life [6,41–45].

Second, the technology system used in the study was accurate in discriminating the boxes with the different objects and activating the encouragement and orientation cues of the rooms where those objects were to be transported and deposited. This role of the technology can be considered crucial to support the performance of people with intellectual and visual disabilities who are unlikely to discriminate many of the objects to be transported and to find the appropriate rooms for them [46–48]. In practice, the technology may be seen as a necessary instrument (a prosthetic means) to help people progress from simply transporting objects to some general destination to distributing them accurately across different (pertinent) destination areas. Using such a prosthetic means in daily contexts would appear to be a realistic prospect.

Third, fixing tags onto the boxes ensured that there was no need to manipulate (attach tags to) the single objects to be transported. This approach was viewed as (a) a practical solution, given that not all objects could be easily fitted with tags (e.g., it could be rather difficult to fit a toothpaste tube or a toothbrush with a tag given the shape and dimensions of the tags), and (b) a time-saving strategy, given that fitting all objects with tags would require a considerable time investment in addition to interfering with the normal use of the objects within the context. Using the boxes was convenient because they allowed the participants to transport several objects at a time. Moreover, the boxes could be recovered after their use and employed across sessions without any additional preparation work or any waste of the tags that were pasted on them.

Fourth, the tag reader used in this study was divided into two sections that were designed to be relatively small so that the participants could wear them without a negative impact on their handling of the boxes [47–49]. A wearable tag reader that automatically proceeds to the identification of the boxes' tags and thus automatically triggers the presentation of instructions and orientation cues may be considered essential for a successful outcome with people like the participants of this study (i.e., people who could have omissions and failures if required to bring a tag reader in contact with the boxes right after collecting them [46,48,50,51].

Fifth, the participants of this study did not have problems wearing the tag reader's components inside their hand and on their wrist. For people who would have problems in doing so, one could find a different position for the tag reader. For example, one could fix it onto the participant's chest. This position would allow the boxes being collected to touch or come close to the tag reader, thus allowing it to identify their tags and consequently activate the presentation of instructions and orientation cues. To ensure the reliable contact (or near contact) of the boxes with the tag reader, one might use boxes larger than those included in this study.

Sixth, while the technology system employed in this study is not a commercially available package, several of its components, such as the smartphone, the mini speakers, and the MacroDroid, are easily accessible and inexpensive, so anyone can purchase them. With regard to the tag reader, it is important to clarify that (a) one of its sections concerns an NFC module that can be readily acquired commercially, and (b) the other section concerns an electronic unit, the design of which can be freely obtained from the authors.

Limitations and Future Research

The main limitations of the study concern the lack of maintenance and generalization data and the lack of assessment of participants' satisfaction and social validation. To counter the first limitation, new studies will have to include follow-up checks to determine performance maintenance over time and also extend the evaluation of the system impact to new settings so as to verify generalization effects (i.e., ascertain whether the system can support the participants' performance within settings not directly involved in the intervention) [52–54].

To counter the second limitation, new studies will need to include an evaluation of participants' satisfaction as part of the assessment process. One of the possible ways to check participants' satisfaction with the sessions could involve the measurement of their indices of happiness (e.g., smiles and other facial or bodily expressions typically associated with happiness) during the sessions with the system and during other (daily) occupational situations [55,56]. A difference in the favor of the sessions would suggest that the participants may have a higher level of satisfaction within those sessions than within conventional occupational situations. A second way to check participants' satisfaction with the sessions may involve the presentation of choice situations in which one of the options is a session with the system and the other option is a daily activity [57,58]. Preference for the session could be taken to suggest that the participants find the sessions more satisfactory than daily activities.

To counter the third limitation, one could apply a social validation procedure in which staff personnel are first asked to watch videos reporting clips of the sessions with the system and then interviewed as to the effectiveness, friendliness, and applicability of the system and the practical/vocational relevance of the participants' performance [59,60]. The interview could also include the use of a conventional questionnaire, such as The System Usability Scale [61,62].

The small number of participants involved might be considered another limitation of this study. In relation to this point, one could make two statements. First, the single-subject research designs used for evaluating the impact of the system appear adequate to support the internal validity of the data reported [63,64]. Second, to determine the external validity of such data, one could rely on single-case replication studies, as well as studies involving both treatment and control groups [65,66].

5. Conclusions

In conclusion, the results show that participants with moderate-to-severe or severe intellectual disabilities and blindness managed to use the technology system to correctly collect, transport, and deposit boxes with objects within an activity context that included six different rooms (i.e., a storage room and five destination rooms). These results, which expand upon previous evidence in the area, appear very encouraging as to the possibility of offering people with significant intellectual disabilities and blindness new occupational opportunities with the potential of being vocationally relevant. Even so, caution is required in drawing conclusions about the robustness and general implications of the findings given the limitations of the study that new research needs to address. New research may also aim to upgrade the technology system so as to make it more easily usable across people and settings.

Author Contributions: Conceptualization, G.E.L.; data curation, G.E.L., G.A., and F.A.; formal analysis, G.E.L., F.P., N.N.S., M.F.O., and J.S.; investigation, G.E.L., G.A., and F.A.; methodology, G.E.L., G.A., F.P., F.A., N.N.S., M.F.O., and J.S.; software, F.P.; validation, G.E.L., G.A., N.N.S., M.F.O., and J.S.; writing—original draft, G.E.L.; writing—review and editing, G.A., F.P., F.A., N.N.S., M.F.O., and J.S. All authors have read and agreed to the published version of the manuscript.

Funding: This research received no external funding.

Institutional Review Board Statement: This study was approved by the Ethics Committee of the Lega F. D'Oro, Osimo (AN), Italy (P090220244). All the procedures performed were in accordance with the ethical standards of the institutional and/or national research committee and with the 1964 Helsinki Declaration and its later amendments or comparable ethical standards.

Informed Consent Statement: Given their intellectual and visual disabilities, the participants could not provide a clear/reliable response as to their interest in the study or read and sign a consent form for it. In view of that, the participants' legal representatives provided written informed consent on their behalf.

Data Availability Statement: The original data contributions presented in the study are reproduced in the graphs of Figures 6 and 7. Datasets are available from the authors on request.

Conflicts of Interest: The authors declare no conflicts of interest. The third author, who developed the tag reader used in this study, makes the design of the reader's electronic circuit available at no cost.

Abbreviations

The following abbreviations are used in this manuscript:

NFC	Near Field Communication
PND	Percentage of Nonoverlapping Data

References

1. Chang, Y.J.; Wang, T.Y. Indoor wayfinding based on wireless sensor networks for individuals with multiple special needs. *Cybern. Syst.* **2010**, *41*, 317–333. [CrossRef]
2. Dijkhuizen, A.; Hilgenkamp, T.I.; Krijnen, W.P.; van der Schans, C.P.; Waninge, A. The impact of visual impairment on the ability to perform activities of daily living for persons with severe/profound intellectual disability. *Res. Dev. Disabil.* **2016**, *48*, 35–42. [CrossRef]
3. Fellinger, J. Intellectual disability and sensory impairment. In *Textbook of Psychiatry for Intellectual Disability and Autism Spectrum Disorder*; Bertelli, M.O., Deb, S., Munir, K., Hassiotis, A., Salvador-Carulla, L., Eds.; Springer: New York, NY, USA, 2022; pp. 849–867. [CrossRef]
4. Jarjoura, W. Disorientation and loss of wayfinding in individuals with congenital blindness and other affecting comorbidities. *Brit. J. Vis. Impair.* **2019**, *37*, 240–247. [CrossRef]
5. Cuturi, L.F.; Aggius-Vella, E.; Campus, C.; Parmiggiani, A.; Gori, M. From science to technology: Orientation and mobility in blind children and adults. *Neurosci. Biobehav. Rev.* **2016**, *71*, 240–251. [CrossRef]
6. Enkelaar, L.; Oosterom-Calo, R.; Zhou, D.; Nijhof, N.; Barakova, E.; Sterkenburg, P. The LEDs move pilot study: The Light Curtain and physical activity and well-being among people with visual and intellectual disabilities. *J. Intellect. Disabil. Res.* **2021**, *65*, 971–988. [CrossRef]
7. Hanzen, G.; Waninge, A.; Vlaskamp, C.; van Nispen, R.M.; van der Putten, A.A. Participation of adults with visual and severe or profound intellectual disabilities: Analysis of individual support plans. *Res. Dev. Disabil.* **2018**, *83*, 132–141. [CrossRef]
8. Lancioni, G.E.; Singh, N.N.; O'Reilly, M.F.; Sigafoos, J.; Campodonico, F.; Zimbaro, C.; Alberti, G.; Trubia, G.; Zagaria, T. Helping people with multiple disabilities manage an assembly task and mobility via technology-regulated sequence cues and contingent stimulation. *Life Span. Disabil.* **2018**, *21*, 143–163.
9. Nair, V.; Olmschenk, G.; Seiple, W.H.; Zhu, Z. ASSIST: Evaluating the usability and performance of an indoor navigation assistant for blind and visually impaired people. *Assist. Technol.* **2022**, *34*, 289–299. [CrossRef]
10. Parker, A. Considering a practical orientation and mobility framework to design communication interventions for people with visual impairments, deafblindness, and multiple disabilities. *Perspect. ASHA Spec. Interest. Groups.* **2017**, *2*, 89. [CrossRef]
11. Desideri, L.; Lancioni, G.; Malavasi, M.; Gherardini, A.; Cesario, L. Step-instruction technology to help people with intellectual and other disabilities perform multistep tasks: A literature review. *J. Dev. Phys. Disabil.* **2021**, *33*, 857–886. [CrossRef]
12. Lancioni, G.E.; Alberti, G.; Filippini, C.; Fiore, A.; Simonetti, C.; Singh, N.N.; O'Reilly, M.F.; Sigafoos, J. Interactive technology to help people with multiple disabilities practice relevant physical responses within an occupational task. *OBM Neurobiol.* **2024**, *8*, 1–15. [CrossRef]
13. Brock, M.E.; Schaefer, J.M.; Seaman, R.L. Self-determination and agency for all: Supporting students with severe disabilities. *Theory Pract.* **2020**, *59*, 162–171. [CrossRef]
14. Gkora, V.; Karabatzaki, Z. Motivation in learning disabilities and the impact of ICTs. *TechHub J.* **2023**, *3*, 14–26. Available online: https://techhubresearch.com/index.php/journal/article/view/79 (accessed on 15 December 2024).
15. Hutzler, Y.; Korsensky, O. Motivational correlates of physical activity in persons with an intellectual disability: A systematic literature review. *J. Intellect. Disabil. Res.* **2010**, *54*, 767–786. [CrossRef]

16. Sahoo, S.; Choudhury, B. Exploring the use of computer vision in assistive technologies for individuals with disabilities: A review. *J. Future Sustain.* **2024**, *4*, 133–148. [CrossRef]
17. Fernandes, H.; Costa, P.; Filipe, V.; Paredes, H.; Barroso, J. A review of assistive spatial orientation and navigation technologies for the visually impaired. *Univ. Access Inf. Soc.* **2019**, *18*, 155–168. [CrossRef]
18. Kuriakose, B.; Shrestha, R.; Sandnes, F.E. Tools and technologies for blind and visually impaired navigation support: A review. *IETE Tech. Rev.* **2020**, *39*, 3–18. [CrossRef]
19. Deverell, L.; Bhowmik, J.; Lau, B.T.; Al Mahmud, A.; Sukunesan, S.; Islam, F.M.A.; McCarthy, C.; Meyer, D. Use of technology by orientation and mobility professionals in Australia and Malaysia before COVID-19. *Disabil. Rehabil. Assist. Technol.* **2020**, *17*, 260–267. [CrossRef]
20. Lancioni, G.E.; Singh, N.N.; O'Reilly, M.F.; Sigafoos, J.; Alberti, G.; Chiariello, V.; Abbatantuono, C.; Taurisano, P.; Desideri, L. Fostering functional occupation and mobility in people with intellectual disability and visual impairment through technology-aided support. *Adv. Neurodev. Disord.* **2023**, *7*, 392–402. [CrossRef]
21. Manzoor, M.; Vimarlund, V. Digital technologies for social inclusion of individuals with disabilities. *Health Technol.* **2018**, *8*, 377–390. [CrossRef]
22. Chavers, T.N.; Schlosser, R.W.; Cheng, C.; Koul, R. Effects of interventions involving speech output technologies on communication outcomes for individuals with developmental disabilities: A scoping review. *Am. J. Speech-Lang. Pathol.* **2022**, *31*, 2248–2267. [CrossRef] [PubMed]
23. Lancioni, G.E.; Singh, N.N.; O'Reilly, M.F.; Sigafoos, J.; Alberti, G.; Troccoli, O.; Orlando, I.; Ricci, C. Enabling people with intellectual and other disabilities to make verbal requests using cardboard chips with mini objects or pictures and a smartphone. *Front. Rehabil. Sci.* **2023**, *4*, 1257493. [CrossRef]
24. Ripat, J.; Verdonck, M.; Gacek, C.; McNicol, S. A qualitative metasynthesis of the meaning of speech-generating devices for people with complex communication needs. *Augment. Altern. Comm.* **2018**, *35*, 69–79. [CrossRef]
25. Burns, J.; Carter, A.; Draper, S.; Foad, A. Engaging and sustaining people with intellectual disabilities in physical activity: A narrative review of existing evidence. *Int. J. Dev. Disabil.* **2022**, *70*, 803–813. [CrossRef] [PubMed]
26. Hassan, N.M.; Landorf, K.B.; Shields, N.; Munteanu, S.E. Effectiveness of interventions to increase physical activity in individuals with intellectual disabilities: A systematic review of randomised controlled trials. *J. Intellec. Disabil. Res.* **2019**, *63*, 168–191. [CrossRef]
27. Rotta, K.; Raaymakers, A.; Poling, A. Using positive reinforcement to increase the physical activity of individuals with developmental disabilities: A review. *J. Dev. Phys. Disabil.* **2023**, *35*, 551–575. [CrossRef]
28. Savage, M.N.; Clark, T.A.; Baffoe, E.; Candelaria, A.E.; Aneke, L.; Gonzalez, R.; Al Enizi, A.; Anguita-Otero, M.; Edwards-Adams, K.; Grandberry, L.; et al. Technology-based physical health interventions for adults with intellectual disability: A scoping review. *J. Dev. Phys. Disabil.* **2024**, *36*, 757–792. [CrossRef]
29. Lancioni, G.E.; Singh, N.N.; O'Reilly, M.F.; Sigafoos, J.; Alberti, G.; Chiariello, V.; Campodonico, F.; Desideri, L. Technology-aided spatial cues, instructions, and preferred stimulation for supporting people with intellectual and visual disabilities in their occupational engagement and mobility: Usability study. *JMIR Rehabil. Assist. Technol.* **2021**, *8*, e33481. [CrossRef]
30. Lancioni, G.E.; Alberti, G.; Filippini, C.; Singh, N.N.; O'Reilly, M.F.; Sigafoos, J.; Orlando, I.; Desideri, L. A technology system to help people with intellectual disability and blindness find room destinations during indoor traveling: Case series study. *JMIR Rehabil. Assist. Technol.* **2024**, *11*, e65680. [CrossRef]
31. Balboni, G.; Belacchi, C.; Bonichini, S.; Coscarelli, A. *Vineland Adaptive Behavior Scales*, 2nd ed.; Vineland-II; Standardizzazione Italiana: Florence, Italy, 2016.
32. Sparrow, S.S.; Cicchetti, D.V.; Balla, D.A. *Vineland Adaptive Behavior Scales*, 2nd ed.; Vineland II; Pearson: New York, NY, USA, 2005.
33. Etikan, I.; Musa, S.A.; Alkassim, R.S. Comparison of convenience sampling and purposive sampling. *Am. J. Theor. Appl. Stat.* **2016**, *5*, 1–4. [CrossRef]
34. Pezzuoli, F.; Corona, D.; Corradini, M.L. Improvements in a wearable device for sign language translation. In *Advances in Human Factors in Wearable Technologies and Game Design*; Ahram, T., Ed.; Advances in Intelligent Systems and Computing; Springer International Publishing: Champaign, IL, USA, 2020; Volume 973, pp. 70–81. [CrossRef]
35. Ledford, J.R.; Gast, D.L. *Single Case Research Methodology: Applications in Special Education and Behavioral Sciences*, 3rd ed.; Routledge: New York, NY, USA, 2018.
36. Strain, P.; Fox, L.; Barton, E.E. On expanding the definition and use of procedural fidelity. *Res. Pract. Pract. Pers. Sev. Disabil.* **2021**, *46*, 173–183. [CrossRef]
37. Parker, R.I.; Vannest, K.J.; Davis, J.L. Effect size in single-case research: A review of nine nonoverlap techniques. *Behav. Modif.* **2011**, *35*, 303–322. [CrossRef]

38. Ashley, D.; Fossey, E.; Bigby, C. The home environments and occupational engagement of people with intellectual disabilities in supported living. *Br. J. Occup. Ther.* **2019**, *82*, 698–709. [CrossRef]
39. Cannella-Malone, H.I.; Schaefer, J.M. A review of research on teaching people with significant disabilities vocational skills. *Career Dev. Transit. Except. Individ.* **2017**, *40*, 67–78. [CrossRef]
40. Luthra, R. Young adults with intellectual disability who are not in employment, education, or daily activities: Family situation and its relation to occupational status. *Cogent Soc. Sci.* **2019**, *5*, 1622484. [CrossRef]
41. Beadle-Brown, J.; Leigh, J.; Whelton, B.; Richardson, L.; Beecham, J.; Baumker, T.; Bradshaw, J. Quality of life and quality of support for people with severe intellectual disability and complex needs. *J. Appl. Res. Intellect. Disabil.* **2016**, *29*, 409–421. [CrossRef]
42. Hobeika, L.; Ghilain, M.; Schiaratura, L.; Lesafre, M.; HuventGrelle, D.; Puisieux, F.; Samson, S. Socio-emotional and motor engagement during musical activities in older adults with major neurocognitive impairment. *Sci. Rep.* **2021**, *11*, 15291. [CrossRef]
43. Kocman, A.; Weber, G. Job satisfaction, quality of work life and work motivation in employees with intellectual disability: A systematic review. *J. Appl. Res. Intellect. Disabil.* **2018**, *31*, 1–22. [CrossRef]
44. Mumbard-Adam, C.; Vicente, E.; Balboni, G. Self-determination and quality of life of people with intellectual and developmental disabilities: Past, present, and future of close research paths. *J. Policy Pract. Intellect. Disabil.* **2024**, *21*, e12460. [CrossRef]
45. Wehmeyer, M.L. The importance of self-determination to the quality of life of people with intellectual disability: A perspective. *Int. J. Environ. Res. Public. Health.* **2020**, *17*, 7121. [CrossRef]
46. Evmenova, A.S.; Graff, H.J.; Genaro Motti, V.; Giwa-Lawal, K.; Zheng, H. Designing a wearable technology intervention to support young adults with intellectual and developmental disabilities in inclusive postsecondary academic environments. *J. Spec. Educ. Technol.* **2019**, *34*, 92–105. [CrossRef]
47. Filippini, C.; Lancioni, G.E.; Alberti, G.; Pezzuoli, F.; Ceccarani, P. A technology aid to help people with blindness and moderate intellectual disability retrieve common objects from storage units: A proof-of-concept study. *Sensors* **2024**, *24*, 4453. [CrossRef] [PubMed]
48. Abdi, S.; Kitsara, I.; Hawley, M.S.; de Witte, L.P. Emerging technologies and their potential for generating new assistive technologies. *Assist. Technol.* **2021**, *33* (Suppl. S1), 17–26. [CrossRef]
49. Nelson, E.C.; Sools, A.M.; Vollenbroek-Hutten, M.M.R.; Verhagen, T.; Noordzij, M.L. Embodiment of wearable technology: Qualitative longitudinal study. *JMIR Mhealth Uhealth* **2020**, *8*, e16973. [CrossRef]
50. Johnson, K.R.; Blaskowitz, M.G.; Mahoney, W.J. Technology for adults with intellectual disability: Secondary analysis of a scoping review. *Can. J. Occup. Ther.* **2023**, *90*, 395–404. [CrossRef]
51. Mishra, S.; Laplante-Lévesque, A.; Barbareschi, G.; Witte, L.D.; Abdi, S.; Spann, A.; Khasnabis, C.; Allen, M. Assistive technology needs, access and coverage, and related barriers and facilitators in the WHO European region: A scoping review. *Disabil. Rehabil. Assist. Technol.* **2024**, *19*, 474–485. [CrossRef] [PubMed]
52. Cooper, J.O.; Heron, T.E.; Heward, W.L. *Applied Behavior Analysis*, 3rd ed.; Pearson: New York, NY, USA, 2019.
53. Pennington, B.; Simacek, J.; McComas, J.; McMaster, K.; Elmquist, M. Maintenance and generalization in functional behavior assessment/behavior intervention plan literature. *J. Behav. Educ.* **2019**, *28*, 27–53. [CrossRef]
54. Pierce, W.D.; Cheney, C.D. *Behavior Analysis and Learning*, 6th ed.; Routledge: New York, NY, USA, 2017.
55. Holyfield, C.; Lorah, E. Effects of high-tech versus low-tech AAC on indices of happiness for school-aged children with multiple disabilities. *J. Dev. Phys. Disabil.* **2022**, *35*, 209–225. [CrossRef]
56. Ramey, D.; Healy, O.; McEnaney, E. Defining and measuring indices of happiness and unhappiness in children diagnosed with autism spectrum disorder. *Behav. Anal. Pract.* **2023**, *16*, 194–209. [CrossRef]
57. Frounfelker, S.A.; Bartone, A. The importance of dignity and choice for people assessed as having intellectual disabilities. *J. Intellect. Disabil.* **2021**, *25*, 490–506. [CrossRef]
58. Stancliffe, R.J.; Wehmeyer, M.L.; Shogren, K.A.; Abery, B.H. *Choice, Preference, and Disability*; Springer: New York, NY, USA, 2020.
59. Stasolla, F.; Caffò, A.O.; Perilli, V.; Boccasini, A.; Damiani, R.; D'Amico, F. Assistive technology for promoting adaptive skills of children with cerebral palsy: Ten cases evaluation. *Disabil. Rehabil. Assist. Technol.* **2019**, *14*, 489–502. [CrossRef] [PubMed]
60. Worthen, D.; Luiselli, J.K. Comparative effects and social validation of support strategies to promote mindfulness practices among high school students. *Child. Fam. Behav. Ther.* **2019**, *41*, 221–236. [CrossRef]
61. Lewis, J.R. The System Usability Scale: Past, preset, and future. *Int. J. Hum-Comp. Inter.* **2018**, *34*, 577–590. [CrossRef]
62. Borsci, S.; Federici, S.; Lauriola, M. On the dimensionality of the System Usability Scale: A test of alternative measurement models. *Cogn. Process.* **2009**, *10*, 193–197. [CrossRef] [PubMed]
63. Kazdin, A.E. *Single-Case Research Designs: Methods for Clinical and Applied Settings*, 3rd ed.; Oxford University Press: New York, NY, USA, 2020.

64. Walker, S.G.; Carr, J.E. Generality of findings from single-case designs: It's not all about the "N". *Behav. Anal. Pract.* **2021**, *14*, 991–995. [CrossRef]
65. Coiera, E.; Tong, H.L. Replication studies in the clinical decision support literature–frequency, fidelity, and impact. *J. Am. Med. Inform. Assoc.* **2021**, *28*, 1815–1825. [CrossRef]
66. Tanious, R.; Manolov, R.; Onghena, P.; Vlaeyen, J.W.S. Single-case experimental designs: The importance of randomization and replication. *Nat. Rev. Methods Primers* **2024**, *34*, 100511. [CrossRef]

technologies

MDPI

Article

A Study on Chatbot Development Using No-Code Platforms by People with Disabilities for Their Peers at a Sheltered Workshop

Sara Hamideh Kerdar [1,2,*], Britta Marleen Kirchhoff [1], Lars Adolph [1] and Liane Bächler [2]

[1] Federal Institute of Occupational Safety and Health, 44149 Dortmund, Germany; kirchhoff.britta@baua.bund.de (B.M.K.); adolph.lars@baua.bund.de (L.A.)
[2] Department of Rehabilitation Sciences, TU Dortmund University, 44227 Dortmund, Germany; liane.baechler@tu-dortmund.de
* Correspondence: hamidehkerdar.sara@baua.bund.de

Abstract: No-code (NC) platforms empower individuals without IT experience to create tailored applications and websites. While these platforms are accessible to a broader audience, their usability for people with disabilities remains underexplored. This study investigated whether, with targeted training, people with disabilities could effectively use NC platforms to develop customized tools for their workplace, and whether these tools would be adopted by their peers. Conducted in collaboration with a sheltered workshop in Germany, the study had three phases. Phase I involved a brainstorming session with employees, which shaped the study design and product development. In Phase II, six participants with disabilities received a one-week training to develop chatbots. Phase III implemented the chatbots in the workshop. In Phase II, each participant successfully developed four chatbots, which increased the participants' skills and motivation. Based on the phase III results, users rated the developed chatbots highly (the System Usability Scale (SUS) questionnaire was delivered in the form of a chatbot), indicating their user-friendliness (M = 88.9, SD = 11.2). This study suggests that with appropriate training, individuals with disabilities can use NC platforms to create impactful, customized tools that are user-friendly and accessible to their peers.

Keywords: low-code/no-code; LCNC; inclusion; disability; work; citizen developer; sheltered workshop; technology; AI

1. Introduction

The development of digital technologies, such as apps and websites, requires substantial time and financial resources. However, low-code and no-code (LCNC) platforms have opened new doors to digitalization, allowing individuals, known as 'citizen developers', with limited or no IT skills to develop apps and websites and customize them according to their needs [1,2]. While no-code (NC) platforms offer ready-made templates and functions that can be modified to some degree, low-code (LC) platforms provide more customization options, requiring some coding for greater flexibility [3,4]. Although LCNC platforms provide "lightweight" digital products, they open new doors for business and industry by offering many opportunities [2,5], such as e-commerce, internal and external communication, workflow management, education, finance, and healthcare. Given the rapid growth and adoption of these platforms in the marketplace [5], more companies are looking for candidates with LCNC skills [2]. Such skills could help companies reduce their costs and dependency on IT specialists [6] and find faster solutions to their immediate needs and requirements. For example, such skills enable employees to create their own digital tools based on the needs of their team or even their organization [5], opening up new opportunities for job crafting.

Even though LCNC platforms are attracting attentions in the job market, the literature stays limited on this subject [2]. While many articles focus on the concept of LCNC, its potentials, and challenges (e.g., ref. [7]), not many studies have focused on their actual implementations in the field. Rajaram et al. [8] used Microsoft Power Apps (a LC platform) to develop an educational application, where both learning and examination were possible. On the subject of education, Mew and Field [9] used an LC platform for further support of the students in a project management course. The impact and introduction of LCNC platforms has been studied in different industries, such as construction [3] or manufacturing [6], showing their potential to enhance digitalization. These platforms, coupled with artificial intelligence (AI) or Augmented Reality (AR), could facilitate work-related processes, such as inventory [10] or job status tracking [11]. In a case study, Takahashi et al. [12] explored the impact of LC tools on 'Diversity, Equity and Inclusion' within a corporate context. Employees of a company with no existing IT expertise learned and developed several applications for their organization, mostly focused on "knowledge sharing". They concluded that, while LC platforms have the potential to harness internal skills to reduce workload and costs, creating a supportive environment is essential.

People with disabilities have less employment possibilities [13]. In Germany, sheltered workshops for disabled people offer the possibility to learn and perform simple tasks, taking a rehabilitation center role. However, the transition rates from the sheltered workshops to the primary labor market remains below 1% [14]. Even though it is argued that many of these individuals are not able to make this transfer due to the demands of the general labor market and their disabilities [15], learning new (digital) skills could facilitate their transition and opportunities. Technologies used at work should demonstrate a high level of fit between the requirements of the task, the characteristics of the users, and the technology. According to the Task-Technology Fit (TTF) Model developed by Goodhue and Thompson, they are also influenced by social norms and facilitating conditions, among other things [16]. Positive impact is possible when technology is aligned with the needs of employees and the task at hand. With the TTF Model in mind, LCNC has the potential to either increase the opportunities for people with disabilities (e.g., cognitive or multiple disabilities) to transition to other jobs, or it could increase their job variety and motivation, and the opportunity to transfer on knowledge to others (e.g., peers) through the design of applications. People with disabilities are also experts in their own field and through LCNC they could have the opportunity to develop job aids (e.g., AI-based apps or chatbots) that are highly suited to their tasks. However, the potential of these platforms for employees with disabilities, especially those working in sheltered workshops, has not yet been studied.

Advancements in artificial intelligence have reshaped human–computer interaction, with chatbots playing a central role. These digital assistants engage in natural language conversations, providing instant support, improving productivity, and enhancing user experience [17]. While developing AI solutions such as chatbots could be costly [18], NC platforms provide more cost-effective alternatives, offering pre-coded tools that make chatbot development accessible even to individuals without coding expertise [19]. The use of chatbots for people with disabilities has been studied in different contexts. For example, Mateos-Sanchez et al. [20] used a chatbot to teach communication skills to people with intellectual disabilities. In a systematic review on the use of chatbots for people with disabilities, only "15 of 192 papers" included the target group in their studies [21]. In a report on AI and occupational inclusion, Touzet [22] highlights 142 AI-based technologies which could assist people with disabilities in the workplace. She argues that more than 75% of these technologies would not be possible without AI. She further concludes that AI has the potential to save money and becomes more easily implemented with different types of assistive technologies (AT). In a review, Beudt et al. [23] found that the majority of AI solutions focus on sensory disabilities (i.e., visual and hearing disabilities) and cognitive disabilities are to some extent ignored. However, similar to other studies, they conclude that AI increases the chance of vocational participation for people with disabilities. Given the benefits of chatbots for people with disabilities and the advantages of NC platforms in facilitating their development, the question remains whether these platforms can support people with disabilities in both creating and utilizing chatbots.

LCNC platforms are rapidly expanding, becoming crucial tools for future innovation [24]. However, questions remain regarding their accessibility for people with disabilities, their alignment with users' roles and needs, and the new opportunities they may offer. This study seeks to bridge this gap by exploring the role of people with disabilities in sheltered workshops as citizen developers in their workplace. Specifically, it aims to address the following aspects:

(a) From the perspective of product development as citizen developers: Are LCNC platforms accessible and usable for people with disabilities working in sheltered workshops? Additionally, what types of training could further support them in utilizing these platforms effectively?
(b) From the end users' perspective: Are the products developed using LCNC platforms (chatbots in this study) accessible and user-friendly for individuals with disabilities working in sheltered workshops?

This study seeks to explore how LCNC platforms can be effectively leveraged to enhance digital and vocational inclusion, fostering greater participation in sheltered work environments.

The remainder of this paper is organized as follows: Section 2 provides an overview of the research methods, including details of the questionnaires used, the study setting, the platform and equipment used, and the phases of the study. Section 3 presents both qualitative and quantitative results. The article concludes with Section 4, which discusses the findings, and Section 5, which presents the conclusions of the study.

2. Materials and Methods

This study used a mixed methods approach. Mixed method studies provide a deeper understanding of research questions by incorporating multiple perspectives [25–27]. This approach is especially valuable for detecting new insights and identifying directions for future research [27]. Therefore, since no previous studies have explored the possibilities of NC platforms for people with disabilities as citizen developers in the work environment, an exploratory approach was first adopted to assess whether these platforms could be used by people with disabilities and how training would assist them. Additionally, a quantitative approach was employed, in which participants answered a series of questions before and after the training to account for individual differences and investigate the individual impact of training and skill acquisition.

This study was ethically evaluated and approved by the ethic commission of the Federal Institute for Occupational Safety and Health (German: Bundesanstalt für Arbeitsschutz und Arbeitsmedizin (BAuA)).

To clarify the structure of the study, the participants, questionnaires used, and study phases are described in detail below.

2.1. Participants

The participants in this study were recruited from a sheltered workshop in Germany and were divided into two groups:

(1) Participants who were trained in the use of the NC platform and developed chatbots (hereafter referred to as Developers). These individuals attended the training sessions for a week at the BAuA. A supervisor female—hereafter referred to as Supervisor 1 accompanied the participants for the first three days and another supervisor male—hereafter referred to as Supervisor 2 accompanied participants for the rest of the week. The change in supervisors was due to the fact that Supervisor 1 worked only part-time at the sheltered workshop and could not be available for the whole week.

(2) Other sheltered workshop employees with disabilities who use the developed chatbots in their daily work at the sheltered workshop (hereafter referred to as End Users).

2.2. Questionnaires (Only for the Developers)

Based on the TTF Model, this study examined three core elements—person, technology, and task characteristics—because the alignment of these factors is believed to influence the effectiveness of technologies such as no-code (NC) platforms. To assess each of these core elements, validated questionnaires in German were used. The questions were translated into simpler language. This made them easier to understand for the participants. The questionnaires were printed with each question on a single page to avoid information overload. As all the questionnaires used a Likert scale for their answers, emojis were also used for better understanding [24] (See Figure 1 for an example). The following questionnaires for each core component of the TTF were used.

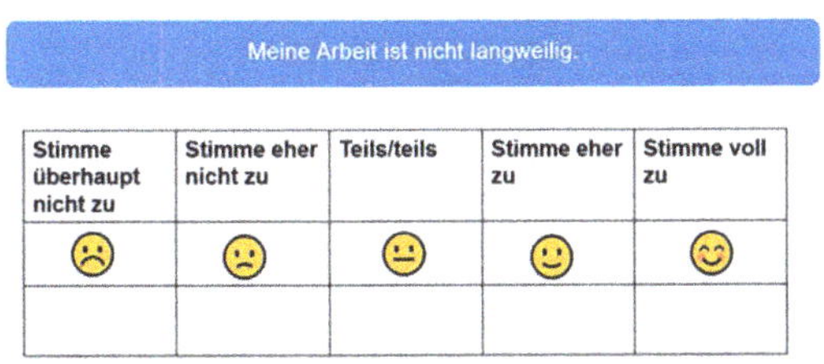

Figure 1. An example of use of emojis for questionnaires (the translation of the question is: 'My work is not boring'. The answers are rated on a scale from 'Strongly Disagree' to 'Strongly Agree').

For the Component "Task"

To evaluate the characteristics of tasks, the German version of The Work Design Questionnaire (WDQ) [28,29] was used. The WDQ items are divided into four main categories: task characteristics, knowledge characteristics, social characteristics, and work context. Each main category has between four and five subcategories, addressing a wide range of subjects, such as ergonomics, social support, and information processing. For the purposes of this study, only the following items were included, as the remaining ones were not relevant to the participants' work tasks or the components of the research: Task Variety and Feedback from Job (from category task characteristic), Problem Solving and Skill Variety (from the category knowledge characteristics), Equipment Use (from the category work context). In total, 18 items were included.

For the Component "Technology"

The Digital Technology Acceptance Scale (DTAS): DTAS evaluates individuals' acceptance of digital technology with 13 items on a 5-point Likert scale (1 = not at all applicable,

5 = fully applicable). The questionnaire is divided into four categories: Ease of Use, Perceived Usefulness, Attitude towards Usage, and Behavioral Intention to Use [30,31].

System Usability Scale (SUS): The German version of the System Usability Scale (SUS) was used to evaluate the usability of the used NC platform (Landbot: https://landbot.io/, accessed on 17 June 2024) from the Developers' point of view [32,33]. The SUS has 10 items with a 5-point Likert scale (1 = strongly disagree, 5 = strongly agree). The score ranges from 0 to 100, with a benchmark (mean score) of 68 [34]. Scores of 100–85 are considered 'the best imaginable', scores of 84–73 'excellent', scores of 72–53 'good', scores of 52–38 'ok/fair', scores of 37–24 'poor', and scores of 25–0 'the worst imaginable' [35,36].

For the Component "Person"

Scale for measuring professional self-efficacy (German: berufliche Selbstwirksamkeitserwartung (BSW-5-Rev)) [37]: The BSW-5-Rev has five items with a four-point scale (1 = strongly disagree, 4 = strongly agree) and measures motivational factors and skills related to occupational self-efficacy.

Technology commitment (German: Kurzskala Technikbereitschaft (TB)) [38]: This 12-item, 5-point Likert scale (1 = strongly disagree, 5 = strongly agree) measures willingness to use technology and is divided into three categories: technology acceptance, technology competence, and technology control convictions.

2.3. Study Phases

The study took place in three main phases, which are explained in this manuscript as follows:

Phase I: study development and brainstorming (i.e., pre-study to adjust ideas tailored to the needs of the sheltered workshop).

Phase II: product development.

Phase III: implementation of the developed products in the sheltered workshop.

In the following sections, the study's phases will be explained, detailing the methodology and data collection. For better understanding, Figure 2 provides an overview of the study.

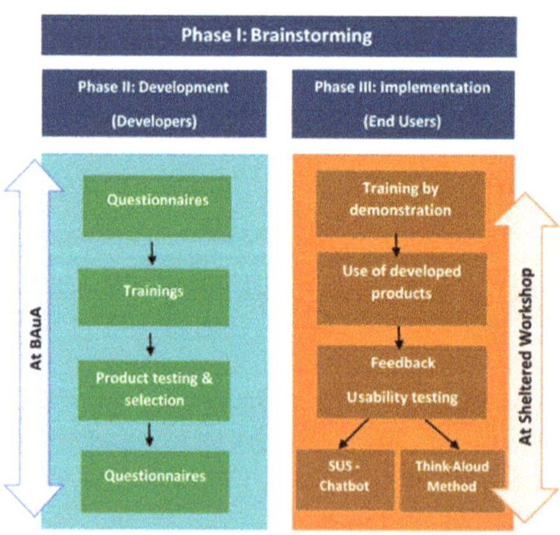

Figure 2. Study overview.

2.3.1. Phase I: Pre-Study

Previous research indicates that successful technology implementation depends on aligning the technology's functionality with the specific requirements of tasks, rather than forcing tasks to adapt to the technology [16,39]. Therefore, in order to adjust the research idea to the specific needs of the sheltered workshop, several steps were taken.

Step 1: Introduction of NC Platforms to the Sheltered Workshop

First, the researchers introduced the concept of LCNC to the sheltered workshop, explaining its functionalities and providing relevant examples. Following an expressed interest in developing the idea further, two field observations were conducted at different locations. The goal of these visits was to gain a deeper understanding of the variety of tasks and technologies used in the sheltered workshops, which primarily involve assembly of products, laundry, catering, and similar activities. The focus of these visits was to engage with the supervisors about the technologies in use, the tasks performed, the challenges faced, and the areas where additional support is needed.

Step 2: Collaborative Brainstorming with Employees and Supervisors in the Sheltered Workshops—Identifying Requirements and Selecting the Product and Platform

Recognizing the importance of directly asking the target group about their needs and desired support, a meeting was held with the staff of the sheltered workshops. In a large hall, employees with disabilities and their supervisors voluntarily participated in a brainstorming session. Around 20 employees and 3 supervisors were asked to consider areas where they needed support or where technology could be helpful. Employees were grouped into teams based on proximity to where they were sitting and exchanged ideas for about 15 min, during which the researchers and the supervisors encouraged them to think by asking them questions regarding what they do, what they would like to have to facilitate their work, etc. The presence of the supervisors was important to facilitate communication, to encourage employees to share their ideas, and to attend to them when assistance was needed. The teams then presented their ideas and all of them were collected on a board. The ideas were read aloud, and participants voted on the most important ones by raising their hands. The ideas with the most votes were selected by the researchers for the study's tasks.

Step 3: Selection of Chatbots for the Study

The choice of a platform for this study was guided by two key considerations. First, the LCNC platform needed to be user-friendly and accessible for the Developers. Second, the final solution (product developed by the Developers) had to be suitable for the specific needs of sheltered workshops while aligning with the requirements of the End Users. Therefore, based on the results of the brainstorming session that identified the needs of sheltered workshops, along with literature supporting the effectiveness of chatbots for the target group (see Section 1: Introduction), chatbots were selected as the product for development. To determine the most suitable platform, various options were evaluated based on their simplicity, ease of use, privacy policies, and features. Given the sensitivity of the data and feedback from the ethics committee, the selection was narrowed to primarily EU-based platforms. As a result, the EU-based NC platform Landbot was chosen for chatbot development.

Step 4: Recruitment

Landbot was presented to the spokesperson (Supervisor 1) of the sheltered workshop to assist with participant recruitment. The supervisor was informed of the inclusion criteria: (1) participation was voluntary, (2) participants must be cognitively capable of logical reasoning, (3) participants should be able to use a mouse and keyboard, and (4) participants must not have severe visual impairment or blindness (as some of the features, such as drag and drop, would have been inaccessible for them). The supervisor then privately spoke to the employees meeting these criteria, explaining the study's methods and aims. Ultimately, six participants voluntarily agreed to participate, with their demographic information presented in Table 1. The disability descriptions are provided by the sheltered workshops based on official medical diagnoses. Participants did not have any training or experience in developing programs or using LCNC platforms. However, all of them had experience working with tablets, smartphones, laptops, and search engines. Additionally, the sheltered workshop staff assess participants' education levels based on their cognitive and physical abilities, determining their eligibility for vocational training at one of the following levels [34]:

- Task-oriented qualification (German: tätigkeitsorientierte Qualifizierung): Focuses on skills required for various tasks across one or more work areas.
- Workplace-oriented qualification (German: arbeitsplatzorientierte Qualifizierung): Focuses on skills needed for specific workplaces within a work area.
- Field-oriented qualification (German: berufsfeldorientierte Qualifizierung): Covers all skills required in a particular work area of the workshop.
- Profession-oriented qualification (German: berufsbildorientierte Qualifizierung): Follows the content of a recognized professional occupation.

Table 1. Developers' demographic information.

Participant	Age (Years)	Gender	Education *	Disability	Tasks at the Sheltered Workshop
P1	18	Female	Field-oriented qualification	Physical and developmental disability	Packaging and assembly of products
P2	19	Male	Workplace-oriented qualification	Intellectual and developmental disability	Packaging and assembly of products
P3	20	Male	Workplace-oriented qualification	Intellectual disability	Packaging and assembly of products
P4	23	Female	Workplace-oriented qualification	Cognitive disability	Packaging and assembly of products
P5	27	Female	Field-oriented qualification	Intellectual disability	Packaging and assembly of products
P6	20	Male	Workplace-oriented qualification	Intellectual and developmental disability	Housekeeping Department

* The education categories are detailed in the Recruitment section (Step 4).

2.3.2. Phase II: Product Development—Developers

Prior to the study, Supervisor 1 read and explained the study information and consent form to the participants. Participants also took home a paper version so that their legal guardians (if applicable) could sign the documents.

For the training week (June 2024), participants met as usual at the sheltered workshop and then used a transfer bus to come together at the study site at the BAuA. Except for one participant who was absent on Day 2 due to illness and another on Day 4 due to missing the bus, all participants attended the training each day.

Setting

The study took place in a training room at the BAuA, designed to accommodate up to 12 participants. For the training session, there were 6 participants, each equipped with an ergonomic table, a chair and a laptop with a mouse. Given the benefits of pair work in software development (e.g., improved quality and time efficiency [40]) and the advantages of team work for people with disabilities [41], the participants were grouped into three pairs. Each pair shared a tablet for accessing training instructions while working independently on their laptops. They assisted each other as needed, and if one participant finished early, they waited for their partner to complete their tasks. In case of difficulties, team members attempted to help each other, and if they could not resolve the issue, the researchers provided indirect assistance by prompting them to identify the problem and possible solutions. If participants still struggled, the researchers would demonstrate where the issue lay and how to resolve it.

Training Material (For Three Pre-Defined Chatbots)

Based on the results of the brainstorming conducted during the pre-study phase (see Section 2.3.1. Step 2) three tasks for three independent chatbots were designed (hereafter referred to as pre-defined chatbots). The chatbots included a Vacation chatbot, a Suggestion Box chatbot, and an online Cookbook chatbot. The researchers designed the conversation flow of the chatbots, defining the questions, responses, and logical progression based on user inputs, ensuring that the chatbots dynamically guide users to different questions depending on their specific answers. Instructions for using the platform to develop these three chatbots were prepared and installed on tablets. PowerPoint was used to develop the instructions, with each slide representing a step in the process. Once participants successfully completed a step, they moved on to the next. The instructions began with screenshots of the platform, accompanied by minimal information explaining the tasks (see Figure 3 for an example). Towards the end of the instructions, or where the process was complicated, videos were prepared where the task and information were again explained using arrows and minimal explanation. It is worth noting that, as will be explained later in Section 3, a fourth chatbot (Sickness Registration) was developed spontaneously within the same week of training, without any instructional guidance. To provide a clearer understanding of the training sessions, Figure 4 presents a detailed overview of each training day.

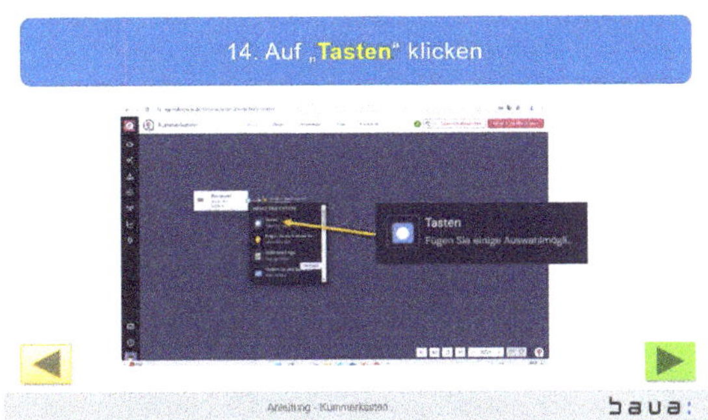

Figure 3. An example of using pictograms for the training instructions (the translation of the instruction title is '14. Click on the "Button"'. Additionally, the screenshot shows the task of clicking on "Tasten" in German, which means "Button" in English, instructing the user to select certain options).

2.3.3. Phase III: Implementation in the Sheltered Workshop

A meeting was organized with the sheltered workshops to present the chatbots developed by the team during the training week. The development team expressed interest in showcasing their chatbots, demonstrating their functionality and potential use cases. In July 2024, the research team, development team, and interested employees from the sheltered workshop gathered in a large hall. Slides introducing what a chatbot is and its applications were displayed on a large screen. The development team then presented live demonstrations of the chatbot flows, with both researchers and development team members available to answer questions from the audience. Presented employees were also informed that they could use the chatbots at any time, using the iPads and tablets available in the sheltered workshop. With the assistance of Supervisor 1, five employees from the sheltered workshop, who had attended the live demonstration, were recruited to test the chatbots immediately afterward. Three researchers conducted interviews with one-to-two participants each, using the think-aloud method [42,43], where participants verbalized their thoughts. Afterward, they completed the SUS questionnaire for the chatbots they tested, with each participant testing two-to-three chatbots.

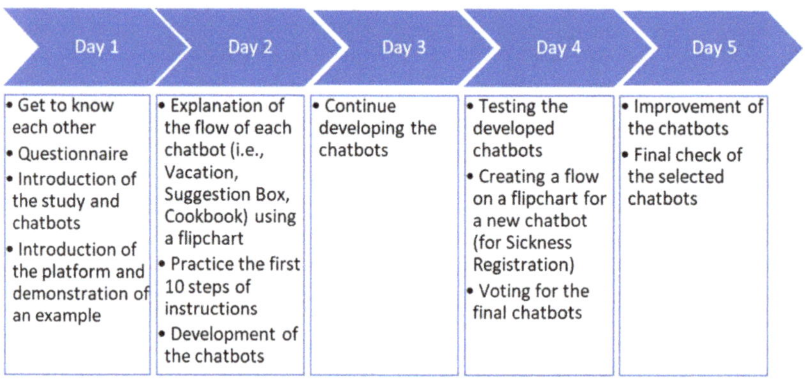

Figure 4. Overview of training days.

At the time of writing, the chatbots are actively being used in the sheltered workshops. The SUS questions are answered at different intervals, based on the availability of Supervisor 1 and participants who have interacted with the chatbots. The SUS questionnaire is presented in a chatbot format, accessible on iPads and tablets available at the workshops. Upon the supervisor's request, employees independently and anonymously answer the questions, without needing the research team present. This approach is effective because participants are familiar with the chatbot interface.

The sheltered workshops have two iPads, with an additional tablet loaned by the research team for the study's duration. One tablet is designated for the online Cookbook chatbot, used exclusively by the housekeeping department, which manages cooking and recipes. For the Sickness Registration (SR) chatbot, small business card-sized flyers with QR codes were printed and distributed for employees to take home. The QR code directs users to the SR chatbot and includes a reminder to use it only for real cases, making it easier to report sickness from home. The remaining chatbots are installed on the other iPads and are accessible at familiar locations within the workshop. To ensure continued use, flyers with QR codes were printed and placed at main stations or distributed among different groups, encouraging employees to use the chatbots.

3. Results

The results related to the Developers and the End Users will be reported in separate sections (Section 3.1. Results—Developers and Section 3.2. Results—End Users).

3.1. Results—Developers

3.1.1. Qualitative Results

Day 1: The first day started with introductions, first the research team and the study, followed by the participants. Then, the questionnaires were distributed among the participants and the supervisor read the questions aloud and explained them if it was unclear to the participants. The researchers then introduced LCNC, including basic knowledge, such as what coding is, along with some examples of their platforms' functionalities. As none of the participants knew what a chatbot was, further explanations, using pictures and videos with examples were given. The pre-defined chatbots were then introduced (see Methods section—chatbots). The schedule for the week was further explained and questions were answered. After the lunch break, the researchers continued to explain important terms, such as what a block, search engine, or drag and drop function and so on are.

To practice and clarify a flow to develop a chatbot, an example was given of how a chatbot could be useful for the sheltered workshop's website. The researchers carried out a brainstorming session with the participants to decide what functions (questions and answers) this chatbot should offer. Based on these ideas, a live demonstration of how to develop a chatbot on Landbot was given. For this purpose, a laptop was connected to a large screen in the room where all participants could watch the demonstration. A researcher demonstrated step by step how to use the platform to develop this chatbot. In this phase, the participants did not practice on their laptops, but only observed how it functioned. Questions were answered and at the end of the day the participants were informed that they would start learning to develop the chatbots the next day.

Day 2: On the second day, the session began with a brief recap of the previous day, without revisiting the platform and its functionalities. Using a flipchart, the flow of the three pre-defined chatbots was outlined, emphasizing the importance of pre-defining key elements during development, such as the questions and corresponding answers. Participants were then invited to provide suggestions, which were incorporated into the chatbot flows, though the core instructions remained unchanged. After presenting each chatbot, participants expressed interest in specific projects and were subsequently divided into three groups based on their preferences.

In order for participants to learn how to use the instructions on the tablet, the first 10 slides were practiced together. Once again, the slides were shown on the room's large screen and, one slide at a time, the participants repeated the step on the tablet and performed the task on their laptops. For example, first slide showed how to open Firefox and second slide showed how to Google search Landbot. Afterwards, participants were asked to work on their own. Table 2 shows the groups and the chatbots they developed on each day.

Table 2. Order of chatbot developments in each group.

	Members	Day 2	Day 3	Day 4
Group 1	P1 and P6	Chatbot 1: Vacation Chatbot 2: Suggestion Box	Chatbot 1: Vacation Chatbot 2: Cookbook	Chatbot 1: Sickness Registration (SR) Chatbot 2: SR
Group 2	P2 and P3	Chatbot 1: Cookbook Chatbot 2: Vacation	Chatbot 1: Vacation Chatbot 2: Suggestion Box	Chatbot 1: SR Chatbot 2: SR
Group 3 *	P4 and P5	Chatbot 1: Suggestion Box Chatbot 2: Vacation	Chatbot 1: Vacation Chatbot 2: Vacation and Suggestion Box	Chatbot 1: SR Chatbot 2: SR

* See method sections for more information. As P4 was absent on day 2, some chatbots were repeated again.

P5 had to work alone, as P4 was absent. Participants were allowed to make minor changes in text or choose different emojis and photos. Only P5 transcribed the exact wording from the slides, completing her first chatbot in approximately 40 min. While testing her chatbot, minor spelling and punctuation errors were found, but the overall flow was correct. In contrast, the other participants took more time, creating their own sentences and adding emojis. Due to P5's speed and proficiency in following the instructions, additional features and improvements were introduced to her. She grasped these quickly, asking for assistance from the researchers when needed. During the development of her second chatbot, 'Suggestion Box', P5 again followed the instructions on the tablet efficiently, finishing within 30 min. In the discussion, the adding of a new feature to the chatbot —an email notification function— was agreed, where the responsible person receives an email each time the 'Suggestion Box' chatbot is used. Although this feature was only taught during the Vacation chatbot, which she had previously developed, P5 initiated the process independently without needing the tablet for guidance. She required minimal help and successfully implemented the new feature.

P1 and P6 (group 1) worked well together as a team. It is important to mention that once the basic functions of Landbot have been learnt, the steps are repetitive. For example, with the "button" function it is possible to create many types of questions. Therefore, after a while, the prepared slides might look repetitive. For instance, P1 was able to perform tasks like creating buttons and editing text with less reliance on the slides, remembering the steps on her own. While her initial attempts were not perfect, she referred back to the slides to refine her process. Notably, some participants were quicker and accomplished more than what the instructions outlined. For example, P1 finished developing the first recipe of the online Cookbook and requested to continue developing more recipes. Independently she googled the required photos, saved them on the laptop and successfully developed the second recipe. She encountered only one issue, where her flow did not appear in the test version. With the researcher's assistance, she identified the mistake and resolved it independently.

In contrast to group 1, P2 and P3 (group 2) were mostly working individually. They initially started developing on their own, without using the tablet or talking with each other. The researchers had to spend time guiding, encouraging them to follow the slides step by step and to wait for each other during the process. This was very important, as without following the instructions, firstly, they were stuck and did not know what to do next and they would not learn different features of Landbot. P3 was very focused on wording, often questioning what the best question or answer would be. He rewrote sentences multiple times, even when he could have simply copied the text from the slides. This process usually took most of his time. However, he had no difficulty in creating the flow and was able to do so easily. It was observed that most of the participants would ask questions when they did not know something or had difficulties or faced errors. P2 and P3, however, never initiated a question. Rather, the researchers or Supervisor 1 had to ask them if they had questions.

Overall, participants seemed to have fun developing chatbots and were very excited. Even though a 15 min break was announced, P3, P1, and P6 started their tasks after 10 min. After the break, within one hour, everyone had finished with the development of their first chatbots. The participants then started to develop their second chatbot, following the instructions on the tablet. By the end of the day, the other participants did not have time to finish their second chatbots. However, they explicitly stated that they wanted to finish these chatbots the next morning. Shortly before concluding the second date, participants were asked about the day's experience. P6 found the work very tiring in the long run. P1 stated that at first, it was difficult to focus but she found the instructions very helpful; she stated that if tasks are repeated often, she does not need instructions and she found the slides with photos better than the ones with videos. P5 found the task quite easy, she did not even notice the videos and did not need them. P3 said he had fun working on the tasks and P2 claimed it was difficult to focus but that he had fun and wanted to continue the next day. For him, it did not matter if the instructions used videos or photos.

Day 3: On the third day, the session began with a brief greeting, and the participants immediately resumed their work from the previous day. Everyone remembered their tasks and continued working independently. At this stage, everyone was developing the Vacation chatbot.

Since P4 was absent the previous day and P5 had already developed two chatbots, P5 was asked to assist P4 in learning to create her first chatbot. The tablet was again used for instructions. P4 followed the slides, with P5 providing guidance only when necessary. It was observed that P5 was able to support P4 independently, without any help from the researchers. P4's chatbot had one issue; a block was not properly connected to the next, disrupting the flow. Unable to identify the problem, P4 worked with the researcher, who helped her review the flow until she recognized the issue. When asked for a solution, P4 successfully resolved it on her own. After developing her second chatbot, the researchers asked P4 about her experience so far. She found the chatbot development enjoyable. Regarding the instructions, she preferred the photos, as she felt the videos moved too quickly. While she considered the instructions somewhat overwhelming, she still found them helpful. Overall, she did not find the practice exhausting or demanding.

When testing her chatbots, P1 was usually able to identify the problems on her own. But she usually needed help to understand why the error occurred. Usually, the researchers would check with her and identify the problem, but P1 would solve the problem herself. The process of testing the chatbot together and thinking aloud about the problem was a helpful way for the participants to recognize their mistakes and fix them. In this way, participants usually understood where the problem was.

To develop the email function (mentioned in the Day 2 section), each question and answer needs a variable that defines it. These variables are placed in the body of the email function at the end. For example, if the chatbot asks where the problem is, a variable such as @Department should be defined and later implemented in the email body. All participants struggled with the concept of variables. The researchers had to assist them in creating several variables they had overlooked, indicating a lack of attention to the slides. To enhance their understanding, the email drafts were displayed on the large screen in the room. Participants could then see what their emails looked like and assess their coherence. After this clarification, everyone completed the development of their Vacation chatbots within 90 min. Only P2 and P3 had some problems with the variables that they could not solve without the help of the researchers, and they decided to work on their improvements instead of starting a new one. The rest of the participants started a new chatbot (P4—second chatbot (online Cookbook); P5—online Cookbook; P1 and P6—3rd chatbot (Suggestion Box)). P1 and P6 had finished developing their 3rd and final chatbot by the lunch break. While P6 decided to go on social media on his phone until lunch break, P1 continued to develop her 3rd recipe (of the online Cookbook). This means that she could independently find her chatbot on the Landbot dashboard and start a new recipe.

Developing a New Chatbot Without Instruction (The 4th Chatbot)

After the lunch break, since the majority of the participants had developed three chatbots, the researcher asked the participants which was their favorite chatbot and why. The Vacation chatbot was mentioned most often because it was the easiest chatbot to create and the topic of vacation was interesting to them. A brainstorming session was held to develop a new chatbot for Sickness Registration (SR) via a chatbot, as the participants had already shown interest and thought such a chatbot would be helpful as anyone could use it from home. To start the process, the researcher drew the process flow on a flipchart while the participants shared their ideas. For example, the researcher asked what the first step should be, and the participants suggested a greeting message. Then, they suggested asking for the person's name. This brainstorming continued until a concrete flow was defined and everyone found it helpful and complete. After a short break, everyone began developing the SR chatbot. Shortly thereafter, P6 announced that he had finished. However, when he attempted to test his chatbot, he discovered a mistake that prevented it from being tested. The researchers guided him in identifying and fixing the problem, after which he was able to work independently on resolving the issue. P1 also had problems with the email variables (how to clearly define them step by step) and a researcher had to help her. However, she did not have any problems with the flow or using the appropriate functions of the Landbot (e.g., button, message, etc.). P2's main difficulty was connecting different blocks and following the logic. Without help from the researchers, he could not finish his work or move on.

It should be noted that the participants developed the 4th chatbot based on the knowledge and experience of the previous days. The tablets were collected, and they did not have access to the instructions. However, once again, the problem with the variables and the email function occurred for all participants. To clarify this better, the researchers explained the concept, step by step, on the large screen of the room. The participants were then asked to continue working. Despite this explanation, some of the participants struggled to implement the function correctly. P6, for example, expressed that he found it easier with the instructions and the slides. Without them, when something is demonstrated or explained, he immediately forgets it.

Once again, the participants were so absorbed in their work that they had to be reminded several times that the workshop was over. When asked if the day had been difficult for them, they all said no and expressed that they had enjoyed it. The participants were usually very involved in their work and did not even ask for a break, commenting that the time went by very quickly compared to the time in the sheltered workshops.

At the end of the third day, after the participants had left, for further planning and performance observation, the researchers reviewed all four developed chatbots of each participant and rated them from 1 (very bad) to 5 (very good). The evaluation criteria included the following: (1) adherence to the steps defined in the flow, (2) correct connection of blocks, (3) coherence and clarity of the text, (4) functionality of the email feature, and (5) overall operational status of the chatbot. These criteria were used to ensure a structured and consistent assessment. Table 3 presents the results of this evaluation.

Table 3. Ratings of the four developed chatbots.

Participant	Suggestion Box	Cookbook	Sickness Registration	Vacation	Voted for Implementation
P1	4	5	5	4.5	Cookbook and SR
P2	5	4	3	3.5	Suggestion Box
P3	5	5	3	4	Vacation
P4	5	5	3	4.5	-
P5	4.5	5	5	5	-
P6	5	5	3	3	-

Day 4: On the fourth day, P5 was absent and a new supervisor (Supervisor 2) accompanied the participants. The day started by asking the participants about their experience of developing a chatbot without the instructions. Participants expressed that overall, it was fun. P2 said that it was a bit difficult for him at the beginning but after some time and practice he could do it. P6 agreed and also said that he would like to have the instructions with him at all times so that he could refer to them when needed and that he would not mind if the instructions were on a tablet or on paper. P1 said she had no problems or difficulties. P3 said that everything was easy for him, but the email function was challenging. P4 agreed with these statements.

Since the second goal of the study was to implement the chatbots in the sheltered workshop, chatbots that were fully functional needed to be selected. Four chatbots were developed by each participant, and the best-performing chatbot for each category was selected through voting. By fully functional, it is meant that the chatbot was able to complete its tasks, where questions led to correct answers and the chatbot worked without problems from start to finish. The email function was also an essential part of the fully functional chatbot, ensuring that the person responsible received a suitable email each time the chatbot was used. This was particularly relevant for the Vacation chatbot, the Sickness Registration chatbot, and the Suggestion Box chatbot, where sending an email to the person responsible was necessary for the effective use of the chatbots in the sheltered workshop. To select the chatbots for implementation, group testing was conducted for each developed chatbot, with participants actively engaging in the testing process. To ensure that the chatbots could be clearly seen by everyone, testing was started on a large screen. The Vacation chatbot was tested first, followed by the testing of each participant's chatbots in their current state. After each chatbot was tested, everyone was asked what the errors or mistakes were, or what could be improved. Many errors, such as issues in the flow or missing blocks, were identified either by the participants themselves or by their peers. However, no one paid attention to spelling and punctuation. So, the researchers had to emphasize this issue. As a tool to improve their dictation, DeepL Write (https://www.deepl.com/de/write (accessed on 17 June 2024)) was introduced. However, none of the participants used it, but continued to ask the researchers. During this testing process, the researchers kept mentioning that mistakes and errors happen during development and it is important to test the chatbots and ask for feedback from peers. They were assured that mistakes are not bad and that they happen to researchers as well. Once everyone received the feedback and the list of needed improvements, time was given to implement them. Most of the problems were again related to the variables and the email function. One last time, one of the researchers explained the concept of a variable in a different format (using the flipchart to draw with examples from daily life) and how it will be used in the email. Although improvements were observed, P3 said that he knew what the problem was, but he did not know what to do or how to make it better. A researcher walked him through his email construction step by step. This helped him understand and implement the changes. In the end, he was able to do it himself without any help. When he sent an email to be checked, he would even suggest improvements in spelling and punctuation. It is worth mentioning that only P1 was able to formulate a perfect email at the end, without any problems or help. Her mistakes were pointed out by the researcher and she would usually say what improvements should be made. Again, participants were so absorbed in their tasks that they did not take a break and when asked, they said they did not need any and continued working.

The initial plan was to view everyone's chatbot on large screen and then vote on it after it had been improved. However, due to time constraints, the participants were asked which of their chatbots should be viewed. The participants were given five minutes to decide if they wanted their chatbot to be tested and later voted on. Initially, P4, P2, and P3 had to be convinced to volunteer because they were too shy or did not trust themselves. However, after one round of testing the chatbots, they also volunteered. Those who volunteered sat in front of their laptops and showed the others how their chatbots worked. Once all the volunteered chatbots had been reviewed, all the participants, including Supervisor 2 and the researchers, voted on which chatbot should be implemented in the sheltered workshop. The names were written on the flipchart and everyone put a colored dot in front of the name they thought should be selected. The chatbots with the most points were chosen (Table 3).

The day was ended with a few short feedback questions as follows:

1. What was good about this week? Everyone said everything together. More explanation was sought and P3 said "developing chatbots", P1 said "learning something new", P2 said "the Vacation chatbot was good", and P4 and P6 said "everything".
2. What did I learn? P3 said: "Put yourself in the developers' shoes and do other tasks for a change".
3. What could be improved? Everyone unanimously said "nothing", apart from P2, who said "more Emojis".
4. What do you take with you? P1 said "new skills" and P3 said "Experience to show the others"
5. What was neglected? P6 said "the breaks" and P3 immediately said "no, the breaks were good, I like it better here than in the workshops, much quieter, many of us go home [from the sheltered workshop] with a headache, I can concentrate well here". P1 added "[at the sheltered workshop] there is a lot of running around, no concentration", P2 added "yes, here is nice", and P1 continued "yes, here you can work well".

Since P4 did not answer any of the questions, the researcher asked her what she said when she went home. She replied, "I told them what we do, what we develop, that we developed chatbots, that we can write". P2 added that he also explains the same things when he goes home. P6 said that he is happy that he can do other things instead of annoying everyone. P3 also added that he "got feedback at home that he is capable of doing more and that his parents saw him on the official job market". Finally, the researcher announced that the work for the day was finished, to which P1 said "sadly".

Day 5: As this was the last day of the training, the participants first answered the same questionnaires as on the first day. A researcher read the questions aloud, and explanations were offered if the questions were not clear to the participants. Afterward, the participants prepared their selected chatbots for implementation in the sheltered workshop. The participants were again divided into groups to speed up the process and to use each other's feedback to improve the selected chatbots; P5 and P2 worked together to improve the Suggestion Box chatbot, P4 and P3 worked together on the Vacation chatbot, and P1 and P6 worked together on the Cookbook chatbot. Since the SR chatbot was almost finished, P1 only spent 2–3 min on it, making minor improvements.

P2 and P5 also needed to improve the email function, but because they had difficulty with the steps and variables, they requested to use the instructions on the tablet again. Although the topic of the instructions (Vacation chatbot) was different from their current chatbot (SR Chatbot), they were still able to complete the task. There were some writing and grammatical issues, and since the participants were unable to correct them, DeepL Write was reintroduced for assistance. Still, the researchers had to point out the mistakes so that they could use DeepL Write to see the correct version. They did not take the initiative to see if all their sentences were correct. At the end of the day, the participants expressed their willingness to introduce their chatbots to their peers at the sheltered workshop when the implementation appointment took place.

A conversation that took place during the break is worth mentioning. During the break, a researcher exchanged ideas with P1 and P6. It was asked how else a chatbot could be helpful for the sheltered workshops. P5 said that a chatbot could look for contact information like a phone number (intern). That way they do not have to call and ask the Central Division first. Sometimes Central Division also has difficulty finding the number or the person. The researcher asked if a chatbot would be helpful to show task steps (how to do a task step by step). P5 thought it would be especially helpful because people keep asking her these questions and she has to help them. But she also has tasks and cannot help them all the time. If a chatbot could show them the steps of the tasks, then she could refer them to the chatbot and save herself time. They were asked if they felt confident in developing a new chatbot without any help. They said that if there were instructions on the tablets (detailed like ones used in the study), then they would not have a problem. They were asked about the flipchart and idea planning. They both said it would be helpful for orientation and guidance.

3.1.2. Quantitative Results

Due to the small sample size, only descriptive analysis was performed on the questionnaires. Table 4 shows the descriptive analysis of the scores.

Table 4. Descriptive analysis of the scores from the questionnaires completed by Developers before and after the training.

Questionnaire	n	Mean	Median	SD
BSW:				
Before training	6	3.06	3.00	0.48
After training	6	3.53	3.70	0.67
TB:				
Before training	6	41.33	40.5	9.99
After training	6	42.67	42.5	7.78
WDQ				
Before training	6			
1. Task variety		3.91	3.87	0.40
2. Feedback from job		4.02	3.83	0.56
3. Problem solving		3.75	3.62	0.31
4. Skill variety		4.25	4.12	0.67
5. Equipment use		3.33	3.33	0.47
After training	6			
1. Task variety		4.12	4.25	0.41
2. Feedback from job		4.11	4.83	1.25
3. Problem solving		3.37	3.50	0.41
4. Skill variety		4.04	4.12	1.04
5. Equipment use		3.44	3.33	1.08
DTAS				
Before training	6			
1. Perceived usefulness		17.67	18.50	2.87
2. Perceived ease of use		14.00	15.50	5.02
3. Attitudes towards usage		12.17	13.50	3.65
4. Behavioral intention to use		9.33	10.00	1.03
after training	6			
1. Perceived usefulness		14.83	16.00	6.01
2. Perceived ease of use		15.50	16.00	4.55
3. Attitudes towards usage		11.83	13.00	4.30
4. Behavioral intention to use		7.17	7.50	3.18

System Usability Scale (SUS)

The developer team's average SUS score for Landbot was 70.83 (SD = 13.66), with the lowest being 55 and the highest being 87.5.

3.2. Results—End Users

3.2.1. Qualitative Results

In the first two months, chatbot usage was minimal, primarily due to the summer holidays in Germany. During this time, many participants were either on vacation or engaged in internships. As a result, the Vacation Chatbot was seldom utilized initially, since vacations had already been approved. However, since the end of the summer holidays, the usage of the Vacation Chatbot has increased. Despite this growth, it has not entirely replaced the paper version that was previously used at the sheltered workshops.

The Suggestion Box chatbot was the least used, despite being requested by employees. After discussing this with Supervisor 1, it was concluded that users need more explanation and time to become accustomed to using it. Currently, users go directly to their group leaders when they have problems. Although using the chatbots could reduce the workload of the group leaders, developing the culture of using the chatbot takes time and practice. Secondly, according to Supervisor 1, there were not many problems to report at the time of the study.

The Cookbook chatbot started with two recipes. However, the idea was welcomed by the housekeeping team and their group leader. So P1 was requested to add more recipes to the chatbot. For example, as the group makes waffles every week for all the staff, they found it helpful to have the recipe. With the help of the group leader and Supervisor 1, photos and measurements were taken and P1 successfully added the new recipe independently (without any instruction or help from the research team). It is important to note that at this time, Landbot had released a new update that changed the position of the features. Based on the Supervisor 1's explanations, P1 had noticed this immediately, but after some time was able to understand and continue the development. One challenge was the malfunctioning translator plugin, which led to Supervisor 1 having to translate for P1.

The SR chatbot is the most used of the chatbots, as it has made it easier for employees to report sickness when they are unable to come to work. This chatbot is the most praised by the personnel as it has reduced their workload. The sheltered workshop is considering the possibility of using this chatbot in all its branches, for all employees and members of staff.

3.2.2. Quantitative Results

SUS results for chatbots: As of now, 14 valid answers have been collected regarding the usability experiences of the developed chatbots implemented in the sheltered workshop. Table 5 shows the demographic information and SUS results.

Table 5. End Users' demographic information and SUS results.

Demographics	N (%)
Gender	
Female	4 (28.6)
Male	9 (64.3)
Missing	1 (7.1)
Age (years)	
18–24	12 (85.7)
25–34	1 (7.1)
45–54	1 (7.1)
Mean (SD)	22.93 (6.9)

Table 5. *Cont.*

Demographics	N (%)
Disability	
Missing	8 (28.6)
Physical disability	1 (7.1)
Developmental disability	1 (7.1)
Mental illness	1 (7.1)
Multiple disability	3 (21.4)
SUS scores	
100–85	12 (85.7)
Under 85	2 (14.3)
Mean (SD)	88.9 (11.2)

4. Discussion

One criticism of knowledge transfer is that insights gained from research often fail to be effectively applied in practice [44]. However, there are various strategies to bridge this gap. One effective approach is to collaborate directly within real (work) environments alongside the research's target group, ensuring that findings are seamlessly integrated into practice and continue to have an impact even after the research concludes [45]. The aim of this study was to give people with disabilities working in sheltered workshops the opportunity to acquire new skills and transfer them to their working environment. To this end, six participants with cognitive disabilities underwent a week-long training to learn how to develop chatbots that could be tailored to their needs and job requirements. In this way, the knowledge gained from the training would not be lost and could be transferred to their peers at the sheltered workshop. In parallel with the knowledge transfer, there was also a peer-to-peer transfer. The Developers introduced the chatbots to their colleagues, where currently the chatbots are used on a daily basis. At the time of writing, the chatbots have been successfully implemented and are being used in the sheltered workshops. Furthermore, the Developers continue to develop the chatbots independently during their work and thus do not forget how to use the NC platform.

One of the primary questions in this study was whether NC platforms are accessible to people with disabilities. The answer, however, is not straightforward, as multiple factors need to be considered. On one hand, the NC platform used in this study was intuitive enough for users to recall key functions and work somewhat independently. However, the significance of targeted training for individuals with cognitive disabilities, particularly those without prior IT experience, cannot be overlooked. In this study, a range of training methods were employed to gradually teach participants how to use the platform. The combination of traditional teaching methods, such as live demonstrations, with modern approaches, including the use of tablets and other interactive technologies, proved to be particularly effective. According to previous research, providing immediate feedback during active learning sessions has been shown to be beneficial in teaching new skills to individuals with cognitive impairments [46,47]. In the current study, direct feedback was provided by reviewing the chatbot's flow with participants and identifying key issues. With this guidance, participants were able to apply their training and resolve the problems effectively. Furthermore, peer learning and guidance from educators have also been found to be highly effective for this group [46]. In this study, it was observed that participants' performance improved when group members communicated and collaborated more effectively. Additionally, having a representative from the sheltered workshop (Supervisor 1), who had deep knowledge of the employees and their tasks, was important and highly beneficial. She actively encouraged and recruited participants, while also providing valuable feedback and support during close collaboration with them. This finding aligns with the study by Schaap et al. [48], which investigated the effects of training for supervisors of people with disabilities in the workplace. Their participants emphasized that having a "good" supervisor—someone who values them and communicates clearly—is crucial and highly supportive. Similarly, Frogner et al. [49] demonstrated the critical role supervisors play in sheltered workshops, noting that they understand the specific needs and abilities of sheltered workers and maintain strong daily working relationships with them. However, it is important to consider that introducing new technologies and tasks could lead to supervisor overload, given the substantial responsibilities they already manage in sheltered workshops.

In her report on AI and occupational inclusion, Touzet [22] explained that minimal support, such as a reliable internet connection and access to appropriate tools, is a prerequisite for effectively using technology. In this study, for instance, P1 faced challenges in developing additional recipes for the Cookbook chatbot at the sheltered workshop due to a weak internet connection and laptop performance. According to Supervisor 1, they often had to be patient and reload the webpage to continue their work. This instability also affected the translation plug-in, requiring Supervisor 1 to take over the translation tasks. Consequently, P1 became dependent on Supervisor 1's availability, despite being capable of managing the tasks independently. Therefore, appropriate funding should be allocated to the sheltered workshop to facilitate the normalization of digitalization within its operations. Additionally, regarding the limitations of LCNC platforms, it has been noted that these platforms often face constraints in terms of customization and the variety of available features. This study acknowledges this limitation. P1 encountered challenges while working in the back-end of Landbot to develop additional recipes for the Cookbook chatbot. As more recipes were added, there was less space available to fit images and steps, which led to increased frustration.

Binzer and Winkler [2] argue that LCNC users should possess a strong professional and academic background, emphasizing that successful use of LCNC tools relies on collaboration, effective communication, and a solid understanding of business functions. This study both agrees and disagrees with this perspective. On one hand, a deep understanding of the workplace was essential, as the chatbots developed needed to meet the specific needs of the sheltered workshop. The Developers' insights and experiences were crucial for the successful implementation of these chatbots, particularly since they are used daily, demonstrating their alignment with the needs of the sheltered workshop employees. On the other hand, this study showed that individuals with disabilities, despite lacking a strong academic or professional background, can effectively use a NC platform with appropriate training and support. However, it should be noted that cases involving LC or more complex platforms may differ, as they may require more advanced IT skills. This highlights the need for further studies with larger sample sizes and additional LCNC platforms. Touzet further notes that "IT literacy" plays a crucial role in utilizing AI-based technologies [22]. The participants in the current study, despite lacking an IT background, were familiar with working with laptops, allowing them to quickly grasp the new features of Landbot. This may be attributed to the younger generations, who have grown up using these technologies and might find it easier to learn new tools, as they likely develop this literacy from an early age.

The second perspective of this study focused on the viewpoints of End Users, namely the employees at the sheltered workshop who have been using chatbots developed by their peers. According to the SUS scores and occasional feedback from Supervisor 1, employees have expressed satisfaction with their use. The chatbots have been tailored to meet the specific needs of the sheltered workshop, making them well-received by the

End Users as well as the supervisors. One notable example is the SR chatbot. Prior to its introduction, employees often relied on their caregivers to notify the workshop's staff when they could not attend work due to illness, a situation that for some individuals frequently arose because of their disabilities. The chatbot has significantly streamlined this process for both employees and staff, leading to discussions about its implementation across all branches. However, it was observed that certain changes require time and effort. For instance, participants have not been using the Suggestion Box chatbot as frequently as expected, and some are using it for unintended purposes. Implementing these changes will necessitate a shift in the organizational culture, along with additional time and resources. These findings are consistent with the study by Oldman et al. [50], which examined the long-term process of transforming sheltered workshops into evidence-based supported employment programs. Their research highlighted critical factors for successful change, such as motivated leadership, adequate financial resources, and a recognized "need for change" among stakeholders. The literature review by Nettles [51] corroborates and builds upon these findings, underscoring additional factors crucial to successful change, such as the roles of families and supervisors in driving the process.

This study has its own limitations. Firstly, the sample size was relatively small, and participants (both Developers and End Users) were selected based on the judgment of Supervisor 1, which introduces a potential bias. Secondly, the research was conducted using only one NC platform, which was limited in its features and capabilities, focusing exclusively on the development of chatbots. There are numerous other LCNC platforms available that offer more complex functionalities and a wider array of products. For example, during the brainstorming phase of the study, the development of an intranet for sheltered workshop employees was discussed. This intranet would allow participants to stay updated on internal news, submit vacation requests, and manage workflows. While such intranet systems could be developed using LCNC platforms, they may require a deeper understanding of programming or more advanced technical knowledge. By not exploring these alternatives, the study may not fully capture the potential benefits and challenges of various LCNC platforms. Furthermore, studies have shown that LCNC platforms present their own set of challenges. For instance, while there is potential to integrate products developed using LCNC platforms into existing systems and tools within companies [18], they are not universally compatible with all systems [52]. In the current study, the chatbots developed using the NC platform were not integrated into the existing systems used in the sheltered workshop, and it remains unclear whether their implementation would create additional challenges or benefits for the workshop. Future research could explore these integrations to assess their long-term feasibility and impact within organizations. In this context, the policies of individual organizations need to be considered. While the implementation of such platforms in the workplace could promote digital inclusion and improve relevant policies, the ethical implications of AI-based LCNC platforms need to be addressed, especially when sensitive personal information is involved. Another limitation of the current study relates to data policies and privacy requirements of LCNC platforms. As previously mentioned, given the sensitivity of the data in the study, platforms were selected based on compliance with EU regulations and the policies of the sheltered workshop. Consequently, the number of platforms available for selection was limited. Future studies would benefit from a larger and more diverse sample, including participants from other sheltered workshops and the exploration of more advanced LCNC platforms for the development of a wider range of products.

5. Conclusions

This study addressed multiple factors that influence the development and implementation of new technologies for people with disabilities in the workplace. By developing tools that are customized to the specific needs, designed by peers, and used on a daily basis, the research offers a comprehensive perspective on inclusion, accessibility, and employment. In line with the existing literature [53], acquiring new skills, such as becoming a citizen developer, can open up new career opportunities, and people with disabilities are no exception. The findings suggest that, with proper training and support, individuals with disabilities can gain new skills and become citizen developers within their organizations. These capabilities have the potential to reduce staff workloads, accelerate digital transformation, and facilitate the transition of people with disabilities into the primary labor market. Usability assessments revealed that End Users found the products intuitive and beneficial across multiple levels. While additional customization to meet individual needs is still required, having in-house developers can simplify the process of development and refinement. This study's results underscore the potential of LCNC platforms and suggest that future research could explore their capabilities in larger sample sizes and more complex platforms.

Author Contributions: Conceptualization, S.H.K. and B.M.K.; methodology S.H.K. and B.M.K.; validation, S.H.K.; formal analysis, S.H.K.; investigation, S.H.K. and B.M.K.; project administration, S.H.K.; resources, S.H.K.; writing—original draft preparation, S.H.K.; writing—review and editing, S.H.K., B.M.K., L.A. and L.B.; visualization, S.H.K.; supervision, B.M.K., L.B. and L.A. All authors have read and agreed to the published version of the manuscript.

Funding: This study is part of a project of the Federal Institute for Occupational Safety and Health in Germany. No external funding was received.

Institutional Review Board Statement: This study was ethically evaluated and approved by the ethic commission of the Federal Institute for Occupational Safety and Health (German: Bundesanstalt für Arbeitsschutz und Arbeitsmedizin (BAuA)-083_2024), approved date: 23 May 2024.

Informed Consent Statement: Informed consent was obtained from all subjects involved in the study.

Data Availability Statement: The datasets generated during and/or analyzed during the current study are not publicly available due to the privacy rights of the participants.

Conflicts of Interest: The authors declare no conflicts of interest.

Abbreviations

The following abbreviations are used in this manuscript:

LCNC	low-code and no-code platforms
LC	low-code
NC	no-code
SR	Sickness Registration chatbot
SUS	System Usability Scale

References

1. El Kamouchi, H.; Kissi, M.; El Beggar, O. Low-code/No-code Development: A systematic literature review. In Proceedings of the 2023 14th International Conference on Intelligent Systems: Theories and Applications (SITA), Casablanca, Morocco, 22–23 November 2023; pp. 1–8.
2. Binzer, B.; Winkler, T. Low-Coders, No-Coders, and Citizen Developers in Demand: Examining Knowledge, Skills, and Abilities Through a Job Market Analysis. In *Transforming the Digitally Sustainable Enterprise: Proceedings of the 18th International Conference on Wirtschaftsinformatik, Paderborn, Germany, 18 September 2023*; Springer: Cham, Switzerland, 2023.

3. Martinez, E.; Pfister, L. Benefits and limitations of using low-code development to support digitalization in the construction industry. *Autom. Constr.* **2023**, *152*, 104909. [CrossRef]
4. Woo, M. The Rise of No/Low Code Software Development—No Experience Needed? *Engineering* **2020**, *6*, 960–961. [CrossRef] [PubMed]
5. Lebens, M.; Finnegan, R.; Sorsen, S.; Shah, J. Rise of the Citizen Developer. *Muma Bus. Rev.* **2021**, *5*, 101–111. [CrossRef] [PubMed]
6. Sanchis, R.; García-Perales, Ó.; Fraile, F.; Poler, R. Low-Code as Enabler of Digital Transformation in Manufacturing Industry. *Appl. Sci.* **2020**, *10*, 12. [CrossRef]
7. McHugh, S.; Carroll, N.; Connolly, C. Low-Code and No-Code in Secondary Education—Empowering Teachers to Embed Citizen Development in Schools. *Comput. Sch.* **2023**, *41*, 399–424. [CrossRef]
8. Rajaram, A.; Olory, C.; Leduc, V.; Evaristo, G.; Coté, K.; Isenberg, J.; Isenberg, J.S.; Dai, D.L.; Karamchandani, J.; Chen, M.F.; et al. An integrated virtual pathology education platform developed using Microsoft Power Apps and Microsoft Teams. *J. Pathol. Inform.* **2022**, *13*, 100117. [CrossRef]
9. Mew, L.; Field, D. A Case Study on Using the Mendix Low Code Platform to Support a Project Management Course. 2018. Available online: https://www.researchgate.net/publication/329488415_A_Case_Study_on_Using_the_Mendix_Low_Code_Platform_to_support_a_Project_Management_Course (accessed on 3 April 2025).
10. Jauhar, S.K.; Jani, S.M.; Kamble, S.S.; Pratap, S.; Belhadi, A.; Gupta, S. How to use no-code artificial intelligence to predict and minimize the inventory distortions for resilient supply chains. *Int. J. Prod. Res.* **2024**, *62*, 5510–5534. [CrossRef]
11. Konin, A.; Siddiqui, S.; Gilani, H.; Mudassir, M.; Ahmed, M.H.; Shaukat, T.; Naufil, M.; Ahmed, A.; Tran, Q.H.; Zia, M.Z. AI-mediated Job Status Tracking in AR as a No-Code service. In Proceedings of the 2022 IEEE International Symposium on Mixed and Augmented Reality Adjunct (ISMAR-Adjunct), Singapore, 17–21 October 2022.
12. Takahashi, N.; Javed, A.; Kohda, Y. How Low-Code Tools Contribute to Diversity, Equity, and Inclusion (DEI) in the Workplace: A Case Study of a Large Japanese Corporation. *Sustainability* **2024**, *16*, 5327. [CrossRef]
13. Teborg, S.; Hünefeld, L.; Gerdes, T.S. Exploring the working conditions of disabled employees: A scoping review. *J. Occup. Med. Toxicol.* **2024**, *19*, 2. [CrossRef]
14. Zukunft der Werkstätten. Perspektiven für und von Menschen mit Behinderung zwischen Teilhabe-Auftrag und Mindestlohn: Schachler, Viviane; Schlummer, Werner; Weber, Roland; 2023. Available online: https://www.pedocs.de/frontdoor.php?source_opus=26510 (accessed on 3 April 2025).
15. BAG WfbM. BAG WfbM zu aktuellen Medienberichten über Werkstätten für Behinderte Menschen 2021. Available online: https://www.bagwfbm.de/article/5199 (accessed on 3 April 2025).
16. Goodhue, D.L.; Thompson, R.L. Task-Technology Fit and Individual Performance. *MIS Q.* **1995**, *19*, 213–236. [CrossRef]
17. Matic, R.; Kabiljo, M.; Zivkovic, M.; Cabarkapa, M. Extensible Chatbot Architecture Using Metamodels of Natural Language Understanding. *Electronics* **2021**, *10*, 2300. [CrossRef]
18. Nguyen Quoc, C.; Nguyen Hoang, T.; Cha, J. Using No-Code/Low-Code Solutions to Promote Artificial Intelligence Adoption in Vietnamese Businesses. *Int. J. Internet Broadcast. Commun.* **2024**, *16*, 370–378.
19. Lorenzo, G.; Elia, G.; Sponziello, A. *Artificial Intelligence Platforms Enabling Conversational Chatbots: The Case of Tiledesk.com*; Springer: Cham, Switzerland, 2025; pp. 119–137.
20. Mateos-Sanchez, M.; Melo, A.C.; Blanco, L.S.; García, A.M.F. Chatbot, as Educational and Inclusive Tool for People with Intellectual Disabilities. *Sustainability* **2022**, *14*, 1520. [CrossRef]
21. de Filippis, M.L.; Federici, S.; Mele, M.L.; Borsci, S.; Bracalenti, M.; Gaudino, G.; Cocco, A.; Amendola, M.; Simonetti, E. Preliminary Results of a Systematic Review: Quality Assessment of Conversational Agents (Chatbots) for People with Disabilities or Special Needs. In *Computers Helping People with Special Needs*; Springer International Publishing: Cham, Switzerland, 2020.
22. Touzet, C. Using AI to support people with disability in the labour market. In *OECD Artificial Intelligence Papers*; OECD Publishing: Paris, France, 2023. [CrossRef]
23. Beudt, S.; Blanc, B.; Feichtenbeiner, R.; Kähler, M. Critical reflection of AI applications for persons with disabilities in vocational rehabilitation. In Proceedings of the DELFI Workshops 2020, Online, 14–15 September 2020; Gesellschaft für Informatik e.V.z.: Bonn, Germany, 2020.
24. Simon, P. *Low-Code/No-Code: Citizen Developers and the Surprising Future of Business Applications*; Racket Publishing: Chicago, IL, USA, 2022.
25. Kajamaa, A.; Mattick, K.; de la Croix, A. How to ... do mixed-methods research. *Clin. Teach.* **2020**, *17*, 267–271. [CrossRef]
26. Dawadi, S.; Shrestha, S.; Giri, R. Mixed-Methods Research: A Discussion on its Types, Challenges, and Criticisms. *J. Stud. Educ.* **2021**, *2*, 25–36. [CrossRef]
27. Creswell, J.W.; Plano Clark, V.L. *Designing and Conducting Mixed Methods Research*, 3rd ed.; SAGE Publications: Thousand Oaks CA, USA, 2017.
28. Morgeson, F.; Humphrey, S. The Work Design Questionnaire (WDQ): Developing and Validating A Comprehensive Measure for Assessing Job Design and the Nature of Work. *J. Appl. Psychol.* **2006**, *91*, 1321–1339. [CrossRef]

29. Stegmann, S.; van Dick, R.; Ullrich, J.; Charalambous, J.; Menzel, B.; Egold, N.; Wu, T.T.-C. Der Work Design Questionnaire—Vorstellung und erste Validierung einer deutschen Version. *Z. Arb. Organ. AO* **2010**, *54*, 1–28.
30. Schorr, A. Skala zur Erfassung der Digitalen Technologieakzeptanz—Weiterentwicklung zum testtheoretisch geprüften Instrument. Digitaler Wandel, Digitale Arbeit, Digitaler Mensch? Bericht zum 66. Arbeitswissenschaftlichen Kongress vom 16.—18. März 2020, Berlin. No. 35, B.20.52020; pp. 1–6. Available online: https://gfa2020.gesellschaft-fuer-arbeitswissenschaft.de/inhalt/B.20.5.pdf (accessed on 3 April 2025).
31. Schorr, A. The Technology Acceptance Model (TAM) and its Importance for Digitalization Research: A Review. *Proc. TecPsy* **2023**, 55–65. [CrossRef]
32. Brooke, J. SUS: A quick and dirty usability scale. *Usability Eval. Ind.* **1995**, *189*, 4–7.
33. Rummel, B. System Usability Scale (Translated into German). 2013. Available online: https://community.sap.com/t5/additional-blogs-by-sap/system-usability-scale-jetzt-auch-auf-deutsch/ba-p/13487686 (accessed on 3 April 2025).
34. Hyzy, M.; Bond, R.; Mulvenna, M.; Bai, L.; Dix, A.; Leigh, S.; Hunt, S. System Usability Scale Benchmarking for Digital Health Apps: Meta-analysis. *JMIR mHealth uHealth* **2022**, *10*, e37290. [CrossRef]
35. Gutiérrez, M.M.; Rojano-Cáceres, J.R. Interpretation of the SUS questionnaire in Mexican sign language to evaluate usability an approach. In Proceedings of the 2020 3rd International Conference of Inclusive Technology and Education (CONTIE), Baja California Sur, Mexico, 28–30 October 2020.
36. Bangor, A.; Kortum, P.; Miller, J. Determining what individual SUS scores mean: Adding an adjective rating scale. *J. Usability Stud.* **2009**, *4*, 114–123.
37. Knispel, J.W.L.S.V.; Arling, V. *Skala zur Messung der Beruflichen Selbstwirksamkeitserwartung (BSW-5-Rev)*; Zusammenstellung sozialwissenschaftlicher Items und Skalen (ZIS): Mannheim, Germany, 2021.
38. Neyer, F.J.F.J.; Gebhardt, C. *Kurzskala Technikbereitschaft (TB, Technology Commitment)*; Zusammenstellung sozialwissenschaftlicher Items und Skalen (ZIS): Mannheim, Germany, 2016.
39. Venkatesh, V.; Morris, M.G.; Davis, G.B.; Davis, F.D. User Acceptance of Information Technology: Toward a Unified View. *MIS Q.* **2003**, *27*, 425–478. [CrossRef]
40. Hannay, J.; Dybå, T.; Arisholm, E.; Sjøberg, D. The effectiveness of pair programming: A meta-analysis. *Inf. Softw. Technol.* **2009**, *51*, 1110–1122. [CrossRef]
41. Roldán-Álvarez, D.; Márquez-Fernández, A.; Rosado-Martín, S.; Martín, E.; Haya, P.A.; García-Herranz, M. Benefits of Combining Multitouch Tabletops and Turn-Based Collaborative Learning Activities for People with Cognitive Disabilities and People with ASD. In Proceedings of the 2014 IEEE 14th International Conference on Advanced Learning Technologies, Athens, Greece, 7–10 July 2014.
42. Noushad, B.; Van Gerven, P.W.M.; de Bruin, A.B.H. Twelve tips for applying the think-aloud method to capture cognitive processes. *Med. Teach.* **2024**, *46*, 892–897. [CrossRef]
43. Ericsson, K.A.; Simon, H.A. Verbal Reports as Data. *Psychol. Rev.* **1980**, *87*, 215–251. [CrossRef]
44. Lundmark, C.; Nilsson, J.; Krook-Riekkola, A. Taking Stock of Knowledge Transfer Studies: Finding Ways Forward. *Environ. Manag.* **2023**, *72*, 1146–1162. [CrossRef]
45. Mohajerzad, H.; Schrader, J. Transfer from research to practice—A scoping review about transfer strategies in the field of research on digital media. *Comput. Educ. Open* **2022**, *3*, 100111. [CrossRef]
46. Matallana, J.; Paredes, M. Teaching methodology for people with intellectual disabilities: A case study in learning ballet with mobile devices. *Univers. Access Inf. Soc.* **2023**, *24*, 409–423. [CrossRef]
47. Gilson, C.B.; Carter, E.W.; Biggs, E.E. Systematic Review of Instructional Methods to Teach Employment Skills to Secondary Students with Intellectual and Developmental Disabilities. *Res. Pract. Pers. Sev. Disabil.* **2017**, *42*, 89–107. [CrossRef]
48. Schaap, R.; Stevels, V.A.; de Wolff, M.S.; Hazelzet, A.; Anema, J.R.; Coenen, P. "I noticed that when I have a good supervisor, it can make a Lot of difference". A Qualitative Study on Guidance of Employees with a Work Disability to Improve Sustainable Employability. *J. Occup. Rehabil.* **2023**, *33*, 201–212. [CrossRef]
49. Frogner, J.; Hanisch, H.M.; Kvam, L.; Witsø, A.E. A Glass House of Care: Sheltered Employment for Persons with Intellectual Disabilities. *Scand. J. Disabil. Res.* **2023**, *25*, 282–294. [CrossRef]
50. Oldman, J.; Thomson, L.; Calsaferri, K.; Luke, A.; Bond, G.R. A Case Report of the Conversion of Sheltered Employment to Evidence-Based Supported Employment in Canada. *Psychiatr. Serv.* **2005**, *56*, 1436–1440. [CrossRef] [PubMed]
51. Nettles, J.L. From Sheltered Workshops to Integrated Employment: A Long Transition. *LC J. Spec. Educ.* **2013**, *8*, 9.

52. Elshan, E.; Siemon, D.; Bruhin, O.; Kedziora, D.; Schmidt, N. Unveiling Challenges and Opportunities in Low Code Development Platforms: A StackOverflow Analysis. In Proceedings of the 57th Hawaii International Conference on System Sciences, Honolulu, HI, USA, 3–6 January 2024.
53. Biedova, O.; Ives, B.; Male, D.; Moore, M. Strategies for Managing Citizen Developers and No-Code Tools. *MIS Q. Exec.* **2024**, *23*, 4.

technologies

MDPI

Article

Neuro-Visual Adaptive Control for Precision in Robot-Assisted Surgery

Claudio Urrea *, Yainet Garcia-Garcia, John Kern and Reinier Rodriguez-Guillen

Electrical Engineering Department, Faculty of Engineering, University of Santiago of Chile, Las Sophoras 165, Estación Central, Santiago 9170020, Chile; yainet.garcia@usach.cl (Y.G.-G.); john.kern@usach.cl (J.K.); reinier.rodriguez@usach.cl (R.R.-G.)

* Correspondence: claudio.urrea@usach.cl; Tel.: +56-2-27-183-350

Abstract: This study introduces a Neuro-Visual Adaptive Control (NVAC) architecture designed to enhance precision and safety in robot-assisted surgery. The proposed system enables semi-autonomous guidance of the laparoscope based on image input. To achieve this, the architecture integrates the following: (1) a computer vision system based on the YOLO11n model, which detects surgical instruments in real time; (2) a Model Reference Adaptive Control with Proportional–Derivative terms (MRAC-PD), which adjusts the robot's behavior in response to environmental changes; and (3) Closed-Form Continuous-Time Neural Networks (CfC-mmRNNs), which efficiently model the system's dynamics. These networks address common deep learning challenges, such as the vanishing gradient problem, and facilitate the generation of smooth control signals that minimize wear on the robot's actuators. Performance evaluations were conducted in CoppeliaSim, utilizing real cholecystectomy images featuring surgical tools. Experimental results demonstrate that the NVAC achieves maximum tracking errors of 1.80×10^{-3} m, 1.08×10^{-4} m, and 1.90×10^{-3} m along the x, y, and z axes, respectively, under highly significant dynamic disturbances. This hybrid approach provides a scalable framework for advancing autonomy in robotic surgery.

Keywords: autonomous robotic surgical assistant; model reference-based neuro-visual adaptive control; surgical instrument detection; CfC-mmRNN; data-driven inverse modeling; visual tracking; YOLO11n

1. Introduction

Minimally invasive robotic surgery has revolutionized surgical procedures, offering benefits to both patients—by reducing recovery time and the risk of complications [1,2]—and surgeons by enhancing their capabilities and providing an ergonomically optimal position. Advances in hardware and software have improved precision and dexterity in tissue and organ manipulation, incorporating advanced features such as tremor reduction in the surgeon's hand, thereby enhancing procedural safety and quality [3,4].

In this context, camera-holding robots have emerged as a solution to improve the stability and quality of intraoperative vision without significantly impacting operation time. These devices minimize unintended movements, reduce the need for endoscope cleaning, and optimize workflow [5]. Over their evolution, they have progressed from basic mechanical systems to intelligent assistant robots integrating computer vision (CV) and machine learning (ML) [6].

However, challenges persist in achieving precise and intuitive control, adapting to dynamic surgical environments, and rejecting external disturbances that negatively affect robot autonomy, field of view (FOV) stability, and procedural fluency. To address these issues, this work proposes a Neuro-Visual Adaptive Control architecture that enhances precision, visual stability, and responsiveness to dynamic environmental variations, thereby promoting robotic autonomy.

Related Work

For a camera-holding robot to assist the surgeon with a degree of autonomy, robust environmental perception and control strategies that adapt to changing conditions are essential. A widely adopted approach to maintaining an appropriate FOV involves dynamically adjusting the vision sensor's position based on the movement of surgical instruments [7–11]. In this context, artificial intelligence (AI) has driven the development of image-guided robotic surgery, often employing hierarchical control architectures. These are characterized by two primary levels: low-level control, responsible for executing movements through robot and tool regulation, and high-level control, tasked with planning and decision-making based on surgical requirements and visual data.

A commercial example is the RoboLens robot, part of the Sina surgical system, which tracks surgical instruments via image processing [6]. Other systems, such as the Smart Tissue Autonomous Robot (STAR), utilize Image-Based Visual Servoing (IBVS) to enhance real-time surgical instrument alignment precision [12]. In [13], a combination of fuzzy adaptive control, disturbance observation, dynamic surface control, and Lyapunov functions improves synchronization and robustness in teleoperation systems with communication delays. Reference [14] proposes an Adaptive Zeroing Neural Network (AZNN) controller to optimize FOV stability and mitigate external disturbances. Meanwhile, Reference [15] introduces an Adaptive Proportional Sliding Mode controller (APSMC) for manipulating an electromagnetically actuated colonoscope.

As surgical environments grow more complex, adaptive control systems have become critical for procedures demanding high precision, such as neurosurgery [16]. For low-level control, various adaptive strategies have been developed alongside hybrid approaches combining classical and advanced controllers. In [17], an Adaptive Fuzzy Control is introduced for flexible robotic endoscopes, adjusting parameters in real time to compensate for friction and nonlinear dynamics without requiring a precise physical model. Reference [18] designs a Fractional-Order Adaptive Fuzzy Sliding Mode Control (AFFOSMC) strategy to enhance trajectory tracking accuracy in surgical manipulators.

Model Reference Adaptive Control (MRAC) stands out as a prominent adaptive control approach, dynamically adjusting its parameters based on a predefined reference model to optimize system performance amid uncertainties and dynamic variations. MRAC has broad applicability in aerospace, renewable energy, and industrial and service robotics [19,20]. In [21], an MRAC based on Robust Fixed Point Transformations (RFPTs) was implemented in a master–slave system for soft tissue surgery, enabling the slave arm to accurately replicate the surgeon's movements.

Cursi et al. reported significant improvements in autonomous trajectory tracking tasks using adaptive modeling with probabilistic networks like Bayesian Neural Networks (BNNs) and Evidential Neural Networks (EvNNs), outperforming Feedforward Artificial Neural Network (ANN)-based adaptive modeling [22,23]. In [24], a hybrid adaptive control was developed for a continuum surgical robot, combining neural network-trained inverse kinematics with online tuning of a PID controller. The authors reported a 50% reduction in maximum tracking error using a neural inverse model, with subsequent integration of the adaptive PID controller yielding further improvements of 74% in maximum error (down to 2.41 mm) and 66% in mean error (down to 1.49 mm). These findings underscore how hybrid strategies and data-driven modeling can effectively compensate for nonlinear system dynamics and manage unpredictable random errors during surgical procedures.

Among visual information processing techniques for surgical tool detection, object detection stands out, with deep learning-based methods excelling in this domain. Algorithms such as Faster Region-based Convolutional Neural Networks (Faster R-CNNs) and the You Only Look Once (YOLO) family have been widely adopted for their real-time processing capabilities and high detection rates [25–27]. Other proposed approaches include anchor-free CNNs [28], URTNet [29], Hourglass modules [30], and Transformer architectures [31], among others.

Despite these advances, challenges remain in validating system performance under more demanding and variable scenarios, applying data-driven control techniques with faster inference and higher precision, and implementing a holistic approach that enhances camera-holding robot autonomy without compromising safety. The future success of these systems hinges on achieving precise, adaptable endoscopic tracking robust to anatomical variations and external disturbances. Furthermore, proposed solutions must be inherently scalable, facilitating their transition from experimental settings to real-world clinical applications, and optimized for efficient operation on devices with limited computational resources without sacrificing performance critical to safe and effective surgical procedures.

In response to these challenges, we propose a Neuro-Visual Adaptive Control (NVAC) architecture, representing a significant advancement in assistive surgical robotics. This approach effectively addresses critical challenges such as real-time surgical tool tracking, adaptation to nonlinear dynamics, and rejection of significant disturbances. The primary contributions of this work are as follows:

- Development of a hybrid Neuro-Visual Adaptive Control architecture integrating a Model Reference Adaptive Controller with Proportional–Derivative terms (MRAC-PD) and Closed-Form Continuous-Time Neural Networks with mixed-memory Long Short-Term Memory architectures (CfC-mmRNN). While hybrid adaptive control and neural network approaches exist, the specific combination of MRAC-PD and CfC-mmRNN in robotic surgery is novel. This integration enables precise and adaptable modeling of dynamic surgical environments, delivering high tracking accuracy, rapid response to variations, optimized inference speed, and smoother control signals, thereby enhancing system stability and efficiency.
- Design and implementation of an optimized visual detection system for robotic surgery, based on YOLO version 11, nano variant (YOLO11n), enabling high-precision real-time tracking with an efficient balance between accuracy and computational load, facilitating improved trajectory planning.
- Experimental validation in simulated environments demonstrating the robustness, precision, and superiority of the controller compared to standard control strategies (e.g., PID, SMC, and baseline MRAC-PD) under complex, nonlinear surgical conditions.
- Comprehensive performance evaluation of the controllers using metrics such as tracking accuracy and external disturbance rejection, including significant forces (up to 15 N), sensor failures, and combined perturbations. These complex, representative scenarios highlight the controller's robustness.
- Establishment of an integrated framework to promote autonomy in robotic surgery, with a scalable approach for complex surgical environments, providing a solid foundation for future research and development in surgical assistant robots.

This article is organized as follows: Section 2 details the methodology, encompassing computational resources, system description, and the design of the control strategy, covering its theoretical basis and practical implementation. Section 3 presents the experimental results, highlighting validation across diverse scenarios. Section 4 discusses the key factors driving the controller's performance, evaluates limitations, and suggests future research directions. Section 5 summarizes the conclusions and main contributions. Finally, Section 6 proposes future work aligned with the study's findings.

2. Materials and Methods

This section outlines the resources, tools, and methodologies employed to develop and validate the proposed Neuro-Visual Adaptive Control system. It details the UR5 robot's dynamic model, simulation platforms, controller design and validation approaches, performance evaluation metrics, and experimental protocols, ensuring reproducibility and scientific rigor.

The methodology adopts an integrated framework to achieve autonomous visual tracking and robotic control in a simulated surgical environment. It comprises three core modules—Simulation Environment, Visual Processing, and Control Design—as depicted in Figure 1.

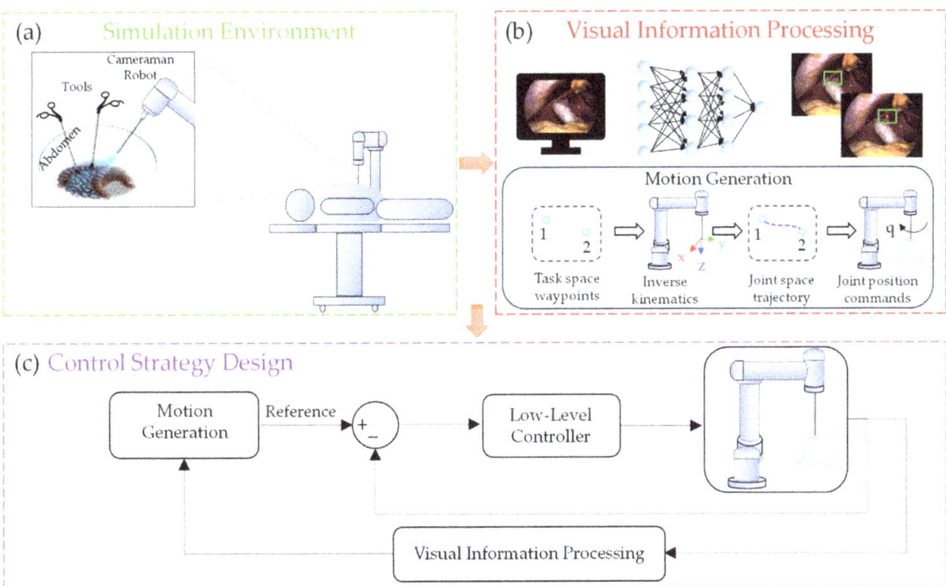

Figure 1. Methodology of the Neuro-Visual Adaptive Controller (NVAC) Operation. (**a**) Simulation Environment: This represents the virtual scenario where the camera-holding robot interacts with surgical tools and the patient. (**b**) Visual Information Processing: In this stage, visual data are interpreted, and motion trajectories for the robot are generated using computer vision models and inverse kinematics. (**c**) Control Strategy Design: The robot's response is defined based on the processed visual information, adjusting its movement through the low-level MRAC-PD-CfC-mmRNN controller.

2.1. Simulation Setup

For the validation of the designed control strategies, CoppeliaSim [32] was employed—a software platform integrating multiple physics engines and enabling advanced modeling of soft tissues, simulation of tissue deformations, physiological movements, rigid body dynamics, and instrument–tissue interactions with high-precision contact models. This capability supports progressive testing as the research advances, within high-fidelity surgical scenarios [9,33].

The simulation environment replicates a controlled surgical setting, wherein the robot interacts with a mannequin featuring real laparoscopic abdominal surgery images from various patients embedded in its abdomen (Figure 2). These images, applied as textures onto a surface, provide a realistic visual foundation for evaluating the control system. The resulting visual fidelity captures the complexity of the surgical field (e.g., variations in lighting and tissue characteristics), exposing the system to natural anatomical variability and enhancing its robustness [34,35].

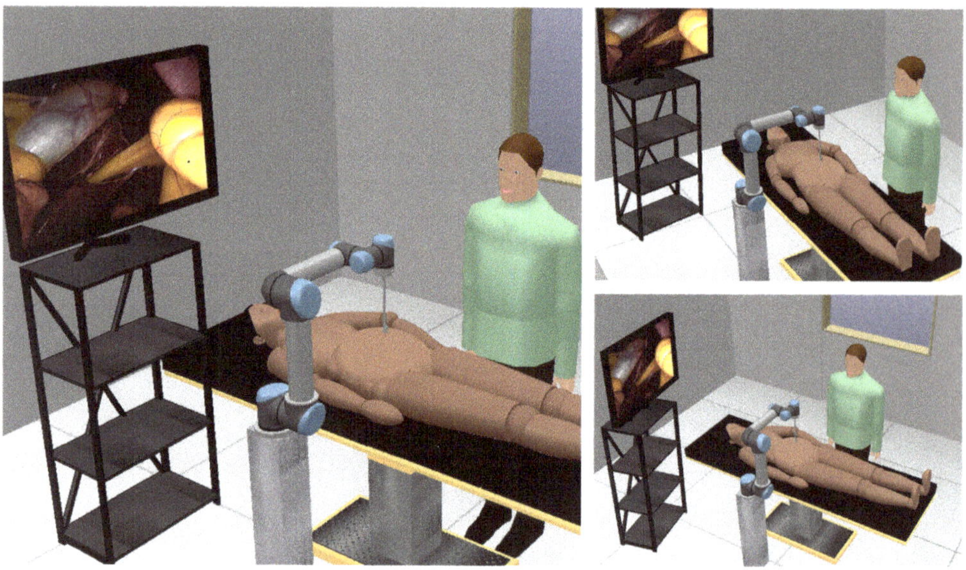

Figure 2. Simulation environment in CoppeliaSim representing a surgical scenario with a human mannequin. A laparoscope equipped with assisted vision is depicted operating within the simulated environment.

To enable dynamic interaction with the images, they are rotated within a range of $\pm 30^\circ$ around the z-axis from their initial position, at an angular velocity of 0.05 rad/s. This mechanism allows assessment of the system's ability to maintain a stable visual reference, facilitating laparoscope guidance. The surgical scenario also incorporates elements of laparoscopic surgery, such as a trocar, through which the robot's end-effector—a passive cylindrical tool with dimensions (0.01 m $\times$ 0.01 m $\times$ 0.262 m)—is inserted to simulate a laparoscope. At its tip, this tool integrates a perspective vision sensor with Legacy OpenGL rendering, a resolution of 270 $\times$ 270 pixels, a 45° field of view, and a detection range of 0.001–0.180 m for short-range visualization.

To ensure surgical safety and fidelity, constraints were established using virtual hyperplanes that delimit the workspace, preventing collisions between the laparoscope and tissues. A fraction of the robot's total operational space was defined with the following dimensions: [x: 0.3769 m to 0.5969 m, y: −0.025 m to 0.245 m, z: 0.9757 m to 1.1547 m]. Additionally, the Remote Center of Motion (RCM) constraint was implemented virtually—a critical element in minimally invasive surgery—enabling surgical instruments to pivot appropriately around the insertion point without causing displacements that could compromise patient safety [35–37].

This methodology ensures the validity of the simulation environment and facilitates the transfer of skills from this setting to real-world surgical practice, as demonstrated in prior autonomous endoscopic positioning systems using CoppeliaSim [38,39]. Thus, the developed environment enables the evaluation of control strategies within a context representative of clinical reality, preparing the system to address surgical scenarios with enhanced precision and safety.

2.1.1. Hardware and Software Tools

The study utilizes MatLab® R2024a [40] and CoppeliaSim Edu 4.8.0 for controller design, implementation, and validation, integrated via the ZeroMQ Remote API with simulation stepping enabled (sim.setStepping(true)) for seamless synchronization. Surgical tool detection leverages the YOLO11n architecture [41], trained in Python 3.9.21, with labeling performed using Roboflow [42]. Simulations were conducted on a high-performance computational platform, with specifications detailed in the Supplementary Materials.

2.1.2. Dataset

The CholecSeg8k dataset [43], comprising 8080 annotated laparoscopic cholecystectomy images (854 × 480 pixels, PNG format), is derived from 17 videos performed by 13 different surgeons (Figure 3). This dataset, an extension of Cholec80 [44], provides extensive diversity in surgical techniques and anatomical variability, while also presenting challenging conditions such as low illumination, blurriness, opacity, smoke presence, and a range of surgical instruments varying in size and depth. This richness of scenarios makes the dataset particularly suitable for our study, as its variability enhances the robustness and generalization capability of the trained detection model.

(a)
(b)
(c)

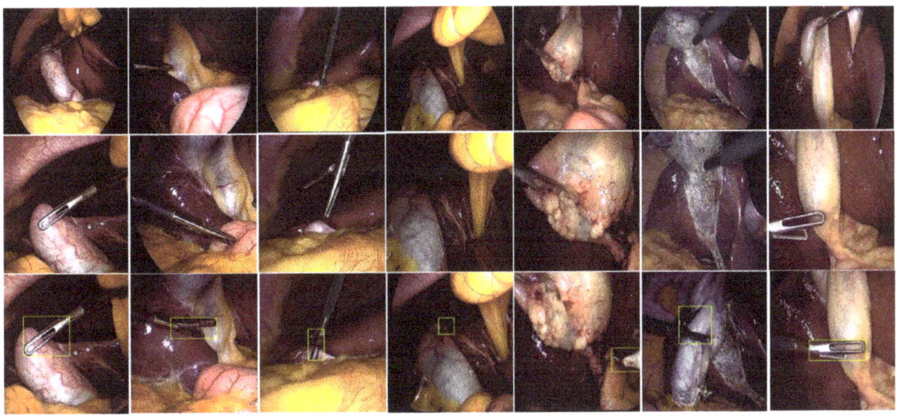

Figure 3. Examples of the dataset used in the study. (**a**) Images from the original CholecSeg8k dataset; (**b**) images captured in MatLab® from the CoppeliaSim environment; (**c**) example of annotations in a subset of images from the original dataset, labeling only the tip of the surgical tool as ground truth.

Since the images from the dataset were loaded as textures in the simulation environment, their resolution was adjusted to 270 × 270 pixels—a process that could invalidate prior labeling. Furthermore, as a strategy to maintain precise focus of the FOV on the operational region, only the tip of the surgical tool was labeled as "tool" in Roboflow, aiming to minimize errors or deviations in the FOV. The labeled images were applied as textures onto a disk-shaped structure in CoppeliaSim and captured via MatLab® to generate the training dataset used in the study. For these reasons, broadly speaking, any dataset employed would have required relabeling to align with the experiment's specific criteria.

2.2. Description of the System Under Study

The UR5 collaborative robot, developed by Universal Robots, was selected to validate the control strategy in robot-assisted surgery due to its versatility and suitability for both industrial and clinical environments. Its key features include a 6 Degrees of Freedom (DoF) configuration for adaptable positioning and seamless integration with external devices, supported by technical specifications such as a 5 kg payload, 850 mm operational radius, and ±0.1 mm positioning accuracy [45]. Figure 4 presents a schematic of the UR5 robot. Detailed modeling of its kinematics and dynamics, including coordinate systems, dimensional parameters, Denavit-Hartenberg (D-H) parameters, and dynamic specifications, as well as the implementation of Remote Center of Motion constraints, are provided in the Supplementary Materials.

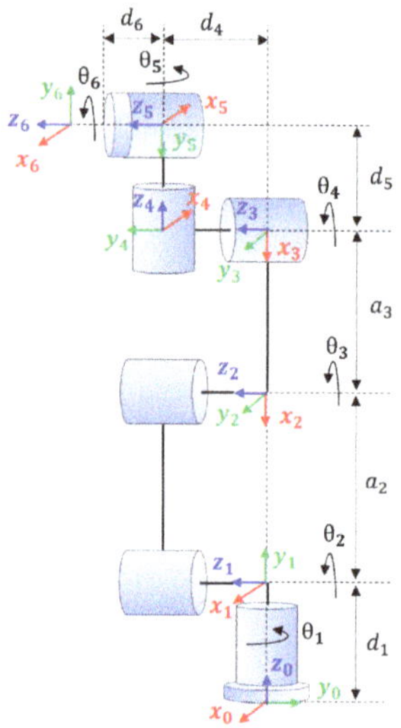

Figure 4. Representation of the structure and joint configuration of the UR5 robot using the Denavit-Hartenberg convention.

2.3. Design of Control Strategy

This section introduces the Neuro-Visual Adaptive Control, an innovative hybrid control architecture designed for the precise guidance of camera-holding robots in laparoscopic surgery. NVAC synergistically integrates advanced visual information processing via the YOLO11n model with adaptive control techniques and neural networks. This combination enables the system to efficiently interpret the complex surgical environment in real time, adapt to anatomical variations and unforeseen disturbances, and maintain optimal camera positioning throughout the procedure. The proposed architecture is conceived to overcome the limitations of conventional approaches, offering enhanced robustness, precision, and responsiveness in challenging environments.

YOLO, first introduced by Redmon and Farhadi in 2015, is renowned for its efficiency in object detection. Developed by Ultralytics under the AGPL-3.0 license, YOLO11 enhances performance across various CV tasks. The YOLO11n variant, utilized in this study, balances high inference speed (9.5 ms) and accuracy with a reduced parameter count, motivating its selection for real-time surgical tool tracking. Figure 5 illustrates the YOLO11 architecture based on [46]. This method generates a continuous sequence of reference points from the centroids of detected bounding boxes, updated periodically through image acquisition and processing, enabling the generation of precise tracking trajectories.

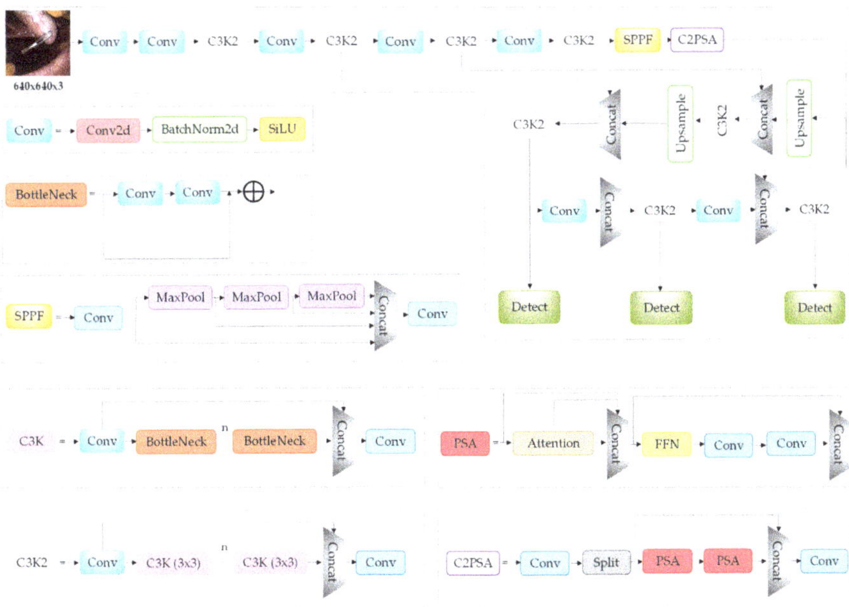

Figure 5. YOLO11 architecture. The diagram illustrates the main components of the model: convolutional layers (Conv) combined with C2PSA blocks at the top, processing pathways featuring BottleNeck and SPPF on the left, and specialized modules such as PSA, FFN, and Detect blocks.

The proposed low-level control consists of a Model Reference Adaptive Control scheme with Proportional–Derivative (PD) terms (MRAC-PD), leveraging its ability to manage nonlinear dynamics without requiring an exact mathematical model of the system. As demonstrated in prior studies [47,48], this configuration maintains accuracy in the presence of parametric uncertainties. The PD component enhances response speed and reduces overshoot, which is critical when manipulating delicate anatomical structures. Unlike conventional controllers such as PID, whose performance degrades significantly under nonlinear conditions, or Sliding Mode Control (SMC), which introduces high-frequency oscillations detrimental to surgical instrumentation, MRAC-PD generates smooth control signals and sustains adaptive robustness.

Additionally, a data-driven robot modeling approach is incorporated—a key strategy in surgical robotics, where analytical models are limited by the mechanical complexity of these systems, dynamic interactions during surgery, and the inherent variability of the surgical environment. The use of data-driven models enhances trajectory tracking accuracy, increases system robustness to sensor failures, and facilitates the integration of kinematic constraints. Furthermore, it enables adaptation to changing operational conditions, rejection of external disturbances, and management of parametric uncertainties. For implementation in real-time control systems, it is essential that such models are computationally efficient, ensuring low latency and optimal dynamic response.

In this context, the architecture of Closed-Form Continuous-Time Neural Networks (CfC) emerges as an ideal solution. Hasani et al.'s Liquid Time-Constant Networks (LTCs) [49] introduced adaptive "liquid" time constants for flexible representation; however, their reliance on Ordinary Differential Equation (ODE) solvers incurs a high computational cost. Closed-Form Continuous-Time Neural Networks (CfC) [47] overcome this limitation by providing a closed-form solution, reducing computational overhead without sacrificing accuracy, thus enabling real-time execution on hardware with limited resources.

The integration of CfC with mixed-memory architectures, such as Long Short-Term Memory (CfC-mmRNN) (Figure 6), effectively mitigates the vanishing gradient problem, which is critical for modeling complex, long-term temporal dependencies. This capability is essential for anticipating tissue movements and proactively responding to environmental changes. Experimental results reported by the authors [47] demonstrate that the CfC-mmRNN architecture achieves superior performance in terms of Mean Squared Error (MSE) when modeling physical dynamics, significantly outperforming architectures such as LTCs and various LSTM variants, as well as achieving an MSE approximately 18% lower than the Transformer architecture.

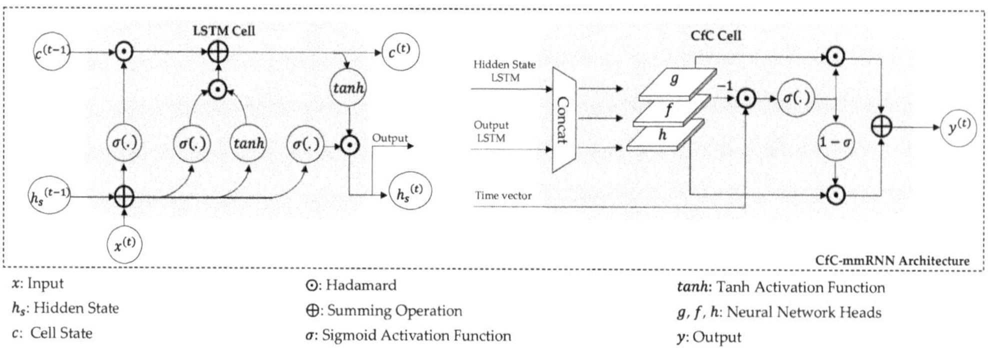

Figure 6. CfC-mmRNN neural network architecture. The figure illustrates the combination of Closed-Form Continuous-Time (CfC) networks with LSTM, forming the CfC-mmRNN architecture. On the left, a traditional LSTM cell is depicted, while on the right, the CfC cell is shown, incorporating a time vector and neural network heads (g, f, h). This integration enhances computational efficiency and the modeling of temporal dynamics.

Even more notable is its computational efficiency, with inference times less than half those of Transformer and LTC architectures, making it an optimal choice for applications requiring real-time processing of temporal sequences with irregularly sampled data. Furthermore, its design—based on a shared backbone that branches into specialized functions (f, g, and h)—facilitates the capture of temporal and structural relationships without compromising the model's expressiveness.

The integration of MRAC-PD with CfC-mmRNN directly addresses the critical requirements of robot-assisted surgery. While MRAC-PD ensures stability, precise tracking, and robustness, CfC-mmRNN enables the modeling of complex nonlinear dynamics without imposing a computational burden that would limit its clinical applicability. This approach optimizes millimeter-level precision, real-time adaptation, and resilience to system disturbances and uncertainties.

2.3.1. Design of the Low-Level MRAC-PD-CfC-mmRNN Adaptive Controller

This subsection provides a detailed overview of the low-level MRAC-PD-CfC-mmRNN controller, which serves as the core of the NVAC and is responsible for regulating the robotic manipulator's dynamic response. The discrete-time dynamics of an n-DoF manipulator—outlined in Supplementary Material, Section 4—are modeled as follows:

$$\mathbf{M}(q[k])\ (q[k+1]-2q[k]+q[k-1])/{T_s}^2+\mathbf{C}(q[k],\dot{q}[k])\dot{q}[k]+\mathbf{G}(q[k])=\tau[k] \quad (1)$$

where

$q[k]$: joint position vector.
$\dot{q}[k] = (q[k] - q[k-1])/T_s$: joint velocity vector.
$\ddot{q}[k] = (q[k+1] - 2q[k] + q[k-1])/{T_s}^2$: joint acceleration vector.
$\mathbf{M}(q[k])$: inertia matrix.
$\mathbf{C}(q[k],\dot{q}[k])\dot{q}[k]$: Coriolis and centrifugal forces matrix.
$\mathbf{G}(q[k])$: gravitational force vector.
$\tau[k]$: control torque vector.
T_s: sampling period.

The controller formulation defines position and velocity errors as follows:

$$e[k]=q_d[k]-q[k] \quad (2)$$

$$\dot{e}[k]=(e[k]-e[k-1])/T_s=\dot{q}_d[k]-\dot{q}[k] \quad (3)$$

where

$q_d[k]$: desired position at step k.
$\dot{q}_d[k]$: desired velocity at step k.
$q[k]$: current position of the robot.

The reference model, specified by Equations (4) and (5), incorporates adaptation gains γ_1 and γ_2 to adjust the reference position $q_r[k]$ and velocity $\dot{q}_r[k]$, facilitating rapid adaptation to system changes.

$$q_r[k]=q_d[k]+\gamma_1 e[k] \quad (4)$$

$$\dot{q}_r[k]=\dot{q}_d[k]+\gamma_2\dot{e}[k] \quad (5)$$

where

γ_1, γ_2: positive diagonal gain matrices.

The adaptation law, given by Equation (6), dynamically updates the adaptive parameters $\Gamma[k]$ to minimize tracking errors between $q_r[k]$ and $q[k]$.

$$\Gamma[k+1]=\Gamma[k]+\gamma_1(q_r[k]-q[k])+\gamma_2(\dot{q}_r[k]-\dot{q}[k]) \quad (6)$$

where

$\Gamma[k] > 0$: vector of adaptive parameters, ensuring convergence of position and velocity errors while compensating for dynamic uncertainties.

The control law, defined in Equation (7), integrates the CfC-mmRNN-based inverse model $\tau_{CfC}[k]$ with PD and adaptive terms for robustness and stability:

$$\tau[k] = \tau_{CfC}[k] + K_p e[k] + K_d \dot{e}[k] + \Gamma[k] \tag{7}$$

where

$\tau_{CfC}[k]$: torque predicted by the inverse model.
K_p, K_d: positive diagonal gain matrices.
$K_p e[k]$: proportional term that reduces the error.
$K_d \dot{e}[k]$: derivative term that improves dynamic stability.

2.3.2. Stability Analysis

A Lyapunov candidate function is proposed in Equation (8) to assess stability:

$$V[k] = \frac{1}{2}\, e[k]^T K_p e[k] + \frac{1}{2}\, \dot{e}[k]^T \mathbf{M}(q[k]) \dot{e}[k] + \frac{1}{2}\, \tilde{\Gamma}[k]^T\, \Pi^{-1} \tilde{\Gamma}[k] \tag{8}$$

where
$\tilde{\Gamma}[k] = \Gamma[k] - \Gamma^*$: adaptive parameter error.
Π^{-1}: inverse adaptive gain matrix.

The Lyapunov difference is computed as

$$\Delta V[k] = V[k+1] - V[k] \tag{9}$$

Substituting the adaptation law (6) and control law (7) into the dynamics (1) yields

$$\Delta V[k] \leq -T_s \dot{e}[k]^T K_d \dot{e}[k] - T_s \dot{e}[k]^T K_p e[k] + T_s \dot{e}[k]^T \tilde{\tau}[k] \tag{10}$$

where

$\tau^*[k]$: actual torque required.
$\tilde{\tau}[k] = \tau^*[k] - \tau_{CfC}[k]$: modeling error, representing the discrepancy between the learned model and the actual system dynamics.

Stability conditions:

(a) The controller gains must satisfy the following:
- $K_p > 0$: ensures that the proportional term contributes to system stability.
- $K_d > T_s K_p / 2$: guarantees adequate damping in the discrete-time system.

(b) Adaptation parameters:
- $\gamma_1, \gamma_2 < 2/T_s$: restricts adaptation gains to prevent excessive oscillations.

(c) The sampling interval must be sufficiently small to satisfy the conditions specified in Equations (11) and (12):

$$\|\mathbf{I} + T_s \mathbf{M}^{-1}(q[k]) K_d\| < 1 \tag{11}$$

$$\|\mathbf{M}^{-1}(q[k])\| < L \tag{12}$$

where
L: a positive constant bounding the inverse of the inertia matrix.

(d) Modeling error:
- $\|\tilde{\tau}[k]\| \leq \xi$, where $\xi > 0$ is an upper bound.

These conditions ensure the asymptotic stability of the system, guaranteeing precise tracking and bounded adaptive parameters:

- Asymptotic convergence of position error: $e[k] \rightarrow 0$ as $k \rightarrow \infty$.

- Velocity error convergence: $\dot{e}[k] \to 0$ as $k \to \infty$.
- Bounded adaptive parameters: $\|\Gamma[k]\| < \infty$.

2.3.3. Trajectory Generation

To select the optimal solution for trajectory generation, a methodology comprising three main components was followed:

1. Constraints: after defining the workspace, the RCM constraint was implemented, ensuring that all movements maintain a fixed fulcrum point.
2. Trajectory generation: smooth and continuous trajectories were generated using the minimum-jerk method between target points, considering maximum velocity, acceleration, and sampling step through interpolation to achieve seamless transitions.
3. Optimal configuration selection: eight inverse kinematics solutions were generated per target position, and the best was selected based on three criteria:
    - Position constraint verification: ensures the end-effector remains within the safe operational volume.
    - Joint limit verification: eliminates configurations exceeding safe joint ranges, preventing collisions or singularities.
    - Minimum configuration distance: prioritizes the solution with the smallest displacement from the current configuration for more efficient movements.

Table 1 lists the control strategy design parameters. The sampling period is $T_s = 0.001$ s, and Figure 7 depicts the NVAC scheme with the MRAC-PD-CfC-mmRNN low-level controller.

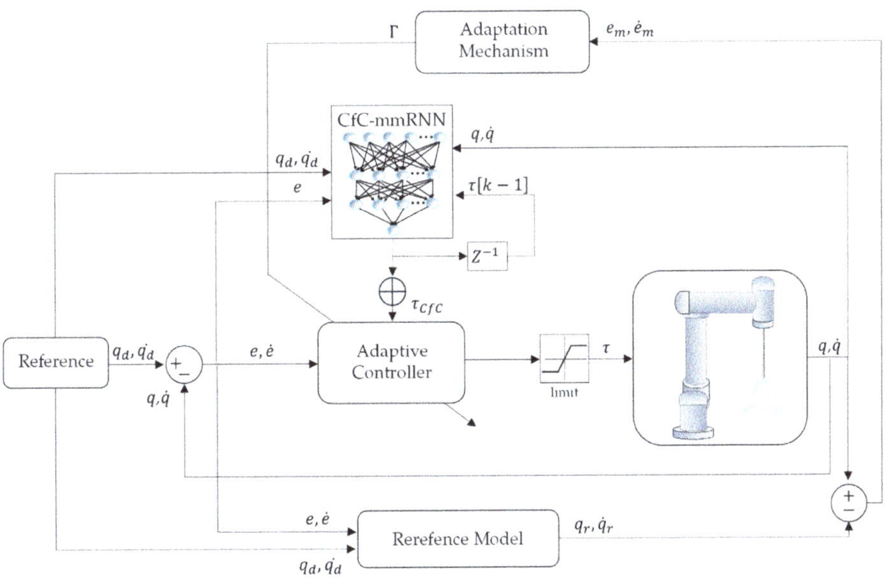

Figure 7. Schematic of the MRAC-PD-CfC-mmRNN low-level controller. The MRAC-PD-CfC-mmRNN controller is responsible for managing the dynamic response of the robotic manipulator within the NVAC framework. The controller accounts for the robot's dynamics and incorporates a reference model that adjusts the desired trajectory using adaptive gains (γ_1, γ_2). The CfC-mmRNN network predicts the inverse torque (τ_{CfC}), supplemented by proportional, derivative, and adaptive terms to enhance control stability and robustness.

Table 1. Design parameters for the NVAC control strategy.

Parameters	Joint 1	Joint 2	Joint 3	Joint 4	Joint 5	Joint 6
K_p	100	3000	320	80	30	2
K_d	100	380	80	20	8	2
γ_1	4	4	4	4	3	3
γ_2	3	3	2	2	3	3

2.4. Neural Network Training

The success of the training process heavily depends on the quantity and quality of input data. In this study, a gray-box approach was adopted, utilizing bounded input signals within a clinically relevant workspace to characterize the robot's dynamics.

To train the inverse model, trajectories were generated within the defined workspace. A Monte Carlo method was employed to identify feasible configurations and exhaustively explore possible trajectories. Notably, training trajectories were intentionally constrained to an "effective space" to establish an operational safety margin, preventing collisions with tissues in the event of transient control errors.

Random configurations were generated within joint limits, and forward kinematics was used to determine the positions and orientations of the end-effector. Each trajectory was designed at varying sampling frequencies (200 Hz, 250 Hz, 400 Hz, and 500 Hz) and comprised a maximum of 10 segments per trajectory. These segments were constructed by connecting selected points according to two possible configurations: straight and/or circular segments. Figure 8a depicts the general workspace of the assistant robot, accounting for the laparoscope's length, while Figure 8b illustrates the restricted working area used for generating training trajectories.

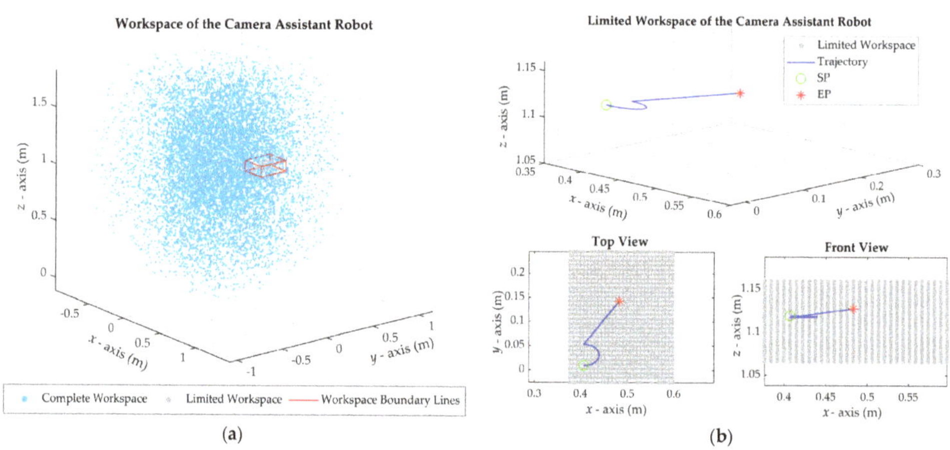

Figure 8. Workspace of the camera-holding robot. (**a**) Representation of the robot's complete workspace, including the laparoscope (blue points), with a restricted operational region in the abdominal area (red lines); (**b**) example of a trajectory within the restricted workspace, showing the starting point (SP, green circle), endpoint (EP, red star), and planned trajectory (blue line). Top and front views enable analysis of the trajectory relative to imposed limits, highlighting compliance with spatial constraints.

Figure 9 presents examples of these trajectories within the restricted workspace.

Table 2 specifies the training parameters for the CfC-mmRNN (system identification) and YOLO11n (tool tip detection) neural networks.

Table 2. Neural network training parameters for system identification and tool tip detection.

Parameters	CfC-mmRNN	Parameters	YOLO11n
Epochs	50	Epochs	300
Initial Learning Rate	0.001	Initial Learning Rate	0.01
Batch Size	64	Batch Size	16
Activation Function	GELU	Optimizer	SGDM
Optimizer	Adam	Momentum	0.937
Weight Decay	6.0×10^{-6}	Weight Decay	5.0×10^{-4}

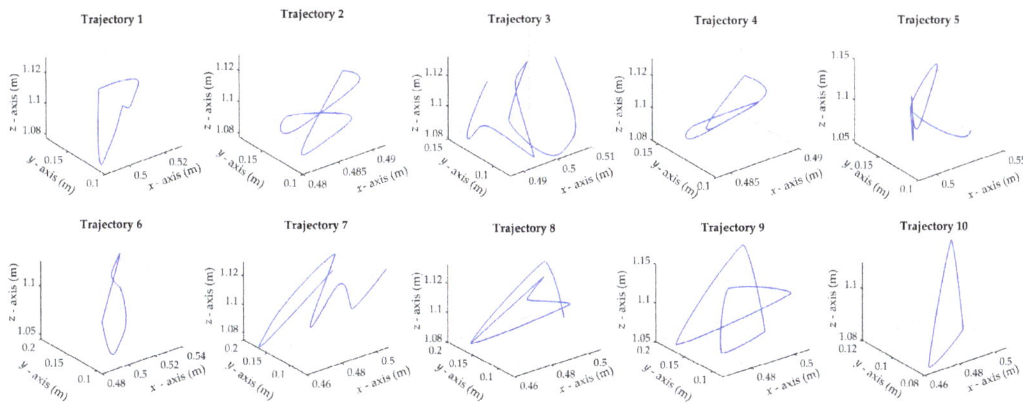

Figure 9. Example of trajectories generated within the restricted workspace for training the robot's inverse model.

2.5. Performance Metrics

The detection performance of the YOLO11n model is evaluated using recall (R), defined in (13), precision (P), defined in (14), and the mean average precision (mAP), which represents the area under the precision–recall curve and is defined in (16) [29].

$$R = \frac{TP}{TP + FN} \quad (13)$$

$$P = \frac{TP}{TP + FP} \quad (14)$$

where

TP (true positive): correct detections of the tool tip as the region of interest.
FP (false positive): incorrect identifications of a region as the tool tip.
FN (false negative): missed detections of the tool tip despite its presence.

$$AP = \int_0^1 P(R)dR \quad (15)$$

$$mAP = \frac{\sum_{i=1}^{N} AP_i}{N} \quad (16)$$

where

N: the total number of classes in the test set.
i: represents class I.
AP_i: the average precision for class i.

The $AP_{0.5}$ refers to the average precision (AP) when the Intersection over Union (IoU) is set to 0.5, enabling measurement of the model's accuracy when a detection is considered correct with 50% overlap between the prediction and the actual tool. The $AP_{0.5:0.95}$ represents the AP across varying IoU thresholds (from 0.5 to 0.95), allowing evaluation of the detection model's performance at different levels of overlap [29].

For the training of the CfC-mmRNN neural network, the Mean Squared Error (MSE) loss function is employed, defined as

$$\mathrm{MSE} = \frac{1}{n}\sum_{i=1}^{n}(y_i - \hat{y}_i)^2 \tag{17}$$

where

n: number of dataset examples.
y_i: actual value for the i-th example.
$\hat{y}_i$: predicted value for the i-th example.

Three performance indices (PIs) quantitatively assess controller performance, each capturing distinct response characteristics:

- Mean Absolute Error (MAE): Robust against outliers and disturbances, MAE offers a balanced measure of average error, making it well suited for dynamic, unpredictable surgical environments:

$$\mathrm{MAE} = \frac{1}{n}\sum_{i=1}^{n}|e_i| \tag{18}$$

- Integral of Time-Weighted Absolute Error (ITAE): By assigning greater weight to persistent errors over time, ITAE is essential for evaluating long-term stability and precision in surgical tracking:

$$\mathrm{ITAE} = \int_0^T t|e(t)|dt \tag{19}$$

- Integral of Time-Weighted Squared Error (ITSE): Combining temporal weighting with quadratic error penalization, ITSE effectively identifies large, late-stage errors and assesses robustness against disturbances:

$$\mathrm{ITSE} = \int_0^T te^2(t)dt \tag{20}$$

These metrics, as detailed in [48–53], provide a comprehensive evaluation of the system's performance under surgical conditions.

3. Results

This section presents the experimental results validating the proposed Neuro-Visual Adaptive Control architecture for the semi-autonomous operation of a camera-holding robot in surgical environments. Overall, the NVAC controller demonstrated exceptional performance across all evaluation metrics, achieving tracking errors of 1.80×10^{-3} m, 1.08×10^{-4} m, and 1.90×10^{-3} m along the x, y, and z axes, respectively, in complex scenarios with significant dynamic disturbances. The YOLO11n-based visual processing system attained a precision of 97.30% and a recall of 94.80% in surgical instrument detection, while the CfC-mmRNN neural network provided accurate system identification with a Mean Squared Error (MSE) of 8.40×10^{-3}.

Comparative analysis with conventional control techniques (PID, SMC, and standard MRAC-PD) confirmed the superior performance of NVAC in trajectory tracking, disturbance rejection, and control signal smoothness. The system maintained robust stability even under challenging conditions, including simulated sensor failures and tissue collisions. These findings underscore the potential of NVAC to significantly enhance precision and safety in robot-assisted surgical applications. The following subsections provide a detailed analysis of these results concerning surgical instrument localization, system identification, and control performance across various simulated surgical scenarios.

3.1. Results of Surgical Tool Localization

To train the YOLO11n model for surgical tool tip detection, a total of 2561 images from the CholecSeg8k dataset were employed, divided into 80% for training (2364 images), 10% for validation (99 images), and 10% for testing (98 images), each resized to 640×640 pixels. Training outcomes, illustrated in Figure 10, exhibit stable and consistent convergence of performance metrics, indicating robust model behavior.

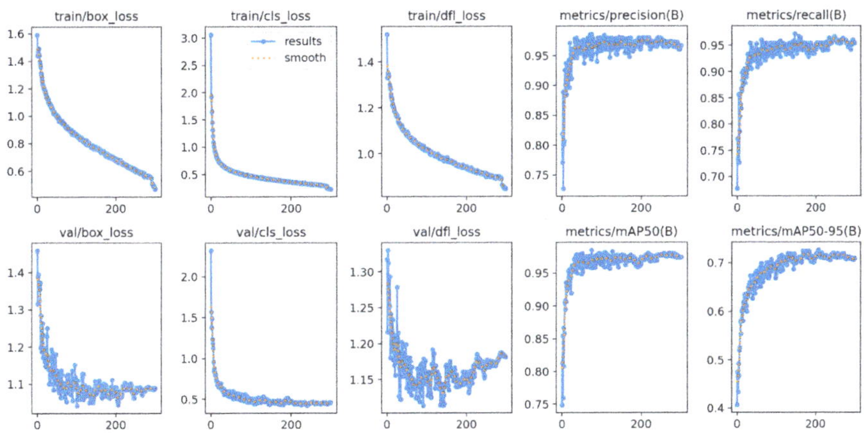

Figure 10. Performance curves of YOLO11 training across training epochs. The top row displays the training losses for box detection (train/box_loss), classification (train/cls_loss), and distribution focal loss (train/dfl_loss), along with precision and recall metrics. The bottom row presents the validation losses (val/box_loss, val/cls_loss, val/dfl_loss) and the mAP_{50} and $mAP_{50\text{–}95}$ metrics. These plots demonstrate the model's effective convergence during training and its ability to generalize on validation data.

The YOLO11n model achieved a precision of 97.30%, recall of 94.80%, an $mAP_{0.5}$ of 97.5%, and an $mAP_{0.5:0.95}$ of 72.7% in detecting surgical instruments. These outcomes are significant given the visual complexity and variability of instruments in surgical settings, highlighting the model's reliability in minimizing false positives that could compromise procedural safety. The elevated recall underscores its ability to rarely miss detectable instruments, a critical factor for continuous tracking during surgery. These results confirm the model's effectiveness for real-world surgical scenarios and its appropriateness for autonomous tool tracking tasks. Figure 10 presents the training performance results for the YOLO11n model.

Figure 11a showcases representative examples of tool tip detection in the test dataset, demonstrating high precision in bounding box placement. Figure 11b depicts the localization of bounding box centroids, calculated in MatLab® from CoppeliaSim data, providing reliable spatial references for robotic control.

3.2. Results of System Identification

System identification utilized the CfC-mmRNN neural network, chosen for its robustness against the vanishing gradient problem in irregularly sampled data, effectively capturing long-term dependencies. A total of 80 trajectories at varying frequencies were employed, sampled at $T_s = 0.001$ s.

Training the inverse dynamics model yielded an MSE of 8.4×10^{-3}, showcasing high precision in predicting the dynamic behavior of the UR5 robot despite its inherent nonlinearities. Figure 12 compares predicted torques with actual values for a test trajectory, revealing strong alignment with minimal deviations, even in regions of significant dynamic variability. This torque curve analysis underscores the model's capability to accurately capture both overarching system dynamics and subtle variations, with minor discrepancies at torque peaks exerting negligible impact on control performance, as confirmed by subsequent tests.

(a)

(b)

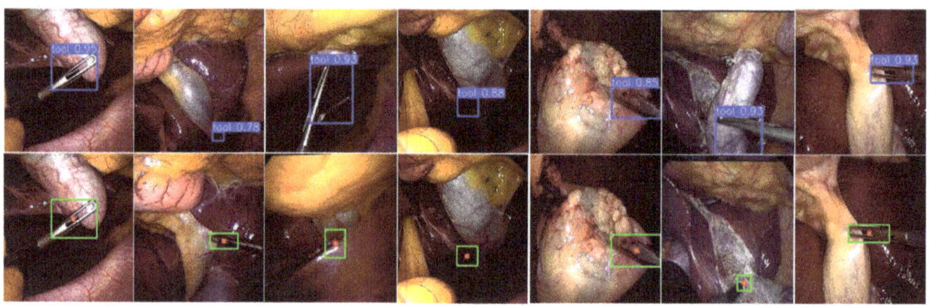

Figure 11. Detection of the surgical tool tip. (**a**) Detection results on the test set using YOLO11n; (**b**) localization of the centroid of the bounding boxes.

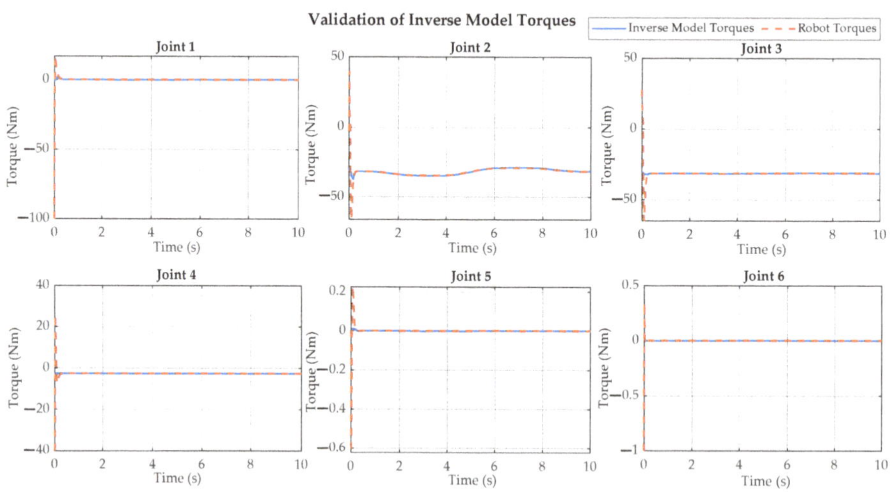

Figure 12. Validation of the inverse model training for a test trajectory. The torques estimated by the inverse model (solid line) are compared with the actual torques applied by the robot (dashed line) across each of the six joints, verifying the model's accuracy in reproducing the system's dynamics.

Table 3 outlines the computational costs of the trained neural networks, confirming their suitability for real-time implementation on resource-constrained hardware.

Table 3. Computational cost of trained neural network models.

Model	Parameters	Memory	Inference Speed
YOLO11x	56,874,931	111.7 MB	34.8 ms
YOLO11n	2,590,035	5.37 MB	9.5 ms
CfC-mmRNN	197,638	798 KB	26 ms

The YOLO11x model, trained with parameters identical to those of YOLO11n, attained a precision of 98% and a recall of 93.5%, closely aligning with YOLO11n's performance. YOLO11n was selected due to its substantially lower computational cost, enhancing its applicability for real-time surgical operations.

3.3. *Simulation Results*

Experiments evaluated the robot's capability to track millimetric trajectories within the abdominal workspace using the NVAC strategy. Reference trajectories were derived from interpolated points captured during instrument tracking at various time instants, ensuring realistic motion profiles. To enhance safety, the robot's torque was restricted according to manufacturer specifications.

3.3.1. Experimental Tests

Four progressively challenging test scenarios were devised to assess the NVAC's performance, extracting key visual points for dynamic camera path planning:

1. Scenario 1: Visual data provided by YOLO11n detects the surgical instrument, generating reference points for a tracking path with moderate geometric transitions.
2. Scenario 2: To simulate estimation errors or sensor signal transmission failures, a controlled disturbance was introduced in joint 6 of the manipulator. Specifically, at the 9 s mark of the simulation, a sudden displacement of 0.06 radians was applied, lasting 0.2 s. This abrupt alteration in the reference mimics an unexpected trajectory deviation, enabling evaluation of the controller's ability to detect discrepancies and recover stability in real time.
3. Scenario 3: The system's robustness is evaluated against an abrupt perturbation simulating a 15 N collision with elements of the surgical environment.
4. Scenario 4: Multiple perturbations are integrated in a challenging scenario: an initial sensor signal failure at the 9 s mark, followed by a 15 N collision at the 10 s mark, assessing real-time path adjustment and tracking accuracy.

The performance of the NVAC was compared against three established controllers—PID, conventional MRAC-PD (with identical tuning parameters), and SMC—using quantitative performance indices.

3.3.2. Trajectory Tracking

Figure 13 showcases the performance of the implemented controllers in tracking the generated trajectories. Figure 13a presents results for Scenario 1, employing a higher density of control points to enhance tracking precision and assess controller behavior under substantial dynamic demands. Figure 13b illustrates performance in Scenario 2, incorporating a perturbation represented by a sudden displacement—a reference value significantly offset from the current workspace—simulating abrupt motion due to estimation errors or sensor signal failures.

For detailed performance analysis, Figures 14–16 present tracking results in Cartesian space (x, y, and z axes) for trajectories 1 and 2, with the first and second columns corresponding to each trajectory, respectively.

Analysis of trajectory tracking highlights the challenges of achieving millimetric precision within the surgical Cartesian space. The proposed NVAC controller demonstrates shorter settling times and superior precision, particularly in regions with steep slopes and curvature. Conversely, the conventional MRAC-PD controller exhibits closely comparable performance but with slightly extended settling times and increased errors. The SMC controller displays intermediate performance, with evident deviations in curved segments and direction changes. The PID controller shows the greatest deviations from the reference, markedly affected by gravitational effects alongside SMC. A comparative analysis of the four controllers confirms that the NVAC delivers the best tracking performance, consistently maintaining close proximity to the reference from the outset.

Table 4 provides performance indices for trajectory 1. Table 5 provides performance indices for trajectory 2, which includes perturbation, facilitating a detailed comparison of controller performance.

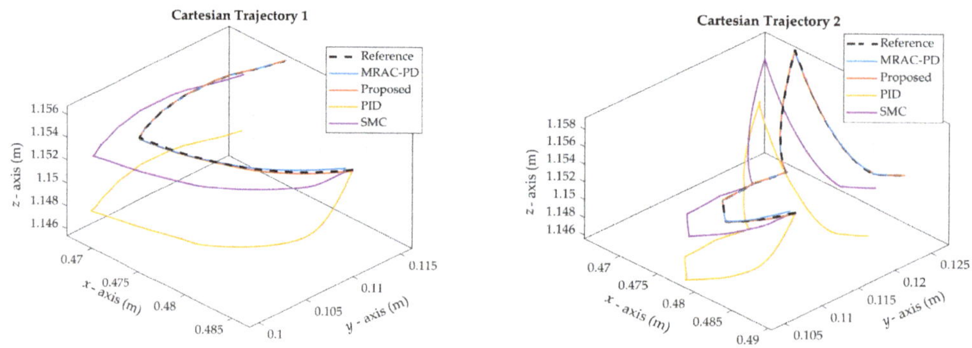

(a) (b)

Figure 13. Trajectory tracking performance of the implemented controllers. (**a**) Desired Cartesian trajectory 1 for Scenario 1. (**b**) Desired Cartesian trajectory 2 for Scenario 2.

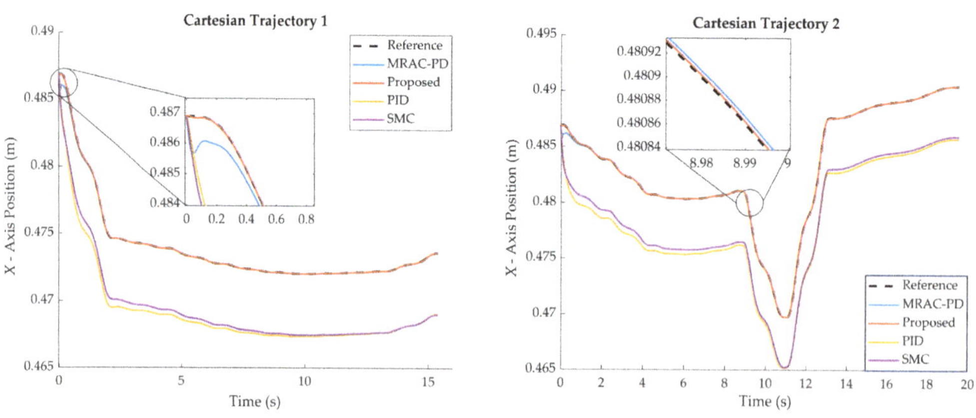

(a) (b)

Figure 14. Simulation results for the implemented control strategies. (**a**) Tracking of the desired Cartesian trajectory 1 on the x-axis; (**b**) tracking of the desired Cartesian trajectory 2 on the x-axis.

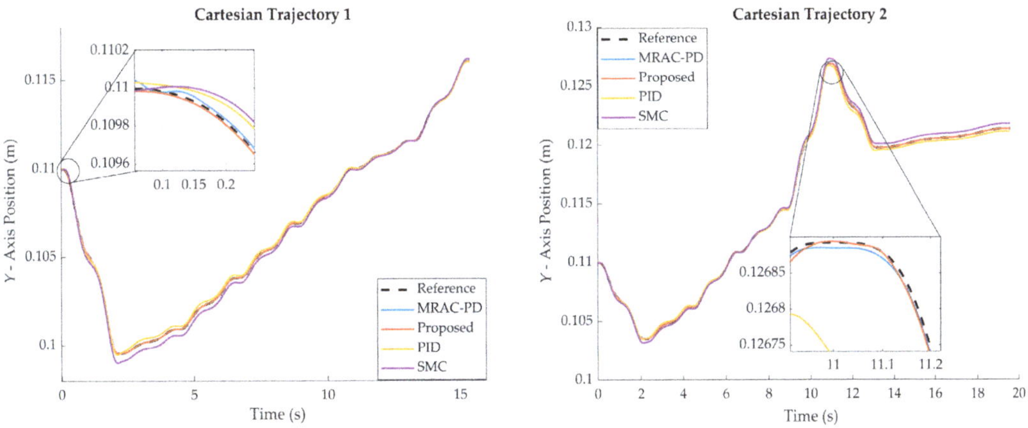

(a) (b)

Figure 15. Simulation results for the implemented control strategies. (**a**) Tracking of the desired Cartesian trajectory 1 on the y-axis; (**b**) tracking of the desired Cartesian trajectory 2 on the y-axis.

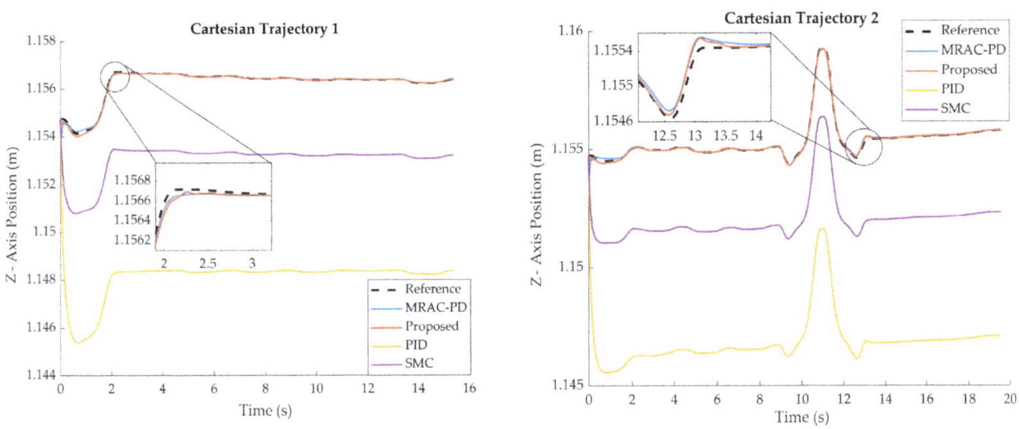

(a) (b)

Figure 16. Simulation results for the implemented control strategies. (**a**) Tracking of the desired Cartesian trajectory 1 on the z-axis; (**b**) tracking of the desired Cartesian trajectory 2 on the z-axis.

Table 4. Performance indexes for Cartesian and joint positions under trajectory 1.

PIs	Controller	x	y	z	Joint 1	Joint 2	Joint 3	Joint 4	Joint 5	Joint 6
MAE	PID	0.0047	9.394×10^{-5}	0.0081	6.71×10^{-5}	0.0065	0.0120	0.0031	0.0008	0.0005
	SMC	0.0045	0.0002	0.0031	3.85×10^{-5}	0.0020	0.0098	0.0027	0.0001	0.0002
	MRAC-PD	2.60×10^{-5}	$\mathbf{3.24 \times 10^{-6}}$	$\mathbf{1.71 \times 10^{-5}}$	1.43×10^{-5}	6.90×10^{-5}	6.82×10^{-5}	$\mathbf{2.00 \times 10^{-5}}$	$\mathbf{2.16 \times 10^{-5}}$	0.0002
	Proposed	$\mathbf{5.22 \times 10^{-6}}$	3.91×10^{-6}	2.11×10^{-5}	$\mathbf{1.36 \times 10^{-5}}$	$\mathbf{3.02 \times 10^{-5}}$	$\mathbf{1.99 \times 10^{-5}}$	2.03×10^{-5}	2.18×10^{-5}	**0.0001**
ITAE	PID	0.5538	0.0084	0.9556	0.0066	0.7814	1.4354	0.3425	0.0709	0.0363
	SMC	0.5383	0.0174	0.3751	0.0028	0.2325	1.1793	0.3337	0.0289	0.0116
	MRAC-PD	**0.0003**	**0.0002**	**0.0008**	0.0015	**0.0014**	0.0013	**0.0008**	0.0023	**0.0105**
	Proposed	**0.0003**	0.0004	0.0012	**0.0013**	0.0021	**0.0010**	**0.0008**	**0.0022**	**0.0105**
ITSE	PID	0.0026	1.01×10^{-6}	0.0077	5.88×10^{-7}	0.0052	0.0174	0.0010	6.73×10^{-5}	2.18×10^{-5}
	SMC	0.0024	4.04×10^{-6}	0.0011	1.75×10^{-7}	0.0004	0.0117	0.0009	7.79×10^{-6}	2.33×10^{-6}
	MRAC-PD	3.93×10^{-8}	$\mathbf{9.27 \times 10^{-10}}$	$\mathbf{1.77 \times 10^{-8}}$	2.54×10^{-8}	2.747×10^{-7}	2.40×10^{-7}	$\mathbf{3.23 \times 10^{-8}}$	5.58×10^{-8}	$\mathbf{1.34 \times 10^{-6}}$
	Proposed	$\mathbf{2.27 \times 10^{-9}}$	2.480×10^{-9}	3.44×10^{-8}	$\mathbf{2.25 \times 10^{-8}}$	$\mathbf{7.79 \times 10^{-8}}$	$\mathbf{3.34 \times 10^{-8}}$	4.09×10^{-8}	$\mathbf{5.52 \times 10^{-8}}$	$\mathbf{1.34 \times 10^{-6}}$

Best performance is denoted in bold.

Table 5. Performance indexes for Cartesian and joint positions under trajectory 2.

PIs	Controller	x	y	z	Joint 1	Joint 2	Joint 3	Joint 4	Joint 5	Joint 6
MAE	PID	0.0049	1.53×10^{-4}	0.0084	1.02×10^{-4}	0.0055	0.0121	0.0031	0.0013	0.0024
	SMC	0.0045	2.45×10^{-4}	0.0033	3.35×10^{-5}	0.0029	0.0098	0.0027	1.95×10^{-4}	**0.0011**
	MRAC-PD	2.49×10^{-5}	**2.86×10^{-6}**	3.362×10^{-5}	1.47×10^{-5}	8.34×10^{-5}	6.70×10^{-5}	4.05×10^{-5}	2.23×10^{-5}	0.0015
	Proposed	**6.68×10^{-6}**	4.63×10^{-6}	**2.81×10^{-5}**	**1.44×10^{-5}**	**3.92×10^{-5}**	**2.78×10^{-5}**	**3.89×10^{-5}**	**2.19×10^{-5}**	0.0013
ITAE	PID	0.9228	0.0373	1.6236	0.0174	1.0312	2.3259	0.5386	0.3276	0.5482
	SMC	0.8693	0.0582	0.6403	0.0046	0.5909	1.8829	0.5075	0.0440	**0.2332**
	MRAC-PD	**0.0012**	**3.89×10^{-4}**	0.0052	**0.0022**	0.0078	0.0054	**0.0073**	0.0034	0.3128
	Proposed	0.0013	7.59×10^{-4}	**0.0048**	**0.0022**	**0.0067**	**0.0051**	0.0078	**0.0033**	0.3126
ITSE	PID	0.0044	8.99×10^{-6}	0.0138	4.96×10^{-6}	0.0056	0.0282	0.0015	6.47×10^{-3}	0.0073
	SMC	0.0039	2.04×10^{-5}	0.0021	2.38×10^{-7}	0.0019	0.0185	0.0013	1.29×10^{-5}	**0.0035**
	MRAC-PD	5.675×10^{-8}	1.93×10^{-9}	3.464×10^{-7}	**6.18×10^{-8}**	9.86×10^{-7}	5.92×10^{-7}	**8.84×10^{-7}**	1.52×10^{-7}	0.0060
	Proposed	**2.02×10^{-8}**	**1.06×10^{-9}**	**2.78×10^{-7}**	6.72×10^{-8}	**5.58×10^{-7}**	**4.23×10^{-7}**	9.83×10^{-7}	**1.44×10^{-7}**	0.0055

Best performance is denoted in bold.

Similar to the images, Table 4 confirms the superior performance of the proposed controller compared to the other controllers, with behavior akin to that of the MRAC-PD. The proposed controller consistently achieved the lowest performance index (PI) values across most metrics. MAE ranges from 10^{-5} to 10^{-6}, indicating exceptional robustness and precision in tracking. ITAE, generally on the order of 10^{-3} for most joints, reflects rapid error convergence. ITSE, ranging from 10^{-6} to 10^{-9}, confirms minimal time-weighted errors. The PI values for Scenario 2, in the presence of a sensor failure disturbance, highlight greater differences among the controllers, with the proposed controller demonstrating a marked improvement over the others.

A critical attribute of control systems is their capacity to reject external disturbances, which is paramount in surgery where precision and stability are essential. In addition to the perturbation in Scenario 2, a further 15 N force impulse was applied to simulate a collision, evaluating performance under extreme conditions. Figure 17 illustrates tracking performance under these disturbances, with Figure 17a representing Scenario 3 and Figure 17b representing Scenario 4.

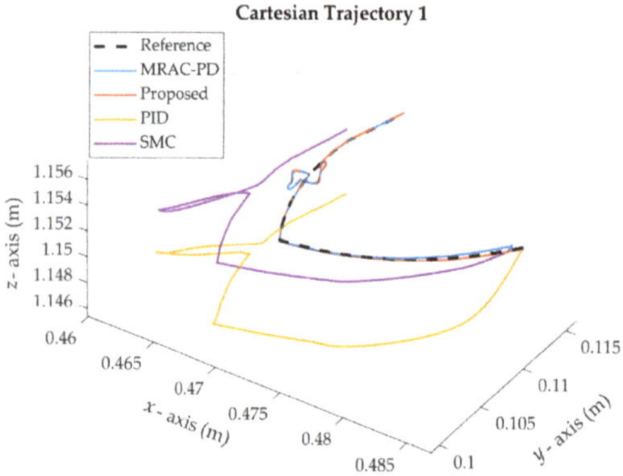

(a)

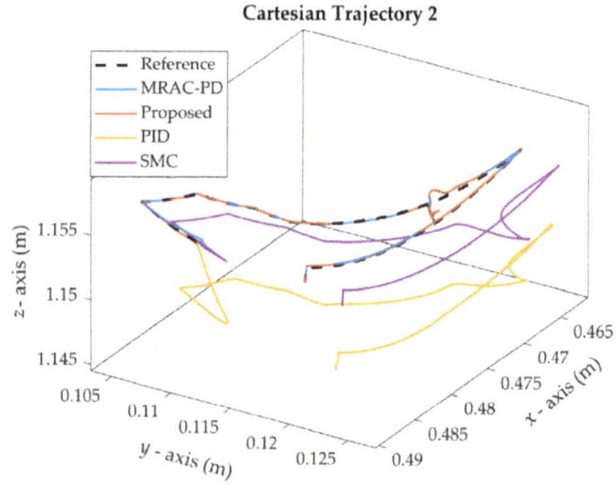

(b)

Figure 17. Cartesian trajectory tracking under external disturbances. (**a**) Trajectory 1, Scenario 3; (**b**) trajectory 2, Scenario 4.

Analysis of the controllers' responses to perturbations reveals distinct recovery capabilities. The proposed NVAC exhibits robust disturbance rejection, with minimal deviation from the desired path and swift recovery, closely resembling the behavior of conventional

MRAC-PD. In contrast, SMC and PID demonstrate greater vulnerability, displaying pronounced deviations and prolonged recovery times. Scenario 4, the most realistic and demanding scenario, integrates an initial perturbation simulating abrupt motion due to estimation errors or sensor failures with a subsequent 15 N collision. Tables 6 and 7 quantitatively compare controller performance for Scenario 3 and 4, respectively, using performance indices.

Table 6. Performance indexes for Cartesian and joint positions under Scenario 3.

PIs	Controller	x	y	z	Joint 1	Joint 2	Joint 3	Joint 4	Joint 5	Joint 6
MAE	PID	6.70×10^{-5}	0.0065	0.0121	6.70×10^{-5}	0.0065	0.0121	0.0033	0.0007	0.0004
	SMC	0.0046	0.0002	0.0032	3.89×10^{-5}	0.0019	0.0100	0.0029	0.0001	0.0002
	MRAC-PD	5.68×10^{-5}	**3.82×10^{-6}**	**4.83×10^{-5}**	1.47×10^{-5}	9.33×10^{-5}	0.0001	**6.75×10^{-5}**	**2.16×10^{-5}**	0.0002
	Proposed	**3.59×10^{-5}**	4.22×10^{-6}	5.24×10^{-5}	**1.40×10^{-5}**	**5.48×10^{-5}**	**6.74×10^{-5}**	6.77×10^{-5}	2.18×10^{-5}	**0.0001**
ITAE	PID	0.0066	0.7860	1.4465	0.0066	0.7860	1.4465	0.3767	0.0708	0.0362
	SMC	0.5538	0.0177	0.3841	0.0028	0.2285	1.1966	0.3613	0.0289	0.0116
	MRAC-PD	**0.0046**	0.0004	**0.0053**	0.0014	**0.0049**	0.0080	0.0077	**0.0022**	**0.0105**
	Proposed	**0.0046**	**0.0003**	0.0057	**0.0013**	0.0057	**0.0078**	**0.0076**	0.0023	**0.0105**
ITSE	PID	5.86×10^{-7}	0.0052	0.0176	5.86×10^{-7}	0.0052	0.0176	0.0016	6.73×10^{-5}	2.18×10^{-5}
	SMC	0.0026	4.21×10^{-6}	0.0012	1.79×10^{-7}	0.0004	0.0121	0.0013	7.82×10^{-6}	2.34×10^{-5}
	MRAC-PD	3.77×10^{-6}	**4.06×10^{-9}**	**3.62×10^{-6}**	2.97×10^{-8}	2.19×10^{-6}	9.69×10^{-6}	**8.62×10^{-6}**	**5.52×10^{-8}**	**1.34×10^{-6}**
	Proposed	**3.72×10^{-6}**	4.49×10^{-9}	3.65×10^{-6}	**2.72×10^{-8}**	**2.08×10^{-6}**	**9.41×10^{-6}**	8.71×10^{-6}	5.58×10^{-8}	**1.34×10^{-6}**

Best performance is denoted in bold.

Table 7. Performance indexes for Cartesian and joint positions under Scenario 4.

PIs	Controller	x	y	z	Joint 1	Joint 2	Joint 3	Joint 4	Joint 5	Joint 6
MAE	PID	0.0049	1.53×10^{-4}	0.0084	1.02×10^{-4}	0.0055	0.0121	0.0032	0.0013	0.0024
	SMC	0.0046	2.53×10^{-4}	0.0033	3.37×10^{-5}	0.0029	0.0099	0.0028	1.95×10^{-4}	**0.0011**
	MRAC-PD	4.86×10^{-5}	**5.02×10^{-6}**	5.05×10^{-5}	1.48×10^{-5}	9.29×10^{-5}	9.93×10^{-5}	7.46×10^{-5}	2.23×10^{-5}	0.0015
	Proposed	**3.01×10^{-5}**	6.89×10^{-6}	**4.58×10^{-5}**	**1.44×10^{-5}**	**4.97×10^{-5}**	**5.99×10^{-5}**	**7.29×10^{-5}**	**2.19×10^{-5}**	0.0013
ITAE	PID	0.9378	0.0376	1.6297	0.0173	1.0364	2.3382	0.5698	0.3276	0.5482
	SMC	0.8863	0.0597	0.6504	0.0046	0.5864	1.9021	0.5380	0.0440	**0.2331**
	MRAC-PD	0.0060	**8.28×10^{-4}**	0.0086	**0.0022**	0.0097	0.0119	**0.0141**	0.0033	0.3128
	Proposed	**0.0059**	0.0012	**0.0083**	**0.0022**	**0.0088**	**0.0115**	0.0145	**0.0032**	0.3126
ITSE	PID	0.0046	9.30×10^{-6}	0.0138	4.95×10^{-6}	0.0056	0.0285	0.0022	6.47×10^{-4}	0.0073
	SMC	0.0041	2.19×10^{-5}	0.0022	2.41×10^{-7}	0.0018	0.0190	0.0017	1.298×10^{-5}	**0.0034**
	MRAC-PD	4.19×10^{-6}	**3.78×10^{-8}**	4.35×10^{-6}	**6.61×10^{-8}**	3.04×10^{-6}	1.09×10^{-5}	**1.06×10^{-5}**	1.52×10^{-7}	0.0060
	Proposed	**4.15×10^{-6}**	5.33×10^{-8}	**4.21×10^{-6}**	7.14×10^{-8}	**2.52×10^{-6}**	**1.07×10^{-5}**	1.08×10^{-5}	**1.44×10^{-7}**	0.0055

Best performance is denoted in bold.

Performance index analysis, as described in the methodology, validates the NVAC's effectiveness and exceptional robustness. These findings confirm superior tracking precision, efficient reduction of persistent errors, and a remarkable capacity to mitigate large errors under substantial perturbations. Figures 18 and 19 illustrate tracking errors for the designed controllers in Scenarios 3 and 4, respectively.

For Scenario 3, the proposed controller achieved maximum errors of 1.80×10^{-3} m on the x- and z-axes and 6.11×10^{-5} m on the y-axis, compared to MRAC-PD's 1.70×10^{-3} m, 6.92×10^{-5} m, and 1.80×10^{-3} m for the x-, y-, and z-axes, respectively. In Scenario 4, the proposed controller recorded maximum errors of 1.80×10^{-3} m, 1.08×10^{-4} m, and 1.90×10^{-3} m across the x-, y-, and z-axes, respectively, with MRAC-PD showing comparable values.

Despite these similarities, comparative torque analysis reveals distinct differences in perturbation response. The proposed NVAC demonstrates faster and more stable recovery with reduced torque oscillations, signifying enhanced disturbance rejection. Its control action is less aggressive than that of MRAC-PD, minimizing abrupt variations while preserving performance. These findings establish the NVAC as a more robust and precise solution, ideally suited for surgical environments where stability is paramount.

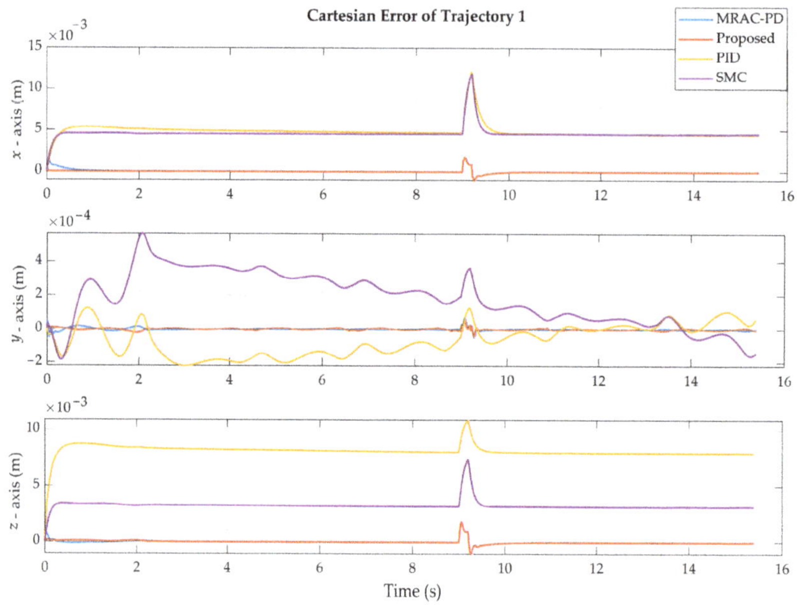

Figure 18. Cartesian tracking errors in surgical instrument tracking for Scenario 3. The figure compares the tracking errors of the designed controllers along the Cartesian axes (x, y, z).

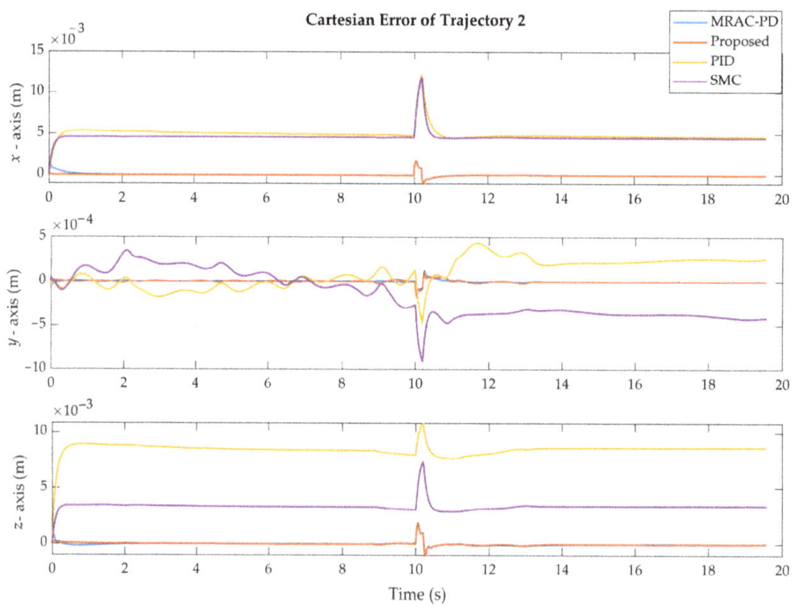

Figure 19. Cartesian tracking errors in surgical instrument tracking for Scenario 4. The figure compares the tracking errors of the designed controllers along the Cartesian axes (x, y, z).

4. Discussion

The results obtained with the NVAC controller demonstrate exceptional performance in terms of surgical precision. In the undisturbed scenario, the maximum errors achieved are submillimeter: 4.87×10^{-5} m (x-axis), 1.22×10^{-5} m (y-axis), and 1.81×10^{-4} m (z-axis). In the most complex scenario, tracking errors increase to 1.80×10^{-3} m (x-axis), 1.08×10^{-4} m (y-axis), and 1.90×10^{-3} m (z-axis), remaining below the clinically acceptable threshold of 2 mm for robotic surgery, as established in the consulted literature [18,24].

Compared to previous studies, such as Wang et al., who reported Mean Absolute Errors of 1.49×10^{-3} m without disturbances and 1.98×10^{-3} m under external perturbations, our approach maintains lower errors even under more demanding conditions. Additionally, the NVAC's ability to recover stability after disturbances is significantly superior. While the controller proposed by Ren et al. [17] requires approximately 2 s to stabilize following disturbances causing angular errors below 1°, the proposed controller achieves recovery times under 0.7 s against 15 N forces—well above typical forces in surgical procedures (e.g., surgical camera: 0.2 N; soft tissue penetration (e.g., liver): 0.08 N; soft tissue resection (e.g., liver): 0.9 N; suturing on soft tissue (e.g., skin): 1.7 N; suturing with knot-tying: 8 N; liver and gallbladder retraction: 6.6 N; general surgical manipulation: 0.5–8 N) [54,55].

This robustness is particularly valuable in surgical environments where involuntary patient movements, accidental collisions, or interactions with denser tissues could introduce unforeseen disturbances. Although a 15 N perturbation exceeds forces commonly encountered in laparoscopic surgery, this test validates the system's ability to maintain stability in critical scenarios, ensuring patient safety under adverse conditions.

The simulated disturbance in Scenario 2, introducing a sudden displacement of 0.06 radians (approximately 3.4°) for 0.2 s, represents a severe sensor failure compared to values reported in the literature. For instance, relative to Ren et al. [17], the NVAC controller demonstrates the ability to manage a larger angular error with a substantially shorter recovery time.

4.1. Study Limitations

While the obtained results are promising, several limitations of this study must be acknowledged. The validation of the NVAC controller was conducted exclusively in simulated environments. Although CoppeliaSim provides a robust platform for modeling complex dynamics, differences exist between simulations and real surgical scenarios, particularly regarding anatomical variability, tissue behavior, fluctuating lighting conditions, and the presence of fluids. For broader acceptance within the medical community, demonstrating results on physical hardware, even in a laboratory setting, would be ideal.

Validation with real cholecystectomy images marks a significant advancement, but comparison with larger clinical datasets could strengthen the model's applicability. Furthermore, although the CholecSeg8k dataset is extensive, it represents a limited subset of potential variations in surgical instruments and visual conditions. The system's ability to detect instruments not represented in the training set may be compromised. While YOLO11n proved efficient for real-time surgical instrument detection, benchmarking against alternatives such as Mask R-CNN or Swin Transformer could confirm its optimality. Additionally, the performance comparison of the proposed controller could be enriched by including modern deep learning-based control approaches.

4.2. Feasibility and Challenges of Transitioning from Simulation to Real-World Clinical Trials

The NVAC system holds potential to enhance visualization in various robotic surgery procedures, such as laparoscopic cholecystectomy, colorectal resection, Nissen fundoplication, and radical prostatectomy. In these procedures, key challenges include frequent camera repositioning, assistant fatigue, difficulty maintaining stable vision in deep spaces, and coordination of multiple instruments.

NVAC addresses these issues through efficient instrument tracking, improved visual stability, submillimeter precision, and real-time adaptation to different anatomical regions. These advantages can enhance surgical safety and efficiency, supporting its potential for future clinical application. Effective transition from simulation-based findings to real-world clinical settings requires rigorous validation and progressive adaptation.

Considerations for Clinical Validation of the NVAC Controller

Developing a Neuro-Visual Adaptive Control system for robotic surgery entails not only validation in simulated environments but also evaluation of its applicability in real clinical contexts. The following sections address critical aspects that would demonstrate its feasibility in an operating room.

1. Enhancements in visual perception: The YOLO11n model delivers high success rates in detecting surgical tool tips, providing rapid computation and accurate reference point acquisition. Additional capabilities of the YOLO family, such as instance segmentation and pose estimation, establish a foundation for future advancements in surgical scene perception. However, despite its effectiveness in real-time detection, YOLO11n exhibits limitations in visual perception, including difficulties in detecting fine details and ensuring precise identification under partial occlusions. Advanced techniques could mitigate these limitations, enhancing precision in complex surgical scenes, although they require greater computational resources, which may be impractical in hardware-constrained operating rooms.

A hybrid approach is recommended, utilizing YOLO11n for rapid detection while supplementing it with semantic segmentation for scenarios demanding greater detail and precision. Figure 20 showcases YOLO11n's performance on complex dataset images, demonstrating robust detection despite limited training data and default parameters. Performance enhancements are achievable by optimizing parameters such as the initial learning rate, optimizer, and loss function. Overall, the YOLO family provides a highly efficient solution for real-time object detection, widely implemented in medical patents.

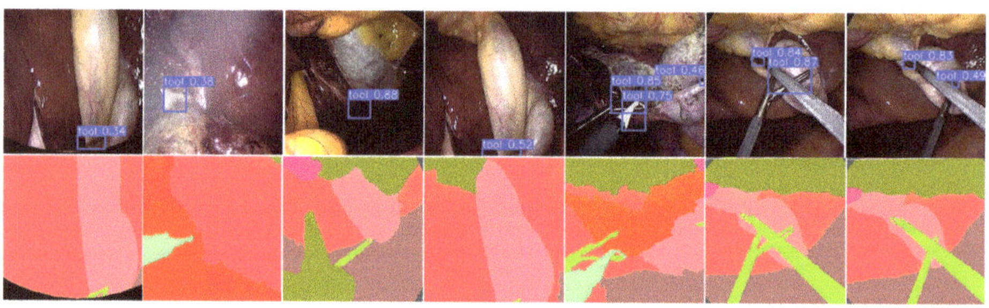

Figure 20. Examples of surgical tool detection with YOLO11n in challenging scenarios, including low lighting, partial occlusion, smoke presence, and small instrument detection.

2. Currently, various commercial platforms have incorporated robotic assistance technologies into laparoscopic procedures. However, these systems primarily rely on manual guidance or servo-control strategies with limited adaptability. In contrast, the proposed NVAC controller offers greater adaptability to intraoperative disturbances, reduced tracking errors, and enhanced stability of the FOV, thereby improving surgical efficiency. To assess its applicability in real-world surgery, integration with certified surgical platforms and verification of compatibility with endoscopic vision systems used in laparoscopy would be necessary. A comparative study with commercial platforms, evaluating precision,

latency, and robustness under varying surgical conditions, would be critical to validate its performance and implementation potential.

Given that these systems operate in environments with resource-constrained hardware, optimization strategies have been explored in three key areas: visual processing, neural model inference, and low-level control. These enhancements would reduce computational latency and ensure execution on medical hardware without delays, facilitating adoption in real clinical settings.

- Computational cost reduction strategies:
  - Model compression: techniques such as quantization (reducing precision from FP32 to INT8) and pruning unnecessary connections reduce memory usage and accelerate inference without sacrificing precision.
  - CfC networks: by eliminating the need for numerical ODE solvers, CfC networks substantially decrease computational overhead, enabling deployment on edge devices; recent studies validate their efficiency on resource-constrained microcontrollers.
- Visual processing optimization:
  - Lightweight YOLO variants: evaluating models like YOLO11n and YOLO-Tiny reduces the number of parameters and layers while maintaining detection accuracy.
  - Inference acceleration: methods such as ONNX and TensorRT conversions optimize model execution, reducing latency and improving detection speed.
- Hardware implementation:
  - Edge-AI frameworks: technologies such as TinyML and TinyEngine support efficient model execution on devices like Jetson Nano or low-power microcontrollers, ensuring real-time processing capabilities.
  - Containerization: deployment in Docker or Singularity containers ensures portability and scalability, facilitating seamless integration across medical hardware [56–58].

3. Evaluation in high-fidelity simulation: to enhance the validity of the experiments, a simulation in CoppeliaSim could be conducted, incorporating tissue modeling that accounts for effects such as breathing, intra-abdominal pressure, variable lighting, and occlusions. This would challenge the robustness of the computer vision system and test the controller's adaptability to unpredictable movements of surgical instruments.

4. Safety and ethical considerations: for future implementation in real surgery, it is critical to address human error management, including unexpected surgeon movements and potential visual detection failures, as well as system fault tolerance, by evaluating recovery mechanisms for sensory feedback errors. A key aspect is the design of intuitive human–robot interaction (HRI) interfaces that integrate haptic, visual, and auditory feedback, enabling early detection of failures or anomalous behavior. Similarly, predictive monitoring of critical parameters—such as force, velocity, and precision—helps reduce the risk of mechanical failures and tissue damage.

5. Compliance with international medical device regulations and ethical considerations is also essential. Partial or full autonomy of the system must remain under surgeon supervision, ensuring that critical decisions stay within human control. Moreover, transparency in algorithms and interpretability of their decisions are vital for building trust in clinical use. Equity in access to these technologies must be addressed to prevent widening healthcare disparities. Legal accountability for potential complications should be clearly defined among manufacturers, medical institutions, and surgeons, with established protocols for intervention in case of failures. This balance between robotic autonomy and human

oversight will be pivotal for the acceptance and integration of these systems into surgical practice, ensuring both patient safety and ethical responsibility in their application.

6. Clinical validation plan:

To transition to a real clinical environment, a three-stage validation plan is proposed:

- Enhanced simulated scenarios: tests in improved simulations modeling tissue dynamics and interactions more realistically, incorporating pre-recorded surgical videos.
- Physical validation: validation using laparoscopic phantoms and pelvitrainers, enabling evaluation in a controlled environment.
- Surgeon evaluation: assessment with surgeons using simulators such as Fundamentals of Laparoscopic Surgery (FLS), gathering feedback on the system's utility in real procedures. The applicability of the NVAC controller could extend to other surgeon-support tasks involving surgical instruments. Performance evaluation with standardized exercises—such as object transfer, cutting precision, and intracorporeal suturing—using abdominal phantoms with realistic tissue properties will demonstrate its applicability.

The MRAC-PD-CfC-mmRNN system represents an advancement in robotic surgery automation, offering more precise and robust adaptive control. However, its applicability in real clinical settings requires further validation, optimization for certified hardware, and compliance with regulatory standards. Developing a testing protocol in collaboration with medical teams will be crucial for its effective implementation in surgical practice.

5. Conclusions

This study marks a significant advancement in hybrid control architectures for assisted robotic surgery. The proposed Neuro-Visual Adaptive Controller innovatively integrates Model Reference Adaptive Control with Proportional–Derivative terms, Closed-Form Continuous-Time Neural Networks, and the YOLO11n model, effectively overcoming the limitations in precision and adaptability inherent in conventional methods. Key findings include the following:

- Exceptional surgical precision, with tracking errors of 1.80×10^{-3} m (x-axis), 1.08×10^{-4} m (y-axis), and 1.90×10^{-3} m (z-axis), considered negligible by clinical standards.
- Robust rejection of external disturbances, ensuring operational stability and heightened safety within the surgical environment.
- Seamless integration of computer vision achieves reliable detection of surgical instruments with a precision of 97.30%, a recall of 94.80%, an $mAP_{0.5}$ of 97.5%, and an $mAP_{0.5:0.95}$ of 72.7%, thereby optimizing real-time visual control.
- Reduced risk of mechanical wear and tissue damage, supported by smooth control signals and stable dynamic responses.

Although the validation of the NVAC was conducted in simulated environments, the results obtained provide a robust foundation for its application in complex clinical scenarios. This work establishes a new benchmark for the integration of neural networks and adaptive control in robotic surgery, paving the way for future transformative advanced applications. However, its implementation in real surgery requires further validation on certified hardware, testing with surgeons, and compliance with medical regulations, representing the next phase of research for its clinical application.

6. Future Works

The findings of this study provide a robust foundation for advancing research in assisted robotic surgery. Nevertheless, several critical areas merit further investigation to fully realize the potential and clinical applicability of the proposed Neuro-Visual Adaptive Controller. The most significant future research directions include the following:

- Enhanced validation in advanced simulated environments: strengthen validation through advanced simulations by incorporating extreme scenarios, such as severe disturbances, variable lighting conditions, and dynamic tissue motion. Furthermore, leveraging clinical databases and pre-recorded surgical videos—without conducting live trials—will refine and validate the NVAC in simulated settings that closely replicate real-world conditions, ensuring a rigorous preparatory phase for clinical deployment.
- Optimization of visual perception models: assess the integration of multimodal vision techniques within simulated environments, incorporating fluorescence and 3D imaging to address current YOLO11n limitations in detecting critical fine details. This enhancement seeks to improve scene perception accuracy, tackling challenges such as occlusions and small instrument detection, while preserving computational feasibility for surgical contexts.
- Enhancement of computational efficiency: implement quantization and pruning techniques to adapt YOLO11n for low-power hardware, complemented by latency and efficiency testing in simulated environments. These optimizations aim to refine the NVAC for seamless integration into resource-constrained clinical devices, ensuring real-time performance without sacrificing precision.
- Integration of reinforcement learning: incorporate reinforcement learning techniques to autonomously optimize robotic trajectories and dynamically adapt to evolving surgical conditions. This approach aims to bolster the NVAC's adaptability, enabling proactive responses to intraoperative variability and enhancing tracking robustness.
- Advancement of robot–surgeon collaboration: develop and evaluate, within simulated environments, a multimodal human–robot collaboration interface integrating visual, auditory, and haptic feedback. This interface seeks to enable intuitive supervision and real-time system adjustments, simulating operational conditions in clinical settings and improving surgeon-robot synergy.

These research directions offer transformative potential for assisted robotic surgery, advancing the frontiers of autonomy and precision beyond current capabilities. By pursuing these developments, the NVAC could address a broader spectrum of clinical applications, significantly improving surgical outcomes and patient experiences.

Supplementary Materials: The following supporting information can be downloaded at: https://www.mdpi.com/article/10.3390/technologies13040135/s1, File S1: Neuro-Visual Adaptive Control in Robot-Assisted Surgery [45,53,59].

Author Contributions: Conceptualization, C.U. and Y.G.-G.; methodology, C.U. and Y.G.-G.; software, C.U. and Y.G.-G.; validation, C.U. and Y.G.-G.; formal analysis, C.U. and Y.G.-G.; investigation, C.U. and Y.G.-G.; resources, C.U. and Y.G.-G.; data curation, C.U. and Y.G.-G.; writing—original draft preparation, C.U. and Y.G.-G.; writing—review and editing, C.U., Y.G.-G., J.K. and R.R.-G.; visualization, C.U.; supervision, C.U. and J.K.; project administration, C.U.; funding acquisition, C.U. All authors have read and agreed to the published version of the manuscript.

Funding: This research received no external funding.

Institutional Review Board Statement: Not applicable.

Informed Consent Statement: Not applicable.

Data Availability Statement: Data are contained within the article.

Acknowledgments: This work was supported by the Faculty of Engineering of the University of Santiago of Chile and the Agencia Nacional de Investigación y Desarrollo de Chile (ANID-Subdirección de Capital Humano/Doctorado Nacional/2022-21220266), Chile.

Conflicts of Interest: The authors declare no conflicts of interest.

Abbreviations

Adam	Adaptive Moment Estimation
AFFOSMC	Adaptive Fuzzy Fractional-Order Sliding Mode Controller
AI	Artificial intelligence
ANN	Artificial Neural Network
AP	Precisión Promedio
APSMC	Adaptive Proportional Sliding Mode controller
AZNN	Adaptive Zeroing Neural Network
BNN	Bayesian Neural Network
CfC	Closed-Form Continuous-Time Neural Network
CfC-mmRNN	Closed-Form Continuous-Time Neural Networks with mixed-memory Recurrent Neural Networks (Combines the CfC's RNN-state with an LSTM)
CNN	Convolutional Neural Network
CV	Computer vision
D-H	Denavit-Hartenberg
DoF	Degrees of freedom
EP	End point
EvNN	Evidential Neural Network
FN	False negative
FOV	Field of view
FP	False positive
GELU	Gaussian error linear unit
GPU	Graphics Processing Unit
HRI	Human–robot interaction
IBVS	Image-Based Visual Servoing
IoU	Intersection over Union
ITAE	Integral of Time-Weighted Absolute Error
ITSE	Integral of Time-Weighted Squared Error
LSTM	Long Short-Term Memory
LTC	Liquid Time-Constant Networks
MAE	Mean absolute error
mAP	media de la Precisión Promedio
ML	Machine learning
MRAC	Model Reference Adaptive Control
MSE	Mean Squared Error
NVAC	Neuro-Visual Adaptive Control
ODE	Ordinary Differential Equations
P	Precision
PD	Proportional–Derivate
PID	Proportional–Integral–Derivate
PIs	Performance indexes
PNG	Portable Network Graphics
R	Recall
RCM	Remote Center of Motion

RFPT	Robust Fixed Point Transformations
RNN	Recurrent Neural Networks
SGDM	Stochastic Gradient Descent with Momentum
SMC	Sliding Mode Control
SP	Start point
STAR	Smart Tissue Autonomous Robot
TP	True positive
YOLO	You Only Look Once
YOLO11n	You Only Look Once, version 11, nano variant

References

1. Mirbagheri, A.; Farahmand, F.; Sarkar, S.; Alamdar, A.; Moradi, M.; Afshari, E. The Sina Robotic Telesurgery System. In *Handbook of Robotic and Image-Guided Surgery*; Elsevier: Amsterdam, The Netherlands, 2020; Chapter 7; pp. 107–121.
2. Dupont, P.E.; Nelson, B.J.; Goldfarb, M.; Hannaford, B.; Menciassi, A.; O'malley, M.K.; Simaan, N.; Valdastri, P.; Yang, G.-Z. A decade retrospective of medical robotics research from 2010 to 2020. *Sci. Robot.* **2021**, *6*, eabi8017.
3. Higgins, R.M.; Gould, J.C. Clinical Applications of Robotics in General Surgery. In *Handbook of Robotic and Image-Guided Surgery*; Elsevier: Amsterdam, The Netherlands, 2020; pp. 211–221.
4. Culmer, P.; Alazmani, A.; Mushtaq, F.; Cross, W.; Jayne, D. Haptics in surgical robots. In *Handbook of Robotic and Image-Guided Surgery*; Elsevier: Amsterdam, The Netherlands, 2020; pp. 239–263.
5. Wan, G.-Y.; Zhou, X.-Y.; Duan, H.-X.; Zou, Z.-Y.; Zhang, M.-M.; Mao, J.-B. Comparison of robotic camera holders with human assistants in endoscopic surgery: A systematic review and meta-analysis. *Minim. Invasive Ther. Allied Technol.* **2023**, *32*, 153–162.
6. Abedin-Nasab, M. *Handbook of Robotic and Image-Guided Surgery*; Elsevier: Amsterdam, The Netherlands, 2020.
7. Li, B.; Lu, B.; Wang, Z.; Zhong, F.; Dou, Q.; Liu, Y.-H. Learning laparoscope actions via video features for proactive robotic field-of-view control. *IEEE Robot. Autom. Lett.* **2022**, *7*, 6653–6660. [CrossRef]
8. Li, J.; Huang, Y.; Zhang, X.; Xie, K.; Xian, Y.; Luo, X.; Chiu, P.W.Y.; Li, Z. An autonomous surgical instrument tracking framework with a binocular camera for a robotic flexible laparoscope. *IEEE Robot. Autom. Lett.* **2023**, *8*, 4291–4298. [CrossRef]
9. Huang, Y.; Li, J.; Zhang, X.; Xie, K.; Li, J.; Liu, Y.; Ng, S.H.; Chiu, P.W.Y.; Li, Z. A surgeon preference-guided autonomous instrument tracking method with a robotic flexible endoscope based on dVRK platform. *IEEE Robot. Autom. Lett.* **2022**, *7*, 2250–2257. [CrossRef]
10. Ou, Y.; Zargarzadeh, S.; Tavakoli, M. Robot Learning Incorporating Human Interventions in the Real World for Autonomous Surgical Endoscopic Camera Control. *J. Med. Robot. Res.* **2023**, *8*, 2340004. [CrossRef]
11. Kong, X.; Mo, H.; Dong, E.; Liu, Y.; Sun, D. Automatic Tracking of Surgical Instruments with a Continuum Laparoscope Using Data-Driven Control in Robotic Surgery. *Adv. Intell. Syst.* **2023**, *5*, 2200188. [CrossRef]
12. Opfermann, J.D.; Leonard, S.; Decker, R.S.; Uebele, N.A.; Bayne, C.E.; Joshi, A.S.; Krieger, A. Semi-autonomous electrosurgery for tumor resection using a multi-degree of freedom electrosurgical tool and visual servoing. In Proceedings of the 2017 IEEE/RSJ International Conference on Intelligent Robots and Systems (IROS), Vancouver, BC, Canada, 24–28 September 2017; IEEE: Piscataway, NJ, USA, 2017; pp. 3653–3660. [CrossRef]
13. Mehrjouyan, A.; Menhaj, M.B.; Hooshiar, A. Safety-enhanced observer-based adaptive fuzzy synchronization control framework for teleoperation systems. *Eur. J. Control* **2023**, *73*, 100885. [CrossRef]
14. Huang, Y.; Li, W.; Zhang, X.; Li, J.; Li, Y.; Sun, Y.; Chiu, P.W.Y.; Li, Z. 4-dof visual servoing of a robotic flexible endoscope with a predefined-time convergent and noise-immune adaptive neural network. *IEEE/ASME Trans. Mechatron.* **2023**, *29*, 576–587. [CrossRef]
15. Li, Y.; Ng, W.Y.; Li, W.; Huang, Y.; Zhang, H.; Xian, Y.; Li, J.; Sun, Y.; Chiu, P.W.Y.; Li, Z. Towards semi-autonomous colon screening using an electromagnetically actuated soft-tethered colonoscope based on visual servo control. *IEEE Trans. Biomed. Eng.* **2023**, *71*, 77–88. [CrossRef]
16. Adjepong, D. Adaptive Control Systems for Medical Robots in Neurosurgery: A Review. *HSOA J. Surg. Curr. Trends Innov.* **2020**, *4*, 030. [CrossRef]
17. Ren, F.; Wang, X.; Yu, N.; Han, J. Adaptive fuzzy control for tendon-sheath actuated bending-tip system with unknown friction for robotic flexible endoscope. *Front. Neurosci.* **2024**, *18*, 1330634. [CrossRef] [PubMed]
18. Sachan, S.; Swarnkar, P. Intelligent fractional-order sliding mode optimised control of surgical manipulator for healthcare system. *Electr. Eng.* **2024**, *106*, 2131–2142. [CrossRef]
19. Kökçam, E.; Tan, N. Comparison of Adaptation Mechanisms on MRAC. *IEEE Access* **2024**, *12*, 31862–31874. [CrossRef]

20. Sánchez–Sánchez, P.; Guillermo Cebada–Reyes, J.; Montiel–Martínez, A.; Reyes–Cortés, F. Optimizing Dehydration Systems: Implementing Model Reference Adaptive Control for Enhanced Efficiency. *Int. J. Adapt. Control Signal Process.* **2025**, *39*, 1–23. [CrossRef]
21. Tar, J.K.; Kovács, L.; Takács, A.; Takács, B.; Zentay, P.; Haidegger, T.; Rudas, I.J. Novel design of a Model Reference Adaptive Controller for soft tissue operations. In Proceedings of the 2014 IEEE International Conference on Systems, Man, and Cybernetics (SMC), San Diego, CA, USA, 5–8 October 2014; IEEE: Piscataway, NJ, USA, 2014; pp. 2446–2451.
22. Cursi, F.; Bai, W.; Yeatman, E.M.; Kormushev, P. Task accuracy enhancement for a surgical macro-micro manipulator with probabilistic neural networks and uncertainty minimization. *IEEE Trans. Autom. Sci. Eng.* **2022**, *21*, 241–256. [CrossRef]
23. Cursi, F.; Bai, W.; Yeatman, E.M.; Kormushev, P. Adaptive kinematic model learning for macro-micro surgical manipulator control. In Proceedings of the 2022 International Conference on Advanced Robotics and Mechatronics (ICARM), Guilin, China, 9–11 July 2022; IEEE: Piscataway, NJ, USA, 2022; pp. 494–501.
24. Wang, Z.; Wang, T.; Zhao, B.; He, Y.; Hu, Y.; Li, B.; Zhang, P.; Meng, M.Q.-H. Hybrid adaptive control strategy for continuum surgical robot under external load. *IEEE Robot. Autom. Lett.* **2021**, *6*, 1407–1414. [CrossRef]
25. Ping, L.; Wang, Z.; Yao, J.; Gao, J.; Yang, S.; Li, J.; Shi, J.; Wu, W.; Hua, S.; Wang, H. Application and evaluation of surgical tool and tool tip recognition based on Convolutional Neural Network in multiple endoscopic surgical scenarios. *Surg. Endosc.* **2023**, *37*, 7376–7384. [CrossRef]
26. Pan, X.; Bi, M.; Wang, H.; Ma, C.; He, X. DBH-YOLO: A surgical instrument detection method based on feature separation in laparoscopic surgery. *Int. J. Comput. Assist. Radiol. Surg.* **2024**, *19*, 2215–2225. [CrossRef]
27. Liu, Z.; Zhou, Y.; Zheng, L.; Zhang, G. SINet: A hybrid deep CNN model for real-time detection and segmentation of surgical instruments. *Biomed. Signal Process. Control* **2024**, *88*, 105670. [CrossRef]
28. Song, H.; Zhao, Z.; Liu, K.; Wu, Y.; Li, F. Anchor-Free Convolutional Neural Network Application to Enhance Real-Time Surgical Tool Detection in Computer-Aided Surgery. *IEEE Trans. Med. Robot. Bionics* **2023**, *6*, 73–83.
29. Peng, C.; Li, Y.; Long, X.; Zhao, X.; Jiang, X.; Guo, J.; Lou, H. Urtnet: An unstructured feature fusion network for real-time detection of endoscopic surgical instruments. *J. Real-Time Image Process.* **2024**, *21*, 190.
30. Benavides, D.; Cisnal, A.; Fontúrbel, C.; de la Fuente, E.; Fraile, J.C. Real-Time Tool Localization for Laparoscopic Surgery Using Convolutional Neural Network. *Sensors* **2024**, *24*, 4191. [CrossRef]
31. Loza, G.; Valdastri, P.; Ali, S. Real-time surgical tool detection with multi-scale positional encoding and contrastive learning. *Healthc. Technol. Lett.* **2024**, *11*, 48–58. [PubMed]
32. Rohmer, E.; Singh, S.P.N.; Freese, M. CoppeliaSim (formerly V-REP): A Versatile and Scalable Robot Simulation Framework. In Proceedings of the 2013 IEEE/RSJ International Conference on Intelligent Robots and Systems, Tokyo, Japan, 3–7 November 2013.
33. Li, W.; Chiu, P.W.Y.; Li, Z. An accelerated finite-time convergent neural network for visual servoing of a flexible surgical endoscope with physical and RCM constraints. *IEEE Trans. Neural Netw. Learn. Syst.* **2020**, *31*, 5272–5284. [CrossRef] [PubMed]
34. Amirthavarshini, G.A.; Thondiyath, A. RCM Constrained Task Space Trajectory Generation for Autonomous Robotic Surgeries. In Proceedings of the 2024 IEEE International Conference on Cyborg and Bionic Systems (CBS), Nagoya, Japan, 20–22 November 2024; IEEE: Piscataway, NJ, USA, 2024; pp. 121–125.
35. Kuo, J.-Y.; Song, K.-T. A Design for Remote Center of Motion Control Using a Software Computing Approach. In Proceedings of the 2020 International Automatic Control Conference (CACS), Hsinchu, Taiwan, 4–7 November 2020; IEEE: Piscataway, NJ, USA, 2020; pp. 1–5.
36. Huang, Y.; Li, J.; Li, W.; Zhang, X.; Sun, Y.; Xie, K.; Hu, Y.; Chiu, P.W.Y.; Li, Z. An Accelerated Anti-Noise Adaptive Neural Network for Robotic Flexible Endoscope With Multitype Surgical Objectives and Constraints. *IEEE Trans. Syst. Man Cybern. Syst.* **2024**, *55*, 990–1003.
37. Colan, J.; Davila, A.; Fozilov, K.; Hasegawa, Y. A concurrent framework for constrained inverse kinematics of minimally invasive surgical robots. *Sensors* **2023**, *23*, 3328. [CrossRef]
38. Iovene, E.; Cattaneo, D.; Fu, J.; Ferrigno, G.; De Momi, E. Hybrid Tracking Module for Real-Time Tool Tracking for an Autonomous Exoscope. *IEEE Robot. Autom. Lett.* **2024**, *9*, 6067–6074.
39. Zinchenko, K.; Song, K.-T. Autonomous endoscope robot positioning using instrument segmentation with virtual reality visualization. *IEEE Access* **2021**, *9*, 72614–72623.
40. *MATLAB*; Mathworks: Natick, MA, USA, 2024; Available online: https://www.mathworks.com (accessed on 25 March 2025).
41. Ultralytics YOLO11. 2024. Available online: https://github.com/ultralytics/ultralytics (accessed on 20 December 2024).
42. Roboflow. 2024. Available online: https://roboflow.com (accessed on 17 December 2024).
43. Kaggle. CholecSeg8k: A Semantic Segmentation Dataset Based on Cholec80. Available online: https://www.kaggle.com/datasets/newslab/cholecseg8k (accessed on 25 March 2025).

44. Twinanda, A.P.; Shehata, S.; Mutter, D.; Marescaux, J.; De Mathelin, M.; Padoy, N. EndoNet: A deep architecture for recognition tasks on laparoscopic videos. *IEEE Trans. Med. Imaging* **2017**, *36*, 86–97.
45. Universal Robots A/S. UR5 Especificaciones Técnicas No. Artículo 110105. Available online: https://www.universal-robots.com/media/50591/ur5_es.pdf (accessed on 25 March 2025).
46. Rao, S.N. YOLOv11 Architecture Explained: Next-Level Object Detection with Enhanced Speed and Accuracy. Medium. Available online: https://medium.com/@nikhil-rao-20/yolov11-explained-next-level-object-detection-with-enhanced-speed-and-accuracy-2dbe2d376f71 (accessed on 25 February 2025).
47. Hasani, R.; Lechner, M.; Amini, A.; Rus, D.; Grosu, R. Liquid time-constant networks. *Proc. AAAI Conf. Artif. Intell.* **2021**, *35*, 7657–7666. [CrossRef]
48. Hasani, R.; Lechner, M.; Amini, A.; Liebenwein, L.; Ray, A.; Tschaikowski, M.; Teschl, G.; Rus, D. Closed-form continuous-time neural networks. *Nat. Mach. Intell.* **2022**, *4*, 992–1003. [CrossRef]
49. Urrea, C.; Garcia-Garcia, Y. Design and Performance Analysis of Level Control Strategies in a Nonlinear Spherical Tank. *Processes* **2023**, *11*, 720. [CrossRef]
50. Kern, J.; Rodriguez-Guillen, R.; Urrea, C.; Garcia-Garcia, Y. Enhancing 3D Rock Localization in Mining Environments Using Bird's-Eye View Images from the Time-of-Flight Blaze 101 Camera. *Technologies* **2024**, *12*, 162. [CrossRef]
51. Hodson, T.O. Root mean square error (RMSE) or mean absolute error (MAE): When to use them or not. *Geosci. Model Dev. Discuss.* **2022**, *2022*, 5481–5487. [CrossRef]
52. Rodriguez-Guillen, R.; Kern, J.; Urrea, C. Fast Rock Detection in Visually Contaminated Mining Environments Using Machine Learning and Deep Learning Techniques. *Appl. Sci.* **2024**, *14*, 731. [CrossRef]
53. Urrea, C.; Garcia-Garcia, Y.; Kern, J. Closed-Form Continuous-Time Neural Networks for Sliding Mode Control with Neural Gravity Compensation. *Robotics* **2024**, *13*, 126. [CrossRef]
54. Leong, F.; Mohammadi, A.; Tan, Y.; Thiruchelvam, D.; Lai, C.Y.; Valdastri, P.; Oetomo, D. Disturbance Rejection in Multi-DOF Local Magnetic Actuation for the Robotic Abdominal Surgery. *IEEE Robot. Autom. Lett.* **2018**, *3*, 1568–1575.
55. Picod, G.; Jambon, A.; Vinatier, D.; Dubois, P. What can the operator actually feel when performing a laparoscopy? *Surg. Endosc. Other Interv. Tech.* **2005**, *19*, 95–100.
56. Le, A.T.; Shakiba, M.; Ardekani, I.; Abdulla, W.H. Optimizing Plant Disease Classification with Hybrid Convolutional Neural Network–Recurrent Neural Network and Liquid Time-Constant Network. *Appl. Sci.* **2024**, *14*, 9118. [CrossRef]
57. Huang, Z.; Contreras, L.F.H.; Leung, W.H.; Yu, L.; Truong, N.D.; Nikpour, A.; Kavehei, O. Efficient edge-AI models for robust ECG abnormality detection on resource-constrained hardware. *J. Cardiovasc. Transl. Res.* **2024**, *17*, 879–892. [CrossRef] [PubMed]
58. Belhaoua, A.; Kimpe, T.; Crul, S. TensorRT-based surgical instrument detection assessment for deep learning on edge computing. In *Medical Imaging 2024: Image-Guided Procedures, Robotic Interventions, and Modeling*; SPIE: Bellingham, WA, USA, 2024; Volume 12928, pp. 368–371.
59. Kufieta, K. Force Estimation in Robotic Manipulators: Modeling, Simulation and Experiments. Master's Thesis, Norwegian University of Science and Technology, Trondheim, Norway, 2014. Available online: https://tomgra.folk.ntnu.no/Diplomer/Kufieta.pdf (accessed on 25 March 2025).

technologies

MDPI

Article

Pneumatically Actuated Rehabilitation Equipment for the Sagittal and Frontal Plane Movements of the Neck Joint

Sarah Mareş, Andrea Deaconescu and Tudor Deaconescu *

Department of Industrial Engineering and Management, Transilvania University of Brasov, 500036 Brasov, Romania; sarah.mares@unitbv.ro (S.M.); deacon@unitbv.ro (A.D.)
* Correspondence: tdeacon@unitbv.ro; Tel.: +40-745-757850

Abstract: The timely reintegration into their daily routine of patients suffering from work-related musculoskeletal disorders is a priority in medical rehabilitation. This can be accomplished by means of certain procedures and adequate medical rehabilitation equipment. Starting from these considerations this paper proposes an original constructive solution of a rehabilitation device designed for the passive mobilization of the neck joint in the sagittal and frontal plane. The constructive solution that is put forward uses a pneumatic muscle as the actuation element, ensuring the adaptability of the equipment to the particular pain tolerance of each patient. The construction and dimensioning calculations of the equipment are presented, followed by the determination of the torsional rigidity and compliance permitted by the system. Based on the results the paper concludes with recommendations for the optimum deployment of the rehabilitation equipment.

Keywords: rehabilitation equipment; neck joint; frontal and sagittal planes; pneumatic muscle; compliance

1. Introduction

The cervical spine forms the complex neck joint and consists of the first seven vertebrae. It supports the weight of the head and enables it to carry out a wide range of movements in the three anatomical planes. Part of the complex neck joint, the atlantooccipital and atlantoaxial joints enable flexion-extension, rotation (to the left and right, respectively) and tilting (to the left and the right, respectively) of the head. Besides the vertebrae the neck joint also includes muscles, nerves, tendons and ligaments, each contributing specifically to its mobility and stabilization.

Due to its extremely complex structure the neck joint is frequently affected consequently to problems of the cervical spine and of the surrounding soft tissue and nerves. Such affections include cervical radiculopathy, cervical degenerative disk disease, cervical spondylosis, cervical spinal fracture, cervical spinal cord compression, neck pain, etc. [1]. Some of the significant causes for these disorders of the musculoskeletal system that affect the neck joint are due to the tasks performed at the workplace and to challenging conditions of the work environment. Such work-related musculoskeletal disorders or WMSDs [2,3] are caused by faulty, nonergonomic postures at work, by repetitive motions, excessive use of body force, vibrations, mechanical compression and temperature.

To date WMSDs have been and remain the most frequent work-related health problem in the European Union. As WMSDs affect all employees from all fields of activity, the consecutive costs to companies and society are high. A study conducted by the European

Agency for Safety and Health at Work reveals that about 42% of workers reporting different musculoskeletal disorders suffer from problems of the neck joint and of the shoulders [4]. The Labour Force Survey conducted in Great Britain on a sample of 470,000 individuals states that the majority of workplace-related complaints concern the neck (45%), back (39%) and lower limbs (16%) [5].

As follows from these studies, it is the neck joint that is most frequently affected by WMSDs, and requires effective rehabilitation solutions. The recovery of this joint needs to cover the motor state (muscle tone), the sensorial state (proprioception) and last but not least the psycho-social and professional status of the patient. The treatment of WMSDs involves several approaches, as appropriate: restricting mobility, applying heat or cold, and stretching that facilitate circulation, ease muscle tension and reduce the need for medication and surgery [6].

Neck affections lend themselves to high success rate rehabilitation, thus enhancing patient chances of swift reintegration into everyday activity. Modern therapeutical methods have shortened recovery periods and reduced the failure rate of the treatments used in such pathologies. A key role in rapid recovery is the utilization of adequate rehabilitation equipment conceived for the neck joint. By causing repetitive controlled movements of the neck joint such equipment have a positive impact on improving muscle force and recovering lost or diminished functions. Continuous Passive Motion–CPM is one of the efficient methods that ensure the rehabilitation of the neck joint that is mobilized by external devices with mechanical, electromechanical or pneumatic actuation. The purpose of such mobilization is to avoid the building up of a fibrous tissue and implicitly to reduce joint stiffness. Some of the essential characteristics CPM-based rehabilitation equipment of the neck joint benefits from are the control of the applied forces, of the movement amplitudes, speeds, accelerations, as well as of the duration and frequency of the exercises. The possibility of modifying all these parameters between certain limits allows adjusting the rehabilitation exercises to the clinical state and the pain threshold of the patients [7].

Variable stiffness, also known as adjustable compliance is another feature required from such rehabilitation equipment. The deployment of actuation systems of this type offers the possibility of minimizing the large forces occurring in collisions (shocks), of safe interaction with the user and of storing and releasing energy into passive elastic elements. A system with adjustable compliance has the capacity of rapidly adapting to the state of the patients and their pain tolerance.

An extensive and detailed survey on the wearable assistive robotic devices used for head and neck rehabilitation is reported by Doss et al. in [8]. The paper presents the latest trends related to rehabilitation equipment, the use of various sensors, actuation devices and control techniques meant to generate an optimum set of movements of the head/neck.

At present there are several variants of neck joint rehabilitation equipment with different operational principles available on the marketplace. One of the variants is the Cervical muscles exerciser G160 provided by David Health Solutions [9]. This equipment mobilizes the neck joint in a transverse plane activating the typically neglected rotating muscles of the head. The electrical actuation of this rehabilitation system allows for testing of mobility and isometric strength in both directions of movement. Variant G140 Cervical Extension/Lateral Flexion Device mobilizes extension and lateral flexion of the cervical spine activating extensor and lateral flexor muscles [10].

Another available equipment is conceived for the recovery of patients suffering from dropped head syndrome (DHS). This manifests by weakness and pain of the neck muscles that are unable to lift or mobilize the head. This dynamic neck rehabilitation system (Car-

Neck) is actuated by means of cable transmission and helps DHS patients to carry out flexion/extension motions [11].

Kim et al. propose in [12] a postural correction system designed for forward head posture (FHP) patients. FHP is typical for longtime computer and smartphone users. The equipment consists of flexibility sensors, a rigid chin support and is actuated by an artificial pneumatic muscle. It is a passive rehabilitation system that while enabling the patient to hold their head in a vertical position does not, however, restore the dynamic movements of the head/neck [12].

Yue et al. propose in [13] a parallel manipulator based cervical exoskeleton developed for mimicking head/neck motions. The system can generate flexion/extension of the neck within a $\pm15^\circ$ range, and of $\pm20^\circ$ for lateral bending, respectively.

BTE Technologies put forward a complex rehabilitation equipment of the neck joint that generates movements in the frontal, sagittal and transverse plane. Called Multi-Cervical Unit (MCU) this equipment is electrically actuated and destined for patients suffering from neck pain, whiplash-associated disorders (WAD), and general cervical spine disorders. All characteristics of the joint movements are matched against reference values and stored in the computer, thus ensuring a good traceability of each patient's evolution [14].

Another manufacturer of neck joint rehabilitation equipment if DBC of Finland. The Multi-Purpose Low-Friction Unit (MLU), Cervical Extension (CE), and Cervical 3-Dimensional Rotation (C3R) are pieces of equipment that enable bidimensional elliptic movements in the sagittal plane or coupled movements of posterior sliding and rotation by the transverse axis [15].

The neck joint rehabilitation devices presented above can be used by patients either at home or in specialist clinics supervised by a physical therapist. They are actuated manually, mechanically, pneumatically, or in most cases electrically. At present pneumatic actuation is less deployed, although using compressed air ensures the compliant behavior of the device, adaptable to the patient's complaint. Worth mentioning though is a wrist-inspired magneto-pneumatic hybrid-driven soft actuator with bidirectional torsion capabilities based on the Kresling origami unit, studied in [16]. The proposed solution can be adapted and used also in medical rehabilitation devices of the neck joint.

The overview of neck joint rehabilitation equipment available on the marketplace has not led to identifying a complex neck joint rehabilitation device that is actuated pneumatically and allows movements along several directions. Against the background offered by this finding this paper presents a novel solution of a neck joint rehabilitation system that generates recovery movements in the sagittal and frontal planes.

The paper is structured in six sections. The introductory part is followed by a Section 2 studying the biomechanics of the neck joint in the frontal and sagittal anatomic planes. This study yields the input data required for designing the rehabilitation equipment. The Section 3 presents the selected constructive solution and the working principle of the rehabilitation equipment. The operational stages of the equipment and the generation of movements in the two planes are presented. The Section 4 of the paper concerns the dimensioning of the rehabilitation equipment, presents the performance of the utilized pneumatic muscle and the calculation of the torques required for the rotation of the neck joint. Further presented is the calculation of torsional rigidity and compliance, two essential properties for medical rehabilitation equipment. The Section 5 includes the discussion of the results and recommendations for the operation of the rehabilitation equipment. The last section of the paper presents the main conclusions of the conducted study.

2. Biomechanics of the Neck Joint in the Sagittal and Frontal Planes

The cervical spine forms the neck skeleton and includes two regions: i. the suboccipital cervical spine consisting of the first two cervical vertebrae: C1–atlas and C2–axis, and ii. the inferior cervical spine from C3 to C7 vertebrae with the same characteristics.

The atlantoaxial joint allows the head to rotate by an angular amplitude of ±30°. Rotations of greater amplitudes, up to ±80° are achieved with the participation of the joints of the subjacent vertebrae.

The atlantooccipital joint allows flexion/extension and the lateral tilting of the head, but does not allow rotations. The flexion amplitude of the head allowed by the atlantooccipital joint is of about 20°, while the extension amplitude is of 30°. An amplitude of flexion/extension up to ±60° is possible only with the participation of the subjacent vertebrae.

The lateral tilting of the head is limited to only ±15° in the atlantooccipital joint, but is increased to ±45° also by the participation of the subjacent vertebrae.

The movements of the neck joint in the three anatomic planes: frontal, sagittal and transverse are shown in Figure 1, while in Table 1 the angular amplitudes of these movements are centralized:

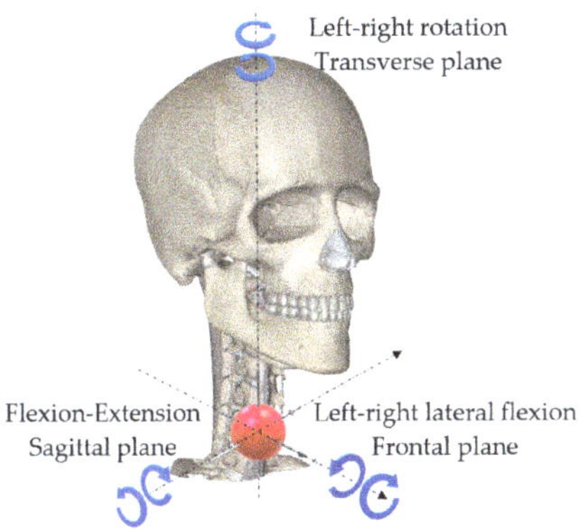

Figure 1. Movements of the neck joint.

Table 1. Movements of the neck joint and their limits.

	Movements	Angular Limits
Sagittal plane	Flexion	50°
	Extension	60°
Frontal plane	Lateral left flexion	45°
	Lateral right flexion	45°
Transverse plane	Left rotation	80°
	Right rotation	80°

This paper aims to present a solution for a piece of rehabilitation equipment of the neck joint in the sagittal and frontal planes, and consequently only the movements in these planes will be analyzed. The design of the neck joint rehabilitation equipment in the sagittal and frontal planes is based on the anthropometric parameters (indices) of the human head. In the case of this joint of interest are the mass, cranial perimeter, the dimensions of the head in the three anatomic planes, etc. Statistically determined, the mass of the adult human head is of approximately 5 kg [17]. Regarding the average circumference of the human head, a study conducted in the United States estimated it to 57 cm in males and 55 cm in females [18]. In paper [19] Newcastle University reports a study that yields an average head circumference of 57.2 cm in males and 55.2 cm in females. Other data concerning the average dimensions of the human head are summarized in Table 2 and Figure 2 [20].

Table 2. Anthropometric indices of the human head and neck.

Maximum width of the head, typically above and behind the ears (A) [cm]	Males	16.5
	Females	15.8
Horizontal distance from the frontmost point of the forehead to the back of the head (B) [cm]	Males	21.7
	Females	20.7
Vertical distance from the lower part of the chin to the top of the head (C) [cm]	Males	25.5
	Females	23.8
Vertical distance from the depression of the nasal root to the top of the head (D) [cm]	Males	12.9
	Females	12.2

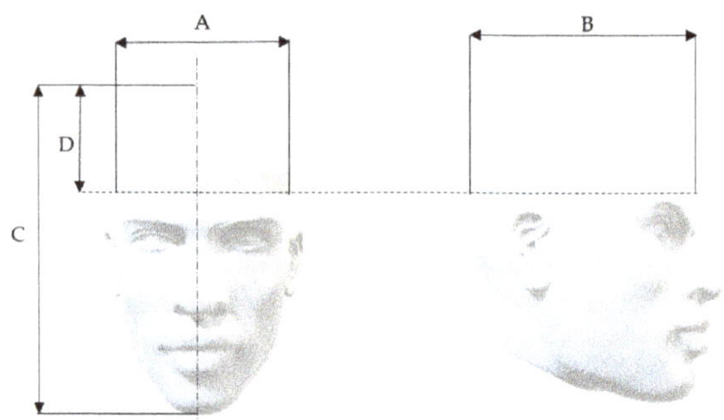

Figure 2. Anthropometric measurements of the human head.

Determining the forces and torques developed by the neck joint is of the essence for dimensioning the proposed rehabilitation equipment. The torques generated by the rotation in the sagittal and frontal planes of the neck joint are of about 12 N·m and 20 N·m, respectively [21–23]. The torques vary over the range of rotation angles of the joint. The previously specified values are the maximum ones to be ennsured by the equipment.

3. Operational Principle of the Rehabilitation Equipment for the Sagittal and Frontal Plane Movements of the Neck Joint

The proposed kinematic diagram for performing the movements in the two anatomic planes is shown in Figures 3 and 4.

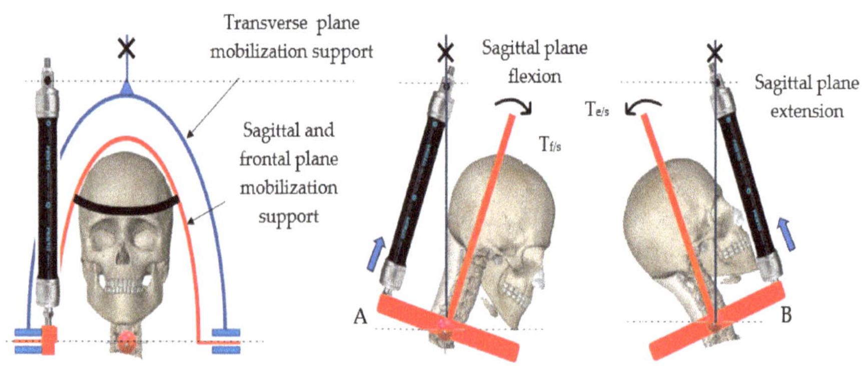

Figure 3. Generating flexion/extension in the sagittal plane.

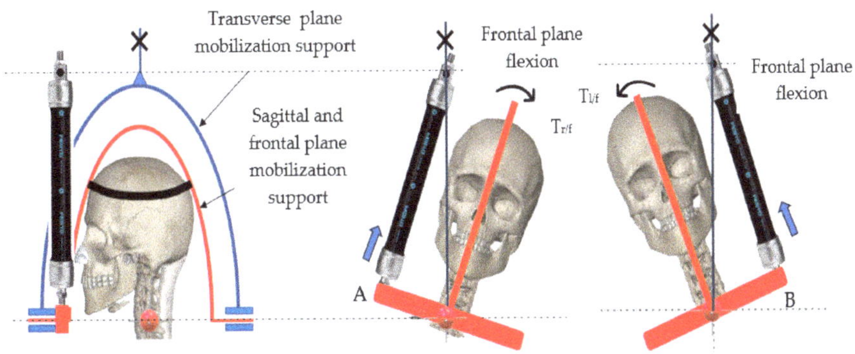

Figure 4. Generating lateral right/left flexion in the frontal plane.

The rotation axis in the two studied anatomical planes is positioned at the interface of vertebrae C4 and C5 [21–23].

The movements of the neck joint are carried out exclusively by the interior mobilization support of the rehabilitation equipment (marked red in the figures above). This support is rotated by means of a single pneumatic muscle of DMSP-20-300N-RM-CR type (manufactured by Festo, Esslingen, Germany), whose dimensions are: interior diameter = 20 mm; length of the active part = 300 mm. The axial contraction of this muscle when charged at a pressure of 6 bar is of $\Delta Lmax$ = 60 mm (20% of its initial length).

The ends of the horizontal lever of the mobilization support in the sagittal and frontal planes are denoted by A and B. Regardless of the plane of movement, the free end of the pneumatic muscle is connected to one of the ends of the support. End A is used in the case of flexion in the sagittal plane or of lateral right flexion in the frontal plane, while end B is used for extension in the sagittal plane or lateral left flexion in the frontal plane.

The limits of the respective movements that have to be reached in the two planes are shown in Table 1, namely:

- In the sagittal plane: flexion: 50°; extension: 60°.
- In the frontal plane: lateral left/right flexion: ±45°.

4. Dimensioning the Movement Generation System in the Sagittal and Frontal Planes

The rotation by an angle ω in one or the other direction in the two anatomic planes takes place when the pneumatic muscle is charged with air at different pressures. The variation of the feed pressure in the muscle causes modification of its length as well as of the developed forces. The connections of the pneumatic muscle to the mobilization support in the (fixed) transverse plane on one hand and to the mobilization support in the (mobile) sagittal and frontal plane, respectively is achieved by means of two spherical joints. Figure 5 shows the assembly of the muscle and the two joints:

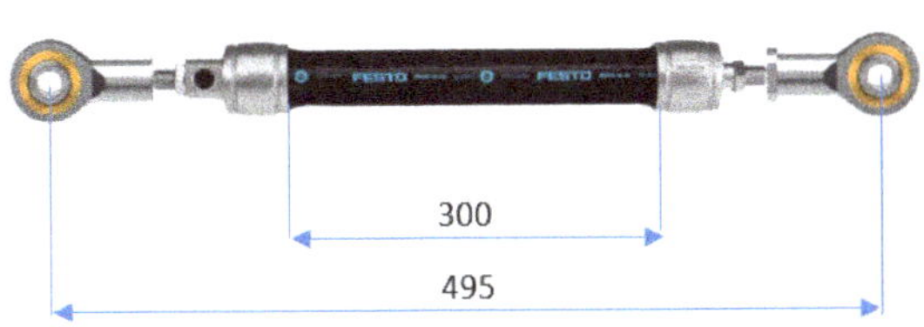

Figure 5. Pneumatic muscle–spherical joints assembly.

The rotation principle of the mobilization support in the sagittal and frontal planes is shown in Figure 6:

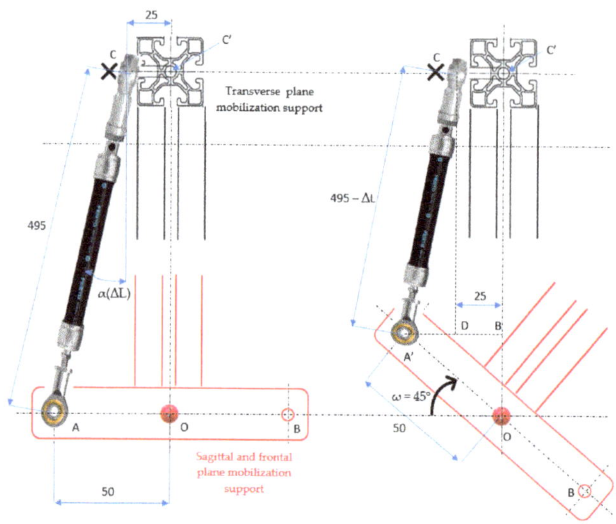

Figure 6. Rotation principle of the mobilization support in the sagittal and frontal planes.

The maximum forces that can be developed by the selected pneumatic muscle are obtained by means of MuscleSim v. 2.0.1.5 program, and the variation diagram of such forces versus compressed air pressure and axial contraction is shown in Figure 7:

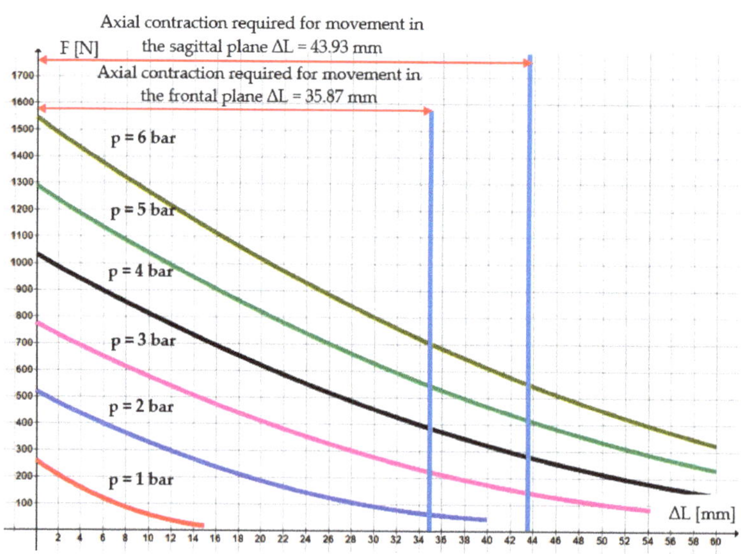

Figure 7. Variation of the force developed by the pneumatic muscle DMSP-20-300N-RM-CR.

Upon carrying out some elementary geometrical calculations it follows that in order to rotate by an angle of $\omega = 45^\circ$ necessary for movement in the frontal plane, the axial contraction of the pneumatic muscle has to be: $\Delta L = 495 - 459.13 = 35.87$ mm. This axial contraction of the pneumatic muscle can be reached by feeding it with compressed air at pressures between 2 and 6 bar. In Figure 7 the operational range is defined within that rotations of the mobilization support up to 45° are possible. Similarly, for movement in the sagittal plane by a maximum angle of $\omega = 60°$, there results $\Delta L = 43.93$ mm. Figure 7 shows the range of working pressures (3 ... 6 bar) at that this angle can be obtained.

The necessary torque for rotation in both planes (sagittal and frontal) is calculated with Equation (1):

$$T = F(\Delta L) \cdot a \cdot \cos(\omega - \alpha(\Delta L)) \tag{1}$$

where $F(\Delta L)$ is the force developed by the pneumatic muscle as a function of its axial contraction, and a is the lever length that rotates the mobilization support. The mounting angle of the pneumatic muscle, $\alpha(\Delta L)$, also depends on the axial contraction. As the angle $\alpha(\Delta L)$ varies only slightly during operation and has small values (1.3 ... 2.9°) it can be neglected. Thus, the previous equation becomes:

$$T = F(\Delta L) \cdot a \cdot \cos(\omega) \tag{2}$$

For the pneumatic muscle DMSP-20-300N-RM-CR fed at $p = 6$ bar, the dependency of the force on the axial contraction is obtained by Graph v.4.4.2 application, namely:

$$F(\Delta L) = 0.148 \cdot \Delta L^2 - 29.28 \cdot \Delta L + 1545.96\ [N] \tag{3}$$

Upon replacing Equation (3) in (2) and considering $a = 0.05$ m it follows that:

$$T(\Delta L, \omega) = \left(0.0074 \cdot \Delta L^2 - 1.464 \cdot \Delta L + 77.298\right) \cdot \cos(\omega)\ [N \cdot m] \tag{4}$$

The graph of this equation is presented in Figure 8. Figure 9 shows the variation of the torque versus the rotation angle of the neck joint:

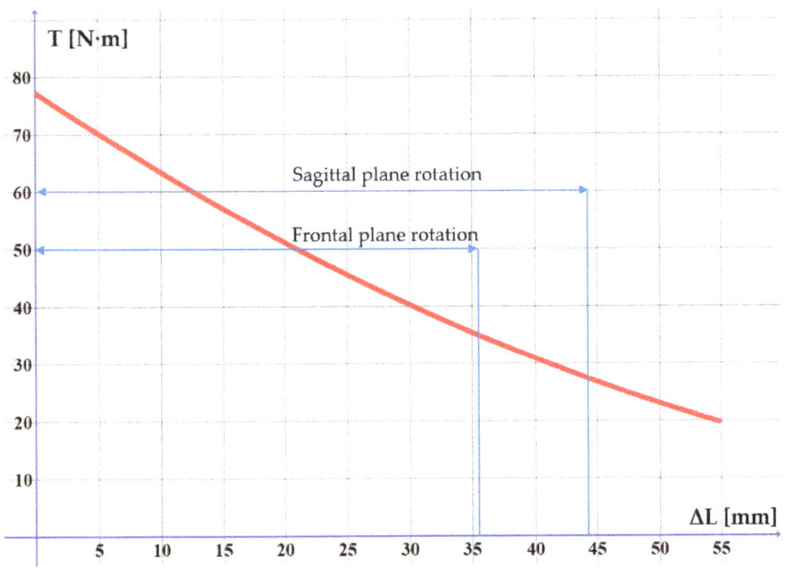

Figure 8. Variation of the torque versus the axial contraction of the pneumatic muscle.

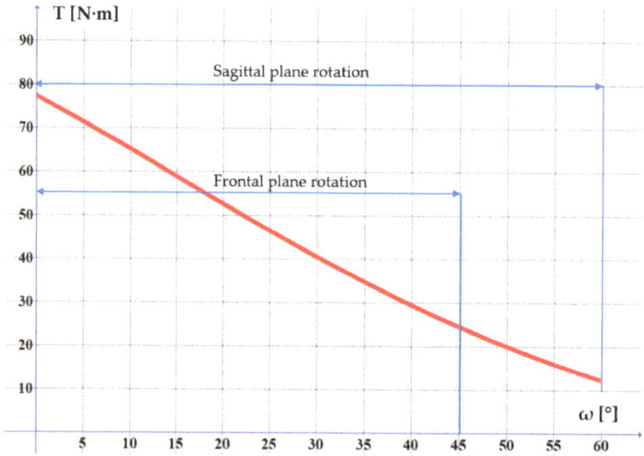

Figure 9. Variation of the torque versus the rotation angle of the neck joint in the sagittal/frontal plane.

By means of the Graph application Equation (5) is obtained:

$$T(\omega) = \left(0.0047{\cdot}\omega^2 - 1.16{\cdot}\omega + 77.29\right)\cdot\cos(\omega)\ [N{\cdot}m] \tag{5}$$

At 6 bar feed pressure the maximum force developed by the muscle is of 703.1 N (from the MuscleSim application provided by de Festo). In this case the torque developed for the movement in the frontal plane is of 24.52 N·m > 20 N·m, and of 12.35 N·m > 12 N·m for the movement in the sagittal plane.

The torsional rigidity of this joint is calculated by Equation (6) and Figure 10 shows its dependency on angle ω.

$$k = -\frac{dT}{d\omega} = -\left[(0.0094{\cdot}\omega - 1.16)\cdot(\cos\omega) + \left(0.0047{\cdot}\omega^2 - 1.16{\cdot}\omega + 77.29\right)\cdot(-\sin\omega)\right]\cdot[\mathrm{N{\cdot}m}/^\circ] \tag{6}$$

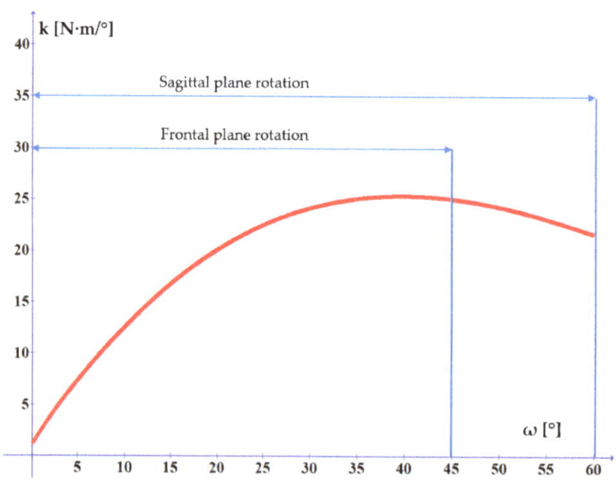

Figure 10. Variation of the torsional rigidity versus the rotation angle of the neck joint.

The torsional compliance is calculated by Equation (7), and was graphically represented in Figure 11:

$$C = k^{-1} = \frac{1}{-[(0.0094\cdot\omega - 1.16)\cdot(\cos\omega) + (0.0047\cdot\omega^2 - 1.16\cdot\omega + 77.29)\cdot(-\sin\omega)]}[^\circ/\text{N}\cdot\text{m}] \quad (7)$$

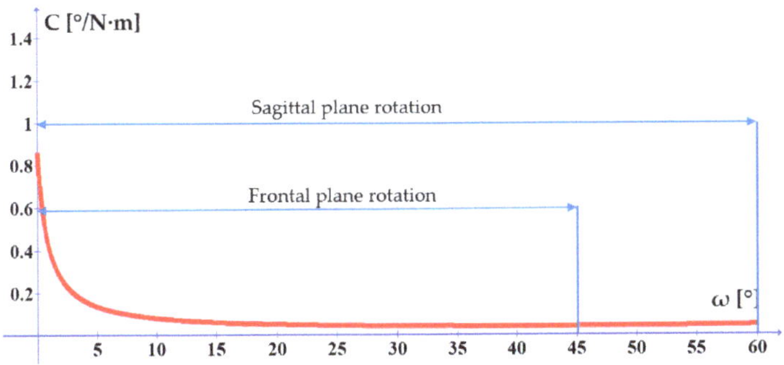

Figure 11. Variation of the torsional compliance versus the rotation angle of the neck joint.

It can be noticed, that as the rotation angle increases, the system's compliance diminishes, initially at a high rate, then tending asymptotically towards minimum values as the angle exceeds 10°.

The study of rotation movements in the sagittal and/or frontal plane the so-called "gravitational test" has to be carried out that considers the influence of the weight of the moving masses. Figure 12 shows the schematic used for calculations. The weight of the mobile assembly is the sum of the weights of the head and the mobilization support [G = (5 + 1.46)·9.81 = 63.37 N]. These data are used to write the equilibrium equation of the torques developed by the pneumatic muscle on one hand and by the weight of the equipment's mobile elements on the other.

$$F_m\cdot 50 = G\cdot 200\cdot sin\omega \quad (8)$$

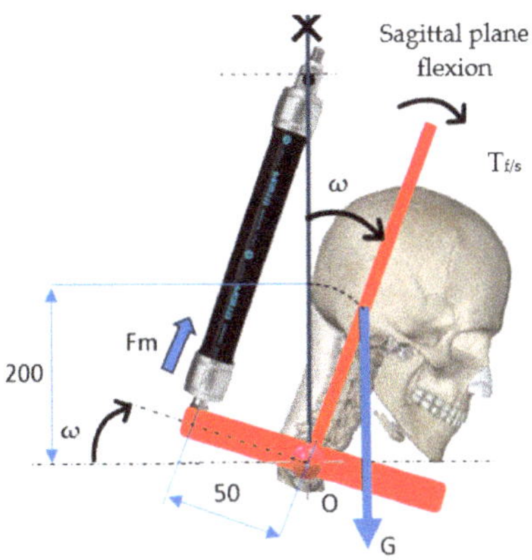

Figure 12. The effect of the moving weights on the rotating module (system).

Upon replacing G = 63.37 N in the above equation there follows:

$$F_m = 253.48\cdot sin\omega\ [N] \quad (9)$$

Figure 13 presents the variation of the force generated by the pneumatic muscle versus the rotation angle of the mobile assembly.

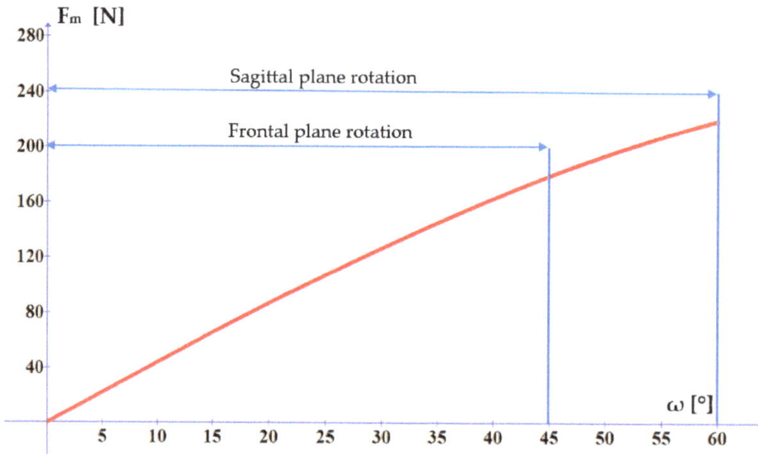

Figure 13. Variation of the force to be generated by the pneumatic muscle in order to rotate the mobile assembly of the equipment.

It can be noticed that the maximum force that has to be developed by the pneumatic muscle in the frontal plane movement is of 180 N. This force is necessary for tilting the head at an angle of $\omega = 45°$. For a tilt of $\omega = 60°$ the necessary force is of 220 N. In Figure 7 it can be observed that the selected pneumatic muscle meets this requirement at a compressed air pressure of 4. . .6 bar.

5. Discussion

The rehabilitation equipment for the sagittal and frontal plane movements of the neck joint has to meet two operational requirements simultaneously: high positioning precision and advanced adaptability to the patient's pain tolerance. This latter requirement entails an adjustable compliance of the actuation system. Concerning these aspects the graphs of the torsional rigidity and compliance lead to two important conclusions:

1. the precise achieving of certain rotation angles and firmly maintaining these requires a high rigidity of the rehabilitation equipment. Figure 10 highlights that the torsional rigidity increases with the rotation angle and that the most rigid behavior manifests in the range of $\omega = 25...60°$;
2. the high adaptability of the rehabilitation equipment to the patient's state requires the intervention of adjustable compliance, as follows from Figure 11. The noticeable positive aspect of this constructive solution is its high compliance in the debut phase of the rehabilitation exercise, which is exactly when the patient's fear of pain and the stiffness of the joint have to be overcome.

The two requirements outlined above are contradictory, thus complicating the possibility of meeting them simultaneously. For this reason, a compromise is called for: at the beginning of the rehabilitation exercising a high compliance has to be prioritized, while subsequently more important is to achieve and maintain precise positioning angles.

In terms of the equipment's safety, the structure of the proposed equipment allows applying the optimum rehabilitation motions to the affected segment of the human body. Regarding the risks patients could be exposed to during testing, such are negligible to a degree of non-existent, given the reduced values of the motion speed and of the actuation forces.

6. Conclusions

This paper has presented a novel solution of rehabilitation equipment for the sagittal and frontal plane movements of the neck joint actuated by a pneumatic muscle. The deployment for actuation purposes of pneumatic muscles that benefit from an inherently compliant behavior ensures the adaptability of the rehabilitation equipment to the concrete circumstances of patient pain tolerance.

The proposed rehabilitation equipment enables rotation movements in the frontal and sagittal plane within the angular limits of the healthy human body, ensuring precise rotation angles and a compliant behavior.

The constructive solution and the operational principle have been described and the torque variation versus the axial contraction of the pneumatic muscle and the rotation angle of the neck joint in the two anatomic planes was calculated. The torsional rigidity and compliance have been determined, and based on the obtained results recommendations have been formulated regarding the optimum deployment of the rehabilitation equipment.

The paper has presented the results of the theoretical study concerning the conception of the pneumatically actuated rehabilitation equipment. The performance characteristics presented in the paper are related to the limits of the movements, the forces and torques, as well as to the torsional compliance, and were obtained only theoretically. At present the prototype of the neck joint rehabilitation system is under construction. Lab tests will be performed on the final prototype, and upon refining the constructive solution, testing will be conducted on human subjects. For this reason, at this time we cannot report experimental results.

Author Contributions: Conceptualization, S.M. and T.D.; methodology, T.D.; validation, A.D.; writing—original draft preparation, S.M. and A.D.; writing—review and editing, S.M., A.D. and T.D.; supervision, T.D. All authors have read and agreed to the published version of the manuscript.

Funding: This research received no external funding.

Institutional Review Board Statement: Not applicable.

Informed Consent Statement: Not applicable.

Data Availability Statement: Data are contained within the article.

Conflicts of Interest: The authors declare no conflicts of interest.

References

1. Cervical Spine. Available online: https://my.clevelandclinic.org/health/articles/22278-cervical-spine (accessed on 7 December 2024).
2. Nunes, I.L.; Bush, P.M. Work-Related Musculoskeletal Disorders Assessment and Prevention. Available online: https://www.intechopen.com/chapters/35811 (accessed on 7 December 2024).
3. Simoneau, S.; St-Vincent, M.; Chicoine, D. *Work-Related Musculoskeletal Disorders. A Better Understanding for More Effective Prevention*; Institut de Recherche Robert Sauvé en Santé et en Sécurité: Quebec, QC, Canada, 1996.
4. de Kok, J.; Vroonhof, P.; Snijders, J.; Roullis, G.; Clarke (Panteia), M.; Peereboom, K.; van Dorst, P.; Isusi, I. *Work-Related Musculoskeletal Disorders: Prevalence, Costs and Demographics in the EU*; European Risk Observatory Report; European Agency for Safety and Health at Work: Luxembourg, 2019.
5. Pratama, A.D.; Farelin, A.D.; Karnadipa, T.; Pahlawi, R.; Noviana, M.; Abdullah, F. The Application of Telerehabilitation for Pain Reduction and Improving Quality of Life in Workers with Work-Related Musculoskeletal Disorders: Systematic Review. *Proceedings* **2022**, *83*, 45. [CrossRef]

6. Work-Related Musculoskeletal Disorders (WMSDs). Available online: https://www.ccohs.ca/oshanswers/diseases/rmirsi.html (accessed on 7 December 2024).
7. Deaconescu, T.; Deaconescu, A. Pneumatic Muscle Actuated Equipment for Continuous Passive Motion. *AIP Conf. Proc.* **2009**, *1174*, 311–321.
8. Doss, A.S.A.; Lingampally, P.K.; Nguyen, G.M.T.; Schilberg, D. A comprehensive review of wearable assistive robotic devices used for head and neck rehabilitation. *Results Eng.* **2023**, *19*, 101306. [CrossRef]
9. David Health Solutions. Cervical Muscles Exerciser G160. Available online: https://www.medicalexpo.com/prod/david-health-solutions/product-92425-836086.html (accessed on 8 December 2024).
10. David Health Solutions. G140 Cervical Extension/Lateral Flexion Device. Available online: https://davidhealth.com/global-content/cervical-extension/ (accessed on 8 December 2024).
11. Shoaib, M.; Lai, C.Y.; Bab-Hadiashar, A. A Novel Design of Cable-Driven Neck Rehabilitation Robot (CarNeck). In Proceedings of the IEEE/ASME International Conference on Advanced Intelligent Mechatronics (AIM), Hong Kong, China, 8–12 July 2019; pp. 819–825. [CrossRef]
12. Kim, H.; Park, H.; Lee, W.; Kim, J.; Park, Y.L. Design of wearable orthopedic devices for treating forward head postures using pneumatic artificial muscles and flex sensors. In Proceedings of the 14th International Conference on Ubiquitous Robots and Ambient Intelligence (URAI 2017), Jeju, Republic of Korea, 28 June–1 July 2017.
13. Yue, D.A.I.; Ping, S.; Hongyu, Z.; Sujiao, L.; Fanfu, F. Design and kinematics analysis of powered cervical exoskeleton based on human biomechanics. *J. Univ. Shanghai Sci. Technol.* **2022**, *44*, 18–26.
14. Multi-Cervical Unit (MCU). Available online: https://www.btetechnologies.com/products/functional-rehabilitation/multi-cervical-unit/ (accessed on 29 July 2024).
15. DBC Active Treatment Devices. Available online: https://www.dbc.fi/additional-device-information (accessed on 29 July 2024).
16. Xu, Y.; Ju, K.; Zhang, C. A Wrist-Inspired Magneto-Pneumatic Hybrid-Driven Soft Actuator with Bidirectional Torsion. *Cyborg Bionic Syst.* **2024**, *5*, 0111. [CrossRef] [PubMed]
17. Human Head. Wikipedia. Available online: https://en.wikipedia.org/wiki/Human_head (accessed on 8 December 2024).
18. Ching, R.P.; (Applied Biomechanics Laboratory, University of Washington, Washington, DC, USA). Technical Brief—Relationship Between Head Mass and Circumference in Human Adults. 20 July 2007.
19. Bushby, K.M.; Cole, T.; Matthews, J.N.; Goodship, J.A. Centiles for adult head circumference. *Arch. Dis. Child.* **1992**, *67*, 1286–1287. [CrossRef] [PubMed]
20. Mareş, S.; Deaconescu, A.; Deaconescu, T. Pneumatically Actuated Torsion Motor for the Transverse Rehabilitation of the Neck Joint. *Actuators* **2024**, *13*, 363. [CrossRef]
21. Berg, H.E.; Berggren, G.; Tesch, P.A. Dynamic neck strength training effect on pain and function. *Arch. Phys. Med. Rehabil.* **1994**, *75*, 661–665. [CrossRef] [PubMed]
22. Choi, H.; Vanderby, R. Comparison of biomechanical human neck models: Muscle forces and spinal loads at C4–C5 level. *J. Appl. Biomech.* **1999**, *15*, 120–138. [CrossRef]
23. Vasavada, A.N.; Li, S.; Delp, S.L. Three-dimensional isometric strength of neck muscles in humans. *Spine* **2001**, *26*, 1904–1909. [CrossRef] [PubMed]

technologies

MDPI

Article

"The Foot Can Do It": Controlling the "Persistence" Prosthetic Arm Using the "Infinity-2" Foot Controller

Peter L. Bishay *, Gerbert Funes Alfaro, Ian Sherrill, Isaiah Reoyo, Elihu McMahon, Camron Carter, Cristian Valdez, Naweeth M. Riyaz, Sara Ali, Adrian Lima, Abel Nieto and Jared Tirone

Department of Mechanical Engineering, California State University, Northridge, CA 91330, USA
* Correspondence: peter.bishay@csun.edu

Abstract: The "Infinity" foot controller for controlling prosthetic arms has been improved in this paper in several ways, including a foot sleeve that enables barefoot use, an improved sensor-controller unit design, and a more intuitive control scheme that allows gradual control of finger actuation. Furthermore, the "Persistence Arm", a novel transradial prosthetic arm prototype, is introduced. This below-the-elbow arm has a direct-drive wrist actuation system, a thumb design with two degrees of freedom, and carbon fiber tendons for actuating the four forefingers. The manufactured prototype arm and foot controller underwent various tests to verify their efficacy. Wireless transmission speed tests showed that the maximum time delay is less than 165 ms, giving almost instantaneous response from the arm to any user's foot control signal. Gripping tests quantified the grip and pulling forces of the arm prototype as 2.8 and 12.7 kg, respectively. The arm successfully gripped various household items of different shapes, weights, and sizes. These results highlight the potential of foot control as an alternative prosthetic arm control method and the possibility of new 3D-printed prosthetic arm designs to replace costly prostheses in the market, which could potentially reduce the high rejection rates of upper limb prostheses.

Keywords: foot control; wrist actuation; robotic arm; 3D-printing

1. Introduction

A recent study was conducted by Salminger et al. [1] in 2020 to assess if new innovations and refinements in prosthetic technology had an impact on the previously reported high upper limb prostheses rejection rates, reported in [2]. Surprisingly, it was found that the advancements of upper limb prosthetics in the last decade had not yet achieved a significant change in prosthetic abandonment. The rejection rate was 44% among 68 individuals with traumatic upper limb loss in Austria. The three major concerns shared by the participants were comfort, device weight, and functionality. Among users, 93% used myoelectric controllers, which reflects the dominance of this control method in controlling powered prosthetic arms. Although academic solutions were proposed to address the patient's complaints, clinical reality has not fully benefited yet from the new advances to cause any improvements in prostheses acceptance rates.

Myoelectric control systems use electromyographic (EMG) signals from residual muscles to control the prosthetic device. Myoelectric controllers have moved from the early single-site EMG sensors to pattern-recognition systems that rely on machine learning to interpret multiple muscle signals [3]. Although this enabled control of multi-degree-of-freedom prostheses, the limitations of this control approach still exist. Myoelectric control systems are affected by the skin condition and cause muscle fatigue. The number of unique control commands is still limited. If the amputation resulted in the absence of muscle function in the residual limb, EMG control would not be an option. This happened with the individual who was not even fitted with a prosthetic arm in the aforementioned recent study [1] due to the absence of muscles in the residual limb. EMG systems are also unreliable and unpredictable according to a recent study by Chadwell et al. [4] that revealed that EMG prostheses users tend to produce undesired activations of the hand or incorrect responses. Franzke's study [5] also proved the dissatisfaction of myoelectric users with the process of switching prosthesis function under conventional control. Pattern recognition was appreciated as an intuitive control that facilitated fast switching between prosthesis functions but was reported to be too unreliable for daily use and require extensive training.

In the state-of-the art review of prosthetic arm systems conducted by Vujaklija et al. [6] in 2016, it was concluded that the current bottleneck of the upper limb prosthetic development seems to be the control of the robotic limbs. Various other non-invasive control approaches were proposed, such as electroencephalography (EEG) [7–9], voice control [9–13], and foot control [14–20]. EEG requires placing multiple brain wave sensors on the head, usually in a headset to be worn by the prosthetic arm user, which is considered a limitation on its own. It also requires significant training and mental concentration during use and is affected by the placement and amount of hair on the head [21]. The reliability level is also lower than other control methods [9]. Despite the current advances in voice recognition technologies, using voice control for prosthetic arms requires the user to talk to the device to control the arm, which would not be desirable in all situations. Noise could affect the reliability of the system [21], and security measures would be needed to prevent others from controlling the user's arm.

Alderson [22] was the first to propose a foot controller for above-the-elbow individuals with upper limb loss of "extreme cases", who have extremely short stump, no stump at all, or a stump of moderate length but with impaired muscular function. The controller included toe contacts in a sole to be worn inside the user's shoe. His patent, that focused mainly on the design of a prosthetic arm, was filed on 10 July 1948, and was granted on 1 January 1952. In 1968, Alderson wrote a chapter on an improved version of his invention in the "Human Limbs and Their Substitutes" book [23]. To resolve the problem of accidental operation of toe controls during walking, he assigned only the little toe to control the motor of the hand, while the big toe and heel were used to select the functions of the motor. This was based on a peculiarity of toe actions he found that the little toe exerts only light pressures in a normal gait but could be pressed down with considerable force when desired. To operate the arm, the little toe should be pressed first followed by the big toe or heel. Control signals from the foot were directed to the arm mechanisms by means of pneumatic bladders embedded in a plastic insole and connected by thin rubber tubing to corresponding bladders in the arm. In 1974, Graupe [24] eliminated the need for three toe movements that were required per limb function in Alderson's invention, and used microelectronic hardware (strain gages) that were unavailable in 1952 to enable control of the prosthetic hand using one toe movement in his proposed controller idea. His system was operational only during sitting, lying, or standing, but was inhibited during walking. Using the natural anatomic and physiologic similarities between the upper and lower extremities, which makes the foot and leg to be an ideal control interface, Luzzio [25], in 2020, developed a stocking laced with multiple sensors to provide input on multiple leg joint positions. The signals were used to control homologous movements in a prosthetic upper extremity. The significant advantage of this form of control, compared to earlier inventions, was the simultaneous activation of multiple joints. Carrozza et al. [26,27] developed a prototype of a wearable insole, called ACHILLE insole, with FSR switches placed at four sensitive areas (heel, big toe, lateral left, and lateral right). The prototype used wireless transmission to control a robotic hand prosthesis with three fingers. Testing it on 10 able-bodied subjects showed a significant decrease in required adaptation and learning from the user's side, compared to EMG control.

Lyons and Joshi [16] conducted an important study in 2015 where EMG sensors were placed on the forearm to record the muscle activity while participants performed gestures with their dominant hand. Then, the sensors were placed on the lower leg while participants performed analogues set of foot gestures. An intuitive mapping between the hand and foot was found and determined to be sufficient for prosthetic control. Accordingly, they used surface EMG (sEMG) sensors placed on the lower leg and mapped the degrees of freedom of the leg to those of the arm to enable noninvasive control of prosthetic elbow, wrist, and hand movements [17,18]. Lee et al. [20] used a wearable fabric sensor on the lower leg to map foot postures to prosthetic hand postures. Their experimental results confirmed that the sEMG signals of the lower limb obtained by using their developed sensors were more distinct than those of the upper limb for eight postures. DEKA Research [28] developed a prosthetic arm along with a foot controller [29] that includes force sensitive resistors (FSRs) in a custom made insole along with inertial measurement units (IMUs). Resnik et al. [19] tested the DEKA foot controller [30] on 36 subjects with upper limb amputation, 77% of whom owned a myoelectric device, 22% owned body-powered devices, and 14% owned a cosmetic arm or no prosthetic device at all. Although some of the subjects described the used FSR or IMU controllers on both feet as "bulky", the subjects' feedback was generally positive. The "Infinity" foot controller developed by Bishay et al. [15] used two push buttons in an insole under the toes to control the fingers of the prosthetic arm, along with a sensor controller unit (SCU) to actuate a two-degree-of-freedom wrist actuation system in the arm. This system relied on the big toe and four lesser toes to control the prosthetic arm fingers in multiple grips, which was shown to be an easy and intuitive control method.

Commercial prostheses are often unaffordable, or inaccessible, to underprivileged individuals (e.g., no health insurance, low incomes, warzone). In addition, each design of a commercial arm has its own limitation. For example, the Hero Arm [31], which is a lightweight, below-the-elbow prosthesis, lacks wrist flexion/extension and pronation/supination movements. Commercial prostheses are also limited in terms of customizability, as they come in standard sizes, and with specific control systems. Some prostheses also require inputs from a natural hand to adjust the orientation of the wrist manually. Piazza et al. [32] presented a state-of-the-art review of artificial hands covering 106 years of engineering (1912–2018). The review included some famous commercial prosthetic arms, such as the Ottobock Michelangelo Hand [33], the i-Limb Quantum [34], the Open Bionics Hero Arm [31], and the BeBionic hand [35]. They concluded that using new fabrication technologies is opening the way to a reduced cost of production of artificial hands. Wendo et al. [36] in 2022 presented a review on open-source 3D-printed upper limb prostheses, as this new fabrication technology offers higher availability and accessibility and can produce complex geometrical and highly customized products, which are essential features for prostheses manufacturing. However, more work is needed to expedite the implementation of 3D-printed prostheses in clinical routines and their acceptance by the healthcare providers community.

In this paper, a modified version of the Infinity foot controller that was originally proposed in [15] is presented. The new features of this controller, named "Infinity-2", include a foot controller sleeve (FCS) that replaces the foot controller insole to enable a more secured fit around the foot when the user is using the controller shoeless. In addition, Bluetooth and Wi-Fi technologies are used in wireless data transmission, leading to high response speeds from the prosthetic arm when the user makes an action with the foot controller. Gradual control of finger deformation has also been achieved through a new control scheme. To demonstrate the capabilities of the foot controller, a new transradial prosthetic arm prototype, named the "Persistence" arm, has been designed. Compared to the Infinity arm reported in [15], this new arm includes a powerful direct drive wrist actuation mechanism, a lightweight forearm core structure with generatively designed mounts, a separate forearm outer shell, four three-digit forefingers that are actuated with carbon-fiber ribbons connected to individual servomotors housed in the palm structure, and a two-degree-of-freedom linkage-based thumb. The whole system has been tested in various tests to prove that the design goals have been successfully achieved. The goal of the whole proposed system is to give the user a simple, effective, reliable, and comfortable way to control their below-the-elbow prosthetic arm utilizing the human's natural connection between the arms and feet.

The rest of the paper is organized as follows: The next section, Materials and Methods, describes all features of the Infinity-2 foot controller, Persistence arm, and the manufacturing and assembly of both. The Results section comes next with details on the performed actuation and gripping tests. This is followed by a Discussion section, and then the paper is concluded in the Conclusions section.

2. Materials and Methods

2.1. Infinity-2 Foot Controller Design

The Infinity-2 foot controller system is shown in Figure 1. It is a two-part system that includes the Foot Controller Unit (FCU) and the Foot Controller Sleeve (FCS).

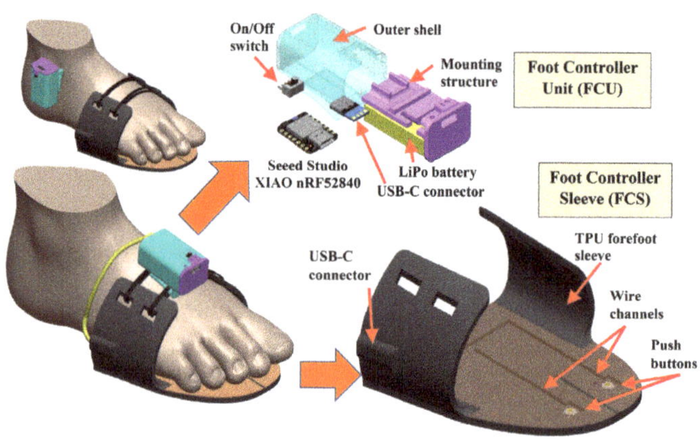

Figure 1. Infinity-2 foot controller system.

The FCU and FCS work together to control a below-the-elbow prosthetic arm that has up to five fingers and two wrist degrees of freedom (DOF), namely wrist flexion/extension and pronation/supination. The FCU contains a Seeeduino XIAO BLE nRF52840 Sense microcontroller (Manufacturer: seeed studio, Shenzhen, China), a rechargeable 400 mAh LiPo battery, an on/off switch, and a USB 3.1 Type C female connector. All these electronic components are secured on the main mounting structure and covered by the outer shell, as shown in Figure 1. The mounting structure and the outer shell are both made of 3D-printed Polylactic Acid (PLA) material. The outer shell has an integrated clip to facilitate attaching the FCU to the FCS, to the collar of a shoe, or to the cuff of a sock. The Seeeduino microcontroller does not only have the 6 DOF Internal Measurement Unit (IMU), which encases an accelerometer and a gyroscope, but it also has a Bluetooth antenna, a battery charger, and a very fast processor to process the IMU data. With an embedded LED, this microcontroller also lets the user know the charge level of the battery. The microcontroller processes all gyroscopic and accelerometer data, which is then sent to the prosthesis and is used to actuate the wrist servomotors. The gyroscope measures the current position of the user's foot. When rotating the foot around the pitch axis (ankle dorsiflexion and plantarflexion), the user can control the wrist extension and flexion, and when rotating the foot around the roll axis (ankle inversion and eversion), the user can control the wrist supination and pronation, as illustrated in Table 1. This allows the user to place their prosthetic palm in multiple different positions for a better grip of objects with various shapes and sizes. Rotation around the yaw axis (ankle abduction and adduction) is negated, as it is used to re-center the device when walking detection is activated.

Table 1. Foot motions and resulting hand motions.

	Ankle dorsiflexion	Ankle plantarflexion	Ankle inversion	Ankle eversion	Big toe press	Lesser toes press	All toe press
Foot motion	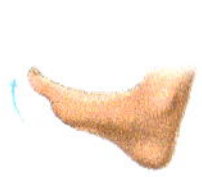	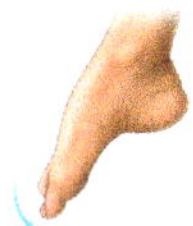	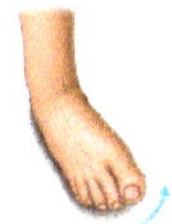	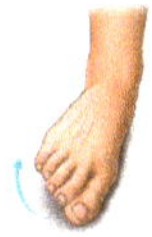	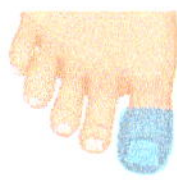	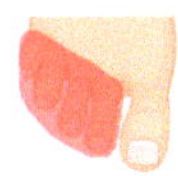	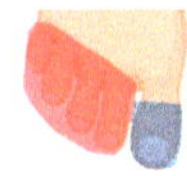
	Wrist extension	Wrist flexion	Wrist supination	Wrist pronation	Fingers flexion	Fingers extension	Grip change
Resulting hand motion	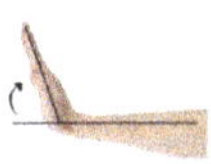	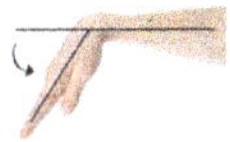	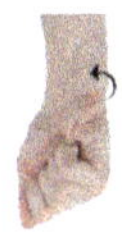	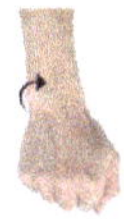	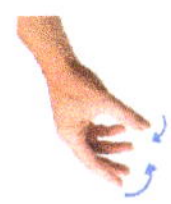	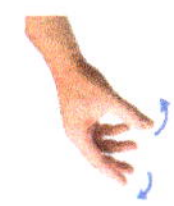	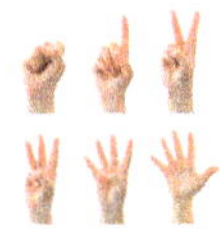

The FCS allows the user to gain finger actuation control as finger flexion and extension in various grip patterns. The FCS consists of four layers, as shown in the exploded view in Figure 2. The forefoot sleeve layer houses all electronics and is 3D-printed of Thermoplastic Polyurethane (TPU), which is a flexible material, to allow the sleeve to deform around the forefoot. This gives a custom fit for the FCS around the user's foot, whether on a barefoot or a sock, or inside a shoe. The sleeve layer is supported by a three-part support layer underneath, which is 3D-printed of Acrylonitrile Butadiene Styrene (ABS) and has channels for push buttons and wires. The button paddles layer is placed above the sleeve layer to increase the surface area of the clickable regions under the tows that can push the buttons placed under them.

This design distributes pressure across the button and its surrounding area, making it easier to press successfully, even if the toes are not perfectly aligned with the button position. The paddles layer is 3D-printed of TPU material. The top layer is made of felt to give comfort to the user. The two push buttons are connected to the USB-C connector through wires routed in the channels. An external USB-C cable is used to connect the FCS to the FCU, as shown in Figure 1. The wiring diagram of the FCU and FCS is shown in Figure A1 in Appendix A.

Each prosthetic arm and FCU have their own set of Universally Unique Identifiers (UUIDs) that are used to pair the devices together. When the FCU is powered on, the device follows the control flowchart shown in Figure 3. First it starts setting up its internal Bluetooth UUID's. Soon after, it enables Bluetooth discoverability. The device then waits for a connection to be established. If the FCU manages to connect to a device, it then closes Bluetooth discoverability, checks its battery level, then moves into a standby mode until an action is done. If the IMU is triggered by motion, the gyroscope then calibrates itself to correctly assign its axes using the yaw axis as the neutral axis. It then checks if the user is walking. If no walking is detected, the action that was done is then transmitted to the prosthetic arm as a corresponding axis value. After checking the battery level, the FCU also processes the button data that comes from the FCS. It checks if the buttons are being pressed or held. If no button has been pressed, it keeps waiting for a button press. If a button is pressed, the FCU goes to the walking detection check, followed by the data transmission step to the prosthetic arm's MAC address.

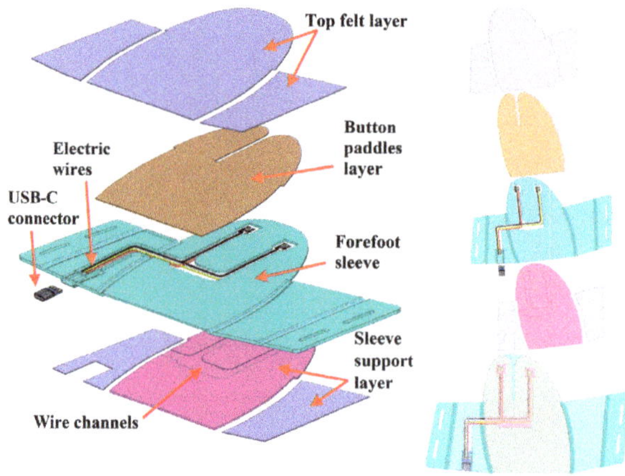

Figure 2. Foot controller sleeve (FCS) in exploded view.

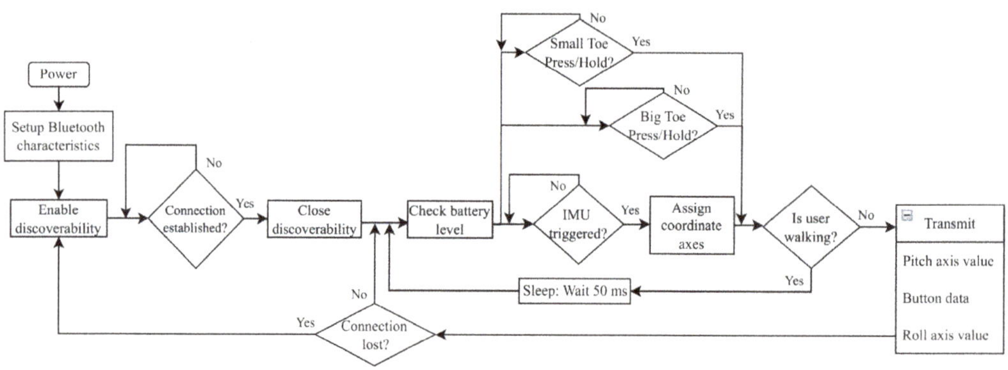

Figure 3. FCU control flowchart.

To determine if the user is walking, the FCU goes through the process shown in Figure 4. This process is done before any data is determined to be ready for transmission. Once the IMU trigger has been determined, the IMU checks all gyroscope axes along with all accelerometer values for all axes. If any two axes are both above their specified threshold for both the gyroscope and accelerometer values, the user is determined to be walking with the device. The threshold values can be adjusted for each user. Testing determined the default values to be used for most users. The threshold was intentionally set to be more sensitive, increasing the likelihood of false-positive walking detections rather than missing actual walking. As a result, the FCU may occasionally classify the user as walking if they rotate their ankle rapidly while attempting to control the wrist. The obtained threshold values allowed different users to utilize the device and confidently walk without worrying about the prosthetic arm actuating while walking.

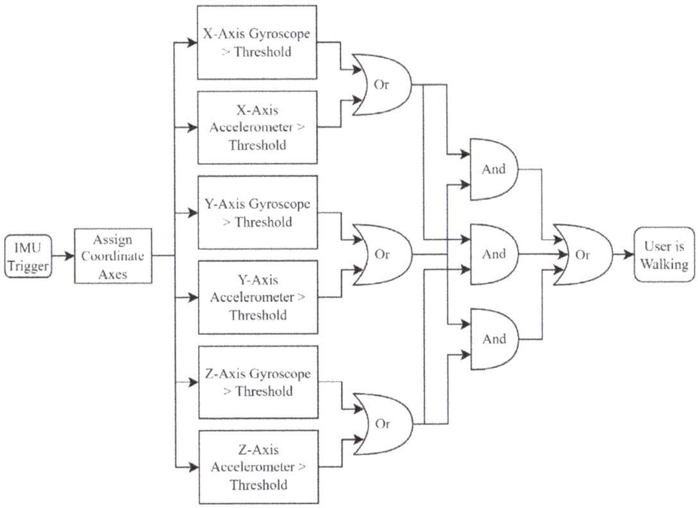

Figure 4. Walking detection system flowchart.

2.2. Persistence Arm

Figure 5 shows the full CAD assembly of the Persistence Arm. The palm contains five lightweight digital servos that actuate the five fingers. The thumb has an additional servomotor to add a second degree of freedom to the thumb actuation. The forearm contains the wrist actuation mechanism as well as the electronics responsible for controlling and supplying power to the arm. The wrist actuation system occupies 50% of the forearm length.

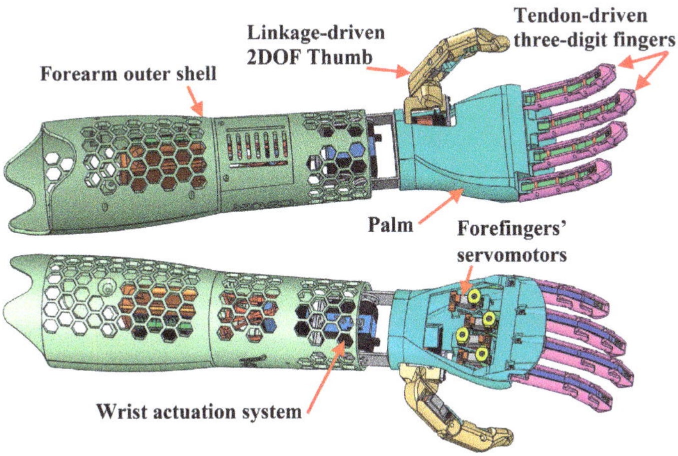

Figure 5. Full CAD assembly of Persistence arm.

The palm was designed to be as biomimetic as possible, taking inspiration from the human hand. The shape, size, and proportions of the Persistence palm were made to resemble an average-sized male hand. However, since the whole CAD model was created parametrically, the size can be reduced to the average female hand size with some adjustments, including reducing the number of forefinger servomotors from 4 to 3, coupling the actuation of the ring and pinky fingers, since they move together in all programmed grips. A similar coupling was done in [15]. The resizing of the CAD model would not affect the components that have standard sizes, such as the servomotors, and locations and dimensions of mounting points. The assembly and exploded views of the palm with its fingers can be seen in Figure 6. The palm has attachment points for each of the fingers. The index, middle, ring, and pinky fingers are secured to the palm using M3 screws that are threaded into heat-set inserts located in the palm. The thumb is attached to a dedicated mount inside the palm, which has its own set of heat-set inserts and a rotating pin at the bottom.

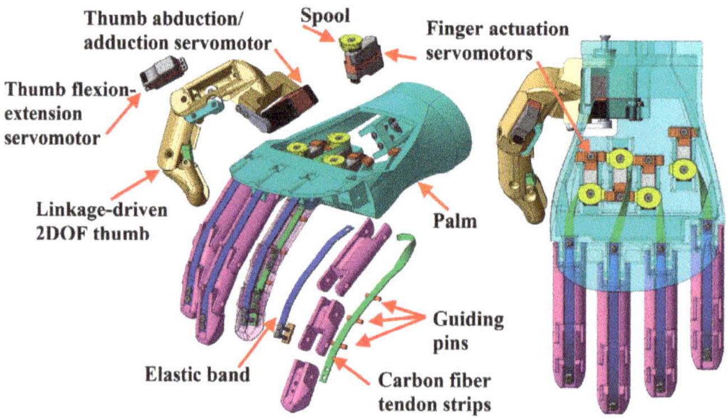

Figure 6. Persistence hand in exploded and assembled views.

The four forefingers are actuated using four KST A08N micro servomotors (stall torque: 3.2 kg.cm at 8.4 V; max. speed: 0.09 s/60°; weight: 7 g; size: 23.5 × 8 × 19 mm). Each servomotor has a spool connected to its shaft. As shown in Figure 7a, a flexible carbon fiber tendon strip, from Carbitex (www.carbitex.com), is attached to each spool and is routed through a special groove in the three finger phalanges. It is then attached to the distal phalange with two retaining screws. When the servomotor operates, it turns its spool, transferring the servomotor's torque into a pulling force on the tendon strip to flex the finger. All three phalanges of the finger move at the same time to close the finger. However, the finger can take different shapes depending on the contour of the object it touches. This compliant behavior enables the hand to grip objects of different shapes and sizes since each finger can deform independently and surround the object in the closest possible way. If the finger does not face any obstacles or objects to grip, it will close on itself. Hence, this design allows for different grips and gestures to be realized by the prosthetic hand, mimicking the human hand's natural deformations.

The spool on the servomotor has a radius of 7 mm, which is big enough to pull the carbon fiber strip just the right amount to fully close the finger. This is done with about 160° rotational movement of the spool by the servomotor. The phalanges of the finger are attached to one another using screws connected to heat-set inserts embedded in the phalanges. Guiding pins are assembled to the phalanges, as shown in Figure 7a, to guide the carbon fiber tendon strip as it slides in its groove when finger flexion happens and to reduce friction. Finger extension is achieved by the elastic band attached and routed through the top side of the finger to allow the finger to fully return to a relaxed position when the servomotor is set to an idle condition. The elastic bands have special channels embedded in the phalanges that allow each band to conform around the finger when it is actuated.

The Persistence arm's thumb has a linkage-based design, different from the design of the forefingers. This design, shown in Figure 7b, enables the thumb to have two degrees of freedom: flexion/extension and abduction/adduction. The flexion/extension servomotor is a KST A08N housed inside the proximal phalange to actuate the middle and distal phalanges via the linkage mechanism. The base of the proximal phalange is connected to the palm, as shown in Figure 8. The base houses the abduction/adduction KST A12-610 servomotor (stall torque: 9 kg.cm at 8.4 V; max. speed: 0.10 s/60°; weight: 20 g; size: 23 × 12 × 27 mm). The thumb base sits on a bearing and a pin inserted in a slot in the palm structure at the location of the metacarpal. This enables the abduction/adduction servomotor to rotate the thumb without friction up to 70°.

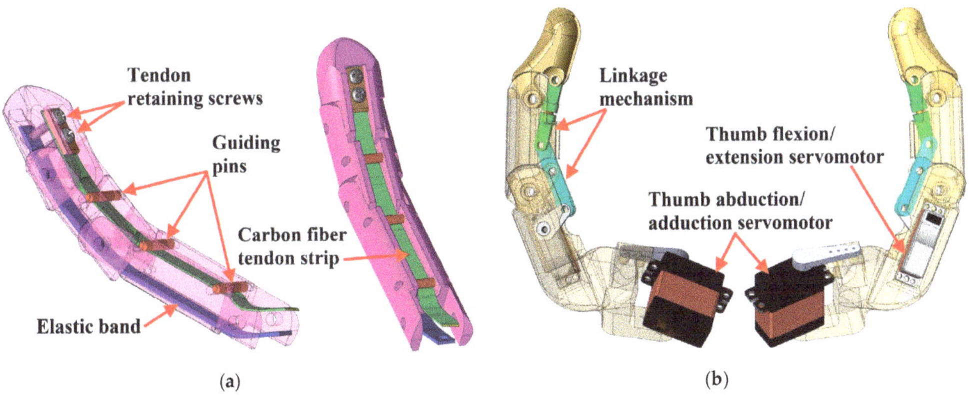

Figure 7. Persistence arm fingers: (**a**) a forefinger, and (**b**) the thumb.

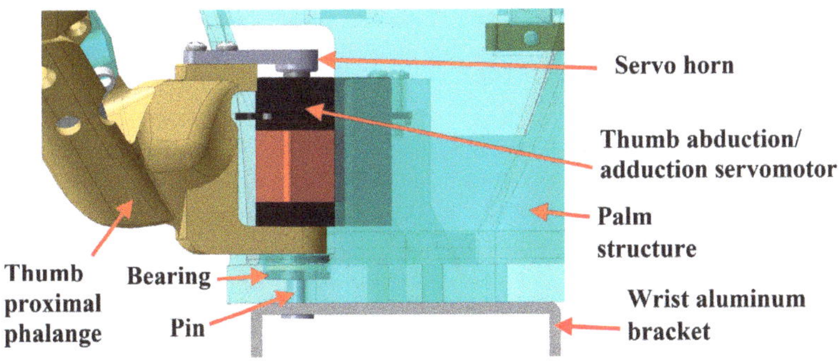

Figure 8. Thumb's connection to the palm structure.

Persistence arm features two wrist degrees of freedom: wrist flexion/extension and wrist pronation/supination. The assembly of the wrist actuation mechanism inside the forearm is shown in Figure 9, with a transparent outer shell to show the internal components. The design features a wrist mount that houses the wrist pronation/supination servomotor, which is a 35 kg DS3235 servomotor (stall torque: 35 kg.cm at 7.4 V; max. speed: 0.11 s/60°; weight: 60 g; size: 40 × 20 × 38.5 mm). An aluminum bracket connects this servomotor to the wrist flexion/extension servomotor, which is a dual bearing 35 kg RDS3235 servomotor (stall torque: 35 kg.cm at 8.4 V; max. speed: 0.11 s/60°; weight: 60 g; size: 40 × 20 × 40 mm). Another aluminum bracket connects this servomotor to the palm structure. This pant-tilt system allows the wrist to rotate 90° in both directions for a 180° range of pronation/supination and to tilt 30° degrees in both directions for a 60° range of wrist flexion/extension.

The control system in the arm includes an ESP-WROOM-32 microcontroller (Manufacturer: Espressif Systems, Shanghai, China), which receives all signals from the foot controller and actuates all servomotors in the arm. A 7.4 V LiPo battery powers all servomotors in the arm through a terminal block. The wiring diagram of the arm is shown in Figure A2 in Appendix A.

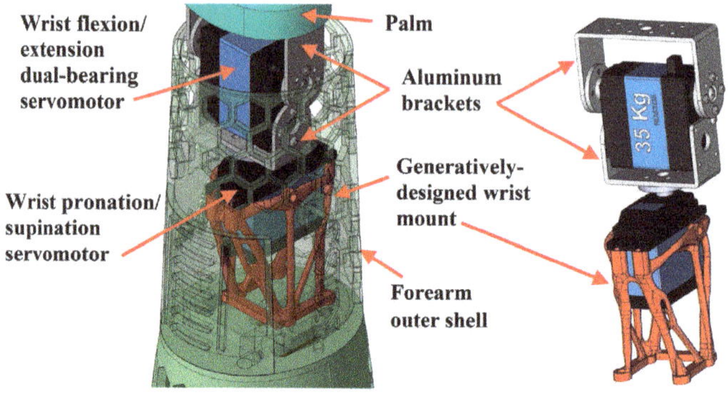

Figure 9. Wrist actuation mechanism in Persistence arm assembled inside the forearm with transparent outer shell.

The Generative Design (GD) tool in Autodesk Fusion was used to design the wrist mount shown in Figure 9. Based on defined preserve regions, obstacle regions, load conditions, material parameters, and manufacturing methods, this tool runs a machine learning (ML) algorithm to iteratively optimize the design. The GD algorithm follows a process of generation, evaluation, and evolution, to optimize the design by reducing mass and maximizing stiffness while still satisfying all defined initial conditions. Appendix B gives more details on the process of creating this mount using the GD tool.

The electronics of the control system are all mounted on a 3D-printed PLA mount in the upper part of the forearm, as shown in Figure 10. ESP-32 is mounted on one side, and the terminal block is mounted on the other. The LiPo battery is placed beside the terminal block. The outer shell of the arm, shown in Figure 5, Figure 9, and Figure 10, is perforated to reduce weight and is made of two parts: the lower part, which surrounds the wrist actuation mechanism, and the upper part, which surrounds the electronics mount. Both parts are connected using four M3 screws that are also securing the wrist mount to the shell. Three M2 alignment screws are also used to strengthen the connection of the upper and lower parts of the forearm shell. Two access points are included in the outer shell. The first is a small door in the lower part, as shown in Figures 5 and 9, and the second is a bigger door in the upper part. The doors are connected to the main body of the shell using M2 screws. The shell is connected to the socket on the residual limb.

Figure 11 shows the Persistence arm's control flowchart. When the arm is powered on, the device checks all motor positions. If any motor is not in its default position, the arm adjusts and resets the motor to bring it back to its default position. Default positions for this arm are as shown in Figure 5: All fingers are fully open, and the wrist is straight with the palm. At the same time, the arm is searching for its designated Foot Controller Unit (FCU) to be paired with via UUID. As a safety measure, a second unique identifier is also used in the pairing procedure to ensure the correct device has been connected. The two devices need to match a password in order to establish a full connection. There is one additional level of security that is built into the transmission. The payload messages have a unique structure that is known to the arm. If the message does not match the structure the arm is expecting, the arm will reject the message. Figure 12 shows the flowchart of the security checks.

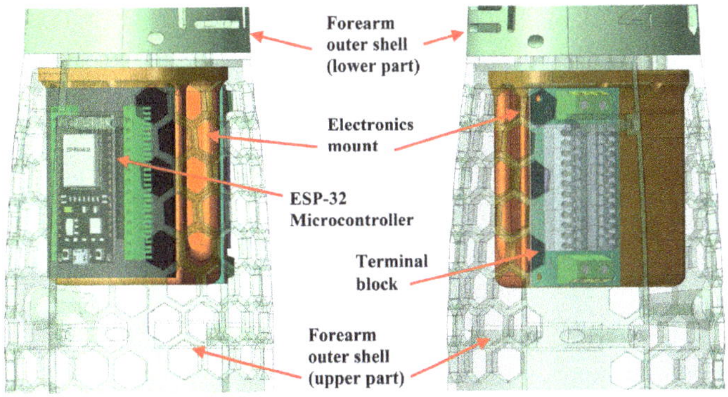

Figure 10. Electronics mount in the upper part of the forearm with transparent outer shell (two sides).

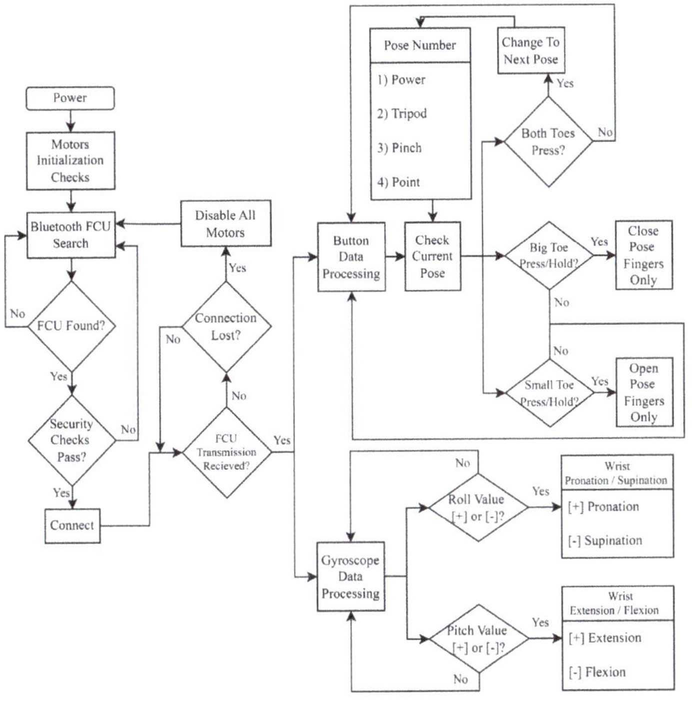

Figure 11. Persistence arm control flowchart.

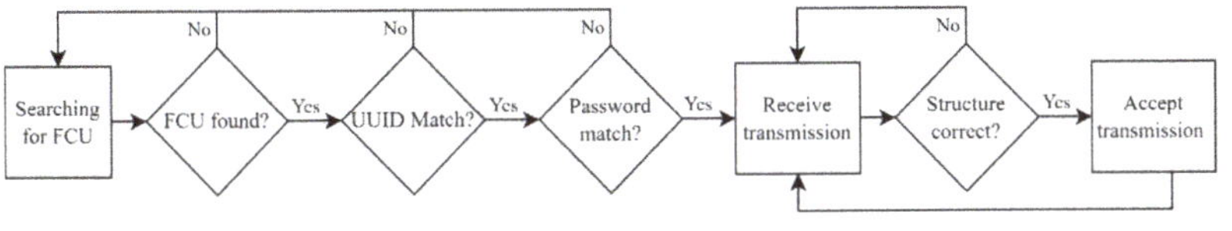

Figure 12. Security checks used in wireless communication between Persistence arm and Infinity-2 foot controller.

After all security checks have passed and the FCU has established a connection, the arm can work as intended. When the raw gyroscope data is received from the FCU, the arm processes this data and translates the received values to their corresponding movements.

Both the roll and pitch values can be positive or negative. If the pitch value is positive, the wrist extends; if it is negative, the wrist flexes. For pronation/supination, if the roll value is positive, the wrist supinates; if it is negative, the wrist pronates. Both wrist flexion/extension and wrist pronation/supination move at a speed of 2° per transmission. Preliminary testing showed that this rate gives the user a good middle ground between speed and precision and allows the user to gradually orient the prosthetic palm in the user's desired position.

Processed button data is sent by the FCU to the arm. When this data is received, the arm performs a check before moving any fingers to find out what pose it is currently going to do. The default starting pose is the "Power" pose. The user can cycle between the four assigned poses by pressing both toe buttons simultaneously. The poses will cycle in the following order: power, tripod, pinch, point. When the pose is identified, the arm moves the appropriate fingers required by that specific pose. If the user presses the big toe button, the arm gradually flexes the desired fingers by 5° for the four forefingers. The thumb metacarpal will adduct by 1°, while the thumb phalanges will flex by 2°. If the user presses the lesser toes button, all fingers extend, and the thumb abducts by the same rate used in closing. This happens once for every single transmission received, allowing the user to hold any of the two buttons down and move the fingers gradually, or get precise movement by simply pressing any of the buttons to move the fingers by just one step to adjust the grip strength to the desired amount. The arm remembers the exact position of each specific finger even if the user switches to a different pose. When the fingers are actuated, all servomotors involved in the selected pose will move gradually as long as the big toe button is pressed. Once the button is released, the fingers stop immediately. If the user changes the pose at this point and then presses the button again, only the servomotors for the newly activated fingers will move, while the others remain in their last known positions until reactivated. If the user then chooses to open the fingers from this new position, all fingers will gradually open together, regardless of the pose. An example of this would be as follows. The user begins with the Power grip, where all five fingers are to be actuated. The fingers gradually close until they reach approximately 35% of their full actuation range. At this point, the user realizes that the object can only be grasped using the tripod grip, which involves the thumb, index, and middle fingers only. They switch to this pose and continue closing these three fingers until they reach around 75%. Meanwhile, the ring and pinky fingers remain at their last known position of 35%. When it is time to release the object, all fingers, regardless of whether the pose is power or tripod, or whether their position was at 35% or 75% of their actuation range, will gradually open until fully extended. If the user starts with a pinch grip (only thumb and index) and then after 40% actuation, switch to power grip, all fingers will move with the same rate until they touch an object or reach their full actuation range. However, in this case, the middle, ring, and pinky fingers will start actuation from their fully extended position, whereas the thumb and index would resume from their 40% actuated positions. Persistence arm can handle parallel processing of the systems discussed: wrist flexion/extension, wrist pronation/supination, and finger gripping. This means that if the user would like to close the fingers while also rotating the wrist, the prosthesis will be able to process both commands and actuate the corresponding servomotors simultaneously.

2.3. Manufacturing and Assembly

All structural components, such as finger phalanges, forearm outer shell, and forearm electronics and wrist mounts, were first 3D-printed of PLA, then electronic components were assembled. Only the palm was 3D-printed of ABS to prevent any possible overheating of the forefingers' servomotors from deforming their mounts in the palm structure, since

ABS performs better in heat resistance scenarios than PLA (the glass transition temperatures of ABS and PLA are 105 °C and 60 °C, respectively). Figure 13 shows the fully assembled proof-of-concept model of the Persistence Arm. Each finger servomotor was secured in its housing inside the 3D-printed palm via a system of heat inserts and screws. Heat inserts were also embedded in all finger phalanges, and then screws were connected to act as joints. 2 mm dia. brass pins were also secured in the fingers to act as guides for the carbon fiber tendons that slide in the finger bottom channels during finger actuation. The flexible Carbitex carbon fiber tendon sheet was cut into strips, and the strips were routed through the fingers to the palm. Within the palm, they were attached to the spools of the servomotors using clamps and screws. The elastic bands were also routed through the top channel of the four forefingers to return the fingers to the neutral position when the fingers are not actuated. The internal links of the thumb were first assembled separately and connected to the flexion/extension servomotor. The thumb with its adduction/abduction mount was then attached to the palm using a thrust ball bearing held in position using a guide screw. Strips of rubber tape were bonded to the fingertips and palmer side of the palm to give the hand additional grip friction.

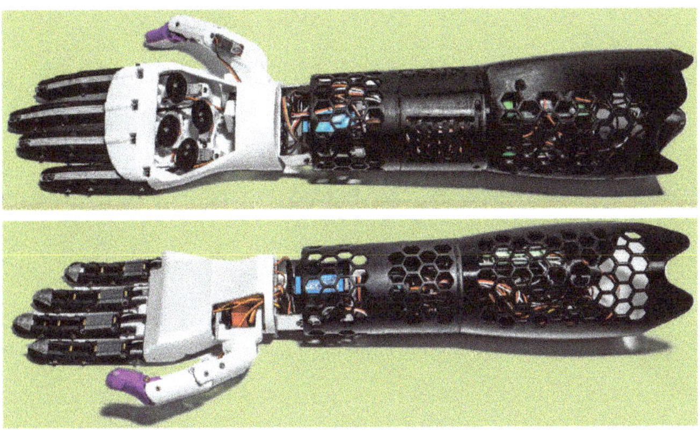

Figure 13. Assembled proof-of-concept model of the Persistence arm.

The wrist actuation servomotors were also assembled and mounted to the generatively designed wrist mount, as shown in Figure 14. The wrist mount and all other electronic components were secured on the forearm core structure and covered with the forearm outer shell. The assembled hand was then connected to the assembled forearm. The total weight of Persistence Arm without a battery is 670 g. The arm with a battery installed weighs 820 g.

The FCS forefoot sleeve and button paddles layers were 3D-printed of TPU material. The three-part support layer was 3D-printed of ABS to provide structural rigidity, and the top felt layer was cut to size. The push buttons were placed snugly in their specified pockets in the forefoot sleeve, and wires were routed through their guide channels and connected to the USB-C connector. All layers were then bonded together using Loctite superglue. The top felt layer gives the user a comfortable, soft feel when they put on the device. Figure 15a shows the assembled foot controller system. A Velcro strap was used to tighten the sleeve around the user's foot securely. The manufactured FCS weighs 31.2 g.

The FCU's outer shell and mounting structure were 3D-printed of PLA. All electrical components were then secured on the mounting structure. Then the outer shell was placed to cover and protect all components, as shown in Figure 15b. The outer shell's integrated clip is used to attach the FCU to the FCS, as shown in Figure 15a, or to the user's shoe collar or sock cuff. The manufactured FCU weighs 51 g. The whole foot controller system, including the short USB-C cable, weighs 96.4 g.

The manufacturing cost of Persistence Arm was $390 and that of the Infinity-2 foot controller was $80. This does not include service charges for 3D-printing, and labor cost for manufacturing and assembly.

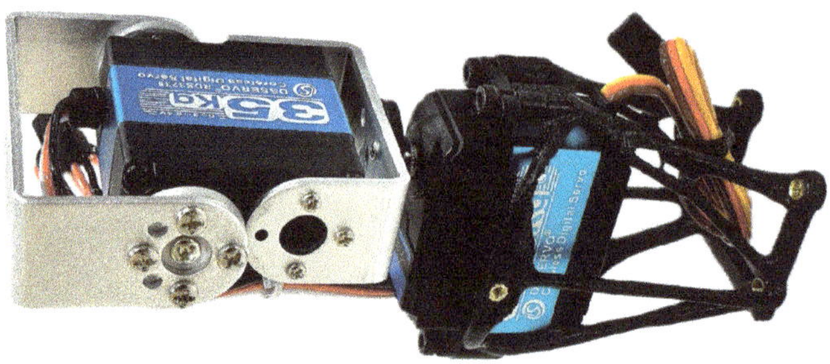

Figure 14. Manufactured wrist actuation mechanism.

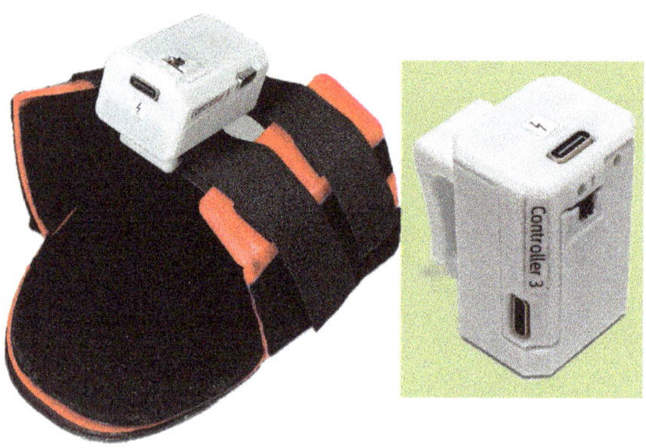

(**a**) (**b**)

Figure 15. (**a**) Assembled foot controller system, (**b**) Foot controller unit (FCU).

2.4. Test Setup

To determine the wireless transmission speed between the foot controller to the arm's ESP32 microcontroller, the devices were connected to a computer via USB connection to log transmission times between both devices using a developed MATLAB code (version R2024a). The goal of the code was to record the time it takes for the arm to receive commands from the controller. Data logging happened in 30 s intervals where all recorded values were compared and averaged out to find the time delay of the device. The FCU had 200 data points and the time delay in all points was plotted (see Section 3.1).

To measure the operating speed of the arm's ESP32 microcontroller when in use, a code was implemented into the arm's control code to log the time delay for each subsystem. Excel Data Streamer was then used to record each trigger that was set in place by this new code. The triggers were sent to Excel, and the time was taken when each trigger was noticed. A start trigger was activated when the device received the transmission from the FCU, and an end trigger was activated once the device finished its current action. For example, if the FCU sent a command to close the fingers by one step, the start trigger would be activated as soon as the message was received, and the end trigger would be activated when the device finishes moving the fingers by one step. Using this method, the time delay for each wrist pronation/supination, wrist flexion/extension, and finger movement was logged and plotted (see Section 3.1).

To measure the gripping force of the proof-of-concept Persistence hand, a BASELINE digital hand dynamometer (Model: 12-0070, capacity: 136 kg, resolution: 0.045 kg, accuracy: 1% of full scale), shown in Figure 16a, was used. The hand was put in the power grip pose and wrapped around the dynamometer to determine the grip strength.

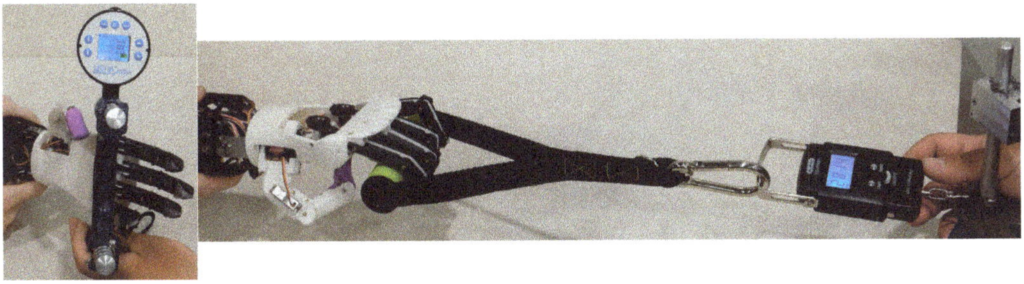

(**a**) (**b**)

Figure 16. (**a**) Grip force test, (**b**) Pulling force test.

To measure the pulling strength of the arm, an exercise handle was attached to a digital scale (Brand and model: Dr. Meter ES-PS01 (Manufacturer: Dr. Meter, Newark, CA, USA), capacity: 50 kg, resolution: 0.010 kg), and the arm was pulled to measure the maximum pulling force, as shown in Figure 16b.

3. Results

3.1. Wireless Transmission Speed Tests

Figure 17 shows the time delay of all data points in the wireless transmission speed test. The "transmissions" in the abscissa refers to the total number of acknowledged messages or data packets successfully sent from one device to another. In this context, "acknowledged" indicates that the receiving device has confirmed receipt of the message, ensuring reliable communication between devices. This metric helps keep track of successful data exchanges and evaluates the efficiency of the communication system. The average transmission delay was 43.4 ms. Using Bluetooth and WiFi wireless transmission protocols proved that these devices are fast enough to get an almost instant response time for the user.

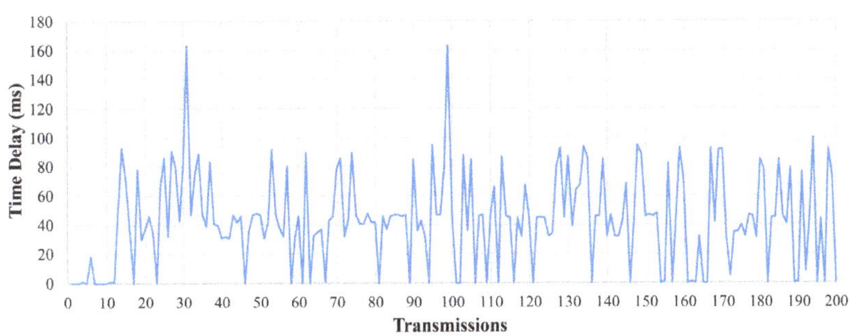

Figure 17. Time delay in wireless transmission of data from the FCU to the prosthetic arm.

The delay in response time of wrist pronation/supination, wrist flexion/extension, and finger movement are shown in Figures 18–20, respectively. Wrist pronation and supination (Figure 18), had average delays of 160.8 μs and 157.0 μs, respectively. Wrist flexion and extension (Figure 19), had average delays of 141.8 and 149.4 μs, respectively. Any finger movement (Figure 20) has a delay of 280.5 μs. These time delays are very short and prove that the arm's microprocessor can handle the current subsystems at adequate speeds.

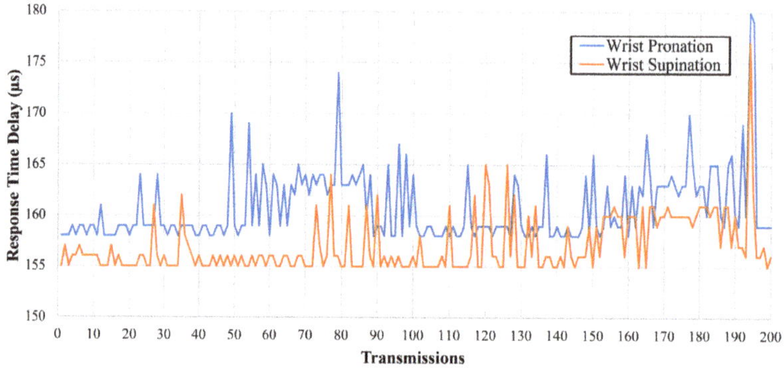

Figure 18. Response time delay in wrist pronation/supination data.

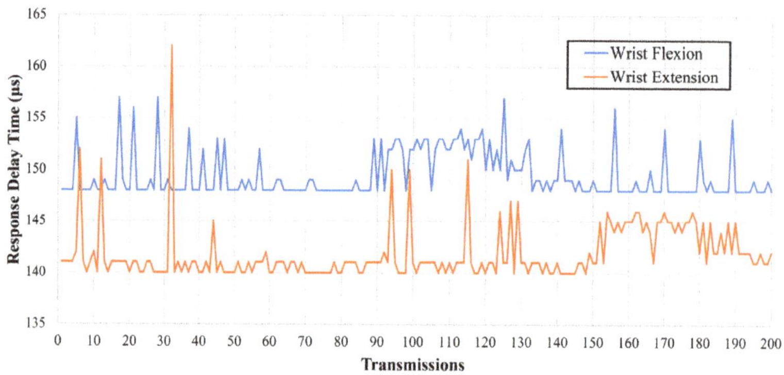

Figure 19. Response time delay in wrist flexion/extension data.

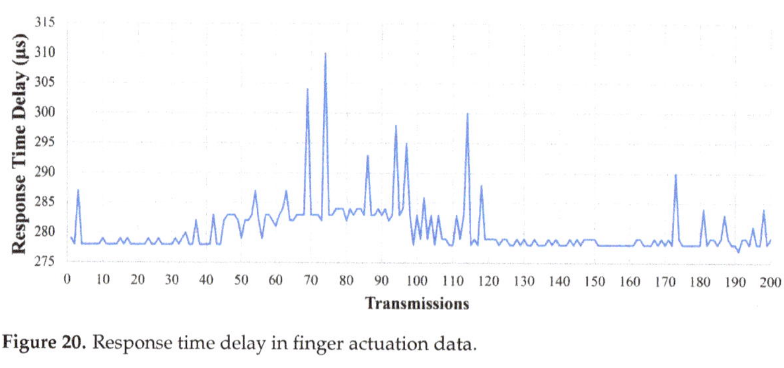

Figure 20. Response time delay in finger actuation data.

3.2. Gripping Tests

The prosthetic arm can possibly perform different grips and gestures that the user desires, but it comes pre-programmed with the five starting poses shown in Figure 21. The user can cycle through the available poses using the FCS by pressing on both push buttons at the same time.

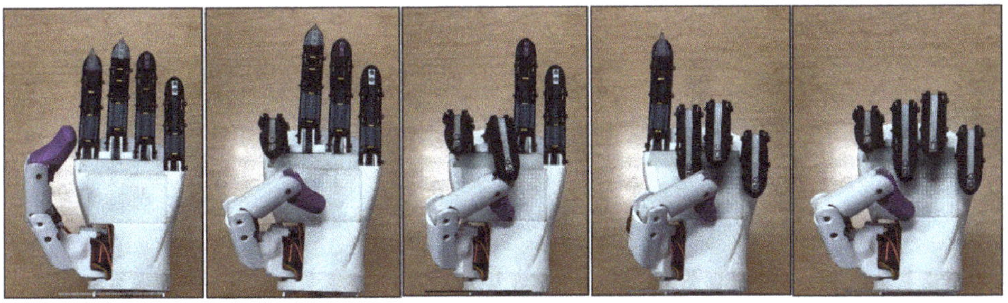

Figure 21. Default grips and gestures in Persistence Arm: Relaxed, pinch, tripod, point, and power.

To have a precise hand orientation adjustment around the object to be gripped, the wrist actuation system enables wrist flexion/extension and pronation/supination in response to the ankle inversion/eversion and dorsiflexion/plantarflexion motions, as demonstrated in Figure 22. In addition, the partial actuation capability allows for more precise control over the wrist orientation and finger actuation to take into consideration the shape and fragility of the object being held. Figure 23 illustrates this feature using wrist supination and power grip as examples.

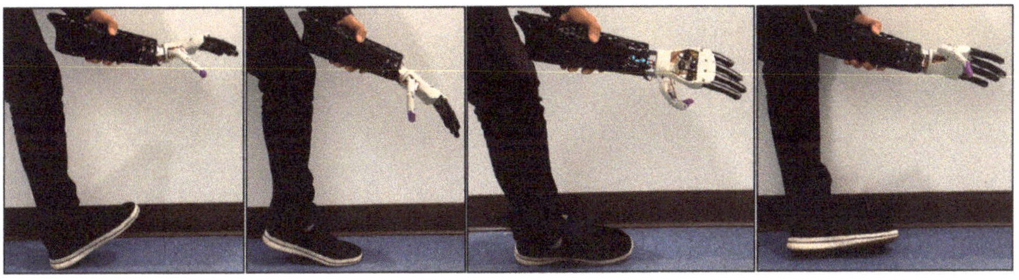

Figure 22. Wrist flexion/extension and pronation/supination.

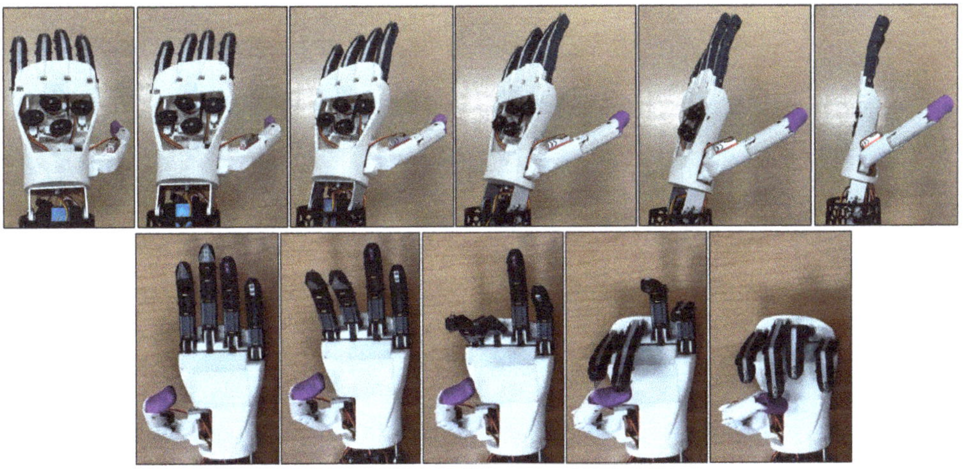

Figure 23. Partial actuation demonstration in wrist supination (**top**) and power grip (**bottom**).

Applying a grip force on the dynamometer has different dynamics than gripping regular household objects because the device requires applying force in one specific direction to measure the force. Despite this challenging requirement, the maximum grip force of the prosthetic arm was found to be 2.8 kg (Figure 16a).

The pull strength test (Figure 16b) showed that the prosthetic fingers started to lose grip at 12.7 kg, giving the prosthesis a maximum vertical holding weight of 12.7 kg. A similar test was performed with just the wrist. In this test, the wrist showed a maximum holding weight of 40.8 kg before the servomotors started to show mechanical failure. In all the tests performed above, mechanical failure of the servomotors was experienced before structural failure of the 3D-printed parts in the arm.

Figure 24 shows Persistence arm gripping different household objects of different shapes, weights, and sizes using power, tripod, and pinch grips. The gripped objects include a hand tool, a Dremel tool, tape rolls of different sizes, plastic cups, empty and full bottles, a screwdriver, an apple, a rubber ball, a wireless computer mouse, a pencil, a small superglue bottle, a USB flash drive, and various 3D-printed objects. Video S1 shows the Persistence arm in action gripping various objects.

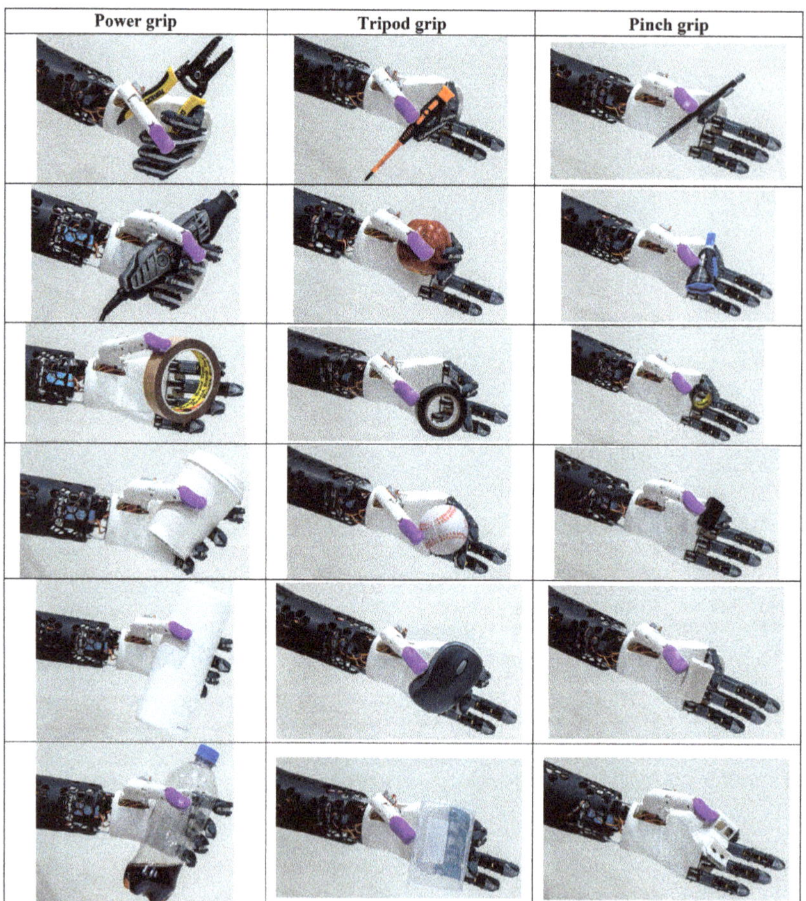

Figure 24. Persistence arm gripping different objects of various shapes, weights, and sizes.

4. Discussion

The Persistence arm has a lot of attractive features. The fact that most structural components are 3D-printed makes it easy for users to replace any part or change the color or material of any component. The flexible carbon-fiber tendons led to a relatively higher grip strength from the fingers. The thumb has two degrees of freedom, leading to a more dexterous gripping capability. The response time delay in actuating all servomotors is very low, as shown in Figures 18–20. However, like any other prosthetic arm design, Persistence arm has some limitations. The arm is suitable for performing daily tasks like gripping various household items and showing specific gestures. The arm is not meant to be used for athletic activities or for carrying heavy weights. The arm is not waterproof, so it cannot operate underwater. A flexible covering of the arm, like the one used on LUKE arm (https://mobiusbionics.com/luke-arm/, accessed on 17 February 2025), is a possible design extension. The arm is also not meant to be used at elevated temperatures. The maximum service temperature of PLA material is around 50 °C, beyond which the PLA components might start to deform. This service temperature can be increased if another material with higher thermal resistance, such as ABS, is used for all parts. The Persistence arm has two wrist degrees of freedom, which are flexion/extension and pronation/supination. However, the radial/ulnar deviation degree of freedom was not considered given its relative low importance compared to the other two wrist degrees of freedom. For users with a long residual limb below the elbow, the whole forearm can be replaced by a shorter version that only includes the essential electronic components, without the wrist actuation mechanism to accommodate for the long residual limb.

Like any other electronic device, the batteries in the arm and the foot controller need to be charged. The estimated approximate operation time with a single full charge of each battery can be estimated as battery capacity (Ah)/current draw (A). For the arm, each finger servomotor draws 0.2 A, except the thumb abduction/adduction KST A12-610 servomotor that draws 1.2 A. Each of the two wrist servomotors draws 2.3 A. This current draw happens when the servomotors are applying the maximum torque they can apply. The arm's 7.4 V LiPo battery has a maximum charge of 5 Ah. If all hand servomotors are actuated to apply the maximum force, while the wrist servomotors are not experiencing any load, the estimated battery life would be 2.27 h (136 min) of constant maximum grip force. In the rare situation that all wrist and hand servomotors are applying their maximum force continuously, the estimated battery life would go down to 0.74 h (44 min). If the servomotors are not continuously experiencing force on them to apply their maximum torque, the current draw would be much smaller, leading to much higher battery life (8–12 h). As for the foot controller, the device draws a maximum current of 20 mA when in use and transmitting. When not in use, the current draw is only 9 mA. The battery capacity of the foot controller is 400 mAh. Hence, when in continuous use, the battery life would be 20 h, and when idle, the battery life would be 44 h, approximately. Although for many users a full charge of each battery would be enough for a single day usage, having a second battery for the arm and the foot controller would ensure that the user can spend a long day with continuous usage of the arm. Replacing the batteries is a simple task that would take a single-handed adult only a few minutes to be done.

Persistence arm's finger design includes three joints per finger actuated with one servomotor, so it is an underactuated mechanism. This gives it the compliance feature, enabling the hand to be adaptive to the shape of the object being gripped. Eliminating the distal interphalangeal (DIP) joint, and replacing the distal and middle phalanges with one pre-deformed distal-middle phalange, like the one used in Infinity arm's fingers [15], would lead to a stiffer finger design.

A recent review paper by Siegel et al. [37] showed that there is a lack of standardization in upper-limb prostheses testing, and that developers often use custom, study-specific tests to validate their novel devices. Clinical settings and research laboratories differ in their time constraints, access to specialized equipment, and testing objectives. Testing of the proposed system was done to assess the performance of the manufactured prototypes focusing on specific engineering aspects. Further tests will be performed in the future, focusing on the standard outcome measures [38], such as the Box and Block (BB) test, University of New Brunswick (UNB) skill and spontaneity tests, Activities Measure for Upper Limb Amputation (AM-ULA) test, Upper Extremity Functional Scale (UEFS) tests, and the Patient-Specific Functional Scale (PSFS) tests, following the works of Resnik et al. [39–41].

The Infinity-2 foot controller also came with new features, compared to the first design reported in [15]. The speed of wireless transmission is extremely high as was shown in Figure 17, thanks to the Bluetooth and Wi-Fi technology enabled in the used microcontroller. The controller can be worn comfortably inside a shoe, on a sock, or barefoot. The controller enables using the toes to fully control the prosthetic arm fingers and simple ankle motions to control wrist actuation. Unlike many other previously documented prostheses' control systems, the proposed controller allows for gradual finger actuation rather than an on/off arrangement. Gradual control of fingers and wrist servomotors enable the user to orient the hand properly around the object being gripped and adjust the grip force precisely to match the weight and structure of the object. This would prevent crushing fragile objects or slippage of smooth or heavy objects. It is known that myoelectric prosthetic hand users have difficulty with, and frequently avoid, grasping fragile objects with their prosthesis [42]. This required Fishel et al. [42] to develop a contact detection reflex system that was integrated into a commercial myoelectric prosthetic hand to adjust the gripping force automatically upon contacting fragile objects. However, such a solution is still depriving the user of fully controlling the grip of the arm. Users might still want to be capable of applying larger gripping forces on some objects than what a reflex system would allow, i.e., to reshape a deformable item or to intentionally crush a plastic cup. Only a system that gives the user full control over the applied gripping force, like the proposed system, could enable that. The controller also offers cycling between different grips and gestures. Preliminary testing done by the developers showed that learning how to use such a controller is significantly easy, requiring a natural toe dexterity. With 15–30 min of practice in the first use, users can be proficient in using the controller. Previous foot controller developers, such as Carrozza et al. [26,27], have also reported ease of adaptation and learning. The controller is independent of the presence of muscles in the residual limb.

Preliminary tests showed that some individuals can significantly increase the chances of success in pressing on the buttons if they raise the big toe slightly up when pressing with the lesser toes and raise the lesser toes slightly up when pressing with the big toe, as shown in Figure 25a. Other individuals preferred to slightly turn the whole foot (inversion or eversion) to press on the left or the right panel, as shown in Figure 25b. Only these simple toe articulations are needed to have full control over the gradual finger deformation.

This controller, however, still has some limitations. First, the user should have at least one functioning foot with the ability to move the ankle and the toes (ankle and toe mobility). Being waterproof was not one of the main goals of the current iteration. However, sealing the FCU and the electronics on the FCS will be a future design extension. The controller has a walking detection system that would freeze the arm during walking. So, the controller can be used only while standing or sitting. A dual control approach can be developed to enable voice control, for example, to control the arm while walking, if there is a need for such a capability. A similar dual control was presented in [9,10]. The code of the proposed foot controller can be easily adjusted to control other prosthetic arms on the market if communication protocols are established between the arm and the controller.

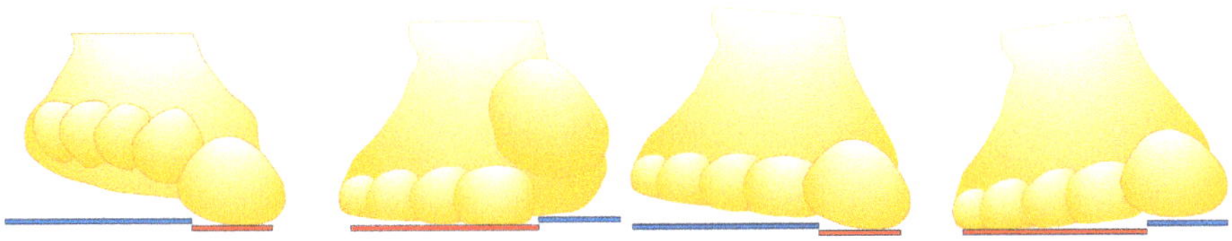

(a) (b)

Figure 25. Toe articulations needed to perform finger opening and closing actuations: (**a**) option 1, (**b**) option 2.

5. Conclusions

Controlling prosthetic arms with foot controllers could be a promising alternative control method to EMG controllers that have a lot of drawbacks, resulting in a high abundance rates of upper limb prostheses. The Infinity-2 foot controller proposed in this work can be used even barefoot because of the new sleeve design that secures the controller around the forefoot. The wireless transmission between the foot controller and the prosthetic arm happens in a fraction of a second, giving almost an immediate effect. The controller can fully control a five-finger prosthetic arm equipped with a two-degree-of-freedom wrist actuation system. It offers gradual control of the fingers to adjust the gripping force based on the fragility, texture, and weight of the object to be gripped. Various grips and gestures that actuate specific groups of fingers can also be performed. Preliminary tests by the developers showed that the system is intuitive, and that training time needed to use the system comfortably is short for most individuals, making it an attractive prosthetic arm control method that does not rely on any remaining muscles in the residual limb. It could also be used by individuals who put on temporary casts after breaking their wrists.

The Persistence arm is a new addition to the transradial 3D-printed prosthetic arm designs that can be used to perform average household daily tasks. It features a two-degree-of-freedom wrist actuation mechanism, and a hand with five fingers individually actuated. The three-phalange underactuated forefinger design and the two-degree-of-freedom linkage-based thumb gave the hand an adaptive performance similar to that of a human hand. Preliminary testing in the current study proved the effectiveness of the proposed designs, offering new alternatives to prosthetic arm users for higher quality of life beyond the trauma of missing the functionality of the human arm.

6. Patents

Utility Patent Application Number: 18/648726, Filing date: 4/29/2024. Title: "Foot Controller for Prosthetic Arms, Their Methods of Production and Use" (Inventors: Peter L. Bishay and Jack Wilgus).

Supplementary Materials: The following supporting information can be downloaded at: https://www.mdpi.com/article/10.3390/technologies13030098/s1, Video S1: Persistence Arm with Infinity-2 Foot Controller System.

Author Contributions: Conceptualization, P.L.B.; methodology, all authors; software, all authors; validation, P.L.B., G.F.A. and I.S.; formal analysis, P.L.B., G.F.A. and I.S.; investigation, all authors; resources, P.L.B.; data curation, P.L.B., G.F.A. and I.S.; writing—original draft preparation, P.L.B., G.F.A. and I.S.; writing—review and editing, P.L.B.; visualization, P.L.B., G.F.A. and I.S.; supervision,

P.L.B.; project administration, P.L.B., G.F.A. and I.S.; funding acquisition, P.L.B. All authors have read and agreed to the published version of the manuscript.

Funding: This research received no external funding.

Institutional Review Board Statement: Ethical review and approval were waived by the CSUN IRB for this study since the preliminary testing was determined not to be human subjects research. No human subjects outside the research team were involved in the preliminary testing of the proposed system.

Informed Consent Statement: Not Applicable.

Data Availability Statement: The data presented in this study is available on request from the corresponding author.

Acknowledgments: This work was performed by the seventh cohort of the "Smart Prosthetics" research-based senior design project at California State University, Northridge (CSUN). The authors acknowledge the Mechanical Engineering Department, the Instructionally Related Activities (IRA) grant, and the Student Travel and Academic Research (STAR) program at CSUN.

Conflicts of Interest: The authors declare no conflicts of interest.

Appendix A

The wiring diagram of the foot controller sleeve and unit is shown in Figure A1, whereas the Persistence arm's wiring diagram is shown in Figure A2.

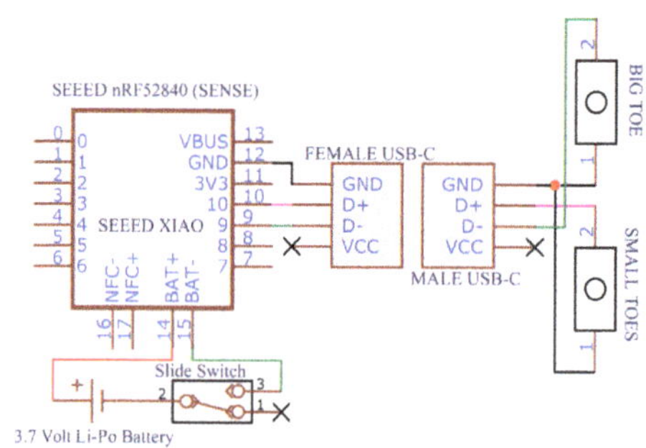

Figure A1. Wiring diagram for FCU and FCS.

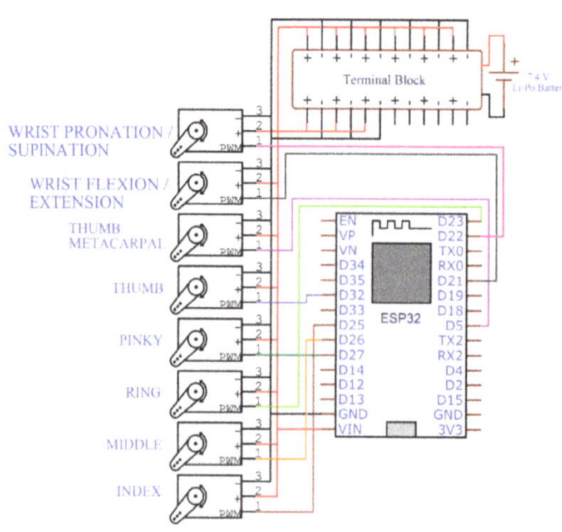

Figure A2. Wiring diagram for Persistence Arm.

Appendix B

The starting shape of the wrist servo mount, shown in Figure A3a, was used in the generative design study. This geometry was reduced to better represent the load conditions. Using a starting shape was an optional step, taken to reduce the number of iterations. Since the main goal of the part was to provide a good mount for the pan-tilt wrist actuation system, the reduced shape was then used to divide the part into different regions. These regions are divided into two categories: preserve regions, where the GD part would connect to the shell of the arm (shown in green in Figure A3b), and obstacle regions, which leave room for both the servo motor to connect and wires to be run through (shown in red in the figure). The load conditions featured an axial load of 180 N in the respective −Z direction distributed among the top screw holes and another 180 N in the respective +Z direction. It also featured a 30 N load upon the side connection to the shell in the respective +Y direction, as well as a mirrored 30 N load upon the other side connection. These values simulated a scenario in which the arm was oriented perpendicular to the ground, and holding 180 N weight. To better represent the strength of the material, the study utilized a custom material profile of Bambu ABS filament with 15% gyroid infill. The profile used tensile strength, yield strength, density, and Young's modulus values that were experimentally determined utilizing a modified ASTM D638 test. The manufacturing method was set to additive manufacturing in the +Z direction and with an overhang angle of 45°. Finally, the goal of the study was set to minimize mass, and a minimum factor of safety of 3.0 was specified. The generated design is shown in Figure A3c. The part was then printed on a Bambu P1P printer with the same settings as the ASTM D638 test coupons.

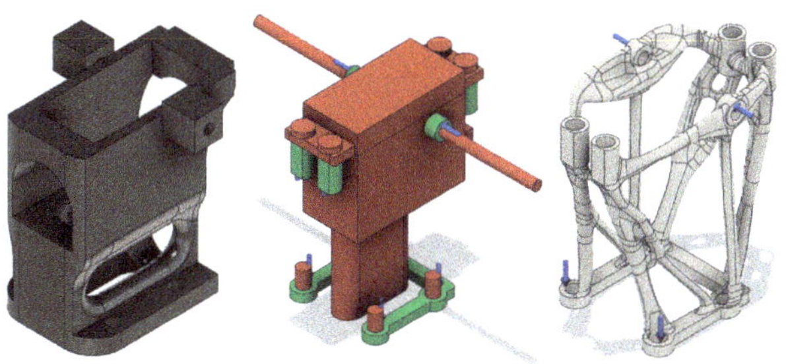

(a) (b) (c)

Figure A3. (**a**) Starting shape of the wrist servo mount with reduced geometry, (**b**) GD model with preserve (green) and obstacle (red) regions, (**c**) Generated design of the mount.

References

1. Salminger, S.; Stino, H.; Pichler, L.H.; Gstoettner, C.; Sturma, A.; Mayer, J.A.; Szivak, M.; Aszmann, O.C. Current rates of prosthetic usage in upper-limb amputees—Have innovations had an impact on device acceptance? *Disabil. Rehabil.* **2022**, *44*, 3708–3713. [CrossRef] [PubMed]
2. Biddiss, E.A.; Chau, T.T. Upper limb prosthesis use and abandonment: A survey of the last 25 years. *Prosthet. Orthot. Int.* **2007**, *31*, 236–257. [CrossRef] [PubMed]
3. Chen, Z.; Min, H.; Wang, D.; Xia, Z.; Sun, F.; Fang, B. A Review of Myoelectric Control for Prosthetic Hand Manipulation. *Biomimetics* **2023**, *8*, 328. [CrossRef] [PubMed]
4. Chadwell, A.; Kenney, L.; Thies, S.; Head, J.; Galpin, A.; Baker, R. Addressing unpredictability may be the key to improving performance with current clinically prescribed myoelectric prostheses. *Sci. Rep.* **2021**, *11*, 3300. [CrossRef]
5. Franzke, A.W.; Kristoffersen, M.B.; Bongers, R.M.; Murgia, A.; Pobatschnig, B.; Unglaube, F.; van der Sluis, C.K. Users' and therapists' perceptions of myoelectric multi-function upper limb prostheses with conventional and pattern recognition control. *PLoS ONE* **2019**, *14*, e0220899. [CrossRef]
6. Vujaklija, I.; Farina, D.; Aszmann, O.C. New developments in prosthetic arm systems. *Orthop. Res. Rev.* **2016**, *8*, 31–39. [CrossRef]

7. Bandara, D.; Arata, J.; Kiguchi, K. Towards Control of a Transhumeral Prosthesis with EEG Signals. *Bioengineering* **2018**, *5*, 26. [CrossRef]
8. Vilela, M.; Hochberg, L.R. Applications of Rain-computer interfaces to the control of robotic and prosthetic arms. In *Handbook of Clinical Neurology*; Elsevier: Amsterdam, The Netherlands, 2020; pp. 87–99. [CrossRef]
9. Bishay, P.L.; Fontana, J.; Raquipiso, B.; Rodriguez, J.; Borreta, M.J.; Enos, B.; Gay, T.; Mauricio, K. Development of a biomimetic transradial prosthetic arm with shape memory alloy muscle wires. *Eng. Res. Express* **2020**, *2*, 035041. [CrossRef]
10. Bishay, P.; Aguilar, C.; Amirbekyan, A.; Vartanian, K.; Arjon-Ramirez, M.; Pucio, D. Design of a Lightweight Shape Memory Alloy Stroke-Amplification and Locking System in a Transradial Prosthetic Arm. In Proceedings of the ASME 2021 Conference on Smart Materials, Adaptive Structures and Intelligent Systems, Virtual, 14–15 September 2021; American Society of Mechanical Engineers: New York, NY, USA, 2021; p. V001T05A015.
11. Arias, L.M.; Iwaniec, M.; Pirowska, P.; Smoleń, M.; Augustyniak, P. Head and Voice-Controlled Human-Machine Interface System for Transhumeral Prosthesis. *Electronics* **2023**, *12*, 4770. [CrossRef]
12. Ozsahin, D.U.; Duwa, B.B.; Idoko, J.B.; Edward, D.; Khorzom, L.; Hussein, O.H.; Alsiba, A.; Hamzah, N.; Ozsahin, I. Voice-controlled prosthetic hand. In *Practical Design and Applications of Medical Devices*; Elsevier: Amsterdam, The Netherlands, 2024; pp. 99–106. [CrossRef]
13. Yang, H.; Tao, Z.; Yang, J.; Ma, W.; Zhang, H.; Xu, M.; Wu, M.; Sun, S.; Jin, H.; Li, W.; et al. A lightweight prosthetic hand with 19-DOF dexterity and human-level functions. *Nat. Commun.* **2025**, *16*, 955. [CrossRef]
14. Resnik, L.; Klinger, S.L.; Etter, K. The DEKA Arm: Its features, functionality, and evolution during the Veterans Af-fairs Study to optimize the DEKA Arm. *Prosthet. Orthot. Int.* **2014**, *38*, 492–504. [CrossRef] [PubMed]
15. Bishay, P.L.; Wilgus, J.; Chen, R.; Valenzuela, D.; Medina, V.; Tan, C.; Ittner, T.; Caldera, M.; Rubalcava, C.; Safarian, S.; et al. Controlling a Below-the-Elbow Prosthetic Arm Using the Infinity Foot Controller. *Prosthesis* **2023**, *5*, 1206–1231. [CrossRef]
16. Lyons, K.R.; Joshi, S.S. A Case Study on Classification of FOOT Gestures Via Surface Electromyography. In Proceedings of the Annual Rehabilitation Engineering and Assistive Technology Society of North America Conference, Denver, CO, USA, 10–14 June 2015; pp. 1–5.
17. Lyons, K.R.; Joshi, S.S. Real-time evaluation of a myoelectric control method for high-level upper limb amputees based on homologous leg movements. In Proceedings of the 2016 38th Annual International Conference of the IEEE Engineering in Medicine and Biology Society (EMBC), Orlando, FL, USA, 6–20 August 2016; pp. 6365–6368.
18. Lyons, K.R.; Joshi, S.S. Upper Limb Prosthesis Control for High-Level Amputees via Myoelectric Recognition of Leg Gestures. *IEEE Trans. Neural Syst. Rehabil. Eng.* **2018**, *26*, 1056–1066. [CrossRef] [PubMed]
19. Resnik, L.; Klinger, S.L.; Etter, K.; Fantini, C. Controlling a multi-degree of freedom upper limb prosthesis using foot controls: User experience. *Disabil. Rehabil. Assist. Technol.* **2014**, *9*, 318–329. [CrossRef] [PubMed]
20. Lee, S.; Sung, M.; Choi, Y. Wearable fabric sensor for controlling myoelectric hand prosthesis via classification of foot postures. *Smart Mater. Struct.* **2020**, *29*, 035004. [CrossRef]
21. Marinelli, A.; Boccardo, N.; Tessari, F.; Di Domenico, D.; Caserta, G.; Canepa, M.; Gini, G.; Barresi, G.; Laffranchi, M.; De Michieli, L.; et al. Active upper limb prostheses: A review on current state and upcoming breakthroughs. *Prog. Biomed. Eng.* **2023**, *5*, 012001. [CrossRef]
22. Alderson, S.W. Electrically Operated Artificial Arm for Above-The-Elbow Amputees. U.S. Patent US2580987A, 1 January 1952.
23. Klopsteg, P.E.; Wilson, P.D. *Human Limbs and Their Substitutes: Presenting Results of Engineering and Medical Studies of the Human Extremities and Application of the Data to the Design and Fitting of Artificial Limbs and to the Care and Training of Amputees*; Hafner: Cleveland, OH, USA, 1968.
24. Graupe, D. Control of upper-limb prostheses in several degrees of freedom. *Bull. Prosthet. Res.* **1974**, *22*, 226–236.
25. Luzzio, C.C. Controlling an Artificial Arm with Foot Movements. *Neurorehabilit. Neural Repair* **2000**, *14*, 207–212. [CrossRef]
26. Carrozza, M.; Persichetti, A.; Laschi, C.; Vecchi, F.; Lazzarini, R.; Tamburrelli, V.; Vacalebri, P.; Dario, P. A Novel Wearable Interface for Robotic Hand Prostheses. In Proceedings of the 9th International Conference on Rehabilitation Robotics, ICORR 2005, Chicago, IL, USA, 28 June–1 July 2005; pp. 109–112.
27. Carrozza, M.C.; Persichetti, A.; Laschi, C.; Vecchi, F.; Lazzarini, R.; Vacalebri, P.; Dario, P. A Wearable Biomechatronic Interface for Controlling Robots with Voluntary Foot Movements. *IEEE/ASME Trans. Mechatron.* **2007**, *12*, 1–11. [CrossRef]
28. Innovations. DEKA, (n.d.). Available online: https://dekaresearch.com/innovations/ (accessed on 28 January 2025).
29. Lanier, G.R., Jr.; Perry, N.C.; Pascoe, A.P.; Van der Merwe, D.A. Method and apparatus for control of a prosthetic. U.S. Patent US20220117759A1, 21 April 2022.
30. Lanier, G.R., Jr.; Perry, N.C.; Pascoe, A.P.; Van der Merwe, D.A. Apparatus for control of a prosthetic. U.S. Patent US9901465B2, 27 February 2018.
31. The Hero Arm Overview is a Prosthetic Arm Made by Open Bionics, (n.d.). Available online: https://openbionics.com/hero-arm-overview/ (accessed on 26 January 2025).

32. Piazza, C.; Grioli, G.; Catalano, M.; Bicchi, A. A Century of Robotic Hands. *Annu. Rev. Control. Robot. Auton. Syst.* **2019**, *2*, 1–32. [CrossRef]
33. Michelangelo Hand | The Michelangelo Hand Helps You Regain Extensive Freedom, (n.d.). Available online: https://www.ottobock.com/en-us/product/8E500 (accessed on 26 January 2025).
34. i-Limb® Quantum Bionic Hand. Ossur.com, (n.d.). Available online: https://www.ossur.com/en-us/prosthetics/arms/i-limb-quantum (accessed on 26 January 2025).
35. bebionic Hand | The Most Lifelike Prosthetic Hand, (n.d.). Available online: https://www.ottobock.com/en-us/product/8E7* (accessed on 26 January 2025).
36. Wendo, K.; Barbier, O.; Bollen, X.; Schubert, T.; Lejeune, T.; Raucent, B.; Olszewski, R. Open-Source 3D Printing in the Prosthetic Field—The Case of Upper Limb Prostheses: A Review. *Machines* **2022**, *10*, 413. [CrossRef]
37. Siegel, J.R.; Battraw, M.A.; Winslow, E.J.; James, M.A.; Joiner, W.M.; Schofield, J.S. Review and critique of current testing protocols for upper-limb prostheses: A call for standardization amidst rapid technological advancements. *Front. Robot. AI* **2023**, *10*, 1292632. [CrossRef]
38. Miller, L.A.P.; Swanson, S.O. Introduction to the Academy's State of the Science Conference on Upper Limb Prosthetic Outcome Measures. *JPO J. Prosthet. Orthot.* **2009**, *21*, 1–2. [CrossRef]
39. Resnik, L.; Borgia, M. Reliability and Validity of Outcome Measures for Upper Limb Amputation. *JPO J. Prosthet. Orthot.* **2012**, *24*, 192–201. [CrossRef]
40. Resnik, L.; Adams, L.; Borgia, M.; Delikat, J.; Disla, R.; Ebner, C.; Walters, L.S. Development and Evaluation of the Activities Measure for Upper Limb Amputees. *Arch. Phys. Med. Rehabil.* **2013**, *94*, 488–494.e4. [CrossRef]
41. Resnik, L.; Borgia, M. Responsiveness of outcome measures for upper limb prosthetic rehabilitation. *Prosthet. Orthot. Int.* **2016**, *40*, 96–108. [CrossRef]
42. Fishel, J.A.; Matulevich, B.; Muller, K.A.; Berke, G.M. The (Sensorized) Hand is Quicker than the Eye: Restoring Grasping Speed and Confidence for Amputees with Tactile Reflexes. In Proceedings of the 2019 International Conference on Robotics and Automation (ICRA), Montreal, QC, Canada, 20–24 May 2019; pp. 5097–5102.

technologies

MDPI

Article

Smart Sport Watch Usage: The Dominant Role of Technology Readiness over Exercise Motivation and Sensation Seeking

Gershon Tenenbaum [1], Tomer Ben-Zion [1], Yair Amichai-Hamburger [1,2], Yair Galily [1,*] and Assaf Lev [3]

[1] School of Psychology, Reichman University, Herzliya 4610101, Israel
[2] The Research Center for Internet Psychology (CIP), Sammy Ofer School of Communication, Reichman University, 8 Ha'Universita st., Herzliya 4610101, Israel
[3] Department of Sports Therapy, Ono Academic College, Kiryat Ono 5545173, Israel; assaf.lev@ono.ac.il
* Correspondence: yg2@runi.ac.il; Tel.: +972-52-4899117

Abstract: The study examines the link between technology readiness/acceptance, motivation for exercising, and sensation seeking and using or avoiding Smart Sport Watches (SSW). A sample of 315 adolescents, *Mage* = 29.6 (SD = 11.01) and healthy male (n = 95, 30.2%) and female (n = 179, 56.85%), completed all the measures of these variables' dimensions via the internet. Multiple followed by univariate analyses of variance (MANOVA, ANOVA) were performed for each of the study's psychological dimensions and single variables. The two categorical factors (e.g., BS factors) were the use of SSW (yes/no) and walk/run (yes/no). Results revealed that adolescents using SSW rated themselves significantly ($p < 0.05$) and substantially higher than their non-SSW users on positive readiness for technology ($d = 0.47$), and specifically on optimism ($d = 0.34$) and innovation ($d = 0.51$). Moreover, users of SSW reported significantly ($p < 0.05$) and substantially lower negative readiness for technology than their non-SSW users' counterparts ($d = -0.49$), and specifically on discomfort ($d = -0.38$) and distrust ($d = -50$), but neither on the overall motivation for exercise dimensions nor on sensation-seeking. Moreover, adolescents who walk/run reported being more internally motivated (d = 0.38), integrated ($d = 0.61$), and identified ($d = 0.34$) than their sedentary counterparts. Discussion centers on the important role of readiness/acceptance in using technological devices and the need to use technology-specific motivation and personality measures to further explore this phenomenon.

Keywords: digital; watches; acceptance; readiness; motivation; exercise; personality

1. Purpose for Using Smart Sport Watches (SSW)

SSW are designed to monitor the physical effort invested in exercising. SSW translate effort output into quantitative measures which are useful for monitoring the person's unfolding physical and health-related activities. In addition, SSW data enable the user to design and monitor his/her exercise regimen and maintain it for some time. SSW users primarily use wearables to guide their training decisions and optimize exercise programming, emphasizing a focus on personal adaptation to their readiness states [1]. The SSW provides information which is useful for both motivational and physical outcomes [2]. The use of wearables in the exercise and health domains has gained a significant momentum in recent years [3]. However, the psychological factors associated with its use are not entirely clear. To capture the underlying motives of SSW use, we consider the person's technology readiness/acceptance, general motivation for exercising, and sensation seeking as predictors of SSW use.

1.1. Technology Readiness/Acceptance

Along with the development and promotion of exercise and health-related technologies, some people experience a threat when using them (i.e., technophobia). Technophobia (i.e., fear of using technology) is prevalent in 30% of the general population, depending on gender, age, education, personality, culture, and ideology [4]. An internet survey among young adults supported the notion that technology readiness moderates the relationships between performance expectancy and attitudes toward wearables [5]. Seifert [6] examined the use of SSW among older adults aged fifty and above and concluded that education, age, technological affinity, and the use of mobile information and communication technology (ICT) devices (e.g., SSW, tablets, radio, TV, computers, and fitness trackers) in particular distinguished SSW users from non-users. However, Wu and Lim [7] identified several key factors influencing older adults' willingness to adopt smart wearable devices. These factors include performance expectancy, effort expectancy, social influence, facilitating conditions, hedonic motivation, price value, and digital health literacy, all of which significantly affect their acceptance.

Technology readiness (TR) is an attitude which pertains to the user's belief towards a technology. It is the user's inclination to engage with a novel technology [8]. TR is a multifaceted concept, dependent on individuals' prominent personality traits relating to technology use. For example, users demonstrate a high level of positive technology readiness, heavily influenced by perceived ease of use, underscoring the importance of ease of operation as a critical factor in their willingness to adopt these technologies [9]. Parasuraman [10] distinguished between positive technology readiness (PTR) and negative technology readiness (NTR). Specifically, PTR comprises factors that motivate acceptance of a new technology such as optimism, control, flexibility, efficiency in peoples' lives, and innovativeness—a tendency to be a technological pioneer and thought leader. In contrast, NTR includes two factors that inhibit acceptance of new technology: (a) discomfort—a perceived lack of control over technology and a feeling of being overwhelmed by it—and (b) insecurity—distrust of technology, stemming from skepticism about its ability to work properly and concerns about its potential harmful consequences [10].

A technology acceptance model was derived from Ajzen and Fishbein's [11] theory of reasoned action (TRA). The TRA model was fundamentally used to predict the degree of acceptance of any new technology [12]. Accordingly, two main antecedents influence the user's intention to adopt a novel technology: (a) perceived usefulness (PU)—"the degree to which a person believes that using a particular system would enhance his or her job performance", and (b) perceived ease of use—"the degree to which a person believes that using a particular system would be free of effort" ([12] p. 32). Yet, according to Ramen and Aashish [13], some of the researchers have indicated that TAM must be broadened and enhanced with supplemental constructs to improve its interpretations and predictive capabilities [14]. Lin et al. [15], for example, included TR in the existing TAM model to better capture the person's intention to use a novel technology. With this integration, the TRAM (technology readiness and acceptance model) emerged. The model simplifies the process by which one adopts a novel technology by considering his/her experience and awareness about using any technology at large. The role of TR in TRAM is to measure a user's perspective regarding any generic technology.

Most of the current work on TR has viewed it as a variable which affects motivation in the domain of information technology [16–18]. Moreover, user's motivation and behavioral intentions depend on technology readiness because utilitarian and hedonic motivations vary in people with different personality dispositions [19,20]. According to Chang and Chen [21], only a few studies have examined the moderating effect of TR on the relationships between motivations and behavioral intentions, and thus, our aim is to further explore its role in determining the use of smart sport watches in people who recreationally walk and/or run.

1.2. Motivation and Sensation-Seeking Related to Using Technologies and SSW

We postulate that people varying in motivational characteristics and approach to exercise will also vary in SSW usage. To operationalize this conceptualization, the self-determination theory (SDT; [22,23]) was used. The SDT classifies people's motivation on a continuum ranging from a complete lack of motivation to be involved in a task through three stages of external motivation. i.e., (identified, introjected, integrated) and finally to internal motivation. The state of motivation depends on satisfying three basic needs—autonomy, competence, and relatedness [24]. Under the regulation of autonomy, people regulate their behaviors according to their values, attitudes, and beliefs and reject external control over their actions [25]. Achieving competence is required to efficiently monitor the actions people are engaged in [26,27], and the need for relatedness regulates people to be in close relations to others as a source of social networks of people with similar interests [28].

According to the SDT, people are completely unmotivated to a task or a mission because they do not value its immediate benefit, do not perceive the outcomes as imperative for them, and feel they lack the self-efficacy which is required to accomplish the task [23]. Pertaining to exercise and wearing SSW, people may wish to be engaged in exercise but not to use SSW. Accordingly, people who walk/run but refrain from wearing SSW may value the psychological and physical health benefits of the exercise but not necessarily value the use of SSW. We test herein the notion that the motivational stages set by the SDT determine the use of SSW and its functions during and outside the realm of walking/running.

According to the SDT, when people are externally motivated, their involvement in the task is governed by an external control which is associated with a lack of personal autonomy. Under such a motivational state, people expect to receive materialistic, monitory, or psychological rewards for their direct involvement in the task. Coercion, fear of failure, not being rewarded, and materialistic passion are associated with this state of mind [22]. Thus, according to our view, people who walk/run may use SSW to overcome negative consequences associated with physical activity and not use it to its full potential because of their lack of autonomy. In contrast, they may use SSW because they wish to relate to others who use SSW and develop competence in the exercise they are engaged in.

It must be noted that the SDT distinguishes among three types of external regulation of motivation. Introjected regulation is a motivation state where the person strives to comprehend the value of his/her involvement in the task but his/her efforts are regulated by the wish to avoid negative consequences such as guilt, rejection, shame, and embarrassment, along with perceived pressure to feel pride, self-confidence, and feel loved and evaluated by others. Identified regulation is evident when the person internalizes the value of his/her actions toward the goal he/she is striving to achieve. Integrated regulation represents the most autonomous state of mind within the external motivation construct. Within this motivational state, one feels a complete integration between one's goals, values, and actions. This motivational state is not yet internalized because it is not yet fully associated with one's desires and self-accomplishment, but shame and guilt feeling are not experienced because of not satisfying other controlling sources. In the current concept, the person may exercise with SSW because he/she identifies with the potential of the technology to accomplish the exercise regimen [27]. When people are regulated by internal motivation, they act to achieve their own goals and do so because it is part of their identity [29]. In the current conceptualization, exercisers use or do not use SSW because of their autonomous state of mind, along with the need to develop physical competence and social relations. They lack the need to satisfy external sources by using SSW when exercising [22].

Motivation to exercise is likely to increase when the runner uses SSW [30]. Using SSW increases the running velocity and its associated heart rate [2,30]. Moreover, motivation was found to positively influence goal orientation, with curiosity and trend-driven motivations significantly enhancing exercise involvement. This suggests that the underlying reasons for using the technology can shape users' goals and increase their engagement in physical activities [31]. In contrast, this technology, and similar ones, may prevent people from directly attending to their body that would be otherwise attended to when running without SSW [32]. It may well be that such devices lead people to depend on technological-biological sensors and prevent them from self-regulating and self-monitoring their physical efforts. Thus, using or avoiding SSW while exercising may be accounted for by different states of motivation by people who exercise.

In addition to the SDT motivational framework, sensation-seeking may also determine the use of or refraining from technology use. Sensation seekers are people searching for exciting, novel, and rich experiences, which sometimes involve significant risk-taking [33]. Such people are likely to feel frustrated when their stimulation is underestimated or not fulfilled. Sensation seeking was related to choosing a high-risk sport [34], to a personal history of sport-related concussion [35], and to sport-related concussion in adolescent and young adult athletes [36]. Thus, it seems that people high on sensation seeking may perceive the SSW as a technology that limits their freedom and are not likely to use it.

2. The Purpose of the Study

Our aim is to study how readiness/acceptance of technology, motivation to exercise, and sensation seeking account for using SSW and its main functions. It is evident that technological attraction and the practical use of other technological devices, such as tablets and smartphone, are related to the technology readiness and acceptance tendency [6]. We therefore predict that the more positive the approach to use technology (i.e., lower technophobia), the more prevalence the use of SSW and its features will be. We also hypothesize that people motivated internally will make greater use of SSW because of feeling more autonomous and competent. Along this line of thought, we hypothesize that users of SSW will be lower on sensation-seeking than non-users of SSW. Specifically, people high in sensation seeking will tend to refrain from using SSW features which provide information about their training program and features which provide information about their bodily information. In contrast, people low in sensation seeking are likely to have less objection to the SSW.

3. Method

3.1. Participants

A sample of 315 was used for this study. Of these, 276 were students and 39 were not engaged academically. They were healthy young males (n = 95, 30.2%) and females (n = 179, 56.85%), $Mage$ = 29.6 (SD = 11.01), who studied in various colleges in Israel. On average, the participant reported being engaged in walk/run activities for 2.60 h (SD = 1.41) per week, exercised for 57.81 min (SD = 48.42) each time, and covered 6.23 km (SD = 3.89) in each practice. They were approached via social media networks such as Instagram, Facebook, Twitter (X), and TikTok and were assured anonymity and confidentiality through the provision of codes rather than names.

3.2. Measures

Demographic Questionnaire. The questionnaire includes the following items: age, gender, occupation, familial status, exercise habits, and details about using a smartwatch.

Exercise Motivation Scale (EMS-SMS-II; [37]). The SMS-II scale was designed to assess the individuals' level of motivation towards sport in adult athletes, relying on the self-determination theory framework. The term "sport" was replaced by the term "exercise" without losing its motivational orientation and semantic meaning. The motivation questionnaire consists of 17 items that are divided into 6 scales: intrinsic (k = 3), integrated, (k = 3), identified (k = 3), introjected (k = 3), external (k = 3), and amotivation (k = 2). Each item is rated on a 7-point Likert-type scale ranging from 1 (strongly disagree) to 7 (strongly agree). The mean of the items' ratings on each scale is considered the score on the respective dimension. Cronbach α reliability coefficients reported by the authors ranged between 0.70 and 0.88. Furthermore, a six-factor CFA model was fitted to the model, χ^2 (120, N = 290) = 258.14, $p < 0.001$, *RMSEA* = 0.07, *CFI* = 0.94, *NFI* = 0.90, *TLI* = 0.92. Item-factor loadings ranged between 0.47 and 0.95. The Cronbach Alpha in the current study ranged between 0.64 and 0.82. The SMS-II was translated into Hebrew and then back to English by five scholars well-versed in both languages. The final questionnaire was set upon full agreement among the researchers.

Brief Sensation Seeking Scale (BSSS; [38]). The BSSS was designed to assess the individuals' level of a biosocial dimension of personality characterized by "the need for varied, novel, and complex sensations and experiences and the willingness to take physical and social risks for the sake of such experiences" ([39] p. 10). The BSSS was created by adapting items from the SSS-V [39] and a set of items derived from the SSS-V which was tailored for adolescents [40]. The questionnaire consists of a single-factor model of 8 items that are divided into 4 scales (2 questions each): experience seeking, boredom susceptibility, thrill and adventure seeking, and disinhibition. Responses are made on a 5-point Likert-type scale labeled, "strongly disagree", "disagree", "neither disagree nor agree", "agree", and "strongly agree". The coefficient alpha was 0.74, and the model fit to the data was χ^2 (18, n = 281) = 215.75, $p < 0.001$, *RMSEA* = 0.042, *CFI* = 0.98. The BSSS was translated into Hebrew and followed similar procedures to those used for the SMS-II. The Cronbach Alphas Coefficients ranged between 0.73 and 0.80 and under 0.70 for "boredom susceptibility" and "Thrill and adventure seeking".

Technology Readiness and Technology Acceptance Questionnaire (TR; [41]) and **Technology Acceptance Measure** (TAM; [12]). The TR operationalizes the model of Lin et al. [15] using the conceptual framework of Parasuraman [10] and Devis [12]. The TRAM Model relates to individuals' beliefs about and propensity for using innovative technology-based products or services [10]. The TRAM is a theoretical framework that explains the process of using and adopting a technological innovation across a variety of contexts [8]. It was established to explain consumers' intentions to use new technology, and understanding people's technology acceptance behaviors [15]. The Technology Readiness (TR) consists of 14 items that are divided into four dimensions: two positive—optimism (k = 4) and innovativeness, (k = 3)—and two negative—discomfort (k = 4) and insecurity (k = 3). Items are rated on a 5-point Likert-type scale ranging from 1 (strongly disagree) to 5 (strongly agree). Cronbach α reliability coefficients reported by the authors were 0.82, 0.82, 0.70, and 0.79, respectively. The technology acceptance measure (TAM) consists of 12 items divided into three dimensions: perceived usefulness (k = 4), perceived ease of use (k = 4), and intention to use (k = 4). Cronbach α reliability coefficients of the scales reported by the authors were 0.87, 0.91, and 0.83, respectively. The factor loadings for the items ranged between 0.66 and 0.91. Convergent validity using Average variance Extracted (AVE) values were well above the required level of 0.50 for all measures. Discriminant validity values using the HeteroTrait-MonoTrait (HTMT) procedure were between two reflective constructs of below 0.90. The Cronbach Alpha Reliability Coefficients in the current Hebrew version ranged between 0.70 and 0.90, with most above 0.85 and only one dimension, "distrust", under 0.70. The TR and TAM were translated into Hebrew and followed identical translation and verification processes as the BSSS and the SMS-II.

3.3. Procedure

At first, permission to approach the students was obtained from the university's IRB. The questionnaire was designed in a quartics format which allowed a quick and identical administration format to all the participants. Following the IRB research proposal approval, informed consent and all the questionnaires were sent electronically to the participants via Qualtrics Software (https://www.qualtrics.com/). Confidentiality was assured prior to data collection. Specifically, participants were informed that only the researchers have access to their responses. The participants were asked to complete the demographics form first followed by a battery of questionnaires including the SMS-II, BSSS, NFC, and TRAM. A counter-balanced order was used to eliminate order effects. At the end of the administration, the participants were thanked.

4. Results

4.1. Preliminary Analyses Testing the Normality Assumption

Along with verifying the Alpha Internal Consistency Reliability Coefficients (ICRC) for each questionnaire and its respective dimension (see method chapter; $\alpha > 0.70$), we tested the normality assumption using the Skewness and Kurtosis coefficients. The analyses revealed that all the variables used in the study were normally distributed, ranging between -2.00 and 2.00 for both coefficients, respectively.

4.2. Multi-Variate and Univariate Analyses of Variance

Multiple followed by univariate analyses of variance (MANOVA, ANOVA) were performed for each of the study's psychological cluster and single variables. The two categorical factors (e.g., BS factors) were the use of SSW (yes/no) and walk/run (yes/no). The analyses revealed no significant effect for gender. Thus, gender was not considered for further analysis. The main and interactional effects of BS factors on the study's variables are presented in Table 1.

Table 1. Two-way ANOVA main and interactional effects for sensation-seeking, motivation, and readiness for technology by using SSW (yes/no) and walk/run (yes/no) for the entire sample, and readiness for SSW for the adolescents who walk/run but refrain from using SSW (*F*—the statistical effect, *p*—significance level, λ^2—accounted variance of the effect).

Variable	A. Smart Watch (Yes/No)			B. Walk/Run (Yes/No)			A by B		
	F	*p*	λ^2	*F*	*p*	λ^2	*F*	*p*	λ^2
Sensation Seeking Total ($n = 242$)	0.49	0.49	0.00	0.04	0.85	0.00	0.240	0.63	0.00
Experience seeking	1.15	0.28	0.01	0.11	0.74	0.00	0.010	0.91	0.00
Boredom susceptibility	0.030	0.87	0.00	81	0.37	0.00	0.250	0.62	0.00
Thrill and adventure seeking	0.22	0.64	0.00	0.01	0.92	0.00	0.430	0.51	0.00
Disinhibition	3.78	0.05	0.02	0.64	0.43	0.00	0.050	0.82	0.00
Motivation-SMS-II ($n = 236$)									
Internal	0.160	0.69	0.00	6.34	0.01	0.03	0.770	0.38	0.00
Integrated	0.22	0.64	0.00	20.18	0.00	0.08	3.21	0.07	0.01
Identified	1.27	0.26	0.01	7.93	0.01	0.03	1.17	0.28	0.01
Introjected	3.58	0.06	0.02	0.01	0.94	0.00	3.56	0.06	0.02
External	1.70	0.19	0.01	0.59	0.44	0.00	0.600	0.44	0.00
Amotivation	0.420	0.52	0.00	0.02	0.89	0.00	0.750	0.39	0.00
Readiness for Technology (TR) ($n = 240$)									
Positive Readiness	7.19	0.01	0.03	0.18	0.69	0.00	0.460	0.50	0.00
Optimism	4.35	0.04	0.02	0.02	0.90	0.00	0.270	0.60	0.00
Innovation	7.89	0.01	0.03	0.84	0.36	0.00	0.510	0.48	0.00
Negative Readiness	12.84	0.00	0.05	1.38	0.24	0.01	0.00	0.96	0.00
Discomfort	12.19	0.00	0.05	4.58	0.03	0.02	0.670	0.41	0.00
Distrust	7.18	0.01	0.03	0.28	0.60	0.00	1.12	0.29	0.01

Table 1. *Cont.*

Variable	A. Smart Watch (Yes/No)			B. Walk/Run (Yes/No)			A by B		
	F	p	λ^2	F	p	λ^2	F	p	λ^2
Readiness for Smart Watch (TAM) (n = 121)									
Total	-	-	-	17.19	0.00	0.12	-	-	-
Perceived usefulness				34.01	0.00	0.22	-	-	-
Perceived ease of use	-	-	-	2.78	0.10	0.02	-	-	-
Intention to use	-	-	-	3.73	0.06	0.03	-	-	-

4.3. *Readiness for Technology*

The MANOVA pertaining to Positive Readiness for Technology resulted in a significant overall SSW use effect, Wilk's $\lambda = 0.96$, $F(2{,}239) = 3.79$, $p < 0.02$, $\eta_p{}^2 = 0.03$, but neither walk/run nor their interaction showed a significant effect ($p > 0.05$). A similar significant SSW use effect was revealed for Negative Readiness for Technology, Wilk's $\lambda = 0.05$, $F(2{,}239) = 6.52$, $p < 0.002$, $\eta^2 = 0.95$. The follow-up ANOVAs revealed significant univariate effects for the four Readiness for Technology dimensions ($p < 0.05$). Figure 1 presents these effects descriptively (means and SDs) along with Cohen's d coefficients.

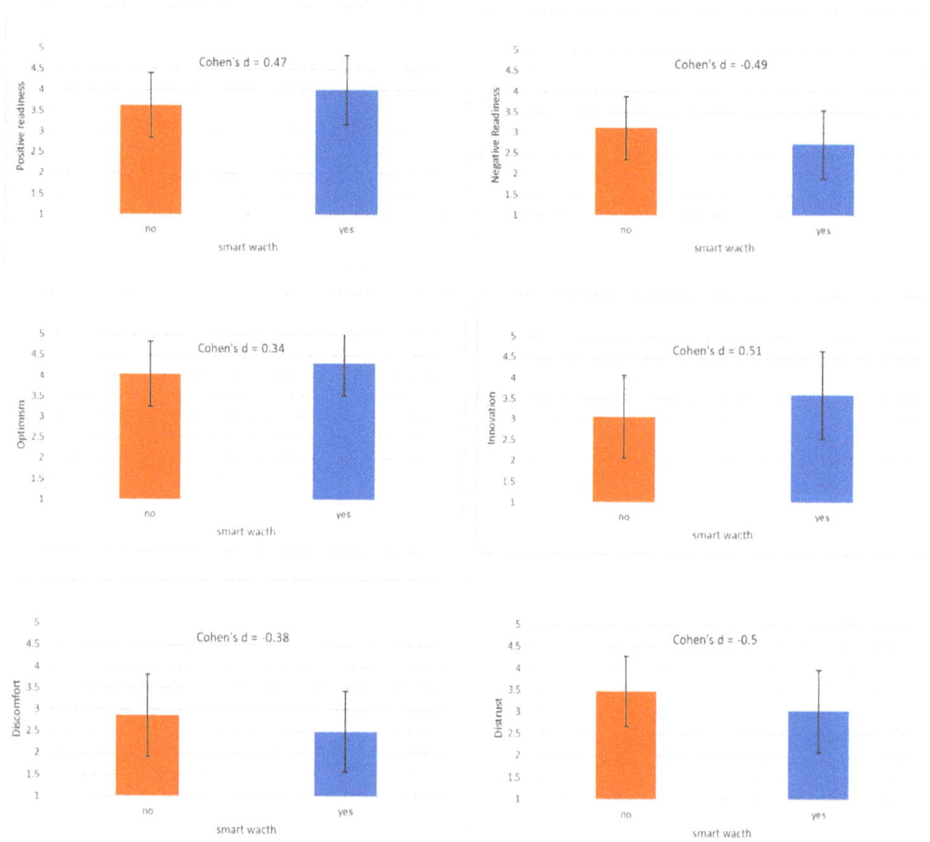

Figure 1. Means and SDs for positive and negative readiness for technology dimensions and total scores in adolescents who use and avoid using SSW.

People using SSW rated themselves significantly ($p < 0.05$) and substantially higher than their non-SSW users on positive readiness for technology ($d = 0.47$), and specifically on optimism ($d = 0.34$) and innovation ($d = 0.51$). Moreover, users of SSW reported significantly ($p < 0.05$) and substantially lower negative readiness for technology than their non-SSW users' counterparts ($d = -0.49$), and specifically on discomfort ($d = -0.38$) and distrust ($d = -50$).

4.4. Motivation for Exercise

The MANOVA performed for the six dimensions of Motivation to Exercise resulted in an overall non-significant effect of SSW use, Wilk's $\lambda = 0.97$, $F(6{,}229) = 0.52$, $p < 0.87$, $\eta^2 = 0.03$. Despite the non-significant effect, we performed six follow-up ANOVAs. Only one tendency for significance of the SSW use effect ($p < 0.06$) emerged for introjected motivation. Adolescents who use SSW reported being lower on introjected motivation than their non-SSW users ($d = -0.35$) (see Figure 2, bottom panel). However, the mean values for both SSW users and non-users were low.

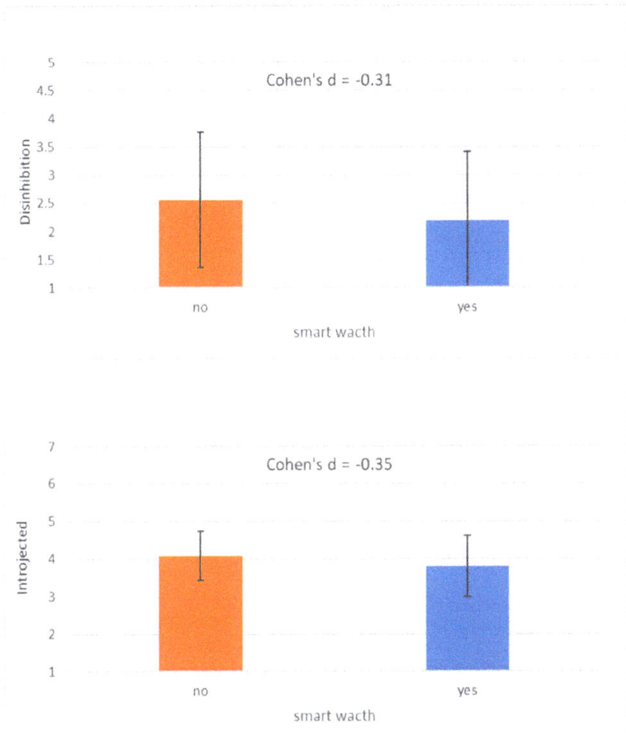

Figure 2. Means and SDs for sensation-seeking disinhibition and for introjected motivation in adolescents who use and avoid using SSW.

The MANOVA also revealed a significant multivariate walk/run effect on the motivation to exercise dimensions, Wilk's $\lambda = 0.92$, $F(6{,}229) = 2.93$, $p < 0.006$, $\eta^2 = 0.08$, and consequently on internal, integrated, and identified motivations (see Table 1 and Figure 3). Adolescents who walk/run reported being more internally motivated ($d = 0.38$), integrated ($d = 0.61$), and identified ($d = 0.34$) than their sedentary counterparts. The mean values of these motivational dimensions were low for both active and sedentary people.

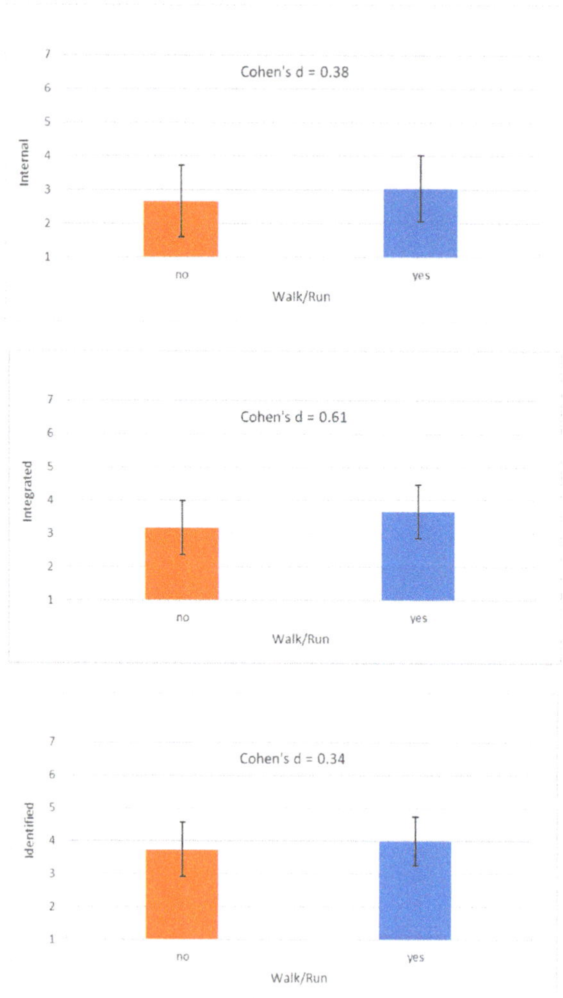

Figure 3. Means and SDs for internal, integrated, and identified motivation dimensions in adolescents who walk/run and adolescents who refrain from walking/running.

4.5. Sensation Seeking

The MANOVA pertaining to sensation-seeking revealed an overall non-significant SSW use effect, Wilk's $\lambda = 0.97$, $F(4{,}239) = 1.69$, $p < 0.15$, $\eta^2 = 0.03$, and follow-up ANOVAs revealed a significant SSW effect ($p < 0.05$) only for disinhibition of the four dimensions. People using SSW reported being lower on disinhibition than people not using SSW ($d = -0.31$, see Figure 2 upper panel). However, the means for disinhibition were low for both SSW users and avoiders.

4.6. SSW and Walk/Run Interaction Effects

Two significant interaction effects of SSW and walk/run emerged (see Table 1); one for integrated motivation and the other for introjected motivation. These two interactions are shown in Figure 4a,b.

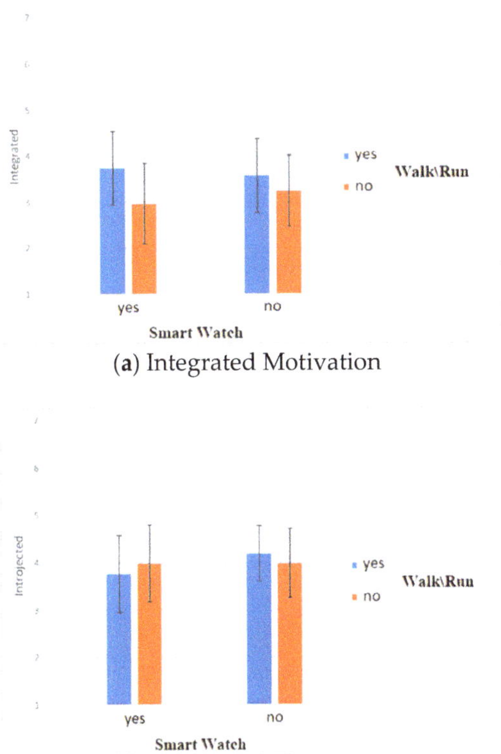

(**a**) Integrated Motivation

(**b**) Intojected Motivation

Figure 4. Mean and SDs for integrated and introjected motivation dimensions in adolescents using and avoiding SSW and walking/running or not.

The first interactional effect is presented in Figure 4a and is assigned to the observation that people using SSW and walking/running reported much higher integrated motivation than those who were sedentary (d = 0.88). Among those who refrained from SSW, this difference was reduced (d = 0.41). As one can notice, walkers/runners reported higher integrated motivation than sedentary adolescents. Different results were obtained for introjected motivation. Users of SSW who refrained from walking/running reported higher introjected motivation than those who walk/run (d = −0.30), but the opposite was true for those who refrain from SSW use. Among them, those who walk/run reported higher introjected motivation than the sedentary (d = 0.29).

4.7. Analyses Pertained to Users of SSW

Additional MANOVA and ANOVA procedures were applied only to users of SSW and pertained to readiness for smart phone use (TAM; in contrast to readiness for technology in general). The MANOVA resulted in a significant main effect for walking/running, Wilk's λ = 0.75, F(3,119), = 13.30, $p < 0.001$, η^2 = 0.25. The follow-up ANOVAs resulted in three main significant ($p < 0.05$) walk/run effects: total readiness for smart phones, perceived usefulness, and a strong tendency toward intention to use them ($p < 0.06$). The descriptive data pertaining to these effects are presented in Figure 5a–c.

Walkers and runners were significantly and substantially higher than those who refrained from walking and running in readiness to use smart phones (total TAM; $d = 0.98$), showed higher usefulness of them ($d = 1.37$), and intended to use them ($d = 0.46$).

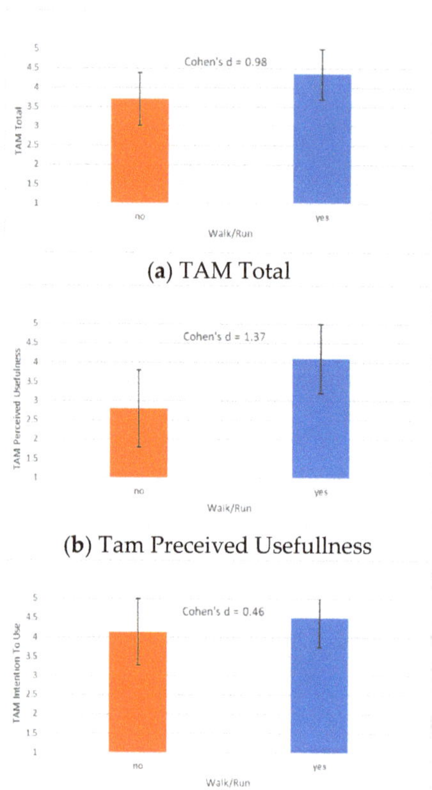

(**a**) TAM Total

(**b**) Tam Preceived Usefullness

(**c**) TAM Intention to Use

Figure 5. Means and SDs for TAM total, perceived usefulness of SSW use, and intention to use SSW for adolescents who walk/run and those who refrain from it.

5. Discussion

Several of the critical factors involved in the adoption of wearable devices, especially watches, have been overlooked in the published research. The current study offers empirical evidence for promoting exploration of the psychological processes involved in the value people hold for technology in general and for SSWs in particular. The study consists of the original Technology Acceptance Model (TAM), extends the profundity of the literature on wearable technologies, and provides applied research references. TAM has been widely opined as a solid base theory for examining users' intentions of using wearable devices. Nevertheless, some scholars critique TAM for insufficiently explaining the users' technology adoption behaviors [15]. Thus, our study was design to explore the psychological determinants, i.e., disposition of readiness/acceptance of technology, motivation for exercise, and sensation seeking, in using SSWs.

By administering both the Technology Readiness and Technology Acceptance Questionnaire (TR; [41]) and the Technology Acceptance Measure (TAM; [12]), we examined our projections that the more positive the approach to using technology is, the more prevalent the use of SSWs and their accompanying features will be. Previous studies demonstrated this link (e.g., [5,6]), and others indicated that young adults' technology readiness moderates the relationships between performance expectancy and attitudes toward wearables [5]. In line with these postulations, our findings indicate that healthy adolescents who are more ready to accept technology are more likely to use SSWs. They were more optimistic and innovative and less negative about, distrustful of, and discomfortable with technology than their non-SSW users.

Positive technology readiness is an attitude which motivates acceptance of a new technology along with optimism, control, flexibility, and efficiency in peoples' lives [10]. In contrast, negative technology readiness results in feelings of discomfort, being overwhelmed by it, and feeling of insecurity and distrust of technology, stemming from skepticism about its ability to work properly and concerns about its potential harmful consequences [10]. We observed that high positive readiness for technology attitude of the study's SSW users (see Figure 1) was reflected by stronger perceived usefulness and higher ease of use than their non-users' counterparts [12]. In previous studies, technology readiness attitude was found to vary in people varying in utilitarian and hedonic motivations ([19,20,42]), which strengthens our assumption that motivation to exercise will be a valuable component in determining the use or avoidance of SSW use. Thus, we assumed that, in line with [22], those motivated internally to exercise will make greater use of their SSWs due to feeling more autonomous and competent and that users of SSWs will score lower on sensation-seeking than non-users.

The findings indicate that adolescents who use SSW reported being regulated by less introjected motivation for exercising than the non-SSW users, though introjected motivation was reported to be low in both cohorts. Specifically, people holding an introjected motivation orientation were more likely to be seeking affirmation from their surroundings or fearing embarrassment by peers. Introjected regulation is a motivation state where the efforts are regulated by the wish to avoid negative consequences such as guilt, rejection, shame, and embarrassment along with perceived pressure to feel pride, self-confidence, and loved and evaluated by others [22]. Refraining from using SSWs was associated with relatively more external, but still low, regulated actions related to exercise. In contrast, adolescents who use SSW were less regulated by external factors and doing it more for their own benefit rather than by conscious effort to impress others and improve their social status. However, we must note that the low ratings given by the SSW user and non-user adolescents to the introjected and other motivation dimensions make these conclusions doubtful.

Our study extended this view by contrasting exercise motivation regulation of users and non-users of SSW who walk/run or refrain from these activities (see Figure 4). Indeed, people may wish to exercise but not use SSW. Accordingly, people who walk/run but refrain from wearing SSW may value the psychological and physical health benefits of the exercise but not necessarily value the use of SSW. We tested herein the notion that the motivational stages set by the SDT [22] determine the use of SSW and its functions during and outside the realm of walking/running. It may well be that people who walk/run may use SSW to overcome negative consequences associated with physical activity and not use it to its full potential because of their lack of autonomy. In contrast, they may use SSW because they wish to relate to others who use SSW and develop competence in the exercise they are engaged in.

The findings also showed that SSW users who walk/run scored higher on integrated motivation than those who refrained from exercising, but both were low on this motivational dimension. A similar, but smaller, difference was noted among non-SSW users. It is therefore clear that it is the exercise which is more associated with the integrated motivational dimension. In other words, integrated motivation for exercising was more related to the mere act of exercising rather than to the SSW use. Relying on Ryan and Deci's [22] SDT, the mean values of the integrated motivation show that people who walk/run feel more integration between their goals, values, and actions than their non-exercise counterparts. This motivational state is not yet internalized, but walkers and runners felt accomplishment of the goals and values more than sedentary exercisers regardless of wearing SSWs. The significant effect of walking/running on the internal, integrated, and identified motivation dimensions where walkers/runners rated themselves higher than those who refrained from exercising (see Figure 3), indicating that motivation for exercise is independent of motivation to use the SSW technology. The low mean values assigned by all the adolescents to these dimensions call for the use of other motivation frameworks to study motivation related to technology use.

Our findings also showed that adolescents who walk/run and use SSW scored the lowest on the introjected motivational dimension. Thus, avoidance of negative feeling is less of a motivated factor for these activities. In sum, the motivation to exercise and use SSW must be further studied using an alternative motivation conceptual framework to better capture the motives which underly the use of SSW alone and without SSW.

We also assumed that the sensation seeking disposition will distinguish between SSW users and avoiders. Specifically, we assumed that adolescents high on sensation seeking will perceive the SSW as a technology that limits their freedom and would not be likely to use it. The findings of this study failed to confirm this view. The sample of adolescents in the current study reported very low ratings of sensation seeking on the four dimensions including disinhibition, which tended to distinguish between SSW users and non-users. Accordingly, SSW users were lower on disinhibition than non-users, meaning they tended to make more decisions free of external constraints than their counterparts, in contrast to our initial assumption. However, the small differences and the low ratings given to sensation seeking by all adolescents makes this psychological concept less valuable to the use of SSW technology.

6. Future Directions

Although the TRAM provides significant data regarding users' intentions for using SSWs, scholars increasingly realize that the focus has shifted from revealing determinants of smartwatch adoption to capturing the factors which cause their long-term usage [43]. On this point, and like Gopinath et al. [44], we argue that perceived ease of use and self-efficacy are undeniably significant. Developers must make concerted efforts to create user-friendly platforms that enhance confidence among users to fully utilize the technological devices. Developers ought to leverage design principles to build a simple watch and mobile interface. They can also introduce tutorials and videos to promote wearable technologies [45], as well as giving importance to specific cultural factors in their creation of apps and manuals. Subsequently, we join Kim and Chiu's [41] recommendation that forthcoming analyses incorporate additional variables in the TRAM, such as perceived trust and enjoyment, to more comprehensively capture the psychological processes involved in the sports wearable technology eco-system. Furthermore, as sports wearables are relatively expensive, users' perceptions of value and quality must be further examined.

Additionally, more research is essential for capturing and tracking the increasing number of wearable technology users. Most wearable technologies are still in their infancy. Challenges including user acceptance, security, ethics, and big data issues must be addressed to enhance the usability and functionality of these devices for practical utilization. The users' preferences must be considered when creating wearable sensing systems. For example, due to the low weight and miniaturization of wearable devices, they are worn close to the body and can be remotely controlled or even bio transplanted, which increases the level of 'interaction' with consumers [46,47]. Furthermore, a combination of heart rate monitoring and positioning can be used to detect whether the user is in a sedentary state. Another possible direction for future studies is to explore whether the usage of SSWs directly influences individuals' physical conditions and active lifestyles [19].

7. Limitations

Our study has three limitations. Firstly, it is based on self-reporting questionnaires, which may create a demand characteristics effect whereby participants in the study do not accurately reflect their real approach to the use of SSW. For example, we can assume that those who bought an expensive SSW but rarely, if ever, use it to measure and improve their exercise activity may feel uncomfortable or guilty about this fact and therefore are more likely to report dishonestly. Secondly, we refrained from measuring people's personality to better capture the intentions for using and benefiting from the use of SSWs. Finally, the study's conclusions refer to a relatively young age cohort (mostly 20–40 years old). Thus, we suggest that younger and older cohorts should also be examined.

Author Contributions: Conceptualization, G.T. and A.L.; methodology, Y.A.-H.; software, T.B.-Z.; validation, Y.G., A.L. and Y.A.-H.; formal analysis, Y.G.; investigation, Y.A.-H.; resources, T.B.-Z.; writing—original draft preparation, G.T.; writing—review and editing, A.L.; supervision, Y.G.; project administration, G.T. All authors have read and agreed to the published version of the manuscript.

Funding: This research received no external funding.

Institutional Review Board Statement: Reichman University IRB 20134/24.

Data Availability Statement: Data Can be obtained by request from the 2nd author.

Conflicts of Interest: The authors declare no conflict of interest.

References

1. Ibrahim, A.H.; Beaumont, C.T.; Strohacker, K. Exploring regular exercisers' experiences with readiness/recovery scores produced by wearable devices: A descriptive qualitative study. *Appl. Psychophysiol. Biofeedback J.* **2024**, *49*, 395–405. [CrossRef]
2. Feng, Y.; Agosto, D.E. Revisiting personal information management through information practices with activity tracking technology. *J. Assoc. Inf. Sci. Technol.* **2019**, *70*, 1352–1367. [CrossRef]
3. Dehghani, M. Exploring the motivational factors on continuous usage intention of smartwatches among actual users. *Behav. Inf. Technol.* **2018**, *37*, 145–158. [CrossRef]
4. Smrke, U.; Špes, T.; Mlakar, I.; Musil, B.; Plohl, N. Technophobia mediates the associations between age, education level, and readiness to adopt new (health) technology among aging adults. *J. Appl. Gerontol.* **2024**, *23*, 7334648241274260. [CrossRef]
5. Aksoy, N.C.; Alan, A.K.; Kabadayi, E.T.; Aksoy, A. Individuals' intention to use sports wearables: The moderating role of technophobia. *Int. J. Sports Mark. Spons.* **2020**, *21*, 225–245.
6. Seifert, A. Smartwatch use among older adults: Findings from two large surveys. In *Human Aspects of IT for the Aged Population. Technologies, Design and User Experience*; Gao, Q., Zhou, J., Eds.; Springer International Publishing: Cham, Switzerland, 2020; pp. 372–385.
7. Chengzhen, W.; Gyoo Gun, L. Investigating older adult users' willingness to adopt wearable devices by integrating the technology acceptance model (UTAUT2) and the technology readiness index theory. *Front. Public Health* **2024**, *12*, 1449594. [CrossRef]
8. Parasuraman, A.; Colby, C.L. *Techno-Ready Marketing: How and Why Your Customers Adopt Technology*; Free Press: New York, NY, USA, 2001.
9. Aripradono, H.W. Analysis technology readiness and acceptance model (TRAM) pada penggunaan sport wearable technology. *Teknika* **2021**, *10*, 68–77. [CrossRef]

10. Parasuraman, A. Technology Readiness Index (TRI): A multiple-item scale to measure readiness to embrace new technologies. *J. Serv. Res.* **2000**, *2*, 307–320. [CrossRef]
11. Ajzen, I.; Fishbein, M.A. Bayesian analysis of attribution processes. *Psychol. Bull.* **1975**, *82*, 261–277. [CrossRef]
12. Davis, F.D. Perceived usefulness, perceived ease of use, and user acceptance of information technology. *MIS Q.* **1989**, *13*, 319–340. [CrossRef]
13. Raman, P.; Aashish, K. To continue or not to continue: A structural analysis of antecedents of mobile payment systems in India. *Int. J. Bank Mark.* **2021**, *39*, 242–271. [CrossRef]
14. Akgül, Y. An analysis of customers' acceptance of internet banking: An integration of E-trust and service quality to the TAM—The case of Turkey. In *E-Manufacturing and E-Service Strategies in Contemporary Organizations*; Gwangwava, N., Mutingi, M., Eds.; IGI Global: Alanya, Turkey, 2018; pp. 154–198. [CrossRef]
15. Lin, C.H.; Shih, H.Y.; Sher, P.J. Integrating technology readiness into technology acceptance: The TRAM model. *Psychol. Mark.* **2007**, *24*, 641–657. [CrossRef]
16. Martens, M.; Roll, O.; Elliott, R. Testing the technology readiness and acceptance model for mobile payments across Germany and South Africa. *Int. J. Innov. Technol. Manag.* **2017**, *14*, 1750033. [CrossRef]
17. Chen, M.F.; Lin, N.P. Incorporation of health consciousness into the technology readiness and acceptance model to predict app download and usage intentions. *Internet Res.* **2018**, *28*, 351–373. [CrossRef]
18. Kaushik, A.K.; Rahman, Z. An empirical investigation of tourists' choice of service delivery options. *Int. J. Contemp. Hosp. Manag.* **2017**, *29*, 1892–1913. [CrossRef]
19. Wang, Y.; So, K.K.F.; Sparks, B.A. Technology readiness and customer satisfaction with travel technologies: A cross-country investigation. *J. Travel. Res.* **2017**, *56*, 563–577. [CrossRef]
20. Ramírez-Correa, P.E.; Grandón, E.E.; Arenas-Gaitán, J. Assessing differences in customers' personal disposition to e-commerce. *Ind. Manag. Data Syst.* **2019**, *119*, 792–820. [CrossRef]
21. Chang, Y.W.; Chen, J. What motivates customers to shop in smart shops? The impacts of smart technology and technology readiness. *J. Retail. Consum. Serv.* **2021**, *58*, 102325. [CrossRef]
22. Deci, E.L.; Ryan, R.M. *Intrinsic Motivation and Self-Determination in Human Behavior*; Plenum Publishing: Rochester, NY, USA, 1985.
23. Deci, E.L.; Ryan, R.M. Self-determination theory and the facilitation of intrinsic motivation, social development, and well-being. *Am. Psychol.* **2017**, *55*, 68–78.
24. Ryan, R.M.; Deci, E.L. *Self-Determination Theory: Basic Psychological Needs in Motivation, Development, and Wellness*; Guilford Publications: New York, NY, USA, 2000.
25. Reeve, J. Teachers as facilitators: What autonomy-supportive teachers do and why their students benefit. *Elem. Sch. J.* **2006**, *106*, 225–236. [CrossRef]
26. Bandura, A. Self-efficacy: Toward a unifying theory of behavioral change. *Psychol. Rev.* **1982**, *84*, 191–215. [CrossRef] [PubMed]
27. Deci, E.L.; Ryan, R.M. Self-determination theory: A macrotheory of human motivation, development, and health. *Can. Psychol.* **2000**, *41*, 178–185. [CrossRef]
28. Vallerand, R.J.; Rousseau, F.L. Intrinsic and extrinsic motivation in sport and exercise: A review using the hierarchical model of intrinsic and extrinsic motivation. *Handb. Sport Psychol.* **2001**, *2*, 389–416.
29. Lev, A. Running through the in-between: Distance runners in a state of liminality. *Leis. Stud.* **2022**, *42*, 648–662. [CrossRef]
30. Tholander, J.; Nylander, S. Snot, sweat, pain, mud, and snow: Performance and experience in the use of sports watches. In Proceedings of the 33rd Annual ACM Conference on Human Factors in Computing Systems, Seoul, Republic of Korea, 18–23 April 2015; pp. 2913–2922.
31. Chin-Cheng, Y.; Shen, C.C.; Lin, Y.S.; Lin, C.T. The relationship between use motivation, target orientation, and sports involvement in sports intelligent wearable equipment. *J. Hum. Sport. Exerc.* **2021**, *16*, 434–443. [CrossRef]
32. Schüll, N.D. Data for life: Wearable technology and the design of self-care. *BioSocieties* **2016**, *11*, 317–333. [CrossRef]
33. Zuckerman, M. Dimensions of sensation-seeking. *J. Consult. Clin. Psychol.* **1971**, *36*, 45–52. [CrossRef]
34. Guszkowska, M.; Bołdak, A. Sensation seeking in males involved in recreational high-risk sports. *Biol. Sport* **2010**, *27*, 157–162. [CrossRef]
35. Veliz, P.; McCabe, S.E.; Eckner, J.T.; Schulenberg, J.E. Concussion, sensation-seeking, and substance use among US adolescents. *Subst. Abuse.* **2019**, *42*, 183–191. [CrossRef]
36. Liebel, S.W.; Edwards, K.A.; Broglio, S.P. Sensation-seeking and impulsivity in athletes with sport-related concussion. *Curr. Psychiatry Rep.* **2021**, *23*, 15. [CrossRef] [PubMed]
37. Pelletier, L.G.; Rocchi, M.A.; Vallerand, R.J.; Deci, E.L.; Ryan, R.M. Validation of the revised sport motivation scale (SMS-II). *Psychol. Sport. Exerc.* **1995**, *14*, 329–341. [CrossRef]

38. Hoyle, R.H.; Stephenson, M.T.; Palmgreen, P.; Lorch, E.P.; Donohew, R.L. Reliability and validity of a brief measure of sensation seeking. *Pers. Individ. Differ.* **2002**, *32*, 401–414. [CrossRef]
39. Zuckerman, M.; Eysenck, S.B.; Eysenck, H.J. Sensation seeking in England and America: Cross-cultural, age, and sex comparisons. *J. Consult. Clin. Psychol.* **1978**, *46*, 139–149. [CrossRef]
40. Huba, G.J.; Newcomb, M.D.; Bentler, P.M. Comparison of canonical correlation and inter-battery factor analysis on sensation seeking and drug use domains. *Appl. Psychol. Meas.* **1981**, *5*, 291–306. [CrossRef]
41. Kim, T.; Chiu, W. Consumer acceptance of sports wearable technology: The role of technology readiness. *Int. J. Sports Mark. Spons.* **2018**, *20*, 109–126. [CrossRef]
42. Jung, Y.; Kim, S.; Choi, B. Consumer valuation of the wearables: The case of smartwatches. *Comput. Human. Behav.* **2016**, *63*, 899–905. [CrossRef]
43. Siepmann, C.; Kowalczuk, P. Understanding continued smartwatch usage: The role of emotional as well as health and fitness factors. *Electron. Mark.* **2021**, *31*, 795–809. [CrossRef]
44. Gopinath, K.; Selvam, G.; Narayanamurthy, G. Determinants of the adoption of wearable devices for health and fitness: A meta-analytical study. *Commun. Assoc. Inf. Syst.* **2022**, *50*, 557–590. [CrossRef]
45. Baudier, P.; Ammi, C.; Wamba, S.F. Differing perceptions of the smartwatch by users within developed countries. *J. Glob. Inf. Manag.* **2020**, *28*, 1–20. [CrossRef]
46. Yau, Y.; Hsiao, C.H. The technology acceptance model and older adults' exercise intentions—A systematic literature review. *Geriatrics* **2022**, *7*, 124. [CrossRef]
47. Wang, Y.; Zhang, X.; Wang, L. Assessing the intention to use sports bracelets among Chinese university students: An extension of technology acceptance model in sports motivation. *Front. Psychol.* **2022**, *13*, 846594. [CrossRef] [PubMed]

technologies

MDPI

Article

Transforming Telemedicine: Strategic Lessons and Metrics from Italy's Telemechron Project (Telemechron Study)

Sara Jayousi [1], Martina Cinelli [1], Roberto Bigazzi [1], Stefano Bianchi [1], Simonetta Scalvini [2], Gabriella Borghi [2], Palmira Bernocchi [2], Sandro Inchiostro [3], Alexia Giovanazzi [3], Marina Mastellaro [3], Maria Adalgisa Gentilini [3], Lorenzo Gios [4], Mauro Grigioni [5], Carla Daniele [5], Giuseppe D'Avenio [5], Sandra Morelli [5] and Daniele Giansanti [5,*]

[1] Local Health Unit, Division of Nephrology and Dialysis, Azienda USL Toscana Nord Ovest, 57124 Livorno, Italy; sarajayousi.eostora@gmail.com (S.J.); martinacinelli99@gmail.com (M.C.); bigazzi53@gmail.com (R.B.); stefanobianchi0205@gmail.com (S.B.)

[2] Continuity of Care Service, Istituti Clinici Scientifici Maugeri IRCCS, Institute of Lumezzane, 25065 Brescia, Italy; simonetta.scalvini@icsmaugeri.it (S.S.); gabriella.borghi@cefriel.com (G.B.); palmira.bernocchi@icsmaugeri.it (P.B.)

[3] Azienda Provinciale per i Servizi Sanitari, Provincia Autonoma di Trento, 38122 Trento, Italy; sandro.inchiostro@apss.tn.it (S.I.); alexia.giovanazzi@apss.tn.it (A.G.); marina.mastellaro@apss.tn.it (M.M.); mariaadalgisa.gentilini@apss.tn.it (M.A.G.)

[4] Trentino Salute 4.0, Competence Center for Digital Health, 38123 Trento, Italy; lgios@fbk.eu

[5] Centro Nazionale Tecnologie Innovative in Sanità Pubblica, Istituto Superiore di Sanità, 00161 Rome, Italy; mauro.grigioni@guest.iss.it (M.G.); carla.daniele@iss.it (C.D.); giuseppe.davenio@iss.it (G.D.); sandra.morelli@iss.it (S.M.)

* Correspondence: daniele.giansanti@iss.it; Tel.: +39-06-49902701

Abstract: *Background:* The Telemechron project addresses critical needs in telemedicine by evaluating technology assessment frameworks and key performance indicators (KPIs), among other objectives. Effective frameworks and KPIs are crucial for assessing telemedicine services, especially in terms of their impact on patient outcomes and service efficiency. *Methods:* This study adopted a dual approach to assess the contributions of the Telemechron project. Firstly, it applied a technology assessment framework to quantitatively evaluate telemedicine services, focusing on measurable improvements and systematic analysis. Secondly, it investigated a set of predefined KPIs using specific metrics and parameters to evaluate their applicability and limitations in telemedicine settings. *Results and Discussion:* The technology assessment framework demonstrated significant utility by providing structured, quantifiable improvements across key aspects of telemedicine services. It was effective in evaluating the alignment of services with strategic goals and their integration with existing healthcare systems. The predefined KPIs, although not developed within this study and not directly used by the different operational units (OUs)—which established their own context-specific KPIs—still provided valuable insights into telemedicine performance. However, the study revealed that these KPIs highlighted a need for further customization to enhance their relevance across various contexts. While the KPIs may offer useful performance indicators, their general applicability necessitated adjustments to better address the specific needs of telemedicine applications. The analysis model for the KPI set, in terms of metrics and parameters, is exportable and generalizable to other national and international telemedicine contexts. *Conclusions:* The study confirms the effectiveness of the framework in delivering measurable improvements in telemedicine services and underscores the importance of adapting KPIs for specific contexts. Future research should focus on further applying and expanding the framework and metrics, refining KPI models, integrating new technologies, and conducting cross-national comparisons to enhance the applicability and effectiveness of telemedicine evaluations.

Keywords: telemedicine; TeleHealth; digital health; technology assessment; KPI; key performance indicator

1. Introduction

1.1. Technology Assessment and Telemedicine

Technology assessment (TA) plays a crucial and strategic role across various sectors, with its importance being particularly pronounced in the healthcare field. Telemedicine, characterized by its complexity and heterogeneity, involves numerous interconnected components. This complexity makes the task of conducting effective technology assessment both particularly challenging and indispensable.

The complexity of telemedicine systems necessitates a thorough and nuanced approach to TA. Given the varied and evolving nature of telemedicine technologies, there is a pressing need for structured and comprehensive assessment frameworks. Such frameworks are essential for evaluating the efficacy, safety, and overall impact of telemedicine interventions, ensuring they meet the diverse needs of patients and healthcare providers effectively.

Various studies have addressed technology assessment (TA) in telemedicine from different perspectives, exploring various domains and highlighting diverse needs [1–20]. The necessity for a structured TA framework is evident from multiple aspects of these studies.

For example, Jacob et al. [2] and Smits et al. [4] underscore the importance of rigorous evaluation frameworks for eHealth tools. They advocate for a comprehensive approach that captures multiple dimensions of technology performance and user experience.

Incorporating stakeholder preferences is another area where a structured framework is crucial. Von Huben et al. [3] emphasize that including stakeholder feedback in TA processes enhances the relevance and acceptability of digital health solutions. This indicates that a structured framework is essential to ensure all relevant perspectives are considered, leading to more effective interventions.

The shift from digital health to digital well-being further reflects the need for a structured framework. Smits et al. [4] highlight that evaluating the impact of digital health technologies on overall well-being requires a framework that goes beyond traditional health metrics, capturing a broader range of effects.

Targeted evaluations of specific health interventions, such as telehealth-based cancer rehabilitation [5], cardiac rehabilitation [13], and telemedicine with clinical decision support for critical care [1], reinforce the importance of a structured framework. These studies show that assessing digital interventions in specialized healthcare domains benefits from an approach that addresses unique needs and challenges.

The application of TA frameworks is a common theme. Von Huben et al. [6,8] and Kitsiou et al. [15] discuss the need for systematic reviews and assessments to analyze the role of digital health in managing chronic diseases. A structured framework facilitates this process, ensuring evaluations are comprehensive and based on evidence.

Innovative approaches, such as the "Sandbox Approach" proposed by Leckenby et al. [7], reflect a proactive stance towards developing structured methodologies. This approach suggests that a flexible yet structured framework can adapt to the evolving landscape of healthcare technology.

Cost-effectiveness analysis, highlighted by Bonten et al. [9] and Jiang et al. [11], demonstrates the importance of incorporating economic considerations into TA. A structured framework that includes cost-effectiveness helps understand the financial implications of digital health interventions and supports informed decision-making. The systematic review by Vis et al. [10] highlights the critical role of health technology assessment frameworks specifically designed for eHealth. Their work emphasizes the need for tailored approaches that can address the unique challenges and opportunities presented by digital health technologies, reinforcing the importance of structured and comprehensive assessment methodologies in this rapidly evolving field.

The focus on peer-to-peer interactions in digital interventions for psychotic disorders [12] emphasizes the importance of including social dimensions in the TA process. A structured framework that considers these aspects ensures a more comprehensive evaluation of digital health interventions.

Critical assessments of home telemonitoring interventions [15] and specific respiratory interventions [16–18] highlight the importance of methodological rigor. Evaluating the quality of existing reviews and exploring evidence-based practices benefit from a structured framework that captures both strengths and limitations.

The evaluation of diagnostic tools, such as portable monitoring devices for diagnosing obstructive sleep apnea [19], and the longitudinal perspective on telemedicine applications [20] further support the need for a structured approach. Longitudinal evaluations and ongoing assessments are crucial for identifying effective applications and addressing evidence gaps over time.

Overall, the studies advocate for a comprehensive and structured approach to TA in digital health and telemedicine. They emphasize the importance of systematic evaluation frameworks that incorporate stakeholder preferences, address a broad range of health impacts, and consider economic and social dimensions. Developing and implementing such frameworks supports a holistic understanding of the strengths and limitations of current digital health evidence, leading to more effective and evidence-based solutions.

1.2. Role of Key Performance Indicators in Telemedicine Tecnology Assessment

Key performance indicators (KPIs) are increasingly discussed for their usefulness in measuring strategic parameters within complex systems, providing tangible and rigorous metrics that are valuable across multiple levels and domains (key performance indicator [21]). These indicators are becoming more commonly applied in the health domain, a rapidly evolving sector (KPIs in the health domain [22]). KPIs offer a structured way to measure and evaluate various parameters, making them essential tools in systems that require precise and multi-level assessment.

Telemedicine, a part of the *health domain*, represents a heterogeneous and complex system where KPIs can play a significant role in technology assessment across various fields of application, particularly where ongoing digitalization drives continuous innovation [23]. KPIs are fundamental in this context, as they provide objective quantifiable metrics, allowing for a clear assessment of how well telemedicine systems function. They enable the identification of both strengths and areas needing improvement, offering valuable insights for technology management and innovation within these dynamic environments. However, it is important to note that KPIs are often very specific and not universally standardized, which presents both opportunities and challenges. The specificity of KPIs means they must be carefully tailored to the unique aspects of each application or domain. For example, in the study by Canning et al. [24], clinical pharmacy quality indicators were found to lack uniformity and fail to measure outcomes directly, illustrating the difficulty of applying standardized KPIs in complex healthcare settings. Despite efforts to establish a consensus on pharmaceutical care bundles and outcome measures, only a limited number of indicators achieved consensus, highlighting the challenge of creating universally applicable KPIs in such a diverse field. Similarly, Garbelli et al. [25] demonstrated that while the implementation of standardized KPIs can lead to significant improvements in patient outcomes, such as reduced mortality, the need for standardization and structured implementation is critical for consistent results. The study found that increased KPI target achievements were linked to better patient survival rates, emphasizing the impact of standardized clinical practice.

In telehealth, Jackson et al. [26] identified variations in the reporting of performance metrics across different telehealth classes and study stages, further underscoring the challenges of KPI standardization. Clinical outcomes and patient satisfaction were commonly reported, but other performance metrics were less frequently documented, reflecting inconsistencies in KPI application.

Similarly, Baughman et al. [27] compared the quality of care between telehealth and in-person office-based care, finding that telehealth exposure led to better performance in specific KPIs related to testing and counseling. This study highlighted the favorable association between telehealth and quality of care, particularly in chronic disease management and preventive care, but also reflected variability in KPI implementation and measurement.

In analyzing the broader implementation of telehealth programs, Avanesova et al. [28] emphasized the importance of consistent KPI collection and routine analysis to support telehealth capacity building and international legislation. This study highlighted the role of KPIs in evaluating patient outcomes and ensuring effective telehealth interventions.

Further studies, such as those by Berlet et al. [29] and Kidholm et al. [30], have shown the importance of KPIs in evaluating new technologies and frameworks. Berlet et al. focused on the usability of a 5G-enabled telemedical system, using KPIs to assess technical performance and clinical applicability. Kidholm et al. assessed the face validity of the Model for Assessment of Telehealth, underscoring the importance of KPIs in evaluating telehealth effectiveness and suggesting areas for improvement.

Other research, including that by Schröder et al. [31] and Vo et al. [32], explored the impact of telehealth on emergency medical services (EMSs) and the integration of telehealth within incentive programs and the related specific KPIs. Schröder et al. [31] highlighted improvements in EMS operations through tele-EMS systems, while Vo et al. proposed an Integrated Telehealth Model (ITM) to incentivize telehealth adoption and quality improvement. Both studies illustrate the role of KPIs in optimizing healthcare delivery and assessing the impact of telehealth interventions.

Overall, while KPIs are integral to technology assessment in telemedicine—driving performance evaluation, supporting strategic decisions, and fostering ongoing enhancements—their specificity and lack of standardization require thoughtful design and implementation. As demonstrated by recent studies, the challenge of applying universally applicable KPIs across diverse healthcare settings remains significant, emphasizing the need for continuous refinement and standardization to enhance their effectiveness.

1.3. Study Context Within a National Project and Key Objectives

In the context of a national Italian project, detailed below in terms of its architecture, roles, and activities, significant emphasis was placed on TA activities and the role of key performance indicators (KPIs) within this framework.

The Italian National Institute of Health (ISS), in accordance with its institutional role within the health domain, collaborated on the project through various supporting activities, particularly focusing on TA and model integration. Among its contributions, the ISS conducted a thorough review of the scientific and documentary literature, which provided essential insights for guiding project partners.

In addition, the ISS developed a well-structured tool for technology assessment tailored to the project's needs. This tool was designed to systematically evaluate various aspects of telemedicine projects, ensuring a comprehensive and rigorous assessment.

The *first review* [33], focusing on TA studies in telemedicine, identified the key characteristics necessary for an effective TA tool. Drawing on these insights, a TA tool was developed and *validated, as detailed in* [34]. This tool consists of five forms with subsections that project development units must complete, ensuring a thorough and consistent evaluation across all project components.

A *second review* [35], which concentrated on KPIs in telemedicine, highlighted the application-specific nature of KPIs and the general lack of standardization. This review revealed that KPIs are often tailored to specific applications, resulting in variability in their use and reporting. It also exposed the diverse and inconsistent KPI proposals from various national and international organizations. This variability in KPI standardization poses challenges for comparing and integrating KPIs across different telemedicine initiatives and emphasizes the need for more uniform KPI development and application.

As the project nears its conclusion, this study aims to achieve several interrelated objectives, with a focus on dissemination across the entire project and team. The first objective is to disseminate detailed information about the project's structure, including partner architecture, roles, and activities. Building on this, the second objective is to quantitatively assess the improvements in TA practices within the project using the validated tool described in [34]. The third objective addresses insights gained from the analysis of KPIs, focusing on their limitations and the need for a structured validation process. Consequently, a KPI model proposed in the national Italian guidelines was examined, and a generalized evaluation model was applied to assess the adequacy of this KPI model based on relevant parameters and metrics.

By achieving these objectives, the study aims to enhance the overall effectiveness of the project, provide valuable insights for future initiatives, and contribute to the standardization and improvement of TA and KPI practices in telemedicine.

2. Methods

In alignment with the proposed objectives, the study design is organized into the following sections:

- *Section 2.1: Project Architecture*
  This section offers a comprehensive overview of the national project's structure. It details how the project was conceptualized and organized, including the integration of the framework used. This part of the study describes the key components of the project, the roles of various participants, and the overarching goals that guided the implementation of the framework. It emphasizes the strategic alignment between the project's objectives and the framework's application, illustrating how the framework was operationalized to address the specific needs and challenges of the project.
- *Section 2.2: Framework and KPI Tabular Schema Application for Enhanced Assessment Structure*
  This section (a) briefly recalls the framework used in this study for the final assessments and (b) reports a detailed tabular schema outlining the KPIs proposed for assessing its application in the project. It includes a list of categorized KPIs in a schema arranged in a structured format for assessing the applicability or non-applicability of each KPI within the context of the project's activities.

2.1. The Project Architecture

The Telemechron project (Telemedicine for Home-based Management of Patients with Comorbidities) was presented under the 2018 targeted research funding call as a network initiative (see funding section).

The Telemechron project represents a significant effort in targeted research focused on the integration of telemedicine in the management of chronic patients. It is a network-based initiative funded by the Ministry of Health, various regional authorities, and an autonomous province. The formal agreement for this project was established on 9 July 2020 under the research code NET-2018-12367206, with a project duration of 36 months, starting on 1 October 2020.

The project involves multiple healthcare institutions, including USL Toscana Nord Ovest in Tuscany, IRCCS Maugeri of Lumezzane in Lombardy, and the Azienda Provinciale per i Servizi Sanitari (Provincial Health Services Company) of the Autonomous Province of Trento. In addition, the Istituto Superiore di Sanità (ISS) is actively collaborating, especially in overseeing quality assurance and technology assessment.

The 36-month project is structured into four main activities, each corresponding to an operative unit (OU) and assigned a specific work package (WP) as follows:

1. OU 1 → WP1: USL Toscana Nord Ovest focuses on the use of telemedicine in managing chronic kidney failure patients. This activity aims to enhance the management of patients through remote monitoring and intervention strategies.
2. OU 3 → WP3: IRCCS Maugeri of Lumezzane addresses the needs of chronic heart failure patients with comorbidities such as diabetes through telemedicine solutions. The goal of this activity is to provide continuous monitoring and personalized care to improve patient outcomes.
3. OU 4 → WP4: Azienda Provinciale per i Servizi Sanitari of the Autonomous Province of Trento works on telemedicine for managing type 2 diabetes mellitus. The activity focuses on home-based care solutions to support diabetes management and to improve long-term health outcomes.
4. OU 2 → WP2: ISS (Istituto Superiore di Sanità) plays a connector/mediator role and leads the technology assessment efforts. This activity is essential for integrating and assessing telemedicine technologies across different domains, ensuring that clinical governance and regulatory standards are met. ISS is also responsible for the development and validation of multidimensional clinical governance indicators to monitor and ensure quality across the project's activities.

By aligning each OU with a WP, the Telemechron project ensures that different aspects of telemedicine for chronic disease management are thoroughly explored while fostering collaboration among healthcare entities. The project aims to build a robust scalable model for the future of healthcare, addressing technological, regulatory, and clinical needs.

Figure 1 reports a sketch of the architecture of the project. There are three operational units (OU1, OU3, OU4) assigned to project development work packages (WP1, WP3, WP4), with one of them (OU1) also responsible for the overall project coordination. Additionally, there is another operational unit (OU2) assigned to WP2, responsible for quality assurance in the integration of the telemedicine model, which includes dynamic and iterative multidimensional technology assessment.

Overall, the Telemechron project represents a significant initiative aimed at enhancing home care for chronic patients through the implementation of telemedicine solutions, contributing to the development and innovation within the healthcare sector. Each partner in the project plays a distinct and complementary role, ensuring the success and effective execution of the initiative. Below is a detailed description of each partner's role.

- USL Toscana Nord Ovest (Tuscany) (OU 1/WP1)
  Role: Coordination of the entire network project and implementation of activities in the Tuscany region.

Focus: Study and experimentation of telemedicine services for patients with chronic kidney failure.
Objective: To coordinate project activities to achieve integration goals and improve home care for patients with chronic kidney failure. This includes evaluating the effectiveness, efficiency, and sustainability of telemedicine solutions.

- IRCCS Maugeri of Lumezzane (Lombardy) (OU 3/WP3)
Role: Study and implementation of telemedicine services within the Lombardy region.
Focus: Patients with chronic heart failure and comorbidities.
Objective: To explore the use of telemedicine to enhance the management and home care of patients with chronic heart failure and associated conditions.
- Azienda Provinciale per i Servizi Sanitari of the Provincia Autonoma di Trento (OU 4/WP4)
Role: Study and implementation of telemedicine services in the Provincia Autonoma di Trento.
Focus: Patients with type 2 diabetes mellitus.
Objective: To test and evaluate telemedicine solutions that improve the monitoring and management of type 2 diabetes in the context of home care.
- ISS (Istituto Superiore di Sanità) (OU 2/WP2)
Role: Coordination of technology assessment activities, multidimensional evaluation, and methodological support to all project partners.
Focus: Technological and multidimensional assessment of telemedicine services.
Objective: To provide an integrated and comprehensive evaluation of the telemedicine services implemented by the other partners, focusing on clinical effectiveness, safety, organizational impact, and financial sustainability.

Together, these competencies and responsibilities aim to cover a broad spectrum of chronic medical conditions, making a significant contribution to the progress and innovation in telemedicine and home care. The collaboration among partners enables a holistic and integrated approach to addressing challenges and maximizing the benefits of the Telemechron project.

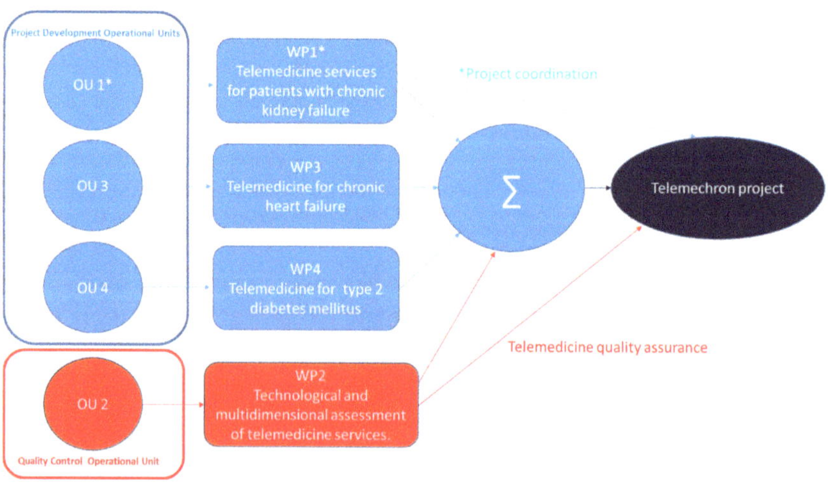

Figure 1. Sketch of the Telemechron project. The asterisk "*" indicates the coordination unit for the entire project, OU 1. Units dedicated to project development are marked in blue. OU 2, dedicated to the technological and multidimensional assessment of telemedicine services, is marked in red. This unit has ensured telemedicine quality assurance throughout the entire project.

2.2. Framework and KPI Tabular Schema Application for Enhanced Assessment Structure

2.2.1. Framework Used for the Assessment

The framework developed by the Italian National Institute of Health (ISS) is a central tool for conducting comprehensive evaluations across various domains of telemedicine services. It provides a structured approach to assess the planning, implementation, and outcomes of these initiatives (see in Box 1 the structure). Designed to address a broad range of necessary areas for successful telemedicine delivery, the framework allows for a thorough review of strategic alignment, organizational design, technical requirements, financial considerations, and service performance.

The framework serves as the primary tool for quality control, ensuring consistency and standardization across all project units. This systematic approach allows all participating units to report on key criteria in a consistent and standardized format, which is essential for maintaining objectivity, transparency, and alignment with national healthcare priorities.

Each OU within the project, while adhering to the overall framework structure, provides its own detailed framework based on the specific context and needs of its telemedicine service. The framework is divided into various sheets (Box 1), each corresponding to different components/aspects of the service, and they are further subdivided into subsections that guide the OUs in providing in-depth analysis and reporting. These sheets cover areas such as service functionality, target population, expected outcomes, and operational needs.

For example, the following can be observed:

- OU 1 (USL Toscana Nord Ovest) focuses on chronic kidney failure and provides a framework for this patient group.
- OU 3 (IRCCS Maugeri of Lumezzane) develops a framework addressing chronic heart failure and comorbidities.
- OU 4 (Azienda Provinciale per i Servizi Sanitari of the Provincia Autonoma di Trento) provides its own framework for telemedicine services for type 2 diabetes mellitus patients.

Each OU's specific framework ensures that the ISS can carry out a detailed and systematic evaluation, as it gathers data and insights directly from the units working on the ground. This collaborative approach ensures that all critical components of the telemedicine services are evaluated and understood in context.

Once the project units complete and submit their responses using their frameworks, the ISS conducts a thorough evaluation, including a detailed audit to confirm the accuracy and completeness of the information. The audit process cross-references the data with established guidelines and best practices, ensuring that the services are both effective and efficient.

After the audit, the ISS provides feedback in the form of a detailed report. This feedback not only serves as an evaluation but also acts as a tool for continuous improvement. The report identifies areas of strength and areas needing improvement, offering actionable recommendations for enhancing the telemedicine services.

The iterative feedback loop fosters a culture of continuous quality improvement, enabling the project units to refine and adjust their services in response to ongoing evaluations. This ensures that telemedicine services remain adaptable and aligned with the evolving needs of healthcare delivery, thus enhancing the long-term success and sustainability of these services.

The framework is not just an evaluation tool; it serves as a dynamic dossier that documents all essential aspects of a telemedicine service. The sheets within the framework act as data collection forms to be completed by the project teams. Each sheet corresponds to a specific component/aspect of the service, such as service profiling, strategic alignment, design and implementation, adoption processes, and evaluation.

The detailed structure allows for a comprehensive documentation process, ensuring that all relevant information is systematically collected and clearly presented. This ensures consistency across all project units, facilitating the analysis of the effectiveness, scalability, and potential for the broader implementation of telemedicine services. The framework also serves as a reference for future projects, helping to identify best practices and key success factors.

Ultimately, this dossier-style framework (Box 1) enables a clear, organized approach to documenting, evaluating, and improving telemedicine services, supporting their effective implementation and fostering innovation and continuous learning throughout the project.

Box 1. Architecture of the framework.

Sheet No. 1: Profile of the Telemedicine Service or Suite of Telemedicine Services

- 1.1 Name of the telemedicine service or suite of services
- 1.2 Healthcare organization and reference region or autonomous province
- 1.3 Operational unit
- 1.4 Service or telemedicine suite manager
- 1.5 Type of telemedicine service or services in the suite

Sheet No. 2: Strategic Framework of the Telemedicine Service or Suite of Telemedicine Services

- 2.1 SWOT analysis of healthcare before introducing the telemedicine service or suite
- 2.2 Care needs addressed by the telemedicine service or suite
- 2.3 Functional description of the telemedicine service or suite
- 2.4 Target population and therapeutic and socio-economic indications
- 2.5 Evidence from the scientific literature

Sheet No. 3: Design and Implementation of the Telemedicine Service or Suite of Telemedicine Services

- 3.1 Organizational and managerial requirements gap analysis
- 3.2 Technical and technological requirements gap analysis
- 3.3 Economic financial evaluations and procurement strategy for acquiring goods and services from the market
- 3.4 Methodology adopted and stakeholders involved in the design and implementation
- 3.5 Regulatory and compliance aspects for implementation
- 3.6 Risk management
- 3.7 Best practices

Sheet No. 4: Adoption of the Telemedicine Service or Suite of Telemedicine Services

- 4.1 Criteria and procedures for service activation and management
- 4.2 Methods and indicators for monitoring service quality and minimum performance thresholds (service level agreement)
- 4.3 Service pricing and cost-sharing rules
- 4.4 Change management
- 4.5 Activation date of the telemedicine service or suite
- 4.6 Volume of services delivered

Sheet No. 5: Evaluation of the Telemedicine Service or Suite of Telemedicine Services

- 5.1 Dimensions and indicators for service evaluation (expectations, KPIs, etc.)
- 5.2 Methods for collecting and analyzing data for service evaluation
- 5.3 Results of service evaluation
- 5.4 Lessons learned, critical success factors, and recommendations for large-scale adoption or transferability of the experience to other contexts

Both in specific phases and at the conclusion of the project, each item of the framework (for example, items 1.1 in the Box 1) was evaluated through both quantitative and qualitative assessments. The quantitative evaluations (objective of this study) involved the use of questions rated on a 6-point Likert scale, which are the focus of this project report. These ratings provided a systematic approach to measuring various aspects of the project based on predefined criteria. Each item was assessed on a scale ranging from "Strongly Disagree" to "Strongly Agree", allowing for nuanced feedback and a comprehensive analysis of the project's performance and outcomes.

In addition to the quantitative evaluations, a detailed report was prepared for submission to the Italian Ministry of Health. This report included a thorough qualitative assessment of the project, offering insights into the implementation processes, challenges encountered, and overall effectiveness. It presented a narrative analysis that contextualized the numerical data, providing a richer understanding of the project's impact and contributions.

2.2.2. Tabular Schema of KPIs with the Structure of Assessment

Participants in the project were given the freedom to define specific key performance indicators (KPIs) based on the project's objectives. This approach aligns with the literature review conducted in [23], which emphasizes the importance of tailoring KPIs to the specific goals of each project. A methodology was proposed to assess the applicability or non-applicability of nationally available KPIs, as proposed in a guideline [36] after comprehensive analysis performed by the ISS working group (WP2).

To facilitate this evaluation, a tabular grid was developed, allowing each work package (WP1, 3, 4) involved in project activity to indicate the priority level of the selected KPIs and further feedback This structured approach enabled a systematic comparison and prioritization of KPIs based on their relevance and importance for each component of the project. Each work package could then rate the KPIs using a defined priority scale.

Experts from the project work packages (WP1, WP3, WP4) and the technology assessment work package (WP2) evaluated the applicability of the proposed key performance indicators (KPIs) within the framework of a national guideline [36]. The goal of this evaluation was to assess how well the KPIs align with and support the objectives and standards outlined in the national telemedicine framework.

WP2 was responsible for developing the evaluation tables and specific metrics. The project units, which had defined specific KPIs for their respective areas, provided valuable input based on their practical experience. Their contributions were crucial in evaluating how effectively the proposed standard KPIs could be integrated into their projects and align with national guidelines. This collaborative approach ensured that both theoretical and practical considerations were addressed, leading to a more thorough assessment of the KPIs.

The tabular grid (Table 1) organizes various indicators into categories for evaluating the performance of telemedicine services.

Table 1. Evaluation metrics for telemedicine services: indicator applicability and prioritization by work packages.

Category	(CODE)/Short Key (Italian Tongue)	Indicator	Applicable for WP (YES/NO)—If NO, Propose an Alternative	Priority for WP (1–5, 1 = min; 5 = max)
DIMENSION Volume of services provided				
	(DIM01)/DIM-Dimensione assoluta	Absolute size: number of users followed/12 months		
	(DIM02)/DIM-Dimensione assoluta dinamica	Dynamic aspect of the size indicator: number of users followed in the last 12 months/number of users followed in the previous 12 months		

Table 1. *Cont.*

Category	(CODE)/Short Key (Italian Tongue)	Indicator	Applicable for WP (YES/NO)—If NO, Propose an Alternative	Priority for WP (1–5, 1 = min; 5 = max)
	(DIM03)/DIM-Copertura del target	Target coverage in %: % of users followed compared to the total number of users affected by the service's targeted condition in the area of interest		
	(DIM04)/DIM-Dimensione media	Average size: average number of contacts/month		
	(DIM05/DIM-Dimensione media/utente	Average dimension: average number of contacts per month per user (applicable for telehealth and televisits in telemonitoring)		
CONTINUITY IN TIME Duration and stability of the service				
	(CON01)/CONTIN_TEMP-Durata	Duration: number of months of activity since service activation		
	(CON02)/CONTIN_TEMP-Stabilità	Stability: dispersion indices (e.g., standard deviation, range) of the average dimension indicator over a reference time period		
COMPLEXITY Organizational complexity of the service				
	(COMPL01)/COMPL-Indicatore qualitativo	Qualitative indicator: type of professionals involved in service delivery (GP, specialist doctor, nurse, etc.)		
	(COMPL02)/COMPL-Indicatore quantitativo	Quantitative indicator: number of operators involved in service delivery (person–months)/number of users		
QUALITY Service response standards and performance				
	(QUAL01)/QUAL-Standard di servizio	Service standard: standard response time		
	(QUAL02)/QUAL-Performance di risposta	Response performance: number of services within the standard time		
EFFICIENCY Service cost				
	(EFFI01)/EFFICIEN-Costo totale annuo	Total annual cost of maintaining the service (staff, equipment, etc.)/number of users followed		
EFFECTIVENESS Comparison with the population of users affected by the condition targeted by the telemedicine service but followed in a conventional manner in the area of interest				

Table 1. *Cont.*

Category	(CODE)/Short Key (Italian Tongue)	Indicator	Applicable for WP (YES/NO)—If NO, Propose an Alternative	Priority for WP (1–5, 1 = min; 5 = max)
	(EFFE01)/EFFICA-Riduzione mortalità	Reduction in mortality: % of deaths in the last 12 months among users followed in telemedicine/% of deaths in the last 12 months among users followed in a conventional manner		
	(EFFE02)/EFFICA-Riduzione incidenza re-ospedalizzazioni	Reduction in the incidence of re-hospitalizations among users: % of re-hospitalizations in the last 12 months among users followed in telemedicine/% of re-hospitalizations in the last 12 months among users followed in a conventional manner		
	(EFFE03)/EFFICA-Riduzione n° giorni degenza	Reduction in the number of hospital days: number of hospital days in the last 12 months per user followed in telemedicine/% of hospital days in the last 12 months per user followed in a conventional manner		
	(EFFE04)/EFFICA-Riduzione tempo trascorso in emergenza	Reduction in the time spent by users in emergency services and number of emergency room visits: time (hours) spent in the last 12 months in emergency services per user followed in telemedicine/time (hours) spent in emergency services in the last 12 months per user followed in a conventional manner		
	(EFFE05)/EFFICA-Miglioramento qualità della vita	Improvement in quality of life: standard measures of quality of life, possibly modified ad hoc (e.g., SF health surveys, SF36, SF12 questionnaires)		
USER SATISFACTION User satisfaction (patients and caregivers)				
	(SAT01)/GRADIM-Indicatore qualitativo	Qualitative indicator: specific questionnaires administered to users (patients, caregivers)		
	(SAT02/GRADIM-Drop-out assoluto	Absolute quantitative indicator (drop-out): number of users who voluntarily leave the telemedicine path/12 months (drop-out)		
	(SAT03) GRADIM-Drop-out relativo	Relative quantitative indicator (drop-out): number of users who voluntarily leave the telemedicine path/12 months/number of users followed (drop-out)		

This method ensured a collaborative and thorough approach to KPI selection, allowing each work package to contribute their insights and expertise. The resulting prioritization helped in focusing efforts on the most relevant and impactful KPIs, ultimately enhancing the project's ability to test in a defined national KPI environment.

3. Results

In line with the study's objectives and utilizing the proposed methodology, this section presents the results obtained within the project.

Through the collaboration of all work packages (WP1–WP4), as outlined in Section 2.1 of the project architecture, both the operational units (OUs) focused on specific projects (WP1, WP3, WP4) and the OU (OU2) responsible for technology assessment (TA) contributed to the project's outcomes. These results are reflected in the evaluation of improvements through the framework validated in [34], which is summarized and referenced here, and in the development and application of a KPI evaluation model using defined and adaptable metrics and parameters within the field of telemedicine.

Section 3.1, "*Quantitative Outcomes from the Framework*", details the final assessment of the three projects and the measure of improvement compared to the initial project position.

Section 3.2, "*Quantitative outcome from the Tabular schema and metrics*", focuses on the definition and application of the KPI evaluation model, detailing the metrics and parameters used. The collaborative approach facilitated effective teamwork. The project OUs operate in three distinct areas of telemedicine—diabetes, cardiology, and nephrology—covering significant sectors of fragility and chronic conditions, providing direct experience with the practicality of KPIs. The TA OU offers mediation and connections between the three domains and intervention models.

3.1. Outcome from the Framework

3.1.1. Quantitative Outcome

Framework Development and Iteration:

Each work package (WP1, WP3, WP4) adhered to this framework (see Box 1), ensuring a comprehensive evaluation of every aspect of the telemedicine service. This included its design, which focused on the service's conceptual framework and operational features, its implementation, which assessed the deployment processes, technical integration, user adoption strategies, and its evaluation, which involved analyzing performance metrics, user satisfaction, clinical outcomes, and overall impact. This approach provided a holistic view, ensuring that both the technical and human-centered aspects of the telemedicine service were thoroughly examined to support its optimization and scalability.

After each initial specific framework is developed, it undergoes several rounds of improvement. Each round involves a cycle of feedback and adjustments to refine the content, ensuring that the framework remains aligned with the overall objectives of the project and incorporates any necessary updates.

Review Cycles:

- Round 1: In the first cycle, each partner submits their initial feedback after compiling their part of the framework. This initial round helps identify any gaps or areas that need clarification or improvement.
- Round 2: After modifications are made based on the feedback from Round 1, the revised framework is reviewed again. Partners provide further input, helping to further refine the methodology and the structure of the framework. This round is focused on making sure the framework is comprehensive and that all elements are well defined.
- Round 3: In the final review round, all previous feedback is consolidated, and any remaining issues or inconsistencies are addressed. This round ensures that the framework is finalized and ready for the next steps.

Final Evaluation:

Once the final version of the framework is complete, it undergoes a quantitative evaluation. This evaluation uses a six-level Likert scale (see as an example the explanation in https://uk.surveymonkey.com/mp/likert-scale/ (accessed on 8 January 2025), a commonly used tool to measure responses across different criteria. In this case, all the items of the framework are assessed.

The six-level Likert scale used in the evaluation ranges from one to six, where

- one represents the lowest score (minimum evaluation);
- six represents the highest score (maximum evaluation).

To interpret the results, a satisfaction threshold is defined as

$$\text{Threshold} = \frac{(1+6)}{2} \tag{1}$$

- Scores above 3.5 reflect positive feedback, with satisfaction increasing as values approach six.
- Scores below 3.5 indicate negative feedback, with dissatisfaction intensifying as values approach one.

The evaluation was conducted systematically across all sheets and their respective items. For illustration, Box 2 highlights the items for sheet 4 assessed by means of the Likert scale.

During each iteration (as explained later), the ISS team performed both analytical and qualitative evaluations using the six-level Likert scale for individual items (e.g., 4.1–4.6). Following this process, an audit feedback report was generated to summarize the findings and provide constructive recommendations.

Box 2. Sheet 4 with the single items assessed using the six-level Likert scale.

4. Adoption of the Telemedicine Service or Suite of Telemedicine Services:

- 4.1 Criteria and procedures for service activation and management
- 4.2 Methods and indicators for monitoring service quality and minimum performance thresholds (service level agreement)
- 4.3 Service pricing and cost-sharing rules
- 4.4 Change management
- 4.5 Activation date of the telemedicine service or suite
- 4.6 Volume of services delivered

Reporting:

The evaluations and measurements were conducted by a team of four experts from WP2, ensuring a comprehensive and objective assessment aligned with the project's objectives.

All experts from WP2 at the ISS brought extensive expertise in technology assessment and had significant experience in health technology assessment (HTA) across multiple domains. Their competencies spanned regulatory aspects, medical devices, and economic and social considerations, ensuring a multidimensional and robust evaluation process.

After the final evaluation is completed, an analytical report is prepared based on the final version of the framework and the feedback received throughout the review cycles. This report synthesizes the evaluation results and outlines key findings, areas for improvement, and recommendations for future adjustments. The report is then submitted to funding and supervising bodies for further review and to ensure that the project aligns with its intended goals.

In summary, this process ensures that the framework is constantly refined through a series of feedback loops, with partners working together to improve its quality. The iterative nature of this approach helps to identify and address issues early, ensuring that the final framework is a robust and effective tool for assessing telemedicine services. The quantitative evaluation provides an objective measure of its effectiveness, while the final reporting ensures transparency and accountability to the funding and supervising bodies.

Figure 2 illustrates the original butterfly diagram in Italian, serving as an example of the evaluation for one work package (WP) based on the six items in sheet 4 during the final round. This statistical graphical tool provides a clear representation of the evaluation outcomes, highlighting both the high level of acceptance and the absence of a tail below zero for any item.

The butterfly diagram, characterized by its symmetrical layout, displays the distribution of responses for each item on a Likert scale, with positive evaluations represented on one side and negative evaluations on the other. The absence of a negative tail indicates that no item received scores falling below the threshold of 3.5, underscoring the overall positive reception.

This visualization is particularly useful in showcasing the convergence of evaluations, as it emphasizes not only the collective agreement on the high scores but also the uniformity in the positive assessment across all items. Such a tool aids in effectively communicating the results, ensuring clarity for stakeholders and facilitating informed decision-making.

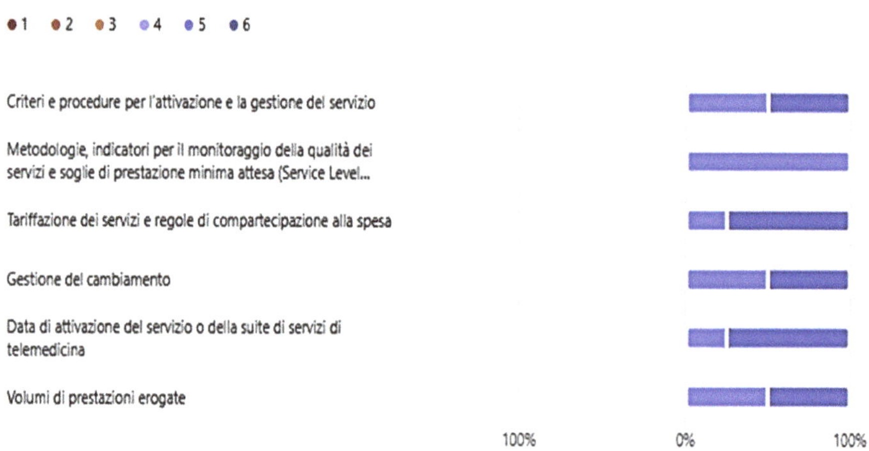

Figure 2. Original butterfly diagram in Italian tongue (see box 2 for the English translation) of one WP evaluation results for sheet 4 in the final round reported as an example.

A similar situation was consistently observed across all five sheets and throughout the three project work packages (WPs). In each case, the evaluations demonstrated a high level of acceptance, with no significant deviations or negative assessments noted for any of the items analyzed. This uniformity across the various WPs highlights the robustness and effectiveness of the methodological approach employed, ensuring that the framework adequately addresses the unique requirements and objectives of each WP while maintaining a cohesive and systematic evaluation process.

Table 2 presents the average scores recorded for each sheet, along with the average improvement compared to the first evaluation round.

Table 2. Average score recorded for each sheet and average increase compared to the first round. The data pertain to all projects (WP1, WP3, WP4) as a whole.

Sheet	Average Score at the End of the Evaluation Process (Round 3)	Average Increase Compared to the Initial Evaluation (Round 1)
No. 1: Personal Data of the Telemedicine Service or Suite of...	5.6	Δ = 1.8
No. 2: Strategic Framework of the Telemedicine Service or Suite of...	5.2	Δ = 1.9
No. 3: Design and Implementation of the Telemedicine Service or Suite of...	5.2	Δ = 1.9
No. 4: Adoption of the Telemedicine Service or Suite of...	5.3	Δ = 2.0
No. 5: Evaluation of the Telemedicine Service or Suite of...	5.3	Δ = 2.1

The data pertains to all WPs (WP1, WP3, WP4) as a whole. The iterative and collaborative nature of this process ensures that the framework continuously evolves to meet the project's needs and expectations effectively.

3.1.2. Further Qualitative Considerations

Family involvement is essential in managing chronic conditions through telemedicine. In cases of chronic kidney failure, telemedicine provides families with tools to assist in managing dialysis, fluid balance, and dietary restrictions, enabling better at-home care and reducing hospital admissions. For type 2 diabetes, it supports families in monitoring blood glucose levels, ensuring medication adherence, and adopting necessary lifestyle changes, leading to improved blood sugar control and fewer complications. In chronic heart failure, telemedicine enhances family participation in tracking symptoms, adhering to treatments, and promoting healthier habits, resulting in better overall condition management.

By offering remote monitoring, real-time access to healthcare professionals, and continuous education, telemedicine empowers families to actively engage in the care process. This involvement improves disease control, minimizes hospitalizations, and enhances patient satisfaction, ultimately leading to a higher quality of life for patients and their families.

However, considering the specific focus of our study, it is important to highlight how the framework, with its tailored items, has contributed and can continue to contribute in these critical areas. Through a structured approach, the framework facilitated a comprehensive understanding of how telemedicine services can support the involvement of families in managing chronic conditions, such as chronic kidney failure, type 2 diabetes, and chronic heart failure.

In the results, it is crucial to highlight that the framework, especially through Sheet No. 2: Strategic Framework of the Telemedicine Service or Suite of Telemedicine Services, has significantly contributed to improving the management of patients with chronic conditions, such as chronic kidney failure, type 2 diabetes, and chronic heart failure, within the family setting. The framework facilitated a deeper understanding of the essential role that families play in managing these complex health conditions. It emphasized that by promoting a greater involvement of family members, telemedicine services can improve patient outcomes and the effectiveness of daily disease management. The framework's design, by focusing on both patients and their families, helped ensure that family members were equipped with the tools and knowledge needed to support patients in managing their conditions at home.

The SWOT analysis (Box 1, item 2.1) conducted within the framework revealed gaps in the traditional healthcare system, particularly in the support for families in managing chronic diseases. It highlighted that prior to the introduction of telemedicine services, there was often inadequate support for families, who are crucial in ensuring adherence to treatment and making necessary lifestyle changes. By identifying these gaps, the framework underscored the potential of telemedicine to directly address these issues and improve family involvement in patient care. This helped improve the daily management of patients with chronic kidney failure, type 2 diabetes, and chronic heart failure by providing families with remote monitoring, education, and guidance.

The section on care needs addressed by the telemedicine service (Box 1 item 2.2) further showed how the service was tailored to meet both the patient's and the family's needs. With telemedicine, families received real-time access to healthcare professionals, educational resources, and reminders about the patient's care plan, which greatly improved their capacity to manage the disease. This functionality ensured that families could monitor patients' health on a daily basis, reinforcing the family's active role in disease management. By addressing these needs, the framework helped to ensure that the families were better prepared to manage their loved ones' conditions, ultimately leading to improvements in patient outcomes.

In the functional description (Box 1 item 2.3), the framework described how the telemedicine service was designed to support both patients and their families. It provided families with easy access to remote consultations, health monitoring tools, and personalized health advice. The framework emphasized that these features were essential in helping families manage the daily care of patients, particularly those with chronic kidney failure, type 2 diabetes, and chronic heart failure. By strengthening the communication between healthcare providers and families, telemedicine services directly contributed to improving the quality of care at home and ensuring more effective disease management.

The target population and therapeutic and socio-economic indications (Box 1 item 2.4) reinforced that the telemedicine service was specifically designed for patients with chronic diseases and their families. The framework recognized that the involvement of family members was critical to achieving positive health outcomes. By targeting families of patients with chronic kidney failure, type 2 diabetes, and chronic heart failure, the telemedicine service ensured that those responsible for daily care were given the support needed to manage their loved one's condition more effectively. This strategic focus on families helped to improve their engagement in healthcare decision-making and better adherence to care plans, resulting in better long-term health outcomes.

Finally, the section on evidence from the scientific literature (Box 1 item 2.5) highlighted the growing body of research that supports family-centered care as an essential component of managing chronic diseases. The framework incorporated evidence showing that when families are actively involved in the care process, patients experience improved adherence to treatment, better management of lifestyle changes, and reduced healthcare utilization. Telemedicine services, as outlined in the framework, directly facilitated this by providing continuous support, education, and monitoring, ensuring that families had the resources they needed to manage their loved ones' conditions effectively.

Overall, the framework has played a pivotal role in improving the daily management of patients with chronic kidney failure, type 2 diabetes, and chronic heart failure, particularly through enhancing family involvement. By identifying and addressing the specific needs of families, the framework has helped ensure that families are empowered to manage their loved ones' health at home. Through improved communication, education, and real-time monitoring, the telemedicine service has contributed to better disease management, improved patient outcomes, and increased satisfaction among both patients and their families. This comprehensive approach has had a lasting impact on chronic disease management, reinforcing the importance of family-centered care in improving health outcomes.

3.2. *Quantitative Outcome from the Tabular Schema of KPIs and Metrics*

Participants in the project were given the freedom to define specific key performance indicators (KPIs) based on the project's objectives (WP1, WP3, WP4). This approach aligns with the literature review conducted in [35], which emphasizes the importance of tailoring KPIs to the specific goals of each project.

In addition to this, experts from the project work packages (WP1, WP3, WP4) and the technology assessment (WP2) assessed the applicability of proposed KPIs within the framework of a national guideline [36], and this is the true outcome of this study aligned with the objectives. This evaluation aimed to determine how effectively these KPIs align with and support the objectives and standards set out in the national telemedicine framework.

WP2 developed the evaluation tables (Table 1) and the metrics described below. In this process, the project units (WP1, WP3, WP4), which had established specific KPIs for their own areas according to the literature trends [35], contributed their practical experience and project-specific insights assessing the set reported in [36].

Their involvement was important for evaluating how well the proposed KPIs fit within the context of their own projects and the national guidelines.

To assess the applicability of the proposed KPIs [36] in Table 1, we decided to develop and implement specific metrics that would allow for precise and large-scale quantification. These metrics are designed to provide a standardized and objective method for evaluating the relevance, applicability, and priority of each KPI within the context of the telemedicine project, ensuring a thorough and systematic assessment process.

The following parameters reported in Table 3 have been defined to assess the applicability and priority of KPIs based on the guidelines [36]:

Table 3. The proposed metrics for assessing the applicability and priority of KPIs.

Parameter	Description
A-match-KPI	This parameter indicates the amount of KPIs in the guidelines deemed applicable.
A-match-KPI by category	This parameter indicates the amount of applicable KPIs within each category of the guidelines.
Priority-KPI	This parameter assigns a priority score to the applicable KPIs.
Priority-KPI by category	This parameter assigns a priority score to the applicable KPIs within each category.
Distance-from-GL-KPI	Considering that the KPIs proposed in the guidelines have a conventional priority of three (medium priority), this parameter expresses the signed distance (based on the assigned priority) from the KPIs proposed in the guidelines.
Distance-from-GL-KPI by category	Considering that the KPIs proposed in the guidelines have a conventional priority of three (medium priority), this parameter expresses the signed distance (based on the assigned priority) from the KPIs proposed in the guidelines, categorized by each category.

The next sections report the applicability and priority (Table 4) assigned by each project and the outcomes (Tables 5–10) based on the metrics assigned in Table 3. *We have chosen to anonymize the projects; thus, Prg1–Prg3 do not directly correspond to WP1-3. This choice is made because there is no direct correlation between the applicability/priority of a KPI and the quality of a specific project activity, as it merely reflects the KPI's suitability within the project context.*

Table 4. Applicability and priority assigned by a single project.

Category	CODE	Indicator	Applicability Score (max = 3 When All the Projects are Applicable; min = 0—When All the Projects Are Not Applicable)	Priority Prg1	Priority Prg2	Priority Prg3
DIMENSION Volume of services provided	DIM01	Absolute size: number of users followed/12 months	2	1	4	5
	DIM02	Dynamic aspect of the size indicator: number of users followed in the last 12 months/number of users followed in the previous 12 months	1	1	5	1
	DIM03	Target coverage in %: % of users followed compared to the total number of users affected by the service's targeted condition in the area of interest	1	1	1	5
	DIM04	Average size: average number of contacts/month	2	1	3	3
	DIM05	Average dimension: average number of contacts per month per user (applicable for telehealth and televisits in telemonitoring)	2	1	4	3
CONTINUITY IN TIME Duration and stability of the service	CON01	Duration: number of months of activity since service activation	3	3	3	4
	CON02	Stability: dispersion indices (e.g., standard deviation, range) of the average dimension indicator over a reference time period	2	3	1	4
COMPLEXITY Organizational complexity of the service	COMPL01	Qualitative indicator: type of professionals involved in service delivery (GP, specialist doctor, nurse, etc.)	3	5	2	4
	COMPL02	Quantitative indicator: number of operators involved in service delivery (person–months)/ number of users	2	5	5	4
QUALITY Service response standards and performance	QUAL01	Service standard: standard response time	2	3	1	3
	QUAL02	Response performance: number of services within the standard time	2	3	1	3
EFFICIENCY Service cost	EFFI01	Total annual cost of maintaining the service (staff, equipment, etc.)/number of users followed	2	5	5	4
EFFECTIVENESS Comparison with the population of users affected by the condition targeted by the telemedicine service but followed in a conventional manner in the area of interest	EFFE01	Reduction in mortality: % of deaths in the last 12 months among users followed in telemedicine/% of deaths in the last 12 months among users followed in a conventional manner	0	1	4	1

Table 4. *Cont.*

Category	CODE	Indicator	Applicability Score (max = 3 When All the Projects are Applicable; min = 0—When All the Projects Are Not Applicable)	Priority Prg1	Priority Prg2	Priority Prg3
	EFFE02	Reduction in the incidence of re-hospitalizations among users: % of re-hospitalizations in the last 12 months among users followed in telemedicine/% of re-hospitalizations in the last 12 months among users followed in a conventional manner	1	1	4	4
	EFFE03	Reduction in the number of hospital days: number of hospital days in the last 12 months per user followed in telemedicine/% of hospital days in the last 12 months per user followed in a conventional manner	0	1	4	1
	EFFE04	Reduction in the time spent by users in emergency services and number of emergency room visits: time (hours) spent in the last 12 months in emergency services per user followed in telemedicine/time (hours) spent in emergency services in the last 12 months per user followed in a conventional manner	0	1	4	1
	EFFE05	Improvement in quality of life: standard measures of quality of life, possibly modified ad hoc (e.g., SF health surveys, SF36, SF12 questionnaires)	1	1	4	5
USER SATISFACTION User satisfaction (patients and caregivers)	SAT01	Qualitative indicator: specific questionnaires administered to users (patients, caregivers)	3	1	4	5
	SAT02	Absolute quantitative indicator (drop-out): number of users who voluntarily leave the telemedicine path/12 months (drop-out)	2	5	5	5
	SAT03	Relative quantitative indicator (drop-out): number of users who voluntarily leave the telemedicine path/ 12 months/number of users followed (drop-out)	2	1	5	5

Table 5. The number of KPIs in the guidelines deemed applicable across different projects.

Project	A-Match-KPI
Prg1	8
Prg2	9
Prg3	16

Table 6. The number of applicable KPIs within each category of the guidelines for each project.

Category	CODES	A-Match-KPI-by-Categ Prg1	A-match-KPI-by-Categ Prg2	A-Match-KPI-by-Categ Prg3
DIM—5 indicators	DIM01-DIM05	0/5	4/5	4/5
CONTIN_TEMP—2 indicators	CON01-CON02	2/2	1/2	2/2
COMPL—2 indicators	COMPL01-COMPL02	2/2	1/2	2/2
QUAL—2 indicators	QUAL01-02	2/2	0/2	2/2
EFFICIEN—1 indicator	EFFI01	1/1	0/1	1/1
EFFECTIVENESS—5 indicators	EFFE01-05	0/5	0/5	2/5
SATISFACTION—3 indicators	SAT01-03	1/3	3/3	3/3

Table 7. The priority scores assigned to the applicable KPIs for each project.

Project	Priority-KPI
Prg1	32/100
Prg2	36/100
Prg3	66/100

Table 8. The priority scores assigned to the applicable KPIs within each category for each project.

Category	CODES	Priority-KPI-by-Categ Prg1	Priority-KPI-by-Categ Prg2	Priority-KPI-by-Categ Prg3
DIM (max value = 5 × 5 indicators = 25)	DIM01-DIM05	NA/25	16/25	16/25
CONTIN_TEMP (max value = 5 × 2 indicators = 10)	CON01-CON02	6/10	3/10	8/10
COMPL (max value = 5 × 2 indicators = 10)	COMPL01-COMPL02	10/10	2/10	8/10
QUAL (max value = 5 × 2 indicators = 10)	QUAL01-02	6/10	NA/10	6/10
EFFICIEN (max value = 5 × 1 indicator = 5)	EFFI01	5/5	5/5	4/5
EFFICACY (max value = 5 × 5 indicators = 25)	EFFE01-05	NA/25	NA/25	9/25
SATISFACTION (max value = 5 × 3 indicators = 15)	SAT01-03	5/15	15/15	15/15

Table 9. The signed distance of the applied KPIs from the conventional priority (priority = 3) proposed in the guidelines.

Project	Distance-KPI (Average Value = 3 × 20 Indicators = 60)
Prg1	32–60 = −28
Prg2	36–60 = −24
Prg3	66–60 = 6

Table 10. The signed distance of the applied KPIs from the conventional priority (priority = 3) proposed in the guidelines, categorized by each category.

Category	CODES	Distance-KPI-by-Categ (Average Value) Prg1	Distance-KPI-by-Categ (Average Value) Prg2	Distance-KPI-by-Categ (Average Value) Prg3
DIM (average value = 3 × 5 indicators = 15)	DIM01-DIM05	NA	16–15 = 1	16–15 = 1
CONTIN_TEMP (average value = 3 × 2 indicators = 6)	CON01-CON02	6–6 = 0	3–6 = −3	8–6 = 2
COMPL (average value = 3 × 2 indicators = 6)	COMPL01-COMPL02	10–6 = 4	2–6 = −4	8–6 = 2
QUAL (average value = 3 × 2 indicators = 6)	QUAL01-02	6–6 = 0	NA	6–6 = 0
EFFICIEN (average value = 3 × 1 indicator = 3)	EFFI01	5–3 = 2	5–3 = 2	4–3 = 1
EFFICACY (average value = 3 × 5 indicators = 15)	EFFE01-05	NA	NA	9–15 = −6
SATISFACTION (average value = 3 × 3 indicators = 9)	SAT01-03	5–9 = −4	15–9 = 6	15–9 = 6

Figure 3 shows a representation with a radar chart associated with the priority of the KPIs. For each KPI, both the CODE and the short keys in Italian defined in Table 1 are reported.

From the table, the following considerations emerge:

All DIMENSION indicators are considered applicable, but not all have been assigned the same priority. In an observational project with few participants, it is logical that DIMENSION indicators have a low priority. Given the highly innovative and complex setting, higher priority was assigned to the COMPLEXITY of service delivery, as well as to EFFICIENCY and SATISFACTION indicators.

However, some DIMENSION indicators are not applicable in certain study contexts. For instance, the "Target coverage in %" indicator is not relevant for a pilot service available only in specific areas of the region. Similarly, the "Dynamic aspect of the dimension indicator" cannot be applied in a project with a limited duration. It was also suggested that the "average number of contacts/month" indicator, which is considered applicable, can help evaluate the resources (time, professionals, etc.) needed to support the offered service.

For TEMPORAL CONTINUITY, the most applicable indicator is the duration indicator, which received an equal priority score of four alongside another indicator.

For COMPLEXITY (organizational complexity of the service), the most applicable indicator is the qualitative one, specifying the types of professionals involved in service delivery. Both complexity indicators received the highest priority score of five.

For SERVICE QUALITY, both proposed indicators are applicable and, when applicable, are considered with medium priority (score of three). They are not applicable in real-time response scenarios.

In one project, the proposed EFFICIENCY indicator ("Total annual cost") is not applicable because it is managed by central management control rather than the project team. When applicable, this efficiency indicator is considered to be of high priority (scores of 4–5).

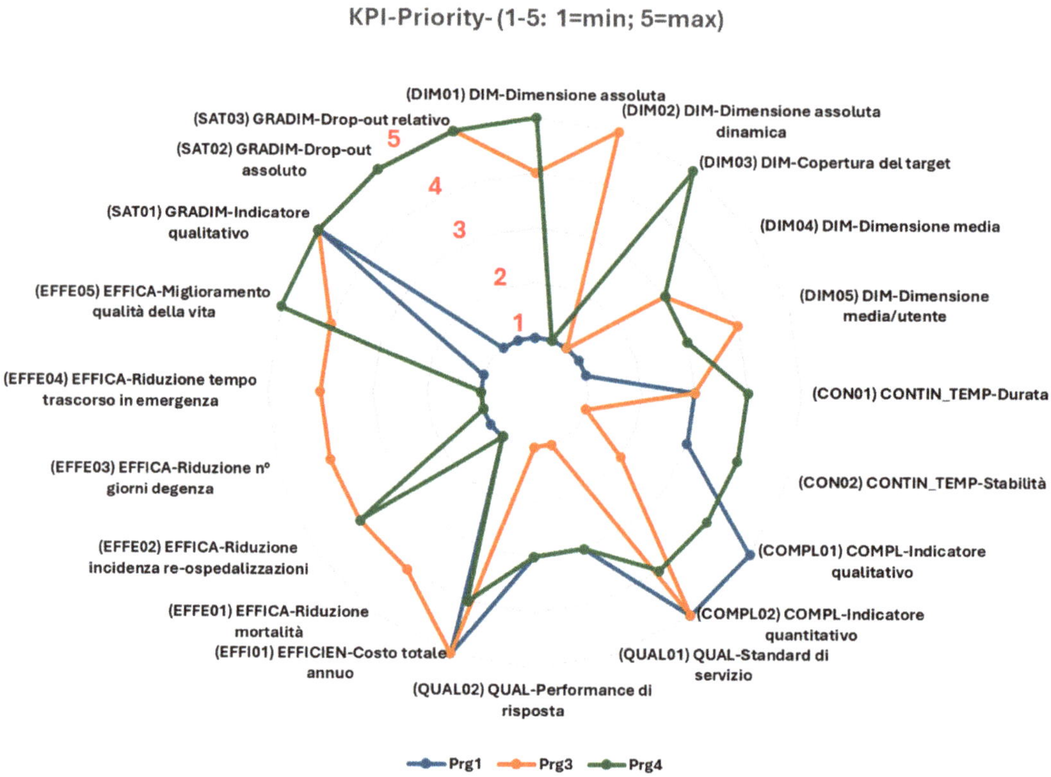

Figure 3. Radar diagram of the assigned priority to the KPIs in each project represented with a different color. Both the CODE and the short description in Italian are reported.

EFFECTIVENESS indicators were mostly deemed not applicable across projects due to their unsuitability for feasibility studies or pilot projects with a limited number of participants. Although not applicable, these indicators received varied priorities depending on the nature of the telemedicine project, with priority 1 for feasibility studies and high priority (4–5) for studies where they are applicable with large numbers. It was noted that the "Improvement in quality of life" indicator was considered to be of high priority (4–5), emphasizing the importance of evaluating whether telemedicine use satisfies the user. If the quality of life does not improve or remain stable, even with cost savings, the service might not be a viable alternative to conventional methods.

In all three projects, a SATISFACTION indicator was considered applicable. The qualitative indicator was the most applicable and received the highest priority (score of five). It was noted that the "Qualitative indicator" provides crucial feedback for building and implementing the service in a real-world context. Meanwhile, the "Absolute quantitative indicator (Drop-Out)" is essential for ensuring the validity of study results and understanding which types of users are less inclined to use telemedicine.

Table 5 reports the number of KPIs in the guidelines deemed applicable across different projects. This table provides an overview of how well each project aligns with the KPIs outlined in the guidelines, showing the overall applicability of the KPIs in each project. The values indicate the extent to which the KPIs recommended in the guidelines are considered relevant and implementable for each project.

Table 6 reports the number of applicable KPIs within each category of the guidelines for each project. This table offers a detailed breakdown of KPI applicability by category, allowing for a more granular view of how well KPIs within specific categories align with the guidelines across different projects. It highlights which categories are better represented and which may require additional focus.

Table 7 reports the priority scores assigned to the applicable KPIs for each project. This table assigns a priority score to each KPI based on its relevance and importance for the project, reflecting how critical each KPI is considered in the context of achieving project goals. It helps in identifying which KPIs are prioritized within each project.

Table 8 reports the priority scores assigned to the applicable KPIs within each category for each project. This table provides insights into the prioritization of KPIs within specific categories, indicating how each category's KPIs are valued in the context of each project. It highlights the relative importance of KPIs within different categories.

Table 9 reports the signed distance of the applied KPIs from the conventional priority (priority = 3) proposed in the guidelines. This parameter expresses how the priority of the KPIs used in each project deviates from the conventional medium priority (3) set in the guidelines. The signed distance indicates whether the priorities are higher or lower compared to the guideline's standard.

Table 10 reports the signed distance of the applied KPIs from the conventional priority (priority = 3) proposed in the guidelines, categorized by each category. This table provides a category-specific view of how the priorities of KPIs in each category deviate from the conventional medium priority (3). It helps to understand deviations in priority on a more granular level, focusing on specific categories within the projects.

This structured approach helps to understand not only the applicability of KPIs but also their prioritization and how closely they align with the guidelines in different project contexts.

Specific considerations

Based on Table 5 that reports the number of KPIs from the guidelines that are deemed applicable across different projects, the following consideration emerges: specifically, Project Prg3 shows the highest applicability with 16 KPIs applicable, indicating that a greater proportion of the recommended KPIs are relevant and can be implemented in this project. In contrast, Project Prg1 shows the lowest applicability, with eight KPIs applicable, suggesting that fewer of the KPIs from the guidelines are considered relevant or feasible in this context. This variation highlights how different projects may vary in terms of the suitability of the KPIs.

By examining the number of applicable KPIs within each category (Table 6), it is possible to identify areas of strength and those requiring additional focus. For example, in Project Prg1, the DIM (dimension) category shows no applicable indicators, while the CONTIN_TEMP (temporal continuity) and COMPL (complexity) categories are better represented. In Project Prg2, the EFFICIEN (efficiency) and EFFECTIVENESS (efficacy) categories have fewer applicable indicators, whereas Project Prg3 shows higher applicability across most categories. This breakdown helps pinpoint which categories of KPIs are effectively addressed and which need further attention in each project.

Table 7 reports the priority scores assigned to the applicable KPIs for each project. This table reflects the relative importance of each KPI in the context of achieving project goals, as assessed through a priority scoring system. A higher priority score indicates that the KPIs are deemed more critical to the project's success. For example, Project Prg3 has the highest priority score of 66 out of 100, suggesting that the KPIs selected for this project are considered highly important for achieving its objectives. Conversely, Projects Prg1 and Prg2 have lower priority scores (32 and 36, respectively), indicating a relatively lower emphasis on these proposed KPIs in those projects.

Table 8 presents the priority scores assigned to the applicable KPIs within each category for each project. This table offers insights into how KPIs are prioritized within specific categories. It shows how each category's KPIs are valued in the context of the project, providing a clear picture of which categories are receiving more focus and which are less prioritized. For instance, Project Prg3 assigns the highest priority to the COMPL (complexity) and CONTIN_TEMP (temporal continuity) categories, while the DIM (dimension) and QUAL (quality) categories receive varying levels of attention. This categorization helps in understanding which aspects of the project are considered most crucial according to the priority scores.

Table 9 reports the signed distance of the applied KPIs from the conventional priority level set by the guidelines (priority = 3). This parameter indicates how the priority of the KPIs in each project deviates from the medium priority standard established in the guidelines. Positive distances suggest that the KPIs are prioritized higher than the conventional level, while negative distances indicate a lower prioritization. For example, Project Prg3 has a positive signed distance (+6), implying that the KPIs in this project are considered more critical than the medium priority level. In contrast, Projects Prg1 and Prg2 have negative distances (−28 and −24, respectively), reflecting a lower priority alignment compared to the standard.

Table 10 shows the signed distance of the applied KPIs from the conventional priority, categorized by each KPI category. This table provides a detailed view of how the priorities of KPIs in each category deviate from the medium priority level set by the guidelines. It helps to understand deviations in priority on a more granular level. For example, the DIM (dimension) category in Project Prg3 shows a positive distance of +1, suggesting a slight increase in priority compared to the medium level. Conversely, the EFFICACY (efficacy) category in Prg3 shows a significant negative distance (−6), indicating a much lower prioritization relative to the guidelines. This category-specific analysis allows for a deeper understanding of how different aspects of the projects align with or diverge from the guideline priorities.

Overall, this structured approach provides a comprehensive understanding of KPIs proposed in [29], encompassing applicability and prioritization across different projects. By examining the overall applicability, category-specific applicability, priority scores, and deviations from the conventional priorities, stakeholders can gain valuable insights into how well the KPIs proposed align with the guidelines and how they are prioritized within each project context. This detailed analysis helps in assessing the effectiveness of the KPI framework and identifying areas for improvement in aligning with the guidelines.

General Comment

The results presented in the tables provide valuable insights into the applicability and prioritization of KPIs across different projects. Analyzing the data reveals the following key observations:

1. Applicability and alignment: The varying numbers of applicable KPIs across projects, as shown in Table 5, indicate that each project aligns differently with the guidelines. Projects like Prg3 demonstrate higher applicability, suggesting a stronger alignment with the recommended KPIs, while others, such as Prg1 and Prg2, show lower applicability. This disparity highlights the need for further tuning of the KPI selection process to ensure that the KPIs are better tailored to the specific contexts of each project.
2. Category-specific insights: The detailed breakdown of KPI applicability by category in Table 6 shows that certain categories, like DIM (dimension) and QUAL (quality),

are not consistently well represented across all projects. This suggests that specific KPIs within these categories may need to be adjusted or more carefully selected to improve their relevance and effectiveness in different project settings.

3. Priority scores and deviations: The priority scores reported in Tables 7 and 8 indicate how critical each KPI is considered within the projects. The discrepancies between the assigned priority scores and the conventional priority levels (as shown in Tables 9 and 10) suggest that there are significant deviations in how KPIs are prioritized. Some projects prioritize KPIs more highly than the conventional medium level, while others fall short. This underscores the need for a reassessment of KPI priorities to ensure they accurately reflect the project's goals and context.
4. Need for tuning: Overall, the results point to a need for tuning the KPI framework to better fit the specific needs of each project. The variation in applicability and priority highlights that a one-size-fits-all approach may not be optimal. Instead, a more tailored approach that considers the unique characteristics and requirements of each project could lead to more effective KPI implementation and evaluation.

In summary, while the analysis provides a comprehensive overview of KPI applicability and prioritization, it also underscores the necessity for refining the KPI selection and prioritization processes. Adjusting and tuning specific KPIs to better align with project goals and contexts will enhance their relevance and utility, ultimately contributing to more successful project outcomes.

4. Discussion

The Telemechron project strategically targets the management of chronic kidney failure, chronic heart failure with comorbidities, and type 2 diabetes mellitus—conditions that not only pose significant health risks but are often accompanied by additional frailties, making their management even more complex. The project underscores the importance of addressing these intertwined chronic conditions and associated frailties, as they require continuous monitoring and multifaceted care strategies. Telemedicine plays a crucial role in this context by offering remote monitoring and timely interventions, which are essential for managing both the primary conditions and their complementary frailties. This approach not only enhances patient outcomes but also helps reduce the burden on healthcare systems by minimizing hospital visits and improving resource allocation. As the project nears its conclusion, the study has focused on the following key areas: sharing detailed insights into the project's structure, analyzing and quantifying improvements in TA practices (*first point of view*), and examining the effectiveness and limitations of KPIs (*second point of view*). By addressing these complex chronic conditions and their related frailties, the Telemechron project highlights the transformative potential of telemedicine in making healthcare more efficient, accessible, and patient-centered.

The discussion is structured into the following four sections:

Section 4.1 "Framing the Contribution of This Study Within the Telemechron Project"

This section contextualizes the study's role in advancing the Telemechron project by highlighting the integration of efforts from all operational units (OUs) and work packages (WPs). It also uses flowcharts to illustrate how the study is positioned within the project's activities and its previous dissemination efforts.

Section 4.2 "Output from the Two Points of View"

This section examines the results derived from the study's analysis of two critical perspectives. It discusses the outcomes from the application of the technology assessment tool and the intervention model for KPIs, providing insights into the metrics and parameters used.

Section 4.3 "Expanded Considerations on the Telemechron Framework for Telemedicine"

This section provides an expanded analysis of the Telemechron project's multidimensional framework, highlighting its innovative approach to telemedicine integration and evaluation.

Section 4.4 "Work in Progress and Suggestions for Future Investigations"

This section reviews the status of the project and outlines areas for future research. It offers recommendations for refining KPI models, integrating advanced technologies, and conducting comparative studies to enhance the overall evaluation framework.

4.1. Framing the Contribution of This Study Within the Telemechron Project

This proposed study serves as a significant contribution from the collaborative efforts of the entire workgroup, which consists of four operational units (OUs) assigned to the four distinct work packages (WPs) of the project. It is specifically focused on technology assessment (TA) and the applicable key performance indicators (KPIs) within the Telemechron project. Highlighting the journey to this project output is crucial, as it is encapsulated in a scientific article.

This contribution was made possible by two critical ongoing *review studies*—one focused on TA [33] and another on KPIs [35]—both conducted by OU 2/WP2. These studies were essential in aligning with the project's goals and in the validation of a pivotal tool, the framework [34], which was conducted by OU 2/WP2. *The review study* on TA [33] was fundamental in pinpointing the appropriate TA framework tool, which was subsequently validated [34] and applied in this project output article.

Similarly, *the review study* on KPIs was indispensable for addressing the nuances of TM metrics within the project and identifying robust metric models. The scientific article we present provides a comprehensive final assessment based on the established framework and introduces a thoroughly evaluated set of proposed KPIs. It elaborates on and applies well-defined parameters for a model of intervention, specifically focusing on the selection and definition of KPIs. This study involved all four OUs/WPs, ensuring a holistic and integrated approach to the assessment through the use of innovative and precisely defined parameters. This detailed methodology ensures that the project's objectives are met with high accuracy and efficiency, providing in-depth insights into the effectiveness and impact of the Telemechron project.

The study presented here constitutes a project report that examines *two key points of view* of technology assessment within the context of telemedicine development. The *first point of view* revolves around the use of a framework introduced in the national Telemechron project [34]. This framework, designed to systematically evaluate telemedicine applications, is based on a comprehensive dossier provided to project partners. This dossier underwent several rounds of review and audit to ensure its robustness and relevance. The report details the final assessment of this framework with a quantitative approach, offering insights into its effectiveness in guiding the evaluation and implementation of telemedicine solutions.

The *second point of view* involved also presenting a set of KPIs to the partners, derived from a nationally relevant document [36]. These KPIs were organized in a tabular format to facilitate their assessment. The purpose of this exercise was to evaluate the applicability of these KPIs to the telemedicine model implemented across three major chronic conditions. This analysis seeks to understand how a generic set of KPIs aligns with or deviates from the specific requirements of telemedicine applications in chronic disease management.

This *second point of view* should be considered using the following three important factors:

1. Framework design and KPI development: The framework required partners to create and propose specific KPIs tailored to their telemedicine applications. These KPIs

were critically assessed within the technology assessment framework and received highly favorable evaluations. This indicates that the framework not only provided a structured approach for assessment but also facilitated the development of relevant and actionable KPIs.

2. Scientific trends and literature review: A review of the scientific literature conducted as part of the project highlighted a trend towards the creation of specific targeted KPIs that align with the unique aspects of telemedicine and its application domains [35]. This trend underscores the need for KPIs that are closely tied to the specific contexts and objectives of telemedicine initiatives rather than relying on generic metrics.
3. Diverse focuses in KPI design: An analysis of national and international reference documents [37–41] shows that different entities prioritize various aspects in their KPI design and proposals. For instance, international organizations such as the WHO [37] and national bodies like the NHS [40] or ATA [38] have different focal points depending on their healthcare system visions and objectives. This variation reflects the broader debate on how to best measure and assess telemedicine effectiveness in different healthcare settings and for diverse patient populations.

4.2. Output from the Two Point of Views

The added value from *the first point of view* of the study is a quantitative final assessment within a telemedicine project, measuring improvement from initial conditions in line with the true and current objective of the study. This includes the demonstrated utility of the proposed tool for technology assessment in the field of telemedicine. All of this has been achieved through a dedicated tool, the framework described and validated in [34].

This technology assessment tool has enabled an evaluation of telemedicine services by providing a comprehensive overview of the service, including its scope, features, and functionalities. It assesses how well the service aligns with strategic goals and integrates with existing healthcare systems. Additionally, the tool reviews the quality of the service's design and the effectiveness of its implementation strategies. It assesses the level of acceptance and usage among patients and healthcare providers and measures performance against established metrics and standards. *Overall, the tool demonstrates its effectiveness by delivering tangible improvements across these areas, offering a structured approach to enhance and optimize telemedicine services.* The framework's strengths are its flexibility and adaptability, which are crucial for assessing various telemedicine contexts. This need for a versatile model aligns with findings from multiple studies and reviews on technology assessment, including Mackintosh et al.'s emphasis on integrating telemedicine with clinical decision support systems [1], Doupi's focus on comprehensive evaluation in health informatics [42], and Ekeland and Grøttland's patient-centered approach using the MAST model [43]. These insights, alongside earlier studies by Giansanti et al. [44,45], underscore the importance of a flexible and systematic evaluation framework that addresses diverse needs and contexts effectively.

The results from the *second point of view* investigated have provided insights into the applicability and limitations of a general set of key performance indicators (KPIs) proposed based on a nationally relevant document [36].

This *second point of view* highlights the following three specific added values:

1. *Evaluation Model and Framework*
   The first added value is the proposed evaluation model based on a schema (Table 1). This schema starts with indicators derived from a national Italian guideline (*columns #1, #2, #3*) and offers an intervention and analysis framework (*columns #4 and #5*). Although this schema is grounded in a national guideline, it can serve as a universal

evaluation model. It is adaptable, allowing for the replacement of categories and dimensions with those from other reference documents as needed. This flexibility ensures that the model remains relevant across various contexts and settings.

2. *Defined Metrics for Applicability*
The second added value is the set of defined metrics (see Table 3) used to assess the applicability and applicability rate of the proposed KPI set. While these metrics are applied within a national context, they possess generalizability and can be utilized with any KPI set derived from other national or international documents. This feature enhances the model's versatility, allowing it to be adapted for diverse evaluation needs.
3. *Alignment with the Literature and Specific KPI Definitions*
The third added value confirms the necessity of defining specific KPIs rather than relying on predefined sets, such as those outlined in the Italian national guidelines [36]. This highlights the importance of developing tailored KPIs that precisely address specific evaluation needs rather than using generic one-size-fits-all measures.

4.3. Expanded Considerations on the Telemechron Framework for Telemedicine

Expanding further on the analysis, it can be emphasized that the framework developed for the Telemechron project addresses multiple domains of interest related to telemedicine and its integration into the healthcare domain (also including aspects related to KPIs). This framework stands out as an innovative tool compared to other telemedicine frameworks previously encountered [33,34], which have primarily focused on metrics. The framework we are referring to here can be defined as a dossier-style framework, offering a holistic and multidimensional approach that goes beyond simple metric analysis and embraces a comprehensive evaluation of all relevant aspects of telemedicine services.

In contrast to frameworks that mainly emphasize technical metrics and service performance, the Telemechron framework incorporates a broader spectrum of dimensions, such as organizational design, strategic alignment, technological requirements, financial considerations, and service outcomes. This multifaceted approach ensures that all critical elements are thoroughly evaluated, allowing for continuous improvement and a better integration of telemedicine services into the healthcare system.

Comparing this approach to a different socially inspired framework, we can look at [46] "A Socially Inspired Framework for Human State Inference Using Expert Opinion Integration". This framework proposes a group decision technique using ordered weighted averaging (OWA) to aggregate opinions from different classifiers, ultimately aiming to infer human states using multiple cues or signals. The study discusses biosensing, which involves two key processes, namely data acquisition and information inference. The socially inspired framework for human state inference works by integrating multiple cues from various experts. The main concept behind this approach is that conventional inference algorithms are treated as inference experts, and the framework utilizes expert opinion elicitation to improve the inference process. The key elements of the socially inspired framework include the following:

Multiple cues: the framework draws on various sources of information.

Multiple experts: different experts contribute, each with different levels of expertise.

Expertise association: experts may have specialized knowledge in different aspects of human states and cues.

Consensus procedures: different procedures are used to arrive at an agreed opinion or outcome, such as identifying the human state in this context.

The paper demonstrates [46] the framework by inferring fatigue as a human state and comparing it with previous studies, showing that this approach leads to better results in terms of accuracy.

Both frameworks—the Telemechron framework and the socially inspired framework for human state inference—share a multidimensional and expert-driven approach, albeit in different fields.

The Telemechron framework focuses on evaluating telemedicine services through a comprehensive lens, covering various aspects of healthcare delivery, from technology to organizational integration. Its use of multiple experts within makes it a collaborative and iterative process for improving telemedicine systems.

The socially inspired framework, on the other hand, is more focused on human state inference, utilizing expert opinion aggregation and various cues to infer human conditions like fatigue. This framework integrates diverse experts (e.g., those with varying expertise in biosensing technologies) to arrive at a consensus on human states.

Both frameworks use expertise and an aggregation of multiple perspectives to produce better outcomes—whether it is for improving telemedicine systems or accurately determining human states. The Telemechron framework offers a comprehensive and systematic approach by integrating multiple dimensions of healthcare, making it suitable for a wide range of telemedicine services. In contrast, the socially inspired framework focuses more specifically on health state inference through signal integration, providing a specialized solution that excels in improving accuracy in specific areas, such as fatigue inference. Both frameworks have their strengths; while Telemechron excels in a holistic approach to telemedicine, the socially inspired framework enhances precision and effectiveness in particular health-related assessments.

Thus, while the domains and specific applications differ, the underlying principles of multidimensional analysis, expert collaboration, and continuous feedback loops provide a solid foundation for innovative and adaptive approaches in both frameworks.

4.4. Work in Progress and Suggestions for Future Investigations

The project is still ongoing, and this study focuses on a portion of the technology assessment activities. Other specific contributions not related to technology assessment but concerning the design and implementation of telemedicine services come from the work packages WP1, WP3, and WP4, which focus on design and protocols, as illustrated by the study reported in [47] proposed by OU3/WP3. This study [47] focuses on evaluating a telemedicine project aimed at improving home-based management of heart failure and type 2 diabetes by promoting lifestyle changes rather than assessing the technology itself. It compares the impact of the project—providing teleconsultations, daily monitoring, and personalized support—against routine care, with the goal of improving outcomes such as physical activity and disease management.

Further developments are anticipated in both technology assessment (OU2/WP2) and the project's specific operational units (OU1/WP1, OU3/WP3, OU4/WP4). Additionally, a detailed analysis of the content of the frameworks completed by the three operational units is planned. The comprehensive and multifaceted results from the analysis of the frameworks will be reviewed in collaboration with project partners and presented through detailed reports to the relevant oversight bodies. Following this, there will be opportunities for further dissemination of the findings at both national and international levels, ensuring that the insights gained from the technology assessment are widely shared, contributing to the broader body of knowledge and potentially influencing future developments in telemedicine.

The developed framework and KPI model have demonstrated their utility in evaluating key aspects of telemedicine, showing concrete improvements and useful metrics for KPI applicability. Future research should focus on the following:

- Enhanced utilization of metrics: exploring the application of metrics in various telemedicine contexts and internationally.
- Refinement of KPI models: continuing to develop context-specific KPIs for deeper insights into telemedicine services.
- Integration with advanced technologies: adapting the framework to include new technologies such as AI and machine learning.
- Cross-national comparisons: comparing the effectiveness of the framework and metrics across different countries and healthcare systems.
- Feedback and iteration: gathering feedback from stakeholders to refine the metrics and model.
- Long-term impact analysis: conducting longitudinal studies to assess the sustainability and effectiveness of the framework and metrics over time.

5. Conclusions

The study represents a significant contribution to the Telemechron project by integrating the collaborative efforts of all four OUs across its distinct WPs. Central to this contribution are advancements in TA and the design and application of a model for assessing a set of KPIs for telemedicine within the project.

The framework, a dedicated tool for TA, has proven effective in quantitatively assessing various aspects of telemedicine services and measuring improvements following three rounds of enhancement initiatives. Thanks to the collaborative input from all OUs, the KPI analysis model has yielded valuable insights into the applicability of the proposed KPI set. It has also provided useful and generalizable metrics and parameters applicable to both national and international telemedicine contexts.

Looking ahead, the project is set to continue evolving. Future research should focus on refining KPI models, exploring their application across different telemedicine settings, and integrating emerging technologies such as AI. Additionally, cross-national comparisons will be essential to evaluate the effectiveness of the framework and metrics across diverse healthcare systems. Collecting stakeholder feedback and conducting longitudinal studies will be crucial for further refining the framework and enhancing its applications in telemedicine.

Author Contributions: Conceptualization, D.G., S.M., G.B. and S.J.; methodology, S.B., S.S., S.I., D.G., R.B. and S.M.; software, All Authors; validation, All authors; formal analysis, D.G., S.M. and S.J.; investigation, All authors; resources, S.B., S.S., S.I., D.G. and R.B.; data curation, S.B., S.S., S.I., D.G., R.B., A.G. and S.M.; writing—original draft preparation, D.G., S.M. and S.J.; writing—review and editing, D.G., S.S., S.I., L.G., S.B., A.G., P.B., G.D., C.D. and G.B.; visualization, C.D., M.G., G.D., M.C., G.B., M.M., M.A.G. and L.G.; supervision, D.G, S.J., S.S., S.I. and S.B.; project administration, S.B. and S.J.; funding acquisition, S.B., S.S., S.I., D.G., R.B. and M.G. All authors have read and agreed to the published version of the manuscript.

Funding: This study is carried out in the framework of the project "Telemedicine for the home management of patients with chronic diseases and comorbidities: analysis of current models and design of innovative strategies to improve the quality of care and optimize the use of resources: TELEMECHRON study" (grant: NET-2018-12367206—Bando della Ricerca Finalizzata 2018 of the Italian Ministry of Health). The article review brings forth a portion of the work conducted by the team of the Istituto Superiore di Sanità, work package 2. The project was funded directly by the

Italian Ministry of Health and by regional institutions (Tuscany and Lombardy Region) and the Provincia Autonoma di Trento. The APC was funded by Daniele Giansanti.

Institutional Review Board Statement: Not applicable, as this study does not involve humans or animals.

Informed Consent Statement: Not applicable.

Data Availability Statement: Data are contained within the article.

Conflicts of Interest: The authors declare no conflicts of interest.

References

1. Mackintosh, N.; Terblanche, M.; Maharaj, R.; Xyrichis, A.; Franklin, K.; Keddie, J.; Larkins, E.; Maslen, A.; Skinner, J.; Newman, S.; et al. Telemedicine with clinical decision support for critical care: A systematic review. *Syst. Rev.* **2016**, *5*, 176. [CrossRef] [PubMed]
2. Jacob, C.; Lindeque, J.; Klein, A.; Ivory, C.; Heuss, S.; Peter, M.K. Assessing the Quality and Impact of eHealth Tools: Systematic Literature Review and NarrativeSynthesis. *JMIR Hum. Factors* **2023**, *10*, e45143. [CrossRef] [PubMed]
3. von Huben, A.; Howell, M.; Norris, S.; Wong, K.C.; Tang, J.; Kazi, S.; Laranjo, L.; Chow, C.K.; Howard, K. Stakeholder preferences for attributes of digital health technologies to consider in health service funding. *Int. J. Technol. Assess. Health Care* **2023**, *39*, e12. [CrossRef]
4. Smits, M.; Kim, C.M.; van Goor, H.; Ludden, G.D.S. From Digital Health to Digital Well- being: Systematic Scoping Review. *J. Med. Internet Res.* **2022**, *24*, e33787. [CrossRef]
5. Brick, R.; Padgett, L.; Jones, J.; Wood, K.C.; Pergolotti, M.; Marshall, T.F.; Campbell, G.; Eilers, R.; Keshavarzi, S.; Flores, A.M.; et al. The influence of telehealth-based cancer rehabilitation interventions on disability: A systematic review. *J. Cancer Surviv.* **2023**, *17*, 1725–1750. [CrossRef]
6. von Huben, A.; Howell, M.; Carrello, J.; Norris, S.; Wortley, S.; Ritchie, A.; Howard, K. Application of a health technology assessment framework to digital health technologies that manage chronic disease: A systematic review. *Int. J. Technol. Assess. Health Care* **2021**, *38*, e9. [CrossRef]
7. Leckenby, E.; Dawoud, D.; Bouvy, J.; Jónsson, P. The Sandbox Approach and its Potential for Use in Health Technology Assessment: A Literature Review. *Appl. Health Econ. Health Policy* **2021**, *19*, 857–869. [CrossRef]
8. von Huben, A.; Howell, M.; Howard, K.; Carrello, J.; Norris, S. Health technology assessment for digital technologies that manage chronic disease: A systematic. *Int. J. Technol. Assess. Health Care* **2021**, *37*, e66. [CrossRef]
9. Bonten, T.N.; Rauwerdink, A.; Wyatt, J.C.; Kasteleyn, M.J.; Witkamp, L.; Riper, H.; van Gemert-Pijnen, L.J.; Cresswell, K.; Sheikh, A.; Schijven, M.P.; et al. Online Guide for Electronic Health Evaluation Approaches: Systematic Scoping Review and Concept Mapping Study. *J. Med. Internet Res.* **2020**, *22*, e17774. [CrossRef]
10. Vis, C.; Bührmann, L.; Riper, H.; Ossebaard, H.C. Health technology assessment frameworks for eHealth: A systematic review. *Int. J. Technol. Assess. Health Care* **2020**, *36*, 204–216. [CrossRef]
11. Jiang, X.; Ming, W.K.; You, J.H. The Cost-Effectiveness of Digital Health Interventions on the Management of Cardiovascular Diseases: Systematic Review. *J. Med. Internet Res.* **2019**, *21*, e13166. [CrossRef] [PubMed]
12. Lawes-Wickwar, S.; McBain, H.; Mulligan, K. Application and Effectiveness of Telehealth to Support Severe Mental Illness Management: Systematic Review. *JMIR Ment. Health* **2018**, *5*, e62. [CrossRef] [PubMed]
13. Shields, G.E.; Wells, A.; Doherty, P.; Heagerty, A.; Buck, D.; Davies, L.M. Cost-effectiveness of cardiac rehabilitation: A systematic review. *Heart* **2018**, *104*, 1403–1410. [CrossRef] [PubMed]
14. Biagianti, B.; Quraishi, S.H.; Schlosser, D.A. Potential Benefits of Incorporating Peer-to-Peer Interactions Into Digital Interventions for Psychotic Disorders: A Systematic Review. *Psychiatr. Serv.* **2018**, *69*, 377–388. [CrossRef] [PubMed]
15. Kitsiou, S.; Paré, G.; Jaana, M. Systematic reviews and meta-analyses of home telemonitoring interventions for patients with chronic diseases: A critical assessment of their methodological quality. *J. Med. Internet Res.* **2013**, *15*, e150. [CrossRef]
16. COPD Working Group. Noninvasive positive pressure ventilation for chronic respiratory failure patients with stable chronic obstructive pulmonary disease (COPD): An evidence-based analysis. *Ont. Health Technol. Assess. Ser.* **2012**, *12*, 1–51.
17. COPD Working Group. Pulmonary rehabilitation for patients with chronic pulmonary disease (COPD): An evidence-based analysis. *Ont. Health Technol. Assess. Ser.* **2012**, *12*, 1–75.
18. Giacomini, M.; DeJean, D.; Simeonov, D.; Smith, A. Experiences of living and dying with COPD: A systematic review and synthesis of the qualitative empirical literature. *Ont. Health Technol. Assess. Ser.* **2012**, *12*, 1–47.

19. Lux, L.; Boehlecke, B.; Lohr, K.N. *Effectiveness of Portable Monitoring Devices for Diagnosing Obstructive Sleep Apnea: Update of a Systematic Review [Internet]*; Agency for Healthcare Research and Quality (US): Rockville, MD, USA, 2004.
20. Roine, R.; Ohinmaa, A.; Hailey, D. Assessing telemedicine: A systematic review of the literature. *CMAJ* **2001**, *165*, 765–771.
21. Available online: https://www.qlik.com/us/kpi#:~:text=KPIsKPI%20Examples-,What%20is%20a%20KPI?,the%20organization%20make%20better%20decisions (accessed on 8 January 2025).
22. Available online: https://hci.care/practical-guidance-for-selecting-key-performance-indicators-in-healthcare/ (accessed on 8 January 2025).
23. Brenner, M.; Weir, A.; McCann, M.; Doyle, C.; Hughes, M.; Moen, A.; Ingvar, M.; Nauwe-laerts, K.; Turk, E.; McCabe, C. Development of the key performance indicators for digital health interventions: A scoping review. *Digit Health* **2023**, *9*, 20552076231152160. [CrossRef] [PubMed] [PubMed Central]
24. Canning, M.L.; Barras, M.; McDougall, R.; Yerkovich, S.; Coombes, I.; Sullivan, C.; Whitfield, K. Defining quality indicators, pharmaceutical care bundles and outcomes of clinical pharmacy service delivery using a Delphi consensus approach. *Int. J. Clin. Pharm.* **2024**, *46*, 451–462. [CrossRef] [PubMed]
25. Garbelli, M.; Ion Titapiccolo, J.; Bellocchio, F.; Stuard, S.; Brancaccio, D.; Neri, L. Prolonged patient survival after implementation of a continuous quality improvement programme empowered by digital transformation in a large dialysis network. *Nephrol. Dial. Transplant.* **2022**, *37*, 469–476. [CrossRef] [PubMed]
26. Jackson, D.E.; McClean, S.I. Trends in telemedicine assessment indicate neglect of key criteria for predicting success. *J. Health Organ. Manag.* **2012**, *26*, 508–523. [CrossRef]
27. Baughman, D.J.; Jabbarpour, Y.; Westfall, J.M.; Jetty, A.; Zain, A.; Baughman, K.; Pollak, B.; Waheed, A. Comparison of Quality Performance Measures for Patients Receiving In-Person vs Telemedicine Primary Care in a Large Integrated Health System. *JAMA Netw. Open* **2022**, *5*, e2233267. [CrossRef] [PubMed]
28. Avanesova, A.A.; Shamliyan, T.A. Worldwide implementation of telemedicine programs in association with research performance and health policy. *Health Policy Technol.* **2019**, *8*, 179–191. [CrossRef]
29. Berlet, M.; Vogel, T.; Gharba, M.; Eichinger, J.; Schulz, E.; Friess, H.; Wilhelm, D.; Ostler, D.; Kranzfelder, M. Emergency Telemedicine Mobile Ultrasounds Using a 5G-Enabled Application: Development and Usability Study. *JMIR Form. Res.* **2022**, *6*, e36824. [CrossRef]
30. Kidholm, K.; Jensen, L.K.; Kjølhede, T.; Nielsen, E.; Horup, M.B. Validity of the Model for Assessment of Telemedicine: A Delphi study. *J. Telemed. Telecare* **2018**, *24*, 118–125. [CrossRef]
31. Schröder, H.; Beckers, S.K.; Borgs, C.; Sommer, A.; Rossaint, R.; Grüßer, L.; Felzen, M. Long-term effects of a prehospital telemedicine system on structural and process quality indicators of an emergency medical service. *Sci. Rep.* **2024**, *14*, 310. [CrossRef]
32. Vo, A.; Shore, J.; Waugh, M.; Doarn, C.R.; Richardson, J.; Hathaway, O.; Bostick, E.; Lippolis, S.; Thomas, M. Meaningful use: A national framework for integrated telemedicine. *Telemed. e-Health* **2015**, *21*, 355–363. [CrossRef]
33. Morelli, S.; D'Avenio, G.; Daniele, C.; Grigioni, M.; Giansanti, D. Under the Tech Umbrella: Assessing the Landscape of Telemedicine Innovations (Telemechron Study). *Healthcare* **2024**, *12*, 615. [CrossRef]
34. Morelli, S.; Daniele, C.; D'Avenio, G.; Grigioni, M.; Giansanti, D. Pioneering a Framework for Robust Tele-medicine Technology Assessment (Telemechron Study). *Technologies* **2024**, *12*, 373. [CrossRef]
35. Morelli, S.; Daniele, C.; D'Avenio, G.; Grigioni, M.; Giansanti, D. Optimizing Telehealth: Leveraging Key Performance In-dicators for Enhanced TeleHealth and Digital Healthcare Outcomes (Telemechron Study). *Healthcare* **2024**, *12*, 1319. [CrossRef] [PubMed]
36. Italian Telemedicine Guidelines. Available online: https://www.salute.gov.it/imgs/C_17_pubblicazioni_2129_allegato.pdf (accessed on 8 January 2025).
37. WHO. Defining Evaluation Indicators for Telemedicine as a Tool for Reducing Health Inequities: Study and Results of a Community of Practice. 2016. Available online: https://iris.paho.org/handle/10665.2/28562 (accessed on 24 June 2024).
38. ATA. 15 Key Performance Indicators to Power Success in Telehealth. 2021. Available online: https://www.americantelemed.org/blog/vitelnet8-5/ (accessed on 15 June 2022).
39. Qaseem, A.; MacLean, C.H.; Tierney, S.; Cross, J.T., Jr.; MacDonald, S.T.; Goldzweig, C.L.; Fitterman, N.; Performance Measurement Committee of the American College of Physicians; Andrews, R.; Basch, P.; et al. Performance Measures for Physicians Providing Clinical Care Using Telemedicine: A Position Paper From the American College of Physicians. *Ann. Intern. Med.* **2023**, *176*, 694–698. [CrossRef]
40. NHS. Integrated Urgent Care: Key Performance Indicators 2023/24. 2024. Available online: https://www.england.nhs.uk/long-read/integrated-urgent-care-key-performance-indicators-2023-24/ (accessed on 24 June 2024).

41. Health Policies and Standards Department, Health Regulation Sector, Government of Dubai. Guidelines for Reporting Telehealth Key Performance. 2021. Available online: https://www.dha.gov.ae/uploads/042022/Guidelines%20for%20Reporting%20Telehealth%20KPIs2022450157.pdf (accessed on 24 June 2024).
42. Doupi, P. Evolving Health IT Systems Evaluation: The Convergence of Health Informatics and HTA. *Stud. Health Technol. Inform.* **2016**, *222*, 220–236.
43. Ekeland, A.G.; Grøttland, A. Assessment of Mast in European Patient-Centered Telemedicine Pilots. *Int. J. Technol. Assess. HealthCare* **2015**, *31*, 304–311. [CrossRef]
44. Giansanti, D.; Morelli, S.; Macellari, V. Telemedicine technology assessment part II: Tools for a quality control system. *Telemed. e-Health* **2007**, *13*, 130–140. [CrossRef]
45. Giansanti, D.; Morelli, S.; Macellari, V. Telemedicine technology assessment part I: Setup and validation of a quality control System. *Telemed. e-Health* **2007**, *13*, 118–129. [CrossRef]
46. Modi, S.; Lin, Y.; Cheng, L.; Yang, G.; Liu, L.; Zhang, W.J. A Socially Inspired Framework for Human State Inference Using Expert Opinion Integration. *IEEE/ASME Trans. Mechatron.* **2011**, *16*, 874–878. [CrossRef]
47. Bernocchi, P.; Giudici, V.; Borghi, G.; Bertolaia, P.; D'Isa, S.; Trevisan, R.; Scalvini, S. Telemedicine home-based management in patients with chronic heart failure and diabetes type II: Study protocol for a randomized controlled trial. *Trials* **2024**, *25*, 333. [CrossRef] [PubMed] [PubMed Central]

technologies

MDPI

Systematic Review

Remote Rehabilitation and Virtual Reality Interventions Using Motion Sensors for Chronic Low Back Pain: A Systematic Review of Biomechanical, Pain, Quality of Life, and Adherence Outcomes

Marina Garofano [1,*], Rosaria Del Sorbo [1,*], Mariaconsiglia Calabrese [1], Massimo Giordano [1], Maria Pia Di Palo [1], Marianna Bartolomeo [1], Chiara Maria Ragusa [1], Gaetano Ungaro [2], Gianluca Fimiani [3], Federica Di Spirito [1], Massimo Amato [1], Michele Ciccarelli [1], Claudio Pascarelli [4], Giuseppe Scanniello [3], Placido Bramanti [5] and Alessia Bramanti [1]

1 Department of Medicine, Surgery and Dentistry, University of Salerno, Via S. Allende, 84081 Baronissi, Italy; macalabrese@unisa.it (M.C.); mgiordano@unisa.it (M.G.); mariapia140497@gmail.com (M.P.D.P.); mbartolomeo@unisa.it (M.B.); chiaramragusa@hotmail.com (C.M.R.); fdispirito@unisa.it (F.D.S.); mamato@unisa.it (M.A.); mciccarelli@unisa.it (M.C.); abramanti@unisa.it (A.B.)

2 University Hospital "San Giovanni di Dio e Ruggi d'Aragona", Via San Leonardo, 84125 Salerno, Italy; gaungaro@unisa.it

3 Department of Computer Science, University of Salerno, Via Giovanni Paolo II, 132, 84084 Fisciano, Italy; gfimiani@unisa.it (G.F.); gscanniello@unisa.it (G.S.)

4 Department of Engineering for Innovation, University of Salento, 73100 Lecce, Italy; claudio.pascarelli@unisalento.it

5 Faculty of Psychology, University eCampus, 22060 Novedrate, Italy; bramanti.dino@gmail.com

* Correspondence: mgarofano@unisa.it (M.G.); rdelsorbo@unisa.it (R.D.S.)

Abstract: Background: Chronic low back pain (CLBP) is a leading cause of disability, impacting quality of life (QoL), function, and work productivity. Traditional rehabilitation faces challenges in accessibility and adherence. Remote rehabilitation and virtual reality (VR) interventions using motion sensors offer real-time movement tracking, biofeedback, and personalized exercises. This systematic review evaluates their effectiveness in pain reduction, functional improvement, adherence, and QoL. Methods: A systematic search was performed across PubMed, Scopus, Web of Science, and PEDro (2015–2025), including randomized controlled trials, observational, and feasibility studies on adults with CLBP undergoing sensor-based digital rehabilitation. The primary outcomes included pain, functional mobility, and movement biomechanics; secondary outcomes included adherence, QoL, and cost-effectiveness. Eight studies involving 7166 participants were included. Overall, sensor-based remote rehabilitation and VR interventions demonstrated positive effects on pain, function, and adherence. Pain reductions ranged from modest short-term decreases to over 60% in long-term programs (e.g., −68.5% in VAS). Functional improvements included lumbar ROM gains up to +9.9° and better movement control. Adherence was consistently high, with some programs reporting completion rates between 73% and 90%, particularly those incorporating gamification or real-time feedback. Selected studies also showed QoL improvements (e.g., +9.10 points on SF-36) and reductions in work impairment by over 60%. A few trials reported significant decreases in inflammatory markers (e.g., CRP −1.16 mg/L, TNF-α −8.9 pg/mL). Conclusions: Motion sensor-based remote rehabilitation and VR interventions show promising results in pain management, mobility, and adherence for individuals with CLBP. Gamification and biofeedback features enhance engagement, addressing a key challenge of conventional rehabilitation. However, more long-term RCTs and economic evaluations are needed to confirm their effectiveness and cost-efficiency.

Keywords: chronic low back pain; remote rehabilitation; virtual reality; motion sensors; digital health; pain management; sensor-based therapy; musculoskeletal disorders

1. Introduction

Low-back pain (LBP) refers to pain or discomfort situated between the lower rib margin and the upper boundary of the gluteal region, with or without radiating symptoms in the legs [1]. When LBP persists for at least 12 weeks, lacks a clear underlying pathology, and varies in intensity, it is classified as chronic and nonspecific [2,3]. Chronic low back pain (CLBP) is one of the most common musculoskeletal disorders worldwide, and it is estimated that a significant percentage of the adult population will experience CLBP at least once in their lifetime [3–5]. Traditionally, the treatment of CLBP has included drug therapies, therapeutic exercise, physiotherapy, and psychological interventions for pain management [6–8]. In recent years, innovative technologies have been incorporated into the rehabilitation of CLBP with the aim of improving the effectiveness of interventions, increasing patient adherence and providing more personalized and accessible treatment options [9–11]. Among these, telerehabilitation, virtual reality (VR), machine learning (ML), and wearable sensors are transforming clinical practice. Several studies, including those by Lara-Palomo et al. [12] and Raiszadeh et al. [13], have shown that telerehabilitation is comparable to traditional physiotherapy in terms of pain reduction and improvement in functional disability [12,14]. VR is used to create immersive environments that facilitate the performance of therapeutic exercises with high levels of engagement, reduce fear of movement (kinesiophobia), and improve proprioception compared to conventional methods [15–17]. Initially developed for engineering applications, VR has been widely adopted in healthcare—particularly in musculoskeletal rehabilitation, and also for CLBP—where it shows promise in improving patient motivation and optimizing functional outcomes [18]. ML algorithms offer new ways to personalize treatment by analyzing data collected from patients to predict rehabilitation progress and optimize treatment strategies [19–21]; additionally, they play a crucial role in movement assessment by identifying pathological movement patterns [22,23]. Finally, wearable sensors such as accelerometers, gyroscopes, and magnetometers, which capture detailed information about the body's dynamics in real time, allow continuous and objective monitoring of movement, providing accurate data on motor performance and enabling real-time feedback [24–27]. Despite the growing use of these technologies, current evidence remains fragmented, with many studies addressing them separately and using inconsistent outcome measures. A comprehensive synthesis of their combined application, particularly wearable sensors within telerehabilitation programs, is still lacking. This systematic review aims to synthesize the available evidence on the effectiveness of wearable motion sensors and telerehabilitation technologies in managing movement-related outcomes for individuals with low back pain. Specifically, it will assess their impact on key clinical parameters such as pain reduction, improved function and mobility, enhanced quality of life (QoL), and optimized patient management. Additionally, this review will identify the main methodological limitations of existing studies and explore future perspectives for the large-scale implementation of these technologies in clinical practice.

2. Materials and Methods

2.1. Study Protocol

The current study protocol was designed in accordance with the PRISMA guidelines (Preferred Reporting Items for Systematic Reviews) [28], ensuring a rigorous methodological approach prior to the literature search and data analysis with a specific focus on the research questions and the clinical effectiveness of innovative technologies, including telerehabilitation, VR, ML, and wearable sensors, in the rehabilitation of CLBP. The analysis focuses on the effects of these technologies in terms of pain reduction, functional improvement, enhanced QoL, and treatment adherence, evaluating their impact on rehabilitation pathways and therapeutic strategies. Before starting the literature search and data analysis, the related study protocol was registered in the International Prospective Register of Systematic Reviews (PROSPERO) database of systematic reviews (identification number: CRD42024608097). The formulation of the research question and the strategy and criteria for study selection were developed using the PICO model [29]. The study question focused on the following:

Population (P): Adults ($\geq$18 years) with low back pain.

Intervention (I): Remote rehabilitation utilizing motion tracking and sensor-based movement monitoring technologies.

Comparison (C): Conventional in-person rehabilitation or no rehabilitation.

Outcomes (O):

Main outcome(s): Evaluation of clinically relevant movement and biomechanical parameters, including lumbar and trunk range of motion (ROM), postural control, movement kinematics, and motor coordination.

Additional outcome(s): Pain, cost-effectiveness, adherence, accessibility, any healthcare outcome measures, and QoL.

2.2. Search Strategy and Study Selection

The literature search was conducted electronically across four databases: PubMed, Scopus, WOS, and PEDro. The database screening was carried out independently by three reviewers (A.B., R.D.S., Marina Garofano) from January 2015 to 1 February 2025, using the following keywords combined with Boolean operators: low back pain, movement analysis, motion tracking, movement monitoring, motion capture, telerehabilitation, remote rehabilitation, and virtual rehabilitation. Complete search strategies are provided in Appendix A. The collected citations were recorded, duplicates were eliminated using EndNote, and the titles and abstracts obtained were independently screened by two reviewers (A.B., R.D.S). The full texts of potentially relevant papers and ambiguous abstracts were reviewed independently by the same authors (A.B., R.D.S.), who resolved disagreements through discussion and consensus and, if necessary, with the involvement of a third reviewer (Marina Garofano).

The inclusion criteria were as follows:

- Source: studies published in the English language from 2015 to 1 February 2025;
- Study design: randomized controlled trial (RCT), observational studies, feasibility studies;
- Study population: Adults (>18) with low back pain (no gender restrictions);
- Study intervention: Remote rehabilitation with the use of movement sensors;
- Study outcomes: Evaluation of movement and biomechanical parameters, including "movement", "motor activity", "movement analysis", "motion tracking", "movement monitoring", "biomechanics", and "kinematics"; and "motion capture", pain, cost-effectiveness, adherence, accessibility, any healthcare outcome measures, and QoL.

The exclusion criteria were as follows:

- Source: studies published before 2015 or after 1 February 2025;

- Study intervention: Studies not involving remote rehabilitation, studies not utilizing movement sensors for assessment or intervention, or interventions focusing solely on pharmacological or surgical treatments.
- Study outcomes: studies not reporting movement-related or biomechanical outcomes; studies without measurable clinical outcomes related to pain, cost-effectiveness, adherence, accessibility, healthcare impact, or QoL.

2.3. Data Extraction and Collection

Two authors (Marina Garofano and R.D.S.) independently screened the titles and abstracts retrieved from the database searches to determine their eligibility based on the inclusion criteria. Studies were included or excluded upon mutual agreement. In cases of disagreement regarding a manuscript's inclusion based on abstract evaluation, discrepancies were resolved through discussion and consensus. If consensus was not reached, a third reviewer (A.B.) was consulted for the final decision. The data extraction process followed established methodologies and was structured to align with the research questions of this review. Extracted data included: (a) author, year, and country; (b) study design; (c) participants; (d) mean age; (e) intervention; (f) control group; (g) technological solution; (h) primary outcomes; (i) secondary outcomes; (j) key results. This systematic approach ensured a rigorous and consistent collection of relevant data, facilitating a comprehensive synthesis of evidence to address the research questions.

2.4. Quality Assessment

Three independent reviewers assessed the methodological quality of the studies in this review, using validated tools for risk of bias analysis. The Risk of Bias 2 (ROB-2) [30] tool was used for RCTs Table 1, while Risk of Bias in Non-randomized Studies (ROBINS-I) [31] was used for non-randomized studies Table 2. The methodological aspects addressed in this evaluation are selection of participants, presence of confounding factors, accuracy in classification of the intervention, fidelity to the intended procedure, handling of missing data, selection of reported outcomes, and reliability in measuring them. The risk of bias was classified into four categories:

Table 1. Cochrane risk of bias tool for the risk of bias in individual studies.

Study	Bias Arising from the Randomization Process	Bias Due to Deviations from Intended Interventions	Bias Due to Missing Outcome Data	Bias in Measurement of the Outcome	Bias in Selection of the Reported Result	Overall
Matheve et al., 2018 [32]	Low	Low	Low	Some concerns	Low	Low
Matheve et al., 2020 [33]	Low	Low	Low	Some concerns	Low	Low
Mueller et al., 2022 [34]	High	High	Some concerns	High	Some concerns	High
Nambi et al., 2023 [35]	Low	Low	High	High	High	High
Shi et al., 2024 [36]	Low	Low	High	High	Some concerns	High

LOW, if all assessed domains were found to have a minimal risk of bias;

MODERATE, if at least one domain with intermediate risk was present, without evidence of high criticality;

SERIOUS, if at least one domain showed a high risk of bias, but no aspect critically compromised the reliability of the study;

HIGH, if the risk of bias was such that it called into question the overall validity of the study.

These analyses determined the level of reliability of the included studies and considered the impact of the risk of bias in interpreting the results of this systematic review.

Table 2. ROBINS-I Tool for non-RCTs; abbreviations: PY (Probably Yes), P (Possibly), PN (Probably No), N (No).

Study	Bias Due to Confounding	Bias in Selection of Participants	Bias in Classification of Interventions	Bias Due to Deviations from Intended Interventions	Bias Due to Missing Data	Bias in Measurement of Outcomes	Bias in Selection of Reported Results	Overall Risk of Bias
Bailey et al., 2020 [37]	PY	P	PN	P	P	PY	PY	SERIOUS
Park et al., 2022 [38]	P	P	PN	P	PY	PY	PN	MODERATE
Shebib et al., 2019 [39]	PN	PN	PN	P	PY	P	P	LOW TO MODERATE

3. Results

3.1. Study Selection and Characteristics

The study selection process followed the PRISMA 2020 guidelines [28]. A total of 4301 records were identified through database searches of PubMed (195 records), Scopus (328 records), Web of Science (3825 records), and PEDro (8 records). After removing 263 duplicate records with EndNote, 4038 records remained for screening. Following the screening, 4016 records were excluded based on the title and abstract, leaving 22 reports for retrieval. All reports were successfully retrieved and assessed for eligibility. Of these, 14 were excluded for various reasons, 3 articles were excluded because they did not address telerehabilitation, 5 did not involve the use of motion sensors, and 3 focused on VR without combining it with telerehabilitation and sensor use. Ultimately, eight studies met the inclusion criteria and were included in the systematic review. These studies were critically appraised to ensure they aligned with the research objectives and provided relevant data for analysis. This selection process is summarized in the PRISMA flow diagram (Figure 1), and in Table 3, there are the descriptive characteristics of the eight included studies, with a focus on: (a) author, year, and country; (b) study design; (c) participants; (d) mean age; (e) intervention; (f) control group; (g) technological solution; (h) primary outcomes; (i) secondary outcomes; and (j) key results.

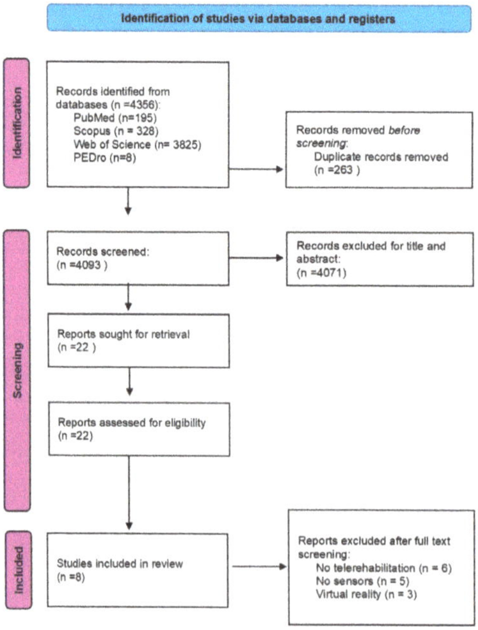

Figure 1. Flow diagram of study selection.

Table 3. Descriptive characteristics of the included studies.

Authors, Year, Country	Study Design	Participants (N, M/F)	Mean Age (SD)	Intervention	Control Group	Technological Solution	Primary Outcomes	Secondary Outcomes	Key Results
Bailey et al., 2020, USA [37]	Longitudinal Observational Study	6468 (M:1487, F:4981, CLBP)	42.58 (10.91)	12-week digital care program with sensor-guided exercise, CBT, and coaching	N/A	Bluetooth motion sensors & mobile app	Pain intensity (VAS)	Depression (PHQ-9), Anxiety (GAD-7), Work productivity (WPAI)	VAS pain −68.45%, Depression −57.5%, Anxiety −58.1%, Work productivity +61.5%
Matheve et al., 2018, Belgium [32]	RCT	108 (54 CLBP–M:24, F:30; 54 Healthy–M:36, F:18)	CLBP: 40 (17), Healthy: 37 (14)	Sensor-based postural feedback to improve movement control	Mirror feedback & No-feedback	Wireless inertial sensors & avatar interface	Lumbopelvic movement control (Kinematic analysis)	NPRS, RMDQ, TSK	Significant movement control improvement in sensor group ($p <$ 0.0001)
Matheve et al., 2020, Belgium [33]	RCT	84 (42 IG–M:15, F:27; 42 CG–M:15, F:27)	IG: 44.1 (12.2), CG: 42.8 (13.4)	VR-based exercise therapy using motion sensors	Conventional exercise therapy	Valedo®Pro motion sensor & VR games	Movement control, Motor learning, Pain reduction (NPRS)	Functional performance, TSK, RMDQ	VR + motion sensor improved movement control & pain reduction ($p < 0.01$)
Mueller et al., 2022, Germany [34]	Randomized cross-over pilot trial	13 CLBP (M:5, F:8)	41 (16)	Game-based real-time biofeedback training via trunk exergame	Cross-over design with rest periods	Sensor-based trunk exergame	Maximum angle in lateral flexion	Angle reproduction & secondary movement planes	No primary movement change but improved control in secondary planes ($p = 0.02$)
Nambi et al., 2023, Saudi Arabia [35]	RCT	60 (30 IG, 30 CG, CNLBP, all male)	IG: 21.6 (2.1), CG: 22.1 (1.9)	VR-based trunk exercises with a moving game chair	Isokinetic & core stabilization exercises	Pro-Kin system with VR feedback	Pain intensity (VAS), Muscle CSA (MRI/ultrasound)	Inflammatory biomarkers (CRP, TNF-α, IL-2, IL-4, IL-6)	Significant pain reduction & muscle CSA increase, VRE improved biomarkers
Park et al., 2022, Korea [38]	Retrospective Case-Control Study	176 (104 IG–M:41, F:63; 72 CG–M:51, F:21)	IG: 36.7 (8.03), CG: 38.3 (7.04)	Mobile exercise coaching app using AI motion tracking	Video-streaming exercise group	Smartphone AI motion tracking	QoL (SF-36), Pain intensity (VAS)	Exercise adherence, Treatment satisfaction	Higher QoL (SF-36: +9.10 vs. +1.09), Greater pain reduction (−0.96 vs. −0.26 VAS)
Shebib et al., 2019, USA [39]	RCT	177 (113 IG–M:71, F:42; 64 CG–M:33, F:31)	43 (11)	12-week digital care program with sensor feedback & CBT	Digital education articles only	Wearable sensors & virtual coaching	Disability (ODI, Korff Pain & Disability Scale)	Pain (VAS), Adherence, Surgery interest	Pain −52–64%, Disability −31–55%, High adherence (90%)
Shi et al., 2024, China [36]	RCT	54 (27 IG–M:12, F:14; 27 CG–M:9, F:18)	IG: 43.5 (10.2), CG: 42.9 (9.8)	Telerehabilitation with motion sensors for remote tracking	Outpatient-based exercise therapy	HIRS motion tracking system	Disability (ODI)	Pain (NPRS), FABQ, QoL (SF-36)	Significant pain & function improvement, no difference vs. conventional rehab

Abbreviations: CBT: Cognitive Behavioral Therapy, CG: Control Group, CLBP: Chronic Low Back Pain, CNLBP: Chronic Non-specific Low Back Pain, CRP: C-Reactive Protein, FABQ: Fear-Avoidance Beliefs Questionnaire, F: Female, GAD-7: Generalized Anxiety Disorder-7, HIRS: Healbone Intelligent Rehabilitation System, IG: Intervention Group, IL-2, IL-4, IL-6: Interleukins (inflammatory biomarkers), M: Male, MRI: Magnetic Resonance Imaging, NLBP: Non-specific Low Back Pain, NPRS: Numeric Pain Rating Scale, ODI: Oswestry Disability Index, PHQ-9: Patient Health Questionnaire-9 (Depression), QoL: Quality of Life, RCT: Randomized Controlled Trial, RMDQ: Roland-Morris Disability Questionnaire, SF-36: 36-Item Short Form Health Survey, TNF-α: Tumor Necrosis Factor-alpha, TSK: Tampa Scale of Kinesiophobia, VAS: Visual Analog Scale, VRE: Virtual Reality Exercise, WPAI: Work Productivity and Activity Impairment Questionnaire.

3.2. Participant Demographics

The studies included in this systematic review analyzed a diverse population of adults with CLBP, with a total of 7166 participants across all studies. Sample sizes varied, ranging from small pilot trials (n = 13) [34] to large-scale observational studies (n = 6468) [37]. The mean age of participants differed across studies, with younger cohorts in sports-related interventions (e.g., soccer players, mean age ~22 years) [17] and older populations in telerehabilitation-based programs (mean age ~43–45 years) [36,39]. Gender distribution was often unbalanced, with some studies predominantly including female participants [37], while others had a more equal representation of males and females [33,36]. Clinical characteristics varied, with most participants experiencing nonspecific or CLBP [32–34,36,37,39],

Meanwhile, some studies specifically targeted subpopulations such as office workers or athletes [17,38]. The demographic variability across studies underscores the generalizability of findings to a broad population of individuals with CLBP undergoing digital rehabilitation interventions.

3.3. Outcome Measures

The studies included in this systematic review assessed a range of outcome measures to evaluate the effectiveness of digital rehabilitation interventions for CLBP. Primary outcomes commonly focused on movement-related parameters, including biomechanical assessments (e.g., range of motion, motor control, and movement kinematics) [17,32–34] and pain intensity, typically measured using the Visual Analog Scale (VAS) or Numeric Pain Rating Scale (NPRS) [17,32–34,36–39]. These biomechanical and movement-based outcomes hold substantial clinical relevance, as they are directly linked to functional impairment, postural instability, and movement inefficiencies commonly observed in individuals with chronic low back pain. Improvements in parameters such as lumbar range of motion, trunk stabilization, and motor coordination are essential for restoring mobility, reducing compensatory patterns, and preventing long-term disability. Several studies also evaluated functional disability through standardized tools such as the Oswestry Disability Index (ODI) and the Roland–Morris Disability Questionnaire (RMDQ) [32,33,36,39]. Secondary outcomes included measures of treatment adherence, QoL (e.g., SF-36, EQ-5D), psychological factors (e.g., depression, anxiety, and fear-avoidance beliefs) [33,36,37], and cost-effectiveness [38,39]. Some studies incorporated wearable motion sensors and ML algorithms to provide real-time movement tracking and biofeedback, allowing for more precise assessment of motor learning and rehabilitation progress. The diversity of outcome measures highlights the multidimensional impact of digital rehabilitation strategies, assessing not only pain relief but also functional improvements, engagement, and broader health-related benefits.

3.4. Biomechanical Assessment

Biomechanical assessment was a fundamental outcome in several studies included in this systematic review, utilizing wearable motion sensors, VR-based systems, and telerehabilitation platforms to objectively measure spinal movement, posture, and motor control. Matheve et al. [32] investigated the impact of sensor-based postural feedback on lumbopelvic movement control, demonstrating a significant improvement in lumbar ROM. Compared to mirror feedback, the sensor-based intervention resulted in an estimated ROM difference of 9.9° (95% CI, 6.1–13.7°; $p < 0.0001$), and compared to no feedback, the difference was 10.6° (95% CI, 6.8–14.3°). The corresponding effect sizes were large (Cohen's d $\approx$ 1.3 for sensor vs. mirror and $\approx$ 1.4 for sensor vs. control), highlighting the superior efficacy of real-time feedback via wireless inertial sensors. Similarly, Matheve et al. [33]

analyzed a VR-based rehabilitation program using motion sensors (Valedo®Pro) during pelvic tilt exercises. Participants in the VR group performed a high number of controlled pelvic tilts (mean = 98.1, SD = 15.6), comparable to that of the control group (mean = 100), indicating consistent motor execution. Participants in the VR group exhibited greater engagement and motivation, reinforcing the potential of gamified rehabilitation to enhance compliance. Mueller et al. [34] explored game-based real-time biofeedback training in a randomized cross-over pilot trial. While no significant changes were observed in trunk lateral flexion range or reproduction accuracy ($p > 0.05$), a small yet significant reduction in trunk extension/flexion range (thoracic segment: mean decrease = 0.9°, $p = 0.02$, d = 0.20) was noted, suggesting reduced compensatory movement and improved control in secondary planes. These findings support the hypothesis that even a single session of sensor-based exergaming may elicit acute improvements in movement efficiency. Nambi et al. [17] examined the effects of a VR-based trunk exercise system using a moving game chair on spinal muscle morphology. After four weeks, significant increases in trunk muscle Cross-Sectional Area (CSA) were reported in the VRE group, with the right psoas major increasing from 8.6 ± 0.4 cm^2 to 9.5 ± 0.3 cm^2 and the multifidus from 5.6 ± 0.6 cm^2 to 7.1 ± 0.5 cm^2 ($p < 0.001$). These changes, although less pronounced than those observed in the isokinetic training group, were accompanied by small-to-moderate effect sizes (e.g., multifidus CSA d = 1.5 right, 1.11 left), suggesting improved muscle engagement and motor recruitment through VR-mediated repetitive movement. Overall, these findings underscore the effectiveness of advanced motion-tracking technologies in delivering precise and objective biomechanical assessments, which are fundamental for optimizing rehabilitation strategies in CLBP management (Table 4).

Table 4. Biomechanical Parameters.

Study	Technology Used	Biomechanical Parameters Assessed	Key Findings	Effect Size (Cohen's d)/ Confidence Interval (CI)	Interpretation
Matheve et al., 2018 [32]	Wireless inertial motion sensors	Lumbar and hip ROM, postural control	Significant improvement in lumbar ROM (+9.9°) with sensor-based feedback vs. mirror ($p < 0.0001$)	Cohen's d ≈ 1.3–1.4; CI: 6.1°–13.7°, 6.8°–14.3°	Large effect
Matheve et al., 2020 [33]	VR-based motion tracking (Valedo®Pro)	Movement control, motor learning	High number of controlled pelvic tilts (mean = 98.1, SD = 15.6); improved engagement and attentional focus, supporting motor learning potential	CI not reported; no direct effect size	Suggests motor learning
Mueller et al., 2022 [34]	Trunk exergame with real-time feedback	Trunk movement control, flexion/extension angles	Reduction in thoracic flexion/extension range ($\Delta = -0.9°$, $p = 0.02$), suggesting improved motion control	Cohen's d = 0.20; CI not reported	Small (acute) improvement

Table 4. *Cont.*

Study	Technology Used	Biomechanical Parameters Assessed	Key Findings	Effect Size (Cohen's d)/ Confidence Interval (CI)	Interpretation
Nambi et al., 2023 [35]	VR-based trunk ex. (Pro-Kin system)	Muscle CSA, spinal mobility	Increase Right psoas major CSA ($8.6 \pm 0.4 \rightarrow 9.5 \pm 0.3$ cm^2); increase in multifidus CSA ($5.6 \pm 0.6 \rightarrow 7.1 \pm 0.5$ cm^2); both $p < 0.001$	Multifidus d = 1.5 (R), 1.11 (L); CI not reported	Moderate–Large improvement

Abbreviations: CI: Confidence Interval, CSA: Cross-Sectional Area, d: Cohen's d (effect size), L: left, R: right, ROM: Range of Motion, SD: Standard Deviation, VR: Virtual Reality, VRE: Virtual Reality Exercise.

3.5. Pain

Pain reduction was a primary outcome across all included studies, with most using the VAS or the NPRS for assessment. Sensor-based rehabilitation programs showed significant pain improvements, particularly in long-term interventions. Bailey et al. [37] reported a 68.45% VAS pain reduction after a 12-week digital care program integrating sensor-guided exercises and remote coaching. This corresponded to a standardized mean difference of 1.37 (95% CI: 1.33–1.40), indicating a large and clinically meaningful effect. Similarly, Shebib et al. [39] found among participants who completed the program that VAS pain scores decreased by 62% (from 43.6 to 16.5) and VAS impact on daily life decreased by 64% (from 37.3 to 13.4), with effect sizes ranging from −23.7 points (95% CI: −31.9 to −15.5; $p < 0.001$). A total of 81% reached a minimally important change in VAS, confirming robust clinical benefit. Matheve et al. [32] evaluated the effects of sensor-based postural feedback on movement control in CLBP patients but did not observe significant changes in pain intensity. NPRS scores remained stable across conditions (baseline: 4.5–4.9; post-intervention mean differences: −0.4 to −0.1), indicating that while movement control improved (ROM differences: 9.9–10.6°, $p < 0.0001$), pain was not directly reduced in the short term. In a follow-up study, they [33] reported significant hypoalgesic effects from a single session of VR-based pelvic tilt exercises: pain intensity decreased during (Cohen's d = 1.29, 95% CI: 0.82–1.76) and immediately after (Cohen's d = 0.85, 95% CI: 0.40–1.29) the session. Additionally, time spent thinking of pain was significantly reduced (d = 1.31, 95% CI: 0.84–1.78), confirming the analgesic potential of interactive and gamified VR interventions.

Mueller et al. [34] investigated game-based real-time feedback training using trunk exergames in a cross-over pilot study. Although the intervention improved trunk motion efficiency and reduced compensatory movements ($p = 0.02$; d = 0.20), no significant pain reduction was observed: VAS decreased from 3.3 ± 2.5 to 2.6 ± 2.5, but this change was not statistically significant ($p > 0.05$). VR-assisted interventions also demonstrated pain relief benefits. Nambi et al. [17] reported significant pain reduction after four weeks of VR-based trunk training: VAS dropped from 7.2 ± 0.4 to 1.8 ± 0.3 ($p = 0.001$). Compared to isokinetic training, the VRE group had a mean difference of 0.7 (95% CI: 0.38–1.07); and compared to conventional training, they had a mean difference of 3.0 (95% CI: 2.68–3.31). The effect size was very large (Cohen's d = 5.37), indicating a robust clinical effect. In a study comparing a motion-detecting exercise coaching app with standard video-based exercise, Park et al. [38] compared a machine-learning-based motion-detecting mobile exercise coaching app with standard video-based coaching. After a 14-day program, the intervention group showed a significantly greater reduction in VAS scores for lower back pain (−0.96 ± 1.82) compared to the control group (−0.26 ± 0.71), with $p < 0.01$ between groups. The improvement was correlated with higher adherence and real-time visual/audio feedback, although the absolute pain reduction was modest. Finally, Shi et al. [36] evaluated the effectiveness of an 8-week telerehabilitation program using a smartphone app and integrated sensors. Although both groups (telerehabilitation and outpatient) showed significant within-group improvements in NPRS (−4.65 points), there were no statistically significant between-group differences (mean difference: −0.39, 95% CI: −2.10 to 1.31; $p = 0.64$), confirming that telerehabilitation was non-inferior to standard care in pain reduction. Overall, these findings suggest that wearable sensors and movement-tracking strategies, combined with VR and telerehabilitation technologies, are effective in reducing pain in individuals with CLBP. However, short-term interventions, such as exergames, may require additional sessions to achieve significant and sustained pain relief (Table 5).

Table 5. Pain.

Study	Pain Outcome Measures	Key Results	Effect Size (Cohen's d)/ Confidence Interval (CI)	Interpretation
Bailey et al., 2020 [37]	VAS	68.45% reduction in pain after 12 weeks of intervention	Cohen's d = 1.37 (95% CI: 1.33–1.40)	Large effect
Matheve et al., 2018 [32]	NPRS	No significant change in pain post-intervention	Not reported	No effect
Matheve et al., 2020 [33]	NPRS	Significant pain reduction during (−1.66) and immediately after VR session ($p < 0.01$)	Cohen's d = 1.29 (95% CI: 0.82–1.76); d = 0.85 (95% CI: 0.40–1.29)	Large short-term effect
Mueller et al., 2022 [34]	VAS	No significant reduction in pain (3.3 ± 2.5 pre, 2.6 ± 2.5 post; $p > 0.05$)	Cohen's d = 0.20	Small effect
Nambi et al., 2023 [35]	VAS	Significant reduction in pain after 4-week intervention ($p < 0.05$)	Cohen's d = 5.37; mean difference vs. conventional = 3.0 (95% CI: 2.68–3.31)	Very large effect
Park et al., 2022 [38]	VAS	Greater pain reduction in MDMECA group (−0.96 vs. −0.26; $p < 0.01$)	Not reported; between-group difference = 0.70 ($p < 0.01$)	Modest group difference
Shebib et al., 2019 [39]	VAS	52–64% reduction in pain post-intervention ($p < 0.001$)	Cohen's d not reported; Δ = −23.7 points (95% CI: −31.9 to −15.5)	Large effect
Shi et al., 2024 [36]	NPRS	Significant within-group improvement; no significant between-group difference ($p = 0.64$)	Between-group Δ = −0.39 (95% CI: −2.10 to 1.31); Cohen's d not reported	Non-inferior to outpatient care

Abbreviations: NPRS: Numeric Pain Rating Scale, VAS: Visual Analog Scale.

3.6. Quality of Life

Two studies in this review evaluated the impact of digital rehabilitation interventions on QoL using SF-36, a standardized measure. Park et al. [38] found a significant improvement in SF-36 scores in participants using a motion-detecting mobile exercise coaching app (+9.10, $p < 0.01$), while the control group showed minimal changes (+1.09, $p = 0.37$). Conversely, Shi et al. [36] observed no statistically significant between-group differences in SF-36 score improvements after 8 weeks of telerehabilitation compared to conventional outpatient rehabilitation. While both groups showed within-group QoL improvements, the mean difference between groups at 8 weeks was −0.38 (95% CI: −8.69 to 7.92; $p = 0.93$), indicating non-inferiority but no superiority of telerehabilitation (Table 6).

Table 6. QoL.

Study	QoL Outcome Measures	Results	Effect Size (Cohen's d)/ Confidence Interval (CI)	Interpretation
Park et al., 2022 [38]	SF-36	Motion-detecting mobile app: +9.10, $p < 0.01$ (significant improvement); Control group: +1.09, $p = 0.37$ (minimal change)	Cohen's d ≈ 0.83; CI not reported	Large effect
Shi et al., 2024 [36]	SF-36	No significant difference, both interventions led to improvement	Effect size not reported; between-group difference Δ = −0.38 (95% CI: −8.69 to 7.92; $p = 0.93$)	No significant difference

Abbreviations: SF-36: 36-Item Short Form Health Survey.

3.7. Adherence

Adherence to remote rehabilitation programs utilizing motion sensors varied across the included studies, with completion rates ranging from 53.1% to 100%. High adherence was observed in interventions that incorporated real-time feedback, structured coaching, and gamification elements. Shebib et al. [39] reported 90% engagement among participants who completed a 12-week digital care program, with an average of 3.8 sensor-guided workouts per week. Similarly, Bailey et al. [37] found a 73.04% completion rate, with higher engagement (exercise sessions, coaching interactions) correlating with better outcomes in pain reduction and QoL. Conversely, interventions with less interactivity or structured support showed lower adherence rates. Park et al. [38] reported that 53.1% of participants completed a 14-day mobile coaching program, significantly higher than the 31.0% completion rate in the control group using standard video-based exercise. Shi et al. [36] further highlighted adherence differences between telerehabilitation-based and conventional exercise programs. The telerehabilitation group (TBEG) demonstrated higher adherence (89%) compared to the conventional outpatient group (81%), suggesting that remote monitoring and motion-tracking technology can enhance compliance with rehabilitation protocols. Finally, Mueller et al. [34] reported 100% adherence in a single-session trunk exergame trial, though this high rate may reflect the short intervention duration rather than long-term engagement trends. Overall, adherence appears to be positively influenced by real-time feedback, structured support, and gamification, whereas less interactive interventions may struggle with participant retention. These findings highlight the need for motivational strategies and personalized rehabilitation approaches to optimize adherence in remote rehabilitation for low back pain (Table 7).

Table 7. Adherence.

Study	Completion/Adherence Rate	Key Findings	Effect Size (Cohen's d)/ Confidence Interval (CI)	Interpretation
Shebib et al., 2019 [39]	90% engagement (3.8 workouts/week)	High adherence with structured support and coaching	Not determined	Not determined
Bailey et al., 2020 [37]	73.04% completion rate	Higher engagement correlated with better pain and QoL outcomes	Not reported	Not reported
Park et al., 2022 [38]	53.1% (mobile app) vs. 31.0% (video-based group)	Real-time motion tracking improved adherence	Not reported	Not reported
Shi et al., 2024 [36]	89% (telerehabilitation) vs. 81% (outpatient)	Remote monitoring enhanced adherence	Not reported	Not reported
Mueller et al., 2022 [34]	100% adherence	Likely due to short intervention duration	Not reported	Not reported

Abbreviations: QoL: Quality of life.

3.8. Any Healthcare Measures

The healthcare outcome measures reported across the included studies varied but primarily focused on pain, which we have already analyzed, and also on psychological well-being, inflammatory biomarkers, and functional disability. Regarding mental health, some improvements were also observed; Bailey et al. [37] reported a 57.5% reduction in depression symptoms and a 58.1% decrease in anxiety levels after 12 weeks of a digital care program. Additionally, reductions in Fear-Avoidance Beliefs Questionnaire (FABQ) scores were noted, with Shi et al. [36] reporting a decrease of 31.92 points (SD 15.07) in the telerehabilitation group and 40.15 points (SD 13.38) in the conventional rehabilitation group ($p = 0.12$), while Matheve et al. found no significant post-intervention differences in FABQ scores (37.0 ± 5.6 vs. 36.2 ± 6.9 at baseline) and also in Tampa Scale of Kinesiophobia (TSK) scores (TSK: 37.0 ± 5.6 in the intervention group vs. 36.2 ± 6.9 in the control group at baseline) [33] (Table 8).

In terms of biological outcomes, Nambi et al. [17] found significant reductions in inflammatory biomarkers in the virtual reality exercise (VRE) group. Specifically, CRP levels decreased from 1.56 ± 0.3 mg/L to 0.4 ± 0.08 mg/L ($p = 0.001$) and TNF-α from 16.6 ± 0.7 pg/mL to 7.7 ± 0.5 pg/mL ($p = 0.001$). The effect sizes were very large, with Cohen's d = 6.66 for CRP and d = 4.54 for TNF-α, indicating extremely strong anti-inflammatory effects. Similar results were observed for other inflammatory markers, such as IL-2 (d = 1.81), IL-4 (d = 1.16), and IL-6 (d = 4.57). These findings support the hypothesis that VR-based rehabilitation may elicit robust systemic anti-inflammatory responses in patients with chronic low back pain, possibly mediated by neuromuscular activation and elevated metabolic demands during interactive tasks (Table 9).

Functional disability is measured through standardized tools such as the ODI and RMDQ. Shebib et al. [39] reported a notable reduction in ODI scores from 19.7 at baseline to 13.5 after a 12-week digital care program, representing a 31.5% improvement in disability. The mean difference between groups was −6.9 points (95% CI: −10.5 to −3.3, $p < 0.001$), indicating a large effect. In contrast, the control group, which only received digital educational content, showed no significant change (18.9 to 19.7). Similarly, Shi et al. [36] found a decrease in ODI scores of 16.42 points (SD 7.30) in the telerehabilitation group compared to

13.18 points (SD 8.48) in the conventional rehabilitation group. However, the difference between groups at 8 weeks was not statistically significant (mean difference: −3.24, 95% CI: −8.65 to 2.17, $p = 0.24$), suggesting noninferiority but no clear superiority. Regarding the RMDQ, Matheve et al. evaluated the impact of sensor-based postural feedback on movement control in CLBP patients, but no significant post-intervention differences in RMDQ scores were observed both in a 2018 [32] study (baseline: 6.6 ± 3.3 in the sensor group, 7.5 ± 4.9 in the mirror feedback group, and 7.7 ± 3.5 in the control group) and 2020 study [33] (RMDQ baseline: 11.4 ± 3.8 in the intervention group vs. 10.9 ± 4.3 in the control group) (Table 10).

Table 8. Psychological Well-Being.

Study	Outcome Measures	Key Findings	Effect Size (Cohen's d)/ Confidence Interval (CI)	Interpretation
Bailey et al., 2020 [37]	Depression Symptoms (PHQ-9)	57.5% reduction in depression symptoms after 12 weeks of digital care program.	Not reported	Not reported
Bailey et al., 2020 [37]	Anxiety Symptoms (GAD-7)	58.1% reduction in anxiety levels after 12 weeks of digital care program.	Not reported	Not reported
Shi et al., 2024 [36]	Fear-Avoidance Beliefs (FABQ)	31.92 points decrease in FABQ (telerehabilitation group). $p = 0.12$.	Not reported	Not reported
Matheve et al., 2020 [33]	Fear-Avoidance Beliefs (FABQ)	No significant change in FABQ scores (VR-based rehabilitation group).	Not reported	Not reported
Matheve et al., 2020 [33]	Fear of Movement (TSK)	No significant change in TSK scores (VR-based rehabilitation group).	Not reported	Not reported

Abbreviations. FABQ: Fear-Avoidance Beliefs Questionnaire, GAD-7: Generalized Anxiety Disorder-7, PHQ-9: Patient Health Questionnaire-9 (Depression), TSK: Tampa Scale of Kinesiophobia, VR: Virtual Reality.

Table 9. Inflammatory Biomarkers.

Study	Outcome Measures	Key Findings	Effect Size (Cohen's d)/Confidence Interval (CI)	Interpretation
Nambi et al., 2023 [35]	CRP (mg/L)	Significant decrease in CRP levels from 1.56 to 0.4 mg/L ($p = 0.001$) after VR-based rehabilitation.	Cohen's d: 6.66	Large effect
Nambi et al., 2023 [35]	TNF-α (pg/mL)	Significant decrease in TNF-α levels from 16.6 to 7.7 pg/mL ($p = 0.001$) after VR-based rehabilitation	Cohen's d: 4.54	Large effect

Abbreviations: CRP: C-Reactive Protein, TNF-α: Tumor Necrosis Factor-alpha, VR: Virtual Reality.

Table 10. Functional Disability.

Study	Outcome Measures	Key Findings	Effect Size (Cohen's d)/ Confidence Interval (CI)	Interpretation
Shebib et al., 2019 [39]	ODI	31.5% improvement in disability (ODI reduction from 19.7 to 13.5).	Not reported; between-group mean difference = −6.9 (95% CI: −10.5 to −3.3; $p < 0.001$)	Large clinical effect
Shi et al., 2024 [36]	ODI	16.42 points decrease in ODI (telerehabilitation group, $p = 0.24$); 13.18 points decrease in ODI (conventional rehabilitation group, $p = 0.24$).	Not reported; between-group difference = −3.24 (95% CI: −8.65 to 2.17; $p = 0.24$)	No significant difference
Matheve et al., 2018 [32]	RMDQ	No significant change in RMDQ scores (baseline: 6.6 ± 3.3 in the sensor group, 7.5 ± 4.9 in the mirror feedback group, and 7.7 ± 3.5 in the control group)	Not reported	Not reported
Matheve et al., 2020 [33]	RMDQ	No significant change in RMDQ scores (baseline: 11.4 ± 3.8 in the intervention group vs. 10.9 ± 4.3 in the control group)	Not reported	Not reported

Abbreviations: ODI: Oswestry Disability Index, RMDQ: Roland-Morris Disability Questionnaire.

3.9. Economic Perspective

The economic perspective was addressed in a limited number of studies included in this systematic review. Bailey et al. [37] reported significant economic benefits associated with a 12-week digital rehabilitation program that combined sensor-guided exercises, cognitive–behavioral support, and remote coaching. Participants experienced a 61.5% reduction in work impairment, as measured by the Work Productivity and Activity Impairment (WPAI) questionnaire, with scores improving from 34.12 ± 26.37 to 12.24 ± 15.58, indicating notable recovery in occupational performance and potential indirect cost savings related to CLBP. Similarly, Shebib et al. [39] highlighted a 52% decrease in surgery interest following participation in a digital care program, suggesting possible reductions in healthcare expenditures by limiting the need for invasive procedures. Regarding willingness to pay, Park et al. [38] evaluated participants' financial acceptability of a motion-detecting mobile exercise coaching application. Although no significant differences were observed between groups, the majority of participants indicated a willingness to pay less than USD 5 per month for the service (45.2% in the intervention group vs. 38.9% in the control group, $p = 0.59$), reflecting a moderate perceived economic value of digital rehabilitation technologies (Table 11).

Table 11. Economic Outcomes.

Study	Economic Outcomes	Key Findings	Effect Size (Cohen's d)/ Confidence Interval (CI)	Interpretation
Bailey et al., 2020 [37]	Work Productivity (WPAI)	61.5% reduction in work impairment (WPAI score from 34.12 ± 26.37 to 12.24 ± 15.58)	Not reported	Not reported
Shebib et al., 2019 [39]	Surgery Interest	52% reduction in surgery interest; potential healthcare cost savings	Not reported	Not reported
Park et al., 2022 [38]	Willingness to Pay	Majority willing to pay < $5/month (45.2% in intervention group; $p = 0.59$)	Not reported	Not reported

Abbreviations: WPAI: Work Productivity and Activity Impairment.

3.10. Discussion

This systematic review aimed to evaluate the effectiveness of remote rehabilitation interventions using motion sensors for individuals with LBP, focusing on key outcomes such as movement improvement, pain reduction, QoL, adherence, healthcare, and economic aspects. The findings suggest that sensor-based digital rehabilitation strategies, often combined with VR, mobile applications, and remote coaching, can provide clinically meaningful improvements across multiple domains of patient care.

From a functional perspective, several studies demonstrated that motion-tracking technologies enhance biomechanical outcomes by improving lumbopelvic movement control, reducing compensatory movements, and promoting motor learning, essential to ensure that movement modifications are retained and successfully transferred to daily life, supporting long-term outcomes in musculoskeletal rehabilitation [40–42]. Additionally, the rapid advancement of markerless and wearable systems has significantly expanded the potential of motion analysis beyond clinical settings, allowing for remote, non-invasive, and automated monitoring of posture and movement [40,43]. Interventions incorporating real-time biofeedback through wearable sensors showed significant improvements in ROM and movement efficiency, highlighting the potential of these technologies to support targeted and personalized rehabilitation approaches. Furthermore, VR-based programs, in particular, contributed to increased engagement and motivation, factors known to enhance adherence and optimize rehabilitation outcomes [44–46].

Pain reduction emerged as a consistent benefit across most included studies, with sensor-guided interventions achieving moderate to large decreases in pain intensity over both short and long-term programs. In general, these benefits are observed across various digital interventions, highlighting their potential in chronic pain management [47]. The Cochrane review by Hayden et al. [48] similarly underscored that structured exercise programs yielded clinically meaningful pain relief compared to no treatment or usual care, particularly when interventions were sustained over time. These findings align with previous research emphasizing the importance of continuous feedback and interactive platforms in sustaining patient participation and addressing chronic musculoskeletal pain [49–52]. However, short-duration interventions, such as single-session exergames, were less effective in producing significant pain relief, suggesting that prolonged and structured programs are necessary to achieve lasting benefits [32,34]. Regarding QoL, the evidence was more limited but promising; improvements were primarily noted in studies utilizing interactive mobile coaching applications, while other interventions showed comparable effects to conventional therapies [36,38]. This variability highlights the need for further high-quality trials to understand the specific contribution of digital rehabilitation to broader health-related QoL metrics. Adherence was generally high across studies, particularly in programs integrating gamification, real-time feedback, and remote supervision. High adherence rates are critical for the success of home-based rehabilitation and are directly linked to improved clinical outcomes. Studies suggest that serious games designed with user-centered principles and motivational strategies, such as real-time feedback and progressive challenges, significantly enhance engagement and adherence [53]. Additionally, multimodal digital care programs have demonstrated high completion rates and engagement, even among socioeconomically disadvantaged groups, reinforcing the importance of accessible and patient-centered rehabilitation strategies [54]. Traditional physiotherapy, by contrast, often suffers from high dropout rates due to factors such as lack of motivation, accessibility barriers, and low patient engagement, highlighting the need for innovative digital solutions to support long-term participation [55,56]. An important limitation of this systematic review lies in the heterogeneity of the included studies, which varied substantially in terms of intervention type (e.g., virtual reality platforms, wearable sensor-based feedback, and mobile coaching applications), program duration (ranging from single-session to 12-week interventions), participant demographics (including age, gender distribution, and clinical profiles), and outcome measurement tools. These differences reflect the diverse landscape of digital rehabilitation approaches for chronic low back pain and underscore the challenge of drawing uniform conclusions. While such heterogeneity limits the comparability of results and precluded formal subgroup analysis due to the small number of included studies (n = 8), it also provides a comprehensive overview of current practices and innovation trends in this domain. Future research should prioritize standardized intervention protocols, consistent outcome measures, and stratified study designs to enable more rigorous comparative analyses and meta-analytic synthesis. Moreover, subgroup analyses based on clinical characteristics (e.g., baseline disability level, age groups, or type of digital platform used) will be essential to better understand which interventions are most effective for specific patient populations.

From an economic perspective, only a few studies directly have addressed cost-related outcomes. Bailey et al. [37] reported a significant reduction in work impairment, reflecting potential indirect cost savings through improved productivity. A Cochrane review [48] highlighted that CLBP leads to a significant number of lost work hours, with 65% of patients still experiencing pain after one year, but exercise-based interventions were linked to lower absenteeism and improved productivity, reinforcing their economic benefits. Similarly, Shebib et al. [39] identified a decreased interest in surgical intervention, suggesting downstream healthcare cost reductions. However, despite these encouraging signals, formal health economic evaluations remain scarce. This limits the ability to draw definitive conclusions regarding the cost-effectiveness and financial sustainability of digital rehabilitation strategies for CLBP. Future studies should incorporate robust economic analyses to assess direct healthcare costs, indirect societal costs, and long-term value.

Overall, this review highlights the promising role of wearable sensors, telerehabilitation, and VR technologies in managing CLBP, with reported improvements in pain, movement control, and adherence. However, some findings, particularly those from small-scale or pilot studies with a higher risk of bias [17,34], should be interpreted with caution. These studies, while innovative, may overestimate treatment effects due to methodological limitations such as lack of blinding or small sample sizes. Future high-quality trials are needed to confirm these preliminary results and to standardize outcome reporting, particularly for biomechanical and adherence-related endpoints.

3.11. Comparison of Digital Rehabilitation Modalities and Implementation Challenges

This review included a range of digital rehabilitation modalities, each with unique characteristics influencing their clinical impact. VR-based interventions provided immersive and gamified environments that enhanced motivation and engagement [32,33]. These programs were particularly effective in improving movement control and reducing pain, especially when coupled with motion-tracking technologies. However, VR systems often require dedicated hardware and infrastructure, which may limit their scalability and accessibility in low-resource settings.

AI-driven mobile coaching applications, on the other hand, offered greater flexibility and ease of access by delivering real-time exercise feedback through smartphones [38]. These interventions showed beneficial effects on pain and quality of life and may be especially suited to patients requiring minimal technical support or remote supervision. While more scalable, these tools may provide less detailed biomechanical feedback than sensor-based systems.

Telerehabilitation platforms with wearable sensors allowed for precise movement analysis, objective tracking of rehabilitation progress, and personalized remote supervision [34,36,37,39]. These approaches demonstrated positive outcomes in terms of adherence, functional improvement, and psychological well-being. Nonetheless, long-term data on sustainability and outcomes beyond the intervention period remain limited.

Taken together, the comparative analysis suggests that each modality has strengths suited to specific patient needs, technological resources, and rehabilitation goals. Future studies should directly compare these approaches to determine optimal implementation strategies for chronic low back pain management.

However, beyond clinical effectiveness, several practical challenges must be considered for the successful implementation of digital rehabilitation strategies. Digital literacy remains a key barrier, especially among older adults or individuals with low technological familiarity, who may struggle to engage with mobile apps, VR systems, or sensor-based platforms [57]. Additionally, limited internet access or unstable connectivity, particularly in rural or underserved regions, may delay the continuity of remote rehabilitation [58]. The acceptance and readiness of healthcare professionals also influence adoption: lack of training, skepticism toward digital tools, and concerns about data security may reduce uptake in clinical practice [59], particularly in the field of musculoskeletal rehabilitation, which has traditionally relied on direct physical contact with patients [60]. In addition, ethical and regulatory issues, such as ensuring informed consent, data privacy, and compliance with telehealth legislation, must be carefully addressed to support the responsible integration of these technologies into clinical care [61].

Addressing these challenges is essential to ensure that digital rehabilitation becomes a truly accessible, inclusive, and sustainable solution for chronic low back pain.

4. Conclusions

This systematic review underscores the growing role of remote rehabilitation and VR interventions using motion sensors in managing CLBP. The findings demonstrate that these innovative digital approaches offer significant benefits in multiple domains, including improved movement control, pain reduction, treatment adherence, and suggestive evidence of improvements in QoL. Motion sensors, particularly when integrated with real-time feedback, gamification, and remote supervision, facilitate a more engaging and personalized rehabilitation experience, which is crucial for maintaining long-term participation and optimizing outcomes. VR-based interventions have also shown promise in enhancing proprioception, reducing kinesiophobia, and increasing motivation compared to conventional therapies. Furthermore, adherence to digital rehabilitation programs was consistently high, particularly in interventions incorporating structured coaching and interactive elements, addressing a well-known limitation of traditional physiotherapy, which often suffers from high dropout rates. The economic impact of these technologies, although supported by preliminary findings, suggests potential cost savings through reduced work impairment, improved productivity, and lower healthcare utilization. The integration of wearable sensors and ML tools further expands the potential for real-time monitoring and adaptive treatment, paving the way for more precise and individualized rehabilitation protocols. Overall, the reviewed evidence highlights the transformative potential of digital rehabilitation for CLBP, offering a viable alternative or complement to conventional physiotherapy. These interventions not only provide clinically meaningful improvements but also increase accessibility, particularly for patients with limited access to in-person rehabilitation services. Moving forward, the continued development and refinement of digital rehabilitation technologies, alongside structured implementation strategies, will be key to optimizing their effectiveness and ensuring widespread adoption in clinical practice.

Limitations and Research Gaps

This review highlights promising results, but several limitations must be considered. The study heterogeneity, including variations in sample sizes, intervention protocols, and follow-up durations, limits direct comparisons. Many studies had short intervention periods and potential biases, particularly in blinding and adherence reporting. Additionally, long-term effects remain unclear due to limited follow-up data. The lack of large-scale RCTs and formal cost-effectiveness analyses prevents definitive conclusions on the financial sustainability of digital rehabilitation. Future studies should adopt standardized reporting frameworks to enhance reproducibility and comparability across trials. Multicentric RCTs are also needed to improve external validity and representativeness of patient populations. Moreover, incorporating robust cost-effectiveness evaluations will be essential to inform health policy decisions and guide the allocation of resources. While pain and biomechanical improvements were well-documented, psychosocial factors and long-term adherence received less attention. Future research should focus on standardized methodologies, longer follow-up periods, and AI-driven personalized rehabilitation models. Exploring multidisciplinary approaches that integrate digital rehabilitation with behavioral strategies could further enhance engagement and long-term outcomes. Addressing these gaps will help optimize the effectiveness and integration of motion sensor-based rehabilitation for CLBP.

Author Contributions: Conceptualization and Study Design: M.G. (Marina Garofano), R.D.S., M.C. (Mariaconsiglia Calabrese), M.G. (Massimo Giordano), M.P.D.P., and M.B. contributed to the study's conceptualization and methodological framework. Data Collection and Analysis: C.M.R., G.U., G.F., F.D.S., M.A., and M.C. (Michele Ciccarelli) performed the literature search, data extraction, and risk of bias assessment. Manuscript Writing and Editing: C.P., G.S., and P.B. contributed to drafting the manuscript, revising it critically for important intellectual content, and ensuring the coherence of the discussion and conclusions. Supervision and Final Approval: A.B. and M.G. (Marina Garofano) supervised all stages of the study, including methodology validation, data interpretation, and final manuscript approval. All authors have read and agreed to the published version of the manuscript.

Funding: Research project titled "RespirAction", identified by CUP B83C22003920001, conducted under the scientific responsibility of Prof. Alessia Bramanti as part of the cascading call for Universities, Institutions, and Research Organizations within the "THE—Tuscany Health Ecosystem" project, issued with D.D. 2004/2023—Prot. 315887 on 22 December 2023.

Institutional Review Board Statement: Not applicable.

Informed Consent Statement: Not applicable.

Data Availability Statement: All data are included in this study.

Conflicts of Interest: The authors declare no conflicts of interest.

Appendix A. Search Strategy

Database	Search Strategy	Filters applied	Date of Search
PubMed	#1: Low Back Pain [Mesh] OR # 2: Back Pain, Low OR Back Pains, Low OR Low Back Pains OR Pain, Low Back OR Pains, Low Back OR Low Back Ache OR Ache, Low Back OR Aches, Low Back OR Back Ache, Low OR Back Aches, Low OR Low Back Aches OR Low Backache OR Backache, Low OR Backaches, Low OR Low Backaches OR Lower Back Pain OR Back Pain, Lower OR Back Pains, Lower OR Lower Back Pains OR Pain, Lower Back OR Pains, Lower Back OR Lumbago OR Low Back Pain, Mechanical OR Mechanical Low Back Pain OR Low Back Pain, Posterior Compartment OR Low Back Pain, Postural OR Postural Low Back Pain OR Low Back Pain, Recurrent OR Recurrent Low Back Pain # 3: # 1 OR #2 AND #4: rehabilitation OR physical therapy modalities OR home exercises AND # 5: motion detection OR motion analysis OR motion capture OR motion detection OR movement analysis OR motion tracking OR movement tracking OR sensor OR camera OR video OR User-Computer Interface[MeSH Terms] OR serious game OR exergame OR kinect OR wii OR virtual reality OR feedback OR biofeedback #6: #3 AND #4 AND #5	Publication years: 2015–2025, Filters: Clinical Trial, English, Adult: 19+ years	1 February 2025
Scopus	TITLE-ABS-KEY("Low Back Pain" OR "Back Pain, Low" OR "Back Pains, Low" OR "Low Back Pains" OR "Pain, Low Back" OR "Pains, Low Back" OR "Low Back Ache" OR "Ache, Low Back" OR "Aches, Low Back" OR "Back Ache, Low" OR "Back Aches, Low" OR "Low Back Aches" OR "Low Backache" OR "Backache, Low" OR "Backaches, Low" OR "Low Backaches" OR "Lower Back Pain" OR "Back Pain, Lower" OR "Back Pains, Lower" OR "Lower Back Pains" OR "Pain, Lower Back" OR "Pains, Lower Back" OR "Lumbago" OR "Low Back Pain, Mechanical" OR "Mechanical Low Back Pain" OR "Low Back Pain, Posterior Compartment" OR "Low Back Pain, Postural" OR "Postural Low Back Pain" OR "Low Back Pain, Recurrent" OR "Recurrent Low Back Pain") AND TITLE-ABS-KEY("rehabilitation" OR "physical therapy modalities" OR "home exercises") AND TITLE-ABS-KEY("motion detection" OR "motion analysis" OR "motion capture" OR "movement analysis" OR "motion tracking" OR "movement tracking" OR "sensor" OR "camera" OR "video" OR "User-Computer Interface" OR "serious game" OR "exergame" OR "kinect" OR "wii" OR "virtual reality" OR "feedback" OR "biofeedback")	Publication years: 2015–2025,	1 February 2025

Database	Search Strategy	Filters applied	Date of Search
Web of Science	TS = ("Low Back Pain" OR "Back Pain, Low" OR "Back Pains, Low" OR "Low Back Pains" OR "Pain, Low Back" OR "Pains, Low Back" OR "Low Back Ache" OR "Ache, Low Back" OR "Aches, Low Back" OR "Back Ache, Low" OR "Back Aches, Low" OR "Low Back Aches" OR "Low Backache" OR "Backache, Low" OR "Backaches, Low" OR "Low Backaches" OR "Lower Back Pain" OR "Back Pain, Lower" OR "Back Pains, Lower" OR "Lower Back Pains" OR "Pain, Lower Back" OR "Pains, Lower Back" OR "Lumbago" OR "Low Back Pain, Mechanical" OR "Mechanical Low Back Pain" OR "Low Back Pain, Posterior Compartment" OR "Low Back Pain, Postural" OR "Postural Low Back Pain" OR "Low Back Pain, Recurrent" OR "Recurrent Low Back Pain") AND TS = ("rehabilitation" OR "physical therapy modalities" OR "home exercises") AND TS = ("motion detection" OR "motion analysis" OR "motion capture" OR "movement analysis" OR "motion tracking" OR "movement tracking" OR "sensor" OR "camera" OR "video" OR "User-Computer Interface" OR "serious game" OR "exergame" OR "kinect" OR "wii" OR "virtual reality" OR "feedback" OR "biofeedback")	Publication years: 2015–2025, Document types: Article, Language: English	1 February 2025
PEDro	Simple search: Telerehabilitation, low back pain		1 February 2025

References

1. Krismer, M.; van Tulder, M.; The Low Back Pain Group of the Bone and Joint Health Strategies for Europe Project. Low back pain (non-specific). *Best Pract. Res. Clin. Rheumatol.* **2007**, *21*, 77–91. [CrossRef] [PubMed]
2. Maher, C.; Underwood, M.; Buchbinder, R. Non-specific low back pain. *Lancet* **2017**, *389*, 736–747. [CrossRef] [PubMed]
3. Custers, P.; Van de Kelft, E.; Eeckhaut, B.; Sabbe, W.; Hofman, A.; Debuysscher, A.; Van Acker, G.; Maes, G. Clinical Examination, Diagnosis, and Conservative Treatment of Chronic Low Back Pain: A Narrative Review. *Life* **2024**, *14*, 1090. [CrossRef] [PubMed]
4. Vos, T.; Lim, S.S.; Abbafati, C.; Abbas, K.M.; Abbasi, M.; Abbasifard, M.; Abbasi-Kangevari, M.; Abbastabar, H.; Abd-Allah, F.; Abdelalim, A.; et al. Global burden of 369 diseases and injuries in 204 countries and territories, 1990–2019: A systematic analysis for the Global Burden of Disease Study 2019. *Lancet* **2020**, *396*, 1204–1222. [CrossRef]
5. Sirbu, E.; Onofrei, R.R.; Szasz, S.; Susan, M. Predictors of disability in patients with chronic low back pain. *Arch. Med. Sci.* **2023**, *19*, 94–100. [CrossRef]
6. Foster, N.E.; Anema, J.R.; Cherkin, D.; Chou, R.; Cohen, S.P.; Gross, D.P.; Ferreira, P.H.; Fritz, J.M.; Koes, B.W.; Peul, W.; et al. Prevention and treatment of low back pain: Evidence, challenges, and promising directions. *Lancet* **2018**, *391*, 2368–2383. [CrossRef]
7. Mauck, M.C.; Aylward, A.F.; Barton, C.E.; Birckhead, B.; Carey, T.; Dalton, D.M.; Fields, A.J.; Fritz, J.; Hassett, A.L.; Hoffmeyer, A.; et al. Evidence-based interventions to treat chronic low back pain: Treatment selection for a personalized medicine approach. *Pain. Rep.* **2022**, *7*, e1019. [CrossRef]
8. Blanco-Giménez, P.; Vicente-Mampel, J.; Gargallo, P.; Baraja-Vegas, L.; Bautista, I.J.; Ros-Bernal, F.; Barrios, C. Clinical relevance of combined treatment with exercise in patients with chronic low back pain: A randomized controlled trial. *Sci. Rep.* **2024**, *14*, 17042. [CrossRef]
9. Palazzo, C.; Klinger, E.; Dorner, V.; Kadri, A.; Thierry, O.; Boumenir, Y.; Martin, W.; Poiraudeau, S.; Ville, I. Barriers to home-based exercise program adherence with chronic low back pain: Patient expectations regarding new technologies. *Ann. Phys. Rehabil. Med.* **2016**, *59*, 107–113. [CrossRef]
10. Matheve, T.; Brumagne, S.; Timmermans, A.A.A. The Effectiveness of Technology-Supported Exercise Therapy for Low Back Pain: A Systematic Review. *Am. J. Phys. Med. Rehabil.* **2017**, *96*, 347–356. [CrossRef]
11. Trost, Z.; Zielke, M.; Guck, A.; Nowlin, L.; Zakhidov, D.; France, C.R.; Keefe, F. The promise and challenge of virtual gaming technologies for chronic pain: The case of graded exposure for low back pain. *Pain Manag.* **2015**, *5*, 197–206. [CrossRef] [PubMed]
12. Lara-Palomo, I.C.; Gil-Martínez, E.; Ramírez-García, J.D.; Capel-Alcaraz, A.M.; García-López, H.; Castro-Sánchez, A.M.; Antequera-Soler, E. Efficacy of e-Health Interventions in Patients with Chronic Low-Back Pain: A Systematic Review with Meta-Analysis. *Telemed. J. E-Health* **2022**, *28*, 1734–1752. [CrossRef] [PubMed]
13. De Cola, M.C.; Maresca, G.; D'Aleo, G.; Carnazza, L.; Giliberto, S.; Maggio, M.G.; Bramanti, A.; Calabrò, R.S. Teleassistance for frail elderly people: A usability and customer satisfaction study. *Geriatr. Nurs.* **2020**, *41*, 463–467. [CrossRef] [PubMed]

14. Raiszadeh, K.; Tapicer, J.; Taitano, L.; Wu, J.; Shahidi, B. In-Clinic Versus Web-Based Multidisciplinary Exercise-Based Rehabilitation for Treatment of Low Back Pain: Prospective Clinical Trial in an Integrated Practice Unit Model. *J. Med. Internet Res.* **2021**, *23*, e22548. [CrossRef]
15. Wang, S.; Sun, J.; Yin, X.; Li, H. Effect of virtual reality technology as intervention for people with kinesiophobia: A meta-analysis of randomised controlled trials. *J. Clin. Nurs.* **2023**, *32*, 3074–3086. [CrossRef]
16. Gür, O.; Başar, S. The effect of virtual reality on pain, kinesiophobia and function in total knee arthroplasty patients: A randomized controlled trial. *Knee* **2023**, *45*, 187–197. [CrossRef]
17. Nambi, G.; Abdelbasset, W.K.; Alrawaili, S.M.; Alsubaie, S.F.; Abodonya, A.M.; Saleh, A.K. Virtual reality or isokinetic training; its effect on pain, kinesiophobia and serum stress hormones in chronic low back pain: A randomized controlled trial. *Technol. Health Care* **2021**, *29*, 155–166. [CrossRef]
18. Corallo, A.; Lazoi, M.; Papadia, G.; Pascarelli, C. Action research on virtual-reality-assisted product and process design. *IEEE Trans. Eng. Manag.* **2020**, *69*, 3292–3309. [CrossRef]
19. Alowais, S.A.; Alghamdi, S.S.; Alsuhebany, N.; Alqahtani, T.; Alshaya, A.I.; Almohareb, S.N.; Aldairem, A.; Alrashed, M.; Bin Saleh, K.; Badreldin, H.A.; et al. Revolutionizing healthcare: The role of artificial intelligence in clinical practice. *BMC Med. Educ.* **2023**, *23*, 689. [CrossRef]
20. Reis, F.J.J.; Carvalho, M.B.L.; Neves, G.A.; Nogueira, L.C.; Meziat-Filho, N. Machine learning methods in physical therapy: A scoping review of applications in clinical context. *Musculoskelet. Sci. Pract.* **2024**, *74*, 103184. [CrossRef]
21. Brons, A.; Wang, S.; Visser, B.; Kröse, B.; Bakkes, S.; Veltkamp, R. Machine Learning Methods to Personalize Persuasive Strategies in mHealth Interventions That Promote Physical Activity: Scoping Review and Categorization Overview. *J. Med. Internet Res.* **2024**, *26*, e47774. [CrossRef] [PubMed]
22. Halilaj, E.; Rajagopal, A.; Fiterau, M.; Hicks, J.L.; Hastie, T.J.; Delp, S.L. Machine learning in human movement biomechanics: Best practices, common pitfalls, and new opportunities. *J. Biomech.* **2018**, *81*, 1–11. [CrossRef] [PubMed]
23. Ross, G.B. The Objective Assessment of Movement Quality Using Motion Capture and Machine Learning. Ph.D. Thesis, Université d'Ottawa/University of Ottawa, Ottawa, ON, Canada, 2022.
24. Morouço, P. Wearable Technology and Its Influence on Motor Development and Biomechanical Analysis. *Int. J. Environ. Res. Public. Health* **2024**, *21*, 1126. [CrossRef] [PubMed]
25. Heikenfeld, J.; Jajack, A.; Rogers, J.; Gutruf, P.; Tian, L.; Pan, T.; Li, R.; Khine, M.; Kim, J.; Wang, J. Wearable sensors: Modalities, challenges, and prospects. *Lab. Chip* **2018**, *18*, 217–248. [CrossRef]
26. Porciuncula, F.; Roto, A.V.; Kumar, D.; Davis, I.; Roy, S.; Walsh, C.J.; Awad, L.N. Wearable Movement Sensors for Rehabilitation: A Focused Review of Technological and Clinical Advances. *Pm&r* **2018**, *10*, S220–s232. [CrossRef]
27. Celletti, C.; Mollica, R.; Ferrario, C.; Galli, M.; Camerota, F. Functional Evaluation Using Inertial Measurement of Back School Therapy in Lower Back Pain. *Sensors* **2020**, *20*, 531. [CrossRef]
28. Page, M.J.; McKenzie, J.E.; Bossuyt, P.M.; Boutron, I.; Hoffmann, T.C.; Mulrow, C.D.; Shamseer, L.; Tetzlaff, J.M.; Akl, E.A.; Brennan, S.E.; et al. The PRISMA 2020 statement: An updated guideline for reporting systematic reviews. *BMJ* **2021**, *372*, n71. [CrossRef]
29. Schardt, C.; Adams, M.B.; Owens, T.; Keitz, S.; Fontelo, P. Utilization of the PICO framework to improve searching PubMed for clinical questions. *BMC Med. Inform. Decis. Mak.* **2007**, *7*, 16. [CrossRef]
30. Sterne, J.A.C.; Savović, J.; Page, M.J.; Elbers, R.G.; Blencowe, N.S.; Boutron, I.; Cates, C.J.; Cheng, H.Y.; Corbett, M.S.; Eldridge, S.M.; et al. RoB 2: A revised tool for assessing risk of bias in randomised trials. *BMJ* **2019**, *366*, l4898. [CrossRef]
31. Sterne, J.A.; Hernán, M.A.; Reeves, B.C.; Savović, J.; Berkman, N.D.; Viswanathan, M.; Henry, D.; Altman, D.G.; Ansari, M.T.; Boutron, I.; et al. ROBINS-I: A tool for assessing risk of bias in non-randomised studies of interventions. *BMJ* **2016**, *355*, i4919. [CrossRef]
32. Mueller, J.; Niederer, D.; Tenberg, S.; Oberheim, L.; Moesner, A.; Mueller, S. Acute effects of game-based biofeedback training on trunk motion in chronic low back pain: A randomized cross-over pilot trial. *BMC Sports Sci. Med. Rehabil.* **2022**, *14*, 192. [CrossRef] [PubMed]
33. Bailey, J.F.; Agarwal, V.; Zheng, P.; Smuck, M.; Fredericson, M.; Kennedy, D.J.; Krauss, J. Digital Care for Chronic Musculoskeletal Pain: 10,000 Participant Longitudinal Cohort Study. *J. Med. Internet Res.* **2020**, *22*, e18250. [CrossRef] [PubMed]
34. Shi, W.; Zhang, Y.; Bian, Y.; Chen, L.; Yuan, W.; Zhang, H.; Feng, Q.; Liu, D.; Lin, Y. The Physical and Psychological Effects of Telerehabilitation-Based Exercise for Patients With Nonspecific Low Back Pain: Prospective Randomized Controlled Trial. *JMIR Mhealth Uhealth* **2024**, *12*, e56580. [CrossRef] [PubMed]
35. Shebib, R.; Bailey, J.F.; Smittenaar, P.; Perez, D.A.; Mecklenburg, G.; Hunter, S. Randomized controlled trial of a 12-week digital care program in improving low back pain. *NPJ Digit. Med.* **2019**, *2*, 1. [CrossRef]

36. Matheve, T.; Bogaerts, K.; Timmermans, A. Virtual reality distraction induces hypoalgesia in patients with chronic low back pain: A randomized controlled trial. *J. Neuroeng. Rehabil.* **2020**, *17*, 55. [CrossRef]
37. Matheve, T.; Brumagne, S.; Demoulin, C.; Timmermans, A. Sensor-based postural feedback is more effective than conventional feedback to improve lumbopelvic movement control in patients with chronic low back pain: A randomised controlled trial. *J. Neuroeng. Rehabil.* **2018**, *15*, 85. [CrossRef]
38. Park, J.; Chung, S.Y.; Park, J.H. Real-Time Exercise Feedback through a Convolutional Neural Network: A Machine Learning-Based Motion-Detecting Mobile Exercise Coaching Application. *Yonsei Med. J.* **2022**, *63*, S34–S42. [CrossRef]
39. Simpson, L.; Maharaj, M.M.; Mobbs, R.J. The role of wearables in spinal posture analysis: A systematic review. *BMC Musculoskelet. Disord.* **2019**, *20*, 55. [CrossRef]
40. Mengis, N.; Schmidt, S.; Ellermann, A.; Sobau, C.; Egloff, C.; Kreher, M.M.; Ksoll, K.; Schmidt-Lucke, C.; Rippke, J.N. A Novel Sensor-Based Application for Home-Based Rehabilitation Can Objectively Measure Postoperative Outcomes following Anterior Cruciate Ligament Reconstruction. *J. Pers. Med.* **2023**, *13*, 1398. [CrossRef]
41. Charlton, J.M.; Eng, J.J.; Li, L.C.; Hunt, M.A. Learning Gait Modifications for Musculoskeletal Rehabilitation: Applying Motor Learning Principles to Improve Research and Clinical Implementation. *Phys. Ther.* **2021**, *101*, pzaa207. [CrossRef]
42. Roggio, F.; Ravalli, S.; Maugeri, G.; Bianco, A.; Palma, A.; Di Rosa, M.; Musumeci, G. Technological advancements in the analysis of human motion and posture management through digital devices. *World J. Orthop.* **2021**, *12*, 467–484. [CrossRef] [PubMed]
43. Bevilacqua, R.; Maranesi, E.; Riccardi, G.R.; Donna, V.D.; Pelliccioni, P.; Luzi, R.; Lattanzio, F.; Pelliccioni, G. Non-Immersive Virtual Reality for Rehabilitation of the Older People: A Systematic Review into Efficacy and Effectiveness. *J. Clin. Med.* **2019**, *8*, 1882. [CrossRef] [PubMed]
44. Sessoms, P.H.; Fraser, J.J.; Bodell, D.M.; Haluch, K.S.; Markham, A.E.; Brookfield, J.S.; Jameson, J.; Gottshall, K.R. Clinical effectiveness of virtual reality versus conventional clinic-based vestibular physical therapy on balance and function in active duty service members. A pilot randomized controlled trial. *Virtual Real.* **2023**, *27*, 263–276. [CrossRef]
45. Brepohl, P.C.A.; Leite, H. Virtual reality applied to physiotherapy: A review of current knowledge. *Virtual Real.* **2023**, *27*, 71–95. [CrossRef]
46. Cui, D.; Janela, D.; Costa, F.; Molinos, M.; Areias, A.C.; Moulder, R.G.; Scheer, J.K.; Bento, V.; Cohen, S.P.; Yanamadala, V.; et al. Randomized-controlled trial assessing a digital care program versus conventional physiotherapy for chronic low back pain. *NPJ Digit. Med.* **2023**, *6*, 121. [CrossRef]
47. Hayden, J.A.; Ellis, J.; Ogilvie, R.; Malmivaara, A.; van Tulder, M.W. Exercise therapy for chronic low back pain. *Cochrane Database Syst. Rev.* **2021**, *9*, Cd009790. [CrossRef]
48. Moore, S.K.; Guarino, H.; Acosta, M.C.; Aronson, I.D.; Marsch, L.A.; Rosenblum, A.; Grabinski, M.J.; Turk, D.C. Patients as collaborators: Using focus groups and feedback sessions to develop an interactive, web-based self-management intervention for chronic pain. *Pain. Med.* **2013**, *14*, 1730–1740. [CrossRef]
49. Takai, Y.; Yamamoto-Mitani, N.; Abe, Y.; Suzuki, M. Literature review of pain management for people with chronic pain. *Jpn. J. Nurs. Sci.* **2015**, *12*, 167–183. [CrossRef]
50. Keogh, E.; Rosser, B.A.; Eccleston, C. E-Health and chronic pain management: Current status and developments. *Pain* **2010**, *151*, 18–21. [CrossRef]
51. Eckard, C.; Asbury, C.; Bolduc, B.; Camerlengo, C.; Gotthardt, J.; Healy, L.; Waialae, L.; Zeigler, C.; Childers, J.; Horzempa, J. The Integration of Technology into Treatment Programs to Aid in the Reduction of Chronic Pain. *J. Pain. Manag. Med.* **2016**, *2*, 118. [CrossRef]
52. Ambros-Antemate, J.F.; Beristain-Colorado, M.D.P.; Vargas-Treviño, M.; Gutiérrez-Gutiérrez, J.; Hernández-Cruz, P.A.; Gallegos-Velasco, I.B.; Moreno-Rodríguez, A. Improving Adherence to Physical Therapy in the Development of Serious Games: Conceptual Framework Design Study. *JMIR Form. Res.* **2023**, *7*, e39838. [CrossRef] [PubMed]
53. Areias, A.C.; Molinos, M.; Moulder, R.G.; Janela, D.; Scheer, J.K.; Bento, V.; Yanamadala, V.; Cohen, S.P.; Correia, F.D.; Costa, F. The potential of a multimodal digital care program in addressing healthcare inequities in musculoskeletal pain management. *NPJ Digit. Med.* **2023**, *6*, 188. [CrossRef] [PubMed]
54. Jack, K.; McLean, S.M.; Moffett, J.K.; Gardiner, E. Barriers to treatment adherence in physiotherapy outpatient clinics: A systematic review. *Man. Ther.* **2010**, *15*, 220–228. [CrossRef] [PubMed]
55. Garofano, M.; Vecchione, C.; Calabrese, M.; Rusciano, M.R.; Visco, V.; Granata, G.; Carrizzo, A.; Galasso, G.; Bramanti, P.; Corallo, F.; et al. Technological Developments, Exercise Training Programs, and Clinical Outcomes in Cardiac Telerehabilitation in the Last Ten Years: A Systematic Review. *Healthcare* **2024**, *12*, 1534. [CrossRef]
56. Kebede, A.S.; Ozolins, L.L.; Holst, H.; Galvin, K. Digital Engagement of Older Adults: Scoping Review. *J. Med. Internet Res.* **2022**, *24*, e40192. [CrossRef]

57. Leochico, C.F.D.; Espiritu, A.I.; Ignacio, S.D.; Mojica, J.A.P. Challenges to the Emergence of Telerehabilitation in a Developing Country: A Systematic Review. *Front. Neurol.* **2020**, *11*, 1007. [CrossRef]
58. Erturan, S.; Burak, M.; Elbasan, B. Breaking barriers: Exploring physiotherapists' willingness and challenges in embracing telerehabilitation in a developing country. *Ir. J. Med. Sci.* **2024**, *193*, 1359–1367. [CrossRef]
59. Dierick, F.; Pierre, A.; Profeta, L.; Telliez, F.; Buisseret, F. Perceived Usefulness of Telerehabilitation of Musculoskeletal Disorders: A Belgium-France Pilot Study during Second Wave of COVID-19 Pandemic. *Healthcare* **2021**, *9*, 1605. [CrossRef]
60. Giansanti, D. The Future of Healthcare Is Digital: Unlocking the Potential of Mobile Health and E-Health Solutions. *Healthcare* **2025**, *13*, 802. [CrossRef]
61. Houser, S.H.; Flite, C.A.; Foster, S.L. Privacy and Security Risk Factors Related to Telehealth Services—A Systematic Review. *Perspect. Health Inf. Manag.* **2023**, *20*, 1f.

technologies

MDPI

Systematic Review

Assistive and Emerging Technologies to Detect and Reduce Neurophysiological Stress and Anxiety in Children and Adolescents with Autism and Sensory Processing Disorders: A Systematic Review

Pantelis Pergantis [1,2,*], Victoria Bamicha [1], Aikaterini Doulou [1,2], Antonios I. Christou [3], Nikolaos Bardis [4], Charalabos Skianis [2] and Athanasios Drigas [1,*]

1 Net Media Lab & Mind & Brain R&D, Institute of Informatics & Telecommunications, National Centre of Scientific Research 'Demokritos', 153 41 Agia Paraskevi, Greece; vbamicha@iit.demokritos.gr (V.B.); katerina.doulou@gmail.com (A.D.)

2 Department of Information & Communication Systems Engineering, University of the Aegean, 832 00 Karlovasi, Greece; cskianis@aegean.gr

3 Department of Special Education, University of Thessaly, 382 21 Volos, Greece; antchristou@uth.gr

4 Mathematics and Engineering Science Sector, Hellenic Army Academy, 166 73 Vari, Greece; nbardis@sse.gr

* Correspondence: pantperg@helit.duth.gr (P.P.); dr@iit.demokritos.gr (A.D.)

Abstract: This systematic review aims to investigate the ways in which assistive and developing technologies can help children and adolescents with autism spectrum disorder (ASD) experience less stress and neurophysiological distress. According to recent CDC data, the prevalence of ASD in the United States has climbed to 1 in 36 children. The symptoms of ASD can manifest in a wide range of ways, and the illness itself exhibits significant variations. Furthermore, it has been closely linked to experiencing stress and worry in one's life, which many people refer to as sensory processing disorder (SPD). SPD is a disorder that describes how people behave when they are exposed to environmental stimuli that they may not normally process by feeling more intense than what is causing them to worry and distress. One of the most significant limiting factors that can prevent someone from engaging in what they need to do in their everyday lives is stress. Individuals with ASD deal with stress on a regular basis, which has a big impact on how they function. In order to address a significant research vacuum concerning the use of assistive and emerging technologies to reduce stress in individuals with ASD, this systematic review aims to investigate performance, measuring techniques, and interventions by gathering data from the past 10 years. In order to determine the research hypothesis, particular research questions, and the inclusion and exclusion criteria for the studies, the research process entails gathering studies through systematic review analysis in accordance with the PRISMA principles. Experimental and observational studies on the use of assistive and emerging technologies for stress and anxiety management in children and adolescents with ASD that were published only in English met the inclusion criteria. Research not directly related to stress and anxiety outcomes, articles published in languages other than English, and research conducted outside of the designated time frame were also excluded. The study's findings demonstrated that the technologies under examination had beneficial impacts on reducing stress; nonetheless, notable limitations were found that could compromise the replication and generalizability of legitimate and dependable applications in their utilization.

Keywords: autism spectrum disorder; sensory processing disorder; assistive technology; neurophysiological stress; anxiety; emerging technologies

1. Introduction

According to the most recent CDC estimates, approximately 1 in 36 children are diagnosed with autism spectrum disorder (ASD), with data pointing to a fourfold higher incidence in boys. The prevalence in Greece among children aged 10 to 11 years is 1.15% [1]. Although each person with the disorder is unique, ASD is characterized by key features, and abnormal early brain development and neuronal reorganization appear to be contributing factors to the cause of ASD. Social interactions are frequently quite challenging for people with ASD. These challenges could include trouble keeping eye contact and facial expressions, adjusting to social norms and expectations, and comprehending the intentions and feelings of others. People with ASD could find it difficult to make and keep friends, they might not comprehend that social interactions are two-way, or they might feel awkward sharing their hobbies and interests [2]. Avoiding eye contact, not responding to names, extreme fear, and a lack of interactive and pretend play are some of the symptoms of ASD, which differ from child to child. Children who receive early diagnosis and intervention have been shown to have better social outcomes and higher independence as adults, which ultimately saves healthcare expenses and lessens family stress. Long-term, substantial cost savings also decreased the demand for special education services and more intense treatments. It has also been demonstrated that an early diagnosis results in early enrollment in specialized educational programs that are designed to meet the particular requirements of children with ASD. For these children, these activities provide enhanced socialization opportunities and enhanced scholastic or educational results [3]. Many researchers have also studied the association between the diet of pregnant mothers and environmental factors that may also contribute to this phenomenon. However, because there are no reliable biomarkers, diagnosis is based solely on behavior [4]. ASD is a highly comorbid disorder that includes anxiety, ADHD, obsessive-compulsive disorder, mood disorders, and other behavioral disorders, which show considerable heterogeneity in the recent literature. A recent meta-analysis of 30 studies measuring the prevalence of anxiety and 29 studies measuring the prevalence of depression by [5] found that 46% of patients had a comorbid behavioral challenging disorder, 8% had mood disorders, and 66% of over 600 patients had more than one concurrent condition. Children with ADHD who sought therapy had a similar incidence of any anxiety illness (42%). Other prevalent health issues include selective eating, gastrointestinal diseases, sleep issues, seizures, obesity, and dietary limitations [6]. In terms of cognitive functioning, individuals with ASD demonstrate a wide range of abilities, from severe cognitive impairment to superior and high intelligence. Studies in people with ASD with and without cognitive impairment have found significant differences between groups in terms of symptom severity and subsequent outcomes. In addition, cognitive impairment may be more common in women, in individuals with known birth defects, and in individuals with dysmorphic features, suggesting that there may be subgroups with different etiologies or risk factors [7]. Since they are frequently the initial point of contact for parents, pediatricians are crucial to the early discovery of an individual with ASD. Because of widespread media coverage and the internet, parents are now much better equipped to identify the early indicators of autism spectrum disorder. If their child exhibits any of the symptoms above, they are more likely to voice their concerns to their child's pediatrician. Pediatricians need to be aware of the symptoms of autism spectrum disorder and have a plan in place for systematically evaluating them. Additionally, pediatricians need to know about local services that can assist them in diagnosing and treating ASD [8]. Although ASD can be diagnosed as young as 18 months of age, recent research has shown that the average age of diagnosis of ASD is between 38 and 120 months. Early detection of ASD can lead to early treatment, which improves later cognitive and language skills and reduces the underlying symptoms. Although there has been some criticism of universal screening of children with ASD due to lack of evidence, it is widely recognized that identification and early intervention are critical to public health priorities. Close monitoring of changes in the age of diagnosis of ASD over time will help us assess whether efforts to improve access to early identification and intervention are successful [9].

Improving the quality of life for children with ASD requires an explanation of the neurological mechanisms underlying their stress and anxiety. Since traditional therapy interventions frequently fail to alleviate symptoms, innovative and creative alternatives are needed. New treatment instruments have lately been made possible by advancements in technology. Emerging and assistive technologies have the potential to offer adaptive support and real-time monitoring that can alleviate stress and address a range of specific requirements in the population with ASD.

A condition known as sensory processing disorder (SPD) affects people with ASD in terms of their ability to interpret information from their surroundings. Although [10] proposed a classification of sensory processing disorders, many therapists prefer to refer to children as having difficulties processing and integrating stimuli; therefore, this term is not widely accepted. Excessive or insufficient responsiveness to normal levels of input from the sensory organs is known as sensory modulation disorder (SMD) [11]. Finding possible sensory stimuli and modifying the nervous system's reaction to them are both parts of the neurological process of sensory control. Sensory regulation is the intricate process of interpreting sensory data and generating reactions that are suitably calibrated or consistent with the circumstances. This ability to regulate and organize reactions to sensory inputs, filtering out unimportant stimuli and concentrating on the crucial ones while preserving the optimal level of arousal, is referred to by this word. A person's general quality of life, ability to overcome obstacles in daily life, and ability to interact with their physical and social environment are all impacted by this basic human functioning skill. SMD offers a crucial dimension for connecting with other categorical diagnostic entities that were previously thought of separately, making it an essential component of stress response physiology. In 2020, according to [12] overprotective and avoidant behaviors, as well as inappropriate reactions to harmless sensory inputs, are common in people with SMD. These actions frequently do not align with the expectations and requirements of the surroundings. According to research conducted on children with SMD, exposing them to sensory stimuli in a lab setting has an impact on their sympathetic and parasympathetic nervous systems from a neurophysiological standpoint. Many unique behaviors, including active sensation seeking and/or extreme sensitivity to sensory inputs, can be displayed by people with SMD. Innocent sensory inputs that provide unpleasant, painful, or annoying feelings can cause defensive reflexes, withdrawal from everyday activities, or elevated stress levels. Other symptoms of SMD include tiredness, apathy, or passivity. It can also manifest as delayed reactions to environmental stimuli of normal intensity. As a result, it is evident that SMD can negatively affect functional and developmental abilities, which hinders effective participation [13,14].

The World Health Organization (WHO) defines assistive technology (AT) as a general term that encompasses all systems and services associated with the use of assistive devices and service delivery [15]. In general, it is defined as "any item, piece of equipment or system, whether acquired, modified or adapted for commercial purposes, that is commonly used to enhance, maintain or improve the functioning of an individual" in accordance with the United States' Assistive Technology Act of 1998 [16]. AT is separated into high-tech (programming-based) technologies, like computers, and low-tech (programming-free) technologies, like pencil grips and magnifying lenses [17]. Researchers such as [18] also classify AT into two types: low or simple technology and high and complex technology. Low or simple technology has been described as equipment that most often has a low cost and is easy to create or acquire. It is, therefore, devices that require a simplified process for their operation (pencils, calculators, paper and laminated communication boards, wheelchairs, etc.). Complex technology refers to equipment that has electronic technology (computers, electronic communication boards, electric wheelchairs, etc.). Thus far, assistive technology has shown to be a useful instrument for enhancing the quality of life for all individuals with disabilities. Through assistive technology, people with disabilities can lead successful, independent, and healthy lives while participating in civic life, the workforce, and education. People frequently experience poverty, loneliness, and marginalization in the absence of assistive technology, which exacerbates the effects of illness and disability on patients, their families, and society at large. Assistive technology tools have a significant impact on the well-being of children with ASD, providing new opportunities for therapeutic approaches to improve various skills that contribute to the social inclusion of these children [19].

Emerging technologies are technologies that are at an early stage of development. This means that certain aspects, such as the characteristics of technology and its context of use or the network configuration of actors and their relative roles, are still uncertain and undefined [20]. They are defined as technologies that have the potential to be relevant to society within the next 10 to 15 years. This means that they are currently in the early stages of their development, but at the same time, they have moved beyond the purely conceptual stage [21]. Emerging technologies can be summarized as the definition of five key elements. These are (1) full innovation, (2) relatively rapid development, (3) consistency, (4) significant impact, and (5) uncertainty and ambiguity. More specifically, we conceive of emerging technology as a completely new and relatively rapidly evolving technology that is characterized by a certain degree of consistency that is maintained over time and has the potential to have a significant impact on socio-economic sectors. Moreover, it is observed in terms of the composition of actors, institutions, and patterns of interaction between them, as well as related knowledge production processes [22]. Emerging technologies include a broad and wide variety of technological developments that include artificial intelligence (AI), computer vision (computer vision), cellular communications, virtual reality (VR) and augmented reality (AR), robotics, drones, exergames, and serious games. This research will examine and synthesize the prevailing knowledge about the importance of technology in the field of combating and managing anxiety and stress in autistic children and adolescents to provide feasible and more effective solutions. For the purpose of this study, emerging technologies will be placed in the category of high-tech AT aids.

2. Materials and Methods

2.1. Study Design

The study design of this research was derived from the application of a systematic review approach followed by the PRISMA statement of systematic reviews and meta-analyses, reassuring rigorous and robust delivery through identification, selection, assessment, and synthesis of the finalized included studies. The Open Science Framework was the platform that was used to register the systematic review protocol (https://osf.io/6fnbj/ accessed on 22 February 2025)

The research was driven by more than one hypothesis, which was derived by applying the following PICO framework:

P: Children and young people from birth to 21 years of age with ASD.
I: Assistive technologies (low-high) and emerging technologies.
C: ASD, with typical development and other neurodevelopmental disorders; other types of interventions.
O: Reduction in stress and anxiety, improvement in ASD behavioral traits, reduction in aggressive behavior, and better concentration and focus.

H1: *Assistive and emerging technologies can effectively reduce stress and anxiety in children with ASD.*

H2: *The application of assistive and emerging technologies in real-world settings will demonstrate significant improvements in the management of stress and anxiety for individuals with ASD.*

H3: *The use of assistive and emerging technologies will lead to improved behavioral outcomes for individuals with ASD.*

Throughout this systematic review, we attempted to answer the following research questions:

- RQ1. What assistive and emerging technologies are used to combat stress in people with ASD?
- RQ2. Can assistive and emerging technologies help people with ASD reduce stress?
- RQ3. What are the measurements used to detect the outcomes?
- RQ4. What are the effect sizes of the studies?

For the purpose of this systematic review, research of the literature was conducted to explore the last ten years, studying the changes that have occurred in the years before and after COVID-19 in conjunction with the development of the Industrial Revolution 4.0 in the daily lives of people with ASD and how new emerging and assistive technologies can be beneficial in combating neurophysiological stress and anxiety.

2.2. Inclusion/Exclusion Criteria

To produce results, principles were used that followed specific criteria for the inclusion and exclusion of specific categories of research and articles, which were included in the final analysis for the main part.

More specifically, the inclusion criteria for the main part include the following:

- IC1: Research conducted between January 2014 and 30 March 2024 will be included.
- IC2: Experimental studies, observational studies, and original research will be included.
- IC3: Research and studies that are published in English only will be included.
- IC4: The use of new, assistive, and emerging technologies exclusively for the management of neurophysiological stress and anxiety will be included.
- IC5: Populations that have research inclusion criteria that are relevant to ASD and may include comorbidities with other conditions will be included.
- IC6: Research samples of children and adolescents up to 21 years of age will be included.

The following were the exclusion criteria for the study:

- EC1: Studies conducted before 2014 and after March 2024 will not be included.
- EC2: Studies of literature, systematic reviews, and meta-analyses of other studies will not be included.
- EC3: Studies published in a language other than English will not be included.
- EC4: Studies that include the use of new technologies or assistive technologies that do not include at least stress and anxiety in the outcome measures will not be used.
- EC5: Studies that include other populations of neurodevelopmental disorders will not be used unless they involve a comorbidity with ASD or suggest a corresponding study in that population.
- EC6: Included studies will not contain a sample of subjects older than 21 years of age.

2.3. Databases Screened and Selection Process

To obtain the finalized sample for analysis, the following databases were processed systematically to analyze the literature, which included PubMed, Web of Science, and Scopus. Google Scholar was used as a supplementary database. Eligibility requirements formed the foundation of the selection process. A keyword list for the database was also generated using Boolean operators and various search algorithms to obtain the best results.

The methodology followed, as previously discussed, was based on PRISMA principles using the snowball method for article selection, and the keywords used were autism spectrum disorder (ASD); assistive technologies (AT); emerging technologies; stress; neurophysiological stress; anxiety and their combination (Table 1).

Table 1. Research data string.

"Autism Spectrum Disorder" OR "ASD" OR "Assistive Technologies" OR "AT" OR "Emerging Technologies" OR "Stress" OR "Neurophysiological Stress" OR "Anxiety"
AND
"Autism Spectrum Disorder" AND ("Assistive Technologies" OR "AT") AND ("Emerging Technologies") AND ("Stress" OR "Neurophysiological Stress") AND ("Anxiety")
AND
"ASD" AND ("Assistive Technologies" OR "AT") AND ("Emerging Technologies") AND ("Stress" OR "Neurophysiological Stress") AND ("Anxiety")
AND
"Autism Spectrum Disorder" AND ("Assistive Technologies" OR "AT") AND ("Emerging Technologies") AND ("Neurophysiological Stress" OR "Physiological Stress" OR "Cortisol Levels" OR "Heart Rate Variability") AND ("Anxiety" OR "Emotional Dysregulation" OR "Mental Health")

An advanced search was then conducted using Boolean operators and filters in the databases. As soon as the candidate studies were selected, we started further processing. During the abstract/title screening step, studies that included the predefined terms in both the abstract and the title were given priority. Duplicate papers were then removed, and references that did not meet the eligibility requirements were excluded. Redundant references were eliminated using Mendeley Desktop 1.19.8.

The remaining studies underwent further processing during the full-text screening phase. Following the next steps, the full-text documents were acquired, and the information was carefully reviewed. The selection process also took into account other factors, such as the methodological practices used in each study. Four reviewers, P.P. and V.B., A.D. (Aikaterini Doulou), and A.C., independently identified the studies that qualified. The reviewers could choose to accept, reject, or remain undecided. In the event that the other reviewers were unsure or disagreed, a discussion was held with the input of the fifth (C.S.), sixth (N.B.), and seventh A.D. (Athanasios Drigas) reviewers. After the research was evaluated, the reviewers collected the relevant data and organized it in tables. After that, the results were combined. The qualitative synthesis offered a critical overview, analysis, and evaluation of the body of evidence discussed in this review.

2.4. Data Extraction

Data collected from the included studies referred to participant demographics, information (authors, year, country), specifics related to the research questions formulated, and aspects of the studies' structure (type of study, aim, conditions, measures, key findings, effect sizes, and longitudinal effects).

2.5. Included Studies

Following processing, inclusion, and representative criteria for the main part (n = 36) in the final selection for additional study and analysis, a total of n = 293 articles were found and screened for the included studies. The literature review included the years 2014–2024. Establishing the eligibility criteria was an initial step in the selection process. A list of keywords was also created to start the database search, which made use of a variety of search filters and Boolean operators in order to optimize the quantity of results. Following the elimination of duplicate studies (n = 73), the selection procedure was conducted using title and abstract screening in compliance with the eligibility criteria (n = 220).

The next step in the process was full-text screening after 95 publications were excluded. The remaining studies (n = 125) were processed thoroughly. Unfortunately, retrieving n = 12 articles for full-text screening was not feasible. The final selection process involved five independent reviewers, as discussed previously, who debated whether the eligibility requirements were applicable while looking over the full texts of (n = 113) papers. The remaining (n = 77) were removed since they did not fit the eligibility criteria. Consequently, (n = 36 items) were included in the final selection (Figure 1).

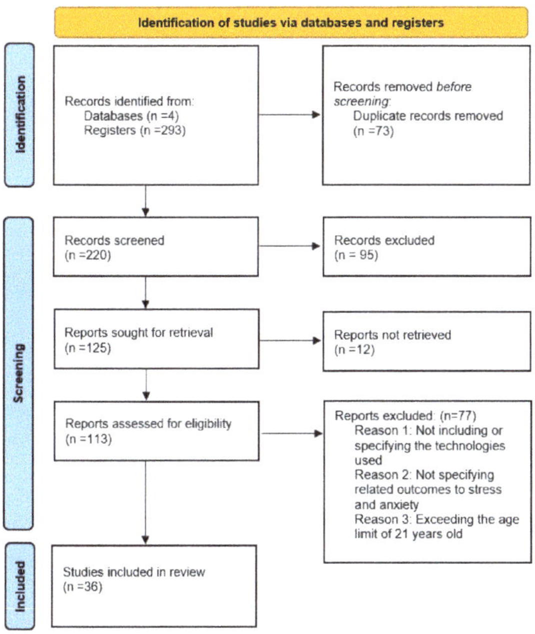

Figure 1. PRISMA 2020 flow diagram.

3. Theoretical Knowledge

3.1. Neurophysiological Stress and Anxiety

In the twenty-first century, stress is the main contributor to health issues. When managed, stress can be good for our physical and mental well-being, but if it persists for an extended period of time, it can cause a number of issues that can significantly affect a person's functioning and general health [23]. Stress might appear as a real or possible threat that necessitates a quick adjustment in behavior. Neural circuits and the brain are essential for the processes of stress response, adaption, and recuperation. More precisely, our nervous system is in charge of deciding what is dangerous and regulating the body's behavior and physiological changes in response to a stressor [24].

In response to stress and other experiences, the growing brain demonstrates notable neuroplasticity (structural and functional plasticity), including synaptic pruning, dendritic remodeling, and neuronal replacement. Stress can cause disruptions in the brain circuits supporting mood, anxiety, judgment, and cognition, which can alter how these behavioral states manifest. This imbalance also impacts systemic physiology through immunological, metabolic, autonomic, and neuroendocrine mediators [25]. To lessen the threat, the stress response triggers a number of defense systems, such as the hormonal messenger system [26].

More precisely, the catecholamines norepinephrine and epinephrine are significant peripheral stressors, while the hypothalamic–pituitary–adrenal (HPA) axis controls glucocorticoids (GCs). Both of these systems are regulated by the autonomic nervous system (ANS), which is composed of the parasympathetic nervous system, sympathetic nervous system, and sympathetic-adrenal cortex. The internal control nerve system's ANS and HPA axes are both intimately related to the autonomic nucleus centers. Following stressor exposure, the central ANS is swiftly activated, peripheral catecholamine production increases rapidly, and the HPA axis is activated immediately thereafter. The anterior pituitary creates and releases adrenocorticotropin hormones into the bloodstream following the first release of corticotropin-releasing hormone (CRH) in the portal pituitary circuit. This, in turn, triggers the pituitary's release of GCs like cortisol. A mostly negative stress response is produced when circulating GCs attach to GC receptors. Additionally, circulating GCs augment certain sympathetically mediated actions. Crucially, the adrenal cortex is directly regulated by the ANS, which could promote the release of GC [27].

3.2. Gut–Brain Axis

An interesting idea in the field of health and disease is that the gut microbiome has the ability to communicate with areas of the brain that can regulate behavior [28]. Examining the interaction between the gut and brain through neurobiological research has revealed a complex system of two-way communication that can maintain homeostasis and proper digestion and impact motivation and higher cognitive function. The brain–gut axis is a bidirectional communication system consisting of neural pathways, such as the enteric nervous system "ENS", vagus, sympathetic and spinal nerves, and chemical pathways, including cytokines, hormones, and neuropeptides as signaling molecules [29].

Emotion-related peripheral patterns, motor activity, excretion, and immunity in the gastrointestinal tract are controlled by both sympathetic and parasympathetic neurosis [30]. Current methods to identify the bacteria that make up the gut microbiota depend on omics analysis using advanced high-tech equipment [29].

Bacteria are essential for normal brain development as well as brain function in adulthood. Neuroplasticity in the adult brain is regulated by the microbiota, which is a critical process involved in neurogenesis and microglia activation. Such discoveries have contributed to a paradigm shift in neuroscience and psychiatry so that early development and subsequent brain function can be altered by targeting the microbiome [31].

The microbiome also affects the structure and function of the amygdala, another key brain region associated with stress. The amygdala is essential for emotional learning and social behavior, as well as for the activation of behavioral and physiological responses to stressful stimuli, particularly those that induce anxiety and/or fear [32]. Disrupted amygdaloid processes have been implicated in a variety of neuropsychiatric disorders, including the autism spectrum [31].

The microbiome contributes to the regulation of neurotransmitters by generating serotonin, dopamine, GABA, histamine, and acetylcholine, both directly and indirectly. The gut microbiota expresses a number of neurotransmitter receptors, which explains the direct influence of the CNS on gut microbiota. All these tasks are performed in coordination with the autonomic, enteric, and neuroendocrine systems, and the HPA axis also contributes [33,34].

3.3. Structural and Functional Differences Caused by Stress in Early Development

Psychosocial stressors, especially when present early in life, contribute to the development of anxiety and depressive disorders. In the cognitive domain, changes have also been observed in children exposed to chronic stress early in life.

Even after controlling for sociodemographic variables like maternal IQ, delivery complications, gender, ethnicity, and birth weight, these effects remained. Language, memory, attention, and executive function are the domains that are engaged. Furthermore, babies that experience stress at a young age frequently have more cognitive biases. For instance, they are less likely to notice positive facial expressions and more prone to perceive social cues as hostile than children who have never experienced psychological distress. Additionally, these children were twice as likely to repeat courses, had poorer work habits, and struggled to build them on their own. They also scored lower on intelligence and academic success assessments and had lower IQ scores. Furthermore, children who experience neglect are more likely to experience behavioral issues. Some of these behavioral issues can be brought on by a decrease in cognitive flexibility. Psychosocial functioning is still impacted. They displayed outcomes linked to decreased social skills and lower behavioral control when their professors evaluated them [35].

The study by [36] examined the relationship between early stress and mesial microstructural integrity in a sample of healthy controls aged 8 to 73 years. Participants were divided into four age groups (8–12, 13–18, 19–50, 51–73). For fractional anisotropy (FA) mesoclavium, a comparison was made between those with three or more morning stress events and those with fewer than three events. During separate analyses, both groups were tested for verbal memory, information processing speed, psychomotor speed, and cognitive flexibility. The results showed that both the younger and older groups of early stressed subjects had significantly lower gender-specific fractional anisotropy than those without early stress. However, no differences were observed between groups for any of the cognitive tasks. Through this research, it was found that early stress is associated with subtle changes in brain structure but not function.

The study by [37], through their systematic literature review, examined how developmental stress, particularly childhood maltreatment, may affect the HPA axis' function and hippocampal structure. In addition, they examined the relationship between HPA axis function and hippocampal volume in healthy states, depression, and other diseases. Evidence was observed that prenatal stress and childhood maltreatment are associated with abnormal development of the HPA system, as well as reduced hippocampal volume.

Reduced hippocampal volume was also associated with increased daily cortisol secretion. The conclusions concluded that a model incorporating child maltreatment, cortisol abnormalities, and hippocampal volume may need to account for other factors such as temperament, genetics, or the presence of depression, providing a holistic explanation of all findings. Also, the role of early-life maltreatment in the impairment of the HPA axis remains unclear.

Ref. [38] study involved the collection of structural MRI scans (n = 61) (32 boys, 29 middle-aged girls, 142.35 ± 21.12 months), using well-validated executive function assessments and in-depth interviews that were conducted to assess stress exposure in humans. Smaller volumes in the prefrontal cortex, namely in the medial frontal gray and white matter and both frontal poles, are linked to cumulative life stress and spatial working memory, according to an analysis of the differences in brain anatomy. The relationship between cumulative life stress and spatial working memory can be explained by individual differences in prefrontal volume, according to mediation analyses. These findings imply that structural alterations in the prefrontal cortex might be a mechanism via which increased cumulative stress results in diminished cognitive function.

The current study's authors [39] looked at how teenagers' brain structures and functional activation to images evoking negative emotions, as well as the stress levels in mothers' self-reported items, affected their cortisol responses to stress. Data on maternal stress perception and salivary cortisol responses to a demanding task were gathered from 66 mothers and adolescents, ages 12 to 14. The teens' brain structure and function were then evaluated by MRI. Adolescent reactivity in the medial prefrontal cortex to negative emotional stress-inducing stimuli was predicted by higher levels of parental perceived stress but not cortisol reactivity, according to whole-brain functional studies. However, no statistically significant correlations were shown for structural analyses. Given the finding that maternal responses to stress are associated with adolescent medial prefrontal cortex function, parental stress may play a role in the development of the neuropsychiatric stress system in adolescence, with potential implications.

In the study by [40], through a systematic review of the literature on functional MRI, as well as a meta-analysis of research regarding structural MRI sensory imaging of brain tumors in pediatric patients with posttraumatic experiences, a possible association between early traumatic experiences and variant brain regions and functions was investigated. A meta-analysis assessing group differences was conducted using all amygdala, hippocampus, brain tumor, and intracranial tumor data that satisfied the inclusion criteria. According to the meta-analysis, PTSD patients had a reduced intracranial volume, total brain volume, and total cortical area. The gray matter volume of the frontal lobe and amygdala and the total gray matter volume of the hippocampus (left and right) were all decreased, although these differences were not statistically significant. Functional investigations showed that the PTSD/PTSD symptom group differed in how different parts of the brain were activated in response to stimuli.

In the study by [41], 27 young subjects with PTSD and 21 typically developing subjects without trauma were assessed at baseline and at a one-year follow-up. During each visit, the youth underwent structural MRI and functional resting MRI at each visit. Areas showing volumetric abnormalities on whole-brain structural analyses were identified and used as seeds in exploratory analyses of intrinsic connectivity. The results showed that young subjects with PTSD showed persistently reduced gray matter volume in the right dorsal prefrontal cortex and a bilateral ventrally arranged prefrontal cortex. Group analyses over time revealed abnormal longitudinal growth of the bilateral prefrontal cortex, with typically developing adolescents showing a normal decrease in the right dorsal prefrontal cortex from baseline to follow-up, whereas adolescents with PTSD showed an increase. Using these regions as seeds, PTSD patients showed atypical longitudinal decreases in intrinsic connectivity of the prefrontal cortex and amygdala as well as with the hippocampus, in contrast to increases in developing adolescents, specifically. Specifically, adolescents with PTSD showed increased ventricular connectivity of the prefrontal cortex and amygdala as well as with the hippocampus over time. Also, volumetric abnormalities of the interventricular PFC and extraventricular PFC were predictive of symptom severity.

3.4. ASD, Sensory Modulation Disorder (SMD), and Stress Due to Hyperreactivity to Stimuli

SMD has been widely recognized and linked in the literature as one of the primary sensory processing issues affecting people with ASD. In their research, [14] clearly identified sensory processing dysfunction in children with ASD and contrasted it with SMD as two distinct characteristics. Thirty-three generally developing children (4–12 years old), thirty-eight children with ASD (5–15 years old), and thirty-one children with ASD problems (5–13 years old) participated in the study. The respondents' arousal and reactivity were examined and quantified by the researchers in a lab setting. The results showed that the two clinical groups differed from one another. Children with ASD exhibited lower initial arousal and reduced reactions when shown a laboratory example of sensory problems. The ASD and SMD clinical groups exhibited considerably more abnormal sensory-related behaviors than children with usual development. In addition, there were three differences between the two groups: the ASD group showed more proprioceptive and vestibular behaviors, which were signs of sensory under-reactivity; the latter group showed more sensation-seeking behaviors; and the former group showed more signs of hyperreactivity to taste and smell.

By comparing sensory processing, social participation, and praxis in a group of 79 children aged 5 to 8 years (M = 6.09), 14 of whom were girls and 65 of whom were boys, ref. [42] added more findings. The children were divided into two groups: the ASD group (n = 41) and the standard development comparison group (n = 38). The researchers assessed the children's sensory profiles using a sensory processing measure (SPM). Details on aspects of their home and classroom modifications were supplied by parents and teachers, respectively. The ASD group received scores suggesting higher levels of dysfunction on all the evaluated measures in both situations, with the biggest differences observed in the variables of the motor act and social involvement. The two senses most impacted in the ASD group were hearing and touch.

Others looked into food selectivity and oral sensitivity to SMD. Ref. [43] evaluated the oral sensory processing of children with SMD (n = 53) and those without SDM (n = 58) who were between the ages of 3 and 11. In addition, the researchers evaluated food in children with ASD according to their preferences, informal oral sensory processing, and fruit and vegetable consumption and how they all related to each other. They discovered that more children with ASD exhibited abnormal sensory processing than those without the disorder. Furthermore, the study revealed that children with ASD who had unusual oral sensory sensitivity ate fewer vegetables and rejected more items. More recent research has found associations between ASD and social difficulties. Ref. [44] study examined the connection between children with ASD's social and adaptive functioning and sensory challenges. The researchers looked at the connections between abnormal sensory processing responses and social skill deficiencies, impaired social cognition, and general adaptive functioning in a group of preschool-aged children with ASD. This study contrasted 36 peer children of similar ages who were generally developing and 64 children with ASD aged 3 to 6 years. Measures of general adaptive functioning, social problems, and sensory processing were gathered from the parents of each child. The results of the study showed that children with ASD who experienced more sensory problems were more likely to struggle in social situations and have lower levels of adaptive functioning. When [45] compared the play activities and sensory information processing of children with ASD (6–10 years old) to those of age and gender-matched (typically developing children), they added more data on social participation. A total of 95 parents of typically developing children and 93 parents of children with ASD were surveyed at daycare facilities, schools, and hospitals. Both the sensory profile (SP) and Participation in Childhood Occupation (PICO) metrics were employed. Boys made up 74% ($n = 72$) of the study's participants (with a 4:1 ratio of boys to girls) in the autistic group. The findings indicated that sensory processing issues are linked to certain childhood participation limits. Children with ASD engaged less frequently, at a lower level, and with less pleasure than typical children their age. Compared to the typical group ($n = 95$), which had sensory processing issues at 21.5% ($p = 0.28$), children with ASD had sensory processing issues at 68.8%. Another study emphasized symptom variability.

In order to ascertain whether cognitive capacity and reported sensory symptoms in the ASD sample explained the sensory processing measure (SPM-2) scores, [46] compared the sensory processing of school-aged children with ASD with that of their normally developing (TD) counterparts. Parents of the two groups—105 children with ASD and 70 children with TD—were given the exam, and the groups were subsequently split into high-functioning and low-functioning groups. The findings demonstrated that children with ASD had higher SPM-2 subscales and overall scores. The hearing, social participation, balance, and movement subscales of the SPM-2 showed a significant difference between children with high and low functioning in the context of ASD, although the total SPM-2 scores did not differ between the two groups of children. This research highlights that the variety of sensory patterns is associated with either high or low cognitive functioning.

3.5. Stress Measurements

The common types of psychological stress commonly measured are major life events, traumatic events, exposure to early life stress, and chronic or current stress. The choice of appropriate stressor exposure to measure depends on the relevance of the population, the research objectives, and the assumption that certain types of stress are associated with relevant outcomes. Capturing a variety of stressors will reduce the likelihood of underestimating an individual's psychological and social stress [47]. Responses to stress can be measured with self-report measures, behavioral coding, or physiological measures. These responses include the emotional, cognitive, behavioral, and physiological responses elicited by stressful stimuli. One of the simplest ways of measuring stress response is a self-report of perceived stress associated with a particular stressor or life situation.

Ref. [48] distinguished three ways in which stress is investigated: (1) The epidemiological tradition focuses on identifying situations and experiences that are considered stressful based on the consensus that they pose a threat to social or physical health. (2) The psychological tradition focuses on individuals' perceptions of stress caused by life events based on their assessment of the threats posed and the availability of effective coping resources. (3) The biological tradition focuses on the brain disruption of physiological systems necessary to regulate homeostasis and normal metabolic control.

Outside of the laboratory, new technologies have improved our ability to record real-time responses to stress in everyday life using mobile phones and handheld devices that are increasingly being implemented by many researchers [49–51]. Examining the impact of stressor exposure and stress responses on health can improve the prediction of health outcomes, as many stress models suggest that these responses also mediate the effects of stress exposure, which may influence health outcomes [47].

The most common ways of measuring and obtaining data on the neurophysiological changes observed are as follows:

- Through GSR (galvanic skin response) by using changes in skin conductance. When stress is present, skin resistance decreases due to increased sweat secretion.
- Electromyography (EMG) measures the electrical activity of muscles. Stress causes differences in muscle contraction, which can be used to determine stress levels.
- Skin temperature changes that correlate to an increase in stress levels.
- Measurement of heart rate and heart rate variability.
- Electrocardiogram (ECG), from which the heart rate and heart rate variability are measured. (Calculation of the variability of heart rate variability [52].

Many physiology-based stress-sensing systems use machine learning and rely on three main types of sensors: wearable sensors, external sensors, and software sensors, where sensor data collected by software do not necessarily require a dedicated hardware sensor [53].

3.6. Measurement of Stress in Individuals with ASD

Individuals with ASD appear to have increased levels of neurophysiological stress and anxiety disorders compared to the neurotypical population and can be categorized into three categories: (1) neurophysiological changes in the presence of a stressor, (2) questionnaires of individuals with ASD and parent caregivers, and (3) those of a mixed type (neurophysiological changes and questionnaires).

From studies conducted by various researchers who have aimed to measure these effects in populations with ASD, we identified a great diversity in the mode of taking; more specifically, [54] measured cortisol in children with ASD who were at rest compared to when faced with a stressor such as blood intake. In addition, the parent questionnaire was given to further the reliability of the child behavioral checklist measurements.

The findings of [55] suggest a distinct neuroendocrine response to social stress in high-functioning autistic children despite similar sympathetic and parasympathetic responses to stress compared to the neurotypical population. This preliminary study examined physiological arousal in children with high-functioning autism (HFA, $n = 19$) compared to a control group ($n = 11$) before, during, and after the Trier Social Stress test (Trier Social Stress). The HFA group was more likely to have decreased salivary cortisol after the stressor, whereas the comparison group was more likely to have increased cortisol ($p = 0.02$); however, no differences in electrodermal activity (a measure of sympathetic arousal) or vagal tone (a measure of parasympathetic activity) were identified between groups.

In their study of a population with ASD compared to a neurotypical sample, [56] measured the skin's temperature, heart rate, and electrodermal activity in a sample of children with ASD ($n = 12$) and those typically developing ($n = 17$) during a stress condition (Stroop task) and baseline condition (surveillance tape). With some regression model adjustments based on the internal period, the recovery period, the stress test, and the remainder of the main level, a comparison of saliva control, heart rate, and heart rate variability was conducted.

Ref. [57] collected behavioral and physiological measures of stress and anxiety during dental cleaning in order to examine the causes and consequences of behavioral and physiological discomfort experienced by children with ASD during normal dental visits. In the control group, which included 44 people aged 6–12 years, there were 22 individuals with ASD and 22 individuals with neurotypical traits. Based on physiological measurements and measures of overt behavioral anxiety, classified by the researchers and dentists, the results indicated that children with ASD were more anxious than the control group. Age was linked to behavioral discomfort in the typical group, while expressive communication and sensory processing issues were linked to behavioral distress in the ASD group. Physiological dysphoria was associated with parent-reported anxiety in the typical group and with sensory processing difficulties in the ASD group. The following assessment measurement tools were used to measure anxiety: Child and Adolescent Symptom Inventory-Anxiety Scale (CASI), Children's Fear Survey Schedule-Dental Subscale (CFSS-DS), Anxiety and Cooperation Scale (A & C Scale), Short Sensory Profile (SSP), Frankl Scale, and the Children's Dental Behavioral Rating Scale (CDBRS) from the questionnaires used to measure neurophysiological changes, such as electrodermal activity (EDA).

The aim of [58] study was to determine if Zen Shiatsu can reduce short and long-term stress levels in children with ASD. The PEDS QL 4.0 Young Child Questionnaire was used to measure stress on the impact of intervention implementation by parents [59].

Ref. [60] conducted a preliminary investigation to evaluate the physiological stress (cortisol) and regulation (respiratory sinus arrhythmia, RSA) of children aged 10 to 12 who were either normally developing (TD) (n = 25) or who had ASD (n = 31) after they were subjected to two social stress protocols. The extent to which cognitive emotions (emotional knowledge) and stress (state and trait) mediate stress responses was also investigated. Depending on the type of stressor, the results displayed distinct stress response patterns. Both groups regularly displayed adaptive and synergistic cortisol and RSA responses during cordial social interactions. However, in response to social appraisal, the ASD group did not show any correlated responses across the physiological systems, which may be due to an attenuated stress response from the evaluative social stressor. The following instruments were used in the present study: the Trier Social Stress Test (TSST)-Child Version, the TSST-friendly pre-baseline, salivary cortisol test, respiratory sinus arrhythmia (RSA), and the Stress Inventory for Children (STAIC).

The study by [8] investigated the relationship between stress and symptoms of ASD in this population in n = 22 without ASD and n = 24 with ASD (with a mean age of 35.7 and 31.8 each), who were individuals with both sensory and cognitive disabilities. Physiological stress levels were determined using salivary cortisol according to the protocol of [61]. No additional self-report or parent and caregiver questionnaires were administered in this study. Participants with and without ASD showed no differences in cortisol levels, as well as differences between the OASIS test day and control day. In contrast, cortisol levels were positively associated with the presence of stereotypical and repetitive behaviors.

Ref. [62] gathered and categorized the scales used in their systematic review in order to create a framework for researching stress in people with OASIS using self-report measures. More precisely, two primary scale categories were reported: a moment-specific state-like questionnaire and general trait-like stress surveys. The following subcategories, which comprised the stress-specific questionnaires, were developed from these in the first category: (1) Chronic Stress Questionnaire for Children and Adolescents, (2) Perceived Stress Scale, (3) Stress in Children Questionnaire, and (4) Adjusted Stress Survey Schedule, and in the second group, these were self-made questionnaires and Depression Anxiety Stress Scale questionnaires. Lastly, the Subjective Units of Distress Survey, a compliance questionnaire, was likewise found in the second category. Only the SSS, which asks the subject to score the severity of their stress responses in eight scenarios, was created for use with individuals with ASD from the first category listed. (1)Threats and changes, (2) expectation and uncertainty, (3) unpleasant experiences, (4) enjoyable experiences (like birthday celebrations or presents), (5) sensory and interpersonal contact, (6) food-related activities, (7) social and environmental connections, and (8) stress associated to rituals were considered [63]. Ref. [64] used resting heart rate variability (HRV) in combination with the Emotional Dysregulation Inventory to measure resting heart rate variabilities in adolescents with ASD compared to neurotypical subjects.

4. Results

4.1. Studies Characteristics

The present study gathered results from a comprehensive summary of $n = 36$ studies that were finally pooled into this systematic review for further analysis. The included studies examined assistive and emerging technologies as mediators to detect and reduce neurophysiological stress and anxiety in children and adolescents with ASD and sensory processing disorders, which were published from 2015 to 2024 (Figure 2).

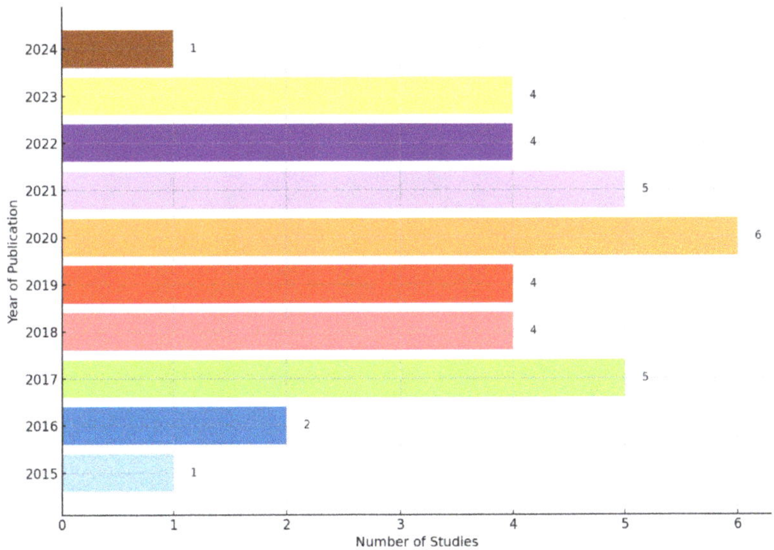

Figure 2. Distribution of studies by year of publication.

The included studies utilized a diverse set of research methodologies, including randomized control trials (RCTS) in $n = 7$ studies, employing a rigorous experimental design to evaluate intervention effectiveness [65–71]. Further studies ($n = 7$) utilized comparative designs without full randomization (quasi-experimental studies) [72–78]. $n = 8$ more studies (pilot and feasibility) focused on assessing the feasibility and preliminary effects of interventions [79–86]. Finally, in $n = 5$ studies (single-subject and case studies), the researchers presented detailed individual analyses of the interventions' impacts [87–91]. Moreover, in $n = 9$ (observational and exploratory), they tried to examine real-world interactions with these types of technologies [92–100] (Figure 3).

According to the study populations, we observed a wide variety of data collected. More specifically, the sample size studies ranged from single-subject case studies up to 201 participants [71,72,97]. The age range of the pool was primarily children and adolescents 3 years of age to 19 years, with some of them including young adults [65–67]. Regarding gender distribution, most of the studies reported more male samples (~80–90%), reflecting ASD prevalence trends [73,75,87].

Finally, the studies were performed across different countries (some uniquely, some co-organized, and some jointly), providing a wider approach to the interpretation of the data acquired. More specifically n = 7 were from the USA [75,79,80,85,87,90,100], n = 3 were from Canada [66,71,76], n = 3 were from China [65,72,77], n = 3 were from Indonesia [68,69,82], n = 3 were from Qatar [81,89,91], n = 3 were from UK [70,96,97], n = 2 were from India [86,98], n = 2 were from Italy [73,95], n = 2 were from Japan [84,99], n = 1 was from Australia [88], n = 1 was from Belgium [83], n = 1 was from Netherlands [92], n = 1 was from Sweden [74], n = 1 was from Israel [94] and n= 3 were studies that were performed in multiple countries, i.e., Israel, the UK, and Sweden [67], France and Italy [78], as well as Turkey, Macedonia, the UK, and Poland [93] (Figure 4).

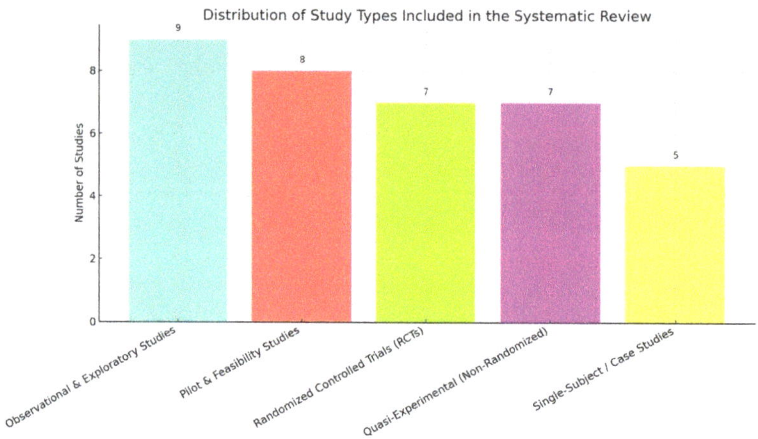

Figure 3. Distribution of study types in the systematic review.

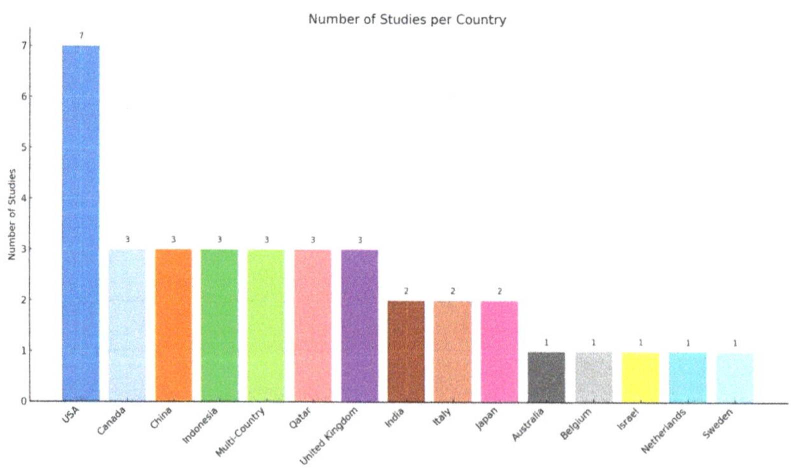

Figure 4. Studies distribution by countries.

4.2. Assistive and Emerging Technologies for Children and Adolescents with ASD on Stress Management (Low Technology)

4.2.1. Visual Programs/Schedules

Stress and anxiety are common among persons with ASD, and they are frequently brought on by the challenges they encounter on a daily basis. Visual programs are a type of low technology that has shown promise when used in any situation where people frequently encounter difficulties. A visual program is a set of pictures or words intended to motivate someone to carry out various duties. They provide abstract ideas like time and action in a concrete form by using words, pictures, and other visual elements to explain what will happen, when it will happen, and where it will happen. They have been effectively utilized to treat issues with sequential memory, time management, and language understanding, as well as to lower anxiety in a range of contexts (classrooms, homes, private gyms, dental offices, etc.) [101].

Ref. [76] conducted a pilot study to investigate whether a visual design system using pictorial communication symbols can help children with autism achieve daily oral hygiene. The study involved 14 boys with ASD, ages 3 to 8, who attended a dental clinic for four consecutive weekly dental appointments. The patients were randomly assigned to either the experimental group, which received a visual program system in addition to standard care, or the control group, which received a "Tell-Show-DO" approach (standard care). The results showed that the combination of a visual teaching program and repeated weekly visits seemed to have helped children with autism reach more milestones by showing higher levels of reduced behavioral distress during dental exams and cleanings.

Ref. [69] compared the effectiveness of using a visual training module to reduce anxiety during dental treatment with that of video modeling in a population of children with ASD. Twenty children with ASD, ages 6 to 10, participated in this experimental clinical investigation. They were split into two groups: the PV-BDG module's visual intervention group (n = 10) and the video modeling group. To quantify salivary immunoglobulin A (sIgA) concentrations, patients' saliva was taken both before and after the intervention. The Shapiro–Wilk normality test and the independent t-test were used to analyze the data and compare how much stress was reduced in the two groups. The findings demonstrated that, as indicated by changes in the sIgA levels, video modeling and visual teaching modules might effectively lower the stress levels of children with ASD while receiving dental care.

Ref. [68] found similar results regarding the efficacy of visual methods when comparing the Berkunjung ke Dokter Gigi Visual Pedagogical Module intervention method (VPM-BDG) and the Berkunjung ke Dokter Gigi Video Modeling intervention method (VM-BDG) in lowering anxiety levels in children with ASD while receiving dental care. Twenty children with ADHD, ages six to ten, participated equally in this clinical study and experimental trial. Following that, they were split into two groups based on the type of intervention: VPM-BDG and VM-BDG. The children's saliva was taken both before and after the intervention, and the delta values of their salivary cortisol concentrations were measured in a lab. The Mann–Whitney test was used to analyze the effectiveness of the two interventions. The mean value in the two intervention groups was -0.006 and 0.0005. The delta values of the salivary cortisol concentrations showed that VM-BDG and VPM-BDG effectively reduced stress levels in the tested sample of subjects.

The study by [88] evaluated the use of visual schedules and task systems to help four students with ASD stay on task and work independently in a typical classroom environment. These strategies were implemented by teachers as inclusive practices and were evaluated by observation in physical classroom environments to test their feasibility in general contexts. All participants demonstrated improvement in their behavior during the task. The results for other secondary dependent variables were mixed, with some students demonstrating decreased off-task behavior and increased productivity.

4.2.2. Sensory Modalities and Wearables

Children and adults with ASD frequently struggle with sensory processing and modulation [102]. According to [14,42,44], a person with ASD may have hyper-responsiveness (touch, hearing, smell, etc.) to the various stimuli they encounter in their surroundings. This can activate the ANS and, more specifically, the sympathetic system, which can lead to an increase in stress levels in the body. The term "wearables" refers to a wide range of items that users can wear to offer biometric information about their homeostatic condition or to normalize their level of arousal by using their features to provide input (biofeedback). The following is a list of topics that have been studied for their qualities as low- or medium-tech aids.

Ref. [99], in their pilot study, investigated the effectiveness of earplugs and noise-canceling (NC) earplugs in relation to behavioral control of problems caused by over-reactivity to auditory inputs in children with ASD. The results showed that the T-scores on the Goal Attainment Scale (GAS) were significantly higher during the use of acoustic noise cancelation compared to baseline. During the baseline time frame, five children with DSA demonstrated improved behavior from those with normal headphone (NC) use; however, there were no differences in the GAS T-Goal scores between the headphone (NC) phase and the baseline phase or between the headphone and NC headphone phases. NC headphones were given to 21 children aged 4 to 16 years who had not used the sound isolator for two weeks and received normal earplugs as a sample after random selection. Participants' responses to auditory stimulation were assessed by their parents or teachers.

Six children with ASD, ages 8 to 16, were examined using a multi-item treatment method in a related study by [75]. As part of their treatment, participants were randomized to wear either over-ear (above the ears) or in-ear (within the ears) hearing aids for two periods. Every child underwent four stages of investigation. The reference week was the first week of data collection; then came the intervention week, the non-intervention week, and the alternative intervention week (as is customary). The Empatica E4 bracelet was used to gather data on electrodermal activity (EDA). Five measurements were taken throughout each of the 16–20 data collection periods that the participants underwent. The purpose of this study was to determine whether there is proof that therapies that lower children's sympathetic activity can effectively treat both hypersensitive and autistic children. The current study used skin conductance measurements to analyze these findings. Separate analyses for paired study periods revealed that the use of noise-isolating headphones led to statistically significant variations in skin conductance levels and the frequency of non-specific conductance responses between baseline and post-study periods. The researchers came to the conclusion that in individuals with ASD and auditory hyper-responsiveness, noise-isolating auditory sensitivity may lessen sympathetic activity.

Ref. [77], in their study, took into account the heterogeneity of auditory perception in children with ASD and how it differs compared to conventional isolation hearing aids. For the purpose of this study, they designed appropriate noise control functions in hearing aids to meet the needs of children with ASD who have different auditory perceptions through a series of auditory perception and electroencephalogram tests, in which children with ASD and with auditory hypersensitivity listened to sounds of different frequencies and amplitudes which were analyzed through the subjects' responses. Appropriate noise reduction targets were determined based on acoustic perception curves constructed from mean acoustic perception values and noise levels using an appropriate power function. A hybrid active noise cancelation (ANC) system based on acoustic perception was then developed and validated. The results showed that frequencies of 250 Hz and 8 kHz were considered the most unpleasant by the majority of autistic children. Participants were divided into five groups using the K-means algorithm. It was found that each group had its own characteristic auditory perceptual response. Finally, improvements in auditory perceptual response were observed when children used this type of headphones, with their auditory perceptual characteristics consistent with different groups of children with autism.

Ref. [87] used an alternating treatment design that assessed the engagement of a 5-year-old child with ASD during math in a general education kindergarten classroom using a weighted blanket and structured work boxes as objects. The results showed that the weighted blanket did not lead to changes in therapeutic behavior, and it was observed that the student's engagement was lower than the baseline. More specifically, the subject sat on the mat more often when using the blanket compared to the baseline sessions but often engaged in behaviors that were not functional (touching the blanket) or were not consistent with engagement in an academic response (e.g., pulling the blanket over his head).

Ref. [85], through their research, examined children with ASD who exhibited behavioral symptoms of sensory processing deficits and whether weighted blankets improved sleep quality. A single-subject design study was conducted with two 4-year-old children who had been diagnosed with both ASD and sleep disorders. An 8-day baseline phase, a 14-day total intervention with weighted blankets, and a 7-day removal period were used to examine the objective sleep measurements and caregiver surveys. Visual analysis and the rate of non-overlap techniques were used to evaluate the caregivers' accounts and objective data. The weighted blanket intervention had little effect on sleep patterns, according to the results. However, by considerably shortening the time it took for participants to fall asleep, the usage of weighted blankets improved their morning mood and decreased stress after nighttime use.

The study by [74] sought to ascertain whether using weighted blankets improved sleep and day-to-day functioning in individuals with ASD and/or ADHD. A total of 85 participants with an ADHD or ASD diagnosis, 48 children (57%) and 37 adults (44%), who were at least 18 years old, were given a weighted blanket to utilize. The participants answered over the phone. The weighted blanket enhanced sleep-related skills, sleep quality throughout the night, and relaxation during the day, according to the results. In children and adults with ASD and/or ADHD, the use of a weighted blanket enhanced their daily morning/evening routines, including getting ready for bed and waking up early.

4.3. Assistive and Emerging Technologies for Children and Adolescents with ASD on Stress Management (High-Tech and Emerging Technologies)

4.3.1. High-Tech Wearables

Ref. [80], through their study, demonstrated a machine learning approach using data from wearable devices to discriminate physiological states associated with stressful and non-stressful conditions in children with ASD in a controlled laboratory setting, where the heart rate and resting rate interval measurements were collected during rest and during activities designed to simulate stress using a consumer (wearable) device. The analysis included 38 children (22 children with ASD and 16 children without ASD). After removing the outliers, 20 statistical features were explained from the data collected during the rest and stress periods of each subject. Using nested cross-validation across 76 sample periods (38 rest periods/38 stress periods), logistic regression (LR) and support vector machine (SVM) classifiers were trained and evaluated to classify each validation sample as a rest or stress period. The SVM and LR models achieved an accuracy of 93% and 87%, respectively. The results of the study showed that the machine learning model combined with mobile device data can support real-time health intervention applications, helping to detect and reduce stress.

In contrast to children with a language impairment (LD), the study by [95] assessed the heart rate (HR) as a possible indicator of stress reactivity in children with ASD. A total of 24 patients (mean age = 42.62 months; SD = 8.14 months) participated in the study; 12 children with ASD and 12 children with LD received physiological evaluations (HR monitoring) and clinical trials while donning HR measurement devices during five interaction activities. An increase in HR during the third activity (ADOS-2 bubble game) was significantly associated with autism symptoms ($r = 0.415$; $p = 0.044$), whereas the association between total ADOS-2 and HR during the first activity (ADOS-2 free play; $r = 0.368$; $p = 0.077$), the second activity (baseline subscale of the Leiter-R scheme; $r = 0.373$; $p = 0.073$), and the fifth dynamic (predicting ADOS-2 of an object procedure; $r = 0.368$; $p = 0.076$) did not quite reach statistical significance. Using a linear regression model, it was found that the total ADOS-2 score significantly influenced heart rate variability ($p = 0.\ 023$). Heart rate monitoring may provide information about stressful situations in children with ASD. In addition, it may help clinicians detect the impact of stress on the core of autism and develop treatment strategies.

The E4 wristband is a portable research tool that offers physiology data, analysis, and real-time imaging software. The E4 has four sensors installed to track and record the heart rate, heart rate variability, skin temperature, sympathetic nervous system activity, and blood volume pulses. Studies on the IBI and mean heart rate have demonstrated the validity and reliability of the E4, which has been used to quantify stress and anxiety in particular populations, including the IBI [75]. In comparison to the Mindwave mobile impedance cardiography device, the study by [103] looked at the instrument's suitability as a pure research tool. Its behavior was examined through naturalistic observation that included gestures and face-to-face interaction. Thirty participants were included in the sample collection; they were connected to both devices and split into pairs to rest and converse with one another. The HRV devices' correlations ranged from modest to high, with the resting values being greater than talking ones. The E4 is unable to deliver precise EDA data, nevertheless.

In order to capture and analyze data, the Hexoskin Shirt (HS), a smart shirt with sensors that assess changes in the body's physiology, including the heart rate, respiration rate, and blood oxygen level, is connected to a health platform. In terms of the validity of Hexoskin's findings, its application has primarily been assessed in groups that do not include individuals with ASD, and it is generally regarded as valid and trustworthy. Nevertheless, it poses challenges associated with connection issues that are seen during physical activity. In a recent study, ref. [94] employed it as a research tool to measure physiological variations in a community of adults with ASD. Three stages of research were carried out. The HS was used in the first phase to measure the physiological differences between adults with high-functioning ADHD and those who were neurotypical. The creation of a particular machine learning algorithm to forecast challenging behavior (CB) in real time, in combination with a smartphone app that notifies users when CB is likely to occur, was the focus of the second phase. In the last phase, individuals with CB and their caretakers were asked to test the system's acceptability and efficacy. According to the sample size estimates, 20 high-functioning individuals with ASD, aged 20 to 40, who lived at home and were part of the observation group, and 20 additional neurotypical individuals of the same age who worked in the control group were part of the first phase of the study. Ten persons with ASD, ages 20 to 40, who displayed extremely violent or disruptive conduct, as well as their caregivers, were recruited for the second phase. One individual with ASD who was between the ages of 20 and 40 and had disruptive or aggressive traits was included in the final phase. Participants with ASD accepted the usage of the SWS and did not find it bothersome.

Users can learn basic social and emotional skills using Empower Me Brain Power (EMBP), available for Google Glass Explorer Edition and other smart glasses. BPS smart glasses are social communication training devices that use augmented reality. Studies on the feasibility, acceptability, safety, and clinical impact of BPS have been conducted. In particular, EMBP glasses were used in a two-week study of a 13-year-old high school student with ASD in Massachusetts in order to develop an intervention targeting attention issues and social learning factors that can cause anxiety in children with ASD in school educational settings [90]. Twice daily, the intervention was given. Participating in the intervention's implementation were student health professionals, special education teachers, and general education teachers. Teachers' opinions, the value of technology, and its effects on students and classrooms were recorded through a series of one-on-one interviews and digital journals. Both teachers and students found the use of smart glasses to be practical and easy to use, needing little time for implementation or learning. Teachers also reported that pupils improved their verbal and nonverbal communication abilities and loved the experience. Furthermore, there was no indication that the technology was distracting or had a detrimental effect on the classroom or other students. According to these findings, social skills therapies that are given via smart glasses may be beneficial, realistic, and effective in enhancing social communication abilities and lowering anxiety. Ref. [104] conducted a second investigation on a single individual to examine the efficacy of a particular device employing EMBP. Over the course of four weeks, a technician used Brain Power glasses to conduct fifteen intervention sessions in a private office. The subject worked with a technician who wore Google Glasses supplemented with artificial intelligence for 15 min in each session. Measures of efficacy included behavioral rating scales with a pre-test design, qEEG analysis, and a few neuropsychological tests. The results of the neuropsychological tests revealed that social cognition and face memory had significantly improved by at least one standard deviation. Changes in particular regions of interest that may be connected to the brain areas involved in the particular neuropsychological functions assessed were found by a Z-Builder analysis. On the other hand, the instructor said that he did not notice any appreciable behavioral changes in the student.

Ref. [91] examined the feasibility of wrist-worn sensors for detecting challenging behaviors in autistic children prior to overt signs by monitoring children's heart rates, electrodermal activity, and movement, as well as the feasibility of using such sensors on the ankle instead of the wrist to reduce manual impact damage and improve object portability through two pilot trials. The first trial involved a wearable sensor on the wrist of a child with autism. The second experiment studied sensors that could be worn on the wrist and ankle of a child with ASD. The results of both pilots showed that the readings from the body-worn sensors correlated with the children's behavior obtained from videos recorded during the experiment. The results showed that wearable sensors can provide additional information that can be transmitted to social robots or caregivers to mitigate self-injurious behaviors.

4.3.2. AI Machine Learning Predictors

Ref. [89] examined a session in which a child with ASD interacted with various stimuli, such as a social robot that was programmed to exhibit the problematic behaviors they had noticed. A wearable gadget that could record different actions and physiological indications was worn by the youngster. To identify the best combination, various characteristics, and machine learning setups were examined. The study's findings demonstrated that, in addition to conventional kinematic measurements, physiological signals also result in more precise predictions. 97% accuracy was attained using the optimal feature and learning model combination. The findings of this study contribute to the development of early detection techniques for problematic behaviors, which may enable prompt intervention by social robots and caregivers.

In their most recent study, ref. [81], the same research team, also investigated the impact of sensors using a variety of machine learning techniques and data methods obtained from children with ASD wearable sensors during their interactions with social games and robots that could identify challenging behavior. Every child wore a wearable gadget that gathered information. The occurrence of problematic behaviors was identified through the use of video comments of the sessions. To identify problematic behavior, four machine learning algorithms were applied in conjunction with extracted temporal data (mean, standard deviation, minimum, and maximum). This study also looked into variations in heart rate variability (HRV). The XGBoost algorithm achieved the best performance, with 99% accuracy. Furthermore, the physiological features outperformed the kinematic features, with the heart rate being the main feature contributing to prediction performance. This study highlights the importance of developing tools and methods to detect challenging behaviors in autistic children during social robot support sessions.

4.3.3. Mobile Apps

A data recording system based on mobileHCI, which employs self-assessment and physiological signal collecting, was presented by [79]. In order to achieve this, the Easy-Connect mobile app was created to make it simple for parents of children with ASD to document stressful situations through an online survey. A portable physiology sensor was used concurrently to gather electrodermal activity (EDA) and photoplethysmography (PPG) data. In order to determine whether physiological patterns and self-reported stress were related, these signals were synced with self-reports. The findings gathered from eight families demonstrated that the suggested framework effectively facilitated data collection. In addition, EDA-based stress markers were identified and found to be connected with self-reported stress. Ten families participated, and eight of them completed the data collection. Seven females and one male (mean age (years): 44.5, SD = 3.16) were among the caregivers. The mean age (years) of the eight boys with ASD was 9.92, with a standard deviation of 1.28. The severity of ASD symptoms in children was assessed using the Social Responsiveness Scale (SRS-2).

In order to determine whether Anxiety Monitor, a wearable, real-time anxiety detection device, can help children with ASD become more conscious of their anxiety symptoms and begin practicing anxiety relaxation strategies, ref. [66] carried out a randomized controlled trial. Over the course of three sessions, twenty-eight children with ASD received instruction on how to use the Anxiety Monitor and relaxation methods for diaphragmatic breathing. On the fourth visit, participants were advised to practice deep breathing when they felt uncomfortable and were randomly assigned to either obtain feedback on their anxiety level or no feedback at all from the stress meter while completing a difficult task (speaking in front of an audience). An increased propensity to commence deep breathing in response to stress was linked to the responses from the stress meter.

4.3.4. Social Robots

A social robot is a machine designed to interact and communicate with humans in any compatible way. Social robots are usually relatively simple in appearance, provide specialized verbal and nonverbal communication capabilities, and are commonly used in a variety of application areas. Robots can use speech, eye contact, body language, gestures, head positions, and social media to communicate with humans in situations where they exhibit predictable and unacceptable behavior, providing humans with accountability, positive feedback, and emotional release from anxiety and stress. In the literature, many social robots have been used with people with ASD. Some of those found in the literature that have been used with children with ASD to reduce anxiety include KASPAR, Kiliro, and Paro [105,106].

Kiliro is a robotic parrot with 270-degree vision that is equipped with two wireless AI sphere cameras and a USB connector. It includes seven touch sensors to identify touch interactions by children and can use QR codes to distinguish letters and numbers. Additionally, Kiliro is able to navigate, comprehend, and react to sounds. Regarding its application in children with anxiety and ASD, ref. [86] employed it to provide data on decreases in anxiety symptoms in autistic populations. For 49 days, seven children between the ages of 6 and 16 participated in this study. One method of measuring stress was to measure the biological changes in physiology by taking samples of saliva and urine. The results following interactions with the Kiliro robot demonstrated effectiveness and utility. Specifically, the findings of saliva and urine testing suggested that research participants' stress levels had decreased.

Blow and colleagues developed the KASPAR robot in 2005 with the goal of using it as a study platform for human–robot interaction [107]. Because of its basic human form, KASPAR was used to evaluate whether it could be utilized as a therapy aid for children with ASD. It serves as a social mediator, assisting children in growing and interacting with both adults and other children. It also helps children build their foundational emotional intelligence. It makes use of basic gestures, body language, and facial expressions. Additionally, without the need for outside stimulation, sensors on the face, hands, body, and feet react to touch, assisting children in learning about tactile contact and promoting socializing.

To find out how well the KASPAR robot interacted with children with ASD, ref. [92] carried out pilot research in a special school. Nine children between the ages of eight and twelve participated in a mixed-methods study using an ABAB design for this reason. A total of 36 sessions were recorded, including two sessions with the teacher (normal care) and four sessions with the KASPAR. The primary findings were the teacher's responses, which were captured on videotape, and the children's small activities during the lesson. The findings indicated that during the KASPAR sessions, as opposed to teacher sessions, the children touched the robot more frequently than the teacher (p-value = 0.028), replicated nonverbally more frequently (p-value = 0.012), focused more (p-value = 0.011), and were less distracted (p-value = 0.021). Children gave teachers more positive verbal replies than they did for KASPAR (p-value = 0.028). Children's spontaneous speech usage and the quantity of nonverbal behavior seen both exhibited clinically significant differences favoring the KASPAR condition. According to the findings, KASPAR is better at connecting with children, holding their attention for longer, and providing more targeted guidance than teachers. In addition to lowering fear and fostering an ideal environment for deeper learning, the children appeared at ease and enthusiastic when interacting with the robot.

Using KASPAR, ref. [93] investigated responses to anxiety when engaging with the technology. The current study set out to create a blood volume pulse (BVP) signal-based anxiety detection system for children with ASD. In order to analyze heart rate variability for stress detection, the researchers in this study extracted the HRV features from the raw BVP signals obtained from the E4 wristband while conducting interactive research with the social robot KASPAR. Children with HRV had their facial emotions examined in order to validate the study of low- and high-frequency power features and the results. The study included twenty-one children from three different nations. The study's primary discovery was that the children's interactions with the KASPAR robot appeared to lessen their anxiety-related emotions.

Japan's AIST created a robotic seal pup known as PARO. Similar to reinforcement mechanisms, autonomous mechanisms can pick up new behaviors from user feedback. With its touch, sound, vision, motion, and temperature sensors, PARO can identify what we are holding and use head, flap, and eye movements to convey emotions. In order to assess the efficacy of assistive therapy, ref. [84] looked at a population of individuals with ASD. To assess their mood, anxiety, and impulsivity, nine inpatient psychiatric patients, ages 8 to 19, were watched. The inpatients were allowed to engage with the robot for two months. The findings were not entirely consistent. It is anticipated that this research will assist individuals with ASD in improving their communication abilities or lowering obsessive or nervous behaviors. However, some individuals find it unfavorable due to specific features, like big eyes and high-frequency navigation noise. It has been demonstrated to be successful in reducing stress and anxiety symptoms in those without ASD [108,109].

4.3.5. Serious Games

Concerning people with ASD and stress management, [83], in their research, examined the impact of the New Horizon game and the SpaceControl app, which were developed in collaboration with therapists and followed the empowerment principles of eHealth. The game combined two short games with relaxation techniques. The performance of the game was analyzed, and usability studies were conducted with three families. Parents and children were asked to complete the Spence Children's Anxiety Scale (SCAS) and the Spence Children's Anxiety Scale-Parents (SCAS-P). The results showed that this game had the potential to reduce anxiety and stress in children with ASD.

By mapping the imitation and joint attention (JA) subset of age-appropriate stimuli from the Early Start Denver Model (ESDM) intervention, ref. [78] created GOLIAH, an automated platform of 11 serious home intervention games, to address the need for hours of intensive intervention to treat children with this condition. A total of 14 children (ages 5 to 8) with ASD and 10 controls (matched for gender, age, region, and normal care) participated in a survey in two specialized clinics, which yielded the results of 6-month matched exploratory controlled research. For six months, participants in the experimental group had four 30 min GOLIAH sessions per week at home and one session in the hospital, in addition to their regular treatment. Linear mixed models were used for statistics. Parents and their children participated in 40% of the planned sessions and had access to all 11 games. In addition to experiencing an increase in the imitation scores on the majority of imitation games, the participants who received GOLIAH training saw improvements in their task completion times on the majority of JA games. Parental anxiety index ratings were unaffected by the GOLIAH intervention. Lastly, there were notable improvements in both groups' Vineland socialization scores, autism diagnostic observation program scores, total parental stress index scores, and issues on the child's internal, external, and overall behavior checklists. Ref. [67], through their study, investigated Emotiplay, a serious game, by conducting a cross-cultural evaluation (in the UK, Israel, and Sweden). Emotiplay aims to teach emotion recognition to children with ASD in a fun way and to create internal motivation. Children with high IQs and ASD, ages 6 to 9, participated in the game for 8 to 12 weeks. Parent-reported levels of autistic symptoms and adaptive socializing were measured, along with emotional recognition (ER) activities, including face, voice, body, and integrative socialization. Fifteen children in the UK were placed through tests, both before and after using serious play. Children were randomly assigned to either the waitlist or control group in Sweden ($n = 36$) and Israel ($n = 38$). The results from the UK indicated that 8 weeks of game use greatly enhanced participants' performance on integration, SA, and body language tests. Additionally, parents indicated that their children were less stressed and had better adaptive socialization.

The research team of [73] developed and validated a 3D serious game through virtual training that can be played to help ASD patients practice their shopping while reducing stress. Due to the need for individualized training, many aspects of this game have been adapted to enhance engagement and improve the overall effectiveness. To evaluate the validity of the game, ten subjects (11.9 $\pm$ 2.7 males, 20 years old) with ADHD played ten sessions of serious games once a week. Participants had practical experience before and after training in a real supermarket. Changes in the participants' daily living skills were assessed using specific tools, including a form based on the International Classification of Functioning, Disability, and Health in Children and Adolescents and the Vineland II Adaptive Behavior Scale. Significant improvements ($p < 0.05$) were found in basic skills acquired through serious game play, particularly in understanding the purchase process, attention direction, and problem-solving skills. These results suggest that personalized serious games may be an important tool for improving daily living skills.

According to [71], 201 families—parents and children—participated in the study. Three steps were incorporated in the mixed research design employed in this investigation. Depending on their diagnoses (ASD, ADHD, or neurotypical), participants were randomized to one of three intervention groups: serious play, parental support, or a combination of serious play and parental support. Following that, routine scores, obtained at three time intervals (baseline, mean, and endurance) throughout an 8-week period, were analyzed using latent growth modeling and repeated ANOVAs. The findings indicated that a diagnosis had a moderate impact on the children's daily routine. Two interventions (parental support alone and a combination of serious play and parental support) showed very large clinical effects for participants with ADHD, while only one treatment (a combination of serious play and parental support) showed this effect for children with ASD.

4.3.6. Virtual Reality

VR technology provides digital installations that promote virtual immersion through electronic visual simulation, immersing users in an engaging 3D world full of sensory cues and emotions. As virtual reality becomes increasingly popular as an educational tool in learning environments, there are growing expectations about its effectiveness with people with disabilities. Virtual reality provides a fun, safe, controlled, and motivating educational environment and can be an engaging intervention for people with ASD. Virtual reality educational applications have shown promising results in this regard [110].

Concerning their use to combat stress in children and adolescents with ASD, their use seems to be increasingly explored by researchers. More specifically, in the study by [111], the researchers used a sample of nine boys aged 7 to 13 years old who were verbal and diagnosed with ASD but without learning difficulties to create and evaluate a novel treatment using cognitive behavioral therapy (CBT) and gradual exposure to a virtual reality environment (VRE). Every child was interested in a particular subject. In addition to increasing the child's exposure to the phobia or phobic stimulus as necessary, the VRE participants received behavioral and cognitive therapy from a psychologist, such as breathing exercises. For each child, four sessions lasting 20 to 30 min each were planned. Four participants fully conquered their fear, while eight of the nine children in the study were eventually able to regulate their phobias. The treatment's effects persisted after a year.

These findings demonstrated that CBT, in conjunction with AER, can be a highly successful treatment for phobias, anxiety, or a specific type of fear in certain young people with ASD.

In a dentistry clinic, [98] study sought to determine how well VR distraction worked to lower anxiety and behavior in children with ASD. A total of 68 children between the ages of 8 and 15 who needed routine, non-invasive dental care and had an ASD diagnosis were enrolled in this study. During two appointments spaced three months apart, these children received routine, painless dental care. At each visit, the children were given the Frankel Behavioral Rating Scale and the Venham imaging test to gauge their dental and behavioral anxiety following treatment. Forty children received dental treatment, and data collection and an analysis of the results were subsequently completed. When using VR distraction, patients' reported anxiety scores significantly decreased, and their dental behavior improved equally significantly ($p = 0.042$ and $p = 0.0001$, respectively). The results showed that VR distraction can help children with ASD who receive routine dental care.

An interactive virtual reality game called SoundFields was used by [70] in their research, using exposure-based therapeutic techniques targeting auditory stimulation through binaural spatial sounds. In order to assess the efficacy of SoundFields in lowering anxiety related to the chosen distracting noises, an experiment was carried out on six children and adolescents with ASD, ages 16 to 19, who showed hyper-responsiveness to particular sounds. Throughout the four weeks of the trial, every participant engaged in active VR game play. Significant decreases in anxiety levels related to the targeted auditory stimuli were found when pre- and post-survey data were compared. According to the study's findings, SoundFields could help individuals with ASD manage their aural hypersensitivity.

The City University of Hong Kong's Centre for Applied Innovation in Internet and Multimedia Technology (AIMTech Center) created six virtual reality training scenarios that mirrored the everyday lives of typical Hong Kong children in order to test the efficacy of a VR-based educational program on emotional and social skills. Ninety-four students with ASD from Hong Kong's general primary schools took part in the study, and 72 of them were included for analysis. The children in the training group were more engaged in social issues, had better adjustment after training (M = 21.8, SD = 2.99) than before training (M = 20.2, SD = 3.43, $t(35) = -3.987$, $p < 0.0005$), and had higher emotional expression and regulation (M = 20.2, SD = 3.00) than before training (M = 18.9, SD = 3.57, $t(35) = -2.174$, $p = 0.037$). Additionally, for emotional expressions ($F(1, 70) = 5.223$, $p = 0.025$, partial $\eta^2 = 0.069$) and social reciprocity ($F(1, 70) = 7.769$, $p = 0.007$, partial $\eta^2 = 0.100$), there was a statistically significant interaction between the group and time. Children were able to participate in virtual reality training despite initial difficulties associated with the glasses. Some children declined to participate for programming reasons, which could have been minimized by using a head-mounted monitor as a portable and cost-effective device. The results summarized that virtual reality appears to be a promising addition to traditional education and therapy by aiding emotional regulation by reducing stress in children with ASD [72]. These six scenarios were put to the test by the same team of researchers [65] in a similar experimental study that used virtual reality to address emotional control in children with ASD. With corresponding psychoeducational procedures and protocols, six distinct learning scenarios were created, including one that facilitated reinforcement and conceptual generalization, four that simulated different social situations, and one that focused on relaxation and emotional control techniques. Children were shown the learning scenarios in a four-view interactive virtual reality environment with non-intrusive motion tracking, also known as half-CAVE. The 14-week, 28-session program involved 94 children with a clinical diagnosis of ASD, ages 6 to 12. When comparing the tests conducted before and after training, the study found that children's emotional expression and regulation, as well as the emotional reciprocity of social emotions, had significantly improved.

The preliminary experimental study by [100] examined the application of virtual reality-based functional communication in five children diagnosed with ASD using an iPhone X and a Google Cardboard device, conducting a VR intervention at a frequency of once a week for 3 weeks for each participant. In these interventions, the researchers measured the ability to perform an activity on a four-point scale. During the fourth week, all children participated in a realistic flight rehearsal at San Diego International Airport. Parents were asked to rate their child's ability to travel by airplane before the first week and after the fourth week. All children improved their airport travel skills from pre- to post-intervention, according to the researchers' and parents' observations. All children were able to move independently at the airport, showing reduced stress in the process.

Ref. [96] examined VR use in a classroom of 31 children with ASD aged 6–16 years by examining the subjects' perceptions of their use through mixed methodological approaches. The results showed that costly and technologically advanced VRs were preferred, more specifically, the HTC Vive; also, users described them as enjoyable, physically and visually comfortable, easy to use, and exciting, wanting to use them again. They also highlighted the beneficial effects of VR, including relaxation/feeling calm, the ability to virtually explore a place before visiting it in the real world, and the development of learning opportunities at school. Figure 5 summarizes all the findings of the technologies used.

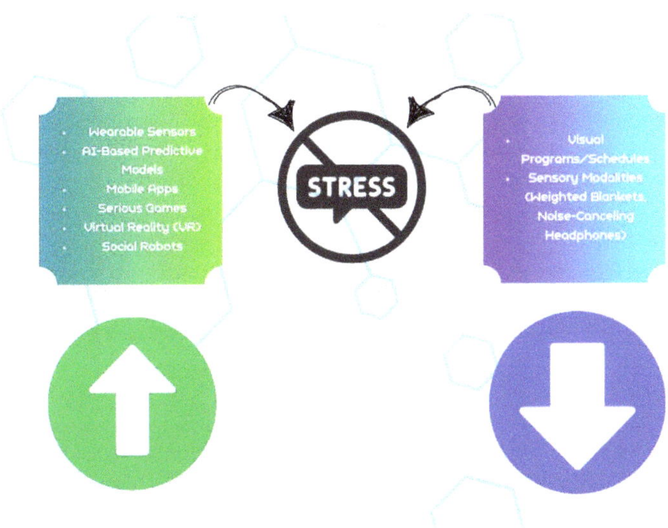

Wearable Sensors
AI-Based Predictive Models
Mobile Apps
Serious Games
Virtual Reality (VR)
Social Robots
STRESS
Visual Programs/Schedules
Sensory Modalities (Weighted Blankets, Noise-Canceling Headphones)

Figure 5. Low and high technologies combating stress.

4.4. Measurement Tools Used

Studies employed a wide range of measurement tools to evaluate stress and anxiety in children and adolescents with ASD. All these measurement tools can be categorized in six key areas, including physiological biomarkers, behavioral observations, psychological and self-reported measures, cognitive and emotional performance metrics, sensory processing assessments, as well as machine learning-based prediction metrics.

Physiological biomarkers were found to be used to evaluate autonomic stress responses. HR and HRV were tracked via wearable devices to determine stress-related changes in ANS. Refs. [66,80], in their studies used HR monitoring as a primary physiological measure, and ref. [81] integrated HR tracking with interbeat interval analysis for stress prediction. EDA and skin conductance in several studies were utilized as key factors to measure sympathetic nervous system activation [75,79]. EDA was also useful in identifying elevated stress responses in real-time settings. Furthermore, cortisol and salivary biomarkers were employed in studies like [68,69] to identify endocrine stress responses pre- and post-intervention.

Regarding behavioral observations, they were utilized to capture an understanding of the engagement and social interaction of individuals related to stressors. More specifically refs. [87,88] applied naturalistic observations to assess engagement in classroom and structure work systems' effectiveness. Others, like [81,92], performed more in-depth micro-behavioral analysis using video tracking and motion data in their studies. These approaches are used to analyze verbal social behaviors, attention shifts, and motor patterns in robot -assisted and interactive interventions.

Psychological and self-reported measures were utilized to capture subjective experiences of stress and anxiety. Studies like [74,79] gathered parent and caregiver reports using structured logs to track stress levels, mostly in natural settings. Similarly, refs. [73,97] evaluated parental perceptions of intervention effectiveness in improving emotional regulation and adaptive behaviors. Self-reported anxiety measures, just like SCAS used in [83], gathered data on a child's perceived anxiety changes.

Related to cognitive and emotional performance, studies focusing on social and emotional learning interventions basically evaluated emotion recognition and social adaption via validated cognitive measures. More specifically, ref. [67] utilized face, body, and voice emotion recognition tasks, while [72] examined measuring affective expressions and social reciprocity using PEP-3 assessments. Others, like [78,88], examined executive functions and cognitive load by integrating them into their interventions involving visual schedules and serious games. More specifically, they analyzed the reaction times in imitation tasks as well as cognitive load reduction in classroom settings.

According to sensory processing and adaptation measures, most of the researchers used sensory profiles and physiological responses to stimuli. Specifically, ref. [97] used SPQ 2 to examine fidget toys' effectiveness in reducing anxiety, and ref. [99] measured auditory sensitivity reduction through the GAS T-scores. Ref. [77] used EEG-based neural monitoring to evaluate adaptive auditory processing responses to stress that was related to adaptive behavior RAAT, and VABS-II was utilized by [71,73], accordingly, to evaluate functional skills and real-life behavioral improvements.

Finally, several studies employed AI and machine learning models to predict stress and challenging behaviors. Ref. [80], as well as [94], utilized classification models to detect physiological stress patterns, presenting high accuracy (AUC > 0.70). Also, ref. [89] used an XGBoost model, achieving 99% accuracy in stress prediction. Aside from the strong demonstration of predictive power, further validation in real-life scenarios is required to confirm their long-term application (Figure 6).

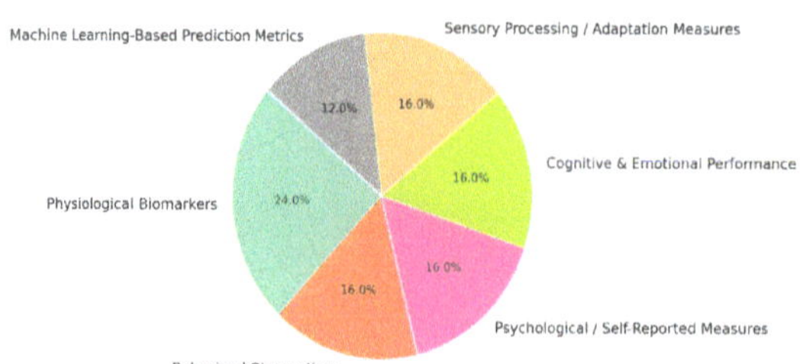

Figure 6. Stress-related measurement tools used across studies.

4.5. Effect Sizes Among Technologies

The present systematic review of $n = 36$ studies revealed important findings regarding the effectiveness of stress and anxiety reduction among children and adolescents with ASD. The results produced a broad spectrum of effect sizes, with some interventions demonstrating strong and significant improvements while others reported modes or inconsistent effects. There was also a significant number of studies that did not explicitly report the effect sizes, creating a critical gap in methodological standardization.

According to the studies analyzed, the most effective were those that provided wearable biofeedback and AI-driven stress detection technologies, demonstrating strong statistically significant effects [66,79,81]. VR interventions produced shared similar findings and presented strong effects, mostly in improving emotional regulation and stress resilience [71,79]. Moderate to large effect sizes were also found in social robotics interventions, supporting their potential for improving social engagement and emotional regulation [67,92]. On the contrary, low-tech assistive technology solutions demonstrated moderate effect sizes, as they were less consistent across different populations and settings in using interventions like weighted blankets [74,87], visual schedules [88], and VR-based distraction techniques [98]. Nonetheless, several studies did not provide explicit effect size calculations and were based on qualitative evaluations, descriptive statistics, as well significance testing without standardized measures of impact magnitude [69,70,84,85,91,93,94,97,99].

Another issue noticed in most of the studies was the limited diversity surrounding the pool of participants. Many studies demonstrated an overreliance on male participants, presenting an imbalance between male and female subjects. Ref. [77] used $n = 75$ boys and only $n = 8$ girls, showcasing unclear results if the effect of auditory interventions was similar across genders.

5. Discussion

The results of this study bring together and demonstrate the benefits and potential of emerging and assistive technologies to reduce neurophysiological stress and anxiety in children and adolescents with ASD and SMD by highlighting both the effectiveness and limitations of these technological interventions. The present research identifies several assistive and emerging technologies that have shown positive effects in reducing anxiety in children with ASD, also offering a unique insight by analysis of various efficacies across different types of technologies (low and high). To the best of our knowledge, this is the first study that collected data and analyzed the whole scope of technologies used (low and high), specifically for targeting stress and anxiety in children and adolescents with ASD, providing valuable pieces of information that can be utilized by researchers for future studies, as well as specialists and educators who work with children and adolescents with ASD and their caregivers. Table 2 summarizes all the data from the studies included.

More specifically, low-tech interventions showed moderate effects in reducing anxiety-related behaviors by supporting individuals with sensory regulation and predictability [76,88]. Aside from the cost-effectiveness as well as availability and usability, their findings were related to several inconsistencies found in several studies [74,87]. On the contrary, high and emerging technology interventions showcased more potential and accuracy in the real-time detection of stress by identifying high-accuracy physiological markers, thus providing feedback for real-time interventions [66,80,94]. AI-based technologies [112], including machine learning models trained on physiological data, have proven to be highly effective in predicting stress-related behaviors in ASD individuals [81,89], showing their growing potential in preventing anxiety episodes and meltdowns. VR-based interventions showcased (in most of the studies) positive effects in improving social skills and emotional regulation [72] while decreasing anxiety levels [70]. Mobile apps were found helpful, providing users with accessible and friendly environments to reduce stress levels and help them to self-report and monitor their state by themselves or their caregivers [66,79]. Similar findings were also identified by the use of Serious Games, which reported a positive impact on emotional regulation and daily routines, especially when they were used in combination with parental support, showcasing a reduction in stress-related behaviors [71]. In addition, parents reported positive effects on autism symptoms in social reciprocity and adaptability while improving their emotion recognition and socializing skills [67]. Finally, social robots were found to be effective in improving social interaction by reducing stress levels in children with ASD [86,92].

Despite the positive effects presented in most of the studies about stress and anxiety reduction as well as detection, several limitations were identified. More specifically, these limitations are related to methodological, technological, participant-related, and longitudinal factors. One of the main limitations reported in a number of studies was the small sample sizes, having a negative impact on statistical power as well as the generalizability of the results. For instance, [87] had one participant, and [81] had only a sample of five children. Furthermore, in several studies [74,95], high dropout rates were identified, reaching 55.6%. In addition, other studies lacked randomized controlled designs, relying only on single-subject feasibility or pilot studies [66,79]. Last but not least, the short duration of many interventions made it difficult to evaluate their true effectiveness [85,86,98].

Table 2. Summary of the included studies for analysis.

Name	Type of Study	Subjects (Age, Gender, Diagnosis)	Intervention	Type of Technology	Measure	Results	Limitations	Effect Sizes	Longitudinal Effects	Country
[99]	Prelimin-ary Study	21 children with ASD, aged 4–16 years (16 boys, 5 girls)	Use of earmuffs and noise-canceling (NC) headphones	Earmuffs, NC headphones	Goal Attainment Scaling (GAS) T-scores	Earmuffs significantly improved Goal Attainment Scaling (GAS) T-scores compared to baseline. NC headphones showed improvement in some children but not significantly overall. Earmuffs were effective in reducing behavioral problems related to hyperreactivity to auditory stimuli. NC headphones were effective for some children but less consistent.	Small sample size; refusal of some participants to wear earmuffs or noise-canceling headphones; limited behavioral data for noise-canceling headphones; lack of control over variables like age, sex, general intelligence, functional level, and frequency of intervention; no examination of adverse or long-term effects; and exclusion of other sound isolation devices like earplugs.	Effect size was calculated with an alpha value of 0.05 and power of 80% for the Goal Attainment Scaling T-score; improvement was set to 1 for the sample size estimation.	No longitudinal effects were assessed; the study primarily focused on immediate behavioral changes using earmuffs and noise-canceling headphones.	Japan
[76]	Pilot Study	14 boys, 3–8 years old, autism spectrum disorder (ASD)	Tell-show-do method + Visual Schedule System (test group) vs. Tell-show-do method (control group)	Visual Schedule System using picture communication symbols	Number of dental steps attempted, completion time per step, behavioral distress levels, physiological arousal (EDA)	Test group completed 1.38 more steps, 35.52 s faster per step, and 18.7% lower distress than the control group.	Small sample size (14 boys). Lack of statistical power to detect significant differences; intervention limited to a single method (visual pedagogy); potential rater bias, as intervention was clearly noticeable; children were not informed about upcoming appointments, which might have influenced anxiety levels.	Patients in the visual pedagogy group completed 1.38 more steps on average, completed steps 35.52 s faster per step, and displayed 18.7% lower levels of behavioral distress. Cohen's d is not explicitly provided, but results indicate a notable clinical effect.	Limited by short study duration. No follow-up to assess long-term retention of improvements. Future research aims to explore more sensitive physiological stress indicators and broader participant demographics.	Canada

Table 2. *Cont.*

Name	Type of Study	Subjects (Age, Gender, Diagnosis)	Intervention	Type of Technology	Measure	Results	Limitations	Effect Sizes	Longitudinal Effects	Country
[88]	Multiple-Baseline, Single-Case Design	4 students, aged 8–11 years, diagnosed with ASD	Use of visual schedules and work systems to increase on-task behavior in mainstream classrooms	low	Observations within a natural classroom environment	Visual schedules and work systems increased on-task behavior in all four students. Mixed results for secondary variables, with some showing reduced off-task behavior and increased productivity. On-task behavior increased from a baseline mean of 20–61% to 53–86% during intervention. Off-task behaviors showed moderate improvement but were not statistically significant. Productivity increased significantly in some students.	Small sample size (4 students); individual variability in teacher implementation of visual schedules and work systems; variability in baseline behaviors due to external classroom factors; limited generalizability due to specific participant demographics; fidelity of implementation was not consistent across all sessions; no follow-up sessions to confirm maintenance of behavior improvements.	Statistically significant improvements in on-task behaviors for three of the four students (Tau-U values ranging from 0.6458 to 1.25; $p <$ 0.05); moderate improvements in productivity for two students (Tau-U = 0.7857, $p = 0.0184$ and Tau-U = 1.5, $p = 0.0015$).	A single maintenance probe was conducted for one student, showing decreased on-task behavior after intervention cessation. No broader longitudinal effects were assessed.	Australia
[87]	Alternating Treat-ments Single Case Research Design	5-year-old male diagnosed with ASD	Weighted blanket and structured work boxes	low	Percentage of 10 s intervals of engagement	SWB resulted in consistently higher levels of engagement. Weighted blanket resulted in lower engagement, often similar to or less than baseline levels.	Single-subject design limits generalizability; short intervention duration (10 min sessions); possible novelty effect of weighted blanket intervention; lack of comparison to other evidence-based sensory interventions; limited reliability of teacher- reported engagement data; and no formal assessment of potential long-term benefits or harms of using weighted blankets.	No effect size was explicitly reported; visual analysis indicates structured work boxes (SWB) showed significant improvements in engagement, while the weighted blanket intervention demonstrated levels of engagement similar to or lower than the baseline.	No longitudinal effects were assessed; outcomes were limited to immediate responses during and after the short intervention period.	USA

Table 2. *Cont.*

Name	Type of Study	Subjects (Age, Gender, Diagnosis)	Intervention	Type of Technology	Measure	Results	Limitations	Effect Sizes	Longitudinal Effects	Country
[85]	Single-Subject Design	Two 4-year-old participants were diagnosed with autism	Weighted blanket intervention for 14 days	Weighted blankets	Objective sleep measures; caregiver surveys	Minimal changes in sleep patterns as a result of the weighted blanket intervention. Enhanced morning mood and significantly decreased time to fall asleep for participants. Findings suggest minimal changes in sleep patterns, enhanced morning mood, and decreased time to fall asleep. Not strong enough to recommend for clinical use.	Very small sample size (2 participants); convenience sampling from a medically underserved region; lack of blinding for caregivers; limited reliability of the Hello Sense Sleep app; potential for caregiver bias in self-reported measures; short intervention duration (14 days); and inability to generalize findings due to the single-subject design.	Effectiveness evaluated using Percentage of Non-Overlapping Data (PND). For participant 1 (John), PND for morning mood was 84% (effective); for participant 2 (Katie), PND for time to fall asleep and night wakings was 84% and 100%, respectively (effective).	No longitudinal effects were assessed; the study focused solely on immediate sleep behavior outcomes during the intervention period.	USA
[75]	Single-Subject Multi-Treatment Design	6 children, aged 8–16 years, diagnosed with ASD	Use of in-ear (IE) and over-ear (OE) noise-attenuating headphones	In-ear (IE) and over-ear (OE) noise-attenuating headphones, Empatica E4 wristbands	Skin conductance levels (SCL), nonspecific skin conductance responses (NS-SCRs)	Noise-attenuating headphones led to a significant decrease in skin conductance levels (SCL) and frequency of nonspecific skin conductance responses (NS-SCRs). SCL and NS-SCR frequency significantly decreased between baseline and the first intervention phase. The intervention provided protection against the negative effects of environmental noise.	Small sample size (6 children); high dropout rate (50%); individual variability in electrodermal activity (EDA) responses; no tracking of 'aware mode' use in in-ear headphones; inability to generalize findings due to single-subject design; and limited data on broader environmental variables like specific noise types or frequencies.	Effect size not directly calculated; intervention showed significant reductions in skin conductance level (SCL) and nonspecific skin conductance responses (NS-SCR) frequency in the intervention phases compared to baseline ($p < 0.05$).	No longitudinal effects were assessed; the study focused on short-term outcomes during and immediately after the intervention.	USA

Table 2. *Cont.*

Name	Type of Study	Subjects (Age, Gender, Diagnosis)	Intervention	Type of Technology	Measure	Results	Limitations	Effect Sizes	Longitudinal Effects	Country
[68]	Clinical and Laboratory Experimental Study	20 children, 6–10 years old, autism spectrum disorder (ASD)	Video Modeling Berkunjung ke Dokter Gigi (VM-BDG) vs. Visual Pedagogy Module Berkunjung ke Dokter Gigi (VPM-BDG)	Video Modeling (VM-BDG), Visual Pedagogy Module (VPM-BDG)	Delta salivary cortisol levels before and after intervention	Both VM-BDG and VPM-BDG effectively reduced stress levels; no significant difference between the interventions.	Small sample size (20 children); no control group without intervention; limited generalizability due to strict inclusion criteria; salivary cortisol measurement may be influenced by external factors; short duration between pre- and post-intervention saliva collection.	Delta salivary cortisol values showed a reduction in stress for both interventions; no statistically significant differences between VM-BDG and VPM-BDG. Both interventions were equally effective in reducing stress but lacked a control comparison for baseline reference.	Short study duration with no long-term follow-up. No assessment of sustained stress reduction over multiple visits. Future research should explore broader demographics and extended data collection periods.	Indonesia
[69]	Clinical Experimental Study	20 children, 6–10 years old, Autism Spectrum Disorder (ASD)	Video Modeling vs. Visual Pedagogical Module	Video Modeling, Visual Pedagogical Module (PV-BDG)	Salivary Immunoglobulin A (sIgA) levels before and after intervention	Both methods reduced stress levels as measured by sIgA; no significant difference between the groups.	Small sample size (20 children); no significant difference in stress reduction between the two interventions; limited generalizability due to specific participant criteria; no control group without intervention; external factors influencing saliva IgA levels were not controlled.	sIgA levels increased after video modeling but decreased with the PV-BDG module; no significant difference in ΔsIgA levels between the two groups; clinical effectiveness was observed but lacks strong statistical significance.	Short study duration with no long-term follow-up; further research is needed to assess sustained stress reduction effects. Future studies should include broader demographics and additional physiological stress markers.	Indonesia

Table 2. *Cont.*

Name	Type of Study	Subjects (Age, Gender, Diagnosis)	Intervention	Type of Technology	Measure	Results	Limitations	Effect Sizes	Longitudinal Effects	Country
[74]	Retrospective Follow-up Study	85 individuals: 48 children aged $\leq$17 (57%), 37 adults $\geq$ 18 years (44%), diagnosed with ADHD and/or ASD	Use of weighted blankets	Weighted blankets (chain-weighted and ball-weighted)	Self-reports via telephone interviews	Weighted blankets improved falling asleep, sleeping through the night, and relaxing during the day. They also improved morning and evening routines, including preparing/going to sleep and waking up. Also, 59% reported improved ability to fall asleep, 81% reported improved sleeping through the night, and 45.8% reported improved daily routines.	Small sample size (8 families); non-randomized design; data collection interruptions due to technological issues; limited diversity in family demographics; inability to capture nuanced stress triggers beyond predefined survey options; and no assessment of real-world generalizability of findings.	Medium to large effect sizes were observed for SCR features (Cohen's d ranging from 0.59 to 2.67) during stress episodes, indicating strong associations between physiological signals and self-reported stress.	No longitudinal effects were assessed; the study focused solely on immediate stress patterns during a short data collection period.	Sweden
[77]	Experimental Study	83 children (75 males; 8 females), 7–12 years old, autism spectrum disorder (ASD)	Development and validation of noise-canceling headphones with aural perception tuning	Hybrid Active Noise Cancelation (ANC) system with EEG-based sound perception tuning	Subjective aural perception ratings, EEG signals for neural responses	Headset effectively reduced auditory hyperreactivity; unpleasant frequencies (250 Hz, 8 kHz) were identified, and noise cancelation improved participants' aural comfort.	Small sample size (83 ASD and 50 TD children); subjective aural perception ratings may introduce bias; external noise factors could impact ANC effectiveness; study limited to specific frequencies (250 Hz–8 kHz); lack of long-term usability testing in real-world environments.	Significant reduction in unpleasant sound perception with ANC headset; frequencies of 250 Hz and 8 kHz were rated as most unpleasant; aural perception ratings significantly correlated with EEG neural responses; different ASD clusters exhibited unique auditory response profiles.	No long-term follow-up on adaptation and behavioral impact; ANC effectiveness in daily settings remains uncertain. Future studies should assess sustained benefits and individual long-term auditory adaptation.	China

Table 2. *Cont.*

Name	Type of Study	Subjects (Age, Gender, Diagnosis)	Intervention	Type of Technology	Measure	Results	Limitations	Effect Sizes	Longitudinal Effects	Country
[84]	Observational Study	9 patients with ASD (4 boys; 5 girls), aged 8–19 years	Interaction with PARO, a baby harp seal-type therapeutic robot	PARO, baby harp seal-type therapeutic robot	Observation of patient interactions with PARO	Effective for some patients in developing good communication and reducing impulsive behaviors or anxiety. Some patients did not like PARO due to its features, like big eyes or drive noise. Some patients treated PARO like a real animal, which helped in communication and reducing anxiety. Other patients disliked PARO for its features.	Small sample size (9 patients); lack of objective indices for measuring effectiveness; potential influence of other concurrent treatments; results may be due to temporary changes in emotional state rather than PARO itself; limited generalizability due to narrow demographic diversity.	Effect size not calculated; observational data indicated some positive changes but lacked quantitative analysis.	No longitudinal effects were assessed; the study focused on short-term behavioral and emotional changes observed during interaction with PARO.	Japan
[86]	Pilot Study with Mixed Methods (Quantitative-Qualitative)	9 children, aged 6–16 years, diagnosed with ASD	Interaction with semi-autonomous parrot-inspired robot KiliRo using the Adapted Model-Rival Method (AMRM) Semi-autonomous parrot-inspired robot	Semi-autonomous parrot-inspired robot (KiliRo)	Facial expressions (Oxford emotion API), informal and semi-formal interviews, closed-format questionnaire	Children appeared attracted and happy to interact with KiliRo. AMRM may help improve learning and social interaction abilities. Participants showed increased happiness and engagement over the study period. Positive feedback from parents, pediatricians, and psychologists on robot's potential.	Small sample size (9 children); short duration of intervention (5 days); simulated autonomy of the robot limits ecological validity; potential bias in qualitative interviews due to group settings; limited diversity in participant demographics; absence of control group for comparison.	Effect size was not explicitly calculated; qualitative and descriptive analyses provided positive indications of emotional engagement and social interaction.	No longitudinal effects were assessed; the focus was on immediate responses and interaction patterns during the short intervention period.	India

Table 2. *Cont.*

Name	Type of Study	Subjects (Age, Gender, Diagnosis)	Intervention	Type of Technology	Measure	Results	Limitations	Effect Sizes	Longitudinal Effects	Country
[67]	Cross-cultural Evaluation with Randomized Controlled Trial	89 children with high-functioning ASC, aged 6–9 years (Israel: 38, Sweden: 36, UK: 15)	Use of Emotiplay serious game for emotion recognition training	Internet-based serious game (Emotiplay)	Emotion recognition tasks (face, voice, body, integrative), SRS-2, VABS-II Socialization scale	Significant improvements in emotion recognition across face, voice, body, and integrative tasks. Parents reported reduced autism symptoms and improved socialization in Israel and Sweden. Children using Emotiplay showed significant improvements in emotion recognition and social skills compared to controls. Parents in Israel reported reduced autism symptoms.	Variation in intervention protocols across countries (UK, Israel, Sweden); inconsistent parental involvement; dropout rates due to lack of motivation and technical issues; potential cultural biases in emotion recognition tasks; short duration of intervention (8 weeks); reliance on parental reporting for generalization and socialization outcomes; and lack of active control groups in certain study sites.	Significant effect sizes were reported for emotion recognition improvements in the intervention group: $\eta^2 = 0.20$ for body tasks, 0.40 for integrative tasks, and 0.30 for country-level differences (MANOVA results).	No longitudinal effects were assessed; improvements were only measured immediately post-intervention with no follow-up period.	UK, Israel, Sweden
[78]	Matched Controlled Exploratory Study	24 children (14 experimental group, 10 control group), 5–8 years old, autism spectrum disorder (ASD), IQ $\geq$ 60	GOLIAH (Gaming Open Library for Intervention in Autism at Home) platform combined with Treatment As Usual (TAU) for 6 months	Automated serious gaming platform (GOLIAH) targeting joint attention and imitation tasks	Performance metrics in imitation and joint attention games; ADOS scores, Vineland socialization, Parenting Stress Index (PSI), Child Behavior Checklist (CBCL)	Improvement in imitation and joint attention performance within GOLIAH games; no significant differences in core ASD symptoms compared to the control group (TAU alone); no increase in parental stress.	Small sample size (14 experimental, 10 control); no randomization due to parental motivation selection; observance rate lower than expected; limited generalizability due to strict inclusion criteria; no web-based version of GOLIAH available at the time of the study.	Significant improvement in 4 out of 6 imitation games; 3 out of 4 joint attention games showed reduced reaction times; no significant group × time interaction for clinical measures; improvements in Vineland socialization, CBCL scores, and parental stress observed in both groups.	No long-term follow-up conducted; study suggests potential for larger randomized controlled trials; future research to focus on younger children and web-based implementation of GOLIAH.	France, Italy

Table 2. *Cont.*

Name	Type of Study	Subjects (Age, Gender, Diagnosis)	Intervention	Type of Technology	Measure	Results	Limitations	Effect Sizes	Longitudinal Effects	Country
[91]	Pilot Study	10-year-old boy with mild autism, 6-year-old neurotypical boy	Use of wearable sensors and social robots for detecting and mitigating meltdowns	Wearable sensors (Empatica E4 wristband), social robots (PARO, toy train)	Physiological signals (HR, EDA, movement), video observations	Wearable sensors effectively detected physiological changes correlating with meltdowns. Sensors on the wrist and ankle showed similar responses. Social robots helped in calming the child. Effective detection of physiological changes during meltdowns. Social robots were effective in calming the child.	Small sample size; pilot study design limits generalizability; sensor placement (wrist vs. ankle) needs further investigation; no long-term data on effectiveness; limited diversity in participant demographics; challenges in controlling for external variables like environmental stimuli.	Effect size not directly calculated; study focused on the correlation of physiological signals (EDA, BVP, accelerometer) with challenging behaviors.	No longitudinal effects were assessed; the focus was on real-time detection of challenging behaviors and immediate intervention possibilities.	Qatar
[65]	Controlled Trial	94 children, 6–12 years old (86 males; 8 females), autism spectrum disorder (ASD) with IQ $\geq$ 60	28-session virtual reality-enabled program using an immersive half-CAVE system to train emotional regulation and social adaptation	Immersive virtual reality (CAVE environment with non-intrusive motion tracking)	Emotion regulation (PEP-3 Affective Expressions), social interaction (PEP-3 Social Reciprocity), emotion recognition (Faces and Eyes Tests), adaptive skills (ABAS-II)	Significant improvement in emotion expression ($p = 0.037$) and social reciprocity ($p = 0.007$); no significant changes in emotion recognition or adaptive skills.	Small sample size (94 children); lack of randomization due to parental selection; no follow-up assessments beyond training period; limited generalizability to diverse ASD populations; no comparison with other VR-based training programs.	Significant improvements in emotion expression and regulation ($p = 0.037$); social reciprocity scores increased significantly ($p = 0.007$); no significant changes in emotion recognition ($p = 0.666$); mixed findings on adaptive skills improvements.	No long-term follow-up was conducted; future studies recommended to assess sustained behavioral improvements; need for broader participant demographics and comparisons with alternative training methods.	China

Table 2. *Cont.*

Name	Type of Study	Subjects (Age, Gender, Diagnosis)	Intervention	Type of Technology	Measure	Results	Limitations	Effect Sizes	Longitudinal Effects	Country
[90]	Single-Subject Study	One 13-year-old male student diagnosed with autism	Smartglasses-based socio-emotional learning intervention using the Empowered Brain system	Smartglasses (Google Glass), Empowered Brain system	Educator logs, video interviews	Educators found the intervention practical and easy to implement. The student demonstrated improved verbal and nonverbal communication skills. No adverse effects on the classroom environment. Positive impact on student's social communication skills. Educators found the technology practical and usable without causing distractions in the classroom.	Single-subject design; limited to one 13-year-old male participant with autism; absence of quantitative validated outcome measures; short intervention period (2 weeks, 16 sessions); findings cannot be generalized due to the specificity of the sample; teacher-reported improvements lack independent verification.	Effect size was not calculated; qualitative teacher-reported improvements in social interaction, eye contact, and classroom participation were observed.	No longitudinal effects were assessed; the study focused on immediate teacher-reported outcomes during the two-week intervention.	USA
[72]	Waitlist Control Design	94 children, mean age 106.3 months (88.9% boys, 11.1% girls), all diagnosed with ASD	VR-based social skills training	Virtual Reality	PEP-3 Affective Expressions and Social Reciprocity	Children showed improved emotional expression, regulation, social interaction, and adaptation post-training, indicating VR training's effectiveness.	Large dropout rate (approximately 20%); limited diversity in demographics (primarily from Hong Kong); difficulty with logistics and scheduling due to reliance on a large, stationary CAVE VR system; some children refused initial participation due to discomfort with VR goggles; absence of long-term data to assess the sustainability of improvements.	Significant effect sizes for improvement in emotional expression and regulation (partial η^2 = 0.069, p = 0.025) and social reciprocity (partial η^2 = 0.100, p = 0.007).	No longitudinal effects were assessed; outcomes were measured immediately post-intervention with no follow-up.	China

Table 2. *Cont.*

Name	Type of Study	Subjects (Age, Gender, Diagnosis)	Intervention	Type of Technology	Measure	Results	Limitations	Effect Sizes	Longitudinal Effects	Country
[80]	Experimental Study	38 children (22 with ASD, 16 without ASD), ages not specified	Machine learning models (SVM, logistic regression) trained on wearables data to differentiate stress and rest states	Consumer-grade wearable device with machine learning algorithms	Heart rate (HR) and RR interval data; accuracy of machine learning models	SVM achieved 93% accuracy; logistic regression achieved 87% accuracy in differentiating stress vs. rest states; similar performance for both ASD and non-ASD groups.	Balanced dataset (equal rest and stress samples) may not reflect real-world class imbalance; small sample size (38 participants); study conducted in a controlled setting, limiting generalizability; movement-induced physiological changes that are not fully accounted for.	The SVM model achieved 93% accuracy; the logistic regression model achieved 87% accuracy; high F1 scores (above 0.84) for stress detection in the ASD group; model performance was stable across ASD and non-ASD groups.	No long-term follow-up to assess real-world applicability. Further research is needed to test effectiveness in social settings. Future studies should address class imbalance in real-world stress exposure scenarios.	USA
[96]	Mixed-Methods Exploratory Study	31 autistic children, 6–16 years old, with autism spectrum disorder (ASD)	Exploration of preferences and usability of three VR head-mounted displays (HTC Vive, ClassVR, Google Cardboard) in school settings	Virtual reality head-mounted displays (HMDs): HTC Vive, ClassVR, Google Cardboard	Questionnaire responses on device preference, enjoyment, physical comfort, and potential uses of VR in classrooms	HTC Vive was most preferred due to the immersive experience, while ClassVR was least preferred; children reported high enjoyment, comfort, and interest in VR for calming, preparing for real-world events, and learning.	Small sample size; limited diversity in participants; narrow age range (6–16 years old); diverse devices with varying functionalities potentially skewed results; lack of longitudinal assessment; only partial utilization of device capabilities; limited software comparability across devices; and subjective preference data.	Effect size not explicitly calculated; results highlighted high preference rates for interactive VR devices (e.g., HTC Vive) over lower-tech options.	No longitudinal effects were assessed; the study focused on the immediate usability and preferences of VR devices.	United Kingdom

Table 2. *Cont.*

Name	Type of Study	Subjects (Age, Gender, Diagnosis)	Intervention	Type of Technology	Measure	Results	Limitations	Effect Sizes	Longitudinal Effects	Country
[98]	Experimental Study	40 children, 8–15 years old, with autism spectrum disorder (ASD)	Virtual reality distraction (VR) during routine non-invasive dental treatments compared to conventional behavior management	Virtual reality (VR) eyeglasses with visual and auditory stimuli	Venham's Picture Test (anxiety), Frankel's Behavior Rating Scale (behavior)	Significant reduction in anxiety ($p = 0.037$) and improvement in dental behavior ($p = 0.0001$) when VR distraction was used.	Small sample size (40 children completed both visits); high dropout rate (58.8%); no randomization due to practical constraints; anxiety and behavior scores may be influenced by prior exposure to dental teams; no physiological stress biomarkers were measured.	Statistically significant reduction in anxiety scores ($p = 0.037$); significant improvement in behavior rating ($p = 0.0001$); negative correlation between anxiety and behavior scores ($p < 0.001$), indicating VR distraction had a positive impact.	No long-term follow-up beyond the second dental visit; future studies should explore extended intervention effects; larger randomized trials are needed to validate VR distraction as a sustained behavior management tool.	India
[83]	Feasibility and Usability Study	3 families, children aged 6–10 years old, autism spectrum disorder (ASD)	New Horizon Serious Game designed for stress and anxiety reduction with relaxation mini-games; parent app SpaceControl for monitoring gaming behavior	Serious Game (mobile-based), relaxation techniques (guided imagery and focused breathing), supporting parent app	Children's mood (Likert scale), SCAS (Spence Children Anxiety Scale), SCAS-P (Parent version), gaming behavior logs	Positive feedback from parents and children. The game showed potential for reducing stress and anxiety, but the results were preliminary due to the small sample size.	Small sample size (3 families); imited generalizability due to pilot study nature; no objective stress biomarkers measured; game impact on actual stress reduction remains unclear; short testing period restricts behavioral adaptation assessment.	Preliminary positive trends were observed in SCAS and SCAS-P scores; no statistically significant effect sizes due to a small sample; parental feedback suggested potential improvements in relaxation effects; engagement levels varied among children.	No long-term follow-up was conducted; future studies aim to assess sustained use over extended periods; need for larger sample size to evaluate longitudinal effectiveness in stress management.	Belgium

Table 2. *Cont.*

Name	Type of Study	Subjects (Age, Gender, Diagnosis)	Intervention	Type of Technology	Measure	Results	Limitations	Effect Sizes	Longitudinal Effects	Country
[95]	Comparative Study	24 children (mean age = 42.62 months; 12 with ASD, 12 with LD)	Use of a wearable heart rate measurement device during interactive activities	Wearable heart rate measurement device (thoracic belt with ECG sensors)	Heart rate (HR) monitoring	HR was significantly higher in children with ASD compared to those with LD during interactive activities. Increased HR correlated with autism severity.	Small sample size (24 children) with a high dropout rate (55.6%); potential biases in interpretation due to unbalanced gender representation; short duration of interactive activities limiting comprehensive HR analysis; reliance on ADOS-2 for stress correlation may miss nuanced non-social stressors; and technical limitations of the wearable device leading to signal inconsistencies in certain activities.	Significant effect sizes were observed for HR differences during stress-inducing activities (ADOS-2 bubble play: Cohen's d = 0.93, $p = 0.026$; anticipation of routine: Cohen's d = 1.06, $p = 0.012$), indicating strong stress responses in children with ASD.	No longitudinal effects were assessed; the study focused solely on short-term physiological responses to structured activities.	Italy
[70]	Pilot Study	6 participants diagnosed with ASD, aged 16–19 years	Use of SoundFields, a virtual reality game with binaural-based spatial audio	Virtual reality game (SoundFields) with binaural-based spatial audio	Self-reported anxiety scores, tracked voluntary interaction time	Significant decrease in anxiety linked to target auditory stimuli after four weeks of intervention. Participants actively engaged and enjoyed the VR environment. Decreased anxiety towards target stimuli, increased voluntary interactions with target auditory stimuli, and positive engagement with the VR environment.	Small sample size (6 participants); lack of a control group to compare results; short intervention duration (4 weeks); potential biases in self-reported anxiety scores; no measures of generalization to real-world auditory hypersensitivity; and reliance on subjective outcome measures rather than physiological or objective behavioral data.	The effect size was not explicitly calculated; the Wilcoxon signed-rank test indicated a significant decrease in self-reported anxiety scores ($p = 0.026$).	No longitudinal effects were assessed; focus was limited to immediate post-intervention outcomes without follow-up evaluations.	UK

Table 2. *Cont.*

Name	Type of Study	Subjects (Age, Gender, Diagnosis)	Intervention	Type of Technology	Measure	Results	Limitations	Effect Sizes	Longitudinal Effects	Country
[100]	Preliminary Controlled Trial	5 children, 4–8 years old (4 males; 1 female), autism spectrum disorder (ASD)	Virtual reality-based air travel training (VR-ATT) with social stories and real-world air travel rehearsal	Google Cardboard VR with iPhone X and narrative-based functional communication activities	Parent-rated air travel ability questionnaire (Likert scale) and clinical activity rubric during intervention	4 out of 5 participants improved by at least 2 points in air travel ability; no significant statistical changes due to the small sample size.	Small sample size (5 children); no control group for comparison; short intervention period (3 weeks); individual differences in VR engagement levels; parent-reported improvements lack objective physiological validation.	Improvement in air travel skills reported by parents; activity completion rubric showed increases in task performance; no statistically significant differences in pre- and post-training scores (p = 0.0625).	No long-term follow-up conducted; future studies are recommended to evaluate real-world transferability; need for a larger sample size and an extended intervention period.	USA
[89]	Feasibility Study	One 10-year-old male child diagnosed with ASD	Use of wearable sensors and social robots to detect challenging behaviors	Wearable sensors (Empatica E4) and social robots (Nao, PARO)	Physiological signals (HR, EDA, IBI, TEMP, BVP), acceleration	Physiological signals combined with kinetic measures led to more accurate predictions of challenging behaviors. Best machine learning model achieved 97% accuracy. Heart rate and interbeat interval were significant predictors of challenging behaviors. Physiological features outperformed kinetic features in prediction accuracy.	Single-subject design (10-year-old male); limited generalizability to other populations; reliance on manually annotated challenging behaviors; absence of long-term or repeated sessions; wearable discomfort or potential harm to the child not thoroughly explored; and the model's dependency on lab settings for data collection.	High accuracy reported for combined physiological and kinetic data (97%) using an MLP classifier; effect size not explicitly calculated, but performance metrics indicated strong model reliability.	No longitudinal effects were assessed; the study was limited to single-session outcomes in a controlled lab environment.	Qatar

Table 2. *Cont.*

Name	Type of Study	Subjects (Age, Gender, Diagnosis)	Intervention	Type of Technology	Measure	Results	Limitations	Effect Sizes	Longitudinal Effects	Country
[92]	Mixed Methods (Quantitative-Qualitative) ABAB Design	9 children, aged 8–12 years, diagnosed with ASD	Interaction with robot KASPAR and usual care with teacher	Semi-autonomous humanoid robot (KASPAR)	Micro behaviors, attention metrics, video recall interviews	Children showed significantly more nonverbal imitation, touched the robot more often, maintained attention longer, and were less distracted during KASPAR sessions compared to teacher sessions. KASPAR was able to make contact with children, hold their attention longer, and engage them in more nonverbal interactions compared to teachers.	Small sample size (9 children); limited generalizability due to the controlled and artificial study setting; absence of long-term follow-up; potential novelty effect of KASPAR; variation in teacher engagement approaches; and limited individual customization of KASPAR for each child's specific needs.	Significant effect sizes were reported for specific micro-behaviors: non-verbal imitation ($r = 0.589$), touching KASPAR ($r = 0.405$), and maintaining attention ($r = 0.545$), demonstrating moderate to large effects.	No longitudinal effects were assessed; the study was limited to immediate outcomes over four weeks with no follow-up evaluations.	Netherlands
[66]	Pilot Randomized Controlled Trial	38 children with ASD, aged 8–18 years, IQ > 50	Use of Anxiety Meter (wearable, real-time anxiety detection technology) with diaphragmatic breathing training	Wearable sensors (Shimmer2) and a tablet display	Proportion of participants initiating deep breathing, heart rate, respiration rate and amplitude, self-reported anxiety	Participants using the Anxiety Meter were more likely to initiate deep breathing and reported feeling calmer. Feedback from the Anxiety Meter increased the likelihood of initiating deep breathing in response to anxiety.	Relatively small sample size (28 children); short intervention period (4 visits); imbalances in IQ and sex between treatment and control groups; controlled-laboratory setting limits real-world generalizability; potential confounding factors such as participant familiarity with stress-eliciting tasks; and reliance on self-reported measures of anxiety reduction and relaxation initiation.	Significant group differences in initiating relaxation techniques: Odds Ratio (OR) = 2.00 (95% CI = [0.340, 1.046], $p = 0.001$). The effect size for physiological signal improvements was not explicitly calculated.	No longitudinal effects were assessed; study outcomes were limited to immediate responses during and after the intervention sessions.	Canada

Table 2. *Cont.*

Name	Type of Study	Subjects (Age, Gender, Diagnosis)	Intervention	Type of Technology	Measure	Results	Limitations	Effect Sizes	Longitudinal Effects	Country
[82]	Pilot Study	20 children with ASD, aged 7–13 years (14 boys; 6 girls)	Use of autism hug machine portable seat (AHMPS) with inflatable wrap and manual pull	Autism hug machine portable seat (AHMPS) with inflatable wrap and manual pull	Conners' Parent Rating Scale-48 (CPRS-48), Galvanic Skin Response (GSR)	Conduct problems significantly decreased in the inflatable group (p = 0.007) compared to the manual pull group. Significant reduction in sympathetic response (p = 0.01) only in the inflatable group. AHMPS with inflatable wrap effectively reduced emotional arousal and neurobiological stress in children with ASD. Conduct problems decreased more in the inflatable wrap group compared to the manual pull group.	Small sample size (20 children); short duration of intervention (3 weeks); limited demographic diversity (Javanese children only); results potentially influenced by parents' subjective ratings; no evaluation of long-term sustainability of behavioral changes; and absence of data on the broader applicability of the portable hug machine in different environments.	Medium effect size was observed for stress reduction in the inflatable wrap group (ηp^2 = 0.396), indicating moderate effectiveness; a small effect size for the manual pull group (ηp^2 = 0.09).	No longitudinal effects were assessed; the study focused on immediate outcomes within the 3-week intervention period.	Indonesia
[93]	Experim-ental Study	21 children, 2–12 years old, ASD	Robot-based intervention using the Kaspar robot combined with physiological monitoring (BVP signals) and facial emotion analysis	Empatica E4 wristband (physiologi-cal monitoring), OpenFace toolkit (facial emotion detection)	Blood volume pulse (BVP), HRV (LF and HF power), facial emotion annotations as stress verification	Overall, children were not stressed during Kaspar robot interactions; stress declined during sessions for some children, as verified by facial emotion analysis.	Small sample size (21 children); lack of real-time data processing; reliance on lab-based settings limits ecological validity; contradictory results between LF and HF stress metrics in certain sessions; no data on individual differences in stress sensitivity; and limited diversity in demographics (participants mostly from specific regions).	Effect size not explicitly calculated; descriptive and session-wise analyses showed reduced stress levels during robot-based interactions, as indicated by decreasing LF and increasing HF values in many cases.	No longitudinal effects were assessed; results were based on session-specific outcomes without follow-up evaluations or broader assessments.	Turkey, Mace-donia, United King-dom, Poland

Table 2. *Cont.*

Name	Type of Study	Subjects (Age, Gender, Diagnosis)	Intervention	Type of Technology	Measure	Results	Limitations	Effect Sizes	Longitudinal Effects	Country
[73]	Pilot Study	10 children and teenagers, 8–16 years old, with autism spectrum disorder (ASD)	ShopAut 2.0, a 3D personalized serious game for training shopping activities with pre- and post-real-life supermarket assessments	3D Serious Game (ShopAut 2.0) with personalized training and individualized features for ASD severity levels	ICF-CY form scores (real-life shopping tasks), Vineland Adaptive Behavior Scale II (VABS-II)	Significant improvements in daily living skills, particularly in shopping procedures, attention, self-control, and problem-solving; VABS-II scores improved in communication, daily living skills, and socialization.	Small sample size (10 ASD participants); no control group for comparison; short intervention period (10 sessions); real-world shopping environment not tested beyond one location; no assessment of long-term retention of skills.	Significant improvements ($p < 0.05$) in shopping procedure, attention, and problem-solving skills; VABS-II scores showed enhanced daily living skills; statistically significant differences in pre- and post-training ICF-CY scores.	Short-term follow-up (6 months) showed sustained improvements; no data on long-term generalization beyond training period; future studies to explore extended intervention and broader sample sizes.	Italy
[94]	Mixed-Methods Design	Phase 1: 40 adults (20 with ASD, 20 without ASD); Phase 2: 10 adults with ASD presenting CB; Phase 3: 1 adult with ASD exhibiting CB	Development and validation of smart wearable shirt (SWS) for real-time prediction of challenging behaviors (CBs)	Smart wearable shirt (Hexoskin SWS)	Physiological parameters (HR, HRV, respiratory rate), behavioral diary	Higher stress levels anticipated in adults with ASD when exposed to stressors. The system was expected to predict CBs with high accuracy using physiological parameters. Higher stress levels were detected in adults with ASD compared to typically developed peers. The system was anticipated to predict CBs with an AUC value above 0.70.	Very small sample size for proof-of-concept phase (1 participant); limited generalizability due to lab-based controlled settings; lack of validated stimuli to elicit consistent stress responses; short duration of study phases (7 days for Phase 2 and proof-of-concept); and the technology's reliance on stable Bluetooth and internet connections may not suit all environments.	Effect size for prediction accuracy not explicitly calculated; expected AUC > 0.70 (fair sensitivity) for predicting challenging behaviors using machine learning models.	No longitudinal effects were assessed; the study focused on short-term proof-of-concept outcomes and immediate data-driven predictions of challenging behaviors.	Israel

Table 2. *Cont.*

Name	Type of Study	Subjects (Age, Gender, Diagnosis)	Intervention	Type of Technology	Measure	Results	Limitations	Effect Sizes	Longitudinal Effects	Country
[81]	Experimental Study	5 male children, aged 7–10 years, diagnosed with ASD	Use of wearable sensors to monitor physiological and kinetic data during interactions	Wearable sensors (Empatica E4), social robots (Nao, PARP)	Heart rate, HRV (RMSSD), acceleration, electrodermal activity, temperature, blood volume pulse	The XGBoost algorithm achieved the best performance, with 99% accuracy in detecting challenging behaviors. Heart rate was the main contributing feature. RMSSD correlated with challenging behaviors. Heart rate (HR) was the most significant feature for detecting challenging behaviors. Physiological features outperformed kinetic features in prediction accuracy.	Very small sample size (5 male children); limited generalizability due to controlled lab environment; manual annotation of challenging behaviors introduces potential human error; no consideration of gender differences; limited long-term data; and reliance on a single wearable sensor, which might miss multi-modal behavioral cues.	High accuracy (99%) was achieved using the XGBoost algorithm for predicting challenging behaviors based on physiological data; effect size was not explicitly reported, but high-performance metrics indicate strong model reliability.	No longitudinal effects were assessed; the study focused on immediate data-driven predictions without long-term monitoring or evaluations.	Qatar
[71]	Combined 3 (intervention) × 3 (diagnosis) × 3 (time) research design with repeated measures	201 families (parents and children), children aged 6–12 years (neurotypical, ADHD, ASD)	Serious game (Kairos) and parental support	Serious game (Kairos) on electronic tablets	Routine Achievement Assessment Tool	For ADHD participants, a significant clinical effect was observed for parental support and a combina- tion of Serious Game and parental support. For ASD children, an effect was observed for a combination of Serious Game and parental support. For neurotypical children, a significant effect was observed for Serious Game alone. Serious Game can improve children's routines. For ADHD and ASD children, adding parental support produces greater clinical improvements.	Significant COVID-19-related methodological adjustments (e.g., allowing parents to choose routines, inconsistent study conditions); lack of standardization in parental support implementation; sample attrition due to pandemic (10%); and variability in reported results due to differences in routines chosen by parents.	For autistic children, significant improvements in routine achievement when using combined intervention (Serious Game and parental support): huge clinical effect (Cohen's d = 2.81) over 8 weeks. For ADHD children, parental support alone yielded a large clinical effect (Cohen's d > 1.2) in the first 4 weeks.	Moderate persistence of effects in neurotypical children but decline observed in ADHD and ASD groups after initial improvement. No formal follow-up data to assess longer-term	Canada

Table 2. *Cont.*

Name	Type of Study	Subjects (Age, Gender, Diagnosis)	Intervention	Type of Technology	Measure	Results	Limitations	Effect Sizes	Longitudinal Effects	Country
[79]	Feasibility Study	8 families, 8 autistic boys (mean age: 9.92 years), caregivers (mean age: 44.5 years)	Self-report stress logging and physiological signal measurement using a mobile app and wearable sensors	Mobile app (EasyConnect) and wearable physiological sensors (Empatica E4)	Self-reports, PPG, and EDA signals	Caregivers and children were able to use the mobile app and sensors effectively to report and measure stress in daily life. Stress indicators from EDA were aligned with self-reports.	Small sample size (8 families); Some families did not use the app despite training; wearable device discomfort, particularly for autistic children; limited options in the stress-reporting questionnaire; external validity concerns due to natural settings.	Medium and large effect sizes were observed in EDA SCR features; higher and wider SCR peaks were found in both autistic children and caregivers during stress-reporting periods; Cohen's d values for stress detection in caregivers were notably high (up to 2.67).	Limited due to the short study duration; no extended follow-up was conducted; future research aims to recruit more families and expand data collection for longitudinal analysis.	USA
[97]	Comparative Survey Study	129 children (53 autistic, 76 neurotypical) aged 3–16 years	Use of fidget toys and fidget spinners	Fidget toys and fidget spinners	Parental survey, Sensory Profile Questionnaire 2 (SPQ 2)	Parents of autistic children perceived fidget toys and spinners as more beneficial compared to NT parents. Higher sensory-seeking scores were associated with greater perceived benefits and reduced anxiety. Autistic children with higher sensory-seeking scores were seen to benefit more from fidget toys in terms of reduced anxiety and increased concentration. NT children with higher sensory-seeking scores also showed similar benefits.	Limited generalizability due to parent-reported data; cultural biases in sensory perception and educational environments; inconsistent frequency and type of fidget toy use between autistic and NT children; small sample sizes for certain subgroup analyses; absence of longitudinal data on sustained outcomes; and potential biases influenced by school policies or media portrayals.	Significant group differences in perceived benefits of fidget toys for anxiety reduction and concentration improvement: χ^2 (4) = 17.478, $p = 0.002$ and χ^2 (4) = 16.148, $p = 0.003$, respectively.	No longitudinal effects were assessed; the study focused on cross-sectional parental perceptions without follow-up data.	UK

According to emerging technologies, many of the studies showcased promising results but also presented several limitations due to technical issues, user discomfort, device limitations, as well as data accuracy. More specifically, wearable sensors, VR interventions, and smart wearable shirts presented discomfort [66,79], difficulty with wearing the equipment [72], as well as technical inconsistencies like Bluetooth and internet connectivity, affecting real-time data collection. Furthermore, data accuracy and algorithm issues were other factors limiting the results, apart from succeeding in high-accuracy levels in stress prediction (up to 99%). Regarding [80,81], their studies were performed only in control lab settings. Ref. [93] also presented findings that made it unclear how biometric stress markers were presented in various sessions. Furthermore, another phenomenon observed in many studies was the overreliance on male subjects, showcasing results that cannot be interpreted without creating gender imbalance issues. Ref. [77] included $n = 75$ boys and only $n = 8$ girls in their samples, making it unclear whether auditory interventions have the same effects across genders. Meanwhile, ref. [66] presented similar findings between experimental groups regarding IQ and gender. No follow-up measurements were also another factor, thus limiting the sustainability of the intervention effects. Most of the studies only measured outcomes immediately post-intervention without measuring the long-term effects [66,71,72,88].

6. Conclusions

Although the findings of this present study are quite encouraging for the application of these technologies in the daily lives of individuals, several limitations were identified that hinder the reliability, validity, and generalizability of the results. Moreover, high diversity was identified concerning the samples tested. ASD, as it is known, presents a wide range, and the samples tested showed high heterogeneity (ranging from low, average, and high functionality, as well as different sensory processing profiles of stimuli), making it difficult to generalize the results.

Regarding the use of these aids in settings such as schools and communities, issues concerning the acceptance and appropriate training of a teacher, therapist, as well as the community itself must be ensured. Cost is another factor that should be considered and is not mentioned in most of the included studies. Also, the majority of the technological tools used in these studies (especially those that are high-tech tools) are not accessible nor available to the general public, assuming that not every socio-economic group can afford to purchase them because they are not provided by the state. Furthermore, the majority of the reported technological devices require specialization and considerable time in training caregivers and users themselves to become familiar with their use. Regarding the methodological elements of the included studies, several limitations were identified regarding the small sample size, which may lead to a type two methodological error, where real effects are not detected, thus preventing the generalizability of the results to the wider population. In addition, most of the studies did not include a control sample and were short in duration (from a few weeks to months), hindering access to long-term changes and making the task of creating specific forms of intervention more difficult. Also, shortcomings were identified in terms of reviewing the data to be able to see if the benefits observed are long-lasting. Finally, an emerging field on gut–microbiome interactions was not identified in any type of study related to the use of any type of technology yet.

Based on the findings of this study, the following observations are noted for future research to improve the methodological factors and to create universal intervention plans in the physical environments of people with ASD experiencing stress.

Initially, the long-term impact of the changes observed from the use of these technologies should be studied. To this end, it is imperative to use experimental models that examine their use over time. In addition, emphasis should be placed on personalizing the needs of each individual. Personalization seems to have a positive effect on the results of the interventions. Also, research should delve into how to build these technologies so that they are more user-friendly. Finally, adequate training should be provided to the user and the person's carers to ensure maximum results.

Author Contributions: Conceptualization, P.P.; methodology, P.P.; software, P.P. and V.B.; validation, P.P., V.B., A.D. (Aikaterini Doulou), A.I.C., C.S., N.B. and A.D. (Athanasios Drigas); formal analysis, P.P.; investigation, P.P.; resources, P.P.; data curation, P.P., V.B., A.D. (Aikaterini Doulou), A.I.C., C.S., N.B. and A.D. (Athanasios Drigas); writing—original draft preparation, P.P.; writing—review and editing, P.P., V.B., A.D. (Aikaterini Doulou), A.I.C., C.S., N.B. and A.D. (Athanasios Drigas); visualization, P.P.; supervision, C.S., N.B. and A.D. (Athanasios Drigas); project administration, P.P. and A.D. (Athanasios Drigas); funding acquisition, A.D. (Athanasios Drigas). All authors have read and agreed to the published version of the manuscript.

Funding: This research received no external funding.

Conflicts of Interest: The authors declare no conflicts of interest.

References

1. Thomaidis, L.; Mavroeidi, N.; Richardson, C.; Choleva, A.; Damianos, G.; Bolias, K.; Tsolia, M. Autism Spectrum Disorders in Greece: Nationwide Prevalence in 10–11 Year-Old Children and Regional Disparities. *J. Clin. Med.* **2020**, *9*, 2163. [CrossRef] [PubMed]
2. Qin, L.; Wang, H.; Ning, W.; Cui, M.; Wang, Q. New advances in the diagnosis and treatment of autism spectrum disorders. *Eur. J. Med. Res.* **2024**, *29*, 322. [CrossRef] [PubMed]
3. Okoye, C.; Obialo-Ibeawuchi, C.M.; Obajeun, O.A.; Sarwar, S.; Tawfik, C.; Waleed, M.S.; Wasim, A.U.; Mohamoud, I.; Afolayan, A.Y.; Mbaezue, R.N. Early diagnosis of Autism Spectrum Disorder: A review and analysis of the risks and benefits. *Cureus* **2023**, *15*, e43226. [CrossRef] [PubMed]
4. Lord, C.; Brugha, T.S.; Charman, T.; Cusack, J.C.; Dumas, G.; Frazier, T.W.; Jones, E.; Jones, R.; Pickles, A.; State, M.W.; et al. Autism spectrum disorder. *Nat. Rev. Dis. Primers* **2020**, *6*, 1–23. [CrossRef]
5. Hollocks, M.J.; Lerh, J.W.; Magiati, I.; Meiser-Stedman, R.; Brugha, T.S. Anxiety and depression in adults with autism spectrum disorder: A systematic review and meta-analysis. *Psychol. Med.* **2019**, *49*, 559–572. [CrossRef]
6. Hodges, H.; Fealko, C.; Soares, N. Autism spectrum disorder: Definition, epidemiology, causes, and clinical evaluation. *J. Clin. Med.* **2020**, *9* (Suppl. S1), S55–S65. [CrossRef]
7. Grzadzinski, R.; Huerta, M.; Lord, C. DSM-5 and autism spectrum disorders (ASDs): An opportunity for identifying ASD subtypes. *Mol. Autism* **2013**, *4*, 12. [CrossRef]
8. Johnson, C.P.; Myers, S.M. Identification and evaluation of children with autism spectrum disorders. *Pediatrics* **2007**, *120*, 1183–1215. [CrossRef]
9. Van 't Hof, M.; Tisseur, C.; van Berckelear-Onnes, I.; van Nieuwenhuyzen, A.; Daniels, A.M.; Deen, M.; Hoek, H.W.; Ester, W.A. Age at autism spectrum disorder diagnosis: A systematic review and meta-analysis from 2012 to 2019. *Autism* **2020**, *25*, 862–873. [CrossRef]
10. Miller, L.J.; Anzalone, M.E.; Lane, S.J.; Cermak, S.A.; Osten, E.T. Concept Evolution in Sensory Integration: A Proposed Nosology for Diagnosis. *Am. J. Occup. Ther.* **2007**, *61*, 135–140. [CrossRef]
11. *Diagnostic and Statistical Manual of Mental Disorders*; American Psychiatric Association: Washington, DC, USA, 2013.
12. Christensen, J.; Wild, H.; Kenzie, E.S.; Wakeland, W.W.; Budding, D.; Lillas, C. Diverse Autonomic Nervous System Stress Response Patterns in Childhood Sensory Modulation. Frontiers in Integrative. *Front. Integr. Neurosci.* **2020**, *14*, 6. [CrossRef] [PubMed]
13. Bar-Shalita, T.; Vatine, J.J.; Parush, S. Sensory modulation disorder: A risk factor for participation in daily life activities. *Dev. Med. Child Neurol.* **2008**, *50*, 932–937. [CrossRef] [PubMed]
14. Schoen, S.A. Physiological and behavioral differences in sensory processing: A comparison of children with Autism Spectrum Disorder and Sensory Processing Disorder. *Front. Integr. Neurosci.* **2009**, *3*, 29. [CrossRef] [PubMed]

15. Sayers, J.V. The World Health Report 2001—Mental Health: New Understanding, New Hope. *Bull. World Health Organ.* **2001**, *79*, 1085.
16. Fernández-Batanero, J.M.; Montenegro-Rueda, M.; Fernández-Cerero, J. Access and Participation of Students with Disabilities: The Challenge for Higher Education. *Int. J. Environ. Res. Public Health* **2022**, *19*, 11918. [CrossRef]
17. Mcculloch, G. Documentary research. In *Routledge eBooks*; CRC Press: Boca Raton, FL, USA, 2004. [CrossRef]
18. Cook, A.M.; Hussey, S.M. *Assistive Technologies: Principles and Practice*; Mosby: St. Louis, MO, USA, 1995.
19. Cañete, R.; Peralta, M.E. ASDesign: A User-Centered Method for the Design of Assistive Technology That Helps Children with Autism Spectrum Disorders Be More Independent in Their Daily Routines. *Sustainability* **2022**, *14*, 516. [CrossRef]
20. Boon, W.; Moors, E. Exploring emerging technologies using metaphors—A study of orphan drugs and pharmacogenomics. *Soc. Sci. Med.* **2008**, *66*, 1915–1927. [CrossRef]
21. Stahl, B.C. What does the future hold? A critical view of emerging information and communication technologies and their social consequences. In *IFIP Advances in Information and Communication Technology*; Springer: Berlin/Heidelberg, Germany, 2011; pp. 59–76. [CrossRef]
22. Rotolo, D.; Hicks, D.; Martin, B.R. What is an emerging technology? *Res. Policy* **2015**, *44*, 1827–1843. [CrossRef]
23. Hostinar, C.E.; Johnson, A.E.; Gunnar, M.R. Parent Support Is Less Effective in Buffering Cortisol Stress Reactivity for Adolescents Compared to Children. *Dev. Sci.* **2015**, *18*, 281–297. [CrossRef]
24. Drigas, A.; Mitsea, E. Metacognition, Stress–Relaxation Balance & Related Hormones. *Int. J. Recent Contrib. Eng. Sci. IT* **2021**, *9*, 4. [CrossRef]
25. Bravou, V.; Driga, A.M.S.; Drigas, A. Emotion Regulation, the Function of Stress Hormones & Digital Technologies. *Tech. BioChemMed* **2022**, *3*, 27–33. [CrossRef]
26. McEwen, B.S. Neurobiological and Systemic Effects of Chronic Stress. *Chronic Stress* **2017**, *1*, 247054701769232. [CrossRef] [PubMed]
27. Makris, G.; Eleftheriades, A.; Pervanidou, P. Early Life Stress, Hormones, and Neurodevelopmental Disorders. *Horm. Res. Paediatr.* **2023**, *96*, 17–24. [CrossRef] [PubMed]
28. Cryan, J.F.; O'Mahony, S.M. The microbiome-gut-brain axis: From bowel to behavior. *Neurogastroenterol. Motil.* **2011**, *23*, 187–192. [CrossRef]
29. Chen, X.; D'Souza, R.; Hong, S. The role of gut microbiota in the gut-brain axis: Current challenges and perspectives. *Protein Cell* **2013**, *4*, 403–414. [CrossRef]
30. Mayer, E.A. Gut Feelings: The Emerging Biology of Gut–Brain Communication. *Nat. Rev. Neurosci.* **2011**, *12*, 453–466. [CrossRef]
31. Foster, J.A.; Rinaman, L.; Cryan, J.F. Stress & the gut-brain axis: Regulation by the microbiome. *Neurobiol. Stress* **2017**, *7*, 124–136. [CrossRef]
32. Stilling, R.M.; Ryan, F.J.; Hoban, A.E.; Shanahan, F.; Clarke, G.; Claesson, M.J.; Dinan, T.G.; Cryan, J.F. Microbes & Neurodevelopment—Absence of Microbiota during Early Life Increases Activity-Related Transcriptional Pathways in the Amygdala. *Brain Behav. Immun.* **2015**, *50*, 209–220. [CrossRef]
33. Puricelli, C.; Rolla, R.; Gigliotti, C.L.; Boggio, E.; Beltrami, E.; Dianzani, U.; Keller, R. The Gut-Brain-Immune axis in Autism Spectrum Disorders: A State-of-Art Report. *Front. Psychiatry* **2022**, *12*, 755171. [CrossRef]
34. Bamicha, V.; Pergantis, P.; Drigas, A. The Effect of Gut Microbiome, Neurotransmitters, and Digital Insights in Autism. *Appl. Microbiol.* **2024**, *4*, 1677–1701. [CrossRef]
35. Banqueri, M.; Méndez, M.; Arias, J. Impact of Stress in Childhood: Psychobiological Alterations. *Psicothema* **2017**, *1*, 18–22. [CrossRef]
36. Seckfort, D.L.; Paul, R.; Grieve, S.M.; Vandenberg, B.; Bryant, R.A.; Williams, L.M.; Clark, C.R.; Cohen, R.A.; Bruce, S.; Gordon, E. Early life stress on brain structure and function across the lifespan: A preliminary study. *Brain Imaging Behav.* **2008**, *2*, 49–58. [CrossRef]
37. Frodl, T.; O'Keane, V. How does the brain deal with cumulative stress? A review with focus on developmental stress, HPA axis function and hippocampal structure in humans. *Neurobiol. Dis.* **2013**, *52*, 24–37. [CrossRef] [PubMed]
38. Hanson, J.L.; Chung, M.K.; Avants, B.B.; Rudolph, K.D.; Shirtcliff, E.A.; Gee, J.C.; Davidson, R.J.; Pollak, S.D. Structural Variations in Prefrontal Cortex Mediate the Relationship between Early Childhood Stress and Spatial Working Memory. *J. Neurosci.* **2012**, *32*, 7917–7925. [CrossRef]
39. Niehaus, C.E.; Chaplin, T.M.; Goncalves, S.F.; Semelsberger, R.; Thompson, J.C. Maternal stress and adolescent brain structure and function. *Brain Behav.* **2019**, *9*, e01311. [CrossRef]
40. Milani, A.C.C.; Hoffmann, E.V.; Fossaluza, V.; Jackowski, A.P.; Mello, M.F. Does pediatric post-traumatic stress disorder alter the brain? Systematic review and meta-analysis of structural and functional magnetic resonance imaging studies. *Psychiatry Clin. Neurosci.* **2017**, *71*, 154–169. [CrossRef]

41. Heyn, S.A.; Keding, T.J.; Ross, M.C.; Cisler, J.M.; Mumford, J.A.; Herringa, R.J. Abnormal prefrontal development in Pediatric posttraumatic stress Disorder: A Longitudinal structural and functional magnetic resonance Imaging study. *Biol. Psychiatry Cogn. Neurosci. Neuroimaging* **2019**, *4*, 171–179. [CrossRef]
42. Fernández-Andrés, M.I.; Pastor-Cerezuela, G.; Sanz-Cervera, P.; Tárraga-Mínguez, R. A Comparative Study of Sensory Processing in Children with and without Autism Spectrum Disorder in the Home and Classroom Environments. *Res. Dev. Disabil.* **2015**, *38*, 202–212. [CrossRef]
43. Chistol, L.T.; Bandini, L.G.; Must, A.; Phillips, S.; Cermak, S.A.; Curtin, C. Sensory Sensitivity and Food Selectivity in Children with Autism Spectrum Disorder. *J. Autism Dev. Disord.* **2018**, *48*, 583–591. [CrossRef]
44. Kojovic, N.; Ben Hadid, L.; Franchini, M.; Schaer, M. Sensory Processing Issues and Their Association with Social Difficulties in Children with Autism Spectrum Disorders. *J. Clin. Med.* **2019**, *8*, 1508. [CrossRef]
45. Loh, S.Y.; Ee, S.I.; Marret, M.J. Sensory processing and its relationship to participation among childhood occupations in children with autism spectrum disorder: Exploring the profile of differences. *Int. J. Dev. Disabil.* **2021**, *69*, 226–237. [CrossRef] [PubMed]
46. Narzisi, A.; Fabbri-Destro, M.; Crifaci, G.; Scatigna, S.; Maugeri, F.; Berloffa, S.; Fantozzi, P.; Prato, A.; Muccio, R.; Valente, E.; et al. Sensory Profiles in School-Aged Children with Autism Spectrum Disorder: A Descriptive Study Using the Sensory Processing Measure-2 (SPM-2). *J. Clin. Med.* **2022**, *11*, 1668. [CrossRef] [PubMed]
47. Crosswell, A.D.; Lockwood, K.G. Best practices for stress measurement: How to measure psychological stress in health research. *Health Psychol. Open* **2020**, *7*, 205510292093307. [CrossRef] [PubMed]
48. Cohen, S.; Gianaros, P.J.; Manuck, S.B. A stage model of stress and disease. *Perspect. Psychol. Sci.* **2016**, *11*, 456–463. [CrossRef]
49. Bravou, V.; Oikonomidou, D.; Drigas, A. Applications of Virtual Reality for Autism Inclusion. A Review. *Retos* **2022**, *45*, 779–785. [CrossRef]
50. Pergantis, P.; Drigas, A. Assistive Technology for Autism Spectrum Disorder Children That Experiences Stress and Anxiety. *Braz. J. Sci.* **2023**, *2*, 77–93. [CrossRef]
51. Moraiti, I.; Drigas, A. Measuring the stress of autistic people with the help of a smartwatch, Internet of Things Technology. *Braz. J. Sci.* **2024**, *3*, 45–56. [CrossRef]
52. Moraiti, I. Examining the stress level of autistic people using a smartwatch integrated with the internet of things technology. *World J. Adv. Res. Rev.* **2023**, *19*, 1372–1389. [CrossRef]
53. Tomczak, M.T. Employees with Autism Spectrum Disorders in the Digitized Work Environment: Perspectives for the Future. *J. Disabil. Policy Stud.* **2021**, *31*, 195–205. [CrossRef]
54. Spratt, E.G.; Nicholas, J.S.; Brady, K.T.; Carpenter, L.A.; Hatcher, C.R.; Meekins, K.A.; Furlanetto, R.W.; Charles, J.M. Enhanced cortisol response to stress in children in autism. *J. Autism Dev. Disord.* **2011**, *42*, 75–81. [CrossRef]
55. Levine, T.P.; Sheinkopf, S.J.; Pescosolido, M.; Rodino, A.; Elia, G.; Lester, B. Physiologic Arousal to Social Stress in Children with Autism Spectrum Disorders: A Pilot Study. *Res. Autism Spectr. Disord.* **2011**, *6*, 177–183. [CrossRef]
56. Kushki, A.; Drumm, E.; Mobarak, M.P.; Tanel, N.; Dupuis, A.; Chau, T.; Anagnostou, E. Investigating the Autonomic Nervous System Response to Anxiety in Children with Autism Spectrum Disorders. *PLoS ONE* **2013**, *8*, e59730. [CrossRef]
57. Stein, L.I.; Lane, C.J.; Williams, M.E.; Dawson, M.E.; Polido, J.C.; Cermak, S.A. Physiological and Behavioral Stress and Anxiety in Children with Autism Spectrum Disorders during Routine Oral Care. *BioMed Res. Int.* **2014**, *2014*, 694876. [CrossRef] [PubMed]
58. Burke, A. Zen shiatsu: A longitudinal case study measuring stress reduction in a child with autism spectrum disorder. *Int. J. Ther. Massage Bodyw.* **2014**, *7*, 23–28. [PubMed] [PubMed Central]
59. Varni, J.W.; Seid, M.; Kurtin, P.S. PEDSQLTM 4.0: Reliability and Validity of the Pediatric Quality of Life InventoryTM Version 4.0 Generic core scales in healthy and patient populations. *Med. Care* **2001**, *39*, 800–812. [CrossRef]
60. Corbett, B.A.; Muscatello, R.A.; Baldinger, C. Comparing stress and arousal systems in response to different social contexts in children with ASD. *Biol. Psychol.* **2019**, *140*, 119–130. [CrossRef]
61. Bloeming-Wolbrink, K.A.; Janssen, M.J.; de Weerth, C.; Ruijssenaars, W.A.; Sweep, F.C.; Eijsbouts, A.; Schuengel, C. Stress in Adults with Congenital Deafblindness and an Intellectual Disability: Information from Their Cortisol Curves. *Br. J. Vis. Impair.* **2012**, *30*, 149–159. [CrossRef]
62. Thoen, A.; Steyaert, J.; Alaerts, K.; Evers, K.; Van Damme, T. A Systematic Review of Self-Reported Stress Questionnaires in People on the Autism Spectrum. *Rev. J. Autism Dev. Disord.* **2021**, *10*, 295–318. [CrossRef]
63. Groden, J.; Diller, A.; Bausman, M.; Velicer, W.; Norman, G.; Cautela, J. The Development of a Stress Survey Schedule for Persons with Autism and Other Developmental Disabilities. *J. Autism Dev. Disord.* **2001**, *31*, 207–217. [CrossRef]
64. Chiu, H.T.; Ip, I.N.; Ching, F.N.Y.; Wong, B.P.-H.; Lui, W.-H.; Tse, C.-S.; Wong, S.W.H. Resting Heart Rate Variability and Emotion Dysregulation in Adolescents with Autism Spectrum Disorder. *J. Autism Dev. Disord.* **2023**, *54*, 1482–1493. [CrossRef]

65. Ip, H.H.; Wong, S.W.; Chan, D.F.; Byrne, J.; Li, C.; Yuan, V.S.; Lau, K.S.; Wong, J.Y. Enhance emotional and social adaptation skills for children with autism spectrum disorder: A virtual reality enabled approach. *Comput. Educ. Comput. Educ.* **2018**, *117*, 1–15. [CrossRef]
66. Nguyen, J.; Cardy, R.E.; Anagnostou, E.; Brian, J.; Kushki, A. Examining the effect of a wearable, anxiety detection technology on improving the awareness of anxiety signs in autism spectrum disorder: A pilot randomized controlled trial. *Mol. Autism* **2021**, *12*, 72. [CrossRef] [PubMed]
67. Fridenson-Hayo, S.; Berggren, S.; Lassalle, A.; Tal, S.; Pigat, D.; Meir-Goren, N.; O'Reilly, H.; Ben-Zur, S.; Bölte, S.; Baron-Cohen, S.; et al. 'Emotiplay': A serious game for learning about emotions in children with autism: Results of a cross-cultural evaluation. *Eur. Child Adolesc. Psychiatry* **2017**, *26*, 979–992. [CrossRef] [PubMed]
68. Rachmani, M.; Rizal, M.F.; Sutadi, H.; Suharsini, M. Comparison of Two Visual Techniques in Decreasing Stress Levels in Children with Autism Spectrum Disorder. *J. Int. Dent. Med. Res.* **2020**, *13*, 1136–1139.
69. Tamany, I.; Rizal, M.F.; Suharsini, M. Comparison of the Effectiveness of Two Intervention Methods in Reducing Stress Levels in Children with Autism. *J. Int. Dent. Med. Res.* **2020**, *13*, 1117–1120.
70. Johnston, D.; Egermann, H.; Kearney, G. SoundFields: A Virtual Reality Game Designed to Address Auditory Hypersensitivity in Individuals with Autism Spectrum Disorder. *Appl. Sci.* **2020**, *10*, 2996. [CrossRef]
71. Lussier-Desrochers, D.; Massé, L.; Simonato, I.; Lachapelle, Y.; Godin-Tremblay, V.; Lemieux, A. Evaluation of the effect of a serious game on the performance of daily routines by autistic and ADHD children. *Adv. Neurodev. Disord.* **2023**, *7*, 566–578. [CrossRef]
72. Yuan, S.N.V.; Ip, H.H.S. Using virtual reality to train emotional and social skills in children with autism spectrum disorder. *Lond. J. Prim. Care* **2018**, *10*, 110–112. [CrossRef]
73. Vallefuoco, E.; Bravaccio, C.; Gison, G.; Pecchia, L.; Pepino, A. Personalized Training via Serious Game to Improve Daily Living Skills in Pediatric Patients with Autism Spectrum Disorder. *IEEE J. Biomed. Health Inform.* **2022**, *26*, 3312–3321. [CrossRef]
74. Baric, V.B.; Skuthälla, S.; Pettersson, M.; Gustafsson, P.A.; Kjellberg, A. The effectiveness of weighted blankets on sleep and everyday activities—A retrospective follow-up study of children and adults with attention deficit hyperactivity disorder and/or autism spectrum disorder. *Scand. J. Occup. Ther.* **2021**, *30*, 1357–1367. [CrossRef]
75. Pfeiffer, B.; Duker, L.S.; Murphy, A.; Shui, C. Effectiveness of Noise-Attenuating headphones on physiological responses for children with autism spectrum disorders. *Front. Integr. Neurosci.* **2019**, *13*, 65. [CrossRef]
76. Mah, J.W.T.; Tsang, P. Visual Schedule System in Dental Care for Patients with Autism: A Pilot Study. *J. Clin. Pediatr. Dent.* **2016**, *40*, 393–399. [CrossRef] [PubMed]
77. Kwong, T.C.; Yuan, H.-L.; Mung, S.W.Y.; Chu, H.K.H.; Chan, C.C.H.; Lun, D.P.K.; Yu, H.M.; Cheng, L.; Choy, Y.S. Healthcare headset with tuneable auditory characteristics control for children with Autism spectrum disorder. *Appl. Acoust.* **2024**, *218*, 109876. [CrossRef]
78. Jouen, A.-L.; Narzisi, A.; Xavier, J.; Tilmont, E.; Bodeau, N.; Bono, V.; Ketem-Premel, N.; Anzalone, S.; Maharatna, K.; Chetouani, M.; et al. GOLIAH (Gaming Open Library for Intervention in Autism at Home): A 6-Month Single Blind Matched Controlled Exploratory Study. *Child Adolesc. Psychiatry Ment. Health* **2017**, *11*, 17. [CrossRef]
79. Yu, Z.; Sherpa, M.T.; Iadarola, S.; Shamlian, K.; Daley, S.; Levine, G.; Bajorski, P.; Zheng, Z. Understanding Stress in Children with ASD and Their Caregivers in Daily Life: A Feasibility Study Using Mobile Devices. In Proceedings of the MobileHCI '23 Companion: 25th International Conference on Mobile Human-Computer Interaction, Athens, Greece, 26–29 September 2023. [CrossRef]
80. Masino, A.J.; Forsyth, D.; Nuske, H.; Herrington, J.; Pennington, J.; Kushleyeva, Y.; Bonafide, C.P. m-Health and Autism: Recognizing Stress and Anxiety with Machine Learning and Wearables Data. In Proceedings of the 2019 IEEE 32nd International Symposium on Computer-Based Medical Systems (CBMS), Cordoba, Spain, 5–7 June 2019; pp. 714–719. [CrossRef]
81. Alban, A.Q.; Alhaddad, A.Y.; Al-Ali, A.; So, W.; Connor, O.; Ayesh, M.; Qidwai, U.A.; Cabibihan, J. Heart Rate as a Predictor of Challenging Behaviours among Children with Autism from Wearable Sensors in Social Robot Interactions. *Robotics* **2023**, *12*, 55. [CrossRef]
82. Afif, I.Y.; Farkhan, M.; Kurdi, O.; Maula, M.I.; Ammarullah, M.I.; Setiyana, B.; Jamari, J.; Winarni, T.I. Effect of Short-Term Deep-Pressure Portable Seat on Behavioral and Biological Stress in Children with Autism Spectrum Disorders: A Pilot Study. *Bioengineering* **2022**, *9*, 48. [CrossRef]
83. Carlier, S.; Van Der Paelt, S.; Ongenae, F.; De Backere, F.; De Turck, F. Empowering Children with ASD and Their Parents: Design of a Serious Game for Anxiety and Stress Reduction. *Sensors* **2020**, *20*, 966. [CrossRef]
84. Nakadoi, Y. Usefulness of Animal Type Robot Assisted Therapy for Autism Spectrum Disorder in the Child and Adolescent Psychiatric Ward. In *Lecture Notes in Computer Science*; Springer Science+Business Media: Berlin/Heidelberg, Germany, 2015; pp. 478–482. [CrossRef]

85. Gee, B.M.; Lloyd, K.; Sutton, J.; McOmber, T. Weighted Blankets and Sleep Quality in Children with Autism Spectrum Disorders: A Single-Subject Design. *Children* **2020**, *8*, 10. [CrossRef]
86. Bharatharaj, J.; Huang, L.; Mohan, R.E.; Al-Jumaily, A.; Krägeloh, C. Robot-Assisted Therapy for Learning and Social Interaction of Children with Autism Spectrum Disorder. *Robotics* **2017**, *6*, 4. [CrossRef]
87. Zimmerman, K.N.; Ledford, J.R.; Severini, K.E. Brief Report: The effects of a weighted blanket on engagement for a student with ASD. *Focus Autism Other Dev. Disabil.* **2018**, *34*, 15–19. [CrossRef]
88. Macdonald, L.; Trembath, D.; Ashburner, J.; Costley, D.; Keen, D. The use of visual schedules and work systems to increase the on-task behaviour of students on the autism spectrum in mainstream classrooms. *J. Res. Spec. Educ. Needs* **2018**, *18*, 254–266. [CrossRef]
89. Alban, A.Q.; Ayesh, M.; Alhaddad, A.Y.; Al-Ali, A.K.; So, W.C.; Connor, O.; Cabibihan, J. Detection of Challenging Behaviours of Children with Autism Using Wearable Sensors during Interactions with Social Robots. In Proceedings of the 2021 30th IEEE International Conference on Robot & Human Interactive Communication (RO-MAN), Vancouver, BC, Canada, 8–12 August 2021. [CrossRef]
90. Keshav, N.U.; Vahabzadeh, A.; Abdus-Sabur, R.; Huey, K.; Salisbury, J.; Liu, R.; Sahin, N.T. Longitudinal Socio-Emotional Learning Intervention for Autism via Smartglasses: Qualitative School Teacher Descriptions of Practicality, Usability, and Efficacy in General and Special Education Classroom Settings. *Educ. Sci.* **2018**, *8*, 107. [CrossRef]
91. Cabibihan, J.; Chellali, R.; So CW, C.; Aldosari, M.; Connor, O.; Alhaddad, A.Y.; Javed, H. Social robots and wearable sensors for mitigating meltdowns in autism—A pilot test. In *Lecture Notes in Computer Science*; Springer: Berlin/Heidelberg, Germany, 2018; pp. 103–114. [CrossRef]
92. Huijnen, C.A.G.J.; Verreussel-Willen, H.A.M.D.; Lexis, M.A.S.; De Witte, L.P. Robot KASPAR as Mediator in Making Contact with Children with Autism: A Pilot Study. *Int. J. Soc. Robot.* **2021**, *13*, 237–249. [CrossRef]
93. Coskun, B.; Uluer, P.; Toprak, E.; Barkana, D.E.; Kose, H.; Zorcec, T.; Robins, B.; Landowska, A. Stress Detection of Children with Autism using Physiological Signals in Kaspar Robot-Based Intervention Studies. In Proceedings of the 2022 9th IEEE RAS/EMBS International Conference for Biomedical Robotics and Biomechatronics (BioRob), Seoul, Republic of Korea, 21–24 August 2022. [CrossRef]
94. Zwilling, M.; Romano, A.; Hoffman, H.; Lotan, M.; Tesler, R. Development and validation of a system for the prediction of challenging behaviors of people with autism spectrum disorder based on a smart wearable shirt: A mixed-methods design. *Front. Behav. Neurosci.* **2022**, *16*, 948184. [CrossRef]
95. Fioriello, F.; Maugeri, A.; D'Alvia, L.; Pittella, E.; Piuzzi, E.; Rizzuto, E.; Del Prete, Z.; Manti, F.; Sogos, C. A wearable heart rate measurement device for children with autism spectrum disorder. *Sci. Rep.* **2020**, *10*, 18659. [CrossRef]
96. Newbutt, N.; Bradley, R.; Conley, I. Using virtual reality head-mounted displays in schools with autistic children: Views, experiences, and future directions. *Cyberpsychology Behav. Soc. Netw.* **2020**, *23*, 23–33.
97. Roche, M.A.; Back, E.; Van Herwegen, J. Parental perspectives on the use of fidget toys and sensory-seeking profiles in autistic and neurotypical children. *Curr. Psychol.* **2023**, *43*, 15872–15882. [CrossRef]
98. Suresh, L.R.; George, C.A. Virtual Reality Distraction on Dental Anxiety and Behavior in Children with Autism Spectrum Disorder. *J. Int. Dent. Med. Res.* **2019**, *12*, 1004–1010.
99. Ikuta, N.; Iwanaga, R.; Tokunaga, A.; Nakane, H.; Tanaka, K.; Tanaka, G. Effectiveness of Earmuffs and Noise-cancelling Headphones for Coping with Hyper-reactivity to Auditory Stimuli in Children with Autism Spectrum Disorder: A Preliminary Study. *Hong Kong J. Occup. Ther.* **2016**, *28*, 24–32. [CrossRef]
100. Miller, I.T.; Wiederhold, B.K.; Miller, C.S.; Wiederhold, M.D. Virtual Reality Air Travel Training with Children on the Autism Spectrum: A Preliminary Report. *Cyberpsychology Behav. Soc. Netw.* **2020**, *23*, 10–15. [CrossRef]
101. Hirano, S.H.; Yeganyan, M.T.; Marcu, G.; Nguyen, D.H.; Boyd, L.A.; Hayes, G.R. vSked: Evaluation of a System to Support Classroom Activities for Children with Autism. In Proceedings of the SIGCHI Conference on Human Factors in Computing Systems, Atlanta, GA, USA, 10–15 April 2010; pp. 1633–1642. [CrossRef]
102. Pergantis, P.; Drigas, A. Sensory Integration Therapy as Enabler for Developing Emotional Intelligence in Children with Autism Spectrum Disorder and the ICT's Role. *Braz. J. Sci.* **2023**, *2*, 53–65. [CrossRef]
103. Milstein, N.; Gordon, I. Validating Measures of Electrodermal Activity and Heart Rate Variability Derived From the Empatica E4 Utilized in Research Settings That Involve Interactive Dyadic States. *Front. Behav. Neurosci.* **2020**, *14*, 148. [CrossRef] [PubMed]
104. Cavallo, F.; Brubaker, H.; Brown, T. Utilizing Individual Z-Scores to Measure Efficacy of the World's First Augmented Reality Glasses for Autism: A Single Case Study. *J. Soc. Sci. Res.* **2020**, *1*, 54–71.
105. Guemghar, I.; Pires de Oliveira Padilha, P.; Abdel-Baki, A.; Jutras-Aswad, D.; Paquette, J.; Pomey, M.-P. Social Robot Interventions in Mental Health Care and Their Outcomes, Barriers, and Facilitators: Scoping Review. *JMIR Ment. Health* **2022**, *9*, e36094. [CrossRef]

106. Rasouli, S.; Gupta, G.; Nilsen, E.; Dautenhahn, K. Potential Applications of Social Robots in Robot-Assisted Interventions for Social Anxiety. *Int. J. Soc. Robot.* **2022**, *14*, 1–32. [CrossRef]
107. Dautenhahn, K.; Nehaniv, C.L.; Walters, M.L.; Robins, B.; Kose-Bagci, H.; Mirza, N.A.; Blow, M. KASPAR—A Minimally Expressive Humanoid Robot for Human–Robot Interaction Research. *Appl. Bionics Biomech.* **2009**, *6*, 369–397. [CrossRef]
108. Aminuddin, R.; Sharkey, A.; Levita, L. Interaction with the Paro Robot May Reduce Psychophysiological Stress Responses. In Proceedings of the 11th ACM/IEEE International Conference on Human-Robot Interaction, Christchurch, New Zealand, 7–10 March 2016; pp. 593–594. [CrossRef]
109. Law, M.; Jarrett, P.; Simpson, M.C.; Holtkamp, H.U.; Giglio, C.; Broadbent, E. The Effects of Interacting with a Paro Robot After a Stressor in Patients with Psoriasis: A Randomised Pilot Study. *Front. Psychol.* **2022**, *13*, 871295. [CrossRef]
110. Doulou, A.; Pergantis, P.; Drigas, A.; Skianis, C. Managing ADHD Symptoms in Children Through the Use of Various Technology-Driven Serious Games: A Systematic Review. *Multimodal Technol. Interact.* **2025**, *9*, 8. [CrossRef]
111. Maskey, M.; Lowry, J.; Rodgers, J.; McConachie, H.; Parr, J.R. Reducing Specific Phobia/Fear in Young People with Autism Spectrum Disorders (ASDs) through a Virtual Reality Environment Intervention. *PLoS ONE* **2014**, *9*, e100374. [CrossRef]
112. Pergantis, P.; Bamicha, V.; Skianis, C.; Drigas, A. AI Chatbots and Cognitive Control: Enhancing Executive Functions Through Chatbot Interactions: A Systematic Review. *Brain Sci.* **2025**, *15*, 47. [CrossRef]

technologies

MDPI

Systematic Review

Indoor Environmental Monitoring and Chronic Respiratory Diseases: A Systematic Review

Patricia Camacho-Magriñán [1,2], Diego Sales-Lerida [1,2], Antonio León-Jiménez [2,3] and Daniel Sanchez-Morillo [1,2,*]

1. Department of Automation Engineering, Electronics and Computer Architecture and Networks, School of Engineering, University of Cadiz, 11519 Puerto Real, Cádiz, Spain; patricia.camachomagri@uca.es (P.C.-M.); diego.lerida@uca.es (D.S.-L.)
2. Instituto de Investigación e Innovación Biomédica de Cádiz (INiBICA), 11009 Cádiz, Spain
3. Pulmonology Department, Puerta del Mar University Hospital, 11009 Cádiz, Spain

* Correspondence: daniel.morillo@uca.es

Abstract: Chronic respiratory diseases (CRD), which include Chronic Obstructive Pulmonary Disease (COPD) and asthma, are significant global health issues, with air quality playing a vital role in exacerbating these conditions. This systematic review explores how monitoring indoor air quality (IAQ) can help manage and reduce respiratory exacerbations in CRD patients. A search of the Web of Science database, yielding 301 articles, was conducted following PRISMA guidelines. Of these, 60 met the inclusion criteria, and after screening, 21 articles were analyzed. The review identified substantial gaps in current research: the lack of standardization in IAQ monitoring; the need for considering geographic variability and for long-term longitudinal studies; and the importance of linking monitored air quality data with respiratory health indicators. It also stressed the importance of considering the heterogeneity of patients in the methodological study design, as well as the convenience of introducing recommendation systems to assess the true impact of corrective measures on indoor air quality in the homes of chronic respiratory patients. The integration of home-based IAQ monitoring with machine learning techniques to enhance our understanding of the relationship between IAQ and respiratory health is emerging as a key area for future research. Addressing all these challenges has the potential to mitigate the impact of CRD and improve the quality of life for patients.

Keywords: indoor air quality; COPD; asthma; machine learning; respiratory diseases; exacerbations

1. Introduction

Chronic respiratory diseases (CRD) pose significant global health challenges, affecting millions and contributing substantially to morbidity and mortality rates worldwide. According to the World Health Organization (WHO), CRD account for approximately 7% of all annual deaths globally, underscoring their critical impact on public health and the urgent need for effective management and prevention strategies [1].

CRD are a major category of non-communicable diseases, with Chronic Obstructive Pulmonary Disease (COPD) and asthma being among the most prevalent and possessing a higher economic burden [2,3]. COPD is characterized by persistent airflow limitation and is one of the leading causes of death, with a prevalence projection of 600 million cases worldwide by 2050 [4]. Asthma, a chronic inflammatory disease that affects the airways, affects over 300 million individuals worldwide and poses a severe overall burden on healthcare systems, due to its high prevalence among children and young adults and associated morbidity [5,6]. Both diseases significantly reduce patients' quality of life and impose a substantial economic burden due to frequent hospitalizations, medical visits, and loss of productivity.

Exacerbation, acute episodes of worsening respiratory symptoms, are critical events in CRD. COPD exacerbations account for most hospitalizations and are a leading cause of death among patients. Similarly, asthma exacerbations can lead to hospitalization and to a decline in lung function over time. Effective management and preventive strategies are crucial for reducing the frequency and severity of exacerbations, which can improve patient's quality of life and reduce the associated economic burden [7–10].

The prevalence of CRD has increased in recent years, with an estimated rise of approximately 40% over the past three decades, largely due to pollution [2]. Despite the significant burden that CRD poses, they have received less public attention and research funding compared to other diseases such as cardiovascular disease, cancer, stroke, diabetes, and Alzheimer's disease. This highlights the need for enhanced research and resource allocation.

A recent body of research highlights the influence of air quality on respiratory health. Epidemiological studies have consistently demonstrated the relationship between exposure to atmospheric pollutants and increased incidence and severity of respiratory diseases. In studying the triggers of exacerbations, some of which are well known, such as allergens or respiratory infections, causal relationships have been found with other factors, such as environmental pollutants [11]. Key outdoor pollutants, including fine particulate matter ($PM_{2.5}$), nitrogen dioxide (NO_2), and ozone (O_3), have been linked to the development and exacerbation of diseases such as COPD and asthma [11–16]. These pollutants primarily originate from anthropogenic outdoor sources such as vehicular traffic, industry, and fossil fuel combustion, emphasizing the importance of public policies to improve air quality.

Indoor air quality (IAQ) is equally important, as individuals spend approximately 90% of their time indoors. Indoor pollutants, including particulate matter, volatile organic compounds (VOCs), carbon dioxide (CO_2), and carbon monoxide (CO), may affect respiratory health [17,18].

Therefore, monitoring and controlling indoor environments is essential to prevent exposure to harmful contaminants. Monitoring technologies, including environmental sensors, play a pivotal role in assessing air quality, both indoors and outdoors [19–22]. These technologies enable the continuous measurement of various parameters such as PM_1, $PM_{2.5}$, PM_{10}, NO_2, O_3, and sulfur dioxide (SO_2) outdoors, as well as VOCs, CO_2, and CO indoors. By providing online data, these sensors support the identification of pollution levels and enable an assessment of their impact on respiratory health, thus facilitating timely interventions.

The integration of AI in healthcare is revolutionizing the management of chronic diseases, including CRD. AI-based predictive models are being developed to forecast exacerbations of COPD and asthma. These models utilize clinical, environmental, and patient behavior data to identify patterns and predict acute episodes. This proactive approach allows for early and personalized interventions that have the potential to improve health outcomes and reduce healthcare costs [5,23]. AI technologies also play a critical role in evaluating the relationship between air quality and respiratory health.

AI-based predictive models which use data from environmental sensors and clinical patient data have shown promising results in predicting the impact of air pollution levels on the incidence and severity of respiratory exacerbations [17,19,21]. This information is crucial for developing effective mitigation strategies and public policies to protect the health of vulnerable populations.

Considering all the above-mentioned, using air quality monitoring technologies and AI in managing CRD offers promising avenues for improving patient outcomes and reducing the economic burden associated with these diseases. Nevertheless, there are gaps in research in this field that are hindering the development of predictive tools to improve the health management of these chronic respiratory patients. These identified gaps include the following:

(a) The lack of methodological standardization in studies.
(b) The need for long-term longitudinal trials that consider the spatial variability, individualized measures of exposure to pollutants, and the heterogeneity in demographic and health characteristics of patients.
(c) The need for linking monitored air quality measurements with respiratory health markers collected from sensors, mobile applications, and the patient's medical history.
(d) The limited research studies focused on how the combination of indoor pollutants and the confounding factors beyond the isolated effects of each pollutant separately affect respiratory health, thus contributing to pro-inflammatory states and genetic and epigenetic alterations.
(e) The lack of personalized early warning and recommendations systems that combine environmental monitoring with artificial intelligence techniques.

This study aimed to build and describe the current perspective on IAQ monitoring in the context of environmental health risks, and to provide a comprehensive guide to current technologies and their potential applications in the field of respiratory health. A multidisciplinary approach combining environmental monitoring with advanced technological solutions is advocated to address the challenges posed by asthma and COPD, the two most prevalent CRD.

This study reviewed scientific literature and identified the extent and gaps available to date on IAQ and its relationship to asthma and COPD progression. Three objectives were drawn up to achieve this task, as follows:

(a) To determine peer-reviewed scientific studies that have been conducted on IAQ monitoring and its effect on the health of patients with asthma or COPD, and to create a synopsis of the empirical knowledge on this field to date.
(b) To provide a focused understanding of the possibilities of monitoring IAQ to predict exacerbations in asthma and COPD and improve respiratory environmental health.
(c) Identify action gaps in indoor monitoring air quality studies and possible actions to mitigate them.

2. Methods

2.1. Search Strategy and Inclusion and Exclusion Criteria

We undertook a systematic review to assess the evidence on the relationship between IAQ, COPD, and asthma. The Preferred Reporting Items for Systematic Reviews and Meta-Analyses (PRISMA) statement was used in this systematic review as a basis for reporting the findings [24]. The search aimed to identify studies with COPD and asthma patients in which IAQ parameters were monitored and linked to disease outcomes, such as acute exacerbation, using artificial intelligence or advanced statistics techniques.

Inclusion criteria covered English-language publications in peer-reviewed journals. Regularly issued conference proceedings, communications abstracts, and non-original articles (e.g., editorials and review papers) were excluded. Nevertheless, the reference list of the reviewed manuscripts was also screened to find potential eligible studies.

A systematic search in the Web of Science (SCI) database was undertaken. The search aimed to identify the evidence from the literature on experiences of IAQ monitoring applied to COPD and asthma. The search was performed on 14 May 2024, and the following search strings were used: (((ALL = ("COPD" OR "ASTHMA")) AND ALL = ("indoor")) AND ALL = ("air quality")). Initially, searches that are more specific were performed, but finally, keywords that are more general were used to ensure the inclusion of potentially relevant studies.

As a first step, the title and abstract of each study were screened for eligibility. The full text of the screened manuscripts was then assessed for eligibility. Two authors conducted the screening, and disagreements were solved by consensus. The resulting eligible articles were included in the review.

2.2. Data Extraction and Quality Assessment

Two reviewers (P.C.-M., D.S.-L.) extracted the data necessary to complete each table, each one-half of the papers.

An agreed data extraction form was used. In case of doubts or discrepancies, a second reviewer was consulted. If discrepancies persisted, they were resolved with the participation of a third reviewer (D.S.-M.). The data items extracted included the following: year of publication, authors, target population (patients with asthma or COPD), study time and sample size, age of patients, clinical data used in the study, a brief description of the objectives and results of the research, pollutants that were monitored, sensors used to gather indoor IAQ data, information about calibration of sensors, data communications, sampling rate, details of data post-processing, and information on the development of predictive models and the application of conventional statistics and machine learning techniques.

Two reviewers assessed all included articles for quality following the Mixed Method Appraisal Tool (MMAT) [25]. The MMAT is an effective tool for quality assessment in mixed-method review studies. MMAT consists of four criteria to assess quantitative (descriptive, randomized, and non-randomized) and qualitative studies. Each study design was evaluated according to its methodological domain (qualitative, quantitative randomized controlled, quantitative non-randomized, quantitative descriptive, fixed methods). The MMAT metric was estimated by assigning 25% to each criterion that was fully addressed. The metric ranged from 0 to 100%. Disagreements were handled with the participation of a third reviewer.

Finally, the narrative synthesis methodology was applied due to the heterogeneity of the findings on study approaches, settings, and intervention factors [26].

2.3. Risk-of-Bias Assessment

Two potential sources of individual studies' bias were identified in this study. First, the eventual omission of systematic reviews of recently completed clinical studies, or other studies not published in journals. Second, the publication's language for studies included in this review was limited to English, which is a potential source of bias that must be considered [27].

3. Results

3.1. Study Selection

The database search revealed 301 records. The title, abstract, and keywords were reviewed and 242 articles that did not meet inclusion criteria were excluded. One article could not be retrieved, and the full text of the remaining 59 potentially relevant articles was assessed. Thirty-seven articles were excluded. Reasons for exclusion included the following: not involving a study on home air quality monitoring ($N = 13$); not focusing on asthma or COPD ($N = 15$); and not correlating IAQ and clinical outcomes ($N = 10$). Finally,

21 articles were included, all published in English. The PRISMA flow diagram illustrated in Figure 1 describes the process followed in this review.

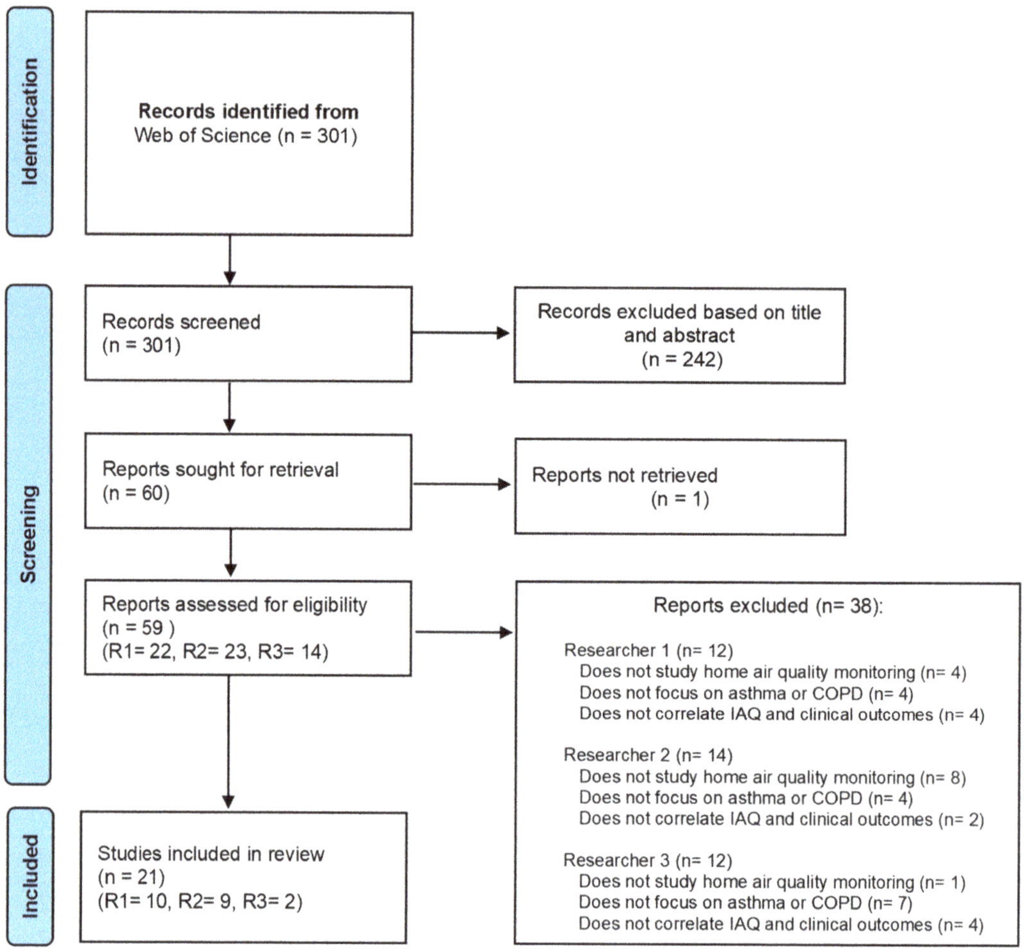

Figure 1. Flow Diagram for study selection following the preferred reporting items for systematic reviews and the meta-analyses (PRISMA) statement.

3.2. *Study Characteristics*

3.2.1. Publication and Study Design Type

Table 1 presents the main characteristics of the selected studies, highlighting key initial information such as their targeted disease and the primary objective. The 21 papers included in this review featured an air quality study linked to outcomes in asthma and COPD. Figure 2 synthesizes the findings.

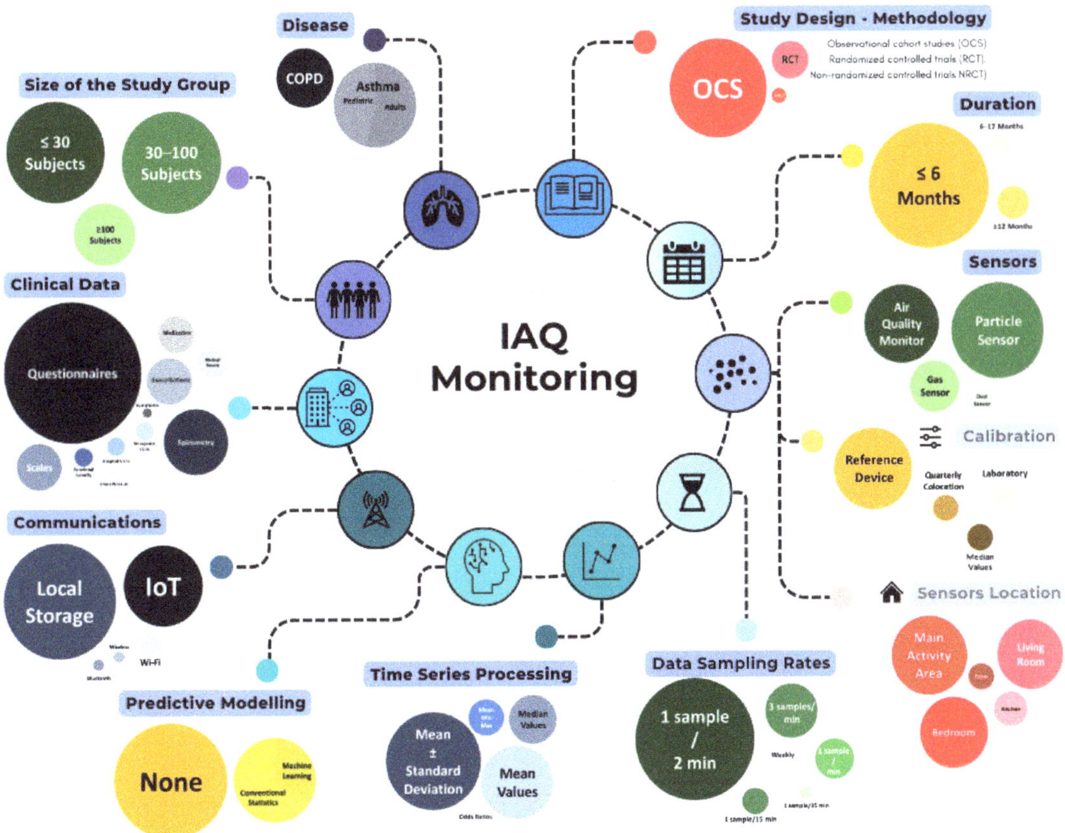

Figure 2. Graphical summary of evaluated aspects in IAQ monitoring.

These studies were categorized based on whether they addressed asthma or COPD. Of the 21 studies, 43% (*N* = 9) focused on COPD [11,12,21,22,28–32], while 57% (*N* = 12) focused on asthma [17,18,33–42].

Regarding the methodology, there were 14 observational cohort studies (OCS), with 9 focused on asthma [17,18,33–36,38,41,42], and 5 on COPD [11,12,21,22,28]. Four asthmas [37,38,40,41] and two COPD studies [29,30] encompassed randomized controlled trials (RCT). Two COPD studies [31,32] performed non-randomized controlled trials (NRCT).

Table 1. Main characteristics of the included studies.

Year	Authors	Country	Disease	Study Design	Study Population	Objective
2023	J. Kang et al. [29]	South Korea	COPD	RCT	Adults	To assess the effectiveness of a behavioral intervention in reducing $PM_{2.5}$ exposure and to improve clinical outcomes in patients with COPD.
2023	N. N. Hansel et al. [30]	USA	COPD	RCT	Adults	To determine whether placement of active portable HEPA cleaners can improve respiratory morbidity in former smokers.
2023	A. McCarron et al. [33].	UK	Asthma	OCS	Adults	To investigate the acute effects of personal exposure to $PM_{2.5}$ on self-reported asthma-related health.
2023	I. Kang et al. [35]	USA	Asthma	OCS	Adults	To examine the joint impacts of exposures to residential indoor and outdoor air pollutants and housing risk factors on asthma-related health outcomes.
2022	G. P. Bălă et al. [28]	Romania	COPD	OCS	Adults	To assess the degree of microparticulate pollution in the houses of COPD patients and to determine whether the values recorded correlate to COPD exacerbations.
2022	B. J. John et al. [22]	Germany	COPD	OCS	Adults	To identify the affected surroundings to take early steps to reduce the risk of COPD and other respiratory illnesses by introducing an AQI real-time device.
2022	U. Rabbani et al. [18]	Pakistan	Asthma	OCS	Adults	To assess the association of formaldehyde, CO, and $PM_{2.5}$ with respiratory symptoms, asthma, and post-bronchodilator reversibility.
2022	J. Woo et al. [37]	South Korea	Asthma	RCT	Pediatric	To predict PEFR with a deep learning algorithm through RNNs and DNNs trained using 4 months of linked data of IAQ and PEFR.
2022	L. Nurhussien et al. [32]	USA	COPD	NRCT	Adults	To study how daily pollutant exposures impact lung function in COPD, considering the influence of eosinophil levels as indicators of airway inflammation and pollution susceptibility.
2021	H. Kim et al. [11]	South Korea	COPD	OCS	Adults	To assess if indoor particulate matter concentration is affected by a life behavior pattern, and if it can be reduced with appropriate lifestyle modification.
2021	C.T. Wu et al. [21]	Taiwan	COPD	OCS	Adults	To develop a prediction system using lifestyle data, environmental factors, and patient symptoms for the early detection of acute exacerbations of COPD in the upcoming 7 days.

Table 1. *Cont.*

Year	Authors	Country	Disease	Study Design	Study Population	Objective
2021	W.D. Bae et al. [17]	South Korea	Asthma	OCS	Adults	To compare ten machine-learning techniques, using imbalanced sampling to improve nine of them in predicting how IAQ affects patients' PEFR.
2021	C.I. Prasasti et al. [34]	Indonesia	Asthma	OCS	Pediatric	To study how VOCs, $PM_{2.5}$, and household environmental exposure relate to respiratory allergic symptoms in children in Surabaya, Indonesia.
2021	A.Y. Lim et al. [42]	South Korea	Asthma	OCS	Adults + Pediatric	To evaluate the IAQ level and daily health symptoms of adults and children living in EEHs compared to conventional buildings over one year.
2020	SE. Guo et al. [31]	Taiwan	COPD	NRCT	Adults	The study explored how educating patients with COPD about particulate matter (PM) affects their knowledge of air pollution prevention, self-care, symptom management, and indoor PM levels.
2020	E.N. Schachter et al. [36]	USA	Asthma	OCS	Pediatric	To study how indoor pollutants and their seasonal changes affect asthma exacerbations in children with moderate to severe asthma.
2020	R. J. Khusial et al. [38]	Netherlands, UK, Greece, and Germany	Asthma	RCT + OCS	Adults	To assess the clinical effectiveness and technology acceptance of myAirCoach-supported self-management on top of usual care in patients with asthma using inhalation medication.
2020	G. H. Lee et al. [39]	South Korea	Asthma	RCT	Pediatric	To study air purifiers' impact on indoor air pollutant levels and asthma control in children, using HEPA filters.
2020	S. Kim et al. [40]	South Korea	Asthma	RCT	Pediatric	To evaluate the effects of indoor $PM_{2.5}$ on children's PEFR, with a daily intervention of air purifiers with filter on, compared with groups with filter off.
2019	R. Chi et al. [12]	China	COPD	OCS	Adults	To compare the effects of outdoor- and indoor-originated $PM_{2.5}$ on cardiopulmonary function in COPD patients and healthy elderly adults.
2019	S. Hussain et al. [41]	UK	Asthma	OCS	Adults	To assess if overnight particulate matter exposure affects daily symptoms, lung function, and inflammation in asthmatic patients sensitive to dust mites.

3.2.2. Subjects, Study Sample and Follow-Up Months

Table 2 provides a more in-depth analysis of the obtained data, focusing on the collected medical information and the experimental duration of the trial. Additionally, the key findings from each study were highlighted. Along with the data from Table 1, the analysis further explores the selected studies, emphasizing the patient population under investigation, as well as sample size and study duration.

Regarding the types of patients studied, a total of six asthma studies [17,18,33,35,38,41] and 100% of studies on COPD [11,12,21,22,28–32] focused on an adult population. Five asthma studies targeted a pediatric population [34,36,37,39,40]. In addition, one asthma study included a mixed approach with both adult and pediatric populations [42]. The sample size of the studies reveals that as the sample size decreases, the number of asthma studies increases. In contrast, studies in COPD tended to have a larger sample size compared to asthma studies.

The duration of the studies varied, with an average length of 5.9 ± 4.4 months. Most of the studies on asthma (67%) [17,18,34,36,37,39–41] and COPD (67%) [11,21,22,30–32] had a duration of less than 6 months.

Table 2. Clinical data, duration, study sample, and main results of the included studies.

Ref.	Clinical Data Gathered During the Study	Follow-Up	Study Sample (Subjects)	Results	MMAT Score
[29]	Questionnaires (SGRQ, CAT), exacerbations	9 months	106	Good adherence to the intervention led to improved CAT scores and lower $PM_{2.5}$ levels compared to poor adherence in the control group. Checking air quality forecasts regularly reduced CAT scores across all activities.	100%
[30]	Questionnaires (SGRQ, CAT), scales (mMRC, BCSS), exacerbations, functional capacity (6 min walk test distance)	6 months	116	The active filter group showed better SGRQ symptom scores, fewer respiratory symptoms, and lower rates of exacerbations and rescue medication use than the sham group. In the active group, a 30–40% reduction in NO_2 and more than 40% in $PM_{2.5}$ was observed.	100%
[33]	Self-reported asthma symptoms, medication use	12 months	28	$PM_{2.5}$ levels varied by location. Higher $PM_{2.5}$ exposure increased asthma symptom likelihood, but it did not affect reliever inhaler use.	75%
[35]	Questionnaires (ACT, HRQoL SF-12), scale (PSS), hospitalizations and emergency department visits	19 months	53	In both cross-sectional and longitudinal analyses, lower ACT scores correlated with higher indoor NO_2 levels, indoor temperature, PM_1, $PM_{2.5}$, and PM_{10}. Emergency department visits were linked to poorer asthma control, physical health, and mental health, as well as higher indoor NO_2 ratios and temperatures.	100%
[28]	Clinical data extracted from medical records, exacerbations	8 months	79	Average PM_1, $PM_{2.5}$, and PM_{10} values were lower in the group of infrequently exacerbating patients than in the group of frequently exacerbating patients.	100%
[22]	Questionnaire (RQ), lung function from medical records	8 days	196	High daily $PM_{2.5}$ levels, especially in smokers, significantly affected COPD patients' health. Indoor $PM_{2.5}$ levels were closely correlated with health conditions, emphasizing the impact of particulate exposure.	50%
[18]	Questionnaire (ATS-DLD-78A), spirometry (FVC, FEV1)	6 months	1629	Formaldehyde and CO levels were associated with cough, phlegm, and wheezing. $PM_{2.5}$ levels were linked to shortness of breath and overall respiratory symptoms and were associated with a lower risk of cough, phlegm, and bronchitis.	100%

Table 2. *Cont.*

Ref.	Clinical Data Gathered During the Study	Follow-Up	Study Sample (Subjects)	Results	MMAT Score
[37]	PEFR	4 months	26	The 10 min RNN model accurately predicted PEFR with an RMSE of 42.5 and MAPE of 14.0, showing how indoor $PM_{2.5}$ levels impacted PEFR over time.	75%
[32]	Questionnaire, spirometry (FVC, FEV1)	4 months	30	Higher personal NO_2 exposure was associated with lower FEV_1 (11.3 mL) and lower forced vital capacity (18.0 mL). $PM_{2.5}$ and NO_2 exposure at personal and community levels were also linked to lower FEV_1 in participants with higher eosinophil levels.	100%
[11]	Questionnaire (inhaler use), exacerbations	3 months	104	Indoor $PM_{2.5}$ levels were influenced by lifestyle and economic status in COPD patients and were significantly linked to acute COPD exacerbations.	75%
[21]	Questionnaire (CAT), scale (mMRC), physiological data, exacerbations	4 months	67	The AECOPD predictive model achieved 92% accuracy, 94% sensitivity, and 90% specificity for 7-day predictions, with an AUC above 0.9. Results show lifestyle and environmental data are highly correlated with health conditions.	100%
[17]	PEFR	6 months	25	Transfer machine learning with imbalanced sampling effectively predicted changes in PEFR linked to IAQ, including $PM_{2.5}$ and carbon dioxide concentrations.	75%
[34]	Questionnaire	3 months	80	The periodic monitoring of IAQ was found to be an effective measure to prevent respiratory allergies among children in an indoor environment.	75%
[42]	Questionnaire, scale	12 months	25 adults + 25 children	Indoor PM_{10}, $PM_{2.5}$, CO_2, and VOCs concentrations were lower in EEH. Seasonal adjustments showed consistent indoor temperature and humidity levels in EEH.	75%
[31]	Questionnaire (CAT), scale (mMRC)	6 months	63	PM education led to improved knowledge in the first and third months but not by the sixth month. The experimental group had greater gains initially, with better physical health in the first month, and better psychological health in the sixth month.	50%

Table 2. *Cont.*

Ref.	Clinical Data Gathered During the Study	Follow-Up	Study Sample (Subjects)	Results	MMAT Score
[36]	Questionnaire, medication use, unscheduled clinic, emergency department visits, hospitalizations, spirometry (FVC, FEV_1)	2 weeks	36	NO_2 and $PM_{2.5}$ elements like Ca, Si, Ni, and Cl were linked to worsened asthma symptoms and increased use of rescue medication in inner-city children with moderate to severe asthma.	100%
[38]	Questionnaires (ACQ, m-AQLQ, EQ-5D-5L), exacerbations, PEFR (FEV_1), FeNO, inhaler use and technique score.	Study 1: 3–6 months Study 2: 3 months	Study 1: 30 Study 2: 12	In study 1, the intervention improved asthma control (ACQ difference 0.70) and reduced exacerbations (HR 0.31). Asthma-related quality of life also improved (mini AQLQ difference 0.53) but forced expiratory volume in 1 s did not change. In study 2, asthma control improved by 0.86 compared to baseline.	100%
[39]	Questionnaire (based on TRACK), PEFR, FeNO	2 months	30	Medication use decreased from 6.9 to 7.12 when using air purifiers, suggesting less medication was needed. Bacterial diversity, measured by the Chao 1 index, was lower with the air purifier on compared to off.	75%
[40]	PEFR, FeNO	1 month, 3 weeks	26	The use of in-home air filtration could be considered as an intervention strategy for IAQ control in asthmatic children's homes.	100%
[12]	Blood pressure, PEFR, FEV_1	7 months	43	During the heating season, COPD patients had a reduction in forced expiratory volume in the first second (FEV_1) associated with $PM_{2.5}$	100%
[41]	Questionnaires (ACQ, AQLQ), PEFR, FeNO, spirometry	3 months	28	No significant associations were observed between overnight particulate matter exposure and clinical outcomes measured daily or at study visits.	100%

3.2.3. Pollutants

Table 3 presents data on the pollutants researched, sensors technologies and location, calibration, communications technologies, sampling rates, data statistical analyses, and information about whether predictive models and/or machine learning techniques were used. Figure 3 provides a summary of the pollutants and environmental conditions examined across the studies.

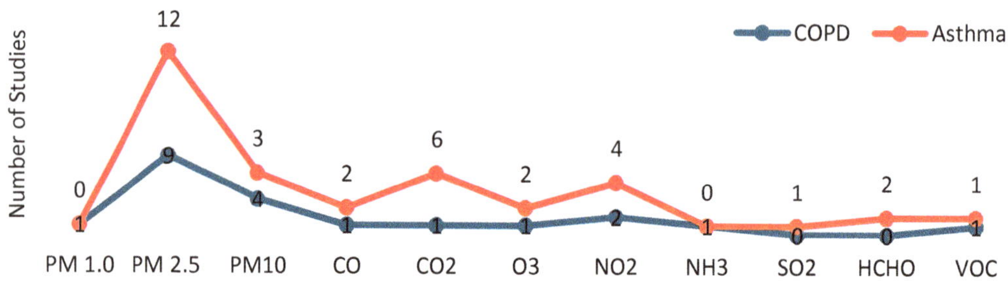

Figure 3. Pollutants that were studied in the selected articles.

Among particulate matter, $PM_{2.5}$ was the most studied pollutant, appearing in all analyzed articles, both in asthma ($N = 12$) [17,18,33–42] and COPD ($N = 9$) [11,12,21,22,28–32].

PM_{10} was studied in four asthma studies [36,38,41,42] and three COPD studies [28,30,31], while PM_1 was only analyzed in one COPD study [28].

Regarding the rest of the pollutants, a total of six studies focused on nitrogen dioxide (NO_2), four of which related to asthma [18,35,36,38] and two to COPD [30,32]. Carbon dioxide (CO_2) was explored in six asthma studies [17,35,37,39,40,42] and in one COPD study [22]. Carbon monoxide (CO) was studied in three studies, two about asthma [18,35], and one about COPD [22]. Ozone (O_3) was analyzed in two asthma studies [35,36] and one COPD study [32]. Formaldehyde (HCHO) was investigated in two asthma studies [18,35]. Finally, volatile organic compounds (VOCs) were studied in one asthma [42] and one COPD study [30]. Sulfur dioxide (SO_2) was analyzed in one asthma study [38], and the relation of ammonia (NH_3) to COPD was explored in a single study [22].

Table 3. Pollutants, sensors, calibration, communications, sampling, and algorithms of the included studies.

Ref.	Pollutants	Sensors	Sensor Location	Calibration	Communications	Sampling	Time Series Processing	Predictive Model	Machine Learning
[29]	$PM_{2.5}$	Particle Sensor	Participants' main area of activity	-	IoT	1 sample/2 min	Mean ± standard deviation	Yes	No
[30]	$PM_{2.5}$, PM_{10}, NO_2, airborne nicotine (VOC)	Particle Sensor, Gas Sensor	Participants' main area of activity	-	Local Storage	1 week in three periods: at months 0, 3, and 6.	-	No	No
[33]	$PM_{2.5}$	Air Quality Monitor	Backpack	Median values for calibration	Local Storage	1 sample/2 min	Min, max, and mean values	Yes	No
[35]	HCHO, CO, CO_2, NO_2, O_3, $PM_{2.5}$	Particle Sensor	Participants' main area of activity	Quarterly colocation calibration	IoT	1 sample/min	Mean ± standard deviation	No	No
[28]	PM_1, PM2.5, and PM_{10}	Air Quality Monitor	Participants' main area of activity	-	Wi-Fi	1 sample/min	Min, max, and mean values	Yes	No
[22]	$PM_{2.5}$, CO, CO_2, NH_3	Particle Sensor, Gas Sensor, Air Quality Monitor	Participants' main area of activity	-	Wi-Fi	1 sample/2 min	Mean values	No	✘
[18]	HCHO, CO, NO_2, $PM_{2.5}$	Air Quality Monitor, Particle Sensor	Living room, bedroom, and kitchen	-	Local Storage	1 sample/5 min	Median values	No	✘
[37]	$PM_{2.5}$, CO_2	Particle sensor, Gas Sensor	Bedrooms/living rooms	With a reference device	Local Storage	1 sample/2 min	Mean values	Yes	Yes
[32]	$PM_{2.5}$, NO_2, O_3	Particle Sensor, Gas Sensor	Living room, bedroom, and kitchen	With a reference device	Local Storage	3 samples/min	Mean ± standard deviation	No	No
[11]	$PM_{2.5}$	Particle Sensor	Center of the participants' houses	-	IoT	1 sample/2 min	Mean ± standard deviation	No	No
[21]	$PM_{2.5}$	Air Quality Monitor	Participants' main area of activity	-	IoT	1 sample/15 min	Mean values	Yes	Yes
[17]	$PM_{2.5}$, CO_2	Particle Sensor, Gas Sensor	Outside, front door, living room, bedroom, and kitchen	-	Local Storage	1 sample/2 min	Mean values	Yes	Yes

Table 3. *Cont.*

Ref.	Pollutants	Sensors	Sensor Location	Calibration	Communications	Sampling	Time Series Processing	Predictive Model	Machine Learning
[34]	$PM_{2.5}$	Dust Sensor	Bedroom	Airflow calibrator	Local Storage	-	Min, max, and mean values	Yes	No
[42]	PM_{10}, $PM_{2.5}$, CO_2, VOCs	Air Quality Monitor	Living room	-	IoT	1 sample/5 min	Mean values	Yes	No
[31]	PM_{10}, $PM_{2.5}$,	Dust Sensor	Outside, front door, living room, bedroom, and kitchen	-	Local Storage	3 samples/min	Mean $\pm$ standard deviation	Yes	No
[36]	PM_{10}, $PM_{2.5}$, NO_2, SO_2, O_3	Dust Sensor, Gas Sensor	Participants' main area of activity	-	Local Storage	3 samples/min	Odds ratios	No	No
[38]	NO_2, SO_2, $PM_{2.5}$, PM_{10}	Air Quality Monitor	Bedrooms	-	Bluetooth	1 sample/2 min	Mean $\pm$ standard deviation and median values	No	No
[39]	$PM_{2.5}$, CO_2	Particle Sensor	Living room	-	IoT	1 sample/2 min	Mean $\pm$ standard deviation	No	No
[40]	$PM_{2.5}$, CO_2	Air Quality Monitor, Particle Sensor	Living room	Laboratory test	IoT	1 sample/2 min	Median values	No	No
[12]	$PM_{2.5}$	Dust Sensor	Participants' main area of activity	-	Local Storage	3 samples/min	Mean $\pm$ standard deviation and median values	No	No
[41]	PM_{10}, $PM_{2.5}$	Air Quality Monitor	Bedroom	-	Wireless	1 sample/min	Mean values	No	No

3.3. Quality Assessment

Of all the studies evaluating the impact of IAQ on asthma and COPD, thirteen studies achieved an MMAT score of 100%, seven scored 75%, and two scored 50% (Table 2). Quality limitations in the cohort observational studies included issues such as insufficient details regarding the selection bias of participants [11,18,22], unclear origins of measurement data [17,33,34], unknown validity of measurement tools [22], or the use of non-standardized instruments [31]. Regarding randomized controlled trials, quality variability was noted in cases where there was no clear description of randomization procedures, lack of detailed reporting on blinding methods [39], incomplete outcome data [37], or a high dropout rate.

3.4. Clinical Data

In most of the selected studies, air quality data was supplemented with symptoms or physiological information collected from patients. Symptoms collected through questionnaires were used for asthma [18,33–36,38,39,41,42] and COPD [11,21,22,29–32].

In COPD, basic vital signs, such as blood pressure or heart rate [12,21], lung function data [12,22,32], medication adherence [11,12], calories and daily steps [21], and 6 min walk test distance [30] were monitored. In asthma, lung function was measured in [17,18,36–41] and medication use was tracked in [33,36,38]. Fractional Exhaled Nitric Oxide (FeNO) was also reported in some asthma studies [38–41].

Finally, exacerbations were tracked and accounted for both asthma [35,36,38] and COPD [11,21,28–30].

3.5. Air Quality Sensors

The sensors used in the various selected studies vary according to the pollutants analyzed, with the following types being the most prominent: IAQ monitors, particle sensors and gas sensors. IAQ monitors collect a range of data from a single point, detecting particulate matter, gases, temperature, and humidity, among other parameters.

A single dust sensor was used in several studies (one study on asthma [34] and four on COPD [11,12,29,31]). Also, a single IAQ monitor was used in some studies (four on asthma [33,38,41,42] and two on COPD [21,28]). One asthma study made use of a particle sensor [39]. The use of multiple sensors was more common, with six studies on asthma [17,18,35–37,40] and three on COPD [22,30,32].

The air quality data recorded by the sensors were either stored locally or transmitted from the patient's home to a central repository. It should be noted that most of the studies did not include details on the protocol for data communication that was used. Data were locally stored in eleven studies (six on asthma [17,18,33,34,36,37] and four on COPD [12,30–32]). In general, Wi-Fi and the Internet of Things (IoT) were the most used protocols in the rest of the studies. IoT was used in four asthma [35,39,40,42] and three COPD studies [11,21,29]. Wi-Fi was used in two studies [22,28] and Bluetooth in only one study on asthma [38].

3.6. Sensors Calibration

Sensor calibration is often a critical step before device deployment. Despite its relevance, the calibration procedure was not reported in 15 out of the 21 reviewed articles (71%). Eleven percent of COPD studies [32] and seventeen percent of asthma-related articles [34,37] utilized a reference device as a calibration standard. Other calibration approaches were only described in asthma studies, with 8% of articles [33] using mean values, 8% quarterly collocation [35], and 8% conducting a laboratory test for calibration purposes [40].

A relevant aspect to consider is the placement of sensors in the different areas of the patient's home (Figure 4). In 17% of asthma articles [35,36] and 78% of COPD articles [11,12,21,22,28–30], sensors were placed in the patient's center or primary activity area, although the criteria for determining this area were not detailed. Sensors were placed in the bedrooms in 50% of asthma articles [17,18,34,37,38,41] and 22% of COPD articles [31,32]. Living rooms were selected in 50% of asthma articles [17,18,37,39,40,42] and 22% of COPD articles [31,32]. To a lesser extent, sensors were placed in kitchens in 17% of asthma articles [17,18] and 22% of COPD articles [31,32]. Other locations for sensors accounted for 17% of asthma [17,33] and 11% of COPD articles [31].

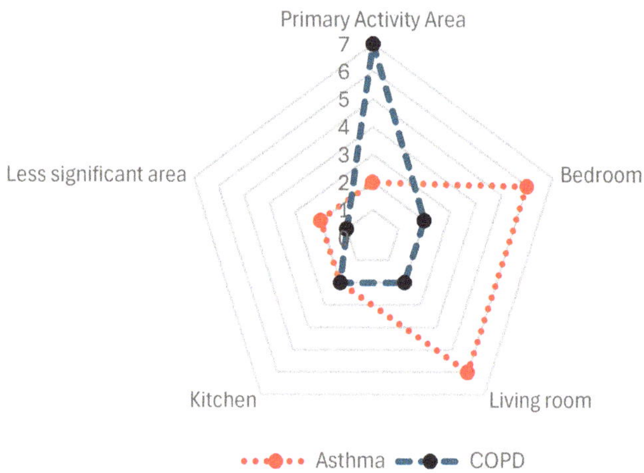

Figure 4. Sensor placement, compiled from the selected studies.

3.7. Data Processing

The data processing and analysis of the information collected through sensors was conducted heterogeneously. When reported, sampling was performed at intervals equal to or greater than one minute in 83% of asthma articles [17,18,33,35,37–42] and in 44% of COPD articles [11,21,22,28]. In asthma studies, the sampling rate was greater than one sample per minute in one (8%) study [36]. In COPD, this happened in three studies (33%) [12,31,32]. The sampling rate was unreported in one asthma [34] and one COPD study [30].

Data samples were processed differently. Mainly, the mean and/or standard deviation were calculated in 75% of asthma articles [17,33–35,37–39,41,42] and in 89% of COPD studies [11,12,21,22,28,29,31,32]. Following this, median values were used in 25% of asthma studies [18,38,40] and in 11% of COPD articles [12]. Odds ratios were reported to be used in 8% of asthma articles [36], while minimum and maximum values were estimated in 16% of asthma articles [33,34] and in 11% of COPD articles [28].

3.8. Predictive Models and Machine Learning

In the scoped studies, 16% of asthma articles [17,37] and 10% of COPD articles [21] developed predictive models using machine learning. Over 25% of asthma articles [33,34,42] and 33% of COPD articles [28,29,31] implemented predictive models using traditional statistics. Seven (58%) of asthma articles [18,35,36,38–41] and five (55%) of COPD articles [11,12,22,30,32] did not include a predictive model.

3.9. Disease Progression and Pollutants

3.9.1. Particulate Matter

In the context of air pollutants, particulate matter is present in various forms depending on its size. These contaminants can significantly affect patients with respiratory diseases, potentially exacerbating their conditions if air quality is poor.

Of the nine studies aimed at exploring indoor particulate matter and its relation to COPD, only one (10%) explored PM_1, one (10%) explored PM_{10}, and nine (100%) analyzed $PM_{2.5}$. In the case of asthma, one article (10%) addressed the influence of PM_1, three (30%) evaluated PM_{10}, and twelve (92%) analyzed $PM_{2.5}$.

3.9.2. Gaseous Pollutants

CO_2 and NO_2 were the most studied gases. The effects of CO_2 were evaluated in 50% of asthma studies [17,35,37,39,40,42] and 11% of COPD studies [22]. Concerning NO_2, it was explored in 33% of the studies on asthma [18,35,36,38] and 22% of studies on COPD [30,32]. The impact of CO on asthma was assessed in 17% of articles [18,35] while its impact on COPD was evaluated in 11% of the reviewed studies [22].

HCHO was only considered in two studies, both on asthma [18,35]. NH_3 was evaluated in the context of COPD in only one article [22]. Finally, the association of SO_2 with respiratory pathologies was explored only on asthma, in two studies [36,38]. The effects of O_3 on asthma progression were evaluated in 16% of the studies [35,36], while its relationship to COPD was studied in 11% of the selected articles [32]. Finally, the link between VOCs and disease progression was studied in two studies, one on asthma [42] and one on COPD [30].

4. Discussion

Worldwide, indoor air pollution contributes to over four million annual deaths [43]. This preventable exposure has significant respiratory health effects. To the best of our knowledge no prior research has explored the application of indoor monitoring technologies, sensors, predictive models, and AI in analyzing COPD and asthma progression.

We conducted a systematic review to describe the evolution of and current research on the potential effects of IAQ on COPD and asthma progression. Specifically, we examined studies that collected and analyzed air quality data, biomedical parameters, and clinical information, to identify links between certain pollutants and the triggering of acute respiratory exacerbations.

To this purpose, we conducted a systematic search and article collection using the PRISMA methodology. This search resulted in 21 studies that met our inclusion criteria, providing a solid evidence base for this analysis.

4.1. IAQ, Asthma, and COPD

The relationship between IAQ and respiratory diseases such as asthma and COPD has been the subject of increasing scientific interest in recent decades. While earlier studies focused primarily on outdoor air pollution, it is now recognized that IAQ significantly impacts respiratory health. Factors such as tobacco smoke, cleaning products, VOCs, dust mites, and fine particulate matter have been identified as key elements that can exacerbate asthma and COPD in vulnerable individuals.

Advances in indoor pollutant measurement and a deeper understanding of the biological mechanisms behind these diseases have driven this field's evolution. Notably, studies on the association between IAQ and asthma and COPD progression have increased since 2019, with a particularly pronounced rise in asthma research.

In asthma, researchers have shown that exposure to certain allergens and pollutants in indoor air can trigger attacks [43,44]. Recent studies have examined how humidity, mold, and chemicals in the home affect the severity of asthma symptoms. It has been observed that children and adults living in environments with poor IAQ are more likely to develop asthma or suffer exacerbations of the disease [18,33–36,38–40,42]. The development of predictive systems that consider IAQ as an input for the early detection of acute episodes has been explored recently [17,33,34,37,42]. This strategy has achieved promising results in the early detection of increased asthma symptoms [33], and in predicting changes in peak expiratory flow rate using artificial intelligence techniques [37].

Also, COPD is affected by IAQ, with a high correlation found between IAQ and COPD acute exacerbations [21,28]. Traditionally, tobacco smoke has been recognized as the main risk factor, but recent research has highlighted the importance of other indoor pollutants, such as the biofuels used for cooking in rural areas or the dust generated in industrial settings [45,46]. Household ultrafine particles have been associated with a greater risk to cardiovascular health [47] and with a decline in cardiopulmonary function in COPD [12]. As with asthma, research efforts in recent years have focused on conducting behavioral interventions to improve COPD clinical outcomes [11,29,31], including the development of predictive models [11,21,29].

4.2. Sensors for IAQ Monitoring

Asthma studies measured significantly fewer indoor air quality (IAQ) parameters, and consequently used fewer sensors, compared to COPD studies. This difference may stem from the distinct disease trajectories. COPD patients often experience gradual and subtle clinical changes, necessitating a wider range of sensors to detect subtle deteriorations. In contrast, asthma exacerbations are typically more abrupt, and patients are often more aware of their triggers, enabling quicker and more direct responses, thus reducing the need for extensive sensor arrays.

Overall, there is a trend towards simplifying device configurations, favoring integrated multi-sensor units with data transmission capabilities [18,28,37,40–42]. The combination of air quality monitors, which integrated multiparameter measurements, and dust and gas sensors were the most frequent approach both in asthma and COPD.

Calibration is a prevalent technique employed to minimize measurement errors. Prior to deployment, sensor performance is evaluated against a reference standard, and a calibration model is developed by identifying and addressing potential error sources. While sensor calibration is fundamental to the accurate assessment of IAQ, a substantial proportion of the reviewed studies (over 70%) failed to provide details regarding calibration procedures. This lack of transparency undermines the reliability of reported pollutant concentrations and hinders the ability to conduct meaningful cross-study comparisons. Consequently, future research efforts must prioritize the implementation and transparent reporting of comprehensive calibration protocols, which should include rigorous pre-deployment validation and a schedule for periodic recalibration to ensure sustained data accuracy.

Furthermore, post-deployment calibration, where the calibration model is periodically evaluated to ensure accuracy, was not detailed in any study. The selection of low-cost air pollutants sensors and the lack of detailed calibration processes were identified as significant gaps, posing a challenging task in this context [48–50].

A limited adoption of the IoT in IAQ monitoring was detected, despite its numerous advantages. While only 33% of reviewed studies utilize IoT for real-time IAQ monitoring, technology offers significant benefits, including continuous data collection, low power consumption, scalability, remote accessibility, cloud integration, and cost-effectiveness. IoT is crucial in building next-generation systems [51] and IoT platforms have the potential to leverage artificial intelligence and machine learning for predictive modeling, early warning systems, and optimize air quality management [52], key for managing CRD. With 50% of studies relying on local data storage, remote and centralized monitoring strategies are also compromised. Therefore, promoting the integration of IoT protocols in future IAQ monitoring studies is vital to overcome these limitations and harness advanced technologies for improved CRD care, aligning with the need for personalized early warning systems and recommendations.

4.3. Disease Progression and Pollutants

4.3.1. Particulate Matter

Airborne particles are a form of air pollution that can have a significant impact on human health, particularly due to particulate matter (PM) [53]. PM was a key in IAQ studies due to its various household sources, including heaters, cooking, cleaning products, personal hygiene products, and tobacco.

PM_1, ultrafine particles smaller than 1 micron, are generated through combustion, cooking, infiltration of outdoor air pollution, household products, HVAC systems, electronic devices, building materials, mold, and resuspension of settled dust caused by movement or cleaning activities. Only one reviewed study [28] has explored the correlation between PM_1 and COPD exacerbations, reporting higher PM_1 levels in homes with frequent exacerbations.

Particulate matter with a diameter of 2.5 microns or smaller ($PM_{2.5}$) shares similar sources with PM1. This pollutant was explored in all reviewed studies, both in asthma and COPD, and was linked to respiratory symptoms, including shortness of breath and decreased Forced Expiratory Volume in one second (FEV1) [12,18,32] as well as to higher eosinophil levels [32]. COPD, a lifestyle that involves living in an environment with varying levels of $PM_{2.5}$, has been associated with a significant impact on patient health [11,12,30]. Exposure to this particulate matter was found to be lower in patients who experience infrequent COPD exacerbations [2]. Furthermore, a decrease in $PM_{2.5}$ exposure improved patient health, whether through medical intervention or the use of filters, among other methods [29,30]. Similarly, studies on asthma found that increased $PM_{2.5}$ concentrations were associated with airway inflammation, exacerbated symptoms, including cough, phlegm, and bronchitis [17,18,33,37], and impacting PEFR [37], as well as deteriorating quality of life [41]. The ability of $PM_{2.5}$ to penetrate deeply into the lungs and affect the respiratory system has been pointed out as a critical factor in asthma exacerbation [17]. Reducing $PM_{2.5}$ levels, both during the day and at night, has proven potential to prevent emergency visits due to uncontrolled symptoms [35,36] and to reduce medication use [39]. Daily monitoring of pollutants, coupled with medical interventions, is considered an effective strategy for asthma management. Daily monitoring of pollutants and patient conditions was revealed as an effective preventive measure for better controlling the patient's asthmatic state [38]. However, research on the association between $PM_{2.5}$ exposure variability and asthma clinical outcomes has yielded inconsistent results, with some studies finding no significant associations. This disparity may be attributed to factors such as natural $PM_{2.5}$ variability, study duration, and specific environmental conditions [35].

PM_{10}, particulate matter with a diameter of 10 microns or smaller, is found indoors due to renovation, construction or demolition activities, cleaning activities, dust, and resuspension of airborne particles. In COPD, lower levels of PM_{10} were associated with fewer exacerbations [28], and better physical and psychological health [31]. In asthma, the effects of PM_{10} on children with moderate to severe asthma were explored, but asthma severity was not associated with this specific indoor pollutant [36].

4.3.2. Gaseous Pollutants

Several selected articles explored the effects of CO_2, NO_2, CO, HCHO, NH_3, SO_2, and O_3 on asthma and COPD progression. Indoor CO, often present in homes using fuels such as natural gas for cooking or heating, have been associated with cough, phlegm, and wheezing in asthma patients [18]. However, no direct evidence was found linking CO to COPD in the reviewed studies.

Most of the selected studies focused on analyzing CO_2 and its effects on asthma. The reviewed studies showed that no significant effects were found on respiratory symptoms or lung function.

NO_2, mainly from gas stoves and heating systems, showed significant associations with asthma symptoms in children. In the reviewed studies, NO_2 was linked to worsened asthma symptoms and increased use of rescue medication in inner-city children with moderate to severe asthma [36], and to increased emergency department visits [35]. In COPD, some studies suggest a possible relationship between NO_2 exposure and symptoms, lung function, and the risk of exacerbation [30,32].

HCHO can be released indoors by pressed wood products, adhesives, paints, varnishes, and lacquers, new carpets or synthetic textiles, emissions from cleaning products and disinfectants, and degradation of building materials. The impact of HCHO on respiratory health is well documented, and its presence indoors has been associated with asthma and respiratory symptoms [35], phlegm, wheezing, and coughing [18].

The main sources of indoor NH_3 are cleaning products, fertilizers, decomposition of organic matter, emissions from pets and humans, and cooking and processed foods. NH_3 was monitored in one study on COPD, but it was not linked to any health outcome [22].

Indoor O_3 originates from electronic devices, photochemical reactions between indoor pollutants and sunlight, ozone-generating air purifiers, and outdoor air infiltration. Irritating effects of O_3 on the respiratory tract can contribute to the exacerbation of asthma conditions [20]. Although ozone forms mainly outdoors, it can penetrate buildings and affect IAQ [54]. In COPD, the studies reviewed did not provide much specific information on the relationship between O_3 exposure and disease progression [32]. In asthma, significant associations between poorly controlled asthma and measures of residential O_3 were reported in [35].

VOCs are very prevalent inside households and are commonly caused by cleaning products, paints, solvents, air fresheners and aerosols, new furniture, carpets, wood products, adhesives, and glues, and use of pesticides and repellents. VOCs have been linked to increased risk and severity of asthma, rhinitis, eczema, and airway inflammation. Sensitivity to VOCs can vary widely among people, and some individuals may experience symptoms at lower exposure levels than others. However, the reviewed sources offered limited specific information on VOCs and disease progression. Only in asthma, a higher risk of allergic rhinitis in adults was associated with VOCs [42].

4.4. Predictive Models and AI

COPD and asthma pose a large burden on healthcare [3,55]. While these CRD cannot be cured, various treatments and approaches can help manage symptoms, improve patient's quality of life, and reduce the risk of adverse outcomes, such as exacerbation. Many severe exacerbations, which contribute to significant morbidity, increased healthcare utilization, disability, and mortality are deemed preventable with appropriate outpatient care [56]. A challenging area of research nowadays is based on the development of AI-based models for predicting severe exacerbations of asthma and COPD. Current models conventionally use physiological information gathered from questionnaires and sensors, but they lack the accuracy needed to reduce severe exacerbations and improve outcomes [23,56]. The identification of novel predictors that can enable the early detection of deterioration has been marked as a goal for home telemonitoring to improve clinical accuracy and prevent hospital admissions, improve the quality of life of patients, and reduce health resource utilization [23].

Machine learning has gained ground in the field of air pollution epidemiology [57]. Over the past decade, research has focused on the impact of outdoor air pollution on respiratory diseases, demonstrating the significant role of outdoor environmental factors in exacerbation prediction [58,59]. Nevertheless, patients may spend much time indoors and consequently can be affected by indoor air pollution levels [59–61].

In this context, machine learning models could use IAQ data to better predict asthma and COPD exacerbations, enabling early interventions and personalized management strategies. However, despite its potential to find interactions between pollutant exposition and disease progression and its potential clinical utility in COPD and asthma [59,62], the application of AI techniques together with IAQ remains underexplored, as evidenced by the low number of studies that addressed this research area. Such developments require the use of interdisciplinary and rigorous methodological approaches, including connecting air quality measurements with health markers during the study period (e.g., through validated health questionnaires, measures of lung function, physiological information gathered using sensors, traceability of exacerbations, medication use and consumption of healthcare resources). Specifically, disease exacerbation episodes were only recorded in 25% of the asthma studies and 50% of the COPD studies. These episodes mark a decline in patient health and account for much of the economic burden on health services [63,64], and their follow-up enables the development of supervised machine learning algorithms [56,65].

4.5. Methodological Considerations

Randomized Controlled Trials (RCTs) are the gold standard in clinical research due to their ability to minimize bias, ensure comparability between groups, and establish causal relationships. However, only 29% conducted randomized controlled studies.

Collecting longitudinal data on IAQ, environmental factors, and health outcomes can be costly and time-consuming, especially for large-scale studies. However, longitudinal studies covering longer periods are needed to assess long-term exposure to different indoor air pollutants and their impact on specific populations, such as children, the elderly, and people with pre-existing respiratory conditions. However, 71% of the studies had a duration of less than 6 months. Most studies were based on point data from surveys or monthly/quarterly measurements of indoor air pollutants, rather than continuous monitoring. A six-month air quality study may miss seasonal variations, limiting its ability to capture long-term trends [66]. Studies of short duration can be influenced by temporary events potentially skewing results. Additionally, geographic and temporal representativeness may be restricted, affecting the study's overall reliability. As a consequence, longitudinal studies of more than one year are needed to better understand the risks of chronic exposure and disease progression.

The distribution of sample sizes within the reviewed literature revealed that 38% of studies (8 out of 21) included 30 or fewer participants. Such limited sample sizes inherently restrict statistical power, potentially compromising the robustness of observed effects and limiting the generalizability of findings. To address these limitations, future research should prioritize larger, multi-center studies to improve the representativeness of study populations and reduce inter-study variability. Regarding the inclusion of spatial variability in the analyses, significant spatial differences in reported health symptoms have been identified in different geographic areas [67]. Geographic variability needs to be considered in future research to understand how regional characteristics, ventilation patterns, and pollution sources influence IAQ and health outcomes [66]. Differences in lifestyle habits, building materials, and sources of pollution can affect the external validity of the results. In addition, the heterogeneity in demographic and health characteristics of participants can limit the generalizability of the findings. Variations in disease severity, age, gender, and other individual factors can influence the response to indoor air pollution. Additionally, the lack of representation of certain socioeconomic or ethnic groups can increase the bias of the results, preventing a comprehensive assessment of the impact of indoor air on the health of all patients.

Finally, from a lower-level technical perspective, the frequency with which air quality data are collected can be a significant limitation. In studies with sporadic measurements, the data may not capture important variations in air quality over time. Pollution peaks and daily or seasonal fluctuations can be overlooked if data are collected only at wide intervals, affecting the accuracy of the assessment of respiratory health impacts.

As a result, there is a clear and compelling need to address the lack of standardization in IAQ monitoring in studies involving patients with CRD. Heterogeneity in measurement protocols, sensor calibration, data communication, sampling rates, and analysis methods makes comparison between studies difficult and limits the ability to draw robust conclusions. To overcome these limitations, a more uniform and rigorous framework for future research is needed, ranging from the definition of unified measurement guidelines (e.g., reaching a consensus on which IAQ parameters should be considered) to the adoption of standardized calibration protocols and the promotion of data interoperability through common communication protocols. In addition, the geographic and socioeconomic variability of the populations under study must be considered.

4.6. Opportunities and Challenges

The applications of air quality sensor-based monitoring technologies to the management of respiratory diseases such as COPD and asthma bring research gaps that must be considered for the further development of this field. The reviewed studies revealed several issues, challenges, opportunities, and limitations that will be discussed in this section.

Several key insights emerged from this review that should be considered in future studies, including the following:

(a) the lack of methodological standardization in studies.
(b) the need for long-term longitudinal trials that consider the spatial variability, individualized measures of exposure to pollutants, and the heterogeneity in demographic and health characteristics of patients.
(c) the key to connecting monitored air quality measurements with respiratory health markers.
(d) the lack of personalized early warning and recommendations systems that combine environmental monitoring with artificial intelligence techniques.

In general, more studies are needed to understand the interaction between exposure to indoor air pollutants and the occurrence of specific respiratory symptoms. It is crucial to identify which pollutants are most associated with specific symptoms so that targeted intervention strategies can be developed. In addition, while the relationship between exposure to pollutants and exacerbation of symptoms has been demonstrated, the exact threshold at which certain pollutants become critical to respiratory health is still unknown. In addition, the study of combinations of pollutants, which are often present in indoor spaces, and their possible synergistic effects, is a challenge yet to be addressed.

The placement of air quality sensors within the home is crucial for obtaining representative data. Sensors placed in specific locations may not accurately reflect conditions in other areas of the home where patients spend time. The lack of standardization in sensor placement can lead to underestimation or overestimation of the levels of pollutants to which patients are exposed. In this regard, monitoring personal exposure, which varies according to microenvironments and individual activities, could have significant implications for improving health outcomes [33]. Portable sensors could provide individualized measures of exposure to pollutants, not only indoors but also outdoors. Currently, advances in sensors and smart devices allow for accurate measurements, but mass deployment of these technologies in homes and work environments remains limited. Developing more accessible and low-cost tools that can be used by the public appears to be a crucial need.

Integrating indoor air pollutant measurements, physiological monitoring devices, patient diaries, and medical records offers a unique opportunity to study exposure-health relationships more accurately. However, this integrated approach was considered only in 33% of the studies.

Finally, a paramount challenge lies in translating scientific knowledge into effective global public policies. Although some countries have adopted regulations to improve IAQ, many regions worldwide, particularly in low- and middle-income countries, face significant limitations in access to healthy housing and IAQ-enhancing technologies.

5. Conclusions

Consistent exposure to certain indoor pollutants has been repeatedly linked to increased symptom severity and exacerbation frequency in vulnerable asthma and COPD patients. This review has examined the impact of air quality on disease management, emphasizing the importance of monitoring and controlling indoor environments to protect respiratory health.

Research on IAQ and its impact on asthma and COPD remains an evolving field with significant open questions and challenges. This systematic review underscores the critical need for larger, multi-center studies and standardized IAQ monitoring protocols in studies involving patients with CRD. The identified research gaps, including the lack of unified measurement guidelines, calibration standards, and data communication protocols, significantly compromise data accuracy and comparability and impede the ability to draw robust conclusions and translate research findings into clinical practice.

Additionally, the relatively short duration of most studies hinders the ability to assess long-term health effects and seasonal pollution variations, while the limited use of technologies such as IoT restricts the potential for real-time monitoring and predictive modeling. Expanding AI applications in IAQ research could improve early detection of health risks and enhance precision medicine. Furthermore, a more comprehensive evaluation of specific sources of indoor pollution (such as emissions from new furniture, home renovations, and allergen exposure) may provide deeper insights into their role in the development of respiratory diseases from early life.

Addressing these limitations and leveraging emerging technological advancements could lead to a more profound understanding of the complex relationship between IAQ and respiratory health. Recent innovations, novel methodologies, and increasing public awareness present promising opportunities to develop effective prevention and management strategies to improve respiratory health. These advances may pave the way for personalized approaches to disease management and support policy and social initiatives aimed at improving the health and well-being of individuals affected by CRD.

Author Contributions: The authors confirm that all listed authors meet the requirements for authorship. P.C.-M.: investigation; methodology; writing—original draft preparation; formal analysis; writing—review and editing; visualization. D.S.-L.: investigation; methodology; formal analysis; writing—review and editing. A.L.-J.: review and editing. D.S.-M.: investigation; methodology; conceptualization; writing—original draft preparation; formal analysis; writing—review and editing; visualization; supervision; project administration; funding acquisition. All authors have read and agreed to the published version of the manuscript.

Funding: This contribution has been supported by grant PID2021-126810OB-I00 funded by MICIU/AEI/10.13039/501100011033 and by ERDF/EU.

Institutional Review Board Statement: This manuscript is a review article and does not involve a protocol requiring approval by the relevant institutional review board or ethics committee.

Informed Consent Statement: Not applicable.

Data Availability Statement: No new data were created or analyzed in this study.

Conflicts of Interest: The authors declare no conflicts of interest. The funders had no role in the design of the study; in the collection, analyses, or interpretation of data; in the writing of the manuscript; or in the decision to publish the results.

Abbreviations

The following abbreviations are used in this manuscript:

ACQ	Asthma Control Questionnaire
ACT	Asthma Control Test
AECOPD	Acute Exacerbation of Chronic Obstructive Pulmonary Disease
AQ	Air Quality
AQI	Air Quality Index
AQLQ	Asthma Quality of Life Questionnaire
ATS-DLD-78A	American Thoracic Society Division of Lung Diseases Questionnaire for Detecting Respiratory Symptoms in Welders
AUC	Area Under the Receive Operating Characteristic Curve
BCSS	Breathlessness, Cough and Sputum Scale
CAT	COPD Assessment Test
CO	Carbon Monoxide
CO_2	Carbon Dioxide
COPD	Chronic Obstructive Pulmonary Disease
CRD	Chronic Respiratory Diseases
DNN	Deep Neural Networks
EEH	Energy-efficient homes
FeNO	Fractional Exhaled Nitric Oxide
FEV1	Forced Expiratory Volume during the first second
FVC	Forced Vital Capacity
HCHO	Formaldehyde
HEPA	High-Efficiency Particulate Air
HRQoL	Health-Related Quality of Life
IAQ	Indoor Air Quality
IoT	Internet of Things
MAPE	Mean Absolute Percentage Error
mMRC	Modified Medical Research Council Dyspnea Scale
NH_3	Ammonia
NO_2	Nitrogen Dioxide
NRCT	Non-randomized Control Trial
O_3	Ozone
OCS	Observational Cohort Study
PEFR	Peak Expiratory Flow Rate
PM	Particulate Matter
RCT	Randomized Control Trial
RH	Relative Humidity
RMSE	Root Mean Square Error
RNN	Recurrent Neural Networks
RQ	Respiratory Questionnaire
SGRQ	St. George's Respiratory Questionnaire
SO_2	Sulfur Dioxide
T	Temperature
VOCs	Volatile Organic Compounds

References

1. World Health Organization. Chronic Respiratory Diseases. Available online: https://www.who.int/health-topics/chronic-respiratory-diseases#tab=tab_1 (accessed on 16 July 2024).
2. Labaki, W.W.; Han, M.K. Chronic respiratory diseases: A global view. *Lancet Respir. Med.* **2020**, *8*, 531–533. [CrossRef] [PubMed]
3. Soriano, J.B.; Kendrick, P.J.; Paulson, K.R.; Gupta, V.; Abrams, E.M.; Adedoyin, R.A.; Adhikari, T.B.; Advani, S.M.; Agrawal, A.; Ahmadian, E.; et al. Prevalence and attributable health burden of chronic respiratory diseases, 1990–2017: A systematic analysis for the Global Burden of Disease Study 2017. *Lancet Respir. Med.* **2020**, *8*, 585–596. [CrossRef]
4. Boers, E.; Barrett, M.; Su, J.G.; Benjafield, A.V.; Sinha, S.; Kaye, L.; Zar, H.J.; Vuong, V.; Tellez, D.; Gondalia, R.; et al. Global Burden of Chronic Obstructive Pulmonary Disease Through 2050. *JAMA Netw. Open* **2023**, *6*, e2346598. [CrossRef] [PubMed]
5. Mattila, T.; Vasankari, T.; Herse, F.; Leskelä, R.-L.; Erhola, M.; Avellan-Hietanen, H.; Toppila-Salmi, S.; Haahtela, T. Contrasting healthcare costs of COPD and asthma in elderly. *Respir. Med.* **2023**, *220*, 107477. [CrossRef] [PubMed]
6. Ahmad, K.; Khanam, R.; Kabir, E.; Jürges, H. The Healthcare Cost Burden of Asthma in Children: A Longitudinal Population-Based Study. *Value Health* **2023**, *26*, 1201–1209. [CrossRef]
7. Wedzicha, J.A. Impact of Chronic Obstructive Pulmonary Disease Exacerbations on Patients and Payers. *Proc. Am. Thorac. Soc.* **2006**, *3*, 218–221. [CrossRef]
8. Halpin, D.M.; Miravitlles, M.; Metzdorf, N.; Celli, B. Impact and prevention of severe exacerbations of COPD: A review of the evidence. *Int. J. Chronic Obstr. Pulm. Dis.* **2017**, *12*, 2891–2908. [CrossRef]
9. Graham, L.M.; Eid, N. The impact of asthma exacerbations and preventive strategies. *Curr. Med. Res. Opin.* **2015**, *31*, 825–835. [CrossRef]
10. Loftus, P.A.; Wise, S.K. Epidemiology and economic burden of asthma. *Int. Forum Allergy Rhinol.* **2015**, *5*, S7–S10. [CrossRef]
11. Kim, H.; Na, G.; Park, S.; Ra, S.W.; Kang, S.-Y.; Kim, H.-C.; Lee, S.W. The impact of life behavior and environment on particulate matter in chronic obstructive pulmonary disease. *Environ. Res.* **2021**, *198*, 111265. [CrossRef]
12. Chi, R.; Chen, C.; Li, H.; Pan, L.; Zhao, B.; Deng, F.; Guo, X. Different health effects of indoor- and outdoor-originated $PM_{2.5}$ on cardiopulmonary function in COPD patients and healthy elderly adults. *Indoor Air* **2019**, *29*, 192–201. [CrossRef] [PubMed]
13. Zhang, Z.; Wang, J.; Lu, W. Exposure to nitrogen dioxide and chronic obstructive pulmonary disease (COPD) in adults: A systematic review and meta-analysis. *Environ. Sci. Pollut. Res. Int.* **2018**, *25*, 15133–15145. [CrossRef] [PubMed]
14. Ghozikali, M.G.; Heibati, B.; Naddafi, K.; Kloog, I.; Conti, G.O.; Polosa, R.; Ferrante, M. Evaluation of Chronic Obstructive Pulmonary Disease (COPD) attributed to atmospheric O_3, NO_2, and SO_2 using Air Q Model (2011–2012 year). *Environ. Res.* **2016**, *144*, 99–105. [CrossRef]
15. Huang, W.; Wu, J.; Lin, X. Ozone Exposure and Asthma Attack in Children. *Front. Pediatr.* **2022**, *10*, 830897. [CrossRef]
16. Agache, I.; Canelo-Aybar, C.; Annesi-Maesano, I.; Cecchi, L.; Rigau, D.; Rodríguez-Tanta, L.Y.; Nieto-Gutierrez, W.; Song, Y.; Cantero-Fortiz, Y.; Roqué, M.; et al. The impact of outdoor pollution and extreme temperatures on asthma-related outcomes: A systematic review for the EAACI guidelines on environmental science for allergic diseases and asthma. *Allergy* **2024**, *79*, 1725–1760. [CrossRef]
17. Bae, W.D.; Kim, S.; Park, C.-S.; Alkobaisi, S.; Lee, J.; Seo, W.; Park, J.S.; Park, S.; Lee, S.; Lee, J.W. Performance improvement of machine learning techniques predicting the association of exacerbation of peak expiratory flow ratio with short term exposure level to indoor air quality using adult asthmatics clustered data. *PLoS ONE* **2021**, *16*, e0244233. [CrossRef]
18. Rabbani, U.F.; Razzaq, S.F.; Irfan, M.F.; Semple, S.; Nafees, A.A.F. Indoor Air Pollution and Respiratory Health in a Metropolitan City of Pakistan. *J. Occup. Environ. Med.* **2022**, *64*, 761–765. [CrossRef]
19. Bhat, G.S.; Shankar, N.; Kim, D.; Song, D.J.; Seo, S.; Panahi, I.M.S.; Tamil, L. Machine Learning-Based Asthma Risk Prediction Using IoT and Smartphone Applications. *IEEE Access* **2021**, *9*, 118708–118715. [CrossRef]
20. Dong, Q.; Li, B.; Downen, R.S.; Tran, N.; Chorvinsky, E.; Pillai, D.K.; Zaghloul, M.E.; Li, Z. A Cloud-Connected NO_2 and Ozone Sensor System for Personalized Pediatric Asthma Research and Management. *IEEE Sens. J.* **2020**, *20*, 15143–15153. [CrossRef]
21. Wu, C.-T.; Li, G.-H.; Huang, C.-T.; Cheng, Y.-C.; Chen, C.-H.; Chien, J.-Y.; Kuo, P.-H.; Kuo, L.-C.; Lai, F. Acute Exacerbation of a Chronic Obstructive Pulmonary Disease Prediction System Using Wearable Device Data, Machine Learning, and Deep Learning: Development and Cohort Study. *JMIR Mhealth Uhealth* **2021**, *9*, e22591. [CrossRef]
22. John, B.J.; Harish, C.; Lawrence, C.C.; Krishnakumar, S.; Divakaran, S.; Premkumar, J.; Kanmani, P.G.; Sabarivani, A.; Jagadeesan, stA.K. Monitoring indoor air quality using smart integrated gas sensor module (IGSM) for improving health in COPD patients. *Environ. Sci. Pollut. Res. Int.* **2023**, *30*, 28889–28902. [CrossRef] [PubMed]
23. Sanchez-Morillo, D.; A Fernandez-Granero, M.; Leon-Jimenez, A. Use of predictive algorithms in-home monitoring of chronic obstructive pulmonary disease and asthma: A systematic review. *Chronic Respir. Dis.* **2016**, *13*, 264–283. [CrossRef] [PubMed]
24. Page, M.J.; McKenzie, J.E.; Bossuyt, P.M.; Boutron, I.; Hoffmann, T.C.; Mulrow, C.D.; Shamseer, L.; Tetzlaff, J.M.; Akl, E.A.; Brennan, S.E.; et al. The PRISMA 2020 statement: An updated guideline for reporting systematic reviews. *BMJ* **2021**, *372*, 71. [CrossRef]

25. Hong, Q.N.; Fàbregues, S.; Bartlett, G.; Boardman, F.; Cargo, M.; Dagenais, P.; Gagnon, M.-P.; Griffiths, F.; Nicolau, B.; O'cathain, A.; et al. The Mixed Methods Appraisal Tool (MMAT) version 2018 for information professionals and researchers. *Educ. Inf.* **2018**, *34*, 285–291. [CrossRef]
26. Popay, J.; Roberts, H.; Sowden, A.; Petticrew, M.; Arai, L.; Rodgers, M.; Britten, N.; Roen, K.; Duffy, S. *Guidance on the Conduct of Narrative Synthesis in Systematic Reviews: A Product from the ESRC Methods Programme*; Peninsula Medical School: Lancaster, UK, 2006.
27. Egger, M.; Zellweger-Zähner, T.; Schneider, M.; Junker, C.; Lengeler, C.; Antes, G. Language bias in randomised controlled trials published in English and German. *Lancet* **1997**, *350*, 326–329. [CrossRef]
28. Bălă, G.-P.; Timar, B.; Gorun, F.; Motisan, R.; Pescaru, C.; Tudorache, E.; Marc, M.; Manolescu, D.; Citu, C.; Oancea, C. The Impact of Air Pollution on Frequent Exacerbations among COPD Patients: An Observational Study on the Population of Western Romania. *J. Clin. Med.* **2022**, *11*, 4352. [CrossRef]
29. Kang, J.; Kim, H.-C.; Jang, Y.; Lee, J.B.; Lee, J.S.; Oh, Y.-M.; Ji, H.W.; Jung, J.Y.; Lee, S.W. Randomised controlled trial of a behavioural intervention to reduce exposure to PM2.5 in patients with COPD. *Environ. Int.* **2023**, *181*, 108286. [CrossRef]
30. Hansel, N.N.; Putcha, N.; Woo, H.; Peng, R.; Diette, G.B.; Fawzy, A.; Wise, R.A.; Romero, K.; Davis, M.F.; Rule, A.M.; et al. Randomized Clinical Trial of Air Cleaners to Improve Indoor Air Quality and Chronic Obstructive Pulmonary Disease Health: Results of the CLEAN AIR Study. *Am. J. Respir. Crit. Care Med.* **2022**, *205*, 421–430. [CrossRef]
31. Guo, S.-E.; Chi, M.-C.; Hwang, S.-L.; Lin, C.-M.; Lin, Y.-C. Effects of Particulate Matter Education on Self-Care Knowledge Regarding Air Pollution, Symptom Changes, and Indoor Air Quality among Patients with Chronic Obstructive Pulmonary Disease. *Int. J. Environ. Res. Public Health* **2020**, *17*, 4103. [CrossRef]
32. Nurhussien, L.; Kang, C.-M.; Koutrakis, P.; Coull, B.A.; Rice, M.B. Air Pollution Exposure and Daily Lung Function in Chronic Obstructive Pulmonary Disease: Effect Modification by Eosinophil Level. *Ann. Am. Thorac. Soc.* **2022**, *19*, 728–736. [CrossRef]
33. McCarron, A.; Semple, S.; Braban, C.F.; Gillespie, C.; Swanson, V.; Price, H.D. Personal exposure to fine particulate matter (PM2.5) and self-reported asthma-related health. *Soc. Sci. Med.* **2023**, *337*, 116293. [CrossRef] [PubMed]
34. Prasasti, C.I.; Haryanto, B.; Latif, M.T. Association of VOCs, PM2.5 and household environmental exposure with children's respiratory allergies. *Air Qual. Atmos. Health* **2021**, *14*, 1279–1287. [CrossRef]
35. Kang, I.; McCreery, A.; Azimi, P.; Gramigna, A.; Baca, G.; Hayes, W.; Crowder, T.; Scheu, R.; Evens, A.; Stephens, B. Impacts of residential indoor air quality and environmental risk factors on adult asthma-related health outcomes in Chicago, IL. *J. Expo. Sci. Environ. Epidemiol.* **2023**, *33*, 358–367. [CrossRef] [PubMed]
36. Schachter, E.N.; Rohr, A.; Habre, R.; Koutrakis, P.; Moshier, E.; Nath, A.; Coull, B.; Grunin, A.; Kattan, M. Indoor air pollution and respiratory health effects in inner city children with moderate to severe asthma. *Air Qual. Atmos. Health* **2020**, *13*, 247–257. [CrossRef]
37. Woo, J.; Lee, J.-H.; Kim, Y.; Rudasingwa, G.; Lim, D.H.; Kim, S. Forecasting the Effects of Real-Time Indoor PM2.5 on Peak Expiratory Flow Rates (PEFR) of Asthmatic Children in Korea: A Deep Learning Approach. *IEEE Access* **2022**, *10*, 19391–19400. [CrossRef]
38. Khusial, R.J.; Honkoop, P.J.; Usmani, O.; Soares, M.; Simpson, A.; Biddiscombe, M.; Meah, S.; Bonini, M.; Lalas, A.; Polychronidou, E.; et al. Effectiveness of myAirCoach: A mHealth Self-Management System in Asthma. *J. Allergy Clin. Immunol. Pract.* **2020**, *8*, 1972–1979.e8. [CrossRef]
39. Lee, G.H.; Kim, J.H.; Kim, S.; Lee, S.; Lim, D.H. Effects of Indoor Air Purifiers on Children with Asthma. *Yonsei Med. J.* **2020**, *61*, 310–316. [CrossRef]
40. Kim, S.; Lee, J.; Park, S.; Rudasingwa, G.; Lee, S.; Yu, S.; Lim, D.H. Association between Peak Expiratory Flow Rate and Exposure Level to Indoor PM2.5 in Asthmatic Children, Using Data from the Escort Intervention Study. *Int. J. Environ. Res. Public Health* **2020**, *17*, 7667. [CrossRef]
41. Hussain, S.; Parker, S.; Edwards, K.; Finch, J.; Jeanjean, A.; Leigh, R.; Gonem, S. Effects of indoor particulate matter exposure on daily asthma control. *Ann. Allergy Asthma Immunol.* **2019**, *123*, 375–380.e3. [CrossRef]
42. Lim, A.-Y.; Yoon, M.; Kim, E.-H.; Kim, H.-A.; Lee, M.J.; Cheong, H.-K. Effects of mechanical ventilation on indoor air quality and occupant health status in energy-efficient homes: A longitudinal field study. *Sci. Total Environ.* **2021**, *785*, 147324. [CrossRef]
43. Raju, S.; Siddharthan, T.; McCormack, M.C. Indoor Air Pollution and Respiratory Health. *Clin. Chest Med.* **2020**, *41*, 825–843. [CrossRef] [PubMed]
44. Eguiluz-Gracia, I.; Mathioudakis, A.G.; Bartel, S.; Vijverberg, S.J.H.; Fuertes, E.; Comberiati, P.; Cai, Y.S.; Tomazic, P.V.; Diamant, Z.; Vestbo, J.; et al. The need for clean air: The way air pollution and climate change affect allergic rhinitis and asthma. *Allergy* **2020**, *75*, 2170–2184. [CrossRef] [PubMed]
45. Bruce, N.; Perez-Padilla, R.; Albalak, R. Indoor air pollution in developing countries: A major environmental and public health challenge. *Bull. World Health Organ.* **2000**, *78*, 1078–1092. [PubMed]
46. Kurmi, O.P.; Semple, S.; Simkhada, P.; Smith, W.C.S.; Ayres, J.G. COPD and chronic bronchitis risk of indoor air pollution from solid fuel: A systematic review and meta-analysis. *Thorax* **2010**, *65*, 221–228. [CrossRef]

47. Raju, S.; Woo, H.; Koehler, K.; Fawzy, A.; Liu, C.; Putcha, N.; Balasubramanian, A.; Peng, R.D.; Lin, C.T.; Lemoine, C.; et al. Indoor Air Pollution and Impaired Cardiac Autonomic Function in Chronic Obstructive Pulmonary Disease. *Am. J. Respir. Crit. Care Med.* **2023**, *207*, 721–730. [CrossRef]
48. Spinelle, L.; Gerboles, M.; Villani, M.G.; Aleixandre, M.; Bonavitacola, F. Field calibration of a cluster of low-cost commercially available sensors for air quality monitoring. Part B: NO, CO and CO_2. *Sens. Actuators B Chem.* **2017**, *238*, 706–715. [CrossRef]
49. Karagulian, F.; Barbiere, M.; Kotsev, A.; Spinelle, L.; Gerboles, M.; Lagler, F.; Redon, N.; Crunaire, S.; Borowiak, A. Review of the Performance of Low-Cost Sensors for Air Quality Monitoring. *Atmosphere* **2019**, *10*, 506. [CrossRef]
50. De Vito, S.; Esposito, E.; Salvato, M.; Popoola, O.; Formisano, F.; Jones, R.; Di Francia, G. Calibrating chemical multisensory devices for real world applications: An in-depth comparison of quantitative machine learning approaches. *Sens. Actuators B Chem.* **2017**, *255*, 1191–1210. [CrossRef]
51. Barot, V.; Kapadia, V. Air Quality Monitoring Systems using IoT: A Review. In Proceedings of the 2020 International Conference on Computational Performance Evaluation (ComPE), Shillong, India, 2–4 July 2020; pp. 226–231. [CrossRef]
52. Ullo, S.L.; Sinha, G.R. Advances in Smart Environment Monitoring Systems Using IoT and Sensors. *Sensors* **2020**, *20*, 3113. [CrossRef]
53. Kumar, A.; Dhawan, S.; Bhatt, S.; Saxena, A.; Khare, M.; Dubey, S.K.; Mehta, D.S. Ambient particulate matter monitoring using bright field imaging-based sensor. *Mater. Today Proc.* **2024**. [CrossRef]
54. Chen, C.; Zhao, B. Review of relationship between indoor and outdoor particles: I/O ratio, infiltration factor and penetration factor. *Atmos. Environ.* **2011**, *45*, 275–288. [CrossRef]
55. Momtazmanesh, S.; Moghaddam, S.S.; Ghamari, S.-H.; Rad, E.M.; Rezaei, N.; Shobeiri, P.; Aali, A.; Abbasi-Kangevari, M.; Abbasi-Kangevari, Z.; Abdelmasseh, M.; et al. Global burden of chronic respiratory diseases and risk factors, 1990–2019: An update from the Global Burden of Disease Study 2019. *eClinicalMedicine* **2023**, *59*, 101936. [CrossRef]
56. Zeng, S.; Arjomandi, M.; Tong, Y.; Liao, Z.C.; Luo, G. Developing a Machine Learning Model to Predict Severe Chronic Obstructive Pulmonary Disease Exacerbations: Retrospective Cohort Study. *J. Med. Internet Res.* **2022**, *24*, e28953. [CrossRef] [PubMed]
57. Bellinger, C.; Jabbar, M.S.M.; Zaïane, O.; Osornio-Vargas, A. A systematic review of data mining and machine learning for air pollution epidemiology. *BMC Public Health* **2017**, *17*, 907. [CrossRef] [PubMed]
58. YoussefAgha, A.H.; Jayawardene, W.P.; Lohrmann, D.K.; El Afandi, G.S. Air pollution indicators predict outbreaks of asthma exacerbations among elementary school children: Integration of daily environmental and school health surveillance systems in Pennsylvania. *J. Environ. Monit.* **2012**, *14*, 3202–3210. [CrossRef]
59. Ratcliff, G.E.; Matheny, M.E.; Brown, J.R.; Sullivan, I.; Richmond, B.W.; Paulin, L.M.; Conger, A.K.; Davis, S.E. Integrating Clinical and Air Quality Data to Improve Prediction of COPD Exacerbations. *AMIA Annu. Symp. Proc.* **2024**, *2023*, 1209–1217. Available online: https://pmc.ncbi.nlm.nih.gov/articles/PMC10785856 (accessed on 14 February 2025).
60. Hansel, N.N.; McCormack, M.C.; Belli, A.J.; Matsui, E.C.; Peng, R.D.; Aloe, C.; Paulin, L.; Williams, D.L.; Diette, G.B.; Breysse, P.N. In-Home Air Pollution Is Linked to Respiratory Morbidity in Former Smokers with Chronic Obstructive Pulmonary Disease. *Am. J. Respir. Crit. Care Med.* **2013**, *187*, 1085–1090. [CrossRef]
61. Klepeis, N.E.; Nelson, W.C.; Ott, W.R.; Robinson, J.P.; Tsang, A.M.; Switzer, P.; Behar, J.V.; Hern, S.C.; Engelmann, W.H. The National Human Activity Pattern Survey (NHAPS): A resource for assessing exposure to environmental pollutants. *J. Expo. Sci. Environ. Epidemiol.* **2001**, *11*, 231–252. [CrossRef]
62. Winquist, A.; Kirrane, E.; Klein, M.; Strickland, M.; Darrow, L.A.; Sarnat, S.E.; Gass, K.; Mulholland, J.; Russell, A.; Tolbert, P. Joint Effects of Ambient Air Pollutants on Pediatric Asthma Emergency Department Visits in Atlanta, 1998–2004. *Epidemiology* **2014**, *25*, 666–673. [CrossRef]
63. Perera, P.N.; Armstrong, E.P.; Sherrill, D.L.; Skrepnek, G.H. Acute Exacerbations of COPD in the United States: Inpatient Burden and Predictors of Costs and Mortality. *COPD J. Chronic Obstr. Pulm. Dis.* **2012**, *9*, 131–141. [CrossRef]
64. Rennard, S.I.; Farmer, S.G. Exacerbations and Progression of Disease in Asthma and Chronic Obstructive Pulmonary Disease. *Proc. Am. Thorac. Soc.* **2004**, *1*, 88–92. [CrossRef] [PubMed]
65. Xiong, S.; Chen, W.; Jia, X.; Jia, Y.; Liu, C. Machine learning for prediction of asthma exacerbations among asthmatic patients: A systematic review and meta-analysis. *BMC Pulm. Med.* **2023**, *23*, 278. [CrossRef]
66. Xydi, I.; Saharidis, G.; Kalantzis, G.; Pantazopoulos, I.; Gourgoulianis, K.I.; Kotsiou, O.S. Assessing the Impact of Spatial and Temporal Variability in Fine Particulate Matter Pollution on Respiratory Health Outcomes in Asthma and COPD Patients. *J. Pers. Med.* **2024**, *14*, 833. [CrossRef] [PubMed]
67. Li, C.; Managi, S. Spatial Variability of the Relationship between Air Pollution and Well-being. *Sustain. Cities Soc.* **2022**, *76*, 103447. [CrossRef]

technologies

MDPI

Review

A Review of Assistive Devices in Synovial Joints: Records, Trends, and Classifications

Filiberto Cruz-Flores [1], Ana L. Sánchez-Brito [1], Rafael Campos Amezcua [1], Agustín Barrera Sánchez [1], Héctor R. Azcaray Rivera [2], Arturo J. Martínez Mata [3] and Andrés Blanco Ortega [1,*]

[1] Departamento de Ingeniería Mecánica, Tecnológico Nacional de México/CENIDET, Interior Int, Palmira s/n. Col. Palmira, Cuernavaca 62490, Morelos, Mexico; d18ce054@cenidet.tecnm.mx (F.C.-F.); ana.sanchez19me@cenidet.edu.mx (A.L.S.-B.); rafael.ca@cenidet.tecnm.mx (R.C.A.); d19ce002@cenidet.tecnm.mx (A.B.S.)

[2] Departamento de Ingeniería Electrónica, Tecnológico Nacional de México-Instituto Tecnológico de Oaxaca, Oaxaca de Juárez 68033, Oaxaca, Mexico; hector.azcaray@itoaxaca.edu.mx

[3] Departamento de Metalmecánica, Tecnológico Nacional de México-Instituto Tecnológico de Zacatepec, Zacatepec 62780, Morelos, Mexico; arturo.mm@zacatepec.tecnm.mx

* Correspondence: andres.bo@cenidet.tecnm.mx

Abstract: This article presents a comprehensive review of assistive devices for synovial joints, addressing their definitions, classifications, and technological advancements. The historical evolution of artificial exoskeletons, orthoses, prostheses, and splints is analyzed, emphasizing their impact on rehabilitation and the enhancement of human mobility. Through a systematic compilation of scientific literature, patents, and medical regulations, the study clarifies terminology and classifications that have often been imprecisely used in scientific discourse. The review examines the biomechanical principles of the musculoskeletal system and the kinematics of synovial joints, providing a reference framework for the optimization and design of these devices. Furthermore, it explores the various types of artificial exoskeletons, and their classification based on structure, mobility, power source, and control system, as well as their applications in medical, industrial, and military domains. Finally, this study highlights the necessity of a systematic approach in the design and categorization of these technologies to facilitate their development, comparison, and effective implementation, ultimately improving users' quality of life.

Keywords: exoskeleton; orthosis; prosthesis; splint; synovial joint; movements; trajectories; origins; records; appearances; definitions; uses; differences; biomechanics

1. Introduction

Low back pain is the leading contributor to the overall burden of musculoskeletal diseases. An analysis of the Global Burden of Disease (GBD) reports 570 million prevalent cases worldwide, responsible for 7.4% of global activities of daily living (ADLs). Other contributors to the overall musculoskeletal disease burden include fractures, which affect 440 million people globally (26 million ADLs), and osteoarthritis, impacting 528 million people (19 million ADLs), neck pain (222 million people; 22 million ADLs), amputations (180 million people; 5.5 million ADLs), rheumatoid arthritis (18 million people; 2.4 million ADLs), gout (54 million people; 1.7 million ADLs), and other musculoskeletal conditions (453 million people; 38 million ADLs) [1]. As a solution, musculoskeletal assistive devices are used, which mimic the behavior of synovial joints to prevent, correct, and predict injuries.

It is incredible that technologies exist that are adapted to human physiology, providing superior characteristics to those we possess. Technologies can enhance and amplify movements and forces, acting as a sort of external bones and muscles. For decades, technologies that resemble animal behavior have been developed [2–4], such as devices that mimic biological nature, including their physiological functions and chemical characteristics [5–7]. Based on this, mechanical and mechatronic adaptations have been made to suit the physiology of the human body, primarily to artificially exploit these characteristics.

This article will address devices that align with joint movement behavior, that is, assisting the movement of one or more synovial joints. Devices such as splints, prostheses, orthoses, and exoskeletons that have been under development for years. Prostheses have existed since the time of the ancient Egyptians [8], splints were crucial in events such as wars, where devices were needed to immobilize areas of the body to transport the wounded [9], or in more recent times, where artificial exoskeletons are of great help for a soldier or a worker in the industry, being especially effective in rehabilitation, just like orthoses. Additionally, the benefits these devices offer are extremely useful, and although still costly, the initiative to focus on technologies designed to assist a person's movement has gained increasing importance. The intricacy of such technology, the complexity of locomotion, and understanding of the movement trajectories in space are key, as this would lead to a better understanding of them and allow for artificial replication.

An artificial exoskeleton, in addition to fulfilling its specific design applications, can perform functions like those of a splint, orthosis, or prosthesis. Although it shares some similar characteristics with an orthosis, its functions and applications vary depending on the type of use. Like a prosthesis, which helps reinforce or replace an affected area, an exoskeleton can also serve as an assistance device, adapting to the user's needs over time, with differences in its use depending on the phase of support required. This creates a competitive environment for innovation, encouraging more and more researchers to take an interest in the topic. Research relies on concepts, definitions, and classifications, which, although not misused, have not been applied correctly based on their definition and intended use. This commonly occurs in article titles, newspapers, brochures, and general publications, causing difficulty for researchers to find information in a relevant way, and leading to a lack of uniformity in public information.

This article is structured into several sections to facilitate understanding. Section 2 presents the materials and methods used in the review. Also, in Section 2 the biomechanical characteristics of synovial joints are presented. Section 3 details the classifications and definitions of assistive devices. Section 4 examines current technological trends and their future implications. Finally, Section 5 presents the conclusions and recommendations for the future development of these devices.

2. Materials and Methods

2.1. Splints, Prostheses, Orthoses, and Artificial Exoskeletons

For a person to perform movements, it must be clarified that these consist of the displacement of limbs at a point in space. To carry out bodily movements, it is important to consider that they are performed with the force generated by the muscles, under the supervision of sensory and mechanical fields, and with the freedoms and restrictions that the joints impose. A study by the World Health Organization from 1990 to 2019 determined that, globally, there were a total of 178 million bone fractures [10]. This represents a 33.4% increase since the 1990s, compared to the analyses provided by the Global Burden of Disease (GBD), which showed that around 1.71 million people worldwide suffer from musculoskeletal conditions, including bone fractures, sprains, osteoarthritis, and amputations, among others [1]. For this reason, devices that correct and prevent injuries are essential for rehabilitation and/or treatment follow-up, to improve reversible injuries or provide temporary or permanent replacements, with the goal of allowing a person to have a dignified life routine.

Devices such as splints, prostheses, orthoses, and artificial exoskeletons were, and continue to be, developed to improve rehabilitation capabilities, ergonomics, and assistance with injuries or limitations of the human body. Lighter devices with greater and better characteristics, and above all, economical accessibility, are necessary. Devices are constantly being evaluated or are being improved with new materials or new sophisticated technologies.

Technologies such as assistive devices provide artificial characteristics for different areas of the body, with some focused on containing, replacing, enhancing, and smoothing movements and loads. The National Library of Medicine of the United States defines a splint as a device used to stabilize a part of the body to reduce pain and prevent further injury [11]. A prosthesis is a device designed to replace a missing body part or to improve the function of an existing body part. Injured or missing eyes, arms, hands, legs, or joints are commonly replaced with prosthetic devices [12]. The University of Michigan Health describes an orthosis as a device designed to improve biomechanical function, encourage proper joint alignment, or protect an existing limb [13]. Garcia, M.A. et al. describe an exoskeleton as a type of assistance/rehabilitation robot that can be worn by a human [14]. According to Urrea, C. et al., an exoskeleton is a structure intended to be worn on the human body as a piece of clothing, i.e., a wearable robot (WR), either to complement the function of a limb or to completely replace it [15]. In summary, the four types of human body movement assistance devices can be defined as:

- Splint: It is based on the immobilization of the joint(s).
- Prosthesis: It has two characteristics: to replace the function of amputated areas or to reinforce damaged areas.
- Orthosis: It is based on limiting the range of motion of a single joint.
- Artificial exoskeleton: It is based on increasing physical resistance and the smoothness of movements in the joint(s).

The idea of creating an information database is supported, covering everything from the biological and biomechanical aspects of a person's movements to their mechanical adaptation in artificial assistive devices, creating classifications based on their etymology and application. To achieve this, the biomechanical study of the musculoskeletal system and the classifications of the different joints in the human body were addressed.

2.2. Musculoskeletal System

The musculoskeletal system, according to Poon, L. et al. (2017), is an organ system that provides the framework, support, stability, and movement to the human body, playing a pivotal role in our daily function [16]. Cathy, S. et al. (2014) describes the composition of the musculoskeletal system with ligaments, bones, tendons, cartilage, and connective tissues [17].

The coordinated work of these systems allows a person to perform movements, but this is merely the force-generating work; however, the nervous system and the joints control muscular movements and determine the range and manner of motion, respectively. The unification of the force generated by the musculoskeletal system, the control of the nervous system, and the freedoms of movement characteristic of the joints allow for actions such as standing, sitting, running, walking, among others. Gordon, J. et al. (2013)

describe the movement of the musculoskeletal system as a series of 6 characteristic types of movements [18]. Hinge, Pivot, Saddle, Condyloid, Bell and Socket, Plane.

In Figure 1, an example of each of the six characteristic movements is provided, indicating the type of movement in the joint. Although this would not be the only movement, as a joint can be uniaxial, biaxial, or multiaxial, this depends on the axis and plane of the specific type of movement of the joints.

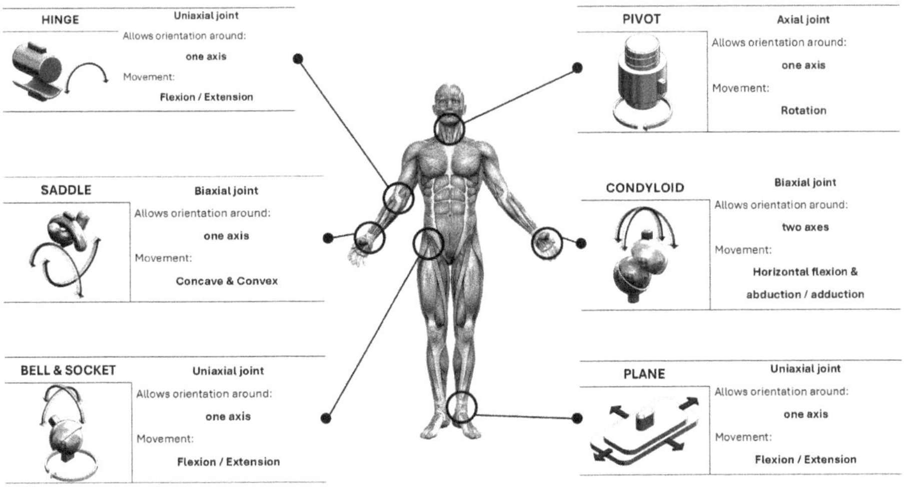

Figure 1. Mechanical movements associated with synovial joints in a person.

The characteristic movements of the joints are essential for understanding movement trajectories and, with this, characterize devices that are more faithful to the movement of the musculoskeletal system. Below, the different types of joints are analyzed, from their biological characteristics to their biomechanical ones.

2.3. *Joints*

A joint is a point where two skeletal elements come into contact [19], allowing movement between them. Joints are essential for mobility and the function of the musculoskeletal system in the human body. There are different types of joints, classified based on their structure and the amount of movement they allow. The main categories of joints are fibrous, cartilaginous, and synovial [19]. Fibrous and cartilaginous joints allow very limited movements, such as those of the skull or the vertebrae in the spine, as they are connected by fibrous connective tissue and cartilage, respectively, while synovial joints are formed by a joint capsule, synovial fluid, and articular surfaces covered with cartilage, such as the knee [19]. Considering that fibrous and cartilaginous joints have very limited movements, they can be considered as fixed or low-mobility joints, while synovial joints allow a wide variety of movements.

Once the structural composition of fibrous, cartilaginous, and synovial joints is understood, it becomes viable to analyze synovial joints, as they possess the mobility required for the behavior of movement trajectories and the range of movements of different body segments. According to the volumes of A. I. Kapandji [20–22], joint physiology is highlighted in three sections: upper limb [20], lower limb [21], and trunk and spine [22]. Due to the limited information available on the trunk and spine in assistive devices, only the joints located in the upper and lower limbs will be addressed.

In Table 1, the joints belonging to each section of the body are broken down. As mentioned earlier, this article will only focus on analyzing the joints belonging to the upper limbs (Elbow, Shoulder, Hand, and Wrist) and lower limbs (Pelvic Girdle, Hip, Gait, Foot, Knee, Ankle).

Table 1. Distribution of joints across the sections of the human body.

Section	Articulation	Segments	Location
Upper limb	Elbow Shoulder Hand Wrist	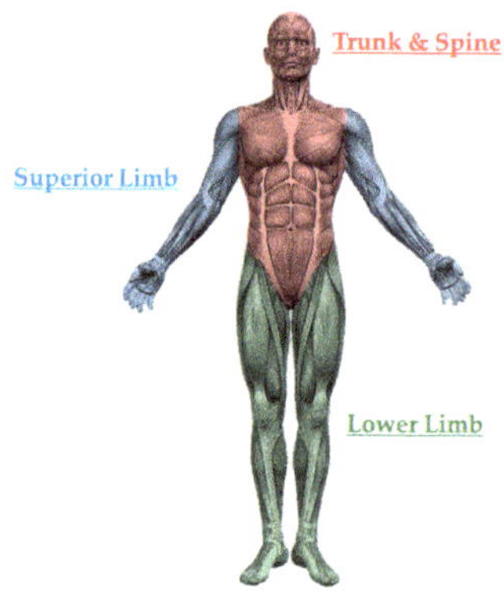	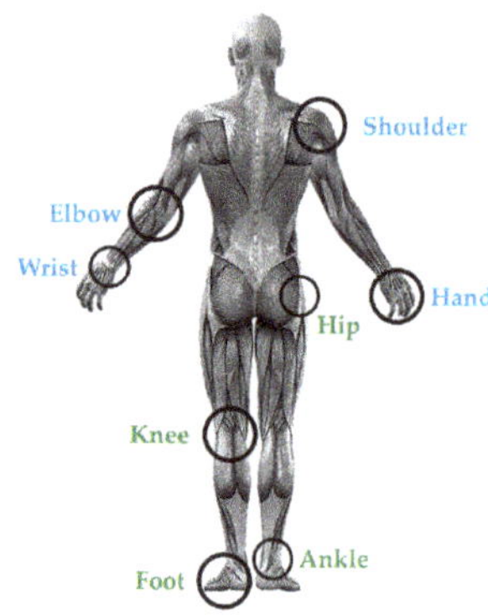
Trunk and spine	Head Pelvic Girdle Spine Cervical Spine Torsal Spine Lumbar Spine Thorax		
Lower limb	Planar Vault Hip Foot Knee Ankle	(**a**)	(**b**)

(**a**) Localization of the three articular segments—blue: upper limb, green: lower limb, red: trunk and spine. (**b**) Localization of the synovial joints of the upper and lower limbs throughout the human body.

There is a movement called "pronation–supination" [20] (pp. 102–145), located between the elbow and wrist joints, known as the "forearm". This movement is used to position the hand when grasping objects. The forearm has one degree of freedom, and its movement occurs along the axis between the elbow and wrist, as these two joints share an axis, the transverse axis, which can be considered the axis for pronation and supination movement [20] (pp. 102–145). In the lower limb, the knee and foot can exhibit a similar movement to pronation–supination; however, this movement originates from the hip, making it an additional movement to that of the hip.

In Table 1 and Figure 2, the distribution of joints throughout the body and their additions, such as the forearm, can be seen. This refers to the movement of the musculoskeletal system, which is essential for the development of technological devices for joint assistance, in this case, synovial joints. By locating the joints, biomechanical analyses can be made, which are useful for calculating ideal trajectories for improvements in assistive devices. Table 2 describes the joints of the upper limb, considering their axes as degrees of mobility and their biomechanical description.

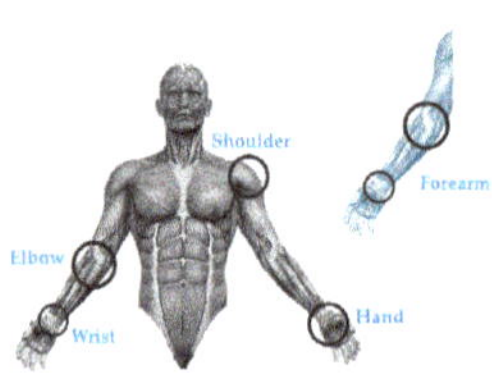

Figure 2. Location of the forearm between the elbow and wrist joints in the upper limb; pronation and supination movement, also known as pronosupination.

Table 2. Description of the upper limb joints.

Articulation	Mobility (Axis)	Description
Shoulder	3	This joint is formed between the humerus, scapula, and clavicle [20] (pp. 2–13). Superficial muscles, such as the deltoid and trapezius, along with deep muscles (supraspinatus, infraspinatus, teres minor, and subscapularis), reinforce this joint. The shoulder is crucial for movements such as abduction, adduction, flexion, and rotation of the arm [20] (pp. 13–74).
Arm	-	The humerus is the main bone in this region. The arm muscles include the biceps brachii, brachialis, and coracobrachialis [20] (pp. 102–145). These muscles are innervated by the brachial plexus and enable movements such as elbow flexion and extension [20] (pp. 102–145).
Elbow	1	The elbow joint involves three bones: the humerus, radius, and ulna [20] (pp. 76–90). It allows for flexion, extension, pronation, and supination movements. The muscles of the anterior compartment (coracobrachialis, brachialis, biceps brachii) and posterior compartment (triceps brachii) are responsible for these movements [20] (pp. 92–102).
Forearm (Elbow–Wrist)	1	In this region, the radius and ulna are the main bones [20] (pp. 104–132). The radial, ulnar, and median nerves innervate the muscles of the forearm. These muscles are divided into anterior compartments (superficial, intermediate, and deep) and posterior compartments (superficial and deep) [20] (pp. 134–144).
Wrist	2	The wrist joint, also known as the radiocarpal joint, is an anatomical structure that connects the bones of the forearm (ulna and radius) with the carpal bones, allowing the connection between the forearm and the hand [20] (pp. 146–150). The joint between the distal radius and the pyramidal bone is indirect and facilitated by the biconcave articular disk, enabling flexion, extension, adduction, and abduction movements [20] (pp. 150–194).
Hand	25	The hand consists of several carpal bones (scaphoid, lunate, pyramidal, pisiform, trapezium, trapezoid, capitate, and hamate), five metacarpals, and phalanges [20] (pp. 198–234). The radial, ulnar, and median nerves also innervate the muscles of the hand, such as the thenar, hypothenar, and metacarpal groups [20] (pp. 238–340).

Body movements are represented in axes and planes [20–23] that describe the characteristic movements of the joints. See Figure 3. The sagittal plane divides the body into right and left halves and allows flexion and extension movements. The frontal plane divides the body into anterior and posterior parts, allowng abduction and adduction movements, and the transverse plane crosses the upper and lower body, allowing rotations [20,23].

In Figure 3, a graphical representation is made for oriental with respect to Table 3 and Figures 4 and 5.

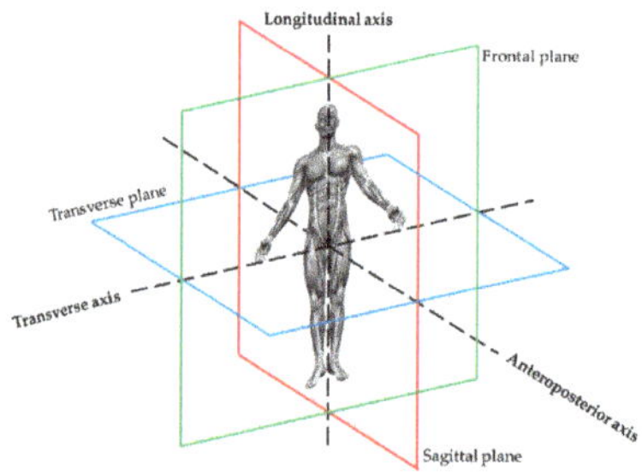

Figure 3. Planes and axes belonging to the spatial references in a person.

Table 3. Characteristic movements in each joint of the upper limb.

<table>
<tr><th>Articulation</th><th>DOF</th><th colspan="2">Axis</th><th>Plane</th><th>Characteristic Movement</th><th>Figure</th></tr>
<tr><td rowspan="3">Shoulder</td><td rowspan="3">3</td><td colspan="2">Transverse</td><td>Sagittal</td><td>F/E</td><td>Figure 4a</td></tr>
<tr><td colspan="2">Anteroposterior</td><td>Frontal</td><td>Ab/Ad</td><td>Figure 4b</td></tr>
<tr><td colspan="2">Longitudinal</td><td>Transverse</td><td>F/E Horizontal</td><td>Figure 4c</td></tr>
<tr><td>Elbow</td><td>1</td><td colspan="2">Transverse</td><td>Sagittal</td><td>F/E</td><td>Figure 5a</td></tr>
<tr><td>Forearm</td><td>1</td><td colspan="2">Longitudinal</td><td>Transverse</td><td>P/S</td><td>Figure 5b</td></tr>
<tr><td rowspan="2">Wrist</td><td rowspan="2">2</td><td colspan="2">Transverse</td><td>Sagittal</td><td>F/E</td><td rowspan="2">Figure 5c</td></tr>
<tr><td colspan="2">Anteroposterior</td><td>Frontal</td><td>Ab/Ad</td></tr>
<tr><td rowspan="8">Hand</td><td rowspan="8">25</td><td>Finger</td><td>DOF</td><td>Axis</td><td>Characteristic movement</td><td rowspan="8">Finger movements produce excessive volume of content. The book A. I. Kapandji is recommended: Physiology, upper limb [20] (pp. 198–340).</td></tr>
<tr><td rowspan="3">Thumb</td><td rowspan="3">5</td><td>Interphalangeal</td><td>F/E</td></tr>
<tr><td>Metacarpophalangeal</td><td>F/E—Ab/Ad</td></tr>
<tr><td>Carpometacarpal</td><td>F/E—Ab/Ad</td></tr>
<tr><td rowspan="4">Index
Middle Ring
Pinky</td><td rowspan="4">5</td><td>Distal Interphalangeal</td><td>F/E</td></tr>
<tr><td>Proximal</td><td>F/E</td></tr>
<tr><td>Metacarpophalangeal</td><td>F/E—Ab/Ad</td></tr>
<tr><td>Carpometacarpal</td><td>F/E</td></tr>
</table>

F/E: Flexion/Extension; Ab/Ad: Abduction/Adduction; P/S: Pronation/Supination.

Given that the information collected for joint movements is extensive, the joints, degrees of freedom, axes, planes, characteristic movements, and illustrative references will be described in independent figures (Figures 4 and 5), as their descriptions cannot be clearly distinguished within the space provided in Table 3.

From Table 1, the joints of the upper limb and their pronosupination were taken as the basis, and in the same table, the joints of the lower limb are described. Like the previous joints, these are analyzed to calculate ideal trajectories for improving assistive devices. In Table 4, the joints of the lower limb are described, considering their axes, degrees of mobility, and biomechanical description. Given that the information collected for joint movements is extensive, the joints, degrees of freedom, axes, planes, characteristic movements, and illustrative references will be described in independent figures (Figures 6 and 7), as their descriptions cannot be clearly distinguished within the space provided in the table.

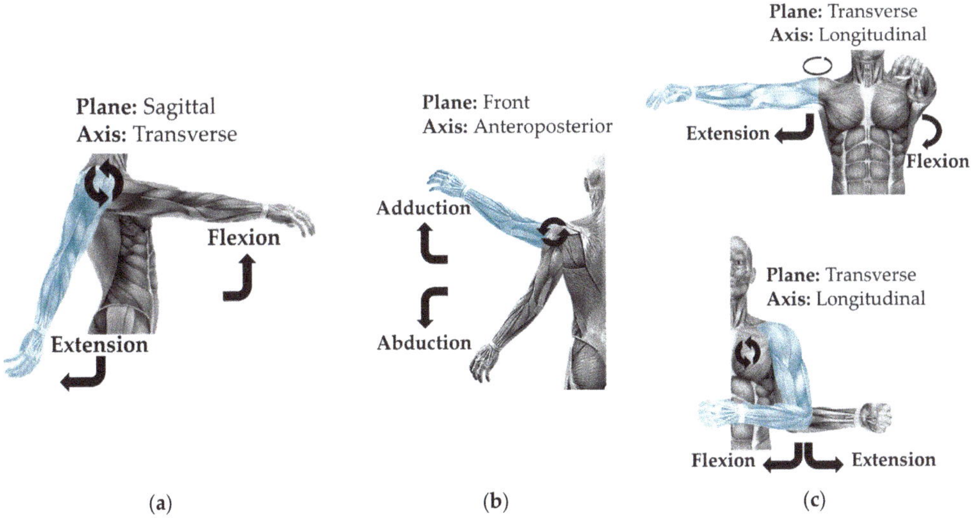

Figure 4. Shoulder movements: (**a**) movement in the transverse axis; (**b**) movement in the anteroposterior axis; (**c**) movement in the longitudinal axis.

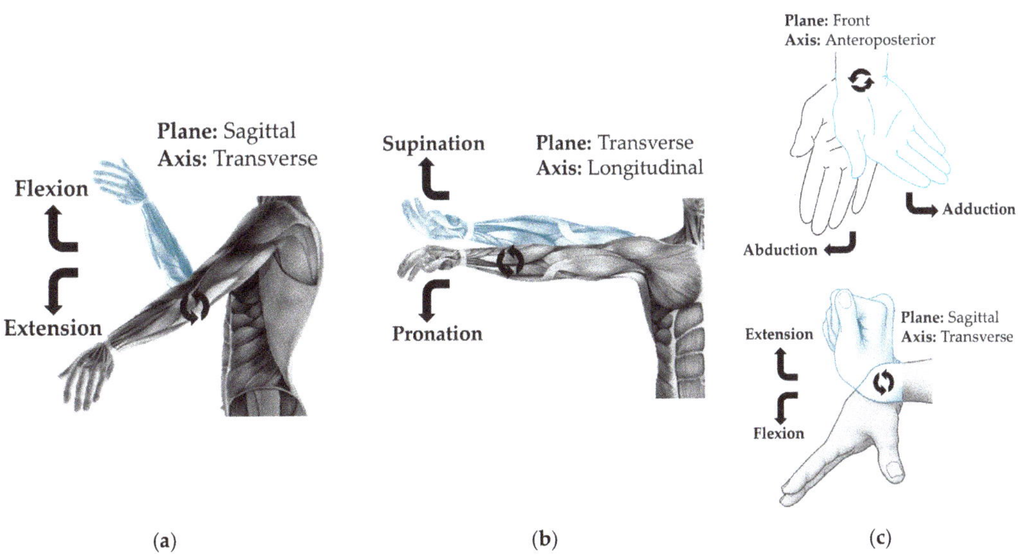

Figure 5. Movements of the elbow, forearm, and wrist: (**a**) movement on the transversal axis; (**b**) movement on the longitudinal axis; (**c**) movement on the anteroposterior and transversal axes.

Table 4. Description of the joints of the lower limb.

Articulation	Mobility (Axis)	Description
Hip	3	It is a type of ball-and-socket joint that connects the hip bone (formed by the ilium, ischium, and pubis) with the femur [21] (pp. 14–32). The joint capsule is strong and fibrous, surrounding the joint. Movements include flexion, extension, abduction, adduction, and rotation [21] (pp. 34–72).
Knee	1	It is a synovial joint that connects the femur with the tibia and the patella. The articular surfaces are the femoral condyles and the tibial surfaces [21] (pp. 76–86). The main movements are flexion and extension. In terms of planes and axes, flexion and extension occur in the sagittal plane around the transverse axis [21] (pp. 88–156).
Ankle	2	It is a joint that connects the tibia and fibula with the talus. The articular surfaces are the tibiofibular mortise and the talus [21] (pp. 160–162). Movements include plantar flexion (pointing the toes downward) and dorsiflexion (lifting the toes). These movements occur in the sagittal plane around the transverse axis [21] (pp. 164–174).
Foot	33	These include the tarsometatarsal, metatarsophalangeal, and interphalangeal joints [21] (pp. 178–182). These allow movements such as flexion, extension, abduction, and adduction of the toes [21] (pp. 184–224).

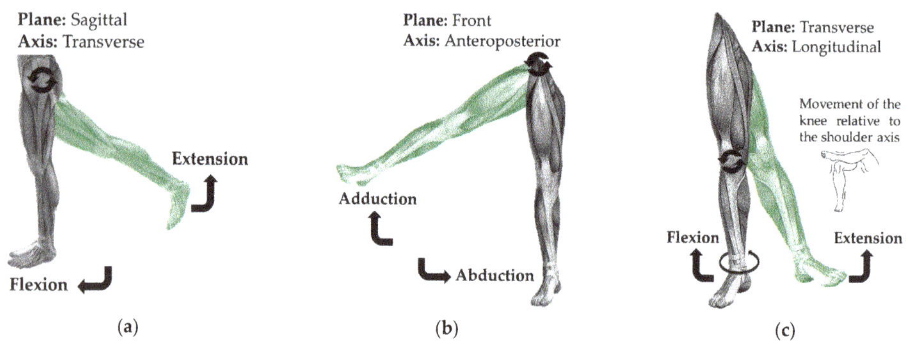

Figure 6. Hip movements: (**a**) movement around the transverse axis; (**b**) movement around the anteroposterior axis; (**c**) movement around the longitudinal axis.

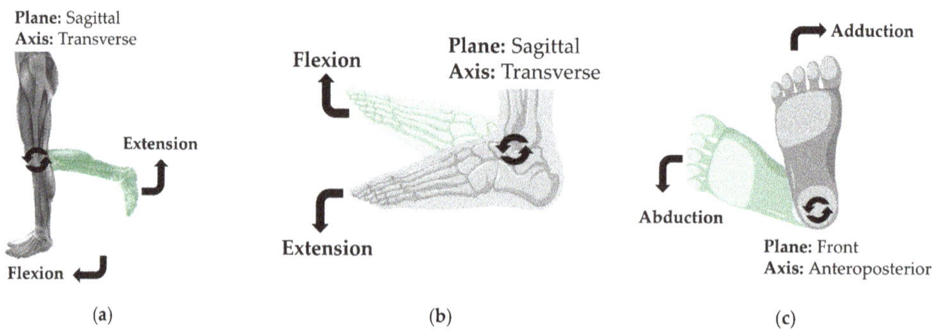

Figure 7. (**a**) Knee movements around the transverse axis; (**b**) ankle movement; (**b**) movement around the transverse axis; (**c**) movement around the anteroposterior axis.

Given that the information collected for joint movements is extensive, the joints, degrees of freedom, axes, planes, characteristic movements, and illustrative references will be described in independent figures (Figures 6 and 7), as their descriptions cannot be clearly distinguished within the space provided in Table 5.

Table 5. Characteristic movements in each joint.

<table>
<tr><th>Articulation</th><th>DOF</th><th>Axis</th><th>Plane</th><th>Characteristic Movement</th><th>Figure</th></tr>
<tr><td>Hip</td><td>3</td><td>Transverse
Anteroposterior
Longitudinal</td><td>Sagittal
Frontal
Transverse</td><td>F/E *
Ab/Ad *
F/E Horizontal</td><td>Figure 6a
Figure 6b
Figure 6c</td></tr>
<tr><td>Knee</td><td>1</td><td>Transverse</td><td>Sagittal</td><td>F/E—P/S *</td><td>Figure 7a</td></tr>
<tr><td>Ankle</td><td>2</td><td>Transverse
Longitudinal</td><td>Sagittal
Transverse</td><td>Fd/Fp *
I/E *</td><td>Figure 7b,c</td></tr>
<tr><td>Foot</td><td>33</td><td colspan="3"><table>
<tr><th>Articulation</th><th>DOF</th><th>Axis</th><th>Characteristic movement</th></tr>
<tr><td>Talocrural</td><td>2</td><td>Transverse</td><td>Fd/Fp</td></tr>
<tr><td>Talocalcaneonavicular</td><td>2</td><td>Anteroposterior</td><td>I/E</td></tr>
<tr><td>Calcaneocuboid</td><td>1</td><td>Anteroposterior</td><td>MD *</td></tr>
<tr><td>Toes</td><td>30</td><td></td><td></td></tr>
<tr><td>Big</td><td>1</td><td>Interphalangeal</td><td>F/E—Ab/Ad</td></tr>
<tr><td rowspan="2">Second, Third, Fourth, Fifth</td><td rowspan="2">2</td><td>Proximal</td><td>F/E—Ab/Ad</td></tr>
<tr><td>Distal</td><td>F/E—Ab/Ad</td></tr>
</table></td><td>Finger movements produce excessive volume of content. The book by A. I. Kapandji is recommended: Physiology, upper limb [21] (pp. 178–224).</td></tr>
</table>

* F/E: Flexion/Extension; Ab/Ad: Abduction/Adduction; P/S: Pronation/Supination; Fd/Fp: Dorsiflexion/Plantar Flexion; I/E: Inversion/Eversion; MD: Gliding Movement.

The movements of the upper and lower limbs are crucial for the design and analysis of robotic devices due to their complexity and variety. These movements are directly related to human biomechanics, involving precise interactions between bones, muscles, tendons, and joints, enabling a wide range of actions and adaptability in various daily tasks. For a robotic device to effectively mimic these movements, it is essential to thoroughly understand how they are performed, both kinematically and dynamically. By studying natural human movements, the kinematics of the exoskeleton or robot can be optimized, improving its ability to replicate human gestures with precision. This not only enhances the device's efficiency and comfort but also allows for better integration into the user's daily activities, ensuring smoother usage and reducing the risk of injury or fatigue. A robot's ability to accurately emulate human movements is also crucial for ensuring that the assistance provided is effective and natural, thus optimizing the device's performance and interaction with the environment.

In the synovial joints of an average person, understanding movement and its behavior is useful, as the trajectories generated by these joints help develop devices that behave more appropriately according to the movement axes of each joint. In Table 6, the function and application area where each device is most used are described, as each device has its own characteristic application. The four devices are illustrated from the elbow joint, located in the upper limb of a person, as this joint has only one degree of freedom and can be described more simply.

Table 6. Description of the functioning of each device.

Device	Function	Application	Figure
Splint	The angle of the joint at which the device is placed will remain in that position until the device is removed.	Medical and Civil	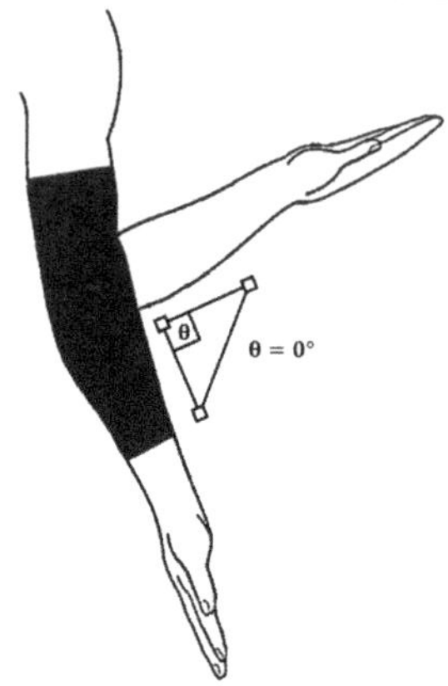
Prosthesis	It replaces or adapts artificial devices in segments with fractures or amputations, substituting the function of the bone, muscle, or joint, or all of them.	Medical and Civil	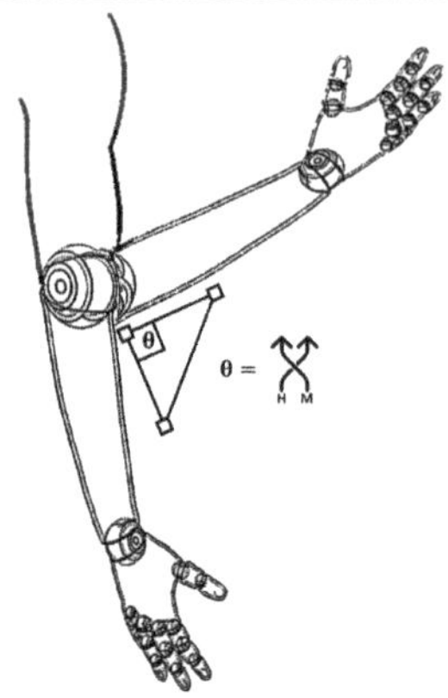
Orthosis	It allows the joint to move within a set range. It can completely stop the movement of the joint.	Medical and Civil	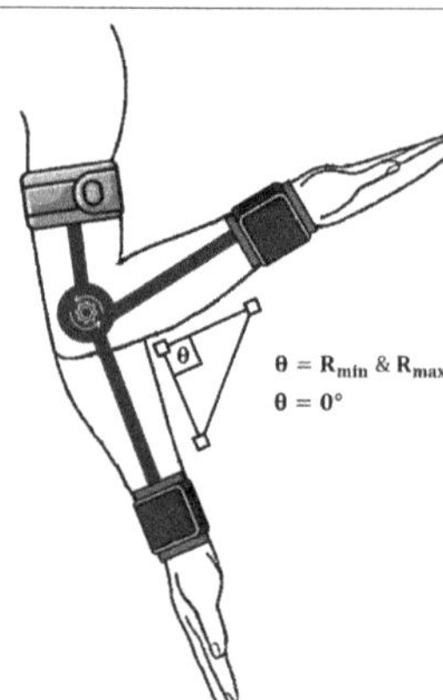

Table 6. *Cont.*

Device	Function	Application	Figure
Artificial exoskeleton	It replaces the function of muscles and joints with mechanical or powered movement. It moves within the biomechanical range of the limb or a smaller range. It allows ergonomic mobility or immobility of the joint.	Medical, Military, Industrial and Civil	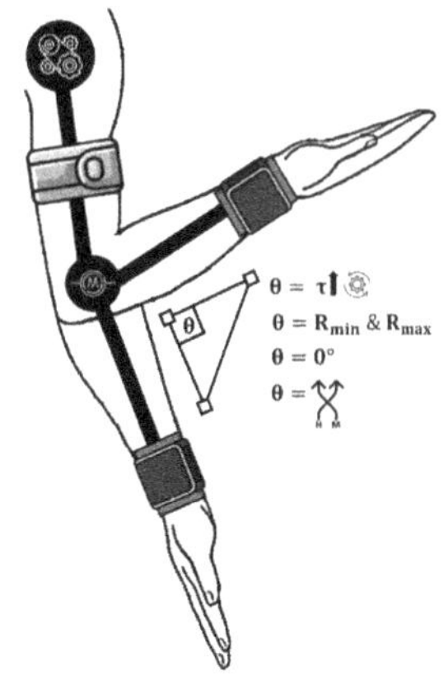

Example: In the case of the elbow representation in Table 6, in the event of an injury where movement needs to be immobilized, it would be feasible to place a common cast. If this had to be both immobile and mobile at different hours of the day, it would be correct to place an orthosis. This would provide immobility for the defined time and could be adjusted to allow movement within a safe range. If the joint is entirely damaged and the only way for the patient to heal is through amputation or internal segment wear such as the bone, the correct option would be to implement a prosthesis to replace the damaged section. Lastly, if the joint presents scenarios where injury could occur, or to prevent one, an artificial exoskeleton with mechanical or robotic quality could be used.

If there was an injury in the joint, this device would have the capability to place it in positions, speeds, and accelerations suitable for optimal recovery. Just like the function of the splint or orthosis, where it can be immobile or mobile, the artificial exoskeleton can immobilize it, limit it, or extend it to reach its natural mobility through actuation. In another case, when substituting the function of the joint due to loss of functionality, with a prosthesis, the normal procedure would be to amputate. However, with this device, since there is a structure surrounding the damaged joint, amputation is unnecessary, as the structure would act to replace the joint's function. Lastly, if the goal is to prevent injury or improve movement and strength characteristics of the joint, the correct option would be to use an artificial exoskeleton with actuation capabilities and a structure that, when surrounding the joint, would replace the muscle's function with mechanical work.

The typology of assistance devices for synovial joints represents the characteristics, functions, and applications of each of the developments and scientific contributions regarding the care of these joints. The dissemination through articles, academia, and private products has a significant influence on the classification of each device. Although there is diversity in these technologies, this article focuses on the analysis of the four most important, as they have been in constant evolution throughout history and continue to be applied today. Tables 7–11 describe the origins, appearances, registrations, definitions, and uses of these technologies. This classification is important because these technologies are often misused in scientific dissemination. While not entirely the case, this causes confusion due to the lack of standardization, leading to new developers having scattered foundations.

Table 7. Description of the origins of the names of the different devices.

Section	Device	Description
Origin of the Word	Splint	The term "splint" likely originates from multiple sources: Middle Low German, referring to a thin piece of iron; Middle Dutch cognate "splinter"; or Swedish, meaning a wooden nail or wedge. All interpretations align with the concept of a plate or strip applied to the skin, typically made from splinters of metal or wood [24].
	Prosthesis	"Prosthesis" has a history spanning thousands of years, with roots in ancient Egypt and Greece, and continues to evolve today with artificial devices for body repair. The term derives from Late Latin, from the Greek "prosthesis," meaning "to add," from "prostithenai" (to add to) and "tithenai" (to place) [25].
	Orthosis	Compared to earlier devices like splints, "orthosis" is relatively modern, having been in use for only a few decades. It comes from the Greek "orthōsis," meaning "to straighten," derived from "orthoun" (to straighten) [26].
	Exoskeleton	The term "exoskeleton" refers to any hardened external structure, such as the shells of crustaceans or the plates of fish and reptiles, particularly when bone-like. It is derived from the Greek "exo-" (outside) and "skeleton," and is grounded in zoological terminology [27].

Table 8. Description of the first record of the different devices.

Section	Device	Year
First Record	Splint	1325 [24]
	Prosthesis	1550 [25]
	Orthosis	1958 [26]
	Artificial exoskeleton	1839 [27]

Table 9. Description of the first appearance of the different devices.

Section	Device	Description
First Appearance	Splint	In the 20th century, during excavations in Egypt, fractures from 5000 years ago were found, bound with bark tablets, wrapped in linen, and secured with bandages. Surgeon Percival Pott standardized the immobilization splint, known as Pott's splint [28]. Later, the Thomas splint emerged to immobilize the lower limb in cases of fractures and chronic bone diseases. During World War I, the splint evolved, and plaster of Paris was used, becoming known as the Tobruk splint, which remains the most used today [29].

Table 9. *Cont.*

Section	Device	Description
	Prosthesis	The University of Basel found a wooden prosthesis belonging to the foot of the daughter of an Egyptian priest in a female burial at Tomb Tebana 95, dating back 3000 years [30].
	Orthosis	The appearance of the first orthotic device dates to the earliest civilizations, when rudimentary forms of splints and supports were used. Over time, orthotics has evolved to become a highly specialized field of medicine, with increasingly complex devices tailored to the individual needs of patients. F. Genêt, F. et al. (2010) describes the importance that a device called an orthosis had in the mid-twentieth century, a disease "Heine–Medin syndrome" (Poliomyelitis) and the poliovirus frequently attacked the respiratory systems and caused paralysis of the upper and lower limbs of those infected. As a result, devices called leather and steel orthoses became quite popular [31].
	Artificial exoskeleton	The oldest exoskeleton-like device known was developed in 1890 by Russian engineer Nicholas Yagn with a patent under the name "Apparatus for facilitating walking, running, and jumping [32]." It was not until 1960 that the first mobile machine with anthropomorphic movements appeared: the Hardiman, a device developed by General Electric and the U.S. government [33].

Table 10. Description of the definitions of the different devices.

Section	Device	Description
Definition	Splint	The word "splint" comes from the noun "to splint." The Cambridge Dictionary defines "to splint" as an object made of rigid or flexible material used to immobilize an area with injury or fracture [34].
	Prosthesis	The Cambridge Dictionary defines "prosthesis" as the science or part of medicine that deals with artificial body parts [35].
	Orthosis	The Cambridge Dictionary defines "orthosis" as a device made to support an injured or malformed part of the body [36].
	Artificial exoskeleton	In biological terms. The Cambridge Dictionary defines "exoskeleton" as a hard outer layer that covers, supports, and protects an invertebrate animal [37]. In medical or military terms. The Cambridge Dictionary defines "exoskeleton" as a suit that supports the body or part of it. It is used by people with injuries to help them walk or by soldiers to help them carry heavy equipment [37].

Table 11. Description of the uses of the different devices.

Section	Device	Description
Utility	Splint	According to the University of Navarra Clinic [38] and the medical dictionary [39], a splint is used to immobilize a fractured, dislocated, or paralyzed body part, which should be kept at rest, in a proper position, or unloaded, as is the case with inflammatory joint diseases, paralysis, dislocation, or fractures.
	Prosthesis	According to Standard UNE 11-909-90/1, adopted from ISO 8549/1, a prosthesis is an external device used to replace, either partially or entirely, a deficient or absent limb segment [40].
	Orthosis	According to Standard UNE 11-909-90/1, adopted from ISO 8549/1, an orthosis is any device applied externally to the human body, used to modify the structural or functional characteristics of the neuromusculoskeletal system, with the purpose of maintaining, improving, or recovering function [41].
	Artificial exoskeleton	According to Standards NTP 1162 and NTP 1163 [42]. Exoskeletons I and II, an exoskeleton is a portable external device placed on the user's body, used to increase ergonomic intervention capabilities and improve working conditions, particularly concerning physical load.

Knowing the first records and early appearances of a technological device is essential for understanding its evolution and historical context. These records allow us to trace the origin of the innovation, identify key advancements that have contributed to its development, and recognize the needs or problems that motivated its creation. Additionally, by reviewing the early versions of a device, it is possible to evaluate how they have improved over time in terms of efficiency, functionality, and accessibility, impacting their role in society and industry regarding the design and development of future technologies, helping to avoid past mistakes and optimize innovation processes.

The etymology of words and their first official appearance are essential for understanding the evolution of concepts and preventing misunderstandings. In the context of robotic devices such as splints, prosthetics, orthoses, and exoskeletons, knowing their origin helps to better understand their function and purpose. Terms like "prosthesis" (replacement) and "exoskeleton" (external support) reflect their specific use and how they have been adapted to medical and technological needs. Thus, etymological knowledge ensures precise and proper use of these terms in the development of technologies.

3. Results

3.1. Artificial Exoskeletons

Diseases, accidents, or the lack of certain attributes in the human body have led us to develop technologies that, while they may not fully facilitate recovery, are valuable for coping with the process, particularly in medical terms. Technologies that enhance, smooth, and/or protect the movements of their users are important not only for safeguarding their physiological integrity but also for implementing artificial characteristics that a regular person does not possess. These characteristics provide security and, most importantly, improve quality of life. Devices such as splints, prostheses, and orthoses are typically limited to one or two tasks. Artificial exoskeletons, on the other hand, serve multiple functions, with applications and features in sectors like medicine, military, industry, and education, among others. They offer added value, as they provide more options for different situations, and this article tracks the records and classifications of this technology.

3.2. From Biological to Artificial

Based on Table 10, the origin of the word "exoskeleton" comes from zoology, describing a hardened structure, mostly of bone nature [27]. In Table 7, it is defined as a hard layer that covers, supports, and protects an invertebrate biological being, which uses the external skeletal structure to support, move, and protect itself [37]. Therefore, an exoskeleton is used for invertebrates, in contrast to vertebrates, which possess an internal skeletal structure called an endoskeleton (Figure 8a). Humans, as well as terrestrial, aerial, or marine animals, have both endo and exoskeletons, and the variety is finite and can be distinguished by their visible characteristics. However, there are animals where the difference is not so clear, such as the terrestrial tortoises, which have both an external and internal skeletal structure (Figure 8b). Their shell and limbs do not share the same line, even though their limbs have an internal bone structure, the containment of their organs is under an external bone structure, making them a hybrid in terms of skeletal composition. This composition is artificially represented when a mechanical structure is placed around a vertebrate.

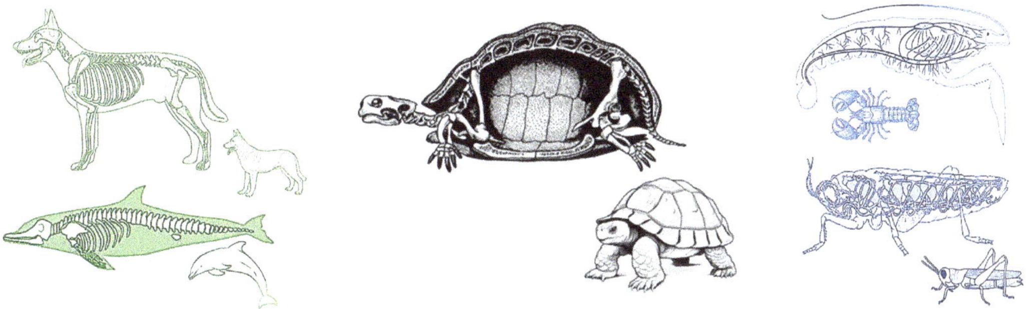

(a) (b) (c)

Figure 8. (**a**) Species with internal bone structures; (**b**) species with both internal and external bone structures; (**c**) species with external bone structures.

An animal like an ant or beetle is known for being able to lift several times its body weight, thanks to having an exoskeleton [43]. The exoskeleton provides greater resistance because its external bone structure absorbs most of the load, in contrast to a vertebrate animal, where the load is absorbed by muscles, joints, and only then reaches the internal skeletal structure. The application of an artificial exoskeleton to a human or animal follows the same principle as species that possess them (Figure 8c); they serve to contain and protect the integrity of the user inside. Based on Table 11, according to standards NTP 1162 and 1163, an artificial exoskeleton is a portable external device that is placed on the user's body, used to increase ergonomic intervention capabilities and improve working conditions, especially regarding physical load [42].

In Figure 9, the concept of the suit's use and the general use of the device is divided into two parts. Here, it is shown that when a user is wearing it, they are covered and protected by it, although this is not always the case. Most artificial exoskeletons are partial, focusing mostly on the upper and lower limbs, but total protection is the primary goal for human exoskeletons.

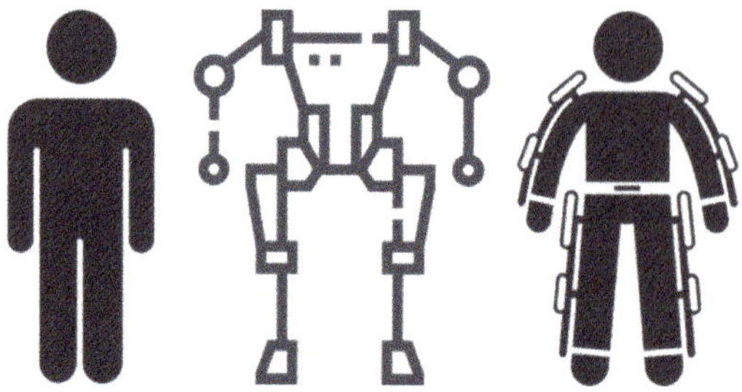

Figure 9. User—Device: artificial exoskeleton on a user.

Based on Figures 9 and 10, and the content from the previous tables, it can be concluded that an exoskeleton is an organic term, in this case, referring to external bone structures. In the case of structural devices developed from non-organic materials such as metals or polymers, it can be referred to as an artificial structure, as it mimics the naturalness of an organic exoskeleton. Therefore, referring to an artificial structure usable by a vertebrate as simply "an exoskeleton" would be incorrect without an adjective to complement it. For example, if it is a mechanical structure made from metal links and assisted by elastic actuators (springs), it can be defined as a Mechanical Exoskeleton. If the structure includes electric motors and its assistance is actuated, controlled, and communicated through instrumental circuits, it can be referred to as a Robotic Exoskeleton. In more recent technologies, like the metaverse, devices that can read movements and translate them into coordinates in cyberspace could be defined as a Haptic Exoskeleton, among others.

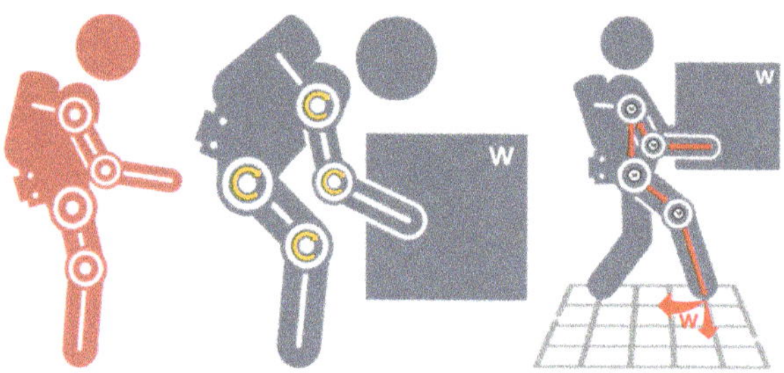

Figure 10. Application: the user does not interact with surrounding loads.

3.3. Classification of Artificial Exoskeletons

Earlier, behaviors related to muscles and joints were analyzed to understand the freedom of movement a typical person possesses, aiming to comprehend the application and behavior of the different devices discussed throughout the article, such as splints, prostheses, orthoses, and artificial exoskeletons. The latter has a wide range of applications and configurations. Therefore, an extensive classification of artificial exoskeletons is proposed, addressing their global and partial configurations. Additionally, the analysis is based on Tables 7–11, which outline the origins, definitions, records, uses, and appearances of this device. According to the tables on etymology, uses, and applications, three basic points should be considered for something to be considered an artificial exoskeleton.

For a satisfactory classificatory analysis of the types of artificial exoskeletons, the de-vice must meet three essential criteria:

- It must be an external structure to the body.
- It must be parallel to the musculoskeletal system.

- It must assist or enhance the forces and movements of the joints.

The analysis of artificial exoskeletons for classification purposes should focus on two main qualities: assistance and enhancement. Based on these two principles, considerations are made regarding the type of structures that resemble the user, the materials that can be used to mold the device, the type of mobility it is designed to employ (which aligns with its application in the medical, military, industrial sectors, among others), the type of energy supply (which is crucial, as it defines the exoskeleton's designation), the type of control used to manage the movement of the structure, the systems that will determine its functionality within its applications, and the types of construction, which can be performed by private sector companies or public sector organizations such as universities or research institutions.

Given that the device may opt for different types of structures, mobilities, power sources, control systems, functional systems, and construction, a global classification of parameters is provided, detailing the characteristics for the different types of developments this device may present [44,45].

Regarding structure, mobility, control, and construction, the most prominent characteristics come from power sources and functional systems. The power supply defines whether the exoskeleton will be mechanical, robotic, pneumatic, or hydraulic. A mechanical exoskeleton, while using elastic actuators as springs, does not provide external energy other than that of the user, making it a passive system. In contrast, an active system involves external energy, with peaks of power input along specific parts of the structure, especially at the actuators. While the structure may not necessarily contain them, the power supply, such as electricity, not only fuels the actuation but also powers the exoskeleton's instrumentation. Pneumatic and hydraulic power supplies, when compared to electrical or non-powered systems, do not provide any other function except actuation of the joints, and are therefore considered pneumatic exoskeletons or hydraulic exoskeletons, as their primary function is to supply movement.

There are four different systems available. Although the literature includes additional variations, two main categories are considered: active and passive systems. Passive systems use gravity compensation and elastic/spring members to store and release energy during movements, assisting users in physical movements. Active systems, on the other hand, rely on one or more actuators to increase the power of the limbs. Once the global characteristics that an artificial exoskeleton may possess have been outlined, an analysis of their behaviors in different configurations is made. Based on this description, in Table 12 each of the various types of behaviors will be described in terms of power supply, structure, and functioning within different applications [46].

Table 12. Components characterize an artificial exoskeleton.

Device	Type	Description
Exoskeletons Artificial	Structure	Rigid Flexible
	Mobility	Mobile Fixed Supported
	Power	Electric Hydraulic Pneumatic No power

Table 12. *Cont.*

Device	Type	Description
	Communication	Control panel Electromyography (EMG) Electroencephalogram (EEG) No communication
	System	Passive Semi-Passive Semi-Active Active
	Construction	Private Public

3.4. *Types of Structure for an Artificial Exoskeleton*

Figure 11 presents a classification of artificial exoskeletons by type of kinematic structure. Table 13 presents a description of these exoskeletons.

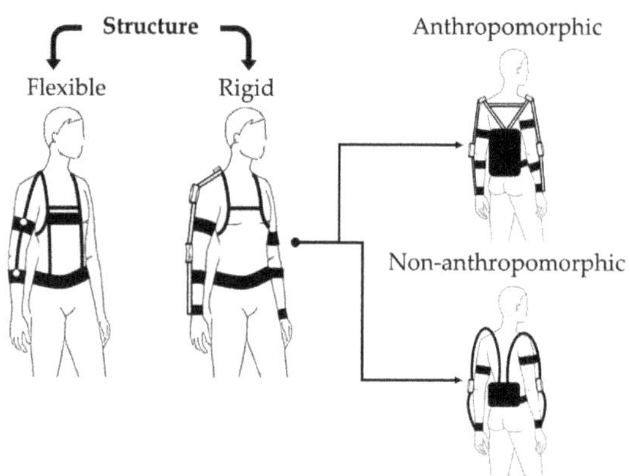

Figure 11. Classification of artificial exoskeletons by kinematic structure type.

Table 13. Description of artificial exoskeletons by kinematic structure type.

Structure	Description	Type	Description
Rigid [44]	It is built with low-flexibility links: metals, polymers, among others. It provides support and stability.	Anthropomorphic	Replicates human joints and proportions.
	These are designed to resist mechanical loads and maintain the integrity of the device.	No anthropomorphic	Prioritizes efficiency and adaptation to perform tasks.
Flexible	It is composed of cables or elastic bands. It provides movement adaptability since it is not a heavy structure. They are designed to collect information or assist with posture during prolonged periods in terms of physical endurance.	This does not apply	This does not apply

3.5. Types of Mobility of an Artificial Exoskeleton

Figure 12 presents a classification of artificial exoskeletons according to their workspace and grounding: mobile, fixed, and anchored. Table 14 presents a description of each of these exoskeleton types.

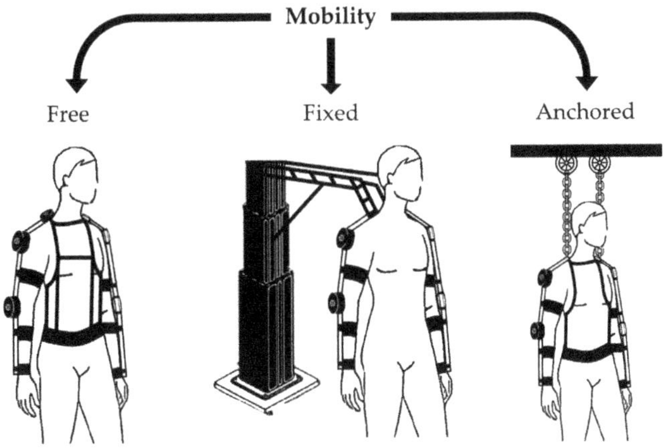

Figure 12. Classification of mobility between a mobile, fixed, and anchored artificial exoskeleton.

Table 14. Description of mobility between a mobile, fixed, and anchored artificial exoskeleton.

Mobility	Description
Free	This type of mobility has no displacement limits. Since the structure is placed on the user, it allows the user to move with it. As it is user-dependent, a battery bank must be implemented if required, or a power supply line, which would limit the user to an area with a range determined by the length of the power system.
Fixed	This type of mobility represents a structure fixed to the ground or a wall. The links are supported by the base, causing the user to have no direct interaction with the structure, only with the movements. The displacement is restricted to the area where it is installed, providing greater stability and power, as it may be connected to a power supply source.
Anchored	This type of mobility suspends the structure with harnesses or cables on a fixed or mobile rail. This allows externally assisted displacement. This type of mobility combines the semi-freedom of a mobile device with the energy efficiency and structural integrity of a fixed device. These types of devices are ideal for companies and rehabilitation of lower limbs.

3.6. Type of Power Supply for an Artificial Exoskeleton

Figure 13 presents a classification of energies according to their performance as electric, pneumatic, or hydraulic motor work. Table 15 describes each energy use for use in an artificial exoskeleton.

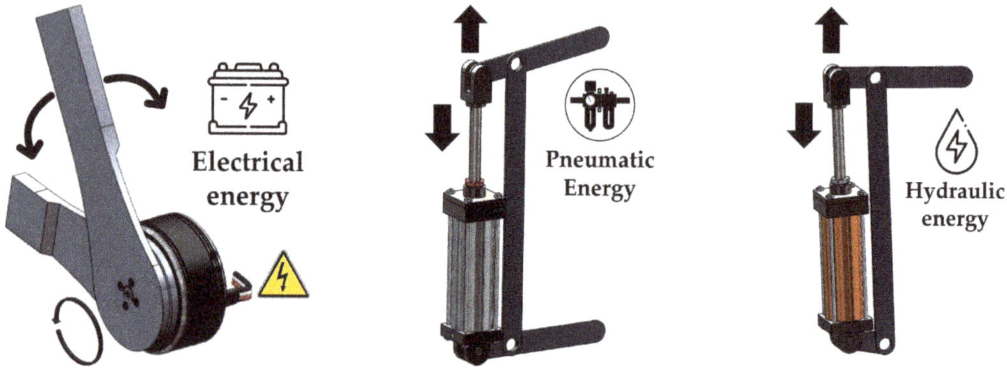

(a) (b) (c)

Figure 13. Classification of artificial exoskeletons according to the type of actuation. (**a**) electric actuator; (**b**) pneumatic actuator; (**c**) hydraulic actuator.

Table 15. Classification of external energies used in an artificial exoskeleton.

Energy	Description	Icon
Electrical (E)	Powers the device hardware Generates the actuation motion	
Hydraulics (H)	Generates the actuation motion	
Pneumatic (N)	Generates the actuation motion	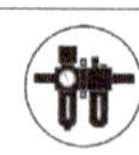
Without power (M)	Movement generated by mechanical components	

3.7. Type of Artificial Exoskeleton System

There are four different systems available. Although the literature includes additional variations, the two main categories are considered: active and passive systems. Passive systems use gravity compensation and elastic/spring members to store and release energy during movements, assisting users in physical movements. Active systems, on the other hand, rely on one or more actuators to increase the power of the limbs. Once the global characteristics that an artificial exoskeleton may possess have been outlined, an analysis of their behaviors in different configurations is made. Based on this description, each of the various types of behaviors will be described in terms of power supply, structure, and functioning within different applications [46]. See Table 16.

Table 16. Classification of exoskeletons according to the type of system.

Exoskeleton	System
Mechanical 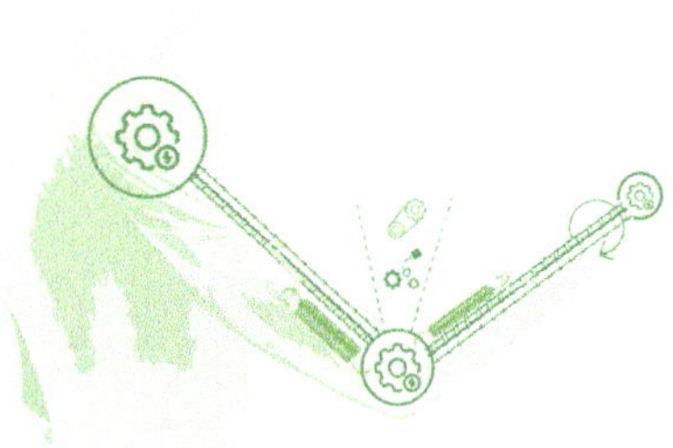	Passive A passive mechanical exoskeleton operates without external energy, processing systems, or actuation. Instead, it relies on mechanical structures such as springs, dampers, and elastic components to assist movement and provide support. Its primary function is to enhance ergonomic intervention capabilities by reducing physical strain, improving posture, and minimizing fatigue during repetitive or physically demanding tasks.
Robotic 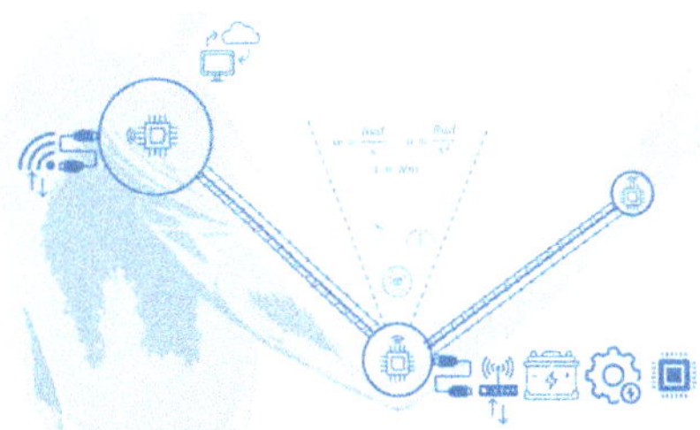	Semi-passive A semi-passive robotic exoskeleton utilizes external energy sources and processing systems but does not incorporate actuation mechanisms. It is designed primarily for data collection, using sensors and computational systems to monitor and analyze limb movement. This type of exoskeleton is commonly used in research and rehabilitation settings to assess biomechanics, track motion patterns, and provide valuable insights for improving assistive technologies.
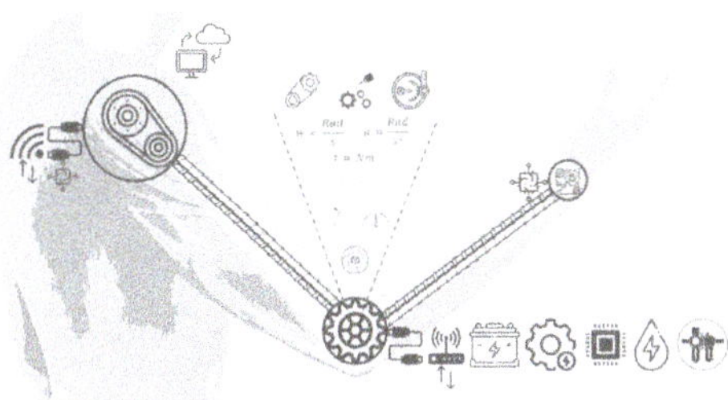	Semi-active An active–passive robotic exoskeleton uses external energy sources, processing systems, and actuation mechanisms for joint rehabilitation, assisting individuals recovering from injuries. It provides controlled assistance to facilitate movement while allowing the user's muscles to engage, or it can actively block joint movement when needed. This combination of external actuation and natural muscle engagement supports gradual recovery and adaptive rehabilitation strategies. Active This active–passive robotic exoskeleton harnesses external energy from hydraulic, pneumatic, electrical, and mechanical sources, incorporating advanced processing systems for data control, reception, and transmission. Its actuation function replaces the user's muscle and joint effort, enhancing ergonomic intervention and absorbing external forces to improve load bearing and mobility. This design enables users to perform physical tasks with greater ease and safety.

Artificial exoskeletons are classified based on their activation level and energy usage. The four main types are passive, semi-passive, semi-active, and active. The choice of system depends on the specific needs and usage conditions of the exoskeleton. This characteristic is where the adjective artificial can be omitted, and the appropriate adjective for the system type being used can be added. See Table 17.

Table 17. Description and classification of the internal features of an artificial exoskeleton.

Dispositive	System	Description	Application
Mechanical Exoskeleton	Passive	• Does not use external energy • Does not use processing systems • Does not use actuation	It is used to enhance ergonomic intervention capabilities.
Robotic Exoskeleton	Semi Passive	• Use external energy ○ (E) (M) * • Use processing systems ○ (Rx) (Tx) * • Does not use actuation	It is used to collect information on limb movement.
	Semi Active	• Use external energy. ○ (H) (N) (E) (M) * • Use processing systems ○ (Ctrl) (Rx) (Tx) * • Use actuation	It is used for the rehabilitation of a joint with injury. It is used to block the movement of the joint with actuation. It uses a percentage of movement provided by the system, with the other percentage coming from the muscle.
	Active	• Use external energy ○ (H) (N) (E) (M) • Use processing systems ○ (Ctrl) (Rx) (Tx) • Use actuation	It replaces the total muscle and joint effort. It is used to increase assisted ergonomic intervention. It is used to absorb all external forces that interact with the user, enhancing their load bearing and mobility capacity.

* E: Electrical energy; M: Mechanical energy; N: Pneumatic energy; H: Hydraulic energy; Ctrl: Application of a control system; Tx: Data transfer; Rx: Data reception.

Based on the description in Table 12, the selected system type can define the behavior of the device. This means that an artificial or mechanical exoskeleton may be considered due to the lack of actuation and instrumentation for control and communication; its function is solely to provide support and stability to the user. On the other hand, a robotic system is characterized as a machine programmed to perform tasks autonomously or which is guided by a third party using external components. Although not necessarily robotic, an exoskeleton requires actuation, as in the case of the semi-active system, as described in Table 16, it can also be considered an electronic exoskeleton or a data collection system.

3.8. Type of Communication of an Artificial Exoskeleton

Table 18 describes the standard communication types that the control card has to activate the operation of an artificial exoskeleton.

Table 18. Classification of communication types in artificial exoskeletons.

Communication	Description	Icon
Sensors	They allow the device to interpret external and internal elements to collaborate with programmed actions to create behaviors and solutions.	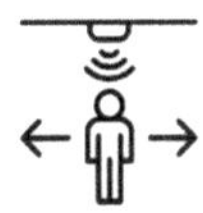
Control Panel	It is a board that changes the system configuration. The user or a third party controls almost everything about the device's behavior and operation.	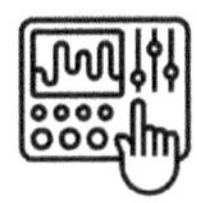
Electromyography (EMG)	These are analog signals coming from the muscles [47] and the nervous system, which are interpreted as operational amplifiers.	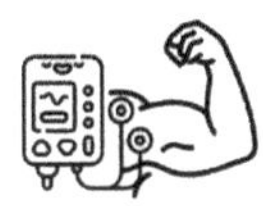
Electroencephalogram (EEG)	These signals come from the electrical activity in the brain [48]. They are amplified signals, as they fall within the micro to millivolt range, interpreted as operational amplifiers.	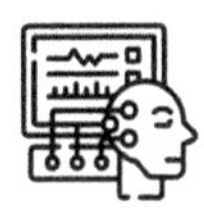
No control	The operation does not require instrumentation.	

3.9. *Types of Robotic Exoskeleton Construction*

Artificial exoskeletons have experienced significant development in both public and private institutions. To innovate more quickly, engineers and researchers have collaborated to create devices that improve the quality of life for individuals. Institutions and companies are innovating with structures, reduced power supply, and increased efficiency. Additionally, some exoskeletons incorporate artificial intelligence to adapt to the user's movement patterns, enhancing their effectiveness. In institutions such as companies, innovation is highly sought after. Below are descriptions of the three most important exoskeletons developed by public institutions and the ninety-six most important developers in the private sector.

- **XoMotion** (Simon Fraser University): Researchers at Simon Fraser University (SFU) created XoMotion, a cutting-edge robotic exoskeleton. This device enables people with mobility disabilities to stand and walk without additional support. It offers a wide range of activities, including walking, climbing stairs, and squatting. XoMotion uses sensors to mimic the human body's logic and generate balanced movement [49].
- **Stanford Ankle Exoskeleton:** Researchers at Stanford University developed an ankle exoskeleton that enables people to walk more efficiently. Training and customization are key to its success. This device connects to the shoe and around the leg, mimicking

a motorized exoskeleton. It helps users push forward while walking and maintain balance [50].

- **Stanford Wireless Exoskeleton:** Another achievement by Stanford University, this is a wireless exoskeleton that increases walking speed by applying torque to the ankle. It facilitates movement during walking and is especially useful for individuals with mobility disabilities [51].

In recent years, the search for private companies dedicated to the research and development of robotic devices, particularly exoskeletons, has seen significant growth. These companies, both emerging and established, are at the forefront of technological innovation, working on the design of exoskeletons aimed at improving the quality of life for individuals with reduced mobility and optimizing physical performance for workers in industrial settings. The development of robotic exoskeletons is divided into various categories, depending on their purpose and application. Assistive exoskeletons, focused on rehabilitation, and power exoskeletons, designed to enhance users' physical abilities, are among the most prominent types. The public sector, universities, research centers, and government agencies collaborate closely on the design of prototypes that aim not only at medical advancements but also at military and rescue applications. In contrast, private companies, driven by the need to commercialize these devices, tend to focus on economic viability and improving technology to meet specific market needs, often allowing them to bring products to practical use more quickly. Collaboration between both sectors is expected to play a crucial role in advancing this technology, combining public resources with the agility and entrepreneurial vision of the private sector.

Below is a selection of the 25 most influential companies in the development of robotic exoskeletons, those that have made a significant impact on the industry thanks to their technological innovations, advances in medical rehabilitation, workplace ergonomics, and general applications. These companies have positioned themselves as leaders in the sector, developing devices that improve human mobility, reduce physical strain in industrial environments, and enhance the recovery of people with motor disabilities. The list includes both established giants and novel startups, all playing a key role in the evolution of this technology that promises to revolutionize human–machine interaction.

1. **ATOUN Inc.**
    - (Nara City, Nara Prefecture, Japan) Exoskeletons for physical task assistance.
2. **Bioness Inc.**
    - (Santa Clarita City, CA, USA) Neuromuscular stimulation devices and exoskeletons.
3. **Bionik Laboratories Corp.**
    - (Toronto City, ON, Canada) Exoskeletons for medical rehabilitation.
4. **Comau**
    - (Grugliasco City, Turin, Italy) Exoskeletons for industrial work assistance.
5. **Cyberdyne Inc.**
    - (Tsukuba City, Ibaraki Prefecture, Japan) Robotic exoskeletons for rehabilitation and mobility.
6. **Ekso Bionics**
    - (San Rafael City, CA, USA) Exoskeletons for medical and industrial rehabilitation.
7. **Exy—Empowering People**
    - (Curitiba City, Paraná, Brazil) Exoskeletons for workplace injury reduction.

8. **Fourier Intelligence**
    - (Xiu Pu Lu City, Shanghai, China) Robotic exoskeletons for rehabilitation.
9. **German Bionic**
    - (Augsburg City, Bavaria, Germany) Smart exoskeletons for industrial assistance.
10. **Honda Motor Co., Ltd.**
    - (Minato City, Tokyo, Japan) Mobility and rehabilitation assistive devices.
11. **Hyundai Motor Company**
    - (Seocho-gu City, Seoul, Republic of Korea) Exoskeletons for mobility and industrial tasks.
12. **INDI**
    - (Monterrey City, Nuevo León, Mexico) Pediatric exoskeletons for walking assistance.
13. **Lockheed Martin Corporation**
    - (Bethesda City, MD, USA) Exoskeletons for military and industrial applications.
14. **Marsi Bionics**
    - (Rivas Vaciamadrid City, Madrid, Spain) Exoskeletons for children with neuromuscular disorders.
15. **Myomo Inc.**
    - (Burlington City, MA, USA) Exoskeletons for neuromuscular injury support.
16. **Ottobock**
    - (Duderstadt City, Niedersachsen, Germany) Exoskeletons and prosthetics for mobility enhancement.
17. **Panasonic Corporation**
    - (Kadoma City, Osaka Prefecture, Japan) Exoskeletons for mobility and industrial tasks.
18. **Parker Hannifin**
    - (Mayfield Heights City, OH, USA) Exoskeletons for rehabilitation and medical assistance.
19. **Raytheon Company**
    - (Arlington City, VA, USA) Exoskeletons for military use.
20. **ReWalk Robotics**
    - (Yokne'am Illit City, Northern District, Israel) Exoskeletons for people with spinal cord injuries.
21. **Rex Bionics**
    - (Auckland City, Auckland Region (North Island), New Zealand) Autonomous exoskeletons for people with reduced mobility.
22. **Sarcos Robotics**
    - (Salt Lake City, UT, USA) Industrial and military exoskeletons.
23. **SuitX**
    - (Emeryville City, CA, USA) Modular exoskeletons for rehabilitation and industry.
24. **Technaid**

- (Arganda del Rey City, Madrid, Spain) Exoskeletons for research and rehabilitation.

25. **Wandercraft SAS**
    - (Paris City, France) Autonomous exoskeletons for personal mobility.

4. Discussion

The research on assistive devices is based on ergonomic adjustment, energy consumption, and adjustable functionality. The latter is one of the aspects most related to the high development and purchase price. This is because they are designed to fit the user's physiological needs or are adjustable but limited to a specific task. On the other hand, energy consumption is only feasible through a continuous power supply, which limits technologies to a specific operational radius, or, if independent, their energy consumption is restricted due to the high demand of the system.

The following discussion points are open to the four devices mentioned in this article, although the correct perspective would be related to artificial exoskeletons and possibly orthoses, since prostheses might exchange their characteristics based on the specific needs and circumstances, while splints are based on the application needs and their low material cost.

- **Structures:** Rigid structures are mostly, if not entirely, made from metal materials due to their high resistance to bending and compression. However, these properties are functional for devices that require excessive physical strength, structural resistance, or conditions that could be dangerous for the user. On the other hand, in the medical field, devices for the rehabilitation of limbs or their segments require lower structural resistance, as the movements are slow and do not usually require prolonged or excessive fatigue. Military devices, while requiring strength, may also require physical resistance for walking or lumbar support, where metallic structures are too heavy for transportation over long distances. Materials with low density and high resistance to bending and compression are ideal to replace the rough and heavy metal structures, which not only are heavy but also have high manufacturing and material costs. Polymers, however, would be ideal for devices that do not require high physical demand. Their use could reduce production costs, given their low manufacturing costs and potential for molding or 3D printing, enabling the creation of complex joints where geometry would help create structures that are both stronger and cheaper with quicker construction timelines.
- **Energy Consumption:** The type of structure impacts energy consumption. Larger structures tend to have greater weight, which translates into higher torque. Large torques require high energy consumption, adding more weight due to the larger actuators. Lighter structures would result in lower torques, allowing the use of smaller actuators, which reduces weight and, in turn, energy consumption. This would be advantageous for mobile devices, as their autonomy would increase significantly with the same battery bank.
- **Energy Efficiency:** Developing energy-efficient actuators and control systems would be essential for enhancing the autonomy of mobile devices. By minimizing energy consumption through smart power management and lightweight designs, manufacturers can extend the operational time of devices between charges, making them more practical for users.
- **Production Times:** Structures would be manufactured with ideal characteristics, since designing in CAD environments allows for complex calculations and geometries

that metal structures could not achieve, all at lower cost and time. With polymers, geometries would not be an issue as they can be created using molds or additive manufacturing at low production costs and considerably faster manufacturing times than conventional or CNC metal pieces.

- **Design Improvements:** Future designs could prioritize lightweight materials with high strength-to-weight ratios, such as advanced polymers or composites, which would significantly reduce the overall weight of devices while maintaining structural integrity. This would allow for greater mobility and usability, particularly in applications where prolonged use is required.
- **Cost Reduction Strategies:** Implementing additive manufacturing techniques, such as 3D printing, could lower production costs and time. This method enables the creation of complex geometries that are difficult or costly to achieve with traditional metal fabrication. By optimizing designs for manufacturability, manufacturers can streamline production processes, reducing material waste and labor costs.
- **Integration of AI and Machine Learning:** The incorporation of artificial intelligence and machine learning algorithms could enhance the adaptability and functionality of assistive devices. Smart systems could learn from user interactions, adjusting in real-time to optimize support and improve user experience. This would enable devices to provide personalized assistance based on the user's specific needs and movements, increasing effectiveness during rehabilitation and daily activities.

5. Conclusions

The development of assistive devices for synovial joints has advanced significantly, incorporating biomechanical and technological innovations that enhance mobility and improve users' quality of life. The proper classification and terminology of these devices—splints, prostheses, orthoses, and artificial exoskeletons—are essential for their design, comparison, and effective application across various fields, including medicine, industry, and the military. Artificial exoskeletons stand out as the most versatile technology in this field, providing support for both rehabilitation and performance enhancement. Their classification based on structure, mobility, power source, and control systems is crucial for their development. Future research should focus on improving ergonomics, reducing energy consumption, and optimizing cost-effectiveness to make these devices more accessible. Ultimately, integrating new technologies and materials into the design of these devices will expand their applications and improve their functionality. However, further biomechanical studies and standardized regulations are necessary to ensure the proper implementation of these technologies for the benefit of users.

Author Contributions: Conceptualization, F.C.-F., A.B.O., A.L.S.-B., A.B.S. and A.J.M.M.; methodology, F.C.-F., A.B.O., A.L.S.-B., R.C.A. and H.R.A.R.; investigation, F.C.-F., A.L.S.-B., A.B.O., A.B.S. and A.J.M.M.; writing—original draft preparation, F.C.-F., A.L.S.-B. and A.B.O.; writing—review and editing, F.C.-F., A.L.S.-B., A.B.O., R.C.A., A.B.S. and H.R.A.R.; supervision, A.B.O. and F.C.-F. All authors have read and agreed to the published version of the manuscript.

Funding: This research received no external funding.

Institutional Review Board Statement: Not applicable.

Informed Consent Statement: Not applicable.

Data Availability Statement: Not applicable.

Acknowledgments: The authors thank the Tecnológico Nacional de México and the Centro Nacional de Investigación y Desarrollo Tecnológico for the support provided to carry out this work. Filiberto Cruz Flores thanks CONACYT for the scholarship granted to carry out his postgraduate studies.

Conflicts of Interest: The authors declare no conflicts of interest.

References

1. World Health Organization (WHO). Musculoskeletal Health. World Health Organization. 2022. Available online: https://www.who.int/news-room/fact-sheets/detail/musculoskeletal-conditions (accessed on 19 February 2025).
2. Tomańska, A.; Stawinoga, M.; Gębarowski, T.; Janeczek, M.; Klećkowska-Nawrot, J.; Goździewska-Harłajczuk, K.; Dobrzyński, M. The musculoskeletal anatomy of the hind limbs of the Komodo dragon (*Varanus komodoensis*, Varanidae). *Animals* **2025**, *15*, 35. [CrossRef]
3. Li, J.; Sun, Z.; Wei, X.; Tan, Q.; He, X. Effect of structure on osteogenesis of bone scaffold: Simulation analysis based on mechanobiology and animal experiment verification. *Bioengineering* **2024**, *11*, 1120. [CrossRef]
4. Mattucci, S.; Speidel, J.; Liu, J.; Kwon, B.K.; Tetzlaff, W.; Oxland, T.R. Basic biomechanics of spinal cord injury: How injuries happen in people and how animal models have informed our understanding. *Clin. Biomech.* **2019**, *64*, 58–68. [CrossRef]
5. André, A.D.; Martins, P. Exoskeletal support devices: Summary of technical aspects. *Bioengineering* **2023**, *10*, 1328. [CrossRef]
6. Garzón, I.; Muñoz-Hurtado, J.; Pereira-Martínez, J.; Ionescu, A.M.; Cardona, J.D.L.C.; Tejada-Casado, M.; Pérez, M.D.M.; Campos, F.; Chato-Astrain, J.; Alaminos, M. Development of new squid gladius biomaterials for corneal tissue engineering. *Mar. Drugs* **2024**, *22*, 535. [CrossRef]
7. Sutton, G.P. Animal biomechanics: A new silent partner in the control of motion. *Curr. Biol.* **2013**, *23*, R651–R652. [CrossRef]
8. Nerlich, A.G.; Zink, A.; Szeimies, U.; Hagedorn, H.G. Ancient Egyptian prosthesis of the big toe. *Lancet* **2000**, *356*, 2176–2179. [CrossRef]
9. Fess, E.E. A history of splinting: To understand the present, view the past. *J. Hand Ther.* **2002**, *15*, 97–132. [CrossRef]
10. World Health Organization (WHO). *Fragility Fractures*; World Health Organization: Geneva, Switzerland, 2024. Available online: https://www.who.int/news-room/fact-sheets/detail/fragility-fractures#:~:text=In%202019,%20there%20were%20178,by%20population%20growth%20and%20ageing (accessed on 19 February 2025).
11. A.D.A.M. Medical Encyclopedia. How to Make a Splint. National Library of Medicine, 2023. [About 3 p.]. Available online: https://medlineplus.gov/ency/article/000040.htm (accessed on 19 February 2025).
12. A.D.A.M. Medical Encyclopedia. Prosthesis. National Library of Medicine. 2023. Available online: https://medlineplus.gov/ency/article/002286.htm (accessed on 19 February 2025).
13. University of Michigan Health. Orthoses (Braces). Rehabilitation Medicine. 2024. Available online: https://www.uofmhealth.org/conditions-treatments/rehabilitation/orthoses#:~:text=An%20orthosis%20is%20a%20device,Muscular%20Dystrophy (accessed on 19 February 2025).
14. Velarde, M.A.G.; Rosado, W.M.A.; Ortega, A.B.; Abúndez, A.; Cortés, C.; Colin, J. Lower limb assistance systems: A state of the art. *Lat. Am. Appl. Res.* **2022**, *52*, 89–99. [CrossRef]
15. Urrea, C.; Agramonte, R. Improving exoskeleton functionality: Design and comparative evaluation of control techniques for pneumatic artificial muscle actuators in lower limb rehabilitation and work tasks. *Processes* **2023**, *11*, 3278. [CrossRef]
16. Lim, P.N.; Wang, Z.; Wang, D.; Konishi, T.; Thian, E.S. Development in additive printing for tissue-engineered bone and tendon regeneration. *Curr. Opin. Biomed. Eng.* **2017**, *2*, 99–104. [CrossRef]
17. Elrod, C.S. Chapter 5—Musculoskeletal system. In *Acute Care Handbook for Physical Therapists*, 4th ed.; Paz, J.C., West, M.P., Eds.; W.B. Saunders: Philadelphia, PA, USA, 2014; pp. 85–122. [CrossRef]
18. Betts, J.G.; Young, K.A.; Wise, J.A.; Johnson, E.; Poe, B.; Kruse, D.H.; Korol, O.; Johnson, J.E.; Womble, M.; DeSaix, P. Chapter 9.4 Synovial joints. In *Anatomy and Physiology*; Ingram: La Vergne, TN, USA, 2013. Available online: https://openstax.org/books/anatomy-and-physiology/pages/9-4-synovial-joints (accessed on 19 February 2025).
19. Betts, J.G.; Young, K.A.; Wise, J.A.; Johnson, E.; Poe, B.; Kruse, D.H.; Korol, O.; Johnson, J.E.; Womble, M.; DeSaix, P. 9.1 Classification of joints. In *Anatomy and Physiology*; Ingram: La Vergne, TN, USA, 2013. Available online: https://openstax.org/books/anatomy-and-physiology/pages/9-1-classification-of-joints (accessed on 19 February 2025).
20. Kapandji, A.I. *Joint Physiology: Commented Diagrams of Human Mechanics, Upper Limb*, 6th ed.; Editorial Medica Panamericana: Madrid, Spain, 2006. Available online: https://www.medicapanamericana.com/es-MX/libros/fisiologia-articular-tomo-1-miembro-superior-tomo-1-miembro-superior-6a-edicion (accessed on 19 February 2025).
21. Kapandji, A.I. *Joint Physiology: Commented Diagrams of Human Mechanics, Lower Limb*, 6th ed.; Editorial Medica Panamericana: Madrid, Spain, 2012. Available online: https://www.medicapanamericana.com/es-MX/libros/fisiologia-articular-tomo-2-miembro-inferior-tomo-2-miembro-inferior (accessed on 19 February 2025).

22. Kapandji, A.I. *Joint Physiology: Commented Diagrams of Human Mechanics, Trunk and Spine*, 6th ed.; Editorial Medica Panamericana: Madrid, Spain, 2012. Available online: https://www.medicapanamericana.com/es-MX/libros/fisiologia-articular-tomo-3-tronco-y-raquis-tomo-3-tronco-y-raquis-6a-edicion (accessed on 19 February 2025).
23. Kong, W.; Sessa, S.; Zecca, M.; Takanishi, A. Anatomical calibration through post-processing of standard motion tests data. *Sensors* **2016**, *16*, 2011. [CrossRef]
24. s.v. "splint, n". In *Oxford English Dictionary*; Oxford University Press eBooks: Oxford, UK, 2023. [CrossRef]
25. s.v. "prosthesis, n". In *Oxford English Dictionary*; Oxford University Press eBooks: Oxford, UK, 2023. [CrossRef]
26. s.v. "orthosis, n". In *Oxford English Dictionary*; Oxford University Press eBooks: Oxford, UK, 2024. [CrossRef]
27. s.v. "exoskeleton, n". In *Oxford English Dictionary*; Oxford University Press eBooks: Oxford, UK, 2024. [CrossRef]
28. Ellis, H. The early days of splints and splinting. *J. Perioper. Pract.* **2011**, *21*, 251–252. [CrossRef]
29. Gray, B.; Santy-Tomlinson, J. The Thomas' splint: Application and patient care. *Int. J. Orthop. Trauma Nurs.* **2018**, *30*, 20–22. [CrossRef]
30. Forssmann, A. Sophistication in Ancient Egypt: A 3000-year-old prosthesis. In *National Geographic History*; National Geographic Partners: Washington, DC, USA, 2017. Available online: https://historia.nationalgeographic.com.es/a/sofisticacion-antiguo-egipto-protesis-hace-3000-anos_11639 (accessed on 19 February 2025).
31. Genêt, F.; Schnitzler, A.; Mathieu, S.; Autret, K.; Théfenne, L.; Dizien, O.; Maldjian, A. Orthotic devices and gait in polio patients. *Ann. Phys. Rehabil. Med.* **2010**, *53*, 51–59. [CrossRef]
32. Yagn, N. Apparatus for Facilitating Walking, Running, and Jumping. United States Patent Office. United States Patent 420,179, 28 January 1890. Available online: https://patents.google.com/patent/US420179A/en (accessed on 19 February 2025).
33. Guan, X.; Ji, L.; Wang, R. Development of exoskeletons and applications in rehabilitation. *MATEC Web Conf.* **2016**, *40*, 02004. [CrossRef]
34. Splint. In *Cambridge Dictionary*; Cambridge University Press: Cambridge, UK, 2024. Available online: https://dictionary.cambridge.org/us/dictionary/english/splint (accessed on 19 February 2025).
35. Prosthesis. In *Cambridge Dictionary*; Cambridge University Press: Cambridge, UK, 2024. Available online: https://dictionary.cambridge.org/us/dictionary/english/prosthesis?q=Prosthesis (accessed on 19 February 2025).
36. Orthosis. In *Cambridge Dictionary*; Cambridge University Press: Cambridge, UK, 2024. Available online: https://dictionary.cambridge.org/us/dictionary/english/orthosis?q=Orthosis (accessed on 19 February 2025).
37. Exoskeleton. In *Cambridge Dictionary*; Cambridge University Press: Cambridge, UK, 2024. Available online: https://dictionary.cambridge.org/us/dictionary/english/exoskeleton (accessed on 19 February 2025).
38. Ferula. Diccionario Médico. (s. f.). Available online: https://www.cun.es/diccionario-medico/terminos/ferula (accessed on 19 February 2025).
39. splint. In *En Merriam-Webster Dictionary*; Merriam-Webster: Springfield, MA, USA, 2025. Available online: https://www.merriam-webster.com/dictionary/splint (accessed on 19 February 2025).
40. Vargas Negrín, F. Indications of orthoses in primary care. *FMC—Contin. Med. Educ. Prim. Care* **2017**, *24*, 465–478. [CrossRef]
41. Manuel, C.B.J. Biomechanics in AFOs: Podopediatric AFOs. *Span. J. Podiatry* **2012**, *23*, 184–194.
42. National Institute for Occupational Safety and Health (INSST). NTP 1162: Exoskeletons I: Definition and Classification. INSST Portal. 2021. Available online: https://www.insst.es/documentacion/colecciones-tecnicas/ntp-notas-tecnicas-de-prevencion/34-serie-ntp-numeros-1152-a-1168-ano-2021/ntp-1162-exoesqueletos-i-definicion-y-clasificacion (accessed on 19 February 2025).
43. Arroyave-Tobon, S.; Drapin, J.; Moretto, P.; Linares, J.-M. Design features of the kinematic chain of the ant exoskeleton. *Procedia CIRP* **2023**, *119*, 855–860. [CrossRef]
44. Crea, S.; Beckerle, P.; De Looze, M.; De Pauw, K.; Grazi, L.; Kermavnar, T.; Masood, J.; O'Sullivan, L.W.; Pacifico, I.; Rodríguez-Guerrero, C.; et al. Occupational exoskeletons: A roadmap toward large-scale adoption. Methodology and challenges of bringing exoskeletons to workplaces. *Wearable Technol.* **2021**, *2*, e11. [CrossRef] [PubMed]
45. Miao, Q.; Zhang, M.; Cao, J.; Xie, S.Q. Reviewing high-level control techniques on robot-assisted upper-limb rehabilitation. *Adv. Robot.* **2018**, *32*, 1253–1268. [CrossRef]
46. Preethichandra, D.M.G.; Piyathilaka, L.; Sul, J.-H.; Izhar, U.; Samarasinghe, R.; Arachchige, S.D.; de Silva, L.C. Passive and active exoskeleton solutions: Sensors, actuators, applications, and recent trends. *Sensors* **2024**, *24*, 7095. [CrossRef] [PubMed]
47. Denby, C.; Stone, T. Chapter 18—Neurological measurement. In *Clinical Engineering*, 2nd ed.; Taktak, A., Ganney, P.S., Long, D., Axell, R.G., Eds.; Academic Press: Cambridge, MA, USA, 2020; pp. 309–319. [CrossRef]
48. Zhao, Y.; He, F.; Guo, Y. EEG signal processing techniques and applications. *Sensors* **2023**, *23*, 9056. [CrossRef] [PubMed]
49. Human In Motion Robotics—Intelligent Innovation in Human Motion. 2014. Available online: https://humaninmotion.com/ (accessed on 19 February 2025).

50. Ankle Exoskeleton Enables Faster Walking. Stanford Report, Stanford University. 2021. Available online: https://news.stanford.edu/stories/2021/04/ankle-exoskeleton-enables-faster-walking (accessed on 19 February 2025).
51. Exoskeleton Makes Walking Faster, Less Tiring. Stanford Report, Stanford University. 2022. Available online: https://news.stanford.edu/stories/2022/10/exoskeleton-makes-walking-faster-less-tiring (accessed on 19 February 2025).

technologies

MDPI

Review

The Landscape of Virtual Reality Use in Mobility Rehabilitation from 2010–2023: A Scoping Review

Danielle T. Felsberg [1,2], Reza Pousti [3], Charlend K. Howard [3], Scott E. Ross [2], Louisa D. Raisbeck [2], Jared T. McGuirt [4] and Christopher K. Rhea [3,*]

1 Department of Physical Therapy, Wingate University, Wingate, NC 28174, USA; d.felsberg@wingate.edu
2 Department of Kinesiology, University of North Carolina at Greensboro, Greensboro, NC 27412, USA; seross@uncg.edu (S.E.R.); ldraisbe@uncg.edu (L.D.R.)
3 Ellmer College of Health Sciences, Old Dominion University, Norfolk, VA 23529, USA; gpous001@odu.edu (R.P.); c1howard@odu.edu (C.K.H.)
4 Department of Nutrition, University of Tennessee, Knoxville, Knoxville, TN 37996, USA; jmcguirt@utk.edu
* Correspondence: crhea@odu.edu

Abstract: Significant advancements in virtual reality (VR) technology have occurred in the past decade, allowing clinical researchers to take advantage of these reduced barriers to explore the use of VR in patient populations. This scoping review on VR interventions to improve mobility in adults and children focuses on the literature from 2010–2023. A total of 2736 articles were screened and 126 articles met the inclusion criteria. Most of the studies were conducted in inpatient clinical settings (n = 41) and investigated VR interventions to improve balance (n = 118). Less immersive (n = 108) products such as Nintendo Wii or Xbox Kinect were primarily used. Additionally, 37.0% of studies (n = 47) used off-the-shelf programs like Wii Fit Plus and 73.2% of studies (n = 93) found statistically significant improvements in motor outcomes following VR intervention. The articles included in this review suggest that the majority of VR research for physical rehabilitation is being performed in clinical settings. Most studies reported statistically significant improvements in their outcome variables following VR intervention. These observations demonstrate that research in this area is moving beyond proof-of-concept and toward translation to clinical applications.

Keywords: scoping review; virtual reality; physical therapy; gait; mobility

1. Introduction

Physical rehabilitation provided by a Physical Therapist (PT) or Physical Therapist Assistant (PTA) aims to address functional deficits and optimize independence. While the scope of rehabilitation addressed by PTs and PTAs can vary by state and country, a common goal is to restore healthy movement. Rehabilitation provided by PTs and PTAs can include a focus on the upper and/or lower body, depending on the patient's needs. Restoring independent mobility is a prevalent therapeutic goal, as it has been shown to be positively associated with quality of life [1]. Therefore, the focus of this scoping review is mobility rehabilitation.

PTs and PTAs create evidence-based treatment protocols to meet a patient's functional goals by utilizing a variety of therapeutic modalities. One such modality is virtual reality (VR), which has been identified as a promising treatment tool to provide effective and meaningful interventions across a variety of human health applications, including cognitive rehabilitation [2], pulmonary rehabilitation [3], pain management [4], intensive care medicine [5], and improvement of motor outcomes [6–9]. VR can be defined as a computer-generated environment which contains sensory information that may be interacted with, visualized, and manipulated to allow natural behaviors to emerge as if the environment were real [10–12]. VR helps meet a clinical need by providing a training modality that can be challenging to recreate in the real world [13,14] and has been shown to enhance psychological motivation to continue the prescribed treatment [15,16]. Previous research investigating the use of VR in rehabilitation has demonstrated significant improvements in mobility outcomes [6–9]; however, most of this research has been conducted in controlled laboratory environments and the translation to clinical practice appears to be limited. As suggested by Cano Porras et al. [8], the merit of VR interventions has continued to be supported (see recent reviews by Góra et al. [17] and Bateni et al. [18]); thus, research in this area should move beyond purely efficacy-based questions and begin to answer questions regarding the efficacy of different types of VR hardware compared to each other and the benefits of using particular types of VR in specific clinical settings or with particular populations, as well as investigating the more deliberate designs of VR intervention.

Research interest in the use of VR as a rehabilitation modality has increased since the introduction of low-cost, commercially available VR hardware around 2010 and has continued as technology has further evolved [11]. While relatively small-scale research studies have explored the utility of VR in physical rehabilitation, there have been few large-scale attempts to identify clinically relevant aspects of these studies. To address this gap, the research questions addressed by our scoping review focused on the following: (1) which populations (healthy and clinical) have been included in this type of research, (2) the geographical location where these studies have occurred, (3) the elements of the study design, (4) the type of VR used, and most importantly, (5) the intervention outcomes. In relation to the latter, it should be noted that the infusion of VR in rehabilitation is not universally positive. For example, it has been shown that older adult dropout rates are higher in randomized study designs that use new technology relative to control interventions [19]. This observation aligns with the finding that older adults' technological acceptance of gamified VR is related to their initial feelings after their first encounter with VR (i.e., was the interaction positive or negative) and their perceived usefulness of the technology [20]. Addressing these research gaps will help to inform research scientists and clinicians of the current evidence for the inclusion of VR in physical rehabilitation.

While VR has been used in several rehabilitation contexts, the purpose of our scoping review was to better understand the research-to-practice landscape of VR for physical rehabilitation interventions to improve mobility. Specifically, we aimed to investigate how VR is being used in physical rehabilitation research to-date, including which clinical populations are being included, the settings and locations of studies, and the types of VR hardware and software being used as a therapeutic tool.

2. Materials and Methods

This scoping review followed the protocol set by the Preferred Reporting Items for Systematic reviews and Meta-Analyses extension for Scoping Reviews (PRISMA-ScR) updated guidance [21]. The PRISMA-ScR checklist can be found in Table S1 in the Supplementary Materials. While our protocol was not pre-registered, the search terms and methods were agreed upon prior to the search. Additionally, to guide the inclusion criteria, a participant, intervention, comparison, outcomes, and study design (PICOS) model was used [22]. The

Zotero citation management system and Excel were used for managing records and data during this review.

A keyword search was performed between 31 July 2023 and 17 August 2023 using the following databases: PubMed, Scopus, and EBSCOhost. Searches were further refined by selecting English-language texts. The keyword searches included all possible combinations of (1) "virtual reality"; (2) "physical therapy", "Physiotherapy", or "rehabilitation"; (3) "gait", "ambulation", "balance", "mobility", "function" or "motor performance". As previously noted, the year 2010 marked a significant transition in the development, usability, and accessibility of VR hardware. Thus, our publication years for the search were constrained to 2010 through the year the search was conducted (2023).

The study selection was guided by a participant, intervention, comparison, outcomes, and study design (PICOS) model, which can be seen in Table 1. The PICOS model was set according to the primary aim of this review, which was to investigate the use of VR as an intervention to improve gait, standing balance, or upright mobility. Using these eligibility criteria, an initial screening of the studies was performed. The full texts of the studies not eliminated during the initial screening were further reviewed for the inclusion and exclusion criteria. The titles, abstracts, and full texts of the articles were assessed independently for eligibility by two reviewers, GP and CH. In cases of disagreement, GP and CH discussed with DF and came to an agreement.

Table 1. PICOS inclusion/exclusion criteria.

Participants	Studies were included if they included human (healthy or clinical) populations. Modeling and animal model studies were excluded.
Interventions	Studies were included if they covered treatment interventions using VR that aimed to improve gait, standing balance, and/or upright mobility. Studies were excluded if they used adjunct therapeutic modalities simultaneously with the VR intervention (robot-assisted gait training, transcranial magnetic stimulation, etc.).
Comparisons	Studies were included if they included pre- and post-treatment assessments and/or comparisons between VR and conventional treatment (i.e., balance training, etc.). Studies were excluded if they did not include these comparisons.
Outcomes	Studies were included if they reported functional or clinical outcome measurements of gross motor abilities, or biomechanical measurements related to gait, balance, or upright mobility. Studies with outcomes outside of this description were excluded.
Study Design	Study designs that employed baseline and post-treatment assessments were included. Studies were excluded if they were case studies or had <10 participants in the experimental group.

Following the database searches and study selection, data extraction was performed to generate the descriptive statistics of the included studies. Data regarding the publication year, patient population, publication location and setting, study protocols, sample size and age, VR hardware and software used, and intervention outcomes were extracted. Information regarding each intervention was also extracted, such as the intervention protocol, objectives, and outcomes. Following the framework used by Campo-Prieto et al. [9], VR was judged as non-immersive, semi-immersive, or fully immersive. Immersion (semi or full) was operationally defined for our study as the feedback provided when interacting with a virtual reality environment.

3. Results

3.1. Study Selection

Figure 1 illustrates the article selection process. The initial database searches led to a total of 3813 articles for initial screening derived from PubMed (n = 2735), Scopus (n = 613), and EBSCOhost (n = 465). Of these 3813 articles, 1022 were duplicates and 55 were removed because they either did not have associated text or were only abstracts (e.g., conference presentations). After removing these articles, 2736 articles were screened for inclusion through their title and abstract. Of these articles, 2413 articles were excluded for not meeting the PICOS criteria due to being a systematic review, meta-analysis, study protocol, case study, or commentary, or because they used an adjunct modality, studied cognitive or psychological factors, did not investigate a gross motor task or did not use gross motor outcomes, were not a VR intervention, or used an upper extremity task. Following the screening process, 323 full-text articles were sought for retrieval for full-text review, and 75 articles were unable to be retrieved as full-text versions were not available at the time of review. This left 248 articles to be assessed for full-text review. Of these 248 full-text articles, 122 were excluded because they did not meet the PICOS eligibility criteria. The 126 remaining articles are included in this review [23–148]. A summary of the demographics of all included studies is presented in Table S2, followed by a summary of their findings in Table S3—both of which are in the Supplementary Materials.

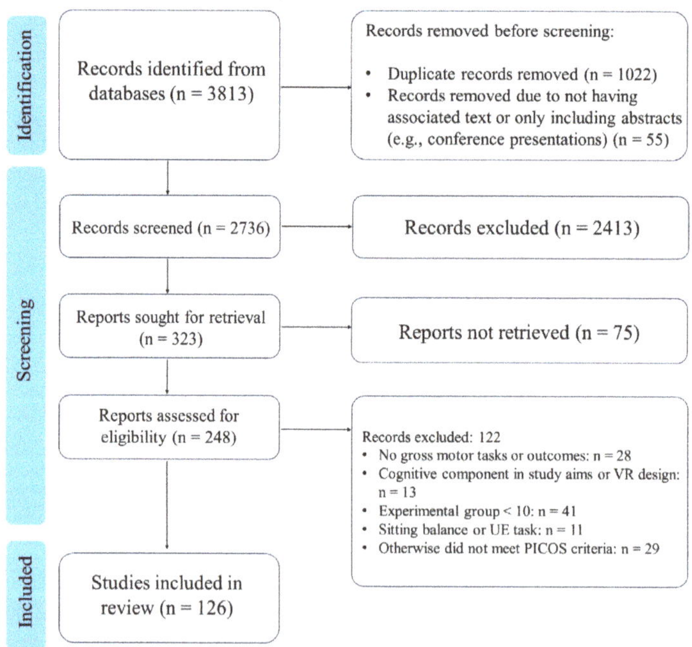

Figure 1. Preferred Reporting Items for Systematic reviews and Meta-Analyses extension for Scoping Reviews (PRISMA-ScR) flow diagram of study selection.

3.2. Publication Year

This search for this review focused on articles published between 2010 and 2023. Of the included articles, none were published in 2010. Over half (n = 66; 52.0%) of the included articles were published in the second half of the last decade, between 2017 and 2021. A table of the distribution of publications between 2011 and 2023 can be seen in Figure 2.

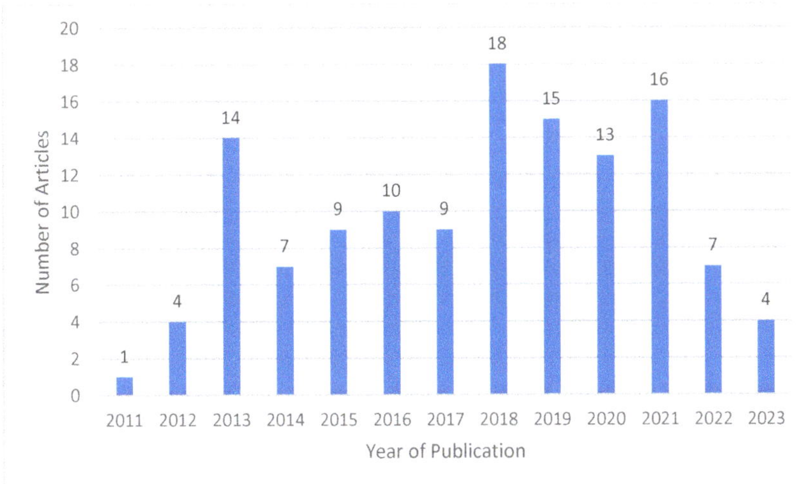

Figure 2. Publications per year.

3.3. Population Studied

The majority of studies (n = 121; 95.3%) used adult populations (mean age: 60.9 ± 13.3 years), with six studies (4.7%) using pediatric participants (mean age: 11.1 ± 2.4 years). Across all 126 included articles, the primary populations studied were stroke survivors (23.6%), Parkinson's disease patients (20.5%), and older adults (13.4%). Figure 3 shows the distribution of all included populations.

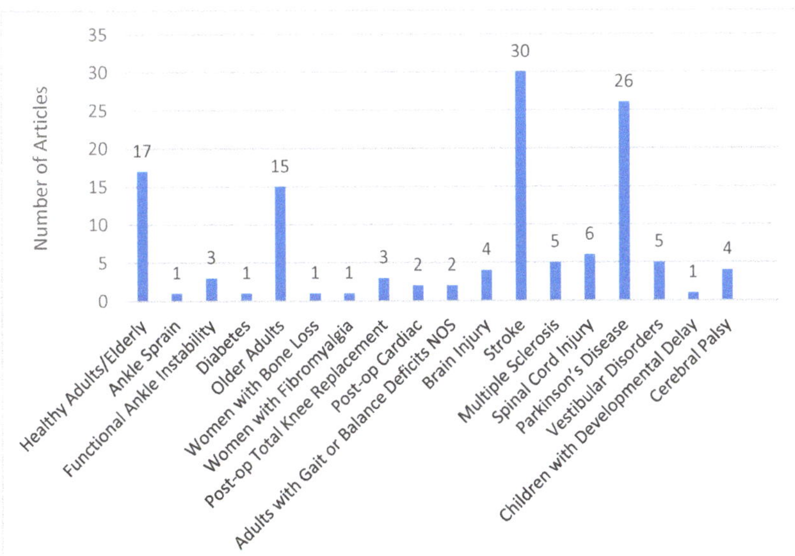

Figure 3. Patient populations of each study.

3.4. Location and Setting

The largest number of studies were conducted in South Korea (n = 23; 18.1%), Italy (n = 14; 11.0%), and Brazil (n = 13; 10.2%). Research conducted in the United States (n = 8; 6.3%) and Spain (n = 6; 4.7%) contributed to the included publications. Four publications each came from Poland (3.1%), Switzerland (3.1%), Israel (3.1%), Taiwan (3.1%), China (3.1%), and Turkey (3.1%). Three publications each came from Australia (2.4%), Malaysia (2.4%), and Pakistan (2.4%). Two publications each came from Canada (1.6%), Egypt (1.6%), France (1.6%), and Japan (1.6%). The remaining countries each produced 0.8% (n = 1, each) of the articles included in this review: Austria, Chile, Germany, India, Jordan, Singapore, Slovenia, and Sweden. Four articles (3.1%) did not provide explicit information regarding the geographic location of their research. The locations of the research conducted for each publication included in this review can be viewed in Figure 4. The largest percentage of studies were conducted in inpatient settings of clinical facilities (n = 37; 29.1%), such as acute rehabilitation centers, hospitals, subacute rehabilitation facilities, and nursing homes. This is followed by laboratory settings (n = 27; 21.3%), community centers (n = 9; 7.1%), outpatient clinical facilities (n = 8; 6.3%), home-based settings (n = 5; 3.9%), telerehabilitation settings (n = 4; 3.2%), and research settings (n = 3; 2.4%). Notably, 24 studies (18.9%) did not explicitly state their research setting.

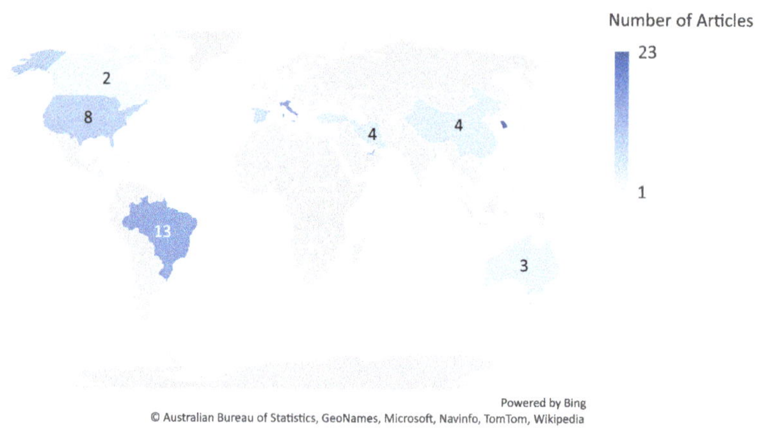

Figure 4. Number of studies per country of 123 articles that included geographic location. Four articles did not report where their study took place.

3.5. Study Protocols

Sixty-seven (52.8%) studies used interventions with the primary aim of improving balance. This is followed in descending order by studies with interventions targeting gait only (n = 18; 14.2%), both gait and balance (n = 17; 13.4%), upright mobility (n = 9; 7.1%), balance and upright mobility (n = 3; 2.4%), and a combination of gait, balance, and upright mobility (n = 4; 3.1%). The total sample size for each study ranged widely from 10 to 195 subjects. The average number of subjects used was 37.0 (±25.7 participants). The majority of studies (n = 108; 85.0%) had a total sample size of 50 or less. The distribution of the sample sizes of the included studies can be seen in Figure 5.

Most studies (n = 76; 59.8%) utilized a two-group study design comparing VR to an active control performing some form of conventional rehabilitation (CR). This is followed by studies with a single, VR-only group (n = 28; 22.0%) or a three-group design comparing VR, CR, and VR + CR (n = 11; 8.7%). The distribution of the study design groups can be viewed in Figure 6. More specifically, the figure shows a breakdown of the intervention types (e.g., VR only, VR + CR, etc.) across the number/type of participant groups (e.g., single group, two-group stratified), illustrating the diversity of study designs in this line of research. A total of 70 studies (55.1%) used study designs with a control group. Of these studies, 48 used a randomized method for allocating their participants, while 22 did not randomize group allocation. The studies employed study designs with various dosages of VR interventions. Intervention length varied from 1 to 12 weeks, with most studies using 6 weeks (n = 23; 18.1%) closely followed by 4 weeks (n = 21; 16.5%). Intervention frequency ranged from once per week to two times per day; the total session number ranged from 5 to 60 sessions. Intervention duration ranged from 15 to 60 min per session. Of note, 25 studies (19.7%) provided a rationale for the design of their VR intervention with empirical support, while 102 studies (80.3%) did not provide an evidence-based rationale for their intervention.

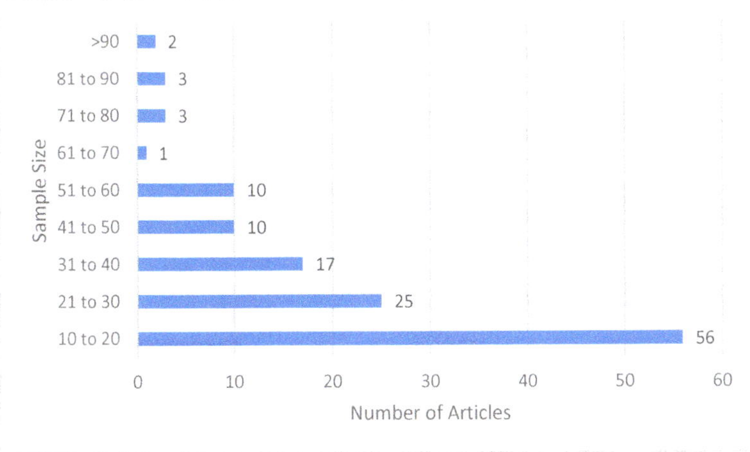

Figure 5. Total sample size.

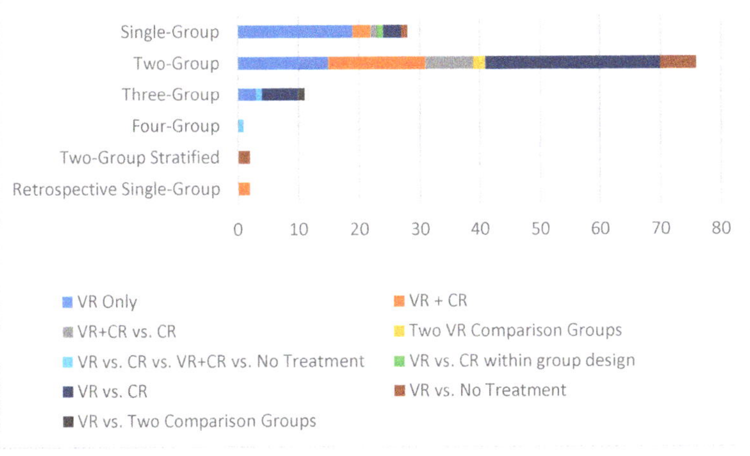

Figure 6. Group study design. VR = virtual reality. CR = conventional reality.

3.6. Virtual Reality Hardware and Software

The majority of studies used less-immersive (n = 44; 34.6%), commercially available VR hardware such as the Nintendo Wii and Xbox Kinect. Thirty-four studies (26.8%) used semi-immersive hardware, including the Computer Assisted Rehabilitation Environment (CAREN) system (n = 2), the Gait Real-time Interactive Lab (GRAIL) system (n = 3), and multi-screen interactive setups (n = 6), which provide increased surroundedness and interactivity over less-immersive VR technologies. Of the thirty-four semi-immersive setups, eight were medical grade hardware (CAREN, GRAIL), and six were custom setups which are not off-the-shelf products. Forty-nine studies (38.3%) used immersive technologies with head-mounted displays (HMD), providing a higher level of immersion due to the full-surroundedness of the display. This immersive VR hardware includes the Oculus Rift (n = 9) and other custom setups (n = 18). Figures 7 and 8 show the distribution of the level of immersion (Figure 7) and the grade (medical, commercial, custom-created, Figure 8) of all VR hardware used in the included publications. One study did not report the details of the VR hardware used for their intervention.

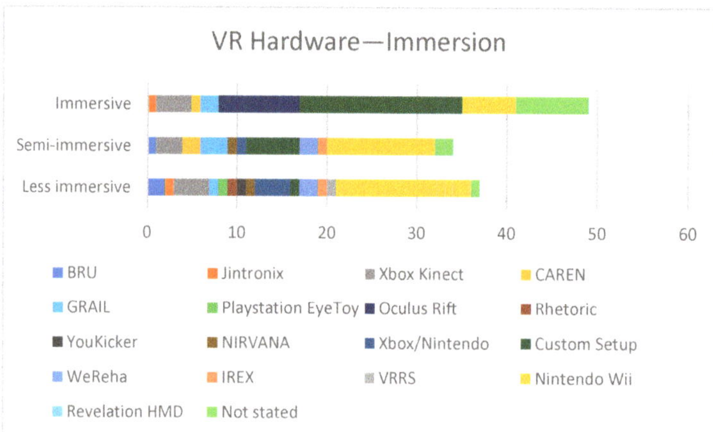

Figure 7. Level of immersion of VR.

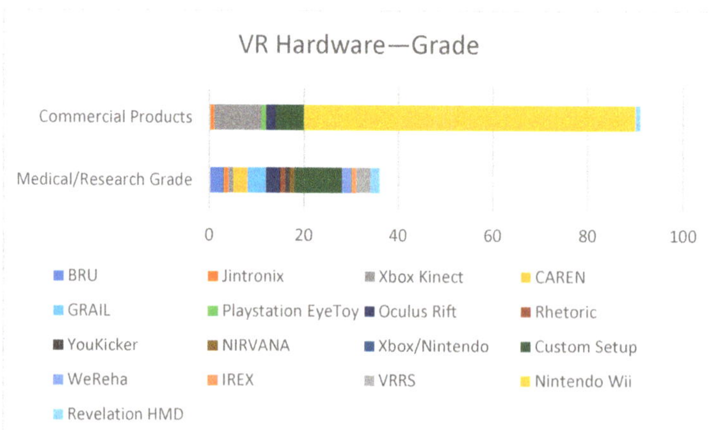

Figure 8. Use of prefabricated VR hardware.

The majority of studies (n = 71; 56.3 %) used off-the-shelf commercial software such as Wii Fit Plus or Kinect Adventures. Twenty-one studies (16.7 %) relied on medical- or research-grade packages (e.g., CAREN, GRAIL). Twenty-nine studies (23.0 %) implemented custom-built programs, typically created in platforms like Unity or 3D Studio Max. Five studies (4.0 %) did not report which software they employed. Figure 9 illustrates the full breakdown of VR software types.

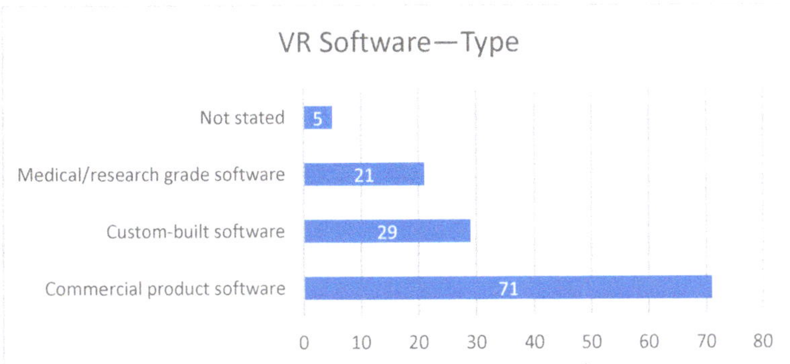

Figure 9. Type of VR software used.

3.7. *Intervention Outcomes*

Most studies (n = 93; 73.2%) reported significant improvements in outcomes related to gait, balance, and upright mobility following their VR intervention. Thirty-six of these studies found a significant improvement in gait, balance, or upright mobility in their VR treatment group compared to the comparison group following VR intervention. Eighteen of the studies (14.2%) that reported between-group differences in favor of the VR group employed study designs in which the VR group also participated in conventional rehabilitation programs. Two studies (1.6%) reported improvements in their VR group; however, these improvements were not statistically significant. None of the included studies reported no change or a decline in function related to gait, balance, or upright mobility following their VR intervention.

4. Discussion

This scoping review aimed to investigate how VR has been used in physical rehabilitation research from 2010 to present. All studies reported improvements in the motor domains of gait, balance, or upright mobility following VR intervention. This is consistent with previous review papers that found that VR interventions provide effective therapeutic outcomes that can be superior to standard care [6–9]. Despite repeated findings that support the effectiveness of VR interventions to improve motor outcomes, it is important to point out the known publication bias toward statistically significant results over those that accept the null hypothesis [149]. Thus, studies finding a degradation, or no change, in motor skills following VR intervention may not be published, which should be taken into consideration when interpreting the results of this review. However, to this point, 1.5% (n= 2) of the studies did publish non-significant results, reporting that the VR group did exhibit improvements in the functional outcomes of their study, but these improvements were not statistically significant.

Prior reviews and meta-analyses regarding VR for rehabilitation have found that studies have limited methodological validity due to small samples, a lack of controls, or the absence of a clear rationale for the development of their intervention [6–9]. In this review, the average sample size was 37 participants, with 101 studies having a total sample size of 50 participants or less. Of these 101 studies, most of them had sample sizes between 10 and 20. This is important to consider, as small sample sizes can lead to low statistical power and an overestimation of the significance of the intervention [150]. It should also be noted that an exclusion criterion for this review was studies with less than 10 subjects in the experimental group. Of the 248 articles included for full-text review, 16.4% (n = 41) were excluded due to having an experimental group smaller than 10.

Previous systematic reviews have cited the lack of a comparison group, a lack of treatment or waitlist control groups, and/or a lack of randomization as methodological shortcomings in this area of research [1,7,151]. Regarding the study design for the articles included in this review, 26.5% of the studies used two-group designs with primarily active control groups participating in CR interventions. The use of a two-group design is the cleanest way to test the efficacy of an intervention and provide a performance comparison to a group not participating in the intervention [152]. Further, including an active control group participating in an intervention considered to be standard care provides a more rigorous comparison than a no-treatment control group [7]. Additionally, the use of active control groups helps to circumvent any ethical dilemmas related to providing no treatment to clinical populations [153]. Regarding group allocation, 37.5% of studies used randomization methods for allocating subjects to their study groups. As previously mentioned, small sample size is a common limitation in this area of research, and small sample sizes can reduce statistical power. However, randomization techniques can help boost statistical power that may be affected by both small sample sizes and between-group analyses [150–152]. The findings of this review suggest that VR researchers adhered to this methodological quality in their study designs, as most studies had an active comparison group and random allocation of participants to each group. Nevertheless, research continues to lack clear rationale regarding the development of interventions. Only 19.5% of the studies in this review provided a rationale with empirical support for at least part of the design of their VR intervention.

Studies continue to focus primarily on adults and predominantly neurological populations. A majority of studies (93.0%) had adult participants, while only nine included pediatric populations. This disparity between adult and pediatric populations could be due to the general composition of the population, which is projected to see considerable growth in the population over 65 years of age [154]. Additionally, the relative ease of recruiting adult subjects compared to obtaining the parental consent for minors could be a contributing factor. More than half of the studies investigated the role of VR interventions in improving gait, balance, or upright mobility in neurologic populations, including those with brain injury, stroke, multiple sclerosis, spinal cord injury, Parkinson's disease, or cerebral palsy. This is possibly due to the extent to which neurological deficits impact a person's overall functional independence and quality of life, making investigating effective treatment interventions a high priority. Injuries to the nervous system can result in a range of deficits, including changes in motor planning and execution, strength, and coordination—all of which can profoundly impact a person's ability to ambulate, balance, or perform everyday activities of daily living [155,156]. Thus, the primary aims of physical rehabilitation interventions for this population align with the primary aim of this review, which was to investigate VR interventions for gait, balance, and upright mobility.

Additionally, physical rehabilitation to improve motor deficits following neurological impairment involves therapy protocols that use high levels of repetition, which can quickly become disengaging for participants [14–16]. To address this barrier, VR has been shown to have psychological benefits for patients in PT, including reducing tension, increasing calmness, easing fatigue, reducing depression, improving motivation, and enhancing the quality of life [156–158]. Aside from neurologic populations, older adults are the next most prominently studied group, comprising 19.5% of the publications included in this review. Aging is associated with frailty, decreased independence, and falls, especially in older adults over the age of 65 [159]. Age-related changes in vision and the vestibular and somatosensory systems, as well as changes in the musculoskeletal system, can influence how older adults maintain balance during movement and upright mobility, again, aligning typical physical rehabilitation treatment plans for this population with the primary outcomes of this review [160]. This is also in line with other reviews that have found VR to be effective in improving mobility, balance, and overall physical functioning in older adults [19,161–163].

Most of the studies included in this review were conducted in more ecologically valid settings than the small portion (17.1%) of studies performed in sterile laboratory environments. It should be noted that 16 publications did not explicitly report their research setting. Despite this, the findings of this review show that the majority of VR research into physical rehabilitation interventions for gait, balance, and upright mobility was conducted in clinical environments, which is in contrast to a previous review which found that VR research is primarily performed in laboratory settings [6]. This could be due to the fact that the previous review was only investigating VR interventions for upright mobility in neurological populations, creating a narrower review of the literature. Additionally, the article searches for the previous review were performed from 2017 to 2018. In the current review, of the studies performed in non-laboratory settings (n = 62), 43.5% of them were published in 2019 or later.

Most of the studies included in this review were conducted outside of the United States, with most being performed in South Korea, followed closely by Brazil and Italy. Regardless of their location, the studies primarily used less immersive and commercially available VR hardware. Additionally, about half of these studies used off-the-shelf software such as Wii Fit or Kinect Adventures. Less than a quarter of the studies used custom-designed software like 3D Studio Max to produce a VR environment tailored to their intervention. This is consistent with previous reviews which have found that most VR interventions utilize hardware that has associated prefabricated environments, and typically these are off-the-shelf programs such as Wii Fit [6,8,162]. Moreover, this speaks to the criticism that research in this area grossly lacks theory-driven VR intervention development [6–9]. The majority of research is being conducted to determine the efficacy level of VR at large and, thus, uses low-cost or time-efficient ways to determine efficacy, such as using ready-to-run programs. This is favorable in a sense, as clinicians may be more likely to use VR technology and games that are easier to access. However, in the case of commercially available VR products, these technologies were created for entertainment, without a priori use of theory-based principles to address the desired motor learning principles, motor deficits, or components of exercise prescription and achieve the specific outcomes of an intervention.

As previously discussed, a limited number of studies provided a rationale for the development of their intervention, including study design, VR hardware and software usage, and intervention dosage. Interventions ranged from 1 to 12 weeks, with the two most common intervention lengths being 4 and 6 weeks. Additionally, intervention frequency and duration ranged from 5 to 60 sessions lasting between 15 and 60 min each. The most common intervention dosage used was a duration of 6 weeks, 3 visits per week, and 30 min for each session. This is consistent with a previous review which found that the most common VR intervention implemented 3 sessions per week for 20–40 min over 4–6 weeks [8].

Of the studies that cited evidence-based rationale for their VR intervention development, eleven of them provided support for either the frequency, intensity, or duration. However, only two articles cited evidence to support their intervention prescription that was specifically related to VR interventions [81,111]. The other nine articles cited support based on empirical evidence related to intervention prescriptions for specific patient populations such as multiple sclerosis patients [71], or recommendations for general physical activity prescriptions from national organizations such as the American College of Sports Medicine (ACSM) [92]. Thus, VR research seems to be applying a more systematic and theory-driven approach to the development of VR interventions; however, more work needs to be done to identify VR-specific recommendations regarding dosage. This is supported by other reviews of VR interventions to improve motor outcomes, as currently a wide range of intervention protocols are being employed, and not always with a priori justification specific to VR training [6,8,164].

VR can be defined as an artificial environment containing sensory information that can be interacted with, visualized, or manipulated to allow natural behaviors to emerge as if the environment were real [10–12]. In the case of VR usage for rehabilitation in the context of the articles included in this review, the natural behaviors elicited are the gross motor functions of gait, balance, and upright mobility. The variety of functionality and customization of VR makes it a promising tool to provide meaningful interventions to improve motor outcomes.

VR can take many forms and continues to evolve as technology advances. With the development of off-the-shelf, commercially available products, VR has been more widely researched for use in a variety of domains, including physical rehabilitation. As can be seen in the publications included in this review, the majority of studies utilize commercially available VR hardware and software. This is consistent with prior systematic reviews which also found that the majority of research is conducted using low-cost VR technologies. This is likely due to the low cost and easy setup being more conducive to use in clinical or home settings. The clinical implications from our scoping review are as follows: (1) VR has become more accessible for clinicians in terms of cost and usability; (2) VR has been integrated into several different settings for rehabilitation purposes, including inpatient/outpatient settings, community centers, and home environments; and (3) infusing VR into a rehabilitation plan has generally led to positive results.

It should be noted that some limitations of this review exist. First, this review was limited to the outcomes of gait, balance, and upright mobility. Other domains of gross motor function, such as upper extremity rehabilitation, and adjacent domains like pain management and cognitive function were not included in this review. Similarly, research that used an adjunctive modality such as transcranial magnetic stimulation, functional electric stimulation, or robot-assisted gait training was also not included in this review. These domains, as they relate to VR research, may be most appropriate to review separately as they have their own critical mass and may reveal interesting insights into the use of VR in these areas. Moreover, VR technology considerably changed, including the accessibility of the technology, across the included years of 2010–2023, which could have impacted the results. It should also be noted that we used the same search string for each database, which is not a best practice method. Each database has a unique coding system (e.g., PubMed uses MeSH terms, SCOPUS uses a TITLE-ABS-KEY format), so tailoring the search to each database's coding system would allow a more optimized return of matching articles. Lastly, the articles were limited to three database searches and do not account for eligible studies that could be acquired through additional databases or grey literature. Despite these limitations, this review included a large sample of research (n = 126) covering a wide range of patient populations, research locations, and research settings, giving a diverse understanding of how VR is being researched for use as an intervention to improve gait, balance, and upright mobility.

5. Conclusions

In conclusion, 58.5% of the studies in this review were conducted outside of a research laboratory. This demonstrates that research in this area is moving beyond proof-of-concept and toward translation to clinical applications. Beyond demonstrating that VR can provide significant improvement in gait, balance, and upright mobility, this also indicates that VR has been implemented in clinical, community, and home environments. What still remains unclear is how this empirical evidence is being utilized by clinical providers. Future research may benefit from assessing the usability from the perspective of the clinical providers assisting with the data collection, as many studies reported that PTs supervised their VR interventions. Additionally, as studies find significant improvement in their desired outcomes, studies regarding the knowledge translation or sustainability of an intervention could be useful for implementing actual use of that VR intervention beyond the boundaries of the study protocol.

Supplementary Materials: The following supporting information can be downloaded at: https://www.mdpi.com/article/10.3390/technologies13050167/s1, Table S1: PRISMA-ScR checklist; Table S2: Demographic information of included studies; Table S3: Summary of findings of included studies. Refs. [23–148,165] are cited in Supplementary Materials file.

Author Contributions: Conceptualization, D.T.F., S.E.R., L.D.R., J.T.M., and C.K.R.; methodology, D.T.F., R.P., C.K.H., S.E.R., L.D.R., J.T.M., and C.K.R.; software, D.T.F., R.P., C.K.H., and C.K.R.; validation, D.T.F., R.P., and C.K.H.; formal analysis, D.T.F., R.P., C.K.H., and C.K.R.; investigation, D.T.F., R.P., and C.K.H.; resources, C.K.R.; data curation, D.T.F., R.P., and C.K.H.; writing—original draft preparation, D.T.F., R.P., C.K.H., and C.K.R.; writing—review and editing, S.E.R., L.D.R., and J.T.M.; visualization, D.T.F., R.P., and C.K.H.; supervision, C.K.R.; project administration, C.K.R. All authors have read and agreed to the published version of the manuscript.

Funding: This research received no external funding.

Institutional Review Board Statement: Not applicable.

Informed Consent Statement: Not applicable.

Data Availability Statement: All the data can be found in the body of the paper and the Supplementary Materials.

Conflicts of Interest: The authors declare no conflicts of interest.

References

1. Bechtold, U.; Stauder, N.; Fieder, M. Let's walk it: Mobility and the perceived quality of life in older adults. *Int. J. Environ. Res. Public Health* **2021**, *18*, 11515. [CrossRef]
2. Despoti, A.; Karatzanos, E.; Patsaki, I.; Tzoumi, D.; Roussou, G.; Leventakis, N.; Papathanasiou, A.; Nanas, S.; Dimitriadi, N. Immersive virtual reality in cognitive rehabilitation: A systematic review. *Health Res. J.* **2022**, *8*, 225–241. [CrossRef]
3. Patsaki, I.; Avgeri, V.; Rigoulia, T.; Zekis, T.; Koumantakis, G.A.; Grammatopoulou, E. Benefits from incorporating virtual reality in pulmonary rehabilitation of COPD patients: A systematic review and meta-analysis. *Adv. Respir. Med.* **2023**, *91*, 324–336. [CrossRef] [PubMed]
4. Goudman, L.; Jansen, J.; Billot, M.; Vets, N.; Smedt, A.D.; Rouland, M.; Rigoard, P.; Moens, M. Virtual reality applications in chronic pain management: Systematic review and meta-analysis. *JMIR Serious Games* **2022**, *10*, e34402. [CrossRef]
5. Kanschik, D.; Bruno, R.R.; Wolff, G.; Kelm, M.; Jung, C. Virtual and augmented reality in intensive care medicine: A systematic review. *Ann. Intensive Care* **2023**, *13*, 81. [CrossRef] [PubMed]

6. Felsberg, D.T.; Maher, J.P.; Rhea, C.K. The state of behavior change techniques in virtual reality rehabilitation of neurologic populations. *Front. Psychol.* **2019**, *10*, 979. [CrossRef] [PubMed]
7. Howard, M.C. A meta-analysis and systematic literature review of virtual reality rehabilitation programs. *Comput. Hum. Behav.* **2017**, *70*, 317–327. [CrossRef]
8. Cano Porras, D.; Siemonsma, P.; Inzelberg, R.; Zeilig, G.; Plotnik, M. Advantages of virtual reality in the rehabilitation of balance and gait: Systematic review. *Neurology* **2018**, *90*, 1017–1025. [CrossRef]
9. Campo-Prieto, P.; Cancela, J.M.; Rodríguez-Fuentes, G. Immersive virtual reality as physical therapy in older adults: Present or future (systematic review). *Virtual Real.* **2021**, *25*, 801–817. [CrossRef]
10. Jerald, J. *The VR Book: Human-Centered Design for Virtual Reality*, 1st ed.; ACM Books: New York, NY, USA, 2016.
11. Rizzo, A.; Koenig, S.T. Is clinical virtual reality ready for primetime? *Neuropsychology* **2017**, *31*, 877–899. [CrossRef]
12. Steinicke, F.; Visell, Y.; Campos, J.; Lécuyer, A. *Human Walking in Virtual Environments*, 1st ed.; Springer: New York, NY, USA, 2013.
13. Adamovich, S.V.; Fluet, G.G.; Tunik, E.; Merians, A.S. Sensorimotor training in virtual reality: A review. *NeuroRehabilitation* **2009**, *25*, 29–44. [CrossRef]
14. Levin, M.F. Can virtual reality offer enriched environments for rehabilitation? *Expert Rev. Neurother.* **2011**, *11*, 153–155. [CrossRef] [PubMed]
15. Levac, D.; Sveistrup, H. Motor learning and virtual reality. In *Virtual Reality for Physical and Motor Rehabilitation*; Weiss, P.L., Keshner, E.A., Levin, M.F., Eds.; Springer: New York, NY, USA, 2014; pp. 25–46.
16. Zimmerli, L.; Jacky, M.; Lunenburger, L.; Riener, R.; Bolliger, M. Increasing patient engagement during virtual reality-based motor rehabilitation. *Arch. Phys. Med. Rehabil.* **2013**, *94*, 1737–1746. [CrossRef]
17. Góra, T.; Tsos, A.; Indyka, S. Bibliometric analysis of the application of digital technology in physical rehabilitation. *Sport Tour. Cent. Eur. J.* **2024**, *7*, 133–146. [CrossRef]
18. Bateni, H.; Carruthers, J.; Mohan, R.; Pishva, S. Use of virtual reality in physical therapy as an intervention and diagnostic tool. *Rehabil. Res. Pract.* **2024**, *2024*, 1122286. [CrossRef] [PubMed]
19. Cieślik, B.; Mazurek, J.; Wrzeciono, A.; Maistrello, L.; Szczepańska-Gieracha, J.; Conte, P.; Kiper, P. Examining technology-assisted rehabilitation for older adults' functional mobility: A network meta-analysis on efficacy and acceptability. *npj Digit. Med.* **2023**, *6*, 159. [CrossRef] [PubMed]
20. Pang, W.Y.J.; Cheng, L. Acceptance of gamified virtual reality environments by older adults. *Educ. Gerontol.* **2023**, *49*, 830–841. [CrossRef]
21. Peters, M.D.; Marnie, C.; Tricco, A.C.; Pollock, D.; Munn, Z.; Alexander, L.; McInerney, P.; Godfrey, C.M.; Khalil, H. Updated methodological guidance for the conduct of scoping reviews. *JBI Evid. Synth.* **2020**, *18*, 2119–2126. [CrossRef]
22. Liberati, A.; Altman, D.G.; Tetzlaff, J.; Tetzlaff, J.; Mulrow, C.; Gøtzsche, P.C.; Ioannidis, J.P.A.; Clarke, M.; Devereaux, P.J.; Kleijnen, J.; et al. The PRISMA statement for reporting systematic reviews and meta-analyses of studies that evaluate healthcare interventions: Explanation and elaboration. *BMJ* **2009**, *154*, 339. [CrossRef]
23. Afridi, A.; Malik, A.N.; Ali, S.; Amjad, I. Effect of balance training in older adults using Wii Fit Plus. *J. Pak. Med. Assoc.* **2018**, *68*, 480–483.
24. Aharoni, M.M.H.; Lubetzky, A.V.; Arie, L.; Krasovsky, T. Factors associated with dynamic balance in people with Persistent Postural Perceptual Dizziness (PPPD): A cross-sectional study using a virtual-reality Four Square Step Test. *J. Neuroeng. Rehabil.* **2021**, *18*, 55. [CrossRef] [PubMed]
25. Alahmari, K.A.; Sparto, P.J.; Marchetti, G.F.; Redfern, M.S.; Furman, J.M.; Whitney, S.L. Comparison of virtual reality-based therapy with customized vestibular physical therapy for the treatment of vestibular disorders. *IEEE Trans. Neural Syst. Rehabil. Eng.* **2014**, *22*, 389–399. [CrossRef] [PubMed]
26. Alhirsan, S.M.; Capó-Lugo, C.E.; Brown, D.A. Effects of different types of augmented feedback on intrinsic motivation and walking speed performance in post-stroke: A study protocol. *Contemp. Clin. Trials Commun.* **2021**, *24*, 100863. [CrossRef]
27. An, C.M.; Park, Y.H. The effects of semi-immersive virtual reality therapy on standing balance and upright mobility function in individuals with chronic incomplete spinal cord injury: A preliminary study. *J. Spinal Cord Med.* **2018**, *41*, 223–229. [CrossRef]
28. Anson, E.; Ma, L.; Meetam, T.; Thompson, E.; Rathore, R.; Dean, V.; Jeka, J. Trunk motion visual feedback during walking improves dynamic balance in older adults: Assessor-blinded randomized controlled trial. *Gait Posture* **2018**, *62*, 342–348.
29. Anwar, N.; Karimi, H.; Ahmad, A.; Mumtaz, N.; Saqulain, G.; Gilani, S.A. A novel virtual reality training strategy for post-stroke patients: A randomized clinical trial. *J. Healthc. Eng.* **2021**, *6598726*.
30. Bang, Y.S.; Son, K.H.; Kim, H.J. Effects of virtual reality training using Nintendo Wii and treadmill walking exercise on balance and walking for stroke patients. *J. Phys. Ther. Sci.* **2016**, *28*, 3112–3115. [CrossRef]

31. Bellomo, R.G.; Paolucci, T.; Saggino, A.; Pezzi, L.; Bramanti, A.; Cimino, V.; Tommasi, M.; Saggini, R. The WeReha project for an innovative home-based exercise training in chronic stroke patients: A clinical study. *J. Cent. Nerv. Syst. Dis.* **2020**, *12*, 117957352097986. [CrossRef]
32. Brachman, A.; Marszałek, W.; Kamieniarz, A.; Michalska, J.; Pawłowski, M.; Juras, G. Biomechanical measures of balance after balance-based exergaming training dedicated for patients with Parkinson's disease. *Gait Posture* **2021**, *87*, 170–176. [CrossRef] [PubMed]
33. Brachman, A.; Marszałek, W.; Kamieniarz, A.; Michalska, J.; Pawłowski, M.; Akbaş, A.; Juras, G. The effects of exergaming training on balance in healthy elderly women—A pilot study. *Int. J. Environ. Res. Public Health* **2021**, *18*, 1412. [CrossRef]
34. Pazzaglia, C.; Imbimbo, I.; Tranchita, E.; Minganti, C.; Ricciardi, D.; Lo Monaco, R.; Parisi, A.; Padua, L. Comparison of virtual reality rehabilitation and conventional rehabilitation in Parkinson's disease: A randomized controlled trial. *Physiotherapy* **2020**, *106*, 36–42. [CrossRef]
35. Cacau, L.D.A.P.; Oliveira, G.U.; Maynard, L.G.; Araújo Filho, A.A.; Silva Jr, W.M.; Cerqueria Neto, M.L.; Antoniolli, A.R.; Santana-Filho, V.J. The use of virtual reality as an intervention tool in the postoperative period of cardiac surgery. *Rev. Bras. Cir. Cardiovasc.* **2013**, *28*, 281–289. [CrossRef] [PubMed]
36. Calabrò, R.S.; Naro, A.; Cimino, V.; Buda, A.; Paladina, G.; Di Lorenzo, G.; Manuli, A.; Milardi, D.; Bramanti, P.; Bramanti, A. Improving motor performance in Parkinson's disease: A preliminary study on the promising use of the computer-assisted virtual reality environment (CAREN). *Neurol. Sci.* **2020**, *41*, 933–941. [CrossRef]
37. Campo-Prieto, P.; Cancela-Carral, J.M.; Rodríguez-Fuentes, G. Feasibility and effects of an immersive virtual reality exergame program on physical functions in institutionalized older adults: A randomized clinical trial. *Sensors* **2022**, *22*, 6742. [CrossRef] [PubMed]
38. Cannell, J.; Jovic, E.; Rathjen, A.; Lane, K.; Tyson, A.M.; Callisaya, M.L.; Smith, S.T.; Ahuja, K.D.K.; Bird, M.-L. The efficacy of interactive, motion capture-based rehabilitation on functional outcomes in an inpatient stroke population: A randomized controlled trial. *Clin. Rehabil.* **2018**, *32*, 191–200. [CrossRef] [PubMed]
39. Cano Porras, D.; Sharon, H.; Inzelberg, R.; Ziv-Ner, Y.; Zeilig, G.; Plotnik, M. Advanced virtual reality-based rehabilitation of balance and gait in clinical practice. *Ther. Adv. Chronic Dis.* **2019**, *10*, 2040622319868379. [CrossRef]
40. Chen, P.J.; Penn, I.W.; Wei, S.H.; Chuang, L.R.; Sung, W.H. Augmented reality-assisted training with selected Tai-Chi movements improves balance control and increases lower limb muscle strength in older adults: A prospective randomized trial. *J. Exerc. Sci. Fit.* **2020**, *18*, 142–147. [CrossRef]
41. Cho, G.H.; Hwangbo, G.; Shin, H.S. The effects of virtual reality-based balance training on balance of the elderly. *J. Phys. Ther. Sci.* **2014**, *26*, 615–617. [CrossRef]
42. Cho, K.H.; Lee, K.J.; Song, C.H. Virtual-reality balance training with a video-game system improves dynamic balance in chronic stroke patients. *Tohoku J. Exp. Med.* **2012**, *228*, 69–74. [CrossRef]
43. Cikajlo, I.; Rudolf, M.; Mainetti, R.; Borghese, N.A. Multi-exergames to set targets and supplement the intensified conventional balance training in patients with stroke: A randomized pilot trial. *Front. Psychol.* **2020**, *11*, 572. [CrossRef]
44. Collado-Mateo, D.; Dominguez-Muñoz, F.J.; Adsuar, J.C.; Merellano-Navarro, E.; Gusi, N. Exergames for women with fibromyalgia: A randomized controlled trial to evaluate the effects on mobility skills, balance, and fear of falling. *PeerJ* **2017**, *5*, e3211. [CrossRef]
45. de Melo, G.E.L.; Kleiner, A.F.R.; Lopes, J.B.P.; Dumont, A.J.L.; Lazzari, R.D.; Galli, M.; Oliveira, C.S. Effect of virtual reality training on walking distance and physical fitness in individuals with Parkinson's disease. *NeuroRehabilitation* **2018**, *42*, 473–480. [CrossRef] [PubMed]
46. de Rooij, I.J.M.; van de Port, I.G.L.; Punt, M.; Abbink-van Moorsel, P.J.M.; Kortsmit, M.; van Eijk, R.P.A.; Visser-Meily, J.M.A.; Meijer, J.-W.G. Effect of virtual reality gait training on participation in survivors of subacute stroke: A randomized controlled trial. *Phys. Ther.* **2021**, *101*, pzab051. [CrossRef] [PubMed]
47. de Vries, A.W.; Faber, G.; Jonkers, I.; Van Dieen, J.H.; Verschueren, S.M.P. Virtual reality balance training for elderly: Similar skiing games elicit different challenges in balance training. *Gait Posture* **2018**, *59*, 111–116. [CrossRef]
48. Feng, H.; Li, C.; Liu, J.; Wang, L.; Ma, J.; Li, G.; Gan, L.; Shang, X.; Wu, Z. Virtual reality rehabilitation versus conventional physical therapy for improving balance and gait in Parkinson's disease patients: A randomized controlled trial. *Med. Sci. Monit.* **2019**, *25*, 4186–4192. [CrossRef] [PubMed]
49. Ferraz, D.D.; Trippo, K.V.; Duarte, G.P.; Neto, M.G.; Bernardes Santos, K.O.; Filho, J.O. The effects of functional training, bicycle exercise, and exergaming on walking capacity of elderly patients with Parkinson's disease: A pilot randomized controlled single-blinded trial. *Arch. Phys. Med. Rehabil.* **2018**, *99*, 826–833. [CrossRef]
50. Finley, J.M.; Gotsis, M.; Lympouridis, V.; Jain, S.; Kim, A.; Fisher, B.E. Design and development of a virtual reality-based mobility training game for people with Parkinson's disease. *Front. Neurol.* **2020**, *11*, 577713. [CrossRef]

51. Fransson, P.A.; Patel, M.; Jensen, H.; Lundberg, M.; Tjernström, F.; Magnusson, M.; Ekvall Hansson, E. Postural instability in an immersive virtual reality adapts with repetition and includes directional and gender-specific effects. *Sci. Rep.* **2019**, *9*, 3168. [CrossRef]
52. Gagliardi, C.; Turconi, A.C.; Biffi, E.; Maghini, C.; Marelli, A.; Cesareo, A.; Diella, E.; Panzeri, D. Immersive virtual reality to improve walking abilities in cerebral palsy: A pilot study. *Ann. Biomed. Eng.* **2018**, *46*, 1376–1384. [CrossRef]
53. Gandolfi, M.; Geroin, C.; Dimitrova, E.; Boldrini, P.; Waldner, A.; Bonadiman, S.; Picelli, A.; Regazzo, S.; Stirbu, E.; Primon, D.; et al. Virtual reality telerehabilitation for postural instability in Parkinson's disease: A multicenter, single-blind, randomized, controlled trial. *BioMed Res. Int.* **2017**, *2017*, 7962826. [CrossRef]
54. Garcia, A.P.; Ganança, M.M.; Cusin, F.S.; Tomaz, A.; Ganança, F.F.; Caovilla, H.H. Vestibular rehabilitation with virtual reality in Ménière's disease. *Braz. J. Otorhinolaryngol.* **2013**, *79*, 366–374. [CrossRef]
55. Gatica-Rojas, V.; Cartes-Velásquez, R.; Guzmán-Muñoz, E.; Méndez-Rebolledo, G.; Soto-Poblete, A.; Pacheco-Espinoza, A.C.; Amigo-Mendoza, C.; Albornoz-Verdugo, M.E.; Elgueta-Cancino, E. Effectiveness of a Nintendo Wii balance board exercise programme on standing balance of children with cerebral palsy: A randomised clinical trial protocol. *Contemp. Clin. Trials Commun.* **2017**, *6*, 17–21. [CrossRef] [PubMed]
56. Gianola, S.; Stucovitz, E.; Castellini, G.; Mascali, M.; Vanni, F.; Tramacere, I.; Banfi, G.; Tornese, D. Effects of early virtual reality-based rehabilitation in patients with total knee arthroplasty: A randomized controlled trial. *Medicine* **2020**, *99*, e19136. [CrossRef] [PubMed]
57. Goffredo, M.; Pournajaf, S.; D'Elia, T.S.; Pellicciari, L.; Bertone, M.; Criscuolo, S.; Damiani, C.; Franceschini, M. Does virtual reality rehabilitation influence postural control after total knee replacement? *Gait Posture* **2019**, *74*, 19–20. [CrossRef]
58. Gómez Álvarez, N.; Venegas Mortecinos, A.; Zapata Rodríguez, V.; López Fontanilla, M.; Maudier Vásquez, M.; Pavez-Adasme, G.; Hernández-Mosqueira, C. Effect of an intervention based on virtual reality on motor development and postural control in children with Down syndrome. *Rev. Chil. Pediatr.* **2018**, *89*, 747–752. [PubMed]
59. Gonçalves, G.B.; Leite, M.A.A.; Orsini, M.; Pereira, J.S. Effects of using the Nintendo Wii Fit Plus platform in the sensorimotor training of gait disorders in Parkinson's disease. *Neurol. Int.* **2014**, *6*, 5048. [CrossRef]
60. Gulcan, K.; Guclu-Gunduz, A.; Yasar, E.; Ar, U.; Sucullu Karadag, Y.; Saygili, F. The effects of augmented and virtual reality gait training on balance and gait in patients with Parkinson's disease. *Acta Neurol. Belg.* **2023**, *123*, 1917–1925. [CrossRef]
61. Gutiérrez, R.O.; Galán del Río, F.; Cano de la Cuerda, R.; Alguacil Diego, I.M.; González, R.A.; Page, J.C.M. A telerehabilitation program by virtual reality-video games improves balance and postural control in multiple sclerosis patients. *NeuroRehabilitation* **2013**, *33*, 545–554. [CrossRef]
62. Hadamus, A.; Białoszewski, D.; Błażkiewicz, M.; Kowalska, A.J.; Urbaniak, E.; Wydra, K.T.; Wiaderna, K.; Boratyński, R.; Kobza, A.; Marczyński, W. Assessment of the effectiveness of rehabilitation after total knee replacement surgery using sample entropy and classical measures of body balance. *Entropy* **2021**, *23*, 164. [CrossRef]
63. Hadamus, A.; Błażkiewicz, M.; Wydra, K.T.; Kowalska, A.J.; Łukowicz, M.; Białoszewski, D.; Marczyński, W. Effectiveness of early rehabilitation with exergaming in virtual reality on gait in patients after total knee replacement. *J. Clin. Med.* **2022**, *11*, 4950. [CrossRef]
64. Holmes, J.D.; Gu, M.L.; Johnson, A.M.; Jenkins, M.E. The effects of a home-based virtual reality rehabilitation program on balance among individuals with Parkinson's disease. *Phys. Occup. Ther. Geriatr.* **2013**, *31*, 241–253. [CrossRef]
65. Ibrahim, M.S.; Mattar, A.G.; Elhafez, S.M. Efficacy of virtual reality-based balance training versus the Biodex balance system training on the body balance of adults. *J. Phys. Ther. Sci.* **2016**, *28*, 20–26. [CrossRef] [PubMed]
66. Imaizumi, L.F.I.; Polastri, P.F.; Penedo, T.; Vieira, L.H.P.; Simieli, L.; Navega, F.R.F.; Monteiro, C.B.M.; Rodrigues, S.T.; Barbieri, F.A. Virtual reality head-mounted goggles increase the body sway of young adults during standing posture. *Neurosci. Lett.* **2020**, *737*, 135333. [CrossRef]
67. Janeh, O.; Fründt, O.; Schönwald, B.; Gulberti, A.; Buhmann, C.; Gerloff, C.; Steinicke, F.; Pötter-Nerger, M. Gait training in virtual reality: Short-term effects of different virtual manipulation techniques in Parkinson's disease. *Cells* **2019**, *8*, 419. [CrossRef] [PubMed]
68. Jelsma, J.; Pronk, M.; Ferguson, G.; Jelsma-Smit, D. The effect of the Nintendo Wii Fit on balance control and gross motor function of children with spastic hemiplegic cerebral palsy. *Dev. Neurorehabil.* **2013**, *16*, 27–37. [CrossRef]
69. Junior, V.A.D.S.; Santos, M.D.S.; Ribeiro, N.M.D.S.; Maldonado, I.L. Combining proprioceptive neuromuscular facilitation and virtual reality for improving sensorimotor function in stroke survivors: A randomized clinical trial. *J. Cent. Nerv. Syst. Dis.* **2019**, *11*, 1179573519863826. [CrossRef] [PubMed]
70. Kafri, M.; Weiss, P.L.; Zeilig, G.; Bondi, M.; Baum-Cohen, I.; Kizony, R. Performance in complex life situations: Effects of age, cognition, and walking speed in virtual versus real-life environments. *J. Neuroeng. Rehabil.* **2021**, *18*, 30. [CrossRef]

71. Kalron, A.; Fonkatz, I.; Frid, L.; Baransi, H.; Achiron, A. The effect of balance training on postural control in people with multiple sclerosis using the CAREN virtual reality system: A pilot randomized controlled trial. *J. Neuroeng. Rehabil.* **2016**, *13*, 13. [CrossRef]
72. Kamińska, M.S.; Miller, A.; Rotter, I.; Szylińska, A.; Grochans, E. The effectiveness of virtual reality training in reducing the risk of falls among elderly people. *Clin. Interv. Aging* **2018**, *13*, 2329–2338. [CrossRef]
73. Kantha, P.; Hsu, W.L.; Chen, P.J.; Tsai, Y.C.; Lin, J.J. A novel balance training approach: Biomechanical study of virtual reality-based skateboarding. *Front. Bioeng. Biotechnol.* **2023**, *11*, 1136368. [CrossRef]
74. Kanyılmaz, T.; Topuz, O.; Ardıç, F.N.; Alkan, H.; Öztekin, S.N.S.; Topuz, B.; Ardıç, F. Effectiveness of conventional versus virtual reality-based vestibular rehabilitation exercises in elderly patients with dizziness: A randomized controlled study with 6-month follow-up. *Braz. J. Otorhinolaryngol.* **2022**, *88* (Suppl. S3), S41–S49. [CrossRef]
75. Karasu, A.U.; Batur, E.B.; Karataş, G.K. Effectiveness of Wii-based rehabilitation in stroke: A randomized controlled study. *J. Rehabil. Med.* **2018**, *50*, 406–412. [CrossRef] [PubMed]
76. Khalil, H.; Al-Sharman, A.; El-Salem, K.; Alghwiri, A.A.; Al-Shorafat, D.; Khazaaleh, S.; Abu Foul, L. The development and pilot evaluation of virtual reality balance scenarios in people with multiple sclerosis (MS): A feasibility study. *NeuroRehabilitation* **2018**, *43*, 473–482. [CrossRef]
77. Kim, J.; Son, J.; Ko, N.; Yoon, B. Unsupervised virtual reality-based exercise program improves hip muscle strength and balance control in older adults: A pilot study. *Arch. Phys. Med. Rehabil.* **2013**, *94*, 937–943. [CrossRef] [PubMed]
78. Kim, K.J.; Heo, M. Comparison of virtual reality exercise versus conventional exercise on balance in patients with functional ankle instability: A randomized controlled trial. *J. Back Musculoskelet. Rehabil.* **2019**, *32*, 905–911. [CrossRef] [PubMed]
79. Kim, K.J.; Heo, M. Effects of virtual reality programs on balance in functional ankle instability. *J. Phys. Ther. Sci.* **2015**, *27*, 3097–3101. [CrossRef]
80. Kim, N.; Park, Y.; Lee, B.H. Effects of community-based virtual reality treadmill training on balance ability in patients with chronic stroke. *J. Phys. Ther. Sci.* **2015**, *27*, 655–658. [CrossRef]
81. Kiper, P.; Luque-Moreno, C.; Pernice, S.; Maistrello, L.; Agostini, M.; Turolla, A. Functional changes in the lower extremity after non-immersive virtual reality and physiotherapy following stroke. *J. Rehabil. Med.* **2020**, *52*, jrm00122. [CrossRef]
82. Kumar, D.; Sinha, N.; Dutta, A.; Lahiri, U. Virtual reality-based balance training system augmented with operant conditioning paradigm. *Biomed. Eng. Online* **2019**, *18*, 90. [CrossRef]
83. Kwon, J.A.; Shin, Y.K.; Kim, D.J.; Cho, S.R. Effects of balance training using a virtual reality program in hemiplegic patients. *Int. J. Environ. Res. Public Health* **2022**, *19*, 2805. [CrossRef]
84. Lee, H.Y.; Kim, Y.L.; Lee, S.M. Effects of virtual reality-based training and task-oriented training on balance performance in stroke patients. *J. Phys. Ther. Sci.* **2015**, *27*, 1883–1888. [CrossRef]
85. Lee, K. Speed-interactive pedaling training using smartphone virtual reality application for stroke patients: Single-blinded, randomized clinical trial. *Brain Sci.* **2019**, *9*, 295. [CrossRef] [PubMed]
86. Lee, K. Virtual reality gait training to promote balance and gait among older people: A randomized clinical trial. *Geriatrics* **2020**, *6*, 1. [CrossRef] [PubMed]
87. Lee, M.M.; Shin, D.C.; Song, C.H. Canoe game-based virtual reality training to improve trunk postural stability, balance, and upper limb motor function in subacute stroke patients: A randomized controlled pilot study. *J. Phys. Ther. Sci.* **2016**, *28*, 2019–2024. [CrossRef] [PubMed]
88. Lee, N.Y.; Lee, D.K.; Song, H.S. Effect of virtual reality dance exercise on the balance, activities of daily living, and depressive disorder status of Parkinson's disease patients. *J. Phys. Ther. Sci.* **2015**, *27*, 145–147. [CrossRef]
89. Lee, S.; Shin, S. Effectiveness of virtual reality using video gaming technology in elderly adults with diabetes mellitus. *Diabetes Technol. Ther.* **2013**, *15*, 489–496. [CrossRef]
90. Lheureux, A.; Lebleu, J.; Frisque, C.; Sion, C.; Stoquart, G.; Warlop, T.; Detrembleur, C.; Lejeune, T. Immersive virtual reality to restore natural long-range autocorrelations in Parkinson's disease patients' gait during treadmill walking. *Front. Physiol.* **2020**, *11*, 572063. [CrossRef]
91. Liao, Y.Y.; Yang, Y.R.; Cheng, S.J.; Wu, Y.R.; Fuh, J.L.; Wang, R.Y. Virtual reality–based training to improve obstacle-crossing performance and dynamic balance in patients with Parkinson's disease. *Neurorehabil. Neural Repair* **2015**, *29*, 658–667. [CrossRef]
92. Lima Rebêlo, F.; de Souza Silva, L.F.; Doná, F.; Sales Barreto, A.; de Souza Siqueira Quintans, J. Immersive virtual reality is effective in the rehabilitation of older adults with balance disorders: A randomized clinical trial. *Exp. Gerontol.* **2021**, *149*, 111308. [CrossRef]
93. Lloréns, R.; Colomer-Font, C.; Alcañiz, M.; Noé-Sebastián, E. BioTrak: Análisis de efectividad y satisfacción de un sistema de realidad virtual para la rehabilitación del equilibrio en pacientes con daño cerebral. *Neurología* **2013**, *28*, 268–275. [CrossRef]
94. Lloréns, R.; Gil-Gómez, J.A.; Alcañiz, M.; Colomer, C.; Noé, E. Improvement in balance using a virtual reality-based stepping exercise: A randomized controlled trial involving individuals with chronic stroke. *Clin. Rehabil.* **2015**, *29*, 261–268. [CrossRef]

95. Malik, A.N.; Masood, T. Effects of virtual reality training on mobility and physical function in stroke. *JPMA J. Pak. Med. Assoc.* **2017**, *67*, 1618–1620.
96. Martelli, D.; Xia, B.; Prado, A.; Agrawal, S.K. Gait adaptations during overground walking and multidirectional oscillations of the visual field in a virtual reality headset. *Gait Posture* **2019**, *67*, 251–256. [CrossRef] [PubMed]
97. McEwen, D.; Taillon-Hobson, A.; Bilodeau, M.; Sveistrup, H.; Finestone, H. Virtual reality exercise improves mobility after stroke: An inpatient randomized controlled trial. *Stroke* **2014**, *45*, 1853–1855. [CrossRef]
98. Meldrum, D.; Herdman, S.; Moloney, R.; Murray, D.; Duffy, D.; Malone, K.; French, H.; Hone, S.; Conroy, R.; McConn-Walsh, R. Effectiveness of conventional versus virtual reality-based vestibular rehabilitation in the treatment of dizziness, gait, and balance impairment in adults with unilateral peripheral vestibular loss: A randomised controlled trial. *BMC Ear Nose Throat Disord.* **2012**, *12*, 3. [CrossRef] [PubMed]
99. Micarelli, A.; Viziano, A.; Micarelli, B.; Augimeri, I.; Alessandrini, M. Vestibular rehabilitation in older adults with and without mild cognitive impairment: Effects of virtual reality using a head-mounted display. *Arch. Gerontol. Geriatr.* **2019**, *83*, 246–256. [CrossRef]
100. Miclaus, R.S.; Roman, N.; Henter, R.; Caloian, S. Lower extremity rehabilitation in patients with post-stroke sequelae through virtual reality associated with mirror therapy. *Int. J. Environ. Res. Public Health* **2021**, *18*, 2654. [CrossRef] [PubMed]
101. Mirelman, A.; Maidan, I.; Herman, T.; Deutsch, J.E.; Giladi, N.; Hausdorff, J.M. Virtual reality for gait training: Can it induce motor learning to enhance complex walking and reduce fall risk in patients with Parkinson's disease? *J. Gerontol. Ser. A Biol. Sci. Med. Sci.* **2011**, *66*, 234–240. [CrossRef]
102. Mohammadi, N.; Hadian, M.R.; Olyaei, G.R. Compare the effect of traditional and virtual reality training on subjective-sense of instability and balance in basketball players with functional ankle instability: Matched randomized clinical trial. *J. Biomed. Phys. Eng.* **2023**, *13*, 269–280. [CrossRef]
103. Morone, G.; Paolucci, T.; Luziatelli, S.; Iosa, M.; Piermattei, C.; Zangrando, F.; Paolucci, S.; Vulpiani, M.C.; Saraceni, V.M.; Baldari, C.; et al. Wii Fit is effective in women with bone loss condition associated with balance disorders: A randomized controlled trial. *Aging Clin. Exp. Res.* **2016**, *28*, 1187–1193. [CrossRef]
104. Nuic, D.; Vinti, M.; Karachi, C.; Foulon, P.; Van Hamme, A.; Welter, M.-L. The feasibility and positive effects of a customised videogame rehabilitation programme for freezing of gait and falls in Parkinson's disease patients: A pilot study. *J. NeuroEng. Rehabil.* **2018**, *15*, 31. [CrossRef]
105. Oh, K.; Stanley, C.J.; Damiano, D.L.; Kim, J.; Yoon, J.; Park, H.S. Biomechanical evaluation of virtual reality-based turning on a self-paced linear treadmill. *Gait Posture* **2018**, *65*, 157–162. [CrossRef] [PubMed]
106. Ortiz-Gutiérrez, R.; Cano-de-la-Cuerda, R.; Galán-del-Río, F.; Alguacil-Diego, I.M.; Palacios-Ceña, D.; Miangolarra-Page, J.C. A telerehabilitation program improves postural control in multiple sclerosis patients: A Spanish preliminary study. *Int. J. Environ. Res. Public Health* **2013**, *10*, 5697–5710. [CrossRef]
107. Park, E.C.; Kim, S.G.; Lee, C.W. The effects of virtual reality game exercise on balance and gait of the elderly. *J. Phys. Ther. Sci.* **2015**, *27*, 1157–1159. [CrossRef] [PubMed]
108. Park, Y.H.; Lee, C.H.; Lee, B.H. Clinical usefulness of the virtual reality-based postural control training on the gait ability in patients with stroke. *J. Exerc. Rehabil.* **2013**, *9*, 489–494. [CrossRef]
109. Pedreira Da Fonseca, E.; Ribeiro Da Silva, N.M.; Pinto, E.B. Therapeutic effect of virtual reality on post-stroke patients: Randomized clinical trial. *J. Stroke Cerebrovasc. Dis.* **2017**, *26*, 94–100. [CrossRef] [PubMed]
110. Peri, E.; Panzeri, D.; Beretta, E.; Reni, G.; Strazzer, S.; Biffi, E. Motor improvement in adolescents affected by ataxia secondary to acquired brain injury: A pilot study. *BioMed Res. Int.* **2019**, *2019*, 8967138. [CrossRef]
111. Phu, S.; Vogrin, S.; Al Saedi, A.; Duque, G. Balance training using virtual reality improves balance and physical performance in older adults at high risk of falls. *Clin. Interv. Aging* **2019**, *14*, 1567–1577. [CrossRef]
112. Punt, I.M.; Armand, S.; Ziltener, J.L.; Allet, L. Effect of Wii Fit™ exercise therapy on gait parameters in ankle sprain patients: A randomized controlled trial. *Gait Posture* **2017**, *58*, 52–58. [CrossRef]
113. Raffegeau, T.E.; Clark, M.; Fawver, B.; Engel, B.T.; Young, W.R.; Williams, A.M.; Lohse, K.R.; Fino, P.C. The effect of mobility-related anxiety on walking across the lifespan: A virtual reality simulation study. *Exp. Brain Res.* **2023**, *241*, 1757–1768. [CrossRef]
114. Rajaratnam, B.S.; Gui, K.J.; Lee, J.K.; Kwek, S.; Sim, F.; Lee, E.; Ang, Y.; Ng, K.; Su, Y.; Woo, W.; et al. Does the inclusion of virtual reality games within conventional rehabilitation enhance balance retraining after a recent episode of stroke? *Rehabil. Res. Pract.* **2013**, *2013*, 649561. [CrossRef]
115. Rendon, A.A.; Lohman, E.B.; Thorpe, D.; Johnson, E.G.; Medina, E.; Bradley, B. The effect of virtual reality gaming on dynamic balance in older adults. *Age Ageing* **2012**, *41*, 549–552. [CrossRef] [PubMed]

116. Rodrigues, E.V.; Gallo, L.H.; Guimarães, A.T.B.; Melo Filho, J.; Luna, B.C.; Gomes, A.R.S. Effects of dance exergaming on depressive symptoms, fear of falling, and musculoskeletal function in fallers and nonfallers community-dwelling older women. *Rejuvenation Res.* **2018**, *21*, 518–526. [CrossRef]
117. Rosiak, O.; Krajewski, K.; Woszczak, M.; Jozefowicz-Korczynska, M. Evaluation of the effectiveness of a virtual reality-based exercise program for unilateral peripheral vestibular deficit. *J. Vestib. Res. Equilib. Orientat.* **2018**, *28*, 409–415. [CrossRef]
118. Shema, S.R.; Brozgol, M.; Dorfman, M.; Maidan, I.; Sharaby-Yeshayahu, L.; Malik-Kozuch, H.; Wachsler Yannai, O.; Giladi, N.; Hausdorff, J.M.; Mirelman, A. Clinical experience using a 5-week treadmill training program with virtual reality to enhance gait in an ambulatory physical therapy service. *Phys. Ther.* **2014**, *94*, 1319–1326. [CrossRef] [PubMed]
119. Sadeghi, H.; Jehu, D.A.; Daneshjoo, A.; Shakoor, E.; Razeghi, M.; Amani, A.; Hakim, M.N.; Yusof, A. Effects of 8 weeks of balance training, virtual reality training, and combined exercise on lower limb muscle strength, balance, and functional mobility among older men: A randomized controlled trial. *Sports Health* **2021**, *13*, 606–612. [CrossRef] [PubMed]
120. Salem, Y.; Gropack, S.J.; Coffin, D.; Godwin, E.M. Effectiveness of a low-cost virtual reality system for children with developmental delay: A preliminary randomized single-blind controlled trial. *Physiotherapy* **2012**, *98*, 189–195. [CrossRef]
121. Sana, V.; Ghous, M.; Kashif, M.; Albalwi, A.; Muneer, R.; Zia, M. Effects of vestibular rehabilitation therapy versus virtual reality on balance, dizziness, and gait in patients with subacute stroke: A randomized controlled trial. *Medicine* **2023**, *102*, e33203. [CrossRef]
122. Santos, P.; Machado, T.; Santos, L.; Ribeiro, N.; Melo, A. Efficacy of the Nintendo Wii combination with conventional exercises in the rehabilitation of individuals with Parkinson's disease: A randomized clinical trial. *NeuroRehabilitation* **2019**, *45*, 255–263. [CrossRef]
123. Sengupta, M.; Gupta, A.; Khanna, M.; Rashmi Krishnan, U.K.; Chakrabarti, D. Role of virtual reality in balance training in patients with spinal cord injury: A prospective comparative pre-post study. *Asian Spine J.* **2020**, *14*, 51–58, Erratum in *Asian Spine J.* **2020**, *14*, 268. https://doi.org/10.31616/asj.2019.0013.e1. [CrossRef]
124. Severiano, M.I.R.; Zeigelboim, B.S.; Teive, H.A.G.; Santos, G.J.B.; Fonseca, V.R. Effect of virtual reality in Parkinson's disease: A prospective observational study. *Arq. Neuropsiquiatr.* **2018**, *76*, 78–84. [CrossRef]
125. Sheehy, L.; Taillon-Hobson, A.; Sveistrup, H.; Bilodeau, M.; Fergusson, D.; Levac, D.; Finestone, H. Does the addition of virtual reality training to a standard program of inpatient rehabilitation improve sitting balance ability and function after stroke? Protocol for a single-blind randomized controlled trial. *BMC Neurol.* **2016**, *16*, 42. [CrossRef] [PubMed]
126. Shema, S.R.; Bezalel, P.; Sberlo, Z.; Yannai, O.W.; Giladi, N.; Hausdorff, J.M.; Mirelman, A. Improved mobility and reduced fall risk in older adults after five weeks of virtual reality training. *J. Altern. Med. Res.* **2017**, *9*, 171–175.
127. Shideler, B.L.; Martelli, D.; Prado, A.; Agrawal, S.K. Overground gait training using virtual reality aimed at gait symmetry. *Hum. Mov. Sci.* **2021**, *76*, 102770. [CrossRef]
128. Singh, D.K.A.; Rajaratnam, B.S.; Palaniswamy, V.; Raman, V.P.; Bong, P.S.; Pearson, H. Effects of balance-focused interactive games compared to therapeutic balance classes for older women. *Climacteric J. Int. Menopause Soc.* **2013**, *16*, 141–146. [CrossRef] [PubMed]
129. Singh, D.K.A.; Nordin, N.A.M.; Abd Aziz, N.A.; Beng Kooi, L.; Li Ching, S. Effects of substituting a portion of standard physiotherapy time with virtual reality games among community-dwelling stroke survivors. *BMC Neurol.* **2013**, *13*, 199. [CrossRef] [PubMed]
130. Song, G.B.; Park, E.C. Effect of virtual reality games on stroke patients' balance, gait, depression, and interpersonal relationships. *J. Phys. Ther. Sci.* **2015**, *27*, 2057–2060. [CrossRef]
131. Takami, A.; Watanabe, K.; Makino, M. Immediate effect of video viewing with an illusion of walking at a faster speed using virtual reality on actual walking of stroke patients. *J. Phys. Ther. Sci.* **2021**, *33*, 560–564. [CrossRef]
132. Tarakci, D.; Ersoz Huseyinsinoglu, B.; Tarakci, E.; Razak Ozdincler, A. Effects of Nintendo Wii-Fit® video games on balance in children with mild cerebral palsy. *Pediatr. Int.* **2016**, *58*, 1042–1050. [CrossRef]
133. Tefertiller, C.; Hays, K.; Natale, A.; O'Dell, D.; Ketchum, J.; Sevigny, M.; Eagye, C.B.; Philippus, A.; Harrison-Felix, C. Results from a randomized controlled trial to address balance deficits after traumatic brain injury. *Arch. Phys. Med. Rehabil.* **2019**, *100*, 1409–1416. [CrossRef]
134. Tsang, W.W.N.; Fu, A.S.N. Virtual reality exercise to improve balance control in older adults at risk of falling. *Hong Kong Med. J.* **2016**, *22* (Suppl. S2), S19–S22. [CrossRef]
135. Valiani, V.; Lauzé, M.; Martel, D.; Pahor, M.; Manini, T.M.; Anton, S.; Aubertin-Leheudre, M. A new adaptive home-based exercise technology among older adults living in nursing homes: A pilot study on feasibility, acceptability, and physical performance. *J. Nutr. Health Aging* **2017**, *21*, 819–824. [CrossRef] [PubMed]

136. Van Dijsseldonk, R.B.; De Jong, L.A.F.; Groen, B.E.; Vos-van Der Hulst, M.; Geurts, A.C.H.; Keijsers, N.L.W. Gait stability training in a virtual environment improves gait and dynamic balance capacity in incomplete spinal cord injury patients. *Front. Neurol.* **2018**, *9*, 963. [CrossRef] [PubMed]
137. Villiger, M.; Liviero, J.; Awai, L.; Stoop, R.; Pyk, P.; Clijsen, R.; Curt, A.; Eng, K.; Bolliger, M. Home-based virtual reality-augmented training improves lower limb muscle strength, balance, and functional mobility following chronic incomplete spinal cord injury. *Front. Neurol.* **2017**, *8*, 635. [CrossRef]
138. Villiger, M.; Bohli, D.; Kiper, D.; Pyk, P.; Spillmann, J.; Meilick, B.; Curt, A.; Hepp-Reymond, M.C.; Hotz-Boendermaker, S.; Eng, K. Virtual reality–augmented neurorehabilitation improves motor function and reduces neuropathic pain in patients with incomplete spinal cord injury. *Neurorehabil. Neural Repair* **2013**, *27*, 675–683. [CrossRef]
139. Wiskerke, E.; Kool, J.; Hilfiker, R.; Sattelmayer, K.M.; Verheyden, G. Determining the optimal virtual reality exergame approach for balance therapy in persons with neurological disorders using a Rasch analysis: Longitudinal observational study. *JMIR Serious Games* **2022**, *10*, e30366. [CrossRef]
140. Wüest, S.; Borghese, N.A.; Pirovano, M.; Mainetti, R.; van de Langenberg, R.; de Bruin, E.D. Usability and effects of an exergame-based balance training program. *Games Health J.* **2014**, *3*, 106–114. [CrossRef]
141. Yaman, F.; Leblebicier, M.A.; Okur, İ.; Kızılkaya, M.İ.; Kavuncu, V. Is virtual reality training superior to conventional treatment in improving lower extremity motor function in chronic hemiplegic patients? *Turk. J. Phys. Med. Rehabil.* **2022**, *68*, 391–398. [CrossRef] [PubMed]
142. Yang, W.C.; Wang, H.K.; Wu, R.M.; Lo, C.S.; Lin, K.H. Home-based virtual reality balance training and conventional balance training in Parkinson's disease: A randomized controlled trial. *J. Formos. Med. Assoc.* **2016**, *115*, 734–743. [CrossRef]
143. Xu, Y.; Tong, M.; Ming, W.K.; Lin, Y.; Mai, W.; Huang, W.; Chen, Z. A depth camera–based, task-specific virtual reality rehabilitation game for patients with stroke: Pilot usability study. *JMIR Serious Games* **2021**, *9*, e20916. [CrossRef]
144. Yeh, S.C.; Chen, S.; Wang, P.C.; Su, M.C.; Chang, C.H.; Tsai, P.Y. Interactive 3-dimensional virtual reality rehabilitation for patients with chronic imbalance and vestibular dysfunction. *Technol. Health Care* **2014**, *22*, 915–921. [CrossRef]
145. Yin, C.; Hsueh, Y.H.; Yeh, C.Y.; Lo, H.C.; Lan, Y.T. A virtual reality-cycling training system for lower limb balance improvement. *BioMed Res. Int.* **2016**, *2016*, 9276508. [CrossRef]
146. Yom, C.; Cho, H.Y.; Lee, B. Effects of virtual reality-based ankle exercise on the dynamic balance, muscle tone, and gait of stroke patients. *J. Phys. Ther. Sci.* **2015**, *27*, 845–849. [CrossRef]
147. Yousefi Babadi, S.; Daneshmandi, H. Effects of virtual reality versus conventional balance training on balance of the elderly. *Exp. Gerontol.* **2021**, *153*, 111498. [CrossRef]
148. Zahedian-Nasab, N.; Jaberi, A.; Shirazi, F.; Kavousipor, S. Effect of virtual reality exercises on balance and fall in elderly people with fall risk: A randomized controlled trial. *BMC Geriatr.* **2021**, *21*, 509. [CrossRef]
149. Greenwald, A.G. Consequences of prejudice against the null hypothesis. *Psychol. Bull.* **1975**, *82*, 1–20. [CrossRef]
150. Lohse, K.; Buchanan, T.; Miller, M. Underpowered and overworked: Problems with data analysis in motor learning studies. *J. Mot. Learn. Dev.* **2016**, *4*, 37–58. [CrossRef]
151. Cheng, L.; Sunzi, K.; Dai, F.; Liu, X.; Wang, Y.; Zhang, B.; He, L.; Ju, M. Effects of virtual reality rehabilitation training on gait and balance in patients with Parkinson's disease: A systematic review. *PLoS ONE* **2019**, *14*, e0224819.
152. Charness, G.; Gneezy, U.; Kuhn, M.A. Experimental methods: Between-subject and within-subject design. *J. Econ. Behav. Organ.* **2012**, *81*, 1–8. [CrossRef]
153. Schwartz, C.E.; Chesney, M.A.; Irvine, M.J.; Keefe, F.J. The control group dilemma in clinical research: Applications for psychosocial and behavioral medicine trials. *Psychosom. Med.* **1997**, *59*, 362–371. [CrossRef] [PubMed]
154. Ortman, J.; Velkoff, V.; Hogan, H. *An Aging Nation: The Older Population in the United States*; U.S. Census Bureau: Washington, DC, USA, 2014.
155. Basford, J.R.; Chou, L.S.; Kaufman, K.R.; Brey, R.H.; Walker, A.; Malec, J.F.; Moessner, A.M.; Brown, A.W. An assessment of gait and balance deficits after traumatic brain injury. *Arch. Phys. Med. Rehabil.* **2003**, *84*, 343–349. [CrossRef] [PubMed]
156. Murray, R.F.; Asghari, A.; Egorov, D.D.; Rutkowski, S.B.; Siddall, P.J.; Soden, R.J.; Ruff, R. Impact of spinal cord injury on self-perceived pre- and postmorbid cognitive, emotional, and physical functioning. *Spinal Cord* **2007**, *45*, 429–436. [CrossRef]
157. Chen, C.H.; Jeng, M.C.; Fung, C.P.; Doong, J.L.; Chuang, T.Y. Psychological benefits of virtual reality for patients in rehabilitation therapy. *J. Sport Rehabil.* **2009**, *18*, 258–268. [CrossRef]
158. Qian, J.; McDonough, D.J.; Gao, Z. The effectiveness of virtual reality exercise on individuals' physiological, psychological, and rehabilitative outcomes: A systematic review. *Int. J. Environ. Res. Public Health* **2020**, *17*, 4133. [CrossRef]
159. Ambrose, A.F.; Paul, G.; Hausdorff, J.M. Risk factors for falls among older adults: A review of the literature. *Maturitas* **2013**, *75*, 51–61. [CrossRef]
160. Alexander, N.B. Postural control in older adults. *J. Am. Geriatr. Soc.* **1994**, *42*, 93–108. [CrossRef]

161. Dermody, G.; Whitehead, L.; Wilson, G.; Glass, C. The role of virtual reality in improving health outcomes for community-dwelling older adults: Systematic review. *J. Med. Internet Res.* **2020**, *22*, e17331. [CrossRef]
162. Molina, K.I.; Ricci, N.A.; de Moraes, S.A.; Perracini, M.R. Virtual reality using games for improving physical functioning in older adults: A systematic review. *J. Neuroeng. Rehabil.* **2014**, *11*, 156. [CrossRef]
163. Neri, S.G.; Cardoso, J.R.; Cruz, L.; Lima, R.M.; de Oliveira, R.J.; Iversen, M.D.; Carregaro, R.L. Do virtual reality games improve mobility skills and balance measurements in community-dwelling older adults? Systematic review and meta-analysis. *Clin. Rehabil.* **2017**, *31*, 1292–1304. [CrossRef]
164. Darekar, A.; McFadyen, B.J.; Lamontagne, A.; Fung, J. Efficacy of virtual reality-based intervention on balance and mobility disorders post-stroke: A scoping review. *J. Neuroeng. Rehabil.* **2015**, *12*, 46. [CrossRef] [PubMed]
165. Tricco, A.C.; Lillie, E.; Zarin, W.; O'Brien, K.K.; Colquhoun, H.; Levac, D.; Moher, D.; Peters, M.D.; Horsley, T.; Weeks, L.; et al. PRISMA Extension for Scoping Reviews (PRISMAScR): Checklist and Explanation. *Ann. Intern. Med.* **2018**, *169*, 467–473. [CrossRef]

technologies

MDPI

Review

Robotic Systems for Hand Rehabilitation—Past, Present and Future

Bogdan Gherman [1], Ionut Zima [1,*], Calin Vaida [1], Paul Tucan [1], Adrian Pisla [1], Iosif Birlescu [1], Jose Machado [1,2] and Doina Pisla [1,3,*]

1 CESTER, Technical University of Cluj-Napoca, Memorandumului 28, 400114 Cluj-Napoca, Romania; bogdan.gherman@mep.utcluj.ro (B.G.); calin.vaida@mep.utcluj.ro (C.V.); paul.tucan@mep.utcluj.ro (P.T.); adrian.pisla@muri.utcluj.ro (A.P.); iosif.birlescu@mep.utcluj.ro (I.B.); jmachado@dem.uminho.pt (J.M.)
2 MEtRICs Research Center, Campus of Azurém, University of Minho, 4800-058 Guimarães, Portugal
3 Technical Sciences Academy of Romania, B-dul Dacia, 26, 030167 Bucharest, Romania
* Correspondence: ionut.zima@mep.utcluj.ro (I.Z.); doina.pisla@mep.utcluj.ro (D.P.)

Abstract: Background: Cerebrovascular accident, commonly known as stroke, Parkinson's disease, and multiple sclerosis represent significant neurological conditions affecting millions globally. Stroke remains the third leading cause of death worldwide and significantly impacts patients' hand functionality, making hand rehabilitation crucial for improving quality of life. **Methods:** A comprehensive literature review was conducted analyzing over 300 papers, and categorizing them based on mechanical design, mobility, and actuation systems. To evaluate each device, a database with 45 distinct criteria was developed to systematically assess their characteristics. **Results:** The analysis revealed three main categories of devices: rigid exoskeletons, soft exoskeletons, and hybrid devices. Electric actuation represents the most common source of power. The dorsal placement of the mechanism is predominant, followed by glove-based, lateral, and palmar configurations. A correlation between mass and functionality was observed during the analysis; an increase in the number of actuated fingers or in functionality automatically increases the mass of the device. The research shows significant technological evolution with considerable variation in design complexity, with 29.4% of devices using five or more actuators while 24.8% employ one or two actuators. **Conclusions:** While substantial progress has been made in recent years, several challenges persist, including missing information or incomplete data from source papers and a limited number of clinical studies to evaluate device effectiveness. Significant opportunities remain to improve device functionality, usability, and therapeutic effectiveness, as well as to implement advanced power systems for portable devices.

Keywords: hand exoskeleton; rehabilitation robotics; stroke rehabilitation; hand rehabilitation; exoskeleton

1. Introduction

Cerebrovascular accident, commonly known as stroke, is a global health challenge that affected 17 million individuals in 2021. Stroke is the third leading cause of mortality worldwide [1] and one of the main contributors to adult physical disability [2], impacting more than a person's health [3]. While stroke remains significant, 1.12 million cases and 9.53 million survivors of which are reported annually in the EU [4], robotic rehabilitation serves a larger patient population, including patients who suffer from Parkinson's disease, 8.5 million cases of which are reported globally [5,6], and patients with neuromuscular conditions like multiple sclerosis, 2.8 million cases of which are reported worldwide [7] as of 2020.

After a stroke, survivors often face various complications including movement problems, speech disorders, visual disturbances, personality alterations, cognitive dysfunction, and post-stroke depression, requiring comprehensive rehabilitation approaches [8,9]. The main motor impairments are represented by spasticity and weakness [10,11], with spasticity manifesting as muscle stiffness and increased resistance to passive movements [12], while weakness affects the motor function of the fingers [13].

The effectiveness of rehabilitation relies on neuroplasticity, the brain's capacity to change, reorganize, and adapt, and to enhance its ability to handle new situations [14,15]. Two phases are involved in neuroplasticity: the transformation of the initial neural network [16,17] and subsequent neuronal connection reestablishment [18], enhanced by physical activity and neural stimulation [19,20]. The rehabilitation process involves three main techniques [21]: passive motion involving a therapist (or the healthy hand of the patient) to guide the motion that the affected hand cannot perform anymore, active motion that involves independent movement of the affected hand to the limits of spasticity, and active-assisted therapy that combines both techniques, involving independent motion of the affected hand to the limits of spasticity and beyond this limit with the help of a therapist or patient healthy hand. Active therapy is essential for muscular strengthening and the neuroplasticity process [22–26].

Motor impairments can vary from individual to individual, and muscle state, stroke phase, and severity [27] must be taken into consideration. Current technology can provide precise therapeutic guidance [28], but not considering individual patient differences can reduce the effectiveness of the rehabilitation process [29]. The current growing demand for rehabilitation therapy faces significant challenges such as an insufficient availability of trained therapists [30,31] and a reduced number of therapy sessions [32–34].The following tools are used to measure the progress of the rehabilitation process: the CAHAI (Chedoke Arm and Hand Activity Inventory) [35,36], BBT (Box and Block Test) [37–39], 9-HPT (9-Hole Peg Test) [40,41], and Ad-AHA (Adult Assisting Hand Assessment stroke) [42,43], complemented by patient-reported outcomes through the MHQ (Michigan Hand Outcomes Questionnaire) [44,45], JHFT (Jebsen–Taylor Hand Function Test), which simulates daily activities for unilateral hand function assessment [46,47], DHI (Dizziness Handicap Inventory) [48–52], and the ABILHAND questionnaire [53–55].

The need for new methods to deliver care to the affected patients is reflected in the growing rehabilitation robotics market, which reached approximately USD 500 million in North America in 2020 [56], with expected growth in Asia and Europe [57]. This combination of high neurological disorder prevalence, limited healthcare professional availability, and proven benefits of consistent rehabilitation necessitates the development of hand exoskeletons to supplement traditional therapy methods and address the growing gap between patient needs and available care.

This paper presents a systematic review of rehabilitation hand exoskeletons. Section 1 presents the global impact of neurological disorders, stressing the most important ones, such as stroke, Parkinson's disease, or multiple sclerosis, and discusses rehabilitation needs, neuroplasticity importance, and growing market demand for rehabilitation robotics. Section 2 presents human hand biomechanics, joint types, and motions, and outlines systematic review methodology including database searches, inclusion criteria, and analysis frameworks for over 300 devices. Section 3 categorizes devices into orthoses, exoskeletons, and end-effector types, discusses design requirements including safety, comfort, force transmission, and affordability, and compares mechanical approaches and clinical considerations. Section 4 classifies exoskeletons by type (soft/rigid/hybrid), mobility, mechanism position, actuation, and transmission systems. Section 5 analyzes a database of 300+ devices, presenting trends in publication, geographic distribution, design approaches, and technical specifications, and includes statistical analysis of actuator types and device configurations. Section 6 summarizes findings showing that rigid exoskeletons dominate (50%), with soft (35%) and hybrid (15.5%) following. The section also notes electric actuation prevalence (55.8%) and identifies future research opportunities for improving functionality and therapeutic effectiveness.

2. Materials and Methods

The human hand is one of the most complex and highly versatile parts of the human body, with many degrees of freedom (DoF) that allow a wide range of movement. Various types of joints contribute to the overall dexterity of the human hand; however, the large number of DoF constitutes the main challenge in creating accurate models of the hand's biomechanics [58].

2.1. Skeletal Model of the Human Hand

The skeletal model of the human hand is illustrated in Figure 1. The OpenSim [59] library's hand skeleton model provides insight into the hand's structure. The hand skeleton consists of the capitate bone near the wrist, metacarpals, and phalanges. Each digit contains one metacarpal segment. The four fingers consist of three segments: proximal, intermediate, and distal phalanges. In contrast, the thumb has only two phalanx segments: proximal and distal.

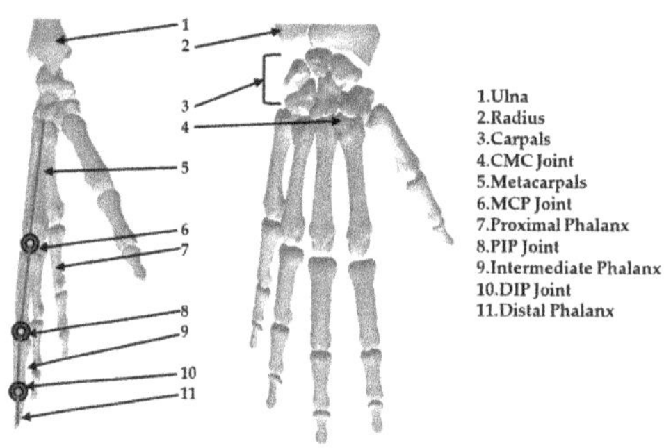

Figure 1. Skeletal model of the human hand.

The names of the hand joints are based on the bones they connect. Each of the four fingers consists of one metacarpophalangeal joint (MCP), one distal interphalangeal joint (DIP), and one proximal interphalangeal joint (PIP). The thumb consists of a MCP and one DIP joint. Near the wrist, each digit connects through a carpometacarpal joint (CMC). The joint that connects the phalanges can be considered a 1 DoF hinge joint because each pair of phalanges can only perform bending and extending movements.

The MCP joint is more complex and can be considered a 2 DoF joint. It can be modeled as a ball-and-socket joint that allows for rotation along two different directions.

The CMC joints, positioned near the wrist, can be considered 2 DoF saddle joints.

2.2. Motions of the Human Hand

Precise terminology is mandatory in the study of human hand biomechanics to describe the various movements of the digits and joints. Flexion and extension motions refer to the decrease and increase of joint angles, respectively. Abduction and adduction describe the movements of fingers away from and towards the middle finger, except for the middle finger itself, which can perform only bilateral abduction [60,61].

Due to its unique anatomical structure, the thumb possesses a more complex range of motion. The abduction of the thumb can be defined as anterior movement perpendicular to the palm, while adduction returns it to the palmar plane.

Circumduction refers to the thumb's movement in a conical pattern at the TMC joint. Pronation represents the movement of the thumb along its longitudinal axis inward toward the index finger. The outward rotation of the thumb is termed supination. The terminology described above provides an accurate description of finger movement. Finger motions, flexion, extension, abduction, adduction, and circumduction are illustrated in Figure 2.

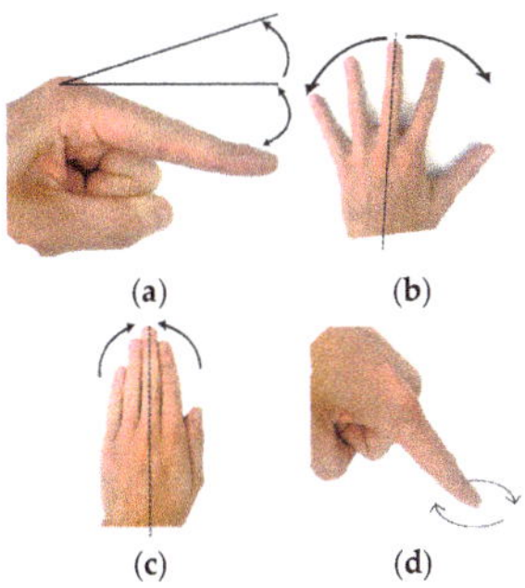

Figure 2. Finger motions: (**a**) Hyperextension-extension-flexion, (**b**) Abduction, (**c**) Adduction, (**d**) Circumduction.

2.3. Predominant Human Hand Postures

The main movements of the human hand are illustrated in Table 1 and are in-depth analyzed in reference [62].

Table 1. Predominant human hand movements.

Movement	Illustration of the Movement	Movement	Illustration of the Movement
Thumb up	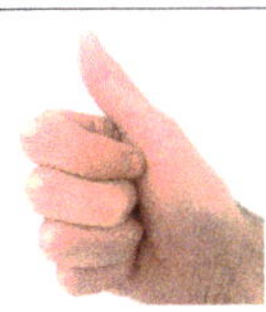	Extension of index and middle, flexion of the other fingers	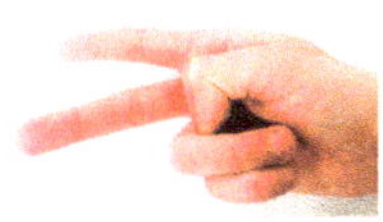
Flexion of ring and little finger extension of the other fingers	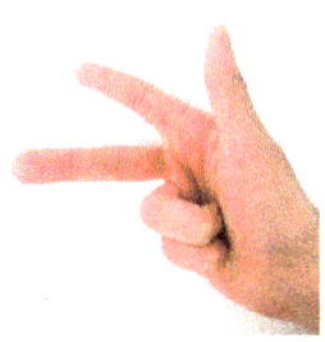	Flexion of fingers except thumb	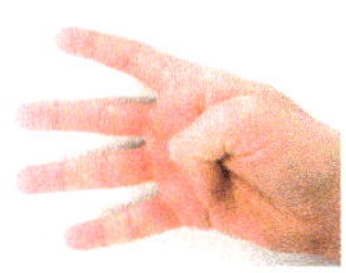
Abduction of all fingers	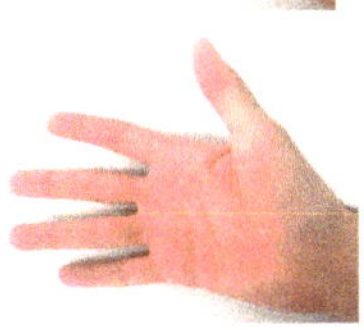	Fingers flexed together in fist	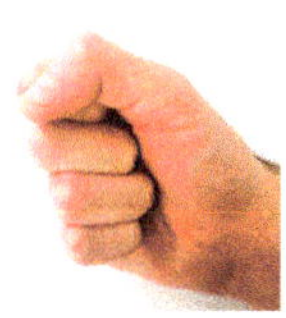

Table 1. *Cont.*

Movement	Illustration of the Movement	Movement	Illustration of the Movement
Pointing index	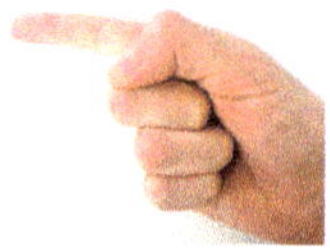	Thumb opposing base of little finger	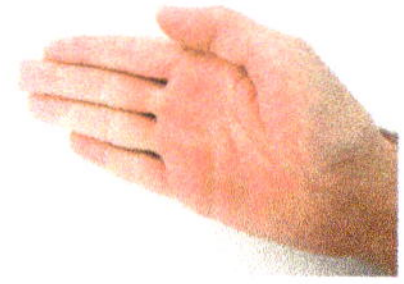

The most common grasp movements of the human hand are depicted in Table 2 and in-depth analyzed in reference [62].

Table 2. Common human hand grasping gestures.

Movement	Illustration of the Movement	Movement	Illustration of the Movement
Large diameter grasp	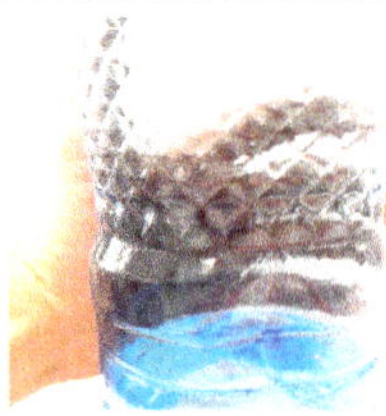	Tripod Grasp	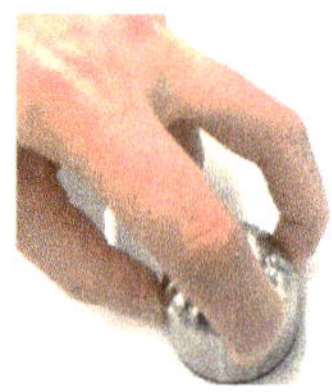
Small diameter grasp	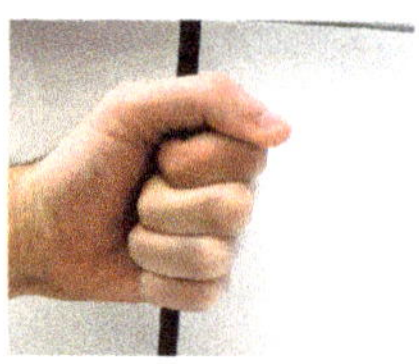	Prismatic pinch grasp	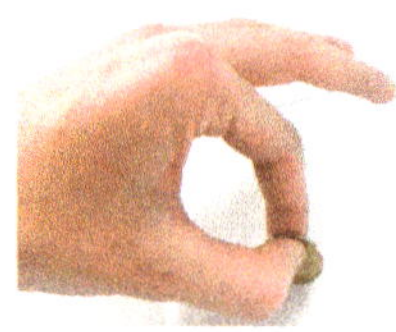
Fixed hook grasp	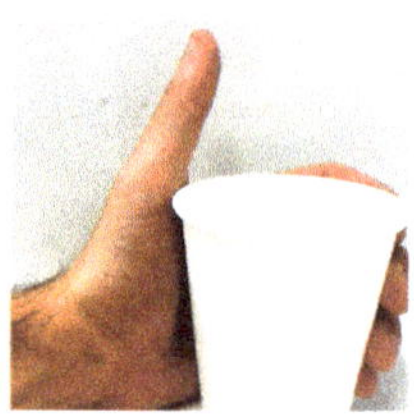	Tip pinch grasp	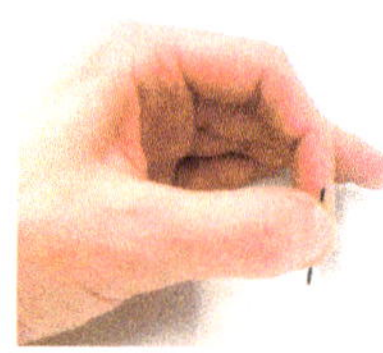
Index finger extension grasp	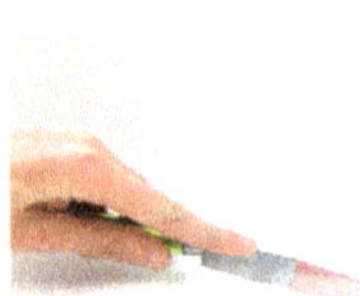	Quadpod grasp	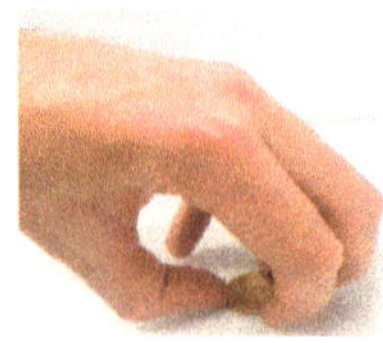
Medium wrap	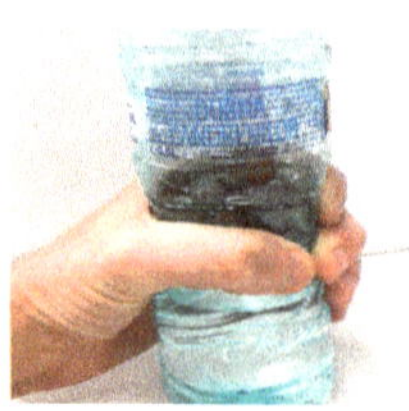	Lateral grasp	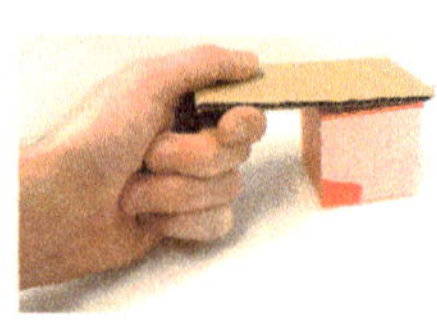

Table 2. *Cont.*

Grasping Movement	Illustration of the Grasping Movement	Grasping Movement	Illustration of the Grasping Movement
Ring grasp	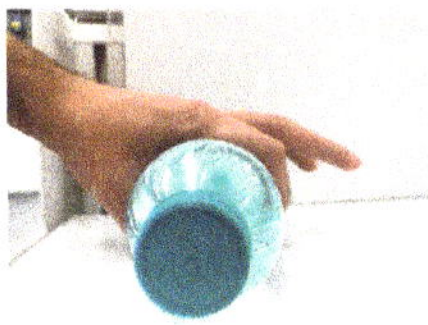	Parallel extension grasp	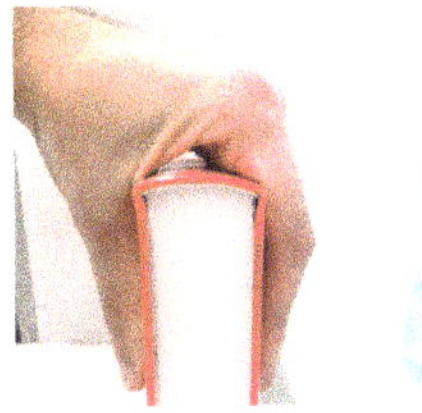
Prismatic four fingers grasp	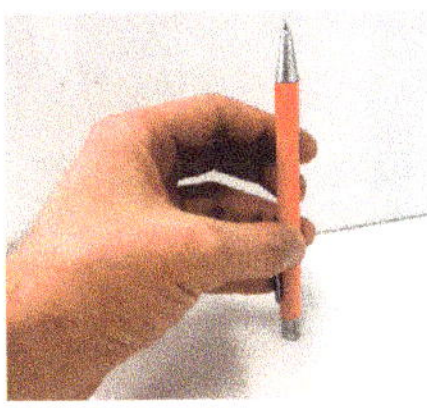	Extension type grasp	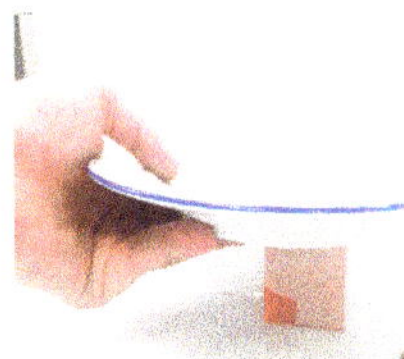
Stick grasp	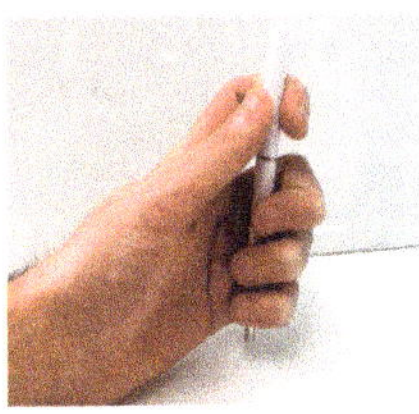	Power disk grasp	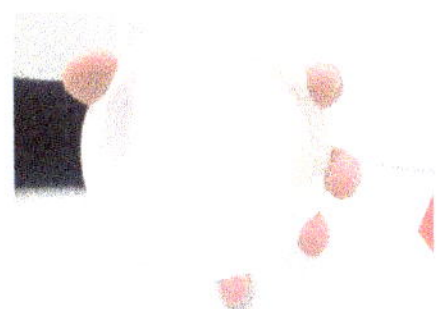
Writing tripod grasp	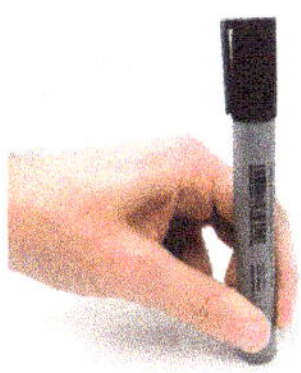	Open a bottle with a tripod grasp	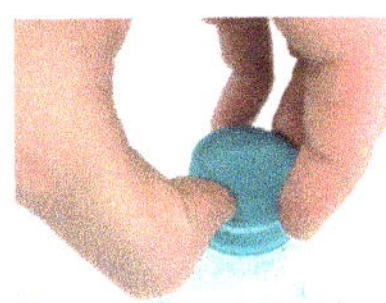

2.4. Data Extraction and Categorization

The protocol illustrated in Figure 3 was used to systematically identify and analyze relevant research articles focusing on hand exoskeleton devices for rehabilitation and assistance.

From each included article, a wide range of data were extracted. This included bibliometric information such as authors, year of publication, country of origin, and publication type (journal article or conference paper). Technical details extracted included the device name (if applicable), type of exoskeleton (rigid, soft, or hybrid), actuation method and type, transmission mechanism, number of actuators, degrees of freedom (total and active), mechanism placement, finger motions assisted, independent vs. coupled finger assistance, number of fingers covered, and range of motion. Additional information on target application, portability, safety features, adaptability features, weight, and any clinical testing was also recorded.

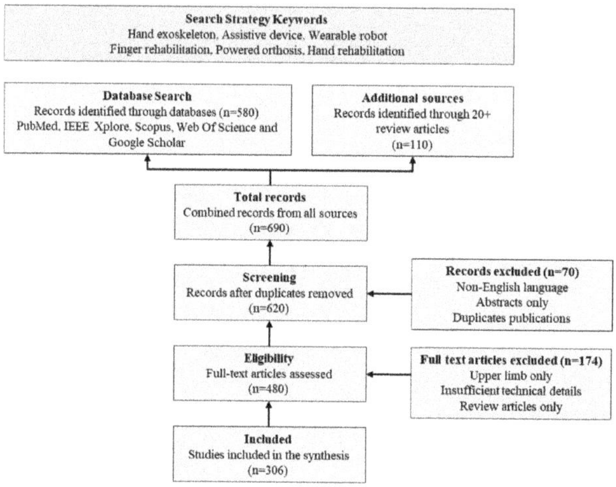

Figure 3. Classification Framework.

2.5. Literature Search and Selection

To identify relevant studies on hand robotic exoskeletons for rehabilitation and assistance, a comprehensive literature search was conducted. The search covered multiple databases including PubMed, IEEE Xplore, Scopus, Web of Science, and Google Scholar, using search terms such as "hand exoskeleton" and "hand rehabilitation robot".

The extracted data was organized into a structured database for analysis as illustrated in Figure 4. Devices were categorized based on their design characteristics, actuation methods, and intended applications, facilitating comprehensive analysis.

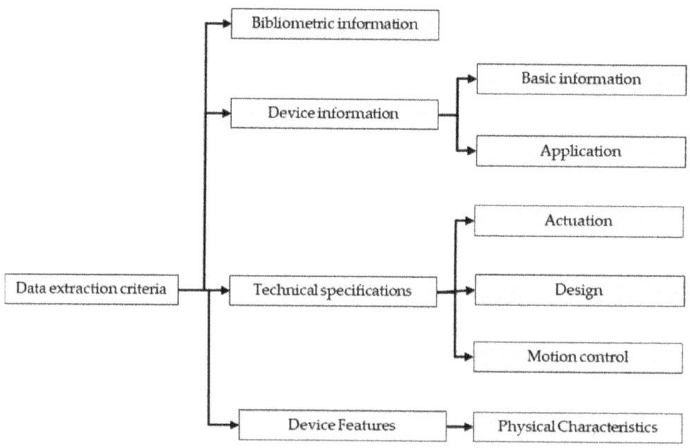

Figure 4. Flow Diagram of Literature Search and Selection Process.

Initially, more articles were identified. After removing duplicates and screening titles and abstracts, articles were selected for full-text review. Following the application of inclusion and exclusion criteria, a final set of 306 articles was included in this review. Additionally, over 20 existing review articles in the field were examined to identify any potentially missing relevant studies.

The inclusion criteria for the review encompassed studies describing hand exoskeleton devices for rehabilitation or assistance, conference proceedings, and articles. Exclusion criteria included studies focused only on upper limb exoskeletons without specific hand components.

2.6. Data Analysis

The analysis of the extracted data involved quantitative approaches. The quantitative analysis utilized descriptive statistics to summarize trends in hand exoskeleton design and functionality. This included examining the distribution of exoskeleton types, distribution of different actuation methods, distribution of transmission mechanisms, average number of DoF, distribution of finger coverage, assisted motions, and weight distribution analysis. Trends in publication types and research output over time, as well as the geographical distribution of research, were also analyzed.

2.7. Limitations

Several limitations of this review were identified. The focus on English-language publications may have excluded relevant studies published in other languages. Despite efforts to be comprehensive, it is possible that some relevant studies were missed due to the specific search terms used or limitations of the databases searched.

3. Hand Rehabilitation Devices

Hand rehabilitation devices (HRDs) can be classified into three main categories: orthoses, exoskeletons, and end-effector devices. Orthoses, similar to traditional hand braces, provide fundamental support. Exoskeletons and end-effector devices go a step further by incorporating powered systems that enable passive exercises. These advanced devices offer crucial support and movement of the fingers through various actuation methods, adding an important dimension to rehabilitation therapy [21,22]. Robot-assisted therapy for upper extremity rehabilitation post-stroke emerged in the 1990s [63] the initial hand rehabilitation robots were designed to take over the physically demanding aspects of therapy from human therapists. The main objectives were to better reproduce the natural motion patterns of human joints and more effectively address the specific needs of rehabilitation. This approach developed better and more flexible robotic systems in hand rehabilitation, leading to the modern devices used today [64].

The field of rehabilitation robotics integrates multidisciplinary knowledge fields, such as anatomy, neuroscience, cognitive and learning sciences, and extensive clinical experience [65].

The development of hand rehabilitation robots requires more than mechanical and engineering considerations; the characteristics of stroke patients, current rehabilitation theories, and methods for assessing therapeutic progress should be taken into consideration [66–74].

Based on mechanical structure, hand rehabilitation devices can be classified into two main categories, exoskeleton devices and end-effector devices.

- Exoskeleton Devices

Exoskeletons are devices that wrap around the target body part, similar to orthoses in their ability to provide safety and support. However, exoskeletons are distinguished by their additional powered components. These extra elements enable exoskeletons to offer active, powered functions to the user. This combination of supportive structure and powered assistance makes exoskeletons particularly useful for rehabilitation, movement augmentation, or other specialized applications where active support is beneficial [21,75].

Finger exoskeletons enable precise actuation of specific joints while providing support, which is crucial for patients with advanced injuries. Their portability makes them valuable for elderly or remote patients, offering consistent rehabilitation or assistance outside clinical settings [75].

- End-Effector Devices

End-effector devices offer a distinct approach to hand rehabilitation compared to exoskeletons. These devices focus on controlling the endpoint or the distal interphalangeal joint of the finger, rather than encompassing and actuating the entire finger structure.

The primary advantages of end-effector devices are their high level of control and feedback precision. By concentrating on the fingertip or the most distal joint, these devices can achieve accurate movement and force application without the complexity of managing multiple joints simultaneously.

4. Exoskeleton Rehabilitation Devices

Exoskeletons are designed to match the shape and the movement of the user's hand. Each degree of freedom in the exoskeletons' design must be precisely aligned with the corresponding human joint. By mimicking human anatomy and joint movements so closely, exoskeletons can provide targeted support and assistance, making them a valuable tool in robotic rehabilitation [75].

Exoskeleton rehabilitation devices can be classified as follows.

4.1. Classification by Type

Exoskeleton hand rehabilitation devices can be divided into three main categories: rigid, soft, and hybrid, as illustrated in Figure 5.

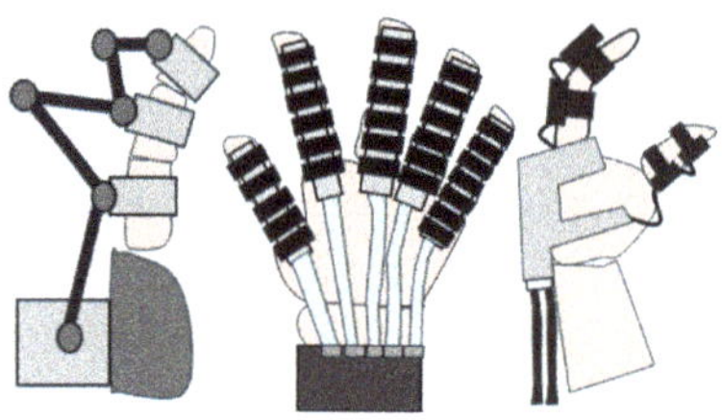

(a) (b) (c)

Figure 5. Schematic representation of the three classes of robotic hand rehabilitation exoskeletons: (**a**) rigid, (**b**) soft, and (**c**) hybrid.

4.1.1. Soft Exoskeletons

In recent years, the development of soft robotics rehabilitation systems based on soft actuation has increased significantly [76].

Soft exoskeletons, sometimes referred to as soft gloves [77], offer unique advantages in rehabilitation. These soft exoskeletons can reduce the overall weight of hand rehabilitation systems and provide better self-alignment between the device and finger joints due to their soft actuation [78,79]. These exoskeletons are typically manufactured using fabric-, plastic-, or silicone-based materials. This flexibility allows the exoskeleton to be customized for each patient's finger size, offering a more personalized rehabilitation experience [78].

4.1.2. Rigid Exoskeletons

Rigid exoskeletons utilize rigid transmission mechanisms, which are systems of rigid links joined together [80]. This is one of the simple ways to translate the movements of the actuator to the intended human joint.

In systems that are fully actuated, both direct and indirect relationships can be established. Using this feature, any measurements taken from the actuator, such as encoder signals, torque, or current, can be used to determine the finger's state. Simple and natural control of the hand is possible due to the direct connection between actuators and hand joints and, as a result, additional tracking systems are not required.

Control algorithms are simplified due to the natural matching of actuator and joint movements, and the overall reliability and precision of the exoskeleton are enhanced. Rigid exoskeletons enable more accurate position control and force transmission, which are crucial for both rehabilitation exercises and assistive applications [76].

Based on the linkage type, the rigid hand exoskeletons can be classified as illustrated in Figure 6. Figure 7 illustrates a schematic representation of each linkage type.

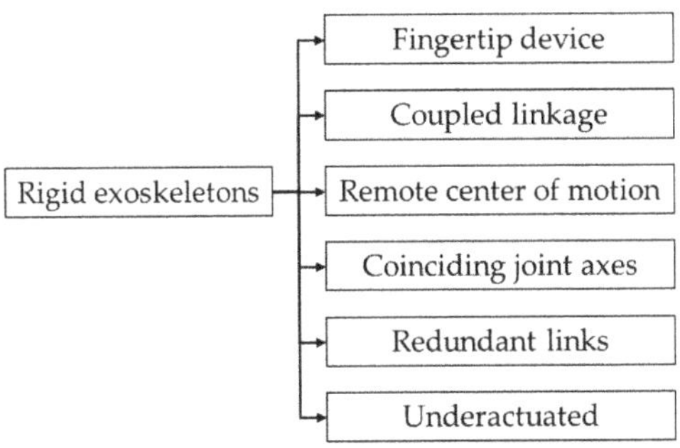

Figure 6. Classification of rigid exoskeletons based on linkage type.

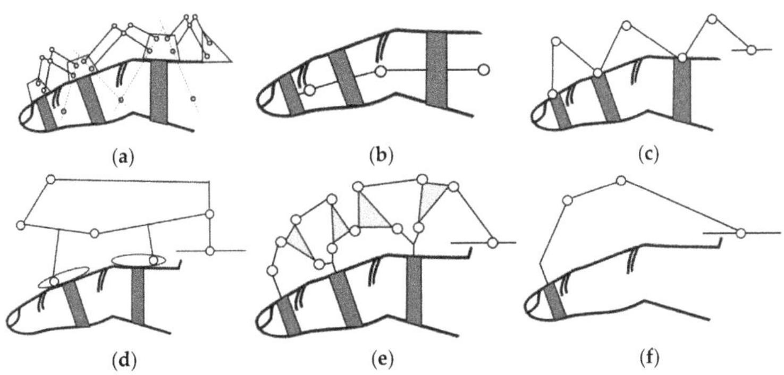

Figure 7. Schematic representation of the main types of linkages. (**a**) Remote center of motion, (**b**) coinciding joint axes, (**c**) redundant links, (**d**) underactuated device, (**e**) coupled linkage device, and (**f**) fingertip device.

Hand exoskeletons can be developed with mechanisms that create remote centers of motion for each link, aligning with the finger joints' natural pivot points, as illustrated in Figure 7a. This type of mechanism has been explored with various potential designs discussed in reference [81]. Popular mechanisms include the parallelogram mechanism and circular prismatic joints [82].

Matched axis types of exoskeletons aim to align joints precisely with those of the human hand, as illustrated in Figure 7b. This method is one of the simplest ways to control hand movements predictably; however, the design presents challenges to implement in practice. The main reason is represented by the placement of the exoskeleton's joints directly next to the finger joints. This type of placement is problematic for multiple fingers due to interference with natural hand movements when fingers need to come close together during grasping. Due to these practical limitations, the matched axes topology is generally not considered a viable option for exoskeletons designed to support multiple fingers simultaneously [82].

An alternative method for connecting the movement of a specific exoskeleton joint to a single hand joint is represented by a redundant linkage. This topology involves the attachment of the system to the digit at points before and after each actuated joint. However, additional linkages and joints should be incorporated between attachment points, as illustrated in Figure 7c. Well-defined relationships between the motions of the exoskeleton and the hand joints are established using this type of mechanism [82].

Multiple finger joints can be controlled using a single actuator through an underactuated mechanism. The main feature of this design is represented by the ability to automatically adjust the forces that act on the different finger phalanges based on the interaction between the device and the user's finger. The adaptive behavior of the device is possible due to the incorporation of passive elements in the mechanism design [72], as illustrated in Figure 7d.

Coupled exoskeleton devices coordinate the movement of different finger joints simultaneously and are designed to interact with the user's finger at multiple contact points, as illustrated in Figure 7e. This type of design allows for more natural finger movement. Through mechanical adjustments of the ratios, these devices can accommodate different motion patterns and adapt to various users without complex control systems [72].

Another type of exoskeleton linkage is represented by the fingertip exoskeleton. Using this type of mechanism, the fingertip's position in space is controlled, regardless of how the individual finger joints move. As illustrated in Figure 7f, this design allows precise fingertip manipulation while enabling natural movement of the finger joints [72]. This type of mechanism is simpler than multi-joint mechanisms. Figure 8 provides visual representations of various linkage types.

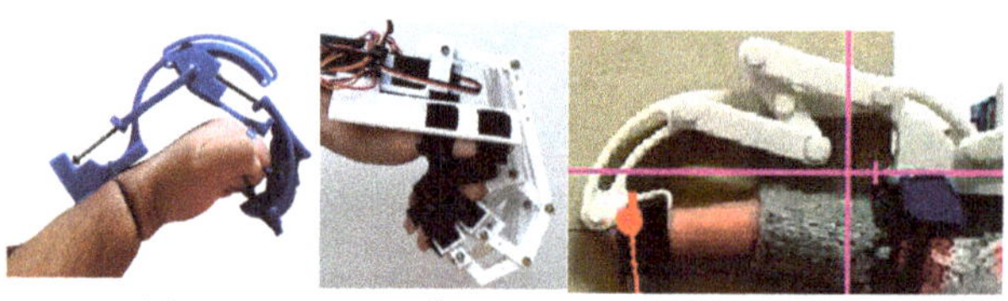

(a) (b) (c)

Figure 8. Exoskeleton types: (**a**) Underactuated device [83], (**b**) coinciding joint axes [84], and (**c**) fingertip linkage device [85].

Prior investigations into redundant linkage exoskeletons include the works of [86–91]. Additional research exploring fingertip linkage devices has been conducted by several authors [92–96]. Investigations into underactuated devices have been studied in [97, 98]. Understanding human hand proportions and exoskeleton connectivity has been explored in [99,100].

A considerable number of studies have investigated coupled devices utilizing a single actuator, for example, the work of [101–106]. Another strand of research has focused on coupled devices employing two actuators [107–111]. The research conducted by [81] introduced an exoskeleton design utilizing a remote center of motion (RCM) mechanism.

4.1.3. Hybrid Exoskeletons

Efficient power transmission, robust force control, and precise kinematics are advantageous characteristics provided by rigid exoskeletons. However, excessive mass, bulky design, and high stiffness are some of the main disadvantages of this type of rigid exoskeleton. To address the disadvantages, researchers developed innovative approaches such as the incorporation of elastic elements within the rigid mechanism to enhance compliance while preserving the advantages of structural rigidity. Hybrid exoskeletons integrate a rigid frame with deformable materials to achieve an optimal balance between mechanical performance and ergonomic consideration [76].

The integration of compliant materials in exoskeleton design significantly enhances device wearability and user comfort. These materials facilitate compatibility with the natural biomechanics of human fingers, improving force output capabilities [112]. Additive manufacturing technologies have facilitated the development of diverse exoskeleton architectures [113]. Some researchers have leveraged these capabilities to create single-unit designs [114–116] while others have explored modular structures [117,118]. An alternative strategy involves the incorporation of elastic spring elements [119]. This approach aims to mitigate the limitations typically associated with rigid structures while preserving their mechanical advantages. Another strategy employs fiber-reinforced soft bending actuators [120–122].

4.2. Classification by Hand Mobility

Exoskeletons can be classified according to hand mobility. Devices can be designed to assist and control different numbers of fingers on the human hand, which typically has five fingers. Figure 9 illustrates various configurations of finger assistance in exoskeleton designs.

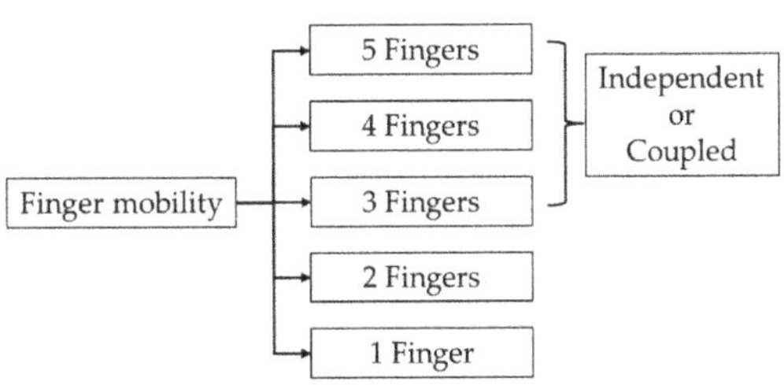

Figure 9. Different configurations based on hand mobility.

Hand exoskeletons can be categorized by the number of actuated fingers. Single-finger designs [13,83,85,95,97,102,103,118,123–155], often focusing on the index finger [13,83,102,118,123,124,144,151,152], serve as initial investigations for multi-finger exoskeletons. Other single-finger exoskeletons target the thumb [142,150,156] or middle finger [133].

Two-finger exoskeletons [157–170], which independently control multiple finger configurations such as thumb–index [103,158,164,167] or index–middle [159,171], have been developed to support targeted hand movements for rehabilitation, such as precision grip tasks. However, most activities of daily living require assistance from at least three fingers [96,98,110,172–184]. Three-finger combinations typically focus on thumb–index–middle configurations [175,176,182,183,185,186].

While three-finger designs can support many tasks, configurations of four fingers [84,88,89,91,112,187–204] offer improved functionality. These include designs assisting all fingers except the thumb [84,106,205], configurations excluding the little finger [189,201,206], and systems actuating thumb–index–middle–ring combinations [89].

Most of the full hand (five fingers) exoskeletons employ independent actuation of all digits [15,93,117,119,120,146,207–231]. These systems enable individual control of each finger, offering maximum dexterity for both rehabilitation and assistive functions. While such designs typically require more complex control systems and a higher number of actuators, they provide the flexibility needed for precise manipulation tasks and personalized rehabilitation strategies.

Some devices implement coupled actuation designs [15,84,109,114,117,119,196,232–246], where certain fingers are mechanically linked to move together. Common coupling strategies include grouping four fingers together with independent control of the thumb [15,114,210,233,235,245,247], using ring–little finger coupling while maintaining independent control of the other digits [232,248,249], or coupling all fingers into a single actuation unit [237,238,250,251]. Some designs implement different coupling combinations for flexion and extension movements [242–244,252], offering a balance between functionality and complexity. These approaches offer advantages in terms of mechanical simplicity and a reduced number of actuators.

4.3. Classification by Mechanism Position

Robotic exoskeletons can be categorized based on the placement of the mechanism. This classification includes palmar, lateral, dorsal, and glove-type configurations, as illustrated in Figure 10. Each placement modality offers distinct biomechanical advantages and constraints, influencing the exoskeleton's functionality [72].

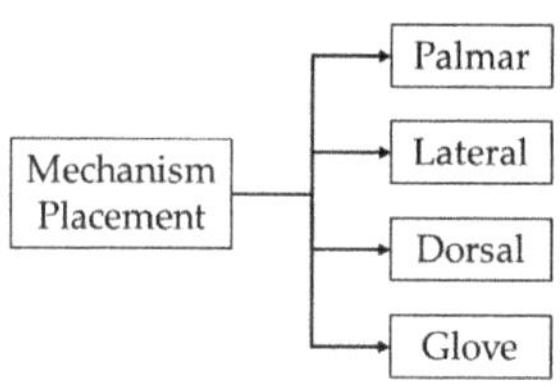

Figure 10. Exoskeletons classification based on mechanism placement.

A schematic representation of each exoskeleton configuration is depicted in Figure 11, illustrating the palmar, lateral, dorsal, and glove-type designs.

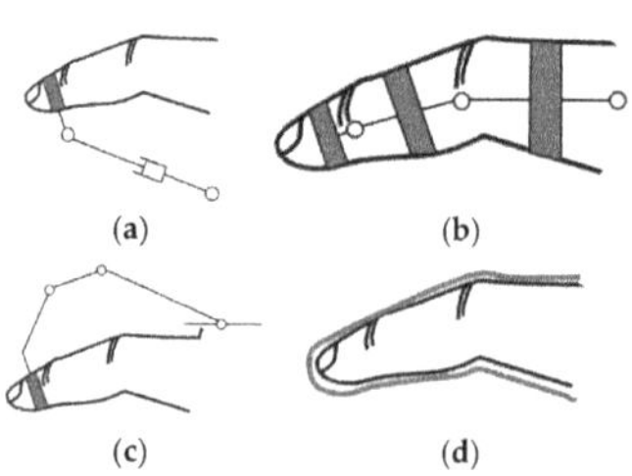

Figure 11. Classification by mechanism placement: (**a**) palmar, (**b**) lateral, (**c**) dorsal, (**d**) glove.

4.3.1. Palmar

Palmar devices are characterized by the placement of mechanical or transmission components within the palmar region of the hand, as illustrated in Figure 11a. This type of mechanism placement has been studied in papers [190,253–256]. However, this configuration presents a limitation for assistive applications.

4.3.2. Lateral

Lateral devices are characterized by the positioning of mechanical or transmission components along the lateral aspects of finger phalanges, as depicted in Figure 11b, and were studied in [85,90,103,129,132,157,158,201,209,234,237,239,256–258]. An important advantage of lateral devices is the preservation of palmar surface availability for tactile interactions with the environment. However, lateral configurations present certain limitations; in multi-finger implementations, there is a potential for inter-digit collisions [72].

4.3.3. Dorsal

Dorsal devices are characterized by the placement of mechanical transmission above the finger phalanges, as illustrated in Figure 11c [59,83–85,87–96,98,101,102,105–114,117, 120,123–128,130,131,134–137,139–151,153,154,156,158,160–164,166,169,173,181–183,185,188, 195–207,210–214,217,219–222,224–227,230,233,235,236,238,240,242,244,245,247,250,251,259–357]. This configuration minimizes inter-digit collisions while preserving palmar surface availability.

4.3.4. Glove

Glove exoskeletons depicted in Figure 11d are characterized by their flexible, fabric-like construction that envelops the hand, with actuation components integrated into or attached to the glove material. This type of design offers several advantages. The soft, pliable nature of these devices allows for extended wear without causing discomfort or restricting natural hand movements. Soft gloves can conform to various hand sizes and shapes, making them suitable for a wider range of users without extensive customization. By using thin, flexible materials, soft gloves preserve much of the user's natural tactile sensation, allowing for better interaction with objects during rehabilitation exercises.

Soft glove exoskeletons have been the subject of extensive research and development in recent years, with significant contributions from various studies [121,133,173–176,180, 184,186,189,191–193,222,228,229,240,243,248,249,262,358–388]. These investigations have explored diverse aspects of glove design, fabrication, and implementation, advancing the field of wearable rehabilitation technology. Figure 12 illustrates each type of mechanism placement with examples from the literature.

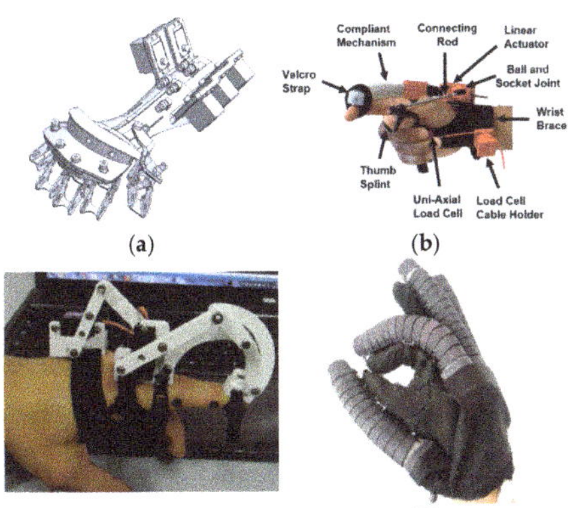

Figure 12. Classification by mechanism placement: (**a**) Palmar [146], (**b**) lateral [132], (**c**) dorsal [144], (**d**) glove [358].

4.4. *Classification by Actuator Type*

Exoskeleton actuation modalities can be classified into electromechanical, pneumatic, shape memory alloy-based, hydraulic, contralateral extremity-driven, human muscle, series elastic actuators, and other approaches as depicted in Figure 13.

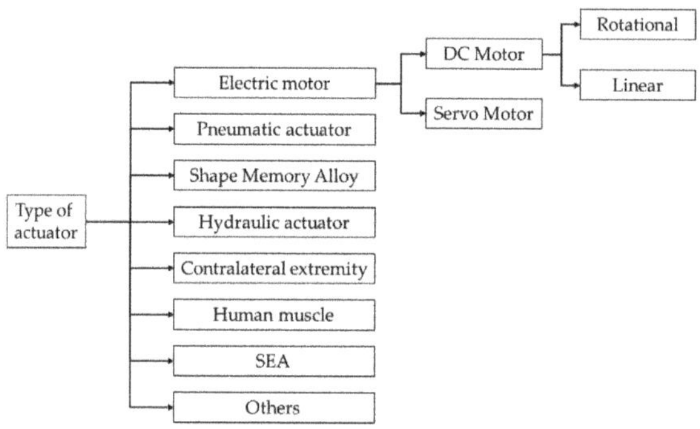

Figure 13. Classification by actuator type.

4.4.1. Electric Motors

Exoskeletons that use rotary DC motors as their actuation method have been the subject of extensive research in recent years, and numerous studies have explored various aspects of implementing this type of motor in exoskeleton systems [13,15,83,87,90,92–97,101, 103,106,108,110,121–123,125,126,128–130,133,135–143,154,157,158,160–162,164,167,170,173,175, 184–186,189,192,194,195,202,204,208,211,227,228,231,234,237,239,240,244,247,248,250,251,255, 256,261–264,273,279,306,308,311,321,324,338,340,361,365,366,370,376,384,387,389–395]. Linear motors are a good choice for controlling finger movements in exoskeleton hands. They can be easily placed on top of the hand and can open and close multiple fingers together [15,59,84,98,104,112,117,132,144–146,150,156,159,171,180,196,197,200,207,212–214,217,231–233,253,260,269,281,283–286,288,299,310,331,367,368,372,376,383,396,397]. Servomotors represent another type of electric actuator that is used in exoskeleton design. These types of motors offer precise position control and rapid response, making them suitable for accurate joint angle manipulation. Several researchers used servomotors in their exoskeleton prototypes, as documented in various publications [84,91,107,119,127, 144,145,171,174,188,190,197,205,212,229,235,254,280,282–287,309,325,337,339,396,398].

4.4.2. Pneumatic Actuators

Pneumatic actuators [132,134,152,153,163,180,191,193,198,201,203,206,217,219,221,222,224, 225,241,243,249,252,257,270–272,289–294,312,313,316,318,319,323,326,328,330,342,358–360,363, 364,371–375,377,378,380,382,385,386,388,399–402] are widely used in hand rehabilitation robots due to their advantages in force generation, control, and weight-to-torque ratio [214,288]. They operate using air flow through various mechanisms such as pneumatic cylinders [102,109,187], air balloons [238], air bladders [241,359], flexible thermoplastic fabrics [249,360], or pneumatic artificial muscles [88,124,203,262,272,318,330,402]. Different categories of soft pneumatic actuators have been developed. Pneu-nets soft actuators (PNSAs) [198,221], made of elastomers, move finger joints directly. Optimized designs use semicircular chambers for better performance [217]. Fiber-reinforced actuators generate higher forces compared to PNSAs and allow for better designs [163,220,289,290,403]. Positive-negative pneumatic actuators allow active control of both flexion and extension [291,292]. Soft tissue-based pneumatic actuators use flexible, lightweight tissues and can achieve high forces [252,293]. McKibben-type pneumatic artificial muscles, made of a rubber inner tube with a braided shell, inflate and contract when pressurized [404]. Manufacturing processes for these actuators include casting in molds, direct 3D printing, and monolithic molding techniques [134].

The main advantages of pneumatic actuators include high, adjustable force and speed at a low cost, good weight-to-torque ratio [214], less maintenance [66,405–407], and the ability to stop under load without damage [69,405]. Some alternative approaches include EMG-controlled systems [226] and various mechanical design configurations [408], each offering distinct benefits for rehabilitation applications.

However, pneumatic actuators have several limitations. These include size constraints due to compressors and air storage chambers, noise, control difficulties due to time variability and nonlinearity, and slower response times in some cases [29,32].

Other studies on pneumatic actuation explored various designs for hand exoskeletons, for example, the work of [295,380]. These designs include soft actuators [198,218], fabric-based systems [216,249,252,293,312,400], and fiber-reinforced silicone actuators [380]. Specialized approaches like thin McKibben muscles [401] and bending-type pneumatic muscles [294] were also investigated. Research has focused on soft exoskeletons for rehabilitation and assistance [193,271,272,358,364,371,374,378] and incorporating various materials such as silicone rubber [134,152,153,163,191,193,206,217,219,220,224,225,290–292,313,316,319,328,342,358,360,363,364,371,373,375,377,380,385,390], flexible 3D-printed materials [270,333,374], and custom pneumatic actuators [270,271].

4.4.3. Shape Memory Alloys

SMAs have two key properties: shape memory effect and super elasticity [409,410]. The shape memory effect is the property of recovering the original shape upon heating to a critical temperature when it is deformed in the low-temperature phase [411]. SMAs work on the principle of phase transformation between two crystalline structures: martensite, the low-temperature phase, and austenite, the high-temperature phase [412]. After plastic deformation, SMA wire can return to its original shape when heated to a certain temperature. Additionally, under isothermal conditions, it can undergo great deformation, consume and absorb mechanical energy, and return to its original shape after removing the load, demonstrating a good damping effect [409,410].

Common materials used for SMAs include Ni–Ti and Cu–Al–Ni, among other combinations. The actuation is typically achieved by heating the SMA wire or rod by applying an electric current through it.

SMAs have been explored by several researchers [296–298,381,413–415] and have several advantages, including a high power-to-weight ratio [266]. This makes them suitable for a wide range of applications as both actuators and sensors.

SMA actuators also present several challenges. Their output motion is characterized by hysteresis, high nonlinearity, and saturation, making precise control difficult [416]. Additionally, SMA wires or rods produce significant heat during operation, thus safety considerations must be implemented when used in exoskeleton systems.

4.4.4. Hydraulic Actuators

Hydraulic actuators operate on a principle similar to pneumatic systems, but they use an incompressible liquid instead of air [277]. These actuators are known for their excellent performance characteristics [32]. Various hydraulic devices have been explored for power transfer in exoskeleton applications, including hydraulic cylinders [417], flexible inflatable materials [265], and certain types of artificial muscles [362]. However, hydraulic actuators have some limitations that affect their use in certain applications. The primary drawback is the requirement for a wider space to accommodate the liquid-transmitting pipes [32]. This spatial requirement makes hydraulic actuators less commonly used in hand rehabilitation robots [418].

4.4.5. Human MUSCLE

An innovative approach involves harnessing the power of the patient's own muscles. This method, which can be broadly categorized as a form of actuation, utilizes functional electrical stimulation, FES, to activate impaired hand muscles [417]. This hybrid approach combines the benefits of electrical muscle stimulation with robotic assistance, potentially improving the effectiveness of hand rehabilitation. A notable example of this combined strategy is the FES and robotic glove system developed by Rong et al. [419].

4.4.6. Contralateral Extremity

In the field of hand rehabilitation, another approach involves utilizing the unaffected limb as a form of actuation for the impaired hand. This method, known as contralateral extremity actuation, is particularly relevant in rehabilitation systems that employ bilateral training strategies [419]. There are two primary ways in which the healthy extremity can drive the rehabilitation of the impaired hand. The first, which remains largely theoretical, involves direct force transfer from the unaffected hand to actuate devices on the impaired side. The second, and more researched approach, uses signals or data from the healthy hand to indirectly control rehabilitation devices on the affected side [420].

4.4.7. Series Elastic Actuators

Series elastic actuators (SEAs) represent an innovative approach to exoskeleton design, combining the power of electric motors with the compliance of spring elements. Unlike traditional actuators that prioritize joint stiffness, SEAs intentionally reduce it, opening new possibilities in rehabilitation robotics [165]. The incorporation of a spring element between the motor and the load in SEAs offers several advantages such as enhanced shock absorption and improved force control accuracy and stability. While SEAs seem to present an ideal solution for hand exoskeletons, they come with some disadvantages; the intentional reduction in joint stiffness limits the magnitude of the force that can be transferred to the exoskeleton and mechanical complexity. Some researchers have explored the potential of SEAs in hand rehabilitation devices [165,199].

4.4.8. Other Types of Actuators

Research into alternative actuator technologies continues, as engineers and researchers develop more efficient and effective solutions. Among the emerging solutions being explored are electroactive polymers and ultrasonic motors [421].

Figure 14 illustrates different types of hand exoskeletons using various actuation methods.

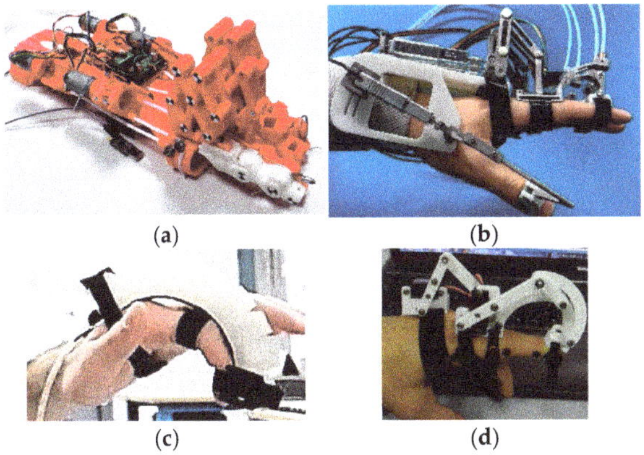

Figure 14. Classification by type of actuator: (**a**) DC Motor [194], (**b**) linear actuator [354], (**c**) pneumatic [134], (**d**) servomotor [144].

4.5. Classification by Transmission Type

An alternative classification method is based on power transmission mechanisms. This approach categorizes systems into several types: geared systems, linkage mechanisms, cable-driven systems, compliant structures, and restorative springs. Figure 15 illustrates these various transmission types.

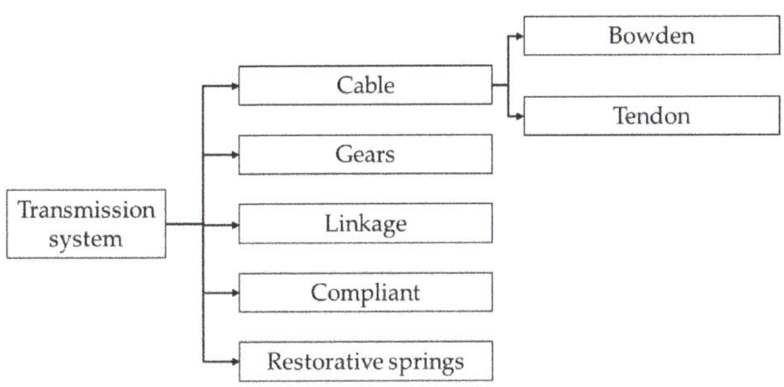

Figure 15. Classification by transmission system.

4.5.1. Linkage

Linkage-based devices are a popular choice in hand rehabilitation robotics. These devices use mechanical links to form finger components and can be categorized based on their control mechanisms and structural designs.

Linkage-based actuation offers several advantages. It can be implemented with various control methods. By combining actuators with rigid exoskeletons, these devices can secure the range of motion and prevent out-of-plane flexion or extension [422,423].

This type of device also presents challenges. Motors and translational linkages can add weight to the system, even for simple motions, and compact designs require more expensive actuators [424–426]. The addition of linkages complicates the exoskeleton's kinematics, with each link's mass, inertia, and center of gravity changing for different hand sizes. Simplified designs with fewer actuators limit mobility and task adjustability.

Several studies have expanded our understanding of linkage-based devices [59,83–85,87,90,91,94–98,110,137,139,140,144,146,147,149–151,156,159,160,162,166,170,171,200,

207,211,212,214,233,236,245,247,250,260,269,273,280–282,286–288,297,299–301,305,306, 309,310,321,322,332,376,392,396,399].

4.5.2. Gears

Gear-motor actuation, while often considered a direct approach, can be expensive and challenging to implement. With a human hand, several gears and gear trains would be used to provide actuation. Designs that use gear-motor actuation face similar weight issues experienced by linkage-based actuation.

There is a fine line between direct drive and gear assembly. Some devices [279,311] are classified as geared systems because the motor is connected through a gear train to the structure. The idea behind a direct drive or geared system is for the actuators to be as close to the structure as possible, typically mounted on the dorsal side of the hand. This type of transmission enables the devices to be portable and less complex, simultaneously minimizing the power or transmission losses, but increasing the weight on the hand.

4.5.3. Cable

Cable-driven exoskeletons [13,15,88,93,120,124,127,130,131,133,138,154,158,161,164,167, 168,173–176,178–182,184–186,189,190,195,197,204,205,208,209,213,222,223,230,234,235,237,240, 242,244,248,251,254–256,277,284,285,296,298,317,325,327,329,334,335,337–340,365,367–370,372, 381,383,384,386,387,390,393–395,397,427–429] are a popular choice for hand rehabilitation, using servo or rotary motors. These systems utilize cables to achieve low-weight solutions. The main advantage of cable-driven systems is their ability to shift the weight of actuation components away from the hand, resulting in lighter devices. Cable mechanisms can be categorized into two types: Bowden cable-driven devices and tendon-driven devices [256]. Bowden cable transmission involves routing cables or rigid rods through low-friction tubes to connect the actuating unit with the hand exoskeleton. This allows for remote placement of the actuating unit, making it suitable for stationary rehabilitation or wheelchair-mounted systems [160,251,256,275,393,430,431]. Another advantage of cable-driven systems is their use of soft exoskeletons, which provide an adaptable design that can adjust to various hand shapes and sizes [432]. This flexibility is particularly beneficial given the diverse dimensions of patients' hands.

Cable-driven systems present several challenges; one major disadvantage is the loss of power and control issues; the actuation experiences transmission losses as the device performs exercises, mainly due to friction.

The main difference between tendon and Bowden cable systems is that tendon cables mimic the hand anatomy structure by flexing and extending the fingers with a cable routed in a glove, whereas Bowden cables use a rigid structure to transfer the cable forces to the fingers, as mentioned previously. Tendon cables are usually connected to the distal part of the finger and flex or extend the finger by applying tension to the cable. This type of transmission is normally unidirectional, meaning only one cable can execute a single task such as flexion or extension. A second cable is required to have a bidirectional actuation, which means another actuator is generally required. These types of developed hand exoskeletons are usually underactuated systems where a single actuator can flex or extend multiple fingers such as in [56–58] using a single cable routed in a loop across or between the fingers.

Tendon cables can suffer from cable breakage, and the routing paths are sometimes complex and can cause power losses due to friction, but they can apply the required forces to the digit itself instead of the joints.

Tendon actuation has been explored and implemented in other numerous studies, as evidenced by the research presented in [34,35,133,173,175–177,179,182,183,186,189,190, 208,222,234,240,242,248,296,298,325,327,365–367,370,383,386,390,397,428,433–435]. Despite these challenges, cables remain an attractive option for hand rehabilitation robots due to their similarity to hand muscles [158,376].

Bowden cable mechanisms have been studied in the following studies [154,159,164, 181,202,223,227,254,308,329,335,337,394,395]. Bowden cables offer more flexibility due to their cable conduit but suffer from variable and high friction forces caused by curves [125].

Pulley cables require continuous tension to maintain traction, limiting their use [128,436]. Examples of devices using pulley cables include the work of [88,235,251,393].

4.5.4. Restorative Springs

Springs, despite being passive components, are commonly integrated into hand exoskeletons that primarily use unidirectional actuation. They are often paired with either tendons or pneumatic cylinders, which typically control only flexion or extension. The springs serve to passively facilitate the opposite motion, complementing the active actuator. Numerous studies have explored and implemented spring-based actuation mechanisms in hand exoskeletons [83,197,232,274,276,284].

4.5.5. Compliant Transmission

Artificial muscles and flexible jointless structures represent innovative approaches in the field of soft robotics, offering compliant and adaptable solutions for finger flexion and extension [437].

Artificial muscles, typically driven by pneumatic or hydraulic systems, consist of a flexible material encased in a braided sheath. When fluid is injected, the muscle contracts, and when pressure is released, it extends [201,203,257,265,272,318,319,330,402]. These systems provide a high degree of flexibility [438]. However, they can face challenges such as ballooning, where excessive pressure causes the flexible material to expand beyond its functional range. Researchers have addressed this issue through careful selection of braiding materials and design optimizations [201,265].

Flexible jointless structures represent an evolution of the artificial muscle concept. These devices, often made from silicone rubber, are molded in specific configurations to achieve bending motions without the need for a braided sheath [302,360]. These structures offer the advantages of simplicity and potentially lower manufacturing costs, as they can be custom-designed for individual users using relatively inexpensive materials.

Further research on flexible jointless structures has been extensively conducted, as evidenced by numerous studies, for example [72,134,153,163,191,193,198,206,217,219–221,225,270,290,292,313,316,328,342,358,360,362–364,371,373–375,377,380,385]. These investigations have significantly contributed to the advancement of this technology, exploring various design configurations, materials, and applications in the field of soft robotics for rehabilitation.

Figure 16 illustrates different types of hand exoskeletons using various transmission systems.

Hand exoskeletons use a wide variety of transmission combinations to achieve optimal performance and functionality. Researchers often combine multiple transmission elements to leverage the strengths of each and address the complex requirements of hand rehabilitation and assistance.

Hand exoskeletons utilize various transmission combinations like cable and steel wire systems [119]. Some designs incorporate cable and spring mechanisms [127] while others explore linkage and spring combinations [281].

The linkage and cable combination appears to be particularly popular among researchers [91,102,103,106,109,118,123,125,130,135,136,141–143,148,157,159,160,169,194,196,202,227,231,259,261,278,303,391].

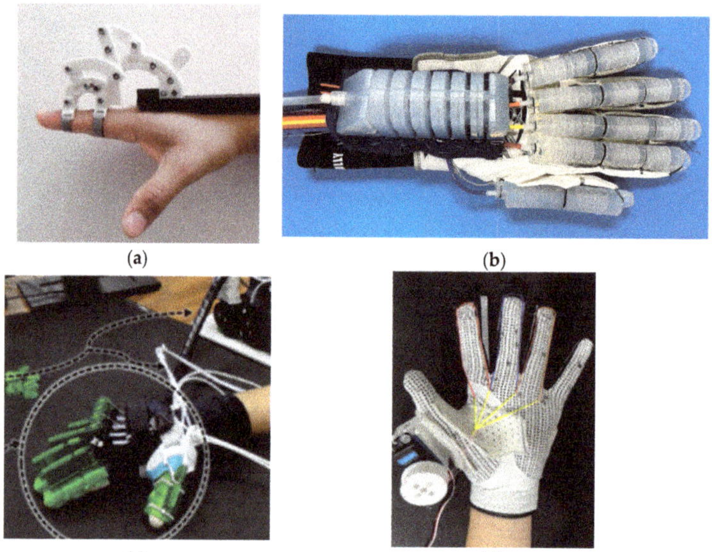

(a) (b) (c) (d)

Figure 16. Classification by type of transmission: (**a**) Linkage [144], (**b**) silicone-rubber [364], (**c**) cable [285], (**d**) tendon [178].

5. Results and Discussion

A comprehensive database was developed to catalog and analyze hand rehabilitation devices reported in the literature. The database contains over 300 devices, each of them characterized by 45 criteria. The criteria were defined in such a way to cover the technical specifications of each device.

5.1. Database Parameters Organization

To facilitate the analysis of the papers, the database was structured into six primary categories. The bibliometric information category contains fundamental publication data including author details, publication year, and article identification.

The database core structure is represented by technical specifications that include information about actuation systems, transmission mechanisms, motion characteristics such as DoF, and range of motion.

Another significant category is represented by control and sensing criteria that include the implementation of different sensors, control methods, intention detection methodologies, feedback, and the interface between the device and the patient.

Each device was documented with its practical features, covering portability, safety, weight, and how well it could adapt to different uses.

Regarding the validation of each device, implementation details were recorded such as test status and commercial availability. The information can be used to evaluate the transition from research prototype to practical application.

5.2. Database Population Process

Each device was analyzed across all six primary categories, with careful attention to maintaining uniform terminology. Missing information was explicitly noted to maintain database integrity and facilitate future updates.

The information organization enables easy access to specific device characteristics, while the structure supports detailed examination of individual devices.

5.3. Limitations and Constraints

During the development of the database, several limitations were identified such as incomplete reporting in original sources, variations in measurements, and incomplete information regarding all criteria that were used.

5.4. Discussions

The systematic data visualization conducted in this study covers design characteristics, technological implementations, and performance metrics across different hand exoskeleton configurations. The following graphs explore these findings in detail.

Figure 17a illustrates the temporal distribution of publications related to hand exoskeleton rehabilitation devices from 2002 to 2024, grouped in 5-year intervals. An important peak research output was observed in the 2016–2020 interval. This trend suggests a growing interest and investment in the field.

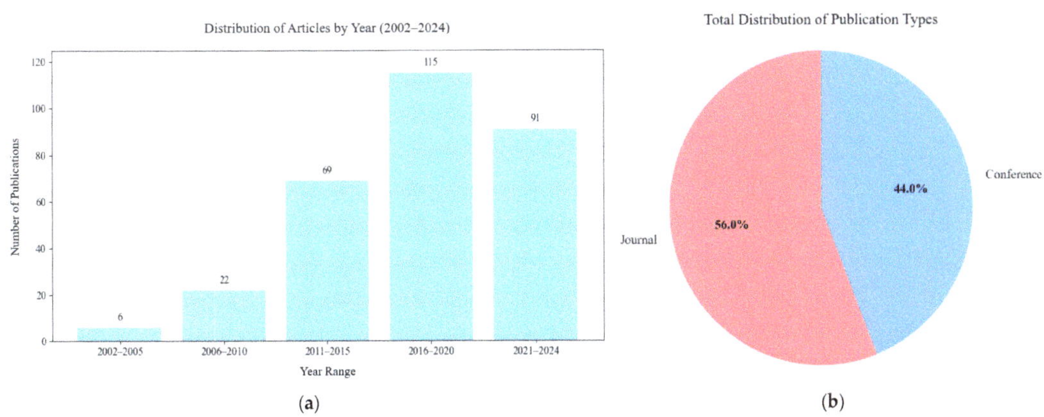

Figure 17. Distribution of publication types (**a**) temporal distribution of publications related to hand exoskeleton rehabilitation devices, (**b**) distribution of publication types.

Figure 17b provides a concise overview of overall distribution of publication types across all years. Journal articles account for 56% of total publications while conference papers account for 44% of total publications.

Figure 18 illustrates the top ten countries that contribute to hand exoskeleton device research based on their publication output. The United States leads, followed by China and Italy.

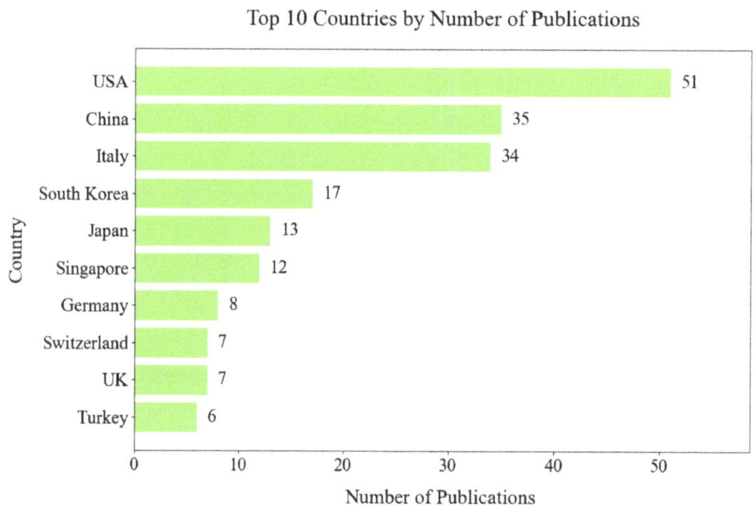

Figure 18. Country contribution based on publication output.

Figure 19 illustrates the evolution of publication types across time. In the early years of the study period, conference papers were more prevalent, but a shift towards journals can be observed in recent years.

The distribution of hand exoskeleton applications across categories is illustrated in Figure 20. Rehabilitation made up 66% of the total, followed by devices used for both rehab and assistance.

The distribution of primary actuation types used in hand exoskeletons is illustrated in Figure 21. The chart categorizes actuation mechanisms into four main groups: electric, pneumatic, other, and not specified.

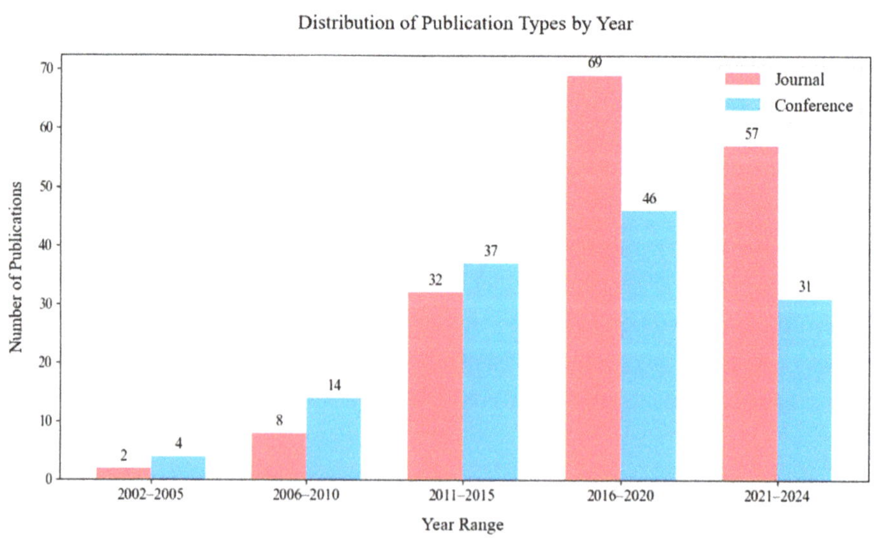

Figure 19. Overall distribution of publication types across all years.

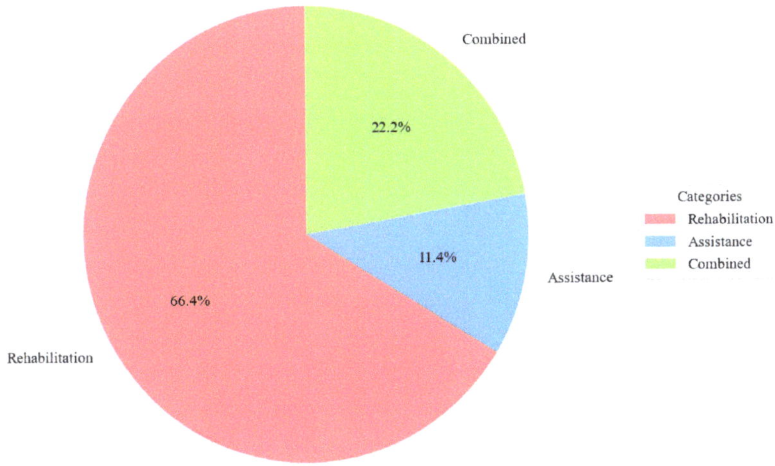

Figure 20. The distribution of hand exoskeleton applications across categories.

Electric actuation represents 55.8% of the studied exoskeletons, followed by pneumatic actuation and other types of actuation. A notable "other" category stands for 12.9% of the total studied exoskeletons.

Electric actuation represents 55.8% of the studied exoskeletons, followed by pneumatic actuation and other types of actuation.

Figure 22 breaks down the types of electric motors found in hand exoskeletons. DC motors are the predominant choice, followed by linear actuators and servomotors. Unspecified electric motors account for 8.3% of the actuators used.

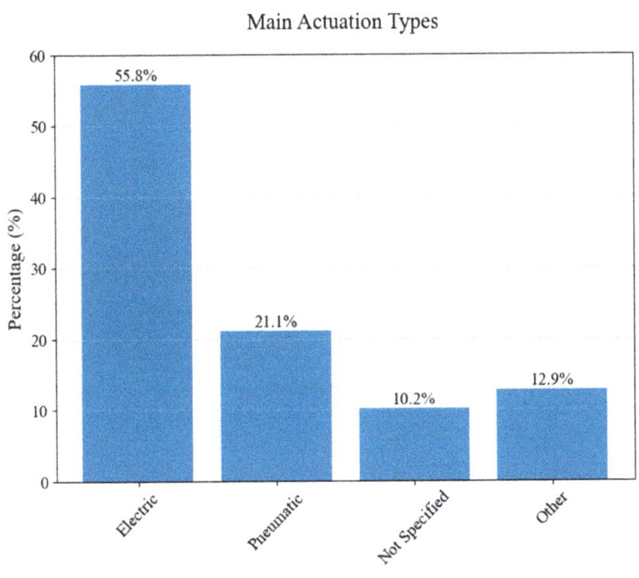

Figure 21. The distribution of actuation types.

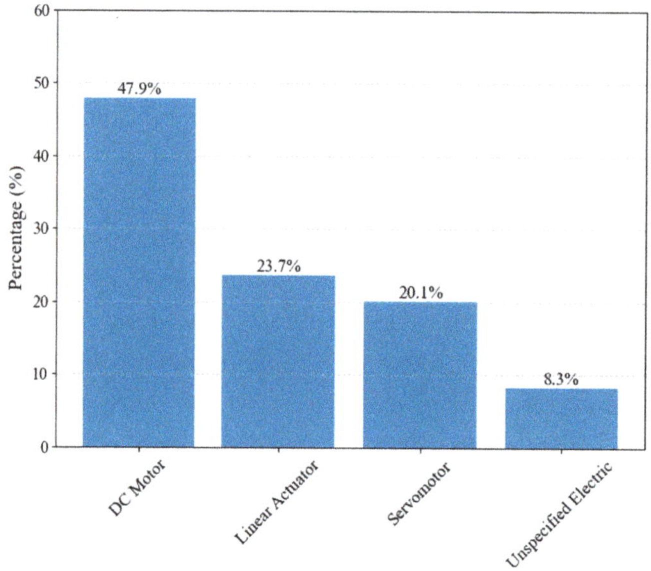

Figure 22. The distribution of electric actuator types.

Figure 23a illustrates the distribution of the main transmissions in hand exoskeleton designs. Combined mechanisms stand in the first place, followed by cable-based solutions, compliant, and linkage-based solutions. Figure 23b describes the combined transmission systems. Cable–linkage combinations are the most frequently used solution, followed by cable–spring, linkage–spring, and gear–linkage configurations.

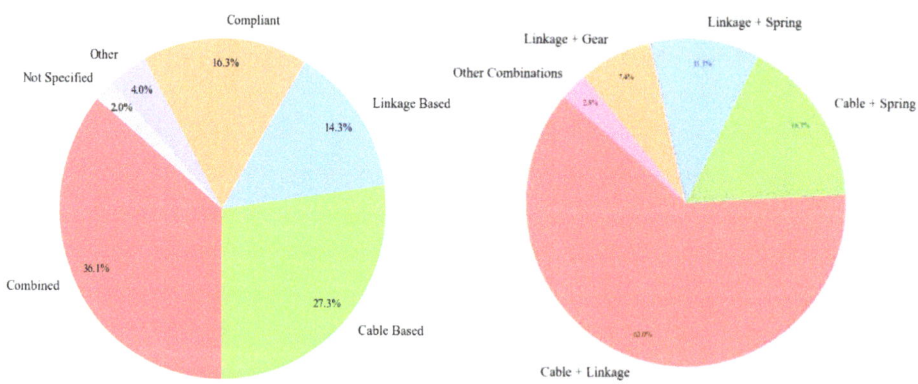

(**a**) (**b**)

Figure 23. Transmission types (**a**) distribution of main transmission, (**b**) combined transmission systems.

Figure 24 breaks down the different types of hand exoskeleton designs. The study categorized exoskeletons into three main categories: rigid, soft, and hybrid. The distribution reveals that rigid designs dominate the field, accounting for approximately 50% of analyzed exoskeletons; soft designs represent a significant proportion of the dataset, comprising 35.0% of the total studied hand exoskeletons. This presence reflects the growing interest in soft robotics. Hybrid designs combine elements of both rigid and soft structures and constitute 15.5% of the studied exoskeletons.

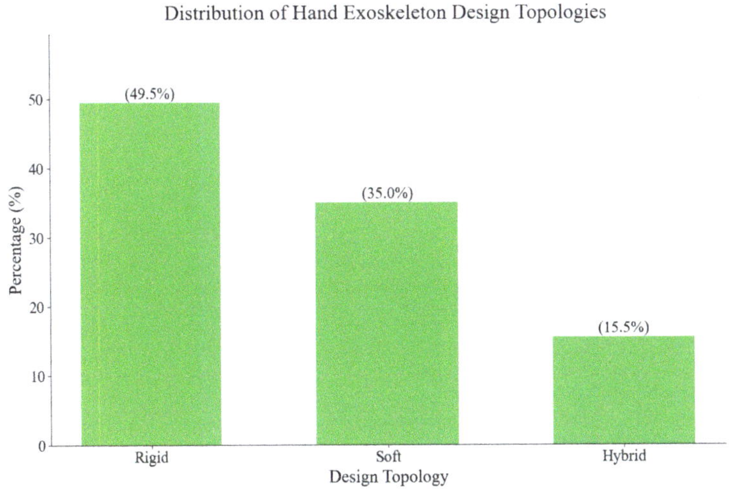

Figure 24. Distribution of the design topologies.

Figure 25 illustrates the distribution of the number of actuators used. The chart reveals a various range of actuator configurations; 29.4% utilize five or more actuators, while 24.8% use only one to two actuators, indicating the prevalence of underactuated, coupled mechanisms or hand exoskeletons that are used for a limited number of fingers. A substantial percentage of 33.9% of the studied papers did not specify the number of actuators that were used.

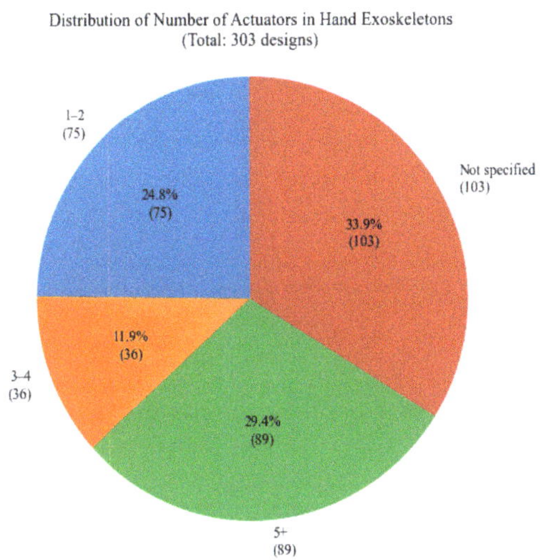

Figure 25. Distribution of actuators number.

In Figure 26, the distribution of mechanism placements is illustrated. Dorsal placement constitutes the majority of the studied hand exoskeletons, followed by glove-based, lateral, and palmar configurations.

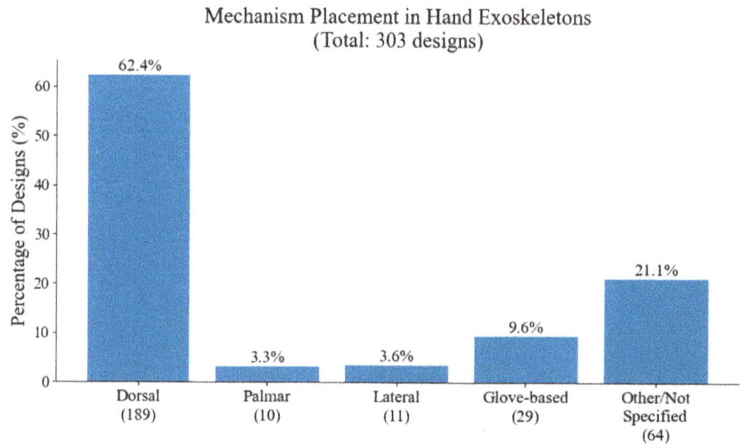

Figure 26. Distribution of mechanism placement.

Figure 27a presents the types of finger motions assisted by the studied hand exoskeleton designs. Most designs focus on both flexion and extension, aiming to provide a full range of motion. Figure 27b illustrates the distribution of independent vs. coupled finger assistance in studied hand exoskeleton designs. A significant majority implement independent finger actuation, allowing for more precise and versatile hand movements. Coupled designs and partially independent designs represent alternative approaches.

Figure 28 illustrates the distribution of finger coverage across the studied hand exoskeletons. The majority of designs aim to assist all five fingers. There is a notable diversity in approaches, with 12.5% of designs focusing on single-finger assistance.

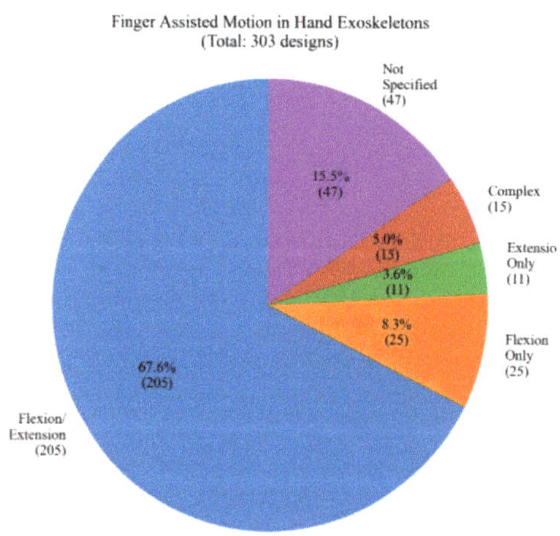

(a)

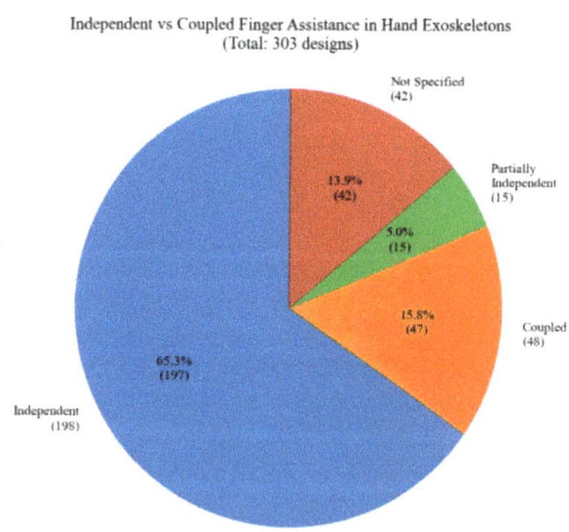

(b)

Figure 27. Type of motions: (**a**) Finger assisted motion, (**b**) independent or coupled.

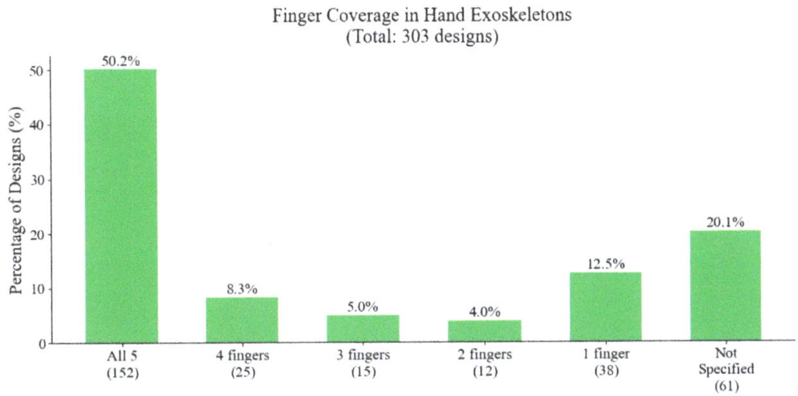

Figure 28. Distribution of finger coverage.

In Figure 29, the distribution of range of motion (ROM) is illustrated. The graph shows data for the metacarpophalangeal (MCP), proximal interphalangeal (PIP), and distal interphalangeal (DIP) joints of each finger. Across all fingers, MCP joints show a preference for ROMs in the 31–90° range, with the highest concentration in the 61–90° category. This aligns with the natural ROM of MCP joints in functional tasks. PIP joints demonstrate the widest range of motion, with significant representations in the 61–90° and 91–120° ranges. DIP joints consistently show smaller ROMs compared to MCP and PIP joints, with most designs in the range of 0–60°.

In Figure 30, the ROM distribution for the thumb joints of the studied exoskeletons is illustrated. The CMC joint, responsible for thumb opposition, shows a preference for smaller ROMs, primarily in the 0–60° range. The thumb MCP joint displays a slightly wider range, with most designs falling in the 31–60° category. The PIP joint shows the widest distribution among thumb joints, with a significant number of designs in the 31–60° and 61–90° ranges.

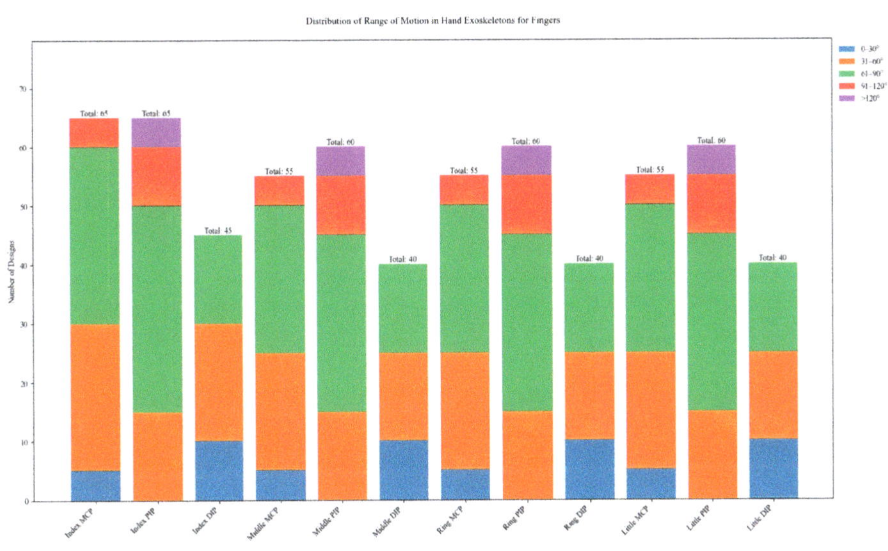

Figure 29. Range of motion (ROM) for finger joints.

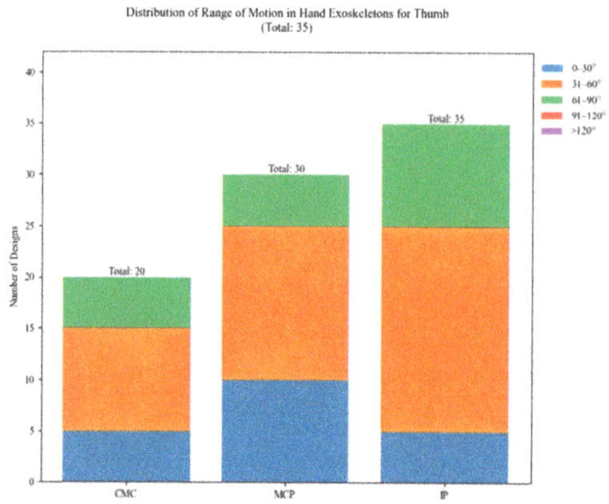

Figure 30. Range of motion (ROM) for thumb joints.

The total DoF distribution is illustrated in Figure 31. Most designs feature 1–5 DoF, followed by 6–10 DoF, corresponding to designs targeting multiple fingers and more complex movements. The presence of designs with 11–15 DoF and 16+ DoF indicates the development of complex systems.

Figure 32 presents the distribution of safety features implemented in hand exoskeleton designs. Mechanical stops are the most common safety feature, closely followed by inherent compliance. Emergency stops and software limits are frequently used.

The distribution of adaptability features in hand exoskeleton designs is illustrated in Figure 33. Most of the designs are adjustable for different sizes of hands. Customizable components and modular designs contribute to the adaptability criterion.

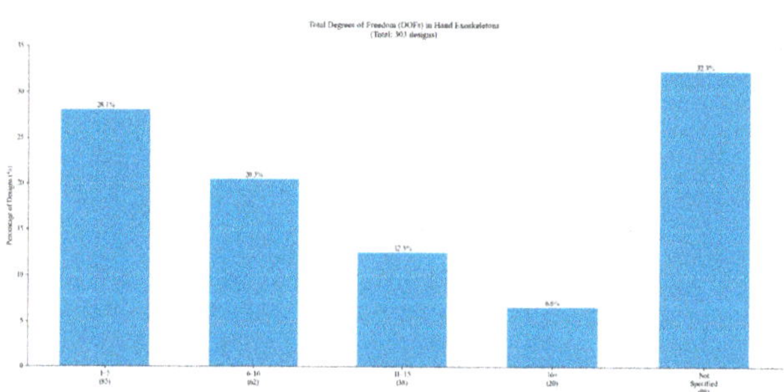

Figure 31. Distribution of Total DoF.

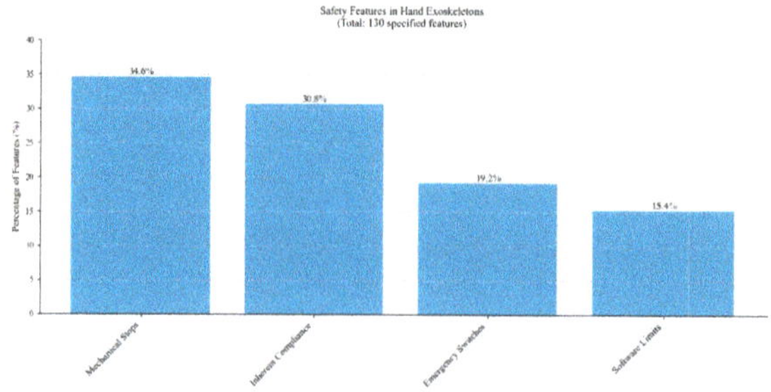

Figure 32. Distribution of safety features across studied hand exoskeletons.

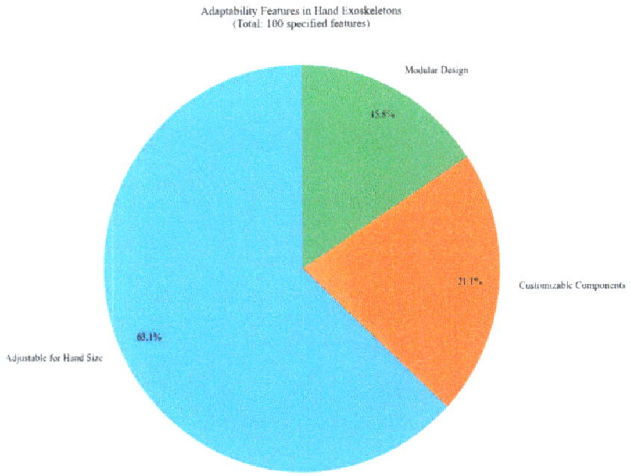

Figure 33. Distribution of adaptability features across studied hand exoskeletons.

Box plot analysis illustrated in Figure 34 reveals a systematic relationship between device complexity, functionality, and weight across studied hand exoskeleton designs. The observed weight range, from 25 g to 3700 g, demonstrates significant variation across designs, with median values showing progressive increases from single-finger configurations with a mass of 138 g to five-finger configurations with a mass of 320 g. Single-finger devices exhibit minimal weight variance, whereas five-finger systems display broader distribution patterns, reflecting diverse design approaches from assistive to rehabilitation applications. Mechanical complexity represents a key weight determinant.

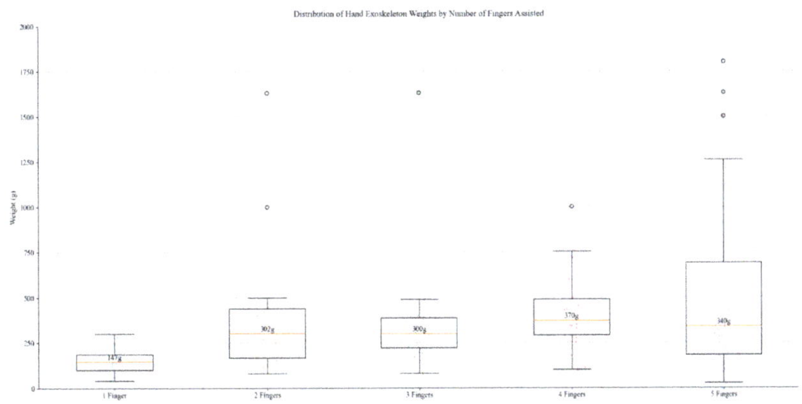

Figure 34. Distribution of weights by number of fingers assisted.

The boxplot analysis depicted in Figure 35 demonstrates distinct weight characteristics between soft and rigid/hybrid hand exoskeletons across different finger assistance configurations. Soft exoskeletons maintain consistently low weights, predominantly below 300 g, regardless of assisted finger count, with five-finger designs ranging from 25 g to 300 g. In contrast, rigid/hybrid systems show substantially higher weights and broader distribution patterns, particularly in multi-finger configurations. While soft exoskeletons maintain relatively stable weights across categories, rigid/hybrid devices exhibit marked weight increases with additional finger assistance, suggesting a direct correlation between mechanical complexity and mass.

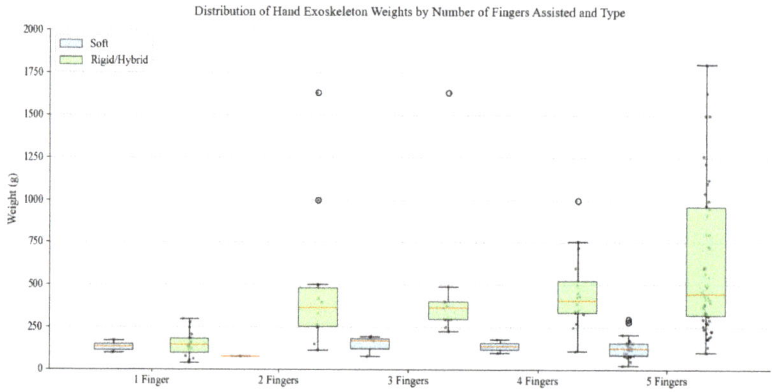

Figure 35. Distribution of Hand exoskeleton weights by number of fingers assisted and type.

6. Conclusions

This paper presents a detailed analysis of hand rehabilitation devices based on a review of over 300 systems developed between 2002 and 2024, aiming to reveal the most relevant trends in the development of such devices. The analysis demonstrates a clear trend toward more complex and user-centered designs, with research output peaking between 2016 and 2020. While rigid exoskeletons remain dominant, representing 50% of all designs, there has been substantial growth in soft (35%), and hybrid (15.5%) systems, reflecting increasing attention to user comfort and natural movement patterns and revealing future possible development trends.

In terms of technical implementation, electric actuation remains the predominant choice, representing 55.8% of all systems, with DC motors being the most common actuator type. This might be because of their simpler control systems and their size, which allow these devices to be wearable. The required actuation torque is not high, which is one of the reasons for which the preference for electric actuation is followed by pneumatic systems. Device complexity varies significantly, with 29.4% of designs using five or more actuators while 24.8% employ only one or two actuators, indicating diverse approaches to movement assistance. It also shows that hand rehabilitation can be performed, at least in the initial stages, using underactuated devices, with several fingers performing the same motion together. This approach seems sometimes preferred for practical reasons. Dorsal mechanism placement emerged as the most common configuration, followed by glove-based designs, with most systems implementing independent finger actuation to enable precise control and versatile movements.

Weight analysis demonstrated a clear correlation between functionality and mass. Lighter soft exoskeletons prioritize comfort and mild impairment assistance, while heavier rigid designs offer higher force output and more complex joint control for severe rehabilitation needs.

Analysis of the rehabilitation devices revealed clear relationships between mechanism design choices and clinical applications. Rigid designs usually deliver higher forces that are suitable for severe impairments requiring substantial assistance, while soft systems are suitable for mild to moderate conditions. Hybrid approaches offer moderate force capabilities while maintaining acceptable comfort for medium-term rehabilitation sessions.

Despite these advances, several challenges remain to be addressed in future research. There is a clear need for further investigation into optimal actuation strategies, such as assistive, active-assistive, or resistive ones, targeting different rehabilitation scenarios and the development of standardized evaluation metrics for device performance and therapeutic effectiveness. Integration of advanced sensing and control systems for more personalized rehabilitation approaches represents another crucial area for development.

The field has key challenges that need to be addressed, with missing or incomplete data from source materials being a major concern, a lack of standardized terminology and metrics for direct comparisons, limited long-term clinical studies evaluating therapeutic effectiveness, and the ongoing challenge of developing improved power sources for portable devices. These findings suggest that while significant progress has been made in hand rehabilitation robotics, substantial opportunities remain for improving device functionality, usability, and therapeutic effectiveness.

Author Contributions: Conceptualization, D.P. and C.V.; Methodology, I.B.; Software, P.T.; Validation, D.P. and J.M.; Formal Analysis, B.G.; Investigation, I.Z.; Resources, B.G.; Data Curation, A.P.; Writing—Original Draft Preparation, I.Z.; Writing—Review and Editing, I.Z. and B.G.; Visualization, C.V.; Supervision, D.P.; Project Administration, C.V.; Funding Acquisition, J.M. All authors have read and agreed to the published version of the manuscript.

Funding: This research was supported by the project New Frontiers in Adaptive Modular Robotics for Patient-centered Medical Rehabilitation—ASKLEPIOS, funded by the European Union—NextGenerationEU, and the Romanian Government under the National Recovery and Resilience Plan for Romania, contract no. 760071/23 May 2023, code CF 121/15 November 2022, with the Romanian Ministry of Research, Innovation and Digitalization within Component 9, investment I8.

Institutional Review Board Statement: Not applicable.

Informed Consent Statement: Not applicable.

Data Availability Statement: The raw data supporting the conclusions of this article will be made available by the authors on request.

Conflicts of Interest: The authors declare no conflicts of interest.

References

1. The Top 10 Causes of Death. Available online: https://www.who.int/news-room/fact-sheets/detail/the-top-10-causes-of-death (accessed on 9 November 2024).
2. Murray, C.J.L.; Vos, T.; Lozano, R.; Naghavi, M.; Flaxman, A.D.; Michaud, C.; Ezzati, M.; Shibuya, K.; Salomon, J.A.; Abdalla, S.; et al. Disability-adjusted life years (DALYs) for 291 diseases and injuries in 21 regions, 1990–2010: A systematic analysis for the Global Burden of Disease Study 2010. *Lancet* **2012**, *380*, 2197–2223. [CrossRef] [PubMed]
3. Major, Z.; Vaida, C.; Major, K.; Tucan, P.; Brusturean, E.; Gherman, B.; Birlescu, I.; Craciunas, R.; Ulinici, I.; Simori, G.; et al. Comparative Assessment of Robotic versus Classical Physical Therapy Using Muscle Strength and Ranges of Motion Testing in Neurological Diseases. *J. Pers. Med.* **2021**, *11*, 953. [CrossRef]
4. Wafa, H.A.; Wolfe, C.D.A.; Emmett, E.; Roth, G.A.; Johnson, C.O.; Wang, Y. Burden of Stroke in Europe: Thirty-Year Projections of Incidence, Prevalence, Deaths, and Disability-Adjusted Life Years. *Stroke* **2020**, *51*, 2418–2427. [CrossRef] [PubMed]
5. Vaida, C.; Carbone, G.; Major, K.A.; Major, Z.; Plitea, N.; Pisla, D. On Human Robot Interaction Modalities in the Upper Limb Rehabilitation After Stroke. *Acta Tech. Napoc. Ser. Appl. Math. Mech. Eng.* **2017**, *60*, 91–102.
6. Yang, Y.; Wang, G.; Zhang, S.; Wang, H.; Zhou, W.; Ren, F.F.; Liang, H.; Wu, D.D.; Ji, X.Y.; Hashimoto, M.; et al. Efficacy and evaluation of therapeutic exercises on adults with Parkinson's disease: A systematic review and network meta-analysis. *BMC Geriatr.* **2022**, *22*, 813. [CrossRef]
7. Selph, S.S.; Skelly, A.C.; Wasson, N.; Dettori, J.R.; Brodt, E.D.; Ensrud, E.; Elliot, D.; Dissinger, K.M.; McDonagh, M. Physical Activity and the Health of Wheelchair Users: A Systematic Review in Multiple Sclerosis, Cerebral Palsy, and Spinal Cord Injury. *Arch. Phys. Med. Rehabil.* **2021**, *102*, 2464–2481. [CrossRef] [PubMed]
8. McKevitt, C.; Fudge, N.; Redfern, J.; Sheldenkar, A.; Crichton, S.; Rudd, A.R.; Forster, A.; Young, J.; Nazareth, I.; Silver, L.E.; et al. Self-reported long-term needs after stroke. *Stroke* **2011**, *42*, 1398–1403. [CrossRef]

9. Wolfe, C.D.A.; Crichton, S.L.; Heuschmann, P.U.; McKevitt, C.J.; Toschke, A.M.; Grieve, A.P.; Rudd, A.G. Estimates of outcomes up to ten years after stroke: Analysis from the prospective South London Stroke Register. *PLoS Med.* **2011**, *8*, e1001033. [CrossRef] [PubMed]
10. *The Burden of Stroke in Europe Report*; King's College London for the Stroke Alliance for Europe: London, UK, 2019; ISBN 978-1-5272-0858-2.
11. Li, S. Spasticity, Motor Recovery, and Neural Plasticity after Stroke. *Front. Neurol.* **2017**, *8*, 120. [CrossRef] [PubMed]
12. Sommerfeld, D.K.; Eek, E.U.-B.; Svensson, A.-K.; Holmqvist, L.W.; von Arbin, M.H. Spasticity After Stroke: Its Occurrence and Association With Motor Impairments and Activity Limitations. *Stroke* **2004**, *35*, 134–139. [CrossRef]
13. Worsnopp, T.T.; Peshkin, M.A.; Colgate, J.E.; Kamper, D.G. An Actuated Finger Exoskeleton for Hand Rehabilitation Following Stroke. In Proceedings of the IEEE 10th International Conference on Rehabilitation Robotics, Noordwijk, The Netherlands, 13–15 June 2007; pp. 896–901. [CrossRef]
14. Demarin, V.; Morovic, S.; Béné, R. Neuroplasticity. *Period. Biol.* **2014**, *116*, 209–211.
15. Alhamad, R.; Seth, N.; Abdullah, H. Initial Testing of Robotic Exoskeleton Hand Device for Stroke Rehabilitation. *Sensors* **2023**, *23*, 6339. [CrossRef]
16. Su, Y.S.; Veeravagu, A.; Grant, G. Neuroplasticity after Traumatic Brain Injury. In *Translational Research in Traumatic Brain Injury*; Laskowitz, D., Grant, G., Eds.; CRC Press/Taylor and Francis Group: Boca Raton, FL, USA, 2016; Chapter 8.
17. Nahmani, M.; Turrigiano, G. Adult Cortical Plasticity Following Injury: Recapitulation of Critical Period Mechanisms? *Neuroscience* **2014**, *283*, 4–16. [CrossRef] [PubMed]
18. Carmichael, S.T. Plasticity of Cortical Projections after Stroke. *Neuroscientist* **2003**, *9*, 64–75. [CrossRef]
19. Keci, A.; Tani, K.; Xhema, J. Role of Rehabilitation in Neural Plasticity. *Open Access Maced. J. Med. Sci.* **2019**, *7*, 1540–1547. [CrossRef] [PubMed]
20. Kleim, J.A. Neural Plasticity and Neurorehabilitation: Teaching the New Brain Old Tricks. *J. Commun. Disord.* **2011**, *44*, 521–528. [CrossRef]
21. Pisla, D.; Tarnita, D.; Tucan, P.; Tohanean, N.; Vaida, C.; Geonea, I.D.; Bogdan, G.; Abrudan, C.; Carbone, G.; Plitea, N. A Parallel Robot with Torque Monitoring for Brachial Monoparesis Rehabilitation Tasks. *Appl. Sci.* **2021**, *11*, 9932. [CrossRef]
22. Kabir, R.; Sunny, M.S.H.; Ahmed, H.U.; Rahman, M.H. Hand Rehabilitation Devices: A Comprehensive Systematic Review. *Micromachines* **2022**, *13*, 1033. [CrossRef]
23. Langhorne, P.; Bernhardt, J.; Kwakkel, G. Stroke Rehabilitation. *Lancet* **2011**, *377*, 1693–1702. [CrossRef]
24. Maceira-Elvira, P.; Popa, T.; Schmid, A.C.; Hummel, F.C. Wearable Technology in Stroke Rehabilitation: Towards Improved Diagnosis and Treatment of Upper-Limb Motor Impairment. *J. Neuroeng. Rehabil.* **2019**, *16*, 142. [CrossRef] [PubMed]
25. Teasell, R.; Salbach, N.M.; Foley, N.; Mountain, A.; Cameron, J.I.; Jong, A.; Acerra, N.E.; Bastasi, D.; Carter, S.L.; Fung, J.; et al. Canadian Stroke Best Practice Recommendations: Rehabilitation, Recovery, and Community Participation following Stroke. Part One: Rehabilitation and Recovery Following Stroke; 6th Edition Update 2019. *Int. J. Stroke* **2020**, *15*, 763–788. [CrossRef]
26. Orthopedic Associates of Hartford. Hand Home Exercises. Available online: https://oahct.com/wp-content/uploads/2020/05/OAH-HAND-EXERCISES.pdf (accessed on 9 November 2024).
27. Peveler, R.; Carson, A.; Rodin, G. ABC of Psychological Medicine: Depression in Medical Patients. *BMJ* **2002**, *325*, 149–152. Available online: http://www.jstor.org/stable/25451876 (accessed on 14 November 2024). [CrossRef]
28. Edwards, D.J. On the Understanding and Development of Modern Physical Neurorehabilitation Methods: Robotics and Non-Invasive Brain Stimulation. *J. Neuroeng. Rehabil.* **2009**, *6*, 3. [CrossRef]
29. Major, Z.Z.; Vaida, C.; Major, K.A.; Tucan, P.; Simori, G.; Banica, A.; Brusturean, E.; Burz, A.; Craciunas, R.; Ulinici, I.; et al. The Impact of Robotic Rehabilitation on the Motor System in Neurological Diseases. A Multimodal Neurophysiological Approach. *Int. J. Environ. Res. Public Health* **2020**, *17*, 6557. [CrossRef]
30. Plitea, N.; Hesselbach, J.; Pisla, D.; Raatz, A.; Vaida, C.; Wrege, J.; Burisch, A. Innovative Development of Parallel Robots and Microrobots. *Acta Teh. Napoc. Ser. Appl. Math. Mec.* **2006**, *49*, 5–26.
31. Pisla, D.; Nadas, I.; Tucan, P.; Albert, S.; Carbone, G.; Antal, T.; Banica, A.; Gherman, B. Development of a Control System and Functional Validation of a Parallel Robot for Lower Limb Rehabilitation. *Actuators* **2021**, *10*, 277. [CrossRef]
32. Yue, Z.; Zhang, X.; Wang, J. Hand Rehabilitation Robotics on Poststroke Motor Recovery. *Behav. Neurol.* **2017**, *2017*, 3908135. [CrossRef]
33. Feine, J.S.; Widmer, C.G.; Lund, J.P. Physical Therapy: A Critique. *Oral Surg. Oral Med. Oral Pathol. Oral Radiol. Endod.* **1997**, *83*, 123–127. [CrossRef]
34. Landry, M.D.; Hack, L.M.; Coulson, E.; Freburger, J.; Johnson, M.P.; Katz, R.; Kerwin, J.; Smith, M.H.; Wessman, H.C.; Venskus, D.G.; et al. Workforce Projections 2010–2020: Annual Supply and Demand Forecasting Models for Physical Therapists Across the United States. *Phys. Ther.* **2016**, *96*, 71–80. [CrossRef]

35. Marek, K.; Redlicka, J.; Miller, E.; Zubrycki, I. Objectivizing Measures of Post-Stroke Hand Rehabilitation Through Multi-Disciplinary Scales. *J. Clin. Med.* **2023**, *12*, 7497. [CrossRef]
36. Gustafsson, L.A.; Turpin, M.J.; Dorman, C.M. Clinical Utility of the Chedoke Arm and Hand Activity Inventory for Stroke Rehabilitation. *Can. J. Occup. Ther.* **2010**, *77*, 167–173. [CrossRef] [PubMed]
37. Ikbali Afsar, S.; Mirzayev, I.; Umit Yemisci, O.; Cosar Saracgil, S.N. Virtual Reality in Upper Extremity Rehabilitation of Stroke Patients: A Randomized Controlled Trial. *J. Stroke Cerebrovasc. Dis.* **2018**, *27*, 3473–3478. [CrossRef] [PubMed]
38. Oliveira, C.S.; Almeida, C.S.; Freitas, L.C.; Santana, R.; Fernandes, G.; Fonseca Junior, P.R.; Moura, R.C.F. Use of the Box and Block Test for the Evaluation of Manual Dexterity in Individuals with Central Nervous System Disorders: A Systematic Review. *Man. Ther. Posturology Rehabil. J.* **2016**, *14*, 436. [CrossRef]
39. Solaro, C.; Di Giovanni, R.; Grange, E.; Mueller, M.; Messmer Uccelli, M.; Bertoni, R.; Brichetto, G.; Tacchino, A.; Patti, F.; Pappalardo, A.; et al. Box and Block Test, Hand Grip Strength and Nine-Hole Peg Test: Correlations Between Three Upper Limb Objective Measures in Multiple Sclerosis. *Eur. J. Neurol.* **2020**, *27*, 2523–2530. [CrossRef]
40. Beebe, J.A.; Lang, C.E. Relationships and Responsiveness of Six Upper Extremity Function Tests During the First Six Months of Recovery After Stroke. *J. Neurol. Phys. Ther.* **2009**, *33*, 96–103. [CrossRef]
41. Moreno-Morente, G.; Hurtado-Pomares, M.; Terol Cantero, M.C. Bibliometric Analysis of Research on the Use of the Nine Hole Peg Test. *Int. J. Environ. Res. Public Health* **2022**, *19*, 10080. [CrossRef]
42. Krumlinde-Sundholm, L.; Lindkvist, B.; Plantin, J.; Hoare, B. Development of the Assisting Hand Assessment for Adults Following Stroke: A Rasch-Built Bimanual Performance Measure. *Disabil. Rehabil.* **2019**, *41*, 472–480. [CrossRef]
43. Brunnstrom, S. Motor Testing Procedures in Hemiplegia: Based on Sequential Recovery Stages. *Phys. Ther.* **1966**, *46*, 357–375. [CrossRef] [PubMed]
44. Arwert, H.; Schut, S.; Boiten, J.; Vliet Vlieland, T.; Meesters, J. Patient Reported Outcomes of Hand Function Three Years After Stroke. *Top. Stroke Rehabil.* **2018**, *25*, 13–19. [CrossRef] [PubMed]
45. Arcidiacone, S.; Panuccio, F.; Tusoni, F.; Galeoto, G. A Systematic Review of the Measurement Properties of the Michigan Hand Outcomes Questionnaire (MHQ). *Hand Surg. Rehabil.* **2022**, *41*, 542–551. [CrossRef]
46. Jebsen, R.H.; Taylor, N.; Trieschmann, R.B.; Trotter, M.J.; Howard, L.A. An Objective and Standardized Test of Hand Function. *Arch. Phys. Med. Rehabil.* **1969**, *50*, 311–319.
47. Resnik, L.; Adams, L.; Borgia, M.; Delikat, J.; Disla, R.; Ebner, C.; Walters, L.S. Development and Evaluation of the Activities Measure for Upper Limb Amputees. *Arch. Phys. Med. Rehabil.* **2013**, *94*, 488–494.e4. [CrossRef] [PubMed]
48. Sezer, N.; Yavuzer, G.; Sivrioglu, K.; Basaran, P.; Koseoglu, B.F. Clinimetric Properties of the Duruoz Hand Index in Patients with Stroke. *Arch. Phys. Med. Rehabil.* **2007**, *88*, 309–314. [CrossRef]
49. Duruöz, M.T.; Poiraudeau, S.; Fermanian, J.; Menkes, C.J.; Amor, B.; Dougados, M.; Revel, M. Development and Validation of a Rheumatoid Hand Functional Disability Scale that Assesses Functional Handicap. *J. Rheumatol.* **1996**, *23*, 1167–1172.
50. Lefevre-Colau, M.M.; Poiraudeau, S.; Fermanian, J.; Etchepare, F.; Alnot, J.Y.; Le Viet, D.; Leclercq, C.; Oberlin, C.; Bargy, F.; Revel, M. Responsiveness of the Cochin Rheumatoid Hand Disability Scale After Surgery. *Rheumatology* **2001**, *40*, 843–850. [CrossRef]
51. Brower, L.M.; Poole, J.L. Reliability and Validity of the Duruoz Hand Index in Persons with Systemic Sclerosis (Scleroderma). *Arthritis Rheum.* **2004**, *51*, 805–809. [CrossRef]
52. Duruöz, M.T.; Cerrahoglu, L.; Dincer-Turhan, Y.; Kürsat, S. Hand Function Assessment in Patients Receiving Haemodialysis. *Swiss Med. Wkly.* **2003**, *133*, 433–438. [CrossRef]
53. Penta, M.; Tesio, L.; Arnould, C.; Zancan, A.; Thonnard, J.L. The ABILHAND Questionnaire as a Measure of Manual Ability in Chronic Stroke Patients: Rasch-Based Validation and Relationship to Upper Limb Impairment. *Stroke* **2001**, *32*, 1627–1634. [CrossRef] [PubMed]
54. Ekstrand, E.; Alt Murphy, M.; Sunnerhagen, K.S. Clinical Interpretation and Cutoff Scores for Manual Ability Measured by the ABILHAND Questionnaire in People with Stroke. *Top. Stroke Rehabil.* **2023**, *30*, 21–31. [CrossRef] [PubMed]
55. Alt Murphy, M.; Resteghini, C.; Feys, P.; Lamers, I. An Overview of Systematic Reviews on Upper Extremity Outcome Measures After Stroke. *BMC Neurol.* **2015**, *15*, 29. [CrossRef]
56. Mordor Intelligence. Rehabilitation Robots Market | 2022-27 | Industry Share, Size, Growth. Available online: https://www.mordorintelligence.com/industry-reports/rehabilitation-robots-market (accessed on 9 November 2024).
57. Fortune Business Insights. Rehabilitation Robots Market Size, Share | Global Analysis 2026. Available online: https://www.fortunebusinessinsights.com/industry-reports/rehabilitation-robots-market-101013 (accessed on 9 November 2024).
58. Ghosh, S. Capturing Human Hand Kinematics for Object Grasping and Manipulation. Master's Thesis, Texas A&M University, College Station, TX, USA, May 2013. Available online: https://oaktrust.library.tamu.edu/items/e966525a-6fa2-4a93-a4e0-7bea33c725ee (accessed on 9 November 2024).

59. Xia, K.; Chen, X.; Chang, X.; Liu, C.; Guo, L.; Xu, X.; Lv, F.; Wang, Y.; Sun, H.; Zhou, J. Hand Exoskeleton Design and Human–Machine Interaction Strategies for Rehabilitation. *Bioengineering* **2022**, *9*, 682. [CrossRef]
60. Suarez-Escobar, M.; Rendon-Velez, E. An Overview of Robotic/Mechanical Devices for Post-Stroke Thumb Rehabilitation. *Disabil. Rehabil. Assist. Technol.* **2018**, *13*, 683–703. [CrossRef] [PubMed]
61. Wang, L.; Meydan, T.; Williams, P.I. A Two-Axis Goniometric Sensor for Tracking Finger Motion. *Sensors* **2017**, *17*, 770. [CrossRef] [PubMed]
62. Jarque-Bou, N.J.; Atzori, M.; Müller, H. A Large Calibrated Database of Hand Movements and Grasps Kinematics. *Sci. Data* **2020**, *7*, 12. [CrossRef] [PubMed]
63. Iqbal, J.; Baizid, K. Stroke rehabilitation using exoskeleton-based robotic exercisers: Mini Review. *Biomed. Res. India* **2014**, *26*, 197–201.
64. Heo, P.; Gu, G.M.; Lee, S.; Rhee, K.; Kim, J. Current Hand Exoskeleton Technologies for Rehabilitation and Assistive Engineering. *Int. J. Precis. Eng. Manuf.* **2012**, *13*, 807–824. [CrossRef]
65. Vaida, C.; Birlescu, I.; Pisla, A.; Carbone, G.; Plitea, N.; Ulinici, I.; Gherman, B.; Puskas, F.; Tucan, P.; Pisla, D. RAISE—An Innovative Parallel Robotic System for Lower Limb Rehabilitation. *Adv. Theory Pract.* **2019**, *4*, 293–302. [CrossRef]
66. Pisla, D.; Plitea, N.; Gherman, B.; Pisla, A.; Vaida, C. Kinematical Analysis and Design of a New Surgical Parallel Robot. In *Computational Kinematics*; Kecskeméthy, A., Müller, A., Eds.; Springer: Berlin/Heidelberg, Germany, 2009. [CrossRef]
67. Vaida, C.; Plitea, N.; Carbone, G.; Birlescu, I.; Ulinici, I.; Pisla, A.; Pisla, D. Innovative Development of a Spherical Parallel Robot for Upper Limb Rehabilitation. *Int. J. Mech. Robot. Syst.* **2018**, *4*, 256. [CrossRef]
68. Brewer, B.R.; McDowell, S.K.; Worthen-Chaudhari, L.C. Poststroke upper extremity rehabilitation: A review of robotic systems and clinical results. *Top. Stroke Rehabil.* **2007**, *14*, 22–44. [CrossRef]
69. Gopura, R.A.R.C.; Bandara, D.S.V.; Kiguchi, K.; Mann, G.K.I. Developments in hardware systems of active upper-limb exoskeleton robots: A review. *Robot. Auton. Syst.* **2016**, *75*, 203–220. [CrossRef]
70. Krebs, H.I.; Hogan, N.; Aisen, M.L.; Volpe, B.T. Robot-aided neurorehabilitation. *IEEE Trans. Rehabil. Eng.* **1998**, *6*, 75–87. [CrossRef]
71. Todorov, E.; Shadmehr, R.; Bizzi, E. Augmented Feedback Presented in a Virtual Environment Accelerates Learning of a Difficult Motor Task. *J. Mot. Behav.* **1997**, *29*, 147–158. [CrossRef]
72. Sarac, M.; Solazzi, M.; Frisoli, A. Design Requirements of Generic Hand Exoskeletons and Survey of Hand Exoskeletons for Rehabilitation, Assistive, or Haptic Use. *IEEE Trans. Haptics* **2019**, *12*, 400–413. [CrossRef] [PubMed]
73. Choi, I.; Hawkes, E.; Christensen, D.; Ploch, C.; Follmer, S. Wolverine: A wearable haptic interface for grasping in virtual reality. In Proceedings of the IEEE/RSJ International Conference on Intelligent Robots and Systems (IROS), Daejeon, Republic of Korea, 9–14 October 2016; pp. 986–993. [CrossRef]
74. Buchholz, B.; Armstrong, T.J. A Kinematic Model of the Human Hand to Evaluate Its Prehensile Capabilities. *J. Biomech.* **1992**, *25*, 149–162. [CrossRef] [PubMed]
75. Aggogeri, F.; Mikolajczyk, T.; O'Kane, J. Robotics for Rehabilitation of Hand Movement in Stroke Survivors. *Adv. Mech. Eng.* **2019**, *11*, 168781401984192. [CrossRef]
76. Achilli, G.M.; Amici, C.; Dragusanu, M.; Gobbo, M.; Logozzo, S.; Malvezzi, M.; Tiboni, M.; Valigi, M.C. Soft, Rigid, and Hybrid Robotic Exoskeletons for Hand Rehabilitation: Roadmap with Impairment-Oriented Rationale for Devices Design and Selection. *Appl. Sci.* **2023**, *13*, 11287. [CrossRef]
77. Tiboni, M.; Amici, C. Soft Gloves: A Review on Recent Developments in Actuation, Sensing, Control and Applications. *Actuators* **2022**, *11*, 232. [CrossRef]
78. Shahid, T.; Gouwanda, D.; Nurzaman, S.G.; Gopalai, A.A. Moving Toward Soft Robotics: A Decade Review of the Design of Hand Exoskeletons. *Biomimetics* **2018**, *3*, 17. [CrossRef]
79. Kang, B.B.; In, H.; Cho, K. Force Transmission in Joint-less Tendon Driven Wearable Robotic Hand. In Proceedings of the 2012 12th International Conference on Control, Automation and Systems, Jeju Island, Republic of Korea, 17–21 October 2012; pp. 1853–1858.
80. Noronha, B.; Accoto, D. Exoskeletal Devices for Hand Assistance and Rehabilitation: A Comprehensive Analysis of State-of-the-Art Technologies. *IEEE Trans. Med. Robot. Bionics* **2021**, *3*, 525–538. [CrossRef]
81. Zong, G.; Pei, X.; Yu, J.; Bi, S. Classification and Type Synthesis of 1-DOF Remote Center of Motion Mechanisms. *Mech. Mach. Theory* **2008**, *43*, 1585–1595. [CrossRef]
82. Ferguson, P.W.; Shen, Y.; Rosen, J. Hand Exoskeleton Systems—Overview. In *Wearable Robotics*; Rosen, J., Ferguson, P.W., Eds.; Academic Press: Cambridge, MA, USA, 2020; pp. 149–175. [CrossRef]
83. Nava-Téllez, I.A.; Elias-Espinosa, M.C.; Cervantes-Culebro, H.; Flores-González, A.E. Parametric Design of a Finger Rehabilitation Mechanism with Double Action and Two Degrees of Freedom. *Appl. Sci.* **2022**, *12*, 10701. [CrossRef]

84. Esposito, D.; Centracchio, J.; Andreozzi, E.; Savino, S.; Gargiulo, G.D.; Naik, G.R.; Bifulco, P. Design of a 3D-Printed Hand Exoskeleton Based on Force-Myography Control for Assistance and Rehabilitation. *Machines* **2022**, *10*, 57. [CrossRef]
85. Hsu, T.-H.; Chiang, Y.-C.; Chan, W.-T.; Chen, S.-J. A Finger Exoskeleton Robot for Finger Movement Rehabilitation. *Inventions* **2017**, *2*, 12. [CrossRef]
86. Dickmann, T.; Wilhelm, N.J.; Glowalla, C.; Haddadin, S.; van der Smagt, P.; Burgkart, R. An Adaptive Mechatronic Exoskeleton for Force-Controlled Finger Rehabilitation. *Front. Robot. AI* **2021**, *8*, 716451. [CrossRef] [PubMed]
87. Troncossi, M.; Mozaffari Foumashi, M.; Carricato, M.; Parenti Castelli, V. Feasibility Study of a Hand Exoskeleton for Rehabilitation of Post-Stroke Patients. In Proceedings of the ASME 2012 International Design Engineering Technical Conferences and Computers and Information in Engineering Conference, Nantes, France, 2–4 July 2012; pp. 137–146. [CrossRef]
88. Wu, J.; Huang, J.; Wang, Y.; Xing, K. A Wearable Rehabilitation Robotic Hand Driven by PM-TS Actuators. In Proceedings of the International Conference on Intelligent Robotics and Applications (ICIRA), Shanghai, China, 10–12 November 2010; pp. 440–450. [CrossRef]
89. Wei, W.; Guo, S.; Zhang, F.; Guo, J.; Ji, Y.; Wang, Y. A Novel Upper Limb Rehabilitation System with Hand Exoskeleton Mechanism. In Proceedings of the 2013 IEEE International Conference on Mechatronics and Automation, Takamatsu, Japan, 4–7 August 2013; pp. 285–290.
90. Gasser, B.W.; Goldfarb, M. Design and Performance Characterization of a Hand Orthosis Prototype to Aid Activities of Daily Living in a Post-Stroke Population. In Proceedings of the 37th Annual International Conference of the IEEE Engineering in Medicine and Biology Society, Milan, Italy, 25–29 August 2015; pp. 3877–3880. [CrossRef]
91. Lince, A.; Celadon, N.; Battezzato, A.; Favetto, A.; Appendino, S.; Ariano, P.; Botta, A.M. Design and Testing of an Under-Actuated Surface EMG-Driven Hand Exoskeleton. In Proceedings of the 2017 International Conference on Rehabilitation Robotics (ICORR), London, UK, 17–20 July 2017; pp. 670–675. [CrossRef]
92. Gosselin, F.; Jouan, T.; Brisset, J.; Andriot, C. Design of a Wearable Haptic Interface for Precise Finger Interactions in Large Virtual Environments. In Proceedings of the First Joint Eurohaptics Conference and Symposium on Haptic Interfaces for Virtual Environment and Teleoperator Systems, Pisa, Italy, 18–20 March 2005; pp. 202–207. [CrossRef]
93. Ben-Tzvi, P.; Ma, Z. Sensing and force-feedback exoskeleton (SAFE) robotic glove. *IEEE Trans. Neural Syst. Rehabil. Eng.* **2015**, *23*, 992–1002. [CrossRef]
94. Fang, H.; Xie, Z.; Liu, H. An Exoskeleton Master Hand for Controlling DLR/HIT Hand. In Proceedings of the 2009 IEEE/RSJ International Conference on Intelligent Robots and Systems, St. Louis, MO, USA, 10–15 October 2009; pp. 3703–3708. [CrossRef]
95. Iqbal, J.; Tsagarakis, N.G.; Caldwell, D.G. A Multi-DOF Robotic Exoskeleton Interface for Hand Motion Assistance. In Proceedings of the 33rd Annual International Conference of the IEEE Engineering in Medicine and Biology Society, Boston, MA, USA, 30 August–3 September 2011; pp. 1575–1578. [CrossRef]
96. Sarakoglou, I.; Brygo, A.; Mazzanti, D.; Hernandez, N.G.; Caldwell, D.G.; Tsagarakis, N.G. HEXOTRAC: A highly under-actuated hand exoskeleton for finger tracking and force feedback. In Proceedings of the 2016 IEEE/RSJ International Conference on Intelligent Robots and Systems (IROS), Daejeon, Republic of Korea, 9–14 October 2016; pp. 1033–1040. [CrossRef]
97. Ertas, I.H.; Hocaoglu, E.; Barkana, D.E.; Patoglu, V. Finger exoskeleton for treatment of tendon injuries. In Proceedings of the 2009 IEEE International Conference on Rehabilitation Robotics (ICORR), Kyoto, Japan, 23–26 June 2009; pp. 194–201. [CrossRef]
98. Sarac, M.; Solazzi, M.; Sotgiu, E.; Bergamasco, M.; Frisoli, A. Design and kinematic optimization of a novel underactuated robotic hand exoskeleton. *Meccanica* **2017**, *52*, 749–761. [CrossRef]
99. Buryanov, A.; Kotiuk, V. Proportions of Hand Segments. *Int. J. Morphol.* **2010**, *28*, 755–758. [CrossRef]
100. Jarrasse, N.; Morel, G. Connecting a Human Limb to an Exoskeleton. *IEEE Trans. Robot.* **2012**, *28*, 697–709. [CrossRef]
101. Tang, Z.J.; Sugano, S.; Iwata, H. A novel, MRI compatible hand exoskeleton for finger rehabilitation. In Proceedings of the 2011 IEEE/SICE International Symposium on System Integration (SII), Kyoto, Japan, 20–22 December 2011; pp. 118–123. [CrossRef]
102. DiCicco, M.; Lucas, L.; Matsuoka, Y. Comparison of control strategies for an EMG controlled orthotic exoskeleton for the hand. In Proceedings of the 2004 IEEE International Conference on Robotics and Automation (ICRA), New Orleans, LA, USA, 26 April–1 May 2004; pp. 1622–1627. [CrossRef]
103. Cempini, M.; Cortese, M.; Vitiello, N.; Giovacchini, F.; Moise, M.; Posteraro, F.; Carrozza, M.C. Kinematics and design of a portable and wearable exoskeleton for hand rehabilitation. In Proceedings of the 2013 IEEE 13th International Conference on Rehabilitation Robotics (ICORR), Seattle, WA, USA, 24–26 June 2013; pp. 1–6. [CrossRef]
104. Rahman, M.A.; Al-Jumaily, A. Design and Development of a Hand Exoskeleton for Rehabilitation Following Stroke. In Proceedings of the 2012 International Conference on Biomedical Engineering (ICBE), Penang, Malaysia, 27–28 February 2012; pp. 1705–1710. [CrossRef]

105. Lu, X.; Yang, Z.; Chen, Y.; Wang, J. Structure Design of a Wearable Device for Hand Rehabilitation. In Proceedings of the 2016 9th International Symposium on Computational Intelligence and Design (ISCID), Hangzhou, China, 10–11 December 2016; pp. 93–96. [CrossRef]
106. Guo, S.; Zhang, W.; Guo, J.; Gao, J.; Hu, Y. Design and kinematic simulation of a novel exoskeleton rehabilitation hand robot. In Proceedings of the 2016 IEEE International Conference on Mechatronics and Automation (ICMA), Harbin, China, 7–10 August 2016; pp. 1125–1130. [CrossRef]
107. Yamaura, H.; Matsushita, K.; Kato, R.; Yokoi, H. Development of hand rehabilitation system for paralysis patient—Universal design using wire-driven mechanism. In Proceedings of the 2009 Annual International Conference of the IEEE Engineering in Medicine and Biology Society, Minneapolis, MN, USA, 3–6 September 2009; pp. 7122–7125. [CrossRef]
108. Fontana, M.; Dettori, A.; Salsedo, F.; Bergamasco, M. Mechanical design of a novel Hand Exoskeleton for accurate force displaying. In Proceedings of the 2009 IEEE International Conference on Robotics and Automation (ICRA), Kobe, Japan, 12–17 May 2009; pp. 1704–1709. [CrossRef]
109. Burton, T.M.W.; Vaidyanathan, R.; Burgess, S.C.; Turton, A.J.; Melhuish, C. Development of a parametric kinematic model of the human hand and a novel robotic exoskeleton. In Proceedings of the 2011 IEEE International Conference on Rehabilitation Robotics (ICORR), Zurich, Switzerland, 29 June–1 July 2011; pp. 1–7. [CrossRef]
110. Wei, Q.; Yang, C.; Bi, Q.; Yang, W. A Grasp Strategy with Flexible Contacting for Multi-fingered Hand Rehabilitation Exoskeleton. In *Wearable Sensors and Robots*; Yang, C., Virk, G., Yang, H., Eds.; Lecture Notes in Electrical Engineering; Springer: Singapore, 2017; Volume 399. [CrossRef]
111. Agarwal, P.; Deshpande, A.D. Impedance and force-field control of the index finger module of a hand exoskeleton for rehabilitation. In Proceedings of the 2015 IEEE International Conference on Rehabilitation Robotics (ICORR), Singapore, 11–14 August 2015; pp. 85–90. [CrossRef]
112. Arata, J.; Ohmoto, K.; Gassert, R.; Lambercy, O.; Fujimoto, H.; Wada, I. A new hand exoskeleton device for rehabilitation using a three-layered sliding spring mechanism. In Proceedings of the 2013 IEEE International Conference on Robotics and Automation (ICRA), Karlsruhe, Germany, 6–10 May 2013; pp. 3902–3907. [CrossRef]
113. Tiboni, M.; Borboni, A.; Vérité, F.; Bregoli, C.; Amici, C. Sensors and Actuation Technologies in Exoskeletons: A Review. *Sensors* **2022**, *22*, 884. [CrossRef]
114. Lin, L.; Zhang, F.; Yang, L.; Fu, Y. Design and Modeling of a Hybrid Soft-Rigid Hand Exoskeleton for Poststroke Rehabilitation. *Int. J. Mech. Sci.* **2021**, *209*, 106831. [CrossRef]
115. Achilli, G.M.; Logozzo, S.; Valigi, M.C.; Dragusanu, M.; Malvezzi, M. Theoretical and Experimental Characterization of a New Robotic gripper's Joint. In *Advances in Italian Mechanism Science*; Niola, V., Gasparetto, A., Quaglia, G., Carbone, G., Eds.; Mechanisms and Machine Science; Springer: Cham, Switzerland, 2022; Volume 122. [CrossRef]
116. Li, M.; Xu, G.; Xie, J.; Chen, C. A Soft Robotic Glove for Hand Rehabilitation Training Controlled by Movements of the Healthy Hand. In Proceedings of the International Conference on Ubiquitous Robots (UR), Kyoto, Japan, 24–27 June 2020; pp. 62–67. [CrossRef]
117. Serbest, K.; Eldoğan, O. Design, Development and Evaluation of a New Hand Exoskeleton for Stroke Rehabilitation at Home. *Politeknik Derg.* **2021**, *24*, 305–314. [CrossRef]
118. Li, G.; Cheng, L.; Sun, N. Design, manipulability analysis and optimization of an index finger exoskeleton for stroke rehabilitation. *Mech. Mach. Theory* **2022**, *167*, 104526. [CrossRef]
119. Bützer, T.; Lambercy, O.; Arata, J.; Gassert, R. Fully wearable actuated soft exoskeleton for grasping assistance in everyday activities. *Soft Robot.* **2021**, *8*, 128–143. [CrossRef]
120. Vertongen, J.; Kamper, D. Design of a 3D printed hybrid mechanical structure for a hand exoskeleton. *Curr. Dir. Biomed. Eng.* **2020**, *6*, 20202003. [CrossRef]
121. Wang, Z.; Wang, D.; Zhang, Y.; Liu, J.; Wen, L.; Xu, W.; Zhang, Y. A Three-Fingered Force Feedback Glove Using Fiber-Reinforced Soft Bending Actuators. *IEEE Trans. Ind. Electron.* **2020**, *67*, 7681–7690. [CrossRef]
122. Rose, C.; O'Malley, M. A Hybrid Rigid-Soft Hand Exoskeleton to Assist Functional Dexterity. *IEEE Robot. Autom. Lett.* **2018**, *3*, 516–523. [CrossRef]
123. Ertas, I.H.; Hocaoglu, E.; Patoglu, V. AssistOn-Finger: An Under-Actuated Finger Exoskeleton for Robot-Assisted Tendon Therapy. *Robotica* **2014**, *32*, 1363–1382. [CrossRef]
124. Sun, Z.; Miao, X.; Li, X. Design of a Bidirectional Force Feedback Dataglove Based on Pneumatic Artificial Muscles. In Proceedings of the 2009 International Conference on Mechatronics and Automation, Changchun, China, 9–12 August 2009; pp. 1767–1771. [CrossRef]
125. Wege, A.; Kondak, K.; Hommel, G. Development and Control of a Hand Exoskeleton for Rehabilitation. In *Human Interaction with Machines*; Hommel, G., Huanye, S., Eds.; Springer: Dordrecht, The Netherlands, 2006; pp. 149–157. [CrossRef]

126. Fu, Y.; Wang, P.; Wang, S.; Liu, H.; Zhang, F. Design and Development of a Portable Exoskeleton Based CPM Machine for Rehabilitation of Hand Injuries. In Proceedings of the IEEE International Conference on Robotics and Biomimetics (ROBIO), Sanya, China, 15–18 December 2008; pp. 1476–1481. [CrossRef]
127. Aubin, P.; Petersen, K.; Sallum, H.; Walsh, C.; Correia, A.; Stirling, L. A pediatric robotic thumb exoskeleton for at-home rehabilitation: The isolated orthosis for thumb actuation (IOTA). *Int. J. Intell. Comput. Cybern.* **2014**, *7*, 233–252. [CrossRef]
128. Jones, C.L.; Wang, F.; Osswald, C.; Kang, X.; Sarkar, N.; Kamper, D.G. Control and kinematic performance analysis of an Actuated Finger Exoskeleton for hand rehabilitation following stroke. In Proceedings of the 2010 3rd IEEE RAS & EMBS International Conference on Biomedical Robotics and Biomechatronics (BioRob), Tokyo, Japan, 26–29 September 2010; pp. 282–287. [CrossRef]
129. Polotto, A.; Modulo, F.; Flumian, F.; Xiao, Z.G.; Boscariol, P.; Menon, C. Index finger rehabilitation/assistive device. In Proceedings of the 2012 4th IEEE RAS & EMBS International Conference on Biomedical Robotics and Biomechatronics (BioRob), Rome, Italy, 24–27 June 2012; pp. 1518–1523. [CrossRef]
130. Wang, J.; Li, J.; Zhang, Y.; Wang, S. Design of an Exoskeleton for Index Finger Rehabilitation. In Proceedings of the 2009 Annual International Conference of the IEEE Engineering in Medicine and Biology Society (EMBC), Minneapolis, MN, USA, 3–6 September 2009; pp. 5957–5960. [CrossRef]
131. Agarwal, P.; Kuo, P.H.; Neptune, R.R.; Deshpande, A.D. A novel framework for virtual prototyping of rehabilitation exoskeletons. In Proceedings of the 2013 IEEE 13th International Conference on Rehabilitation Robotics (ICORR), Seattle, WA, USA, 24–26 June 2013; pp. 1–6. [CrossRef]
132. Sanders, Q.; Reinkensmeyer, D.J. Design and Preliminary Evaluation of a Soft Finger Exoskeleton Controlled by Isometric Grip Force. *Machines* **2024**, *12*, 230. [CrossRef]
133. Abdelhafiz, M.H.; Andreasen Struijk, L.N.S.; Dosen, S.; Spaich, E.G. Biomimetic Tendon-Based Mechanism for Finger Flexion and Extension in a Soft Hand Exoskeleton: Design and Experimental Assessment. *Sensors* **2023**, *23*, 2272. [CrossRef]
134. Tiboni, M.; Loda, D. Monolithic PneuNets Soft Actuators for Robotic Rehabilitation: Methodologies for Design, Production and Characterization. *Actuators* **2023**, *12*, 299. [CrossRef]
135. Sun, N.; Li, G.; Cheng, L. Design and Validation of a Self-Aligning Index Finger Exoskeleton for Post-Stroke Rehabilitation. *IEEE Trans. Neural Syst. Rehabil. Eng.* **2021**, *29*, 1513–1523. [CrossRef] [PubMed]
136. Li, J.; Wang, S.; Wang, J.; Zheng, R.; Zhang, Y.; Chen, Z. Development of a Hand Exoskeleton System for Index Finger Rehabilitation. *Chin. J. Mech. Eng.* **2012**, *25*, 223–233. [CrossRef]
137. Iqbal, J.; Tsagarakis, N.G.; Caldwell, D.G. Design of a Wearable Direct-Driven Optimized Hand Exoskeleton Device. In Proceedings of the International Conference on Advances in Computer-Human Interaction, Gosier, Guadeloupe, France, 23–28 February 2011.
138. Liu, A.; Qiu, J.; Wang, F.; Hou, L. An Adaptive and Jointless Hand Exoskeleton System Design. In Proceedings of the 15th International Conference on Control, Automation, Robotics and Vision (ICARCV), Singapore, 18–21 November 2018; pp. 579–584. [CrossRef]
139. Hong, M.B.; Kim, S.J.; Ihn, Y.S.; Jeong, G.C.; Kim, K. KULEX-Hand: An Underactuated Wearable Hand for Grasping Power Assistance. *IEEE Trans. Robot.* **2019**, *35*, 420–432. [CrossRef]
140. Iqbal, J.; Tsagarakis, N.G.; Caldwell, D.G. A human hand compatible optimised exoskeleton system. In Proceedings of the 2010 IEEE International Conference on Robotics and Biomimetics, Tianjin, China, 14–18 December 2010; pp. 685–690. [CrossRef]
141. Agarwal, P.; Fox, J.; Yun, Y.; O'Malley, M.K.; Deshpande, A.D. An Index Finger Exoskeleton with Series Elastic Actuation for Rehabilitation: Design, Control and Performance Characterization. *Int. J. Robot. Res.* **2015**, *34*, 1747–1772. [CrossRef]
142. Wang, F.; Shastri, M.; Jones, C.L.; Kamper, D.G.; Sarkar, N. Design and Control of an Actuated Thumb Exoskeleton for Hand Rehabilitation Following Stroke. In Proceedings of the IEEE International Conference on Robotics and Automation (ICRA), Shanghai, China, 9–13 May 2011; pp. 3688–3693. [CrossRef]
143. Wege, A.; Hommel, G. Development and Control of a Hand Exoskeleton for Rehabilitation of Hand Injuries. In Proceedings of the IEEE/RSJ International Conference on Intelligent Robots and Systems (IROS), Edmonton, AB, Canada, 2–6 August 2005; pp. 3046–3051. [CrossRef]
144. Carbone, G.; Gerding, E.C.; Corves, B.; Cafolla, D.; Russo, M.; Ceccarelli, M. Design of a Two-DOFs Driving Mechanism for a Motion-Assisted Finger Exoskeleton. *Appl. Sci.* **2020**, *10*, 2619. [CrossRef]
145. Erden, M.S.; McColl, W.; Abassebay, D.; Haldane, S. Hand Exoskeleton to Assess Hand Spasticity. In Proceedings of the 8th IEEE RAS/EMBS International Conference for Biomedical Robotics and Biomechatronics (BioRob), New York, NY, USA, 29 November–1 December 2020; pp. 1004–1009. [CrossRef]
146. Ou, Y.-K.; Wang, Y.-L.; Chang, H.-C.; Chen, C.-C. Design and Development of a Wearable Exoskeleton System for Stroke Rehabilitation. *Healthcare* **2020**, *8*, 18. [CrossRef] [PubMed]

147. Orlando, M.F.; Akolkar, H.; Dutta, A.; Saxena, A.; Behera, L. Optimal Design and Control of a Hand Exoskeleton. In Proceedings of the 2010 IEEE Conference on Robotics, Automation and Mechatronics (RAM), Singapore, 28–30 June 2010; pp. 72–77. [CrossRef]
148. Surakijboworn, M.; Wannasuphoprasit, W. Design of a Novel Finger Exoskeleton with a Sliding Six-Bar Joint Mechanism. In Proceedings of the 6th Augmented Human International Conference (AH'15), New York, NY, USA, 9 March 2015; pp. 77–80. [CrossRef]
149. Bortoletto, R.; Mello, A.N.; Piovesan, D. A Springs Actuated Finger Exoskeleton: From Mechanical Design to Spring Variables Evaluation. In Proceedings of the 2017 International Conference on Rehabilitation Robotics (ICORR), London, UK, 17 July 2017; pp. 1319–1325. [CrossRef]
150. Gabardi, M.; Solazzi, M.; Leonardis, D.; Frisoli, A. Design and Evaluation of a Novel 5 DoF Underactuated Thumb-Exoskeleton. *IEEE Robotics Autom. Lett.* **2018**, *3*, 2322–2329. [CrossRef]
151. Heo, P.; Kim, J. Power-Assistive Finger Exoskeleton With a Palmar Opening at the Fingerpad. *IEEE Trans. Biomed. Eng.* **2014**, *61*, 2688–2697. [CrossRef]
152. Yap, H.K.; Cho, J.; Yeow, R.C.-H. Design and Characterization of Soft Actuator for Hand Rehabilitation Application. *IFMBE Proc.* **2014**, *45*, 367–370. [CrossRef]
153. Zhang, J.; Wang, H.; Tang, J.; Guo, H.; Hong, J. Modeling and Design of a Soft Pneumatic Finger for Hand Rehabilitation. In Proceedings of the 2015 IEEE International Conference on Information and Automation (ICInfA), Lijiang, China, 8–10 August 2015; pp. 2460–2465. [CrossRef]
154. Wang, S.; Li, J.; Zheng, R. Active and Passive Control Algorithm for an Exoskeleton with Bowden Cable Transmission for Hand Rehabilitation. In Proceedings of the 2010 IEEE International Conference on Robotics and Biomimetics (ROBIO), Tianjin, China, 14–18 December 2010. [CrossRef]
155. Vithanage, I.; Wanasinghe, A.; Kavindya, P.; Kulasekera, A.; Chathuranga, D. A Novel Soft Glove for Hand Tremor Suppression: Evaluation of Layer Jamming Actuator Placement. In Proceedings of the 2020 IEEE International Conference on Soft Robotics (RoboSoft), New Haven, CT, USA, 15–19 May 2020; pp. 440–445. [CrossRef]
156. Gu, X.; Zhang, Y.; Sun, W.; Bian, Y.; Zhou, D.; Kristensson, P. Dexmo: An Inexpensive and Lightweight Mechanical Exoskeleton for Motion Capture and Force Feedback in VR. In Proceedings of the CHI Conference on Human Factors in Computing Systems (CHI), San Jose, CA, USA, 7–12 May 2016; pp. 1991–1995. [CrossRef]
157. Cortese, M.; Cempini, M.; Ribeiro, P.; Soekadar, S.; Carrozza, M.; Vitiello, N. A Mechatronic System for Robot-Mediated Hand Telerehabilitation. *IEEE ASME Trans. Mechatron.* **2015**, *20*, 1753–1764. [CrossRef]
158. Cempini, M.; Cortese, M.; Vitiello, N. A Powered Finger–Thumb Wearable Hand Exoskeleton With Self-Aligning Joint Axes. *IEEE ASME Trans. Mechatron.* **2015**, *20*, 705–716. [CrossRef]
159. Taheri, H.; Rowe, J.B.; Gardner, D.; Chan, V.; Gray, K.; Bower, C.; Reinkensmeyer, D.J.; Wolbrecht, E.T. Design and preliminary evaluation of the FINGER rehabilitation robot: Controlling challenge and quantifying finger individuation during musical computer game play. *J. Neuroeng. Rehabil.* **2014**, *11*, 10. [CrossRef]
160. Li, J.; Zheng, R.; Zhang, Y.; Yao, J. iHandRehab: An interactive hand exoskeleton for active and passive rehabilitation. In Proceedings of the 2011 IEEE International Conference on Rehabilitation Robotics (ICORR), Zurich, Switzerland, 29 June–1 July 2011; pp. 1–6. [CrossRef]
161. Hasegawa, Y.; Tokita, J.; Kamibayashi, K.; Sankai, Y. Evaluation of fingertip force accuracy in different support conditions of exoskeleton. In Proceedings of the 2011 IEEE International Conference on Robotics and Automation (ICRA), Shanghai, China, 9–13 May 2011; pp. 680–685. [CrossRef]
162. Moreira, P.; Machado, J.; Vaida, C.; Pisla, D.; Miranda, D.; Martins, N.; Carvalho, V.; Matos, D. Design of Wearable Prostheses: A New Approach. In *Advances in Service and Industrial Robotics*; Pisla, D., Carbone, G., Condurache, D., Vaida, C., Eds.; Springer: Cham, Switzerland, 2024; Volume 157. [CrossRef]
163. Jiralerspong, T.; Heung, H.; Tong, R.K.Y.; Li, Z. A Novel Soft Robotic Glove for Daily Life Assistance. In Proceedings of the IEEE International Conference on Biomedical Robotics and Biomechatronics (BioRob), Enschede, The Netherlands, 26–29 August 2018; pp. 671–676. [CrossRef]
164. Mckinney, Z.; Marconi, D.; Baldoni, A.; Cempini, M.; Crea, S.; Vitiello, N. A Novel Hand Exoskeleton with Series Elastic Actuation for Modulated Torque Transfer. *Mechatronics* **2019**, *61*, 69–82. [CrossRef]
165. Pratt, G.A.; Williamson, M.M. Series Elastic Actuators. In Proceedings of the IEEE/RSJ International Conference on Intelligent Robots and Systems (IROS), Pittsburgh, PA, USA, 5–9 August 1995; pp. 399–406. [CrossRef]
166. Iqbal, J.; Khan, H.; Tsagarakis, N.G.; Caldwell, D.G. A Novel Exoskeleton Robotic System for Hand Rehabilitation—Conceptualization to Prototyping. *Biocybern. Biomed. Eng.* **2014**, *34*, 79–89. [CrossRef]

167. Zhou, Y.; Desplenter, T.; Chinchalkar, S.; Trejos, A.L. A Wearable Mechatronic Glove for Resistive Hand Therapy Exercises. In Proceedings of the 2019 IEEE 16th International Conference on Rehabilitation Robotics (ICORR), Toronto, ON, Canada, 24–28 June 2019; pp. 1097–1102. [CrossRef]
168. Haarman, C.J.W.; Hekman, E.E.G.; Rietman, J.S.; Van Der Kooij, H. Mechanical Design and Feasibility of a Finger Exoskeleton to Support Finger Extension of Severely Affected Stroke Patients. *IEEE Trans. Neural Syst. Rehabil. Eng.* **2023**, *31*, 1268–1276. [CrossRef] [PubMed]
169. Zheng, R.; Li, J. Kinematics and Workspace Analysis of an Exoskeleton for Thumb and Index Finger Rehabilitation. In Proceedings of the 2010 IEEE International Conference on Robotics and Biomimetics (ROBIO), Tianjin, China, 14–18 December 2010; pp. 80–84. [CrossRef]
170. Iqbal, J.; Tsagarakis, N.; Fiorilla, A.; Caldwell, D. A Portable Rehabilitation Device for the Hand. In Proceedings of the 2010 Annual International Conference of the IEEE Engineering in Medicine and Biology Society (EMBC), Buenos Aires, Argentina, 31 August–4 September 2010; pp. 3694–3697. [CrossRef]
171. Tsai, Y.L.; Huang, J.J.; Pu, S.W.; Chen, H.P.; Hsu, S.C.; Chang, J.Y.; Pei, Y.C. Usability Assessment of a Cable-Driven Exoskeletal Robot for Hand Rehabilitation. *Front. Neurorobot.* **2019**, *13*, e00003. [CrossRef]
172. Kim, S.; Lee, J.; Park, W.; Bae, J. Quantitative evaluation of hand functions using a wearable hand exoskeleton system. In Proceedings of the 2017 IEEE International Conference on Rehabilitation Robotics (ICORR), London, UK, 17–20 July 2017; pp. 1488–1493. [CrossRef]
173. In, H.; Lee, D.; Cho, K.-J. Investigation of friction characteristics of a tendon-driven wearable robotic hand. In Proceedings of the ICCAS 2010, Gyeonggi-do, Republic of Korea, 27–30 October 2010; pp. 568–573. [CrossRef]
174. Xu, D.; Wu, Q.; Zhu, Y. Development of a soft cable-driven hand exoskeleton for assisted rehabilitation training. *Ind. Robot* **2021**, *48*, 189–198. [CrossRef]
175. In, H.; Cho, K.-J.; Kim, K.; Lee, B. Jointless structure and under-actuation mechanism for compact hand exoskeleton. In Proceedings of the 2011 IEEE International Conference on Rehabilitation Robotics, Zurich, Switzerland, 29 June–1 July 2011; pp. 1–6. [CrossRef]
176. Kang, B.B.; Lee, H.; In, H.; Jeong, U.; Chung, J.; Cho, K.-J. Development of a polymer-based tendon-driven wearable robotic hand. In Proceedings of the 2016 IEEE International Conference on Robotics and Automation (ICRA), Stockholm, Sweden, 16–21 May 2016; pp. 3750–3755. [CrossRef]
177. Radder, B.; Prange, G.; Kottink, A.; Holmberg, J.; Sletta, K.; Dijk, M.; Meyer, T.; Melendez-Calderon, A.; Buurke, J.; Rietman, J. Home Rehabilitation Supported by a Wearable Soft-Robotic Device for Improving Hand Function in Older Adults: A Pilot Randomized Controlled Trial. *PLoS ONE* **2019**, *14*, e0220544. [CrossRef] [PubMed]
178. Meng, Q.; Shen, Z.; Nie, Z.; Meng, Q.; Wu, Z.; Yu, H. Modeling and Evaluation of a Novel Hybrid-Driven Compliant Hand Exoskeleton Based on Human-Machine Coupling Model. *Appl. Sci.* **2021**, *11*, 10825. [CrossRef]
179. Osuagwu, B.; Timms, S.; Peachment, R.; Dowie, S.; Thrussell, H.; Cross, S.; Shirley, R.; Segura-Fragoso, A.; Taylor, J. Home-Based Rehabilitation Using a Soft Robotic Hand Glove Device Leads to Improvement in Hand Function in People with Chronic Spinal Cord Injury: A Pilot Study. *J. NeuroEng. Rehabil.* **2020**, *17*, 40. [CrossRef] [PubMed]
180. Martinez, L.; Olaloye, O.; Talarico, M.; Shah, S.; Arends, R.; BuSha, B. A Power-Assisted Exoskeleton Optimized for Pinching and Grasping Motions. In Proceedings of the 2010 IEEE 36th Annual Northeast Bioengineering Conference (NEBEC), New York, NY, USA, 26–28 March 2010. [CrossRef]
181. Sierotowicz, M.; Lotti, N.; Nell, L.; Missiroli, F.; Alicea, R.; Zhang, X.; Xiloyannis, M.; Rupp, R.; Papp, E.; Krzywinski, J.; et al. EMG-Driven Machine Learning Control of a Soft Glove for Grasping Assistance and Rehabilitation. *IEEE Robot. Autom. Lett.* **2022**, *7*, 1566–1573. [CrossRef]
182. Kang, B.; Choi, H.; Lee, H.; Cho, K.-J. Exo-Glove Poly II: A Polymer-Based Soft Wearable Robot for the Hand with a Tendon-Driven Actuation System. *Soft Robot.* **2018**, *6*, 214–227. [CrossRef]
183. Jeong, U.; In, H.-K.; Cho, K.-J. Implementation of Various Control Algorithms for Hand Rehabilitation Exercise Using Wearable Robotic Hand. *Intell. Serv. Robot.* **2013**, *6*, 181–189. [CrossRef]
184. Radder, B.; Prange, G.; Kottink, A.; Gaasbeek, L.; Holmberg, J.; Meyer, T.; Melendez-Calderon, A.; Ingvast, J.; Buurke, J.; Rietman, J. A Wearable Soft-Robotic Glove Enables Hand Support in ADL and Rehabilitation: A Feasibility Study on the Assistive Functionality. *J. Rehabil. Assist. Technol. Eng.* **2016**, *3*, 2055668316670553. [CrossRef] [PubMed]
185. Biggar, S.; Yao, W. Design and Evaluation of a Soft and Wearable Robotic Glove for Hand Rehabilitation. *IEEE Trans. Neural Syst. Rehabil. Eng.* **2016**, *24*, 1071–1080. [CrossRef] [PubMed]
186. Xiloyannis, M.; Cappello, L.; Khanh, D.B.; Yen, S.-C.; Masia, L. Modelling and Design of a Synergy-Based Actuator for a Tendon-Driven Soft Robotic Glove. In Proceedings of the 2016 6th IEEE International Conference on Biomedical Robotics and Biomechatronics (BioRob), Singapore, 26–29 June 2016; pp. 1213–1219. [CrossRef]

187. Bouzit, M.; Burdea, G.; Popescu, G.; Boian, R. The Rutgers Master II-new design force-feedback glove. *IEEE-ASME Trans. Mechatron.* **2002**, *7*, 256–263. [CrossRef]
188. Allotta, B.; Conti, R.; Governi, L.; Meli, E.; Ridolfi, A.; Volpe, Y. Development and experimental testing of a portable hand exoskeleton. In Proceedings of the 2015 IEEE/RSJ International Conference on Intelligent Robots and Systems (IROS), Hamburg, Germany, 28 September–2 October 2015; pp. 5339–5344. [CrossRef]
189. Popov, D.; Gaponov, I.; Ryu, J.H. Portable Exoskeleton Glove With Soft Structure for Hand Assistance in Activities of Daily Living. *IEEE/ASME Trans. Mechatron.* **2016**, *22*, 865–875. [CrossRef]
190. Lee, S.W.; Landers, K.A.; Park, H.S. Biomimetic hand exotendon device (BiomHED) for functional hand rehabilitation in stroke. In Proceedings of the 2013 IEEE 13th International Conference on Rehabilitation Robotics (ICORR), Seattle, WA, USA, 24–26 June 2013; pp. 1–4. [CrossRef]
191. Sun, Z.; Guo, Z.; Tang, W. Design of wearable hand rehabilitation glove with soft hoop-reinforced pneumatic actuator. *J. Cent. South Univ.* **2019**, *26*, 106–119. [CrossRef]
192. Setiawan, J.D.; Ariyanto, M.; Nugroho, S.; Munadi, M.; Ismail, R. A soft exoskeleton glove incorporating motor-tendon actuator for hand movements assistance. *IREACO* **2023**, *13*, 1. [CrossRef]
193. Chen, Y.; Yang, Z.; Wen, Y. A Soft Exoskeleton Glove for Hand Bilateral Training via Surface EMG. *Sensors* **2021**, *21*, 578. [CrossRef] [PubMed]
194. Birouaș, F.I.; Țarcă, R.C.; Dzitac, S.; Dzitac, I. Preliminary Results in Testing of a Novel Asymmetric Underactuated Robotic Hand Exoskeleton for Motor Impairment Rehabilitation. *Symmetry* **2020**, *12*, 1470. [CrossRef]
195. Park, S.; Li, J.Z.; Zhang, S.; Zhang, L.Q.; Ding, L.; Zhang, X.; Lan, Y.; Kamper, D.G. User-Driven Functional Movement Training With a Wearable Hand Robot After Stroke. *IEEE Trans. Neural Syst. Rehabil. Eng.* **2020**, *28*, 2265–2275. [CrossRef] [PubMed]
196. Götzelmann, T. A 3D Printable Hand Exoskeleton for the Haptic Exploration of Virtual 3D Scenes. In Proceedings of the 10th International Conference on PErvasive Technologies Related to Assistive Environments (PETRA), Island of Rhodes, Greece, 21–23 June 2017; pp. 63–66. [CrossRef]
197. Pu, S.W.; Tsai, S.Y.; Chang, J.Y. Design and Development of the Wearable Hand Exoskeleton System for Rehabilitation of Hand Impaired Patients. In Proceedings of the IEEE International Conference on Automation Science and Engineering (CASE), Taipei, Taiwan, 18–22 August 2014; pp. 996–1001. [CrossRef]
198. Polygerinos, P.; Lyne, S.; Wang, Z.; Nicolini, L.; Mosadegh, B.; Whitesides, G.; Walsh, C. Towards a Soft Pneumatic Glove for Hand Rehabilitation. In Proceedings of the IEEE/RSJ International Conference on Intelligent Robots and Systems (IROS), Tokyo, Japan, 3–7 November 2013; pp. 1512–1517. [CrossRef]
199. Bianchi, M.; Cempini, M.; Conti, R.; Meli, E.; Ridolfi, A.; Vitiello, N.; Allotta, B. Design of a Series Elastic Transmission for Hand Exoskeletons. *Mechatronics* **2018**, *51*, 8–18. [CrossRef]
200. Arora, A.; Malkin, R. HANDLINK: A Dexterous Robotic Hand Exoskeleton Controlled by Motor Imagery (MI). *J. Adv. Med. Med. Res.* **2022**, *34*, 427–436. [CrossRef]
201. Al-Fahaam, H.; Davis, S.; Nefti-Meziani, S.; Theodoridis, T. Novel Soft Bending Actuator-Based Power Augmentation Hand Exoskeleton Controlled by Human Intention. *Intell. Serv. Robot.* **2018**, *11*, 247–268. [CrossRef]
202. Wege, A.; Kondak, K.; Hommel, G. Force Control Strategy for a Hand Exoskeleton Based on Sliding Mode Position Control. In Proceedings of the 2006 IEEE/RSJ International Conference on Intelligent Robots and Systems (IROS), Beijing, China, 9–15 October 2006; pp. 4615–4620. [CrossRef]
203. Al-Fahaam, H. Power Assistive and Rehabilitation Wearable Robot Based on Pneumatic Soft Actuators. In Proceedings of the 2016 IEEE International Conference on Methods and Models in Automation and Robotics (MMAR), Miedzyzdroje, Poland, 29 August–1 September 2016. [CrossRef]
204. Liu, Z.; Zhao, L.; Yu, P.; Yang, T.; Li, N.; Yang, Y.; Liu, L. A Wearable Bionic Soft Exoskeleton Glove for Stroke Patients. In Proceedings of the 2018 IEEE International Conference on Cyber Technology in Automation, Control, and Intelligent Systems (CYBER), Tianjin, China, 19–23 July 2018; pp. 932–937. [CrossRef]
205. Conti, R.; Meli, E.; Ridolfi, A.; Bianchi, M.; Governi, L.; Volpe, Y.; Allotta, B. Kinematic Synthesis and Testing of a New Portable Hand Exoskeleton. *Meccanica* **2017**, *52*, 2873–2897. [CrossRef]
206. Jamil, B.; Choi, Y. Soft Pneumatic Glove for Grasping Power Improvement. In Proceedings of the 2017 International Conference on Ubiquitous Robots and Ambient Intelligence (URAI), Jeju, Republic of Korea, 28 June–1 July 2017. [CrossRef]
207. Tong, R.K.Y.; Ho, S.K.; Pang, P.; Hu, X.; Tam, W.K.; Fung, K.; Wei, X.J.; Chen, P.; Chen, M. An Intention Driven Hand Functions Task Training Robotic System. In Proceedings of the 32nd Annual International Conference of the IEEE Engineering in Medicine and Biology Society (EMBC), Buenos Aires, Argentina, 31 August–4 September 2010; pp. 3406–3409. [CrossRef]

208. Weiss, P.; Heyer, L.; Munte, T.F.; Heldmann, M.; Schweikard, A.; Maehle, E. Towards a parameterizable exoskeleton for training of hand function after stroke. In Proceedings of the 2013 IEEE International Conference on Rehabilitation Robotics (ICORR), Seattle, WA, USA, 24–26 June 2013; pp. 1–6. [CrossRef]
209. Roccella, S.; Cattin, E.; Vitiello, N.; Giovacchini, F.; Chiri, A.; Vecchi, F.; Carrozza, M.C. Design of a Hand Exoskeleton (Handexos) for the Rehabilitation of the Hand. *Gerontechnology* **2008**, *7*, 197. [CrossRef]
210. Leonardis, D.; Barsotti, M.; Loconsole, C.; Solazzi, M.; Troncossi, M.; Mazzotti, C.; Parenti Castelli, V.; Procopio, C.; Lamola, G.; Chisari, C.; et al. An EMG-Controlled Robotic Hand Exoskeleton for Bilateral Rehabilitation. *IEEE Trans. Haptics* **2015**, *8*, 140–151. [CrossRef]
211. Wang, D.; Meng, Q.; Meng, Q.; Li, X.; Yu, H. Design and Development of a Portable Exoskeleton for Hand Rehabilitation. *IEEE Trans. Neural Syst. Rehabil. Eng.* **2018**, *26*, 2376–2386. [CrossRef]
212. Secciani, N.; Brogi, C.; Pagliai, M.; Buonamici, F.; Gerli, F.; Vannetti, F.; Bianchini, M.; Volpe, Y.; Ridolfi, A. Wearable Robots: An Original Mechatronic Design of a Hand Exoskeleton for Assistive and Rehabilitative Purposes. *Front. Neurorobot.* **2021**, *15*, 750385. [CrossRef] [PubMed]
213. Borboni, A.; Mor, M.; Faglia, R. Gloreha—Hand Robotic Rehabilitation: Design, Mechanical Model, and Experiments. *J. Dyn. Syst. Meas. Control* **2016**, *138*, 111003. [CrossRef]
214. Fischer, H.C.; Triandafilou, K.M.; Thielbar, K.O.; Ochoa, J.M.; Lazzaro, E.D.C.; Pacholski, K.A.; Kamper, D.G. Use of a Portable Assistive Glove to Facilitate Rehabilitation in Stroke Survivors With Severe Hand Impairment. *IEEE Trans. Neural Syst. Rehabil. Eng.* **2016**, *24*, 344–351. [CrossRef]
215. du Plessis, T.; Djouani, K.; Oosthuizen, C. A Review of Active Hand Exoskeletons for Rehabilitation and Assistance. *Robotics* **2021**, *10*, 40. [CrossRef]
216. Chu, C.Y.; Patterson, R.M. Soft Robotic Devices for Hand Rehabilitation and Assistance: A Narrative Review. *J. Neuroeng. Rehabil.* **2018**, *15*, 9. [CrossRef]
217. Wang, X.; Cheng, Y.; Zheng, H.; Li, Y.; Wang, C. Design and Optimization of Actuator for Multi-Joint Soft Rehabilitation Glove. *Ind. Robot* **2021**, *48*, 877–890. [CrossRef]
218. Lim, D.Y.L.; Lai, H.S.; Yeow, R.C.H. A Bidirectional Fabric-Based Soft Robotic Glove for Hand Function Assistance in Patients with Chronic Stroke. *J. Neuroeng. Rehabil.* **2023**, *20*, 120. [CrossRef]
219. Souhail, A.; Vessakosol, P. Low Cost Soft Robotic Gloves for At-Home Rehabilitation and Daily Living Activities. *J. Autom. Mobile Robot. Intell. Syst.* **2019**, *13*, 14–26. [CrossRef]
220. Jiang, Y.; Chen, D.; Que, J.; Liu, Z.; Wang, Z.; Xu, Y. Soft Robotic Glove for Hand Rehabilitation Based on a Novel Fabrication Method. In Proceedings of the IEEE International Conference on Robotics and Biomimetics (ROBIO), Macau, China, 5–8 December 2017; pp. 817–822. [CrossRef]
221. Wang, J.; Fei, Y.; Pang, W. Design, Modeling, and Testing of a Soft Pneumatic Glove With Segmented PneuNets Bending Actuators. *IEEE ASME Trans. Mechatron.* **2019**, *24*, 990–1001. [CrossRef]
222. Radder, B.; Prange, G.; Kottink, A.; Melendez-Calderon, A.; Buurke, J.; Rietman, J. Feasibility of a Wearable Soft-Robotic Glove to Support Impaired Hand Function in Stroke Patients. *J. Rehabil. Med.* **2018**, *50*, 598–606. [CrossRef]
223. Burns, M.; Vinjamuri, R. Design of a Soft Glove-Based Robotic Hand Exoskeleton with Embedded Synergies. In *Advances in Motor Neuroprostheses*; Vinjamuri, R., Ed.; Springer: Cham, Switzerland, 2020; pp. 71–87. [CrossRef]
224. Yun, S.-S.; Kang, B.; Cho, K.-J. Exo-Glove PM: An Easily Customizable Modularized Pneumatic Assistive Glove. *IEEE Robot. Autom. Lett.* **2017**, *2*, 1725–1732. [CrossRef]
225. Guo, Y.; Xu, F.; Song, Y.; Cao, X.; Meng, F. A Soft Robotic Glove for Hand Rehabilitation Using Pneumatic Actuators with Variable Stiffness. In Proceedings of the 2019 International Conference on Intelligent Robotics and Applications (ICIRA), Shenyang, China, 2 August 2019; pp. 119–129. [CrossRef]
226. Zhou, Y.M.; Wagner, D.; Nuckols, R.; Heimgartner, R.; Correia, C.; Clarke, M.; Orzel, D.; O'Neill, C.; Solinsky, R.; Paganoni, S.; et al. Soft Robotic Glove with Integrated Sensing for Intuitive Grasping Assistance Post Spinal Cord Injury. In Proceedings of the 2019 IEEE International Conference on Robotics and Automation (ICRA), Montreal, QC, Canada, 20–24 May 2019; pp. 9059–9065. [CrossRef]
227. Pu, S.-W.; Chang, J.-Y. Robotic Hand System Design for Mirror Therapy Rehabilitation After Stroke. *Microsyst. Technol.* **2020**, *26*, 111–119. [CrossRef]
228. Bernocchi, P.; Mulè, C.; Vanoglio, F.; Taveggia, G.; Luisa, A.; Scalvini, S. Home-Based Hand Rehabilitation with a Robotic Glove in Hemiplegic Patients After Stroke: A Pilot Feasibility Study. *Top. Stroke Rehabil.* **2017**, *25*, 114–119. [CrossRef]
229. Seçkin, M.; Yaman Turan, N. Rehabilitation Glove Device Design. *J. Eng. Technol. Appl. Sci.* **2018**, *3*, 75–81. [CrossRef]

230. Gandolla, M.; Ferrante, S.; Baldassini, D.; Cottini, M.; Seneci, C.; Molteni, F.; Guanziroli, E.; Pedrocchi, A. EMG-Controlled Robotic Hand Rehabilitation Device for Domestic Training. In Proceedings of the XIV Mediterranean Conference on Medical and Biological Engineering and Computing, Paphos, Cyprus, 31 March–2 April 2016; pp. 644–648. [CrossRef]
231. Ben-Tzvi, P.; Danoff, J.; Ma, Z. The Design Evolution of a Sensing and Force-Feedback Exoskeleton Robotic Glove for Hand Rehabilitation Application. *J. Mech. Robot.* **2016**, *8*, 051019. [CrossRef]
232. Randazzo, L.; Iturrate, I.; Perdikis, S.; Millán, J.R. mano: A Wearable Hand Exoskeleton for Activities of Daily Living and Neurorehabilitation. *IEEE Robot. Autom. Lett.* **2018**, *3*, 500–507. [CrossRef]
233. Jo, I.; Lee, J.; Park, Y.; Bae, J. Design of a wearable hand exoskeleton for exercising flexion/extension of the fingers. In Proceedings of the 2017 IEEE International Conference on Rehabilitation Robotics (ICORR), London, UK, 17–20 July 2017; pp. 1615–1620. [CrossRef]
234. Hasegawa, Y.; Mikami, Y.; Watanabe, K.; Sankai, Y. Five-fingered assistive hand with mechanical compliance of human finger. In Proceedings of the 2008 IEEE International Conference on Robotics and Automation (ICRA), Pasadena, CA, USA, 19–23 May 2008; pp. 718–724. [CrossRef]
235. Mulas, M.; Folgheraiter, M.; Gini, G. An EMG-controlled exoskeleton for hand rehabilitation. In Proceedings of the 9th International Conference on Rehabilitation Robotics (ICORR), Chicago, IL, USA, 28 June–1 July 2005; pp. 371–374. [CrossRef]
236. Brokaw, E.B.; Black, I.; Holley, R.J.; Lum, P.S. Hand Spring Operated Movement Enhancer (HandSOME): A portable, passive hand exoskeleton for stroke rehabilitation. *IEEE Trans. Neural Syst. Rehabil. Eng.* **2011**, *19*, 391–399. [CrossRef]
237. Gasser, B.W.; Bennett, D.A.; Durrough, C.M.; Goldfarb, M. Design and preliminary assessment of Vanderbilt hand exoskeleton. In Proceedings of the 2017 IEEE International Conference on Rehabilitation Robotics (ICORR), London, UK, 17–20 July 2017; pp. 1537–1542. [CrossRef]
238. Li, H.; Cheng, L. Preliminary study on the design and control of a pneumatically-actuated hand rehabilitation device. In Proceedings of the IEEE Youth Academic Annual Conference (YAC), Hefei, China, 19–21 May 2017; pp. 860–865. [CrossRef]
239. Refour, E.M.; Sebastian, B.; Chauhan, R.J.; Ben-Tzvi, P. A General Purpose Robotic Hand Exoskeleton With Series Elastic Actuation. *J. Mech. Robot.* **2019**, *11*, 060902. [CrossRef]
240. Lee, S.W.; Landers, K.A.; Park, H.-S. Development of a biomimetic hand exotendon device (BiomHED) for restoration of functional hand movement post-stroke. *IEEE Trans. Neural Syst. Rehabil. Eng.* **2014**, *22*, 886–898. [CrossRef] [PubMed]
241. Coffey, A.; Leamy, D.; Ward, T. A Novel BCI-Controlled Pneumatic Glove System for Home-Based Neurorehabilitation. In Proceedings of the 2014 36th Annual International Conference of the IEEE Engineering in Medicine and Biology Society (EMBC), Chicago, IL, USA, 26–30 August 2014. [CrossRef]
242. Yang, J.; Xie, H.-L.; Shi, J. A Novel Motion-Coupling Design for a Jointless Tendon-Driven Finger Exoskeleton for Rehabilitation. *Mech. Mach. Theory* **2016**, *99*, 83–102. [CrossRef]
243. Kline, T.; Kamper, D.; Schmit, B. Control System for Pneumatically Controlled Glove to Assist in Grasp Activities. In Proceedings of the 2005 IEEE 9th International Conference on Rehabilitation Robotics (ICORR), Chicago, IL, USA, 28 June–1 July 2005; pp. 78–81. [CrossRef]
244. Ochoa, J.; Narasimhan, Y.; Kamper, D. Development of a Portable Actuated Orthotic Glove to Facilitate Gross Extension of the Digits for Therapeutic Training after Stroke. In Proceedings of the 2009 Annual International Conference of the IEEE Engineering in Medicine and Biology Society (EMBC), Minneapolis, MN, USA, 3–6 September 2009; pp. 6918–6921. [CrossRef]
245. Foumashi, M.; Troncossi, M.; Parenti Castelli, V. Design of a New Hand Exoskeleton for Rehabilitation of Post-Stroke Patients. In Proceedings of the Romansy 19-Robot Design, Dynamics and Control, Udine, Italy, 2013; pp. 159–166. [CrossRef]
246. Luo, X.; Kline, T.; Fischer, H.; Stubblefield, K.; Kenyon, R.; Kamper, D. Integration of Augmented Reality and Assistive Devices for Post-Stroke Hand Opening Rehabilitation. In Proceedings of the 2005 Annual International Conference of the IEEE Engineering in Medicine and Biology Society (EMBC), Shanghai, China, 1–4 September 2005; pp. 6855–6858. [CrossRef]
247. Troncossi, M.; Mozaffari, M.; Mazzotti, C.; Zannoli, D.; Parenti Castelli, V. Design and Manufacturing of a Hand-and-Wrist Exoskeleton Prototype for the Rehabilitation of Post-Stroke Patients. In *Quaderni del DIEM–GMA. Atti della Sesta Giornata di Studio Ettore Funaioli*; Asterisco: Rome, Italy, 2012.
248. Gerez, L.; Dwivedi, A.; Liarokapis, M. A hybrid, soft exoskeleton glove equipped with a telescopic extra thumb and abduction capabilities. In Proceedings of the 2020 IEEE International Conference on Robotics and Automation (ICRA), Paris, France, 31 May–31 August 2020; pp. 9100–9106. [CrossRef]
249. Cappello, L.; Meyer, J.T.; Galloway, K.C.; Peisner, A.; Granberry, R.; Wagner, D.A.; Walsh, C.J. Assisting Hand Function After Spinal Cord Injury with a Fabric-Based Soft Robotic Glove. *J. Neuroeng. Rehabil.* **2018**, *15*, 59. [CrossRef]
250. Chang, P.H.; Lee, S.H.; Gu, G.M.; Lee, S.H.; Jin, S.H.; Yeo, S.S.; Seo, J.P.; Jang, S.H. The cortical activation pattern by a rehabilitation robotic hand: A functional NIRS study. *Front. Hum. Neurosci.* **2014**, *8*, 49. [CrossRef] [PubMed]

251. Wege, A.; Zimmermann, A. Electromyography Sensor-Based Control for a Hand Exoskeleton. In Proceedings of the IEEE International Conference on Robotics and Biomimetics, Sanya, China, 15–18 December 2007; pp. 1470–1475. [CrossRef]
252. Ge, L.; Chen, F.; Wang, D.; Zhang, Y.; Han, D.; Wang, T.; Gu, G. Design, Modeling, and Evaluation of Fabric-Based Pneumatic Actuators for Soft Wearable Assistive Gloves. *Soft Robot.* **2020**, *7*, 583–596. [CrossRef]
253. Jo, I.; Bae, J. A Force-Controllable Compact Actuator Module for a Wearable Hand Exoskeleton. *IFAC Proc. Vol.* **2014**, *47*, 4453–4458. [CrossRef]
254. Delph, M.A.; Fischer, S.A.; Gauthier, P.W.; Luna, C.H.M.; Clancy, E.A.; Fischer, G.S. A soft robotic exomusculature glove with integrated sEMG sensing for hand rehabilitation. In Proceedings of the 2013 IEEE 13th International Conference on Rehabilitation Robotics (ICORR), Seattle, WA, USA, 24–26 June 2013; pp. 1–7. [CrossRef]
255. Cheng, L.; Chen, M.; Li, Z. Design and Control of a Wearable Hand Rehabilitation Robot. *IEEE Access* **2018**, *6*, 41884–41896. [CrossRef]
256. Chiri, A.; Vitiello, N.; Giovacchini, F.; Roccella, S.; Vecchi, F.; Carrozza, M.C. Mechatronic Design and Characterization of the Index Finger Module of a Hand Exoskeleton for Post-Stroke Rehabilitation. *IEEE/ASME Trans. Mechatron.* **2012**, *17*, 884–894. [CrossRef]
257. Chua, M.; Lim, J.; Yeow, R.C.-H. Design and Characterization of a Soft Robotic Therapeutic Glove for Rheumatoid Arthritis. *Assist. Technol.* **2017**, *31*, 44–52. [CrossRef] [PubMed]
258. Trott, R.; Kleinig, T.; Hillier, S.; Hobbs, D.; Reynolds, K. A Modular Hybrid Exoskeletal-Soft Glove for High Degree of Freedom Monitoring Capability. In Proceedings of the 2019 IEEE International Conference on Rehabilitation Robotics (ICORR), Toronto, ON, Canada, 24–28 June 2019; pp. 577–582. [CrossRef]
259. Lee, J.; Bae, J. Design of a hand exoskeleton for biomechanical analysis of the stroke hand. In Proceedings of the 2015 IEEE International Conference on Rehabilitation Robotics (ICORR), Singapore, 11–14 August 2015; pp. 484–489. [CrossRef]
260. Cui, L.; Phan, A.; Allison, G. Design and fabrication of a three dimensional printable non-assembly articulated hand exoskeleton for rehabilitation. In Proceedings of the 37th Annual International Conference of the IEEE Engineering in Medicine and Biology Society (EMBC), Milan, Italy, 25–29 August 2015; pp. 4627–4630. [CrossRef]
261. Ferguson, P.W.; Dimapasoc, B.; Shen, Y.; Rosen, J. Design of a Hand Exoskeleton for Use with Upper Limb Exoskeletons. In *Wearable Robotics: Challenges and Trends*; Carrozza, M., Micera, S., Pons, J., Eds.; Biosystems & Biorobotics; Springer: Cham, Switzerland, 2019; Volume 22. [CrossRef]
262. Maeder-York, P.; Clites, T.; Boggs, E.; Neff, R.; Polygerinos, P.; Holland, D.; Stirling, L.; Galloway, K.; Wee, C.; Walsh, C. Biologically Inspired Soft Robot for Thumb Rehabilitation. *J. Med. Devices* **2014**, *8*, 020933. [CrossRef]
263. Fiorilla, A.E.; Tsagarakis, N.G.; Nori, F.; Sandini, G. Design of a 2-finger hand exoskeleton for finger stiffness measurements. *Appl. Bion. Biomech.* **2009**, *6*, 217–228. [CrossRef]
264. Decker, M.; Kim, Y. A hand exoskeleton device for robot assisted sensory-motor training after stroke. In Proceedings of the 2017 IEEE World Haptics Conference (WHC), Munich, Germany, 6–9 June 2017; pp. 436–441. [CrossRef]
265. Polygerinos, P.; Wang, Z.; Galloway, K.C.; Wood, R.J.; Walsh, C.J. Soft Robotic Glove for Combined Assistance and at-Home Rehabilitation. *Robot. Auton. Syst.* **2015**, *73*, 135–143. [CrossRef]
266. Kobayashi, F.; Ikai, G.; Fukui, W.; Nakamoto, H.; Kojima, F. Multipoint haptic device for robot hand teleoperation. In Proceedings of the 2012 International Symposium on Micro-NanoMechatronics and Human Science (MHS), Nagoya, Japan, 4–7 November 2012; pp. 304–309. [CrossRef]
267. Fujimoto, K.; Kobayashi, F.; Nakamoto, H.; Kojima, F. Development of haptic device for five-fingered robot hand teleoperation. In Proceedings of the 2013 IEEE/SICE International Symposium on System Integration (SII), Kobe, Japan, 15–17 December 2013; pp. 820–825. [CrossRef]
268. Triolo, E.; BuSha, B. Design and Experimental Testing of a Force-Augmenting Exoskeleton for the Human Hand. *J. NeuroEngineering Rehabil.* **2022**, *19*, 23. [CrossRef] [PubMed]
269. Hu, X.L.; Tong, K.Y.; Wei, X.J.; Rong, W.; Susanto, E.A.; Ho, S.K. The effects of post-stroke upper-limb training with an electromyography (EMG)-driven hand robot. *J. Electromyogr. Kinesiol.* **2013**, *23*, 1065–1074. [CrossRef] [PubMed]
270. Rojek, I.; Kaczmarek, M.; Kotlarz, P.; Kempiński, M.; Mikołajewski, D.; Szczepański, Z.; Kopowski, J.; Nowak, J.; Macko, M.; Szczepańczyk, A.; et al. Hand Exoskeleton—Development of Own Concept. *Appl. Sci.* **2023**, *13*, 3238. [CrossRef]
271. Jackson, G.; Abdullah, H.A. Development and Testing of a Soft Exoskeleton Robotic Hand Training Device. *Sensors* **2023**, *23*, 8395. [CrossRef]
272. Takahashi, N.; Furuya, S.; Koike, H. Soft Exoskeleton Glove with Human Anatomical Architecture: Production of Dexterous Finger Movements and Skillful Piano Performance. *IEEE Trans. Haptics* **2020**, *13*, 679–690. [CrossRef]

273. Ho, S.K.; Tong, R.K.Y.; Hu, X.; Fung, K.; Wei, X.J.; Rong, W.; Susanto, E. An EMG-driven Exoskeleton Hand Robotic Training Device on Chronic Stroke Subjects: Task Training System for Stroke Rehabilitation. In Proceedings of the IEEE International Conference on Rehabilitation Robotics (ICORR), Zurich, Switzerland, 29 June–1 July 2011; pp. 1–5. [CrossRef]
274. Bertani, R.; Melegari, C.; De Cola, M.C.; Bramanti, P.; Bramanti, A.; Calvo, A. Effects of Robot-Assisted Upper Limb Rehabilitation in Stroke Patients: A Systematic Review with Meta-Analysis. *Neurol. Sci.* **2017**, *38*, 1561–1569. [CrossRef]
275. Zhang, F.; Hua, L.; Fu, Y.; Chen, H.; Wang, S. Design and Development of a Hand Exoskeleton for Rehabilitation of Hand Injuries. *Mech. Mach. Theory* **2014**, *73*, 103–116. [CrossRef]
276. Nazari, V.; Pouladian, M.; Zheng, Y.-P.; Alam, M. A Compact and Lightweight Rehabilitative Exoskeleton to Restore Grasping Functions for People with Hand Paralysis. *Sensors* **2021**, *21*, 6900. [CrossRef]
277. Fu, Y.; Zhang, Q.; Zhang, F.; Gan, Z. Design and Development of a Hand Rehabilitation Robot for Patient-Cooperative Therapy Following Stroke. In Proceedings of the IEEE International Conference on Mechatronics and Automation (ICMA), Beijing, China, 7–10 August 2011; pp. 112–117. [CrossRef]
278. Ma, Z.; Ben-Tzvi, P.; Danoff, J. Hand Rehabilitation Learning System with an Exoskeleton Robotic Glove. *IEEE Trans. Neural Syst. Rehabil. Eng.* **2016**, *24*, 1323–1332. [CrossRef]
279. Sandoval-Gonzalez, O.; Jacinto-Villegas, J.; Herrera-Aguilar, I.; Portilla-Flores, E.A.; Tripicchio, P.; Hernandez-Ramos, M.; Flores-Cuautle, A.; Avila-Vilchis, J.C. Design and Development of a Hand Exoskeleton Robot for Active and Passive Rehabilitation. *Int. J. Adv. Robot. Syst.* **2016**, *13*, 66. [CrossRef]
280. Triwiyanto, T.; Luthfiyah, S.; Pawana, P.; Ahmed, A.A.; Andrian, A. Bilateral Mode Exoskeleton for Hand Rehabilitation with Wireless Control Using 3D Printing Technology Based on IMU Sensor. *HardwareX* **2023**, *14*, e00432. [CrossRef]
281. Abdallah, I.B.; Bouteraa, Y.; Rekik, C. Design and Development of 3D Printed Myoelectric Robotic Exoskeleton for Hand Rehabilitation. *Int. J. Smart Sens. Intell. Syst.* **2017**, *10*, 1–26. [CrossRef]
282. Ceccarelli, M.; Morales-Cruz, C. A Prototype Characterization of ExoFinger, a Finger Exoskeleton. *Int. J. Adv. Robot. Syst.* **2021**, *18*, 172988142110248. [CrossRef]
283. Conti, R.; Meli, E.; Ridolfi, A. A Novel Kinematic Architecture for Portable Hand Exoskeletons. *Mechatronics* **2016**, *35*, 192–207. [CrossRef]
284. Jones, C.L.; Wang, F.; Morrison, R.; Sarkar, N.; Kamper, D.G. Design and Development of the Cable Actuated Finger Exoskeleton for Hand Rehabilitation Following Stroke. *IEEE/ASME Trans. Mechatron.* **2014**, *19*, 131–140. [CrossRef]
285. Ahmed, T.; Assad-Uz-Zaman, M.; Islam, M.R.; Gottheardt, D.; McGonigle, E.; Brahmi, B.; Rahman, M.H. Flexohand: A Hybrid Exoskeleton-Based Novel Hand Rehabilitation Device. *Micromachines* **2021**, *12*, 1274. [CrossRef] [PubMed]
286. Richards, D.; Georgilas, I.; Dagnino, G.; Dogramadzi, S. Powered Exoskeleton with Palm Degrees of Freedom for Hand Rehabilitation. In Proceedings of the 2015 37th Annual International Conference of the IEEE Engineering in Medicine and Biology Society (EMBC), Milan, Italy, 25–29 August 2015. [CrossRef]
287. Wahit, M.A.A.; Ahmad, S.A. Design and Development of Low-Cost Exoskeleton Hand Robot Structure. In Proceedings of the IEEE 15th Student Conference on Research and Development (SCOReD), Putrajaya, Malaysia, 13–14 December 2017; pp. 45–49. [CrossRef]
288. Haghshenas-Jaryani, M.; Nothnagle, C.; Patterson, R.M.; Bugnariu, N.; Wijesundara, M.B.J. Soft Robotic Rehabilitation Exoskeleton (REHAB Glove) for Hand Therapy. In Proceedings of the ASME International Design Engineering Technical Conferences and Computers and Information in Engineering Conference (IDETC-CIE), Cleveland, OH, USA, 6–9 August 2017. Paper No. DETC2017-68291. [CrossRef]
289. Jumphoo, T.; Uthansakul, M.; Duangmanee, P.; Khan, N.; Uthansakul, P. Soft Robotic Glove Controlling Using Brainwave Detection for Continuous Rehabilitation at Home. *Comput. Mater. Contin.* **2021**, *66*, 961–976. [CrossRef]
290. Gerges, F.; Desai, J.; Watkins, J.M.; Burugupally, S.P. Master-Slave Control for a Pneumatically Actuated Low Pressure Soft Robotic Glove to Facilitate Bilateral Training for Stroke Patients. In Proceedings of the 23rd International Symposium on Measurement and Control in Robotics (ISMCR), Budapest, Hungary, 22–24 October 2020; pp. 1–6. [CrossRef]
291. Hu, D.; Zhang, J.; Yang, Y.; Li, Q.; Li, D.; Hong, J. A Novel Soft Robotic Glove with Positive-Negative Pneumatic Actuator for Hand Rehabilitation. In Proceedings of the IEEE/ASME International Conference on Advanced Intelligent Mechatronics (AIM), Boston, MA, USA, 6–9 July 2020; pp. 1840–1847. [CrossRef]
292. Guo, N.; Sun, Z.; Wang, X.; Yeung, E.; To, M.; Li, X.; Hu, Y. Simulation Analysis for Optimal Design of Pneumatic Bellow Actuators for Soft-Robotic Glove. *Biocybern. Biomed. Eng.* **2020**, *40*, 1507–1516. [CrossRef]
293. Feng, M.; Yang, D.; Gu, G. High-Force Fabric-Based Pneumatic Actuators with Asymmetric Chambers and Interference-Reinforced Structure for Soft Wearable Assistive Gloves. *IEEE Robot. Autom. Lett.* **2021**, *6*, 3105–3111. [CrossRef]
294. Noritsugu, T.; Takaiwa, M.; Sasaki, D. Development of Power Assist Wear Using Pneumatic Rubber Artificial Muscles. *J. Robot. Mechatron.* **2009**, *21*, 607–613. [CrossRef]

295. Tjahyono, A.P.; Aw, K.C.; Devaraj, H.; Surendra, W.; Haemmerle, E.; Travas-Sejdic, J. A Five-Fingered Hand Exoskeleton Driven by Pneumatic Artificial Muscles with Novel Polypyrrole Sensors. *Ind. Robot* **2013**, *40*, 251–260. [CrossRef]
296. Hadi, A.; Alipour, K.; Kazeminasab, S.; Elahinia, M. ASR Glove: A Wearable Glove for Hand Assistance and Rehabilitation Using Shape Memory Alloys. *J. Intell. Mater. Syst. Struct.* **2018**, *29*, 1575–1585. [CrossRef]
297. Tang, T.; Zhang, D.; Tao, X.; Zhu, X. An Exoskeleton System for Hand Rehabilitation Driven by Shape Memory Alloy. In Proceedings of the IEEE International Conference on Robotics and Biomimetics (ROBIO), Shenzhen, China, 12–14 December 2013; pp. 756–761. [CrossRef]
298. Whitney, J.P.; Glisson, M.F.; Brockmeyer, E.L.; Hodgins, J.K. A Low-Friction Passive Fluid Transmission and Fluid-Tendon Soft Actuator. In Proceedings of the IEEE/RSJ International Conference on Intelligent Robots and Systems (IROS), Chicago, IL, USA, 14–18 September 2014; pp. 2801–2808. [CrossRef]
299. Rahman, A.; Al-Jumaily, A. Design and Development of a Bilateral Therapeutic Hand Device for Stroke Rehabilitation. *Int. J. Adv. Robot. Syst.* **2013**, *10*, 405. [CrossRef]
300. Chen, T.; Lum, P.S. Hand Rehabilitation After Stroke Using a Wearable, High DOF, Spring Powered Exoskeleton. In Proceedings of the 2016 38th Annual International Conference of the IEEE Engineering in Medicine and Biology Society (EMBC), Orlando, FL, USA, 16–20 August 2016; pp. 578–581. [CrossRef]
301. Casas, R.; Sandison, M.; Chen, T.; Lum, P.S. Clinical Test of a Wearable, High DOF, Spring Powered Hand Exoskeleton (HandSOME II). *IEEE Trans. Neural Syst. Rehabil. Eng.* **2021**, *29*, 1877–1885. [CrossRef] [PubMed]
302. Yap, H.K.; Ang, B.W.K.; Lim, J.H.; Goh, J.C.H.; Yeow, C.-H. A Fabric-Regulated Soft Robotic Glove with User Intent Detection Using EMG and RFID for Hand Assistive Application. In Proceedings of the 2016 IEEE International Conference on Robotics and Automation (ICRA), Stockholm, Sweden, 16–21 May 2016; pp. 3537–3542. [CrossRef]
303. Sun, B.; Xiong, C.; Huang, Y.; Chen, W.; Chen, W. Design of a Compact Finger-Integrated Mechanism with Robust Kinematics for Hand Exoskeleton. In *Intelligent Robotics and Applications*; Liu, H., Kubota, N., Zhu, X., Dillmann, R., Eds.; Lecture Notes in Computer Science; Springer: Cham, Switzerland, 2015; Volume 9246, pp. 211–219. [CrossRef]
304. Pu, S.-W.; Chang, J.-Y.; Pei, Y.-C.; Kuo, C.-C.; Wang, M.-J. Anthropometry-Based Structural Design of a Hand Exoskeleton for Rehabilitation. In Proceedings of the 2016 23rd International Conference on Mechatronics and Machine Vision in Practice (M2VIP), Nanjing, China, 28–30 November 2016; pp. 1–6. [CrossRef]
305. Festo. "ExoHand Festo". 2022. Available online: https://www.festo.com/PDF_Flip/corp/Festo_ExoHand/en/index.html (accessed on 12 November 2024).
306. Ueki, S.; Kawasaki, H.; Ito, S.; Nishimoto, Y.; Abe, M.; Aoki, T.; Ishigure, Y.; Ojika, T.; Mouri, T. Development of a Hand-Assist Robot With Multi-Degrees-of-Freedom for Rehabilitation Therapy. *IEEE/ASME Trans. Mechatron.* **2012**, *17*, 136–146. [CrossRef]
307. Schabowsky, C.; Godfrey, S.; Holley, R.; Lum, P. Development and pilot testing of HEXORR: Hand EXOskeleton Rehabilitation Robot. *J. Neuroeng. Rehabil.* **2010**, *7*, 36. [CrossRef] [PubMed]
308. Zhang, F.; Legeng, L.; Yang, L.; Fu, Y. Design of an Active and Passive Control System of Hand Exoskeleton for Rehabilitation. *Appl. Sci.* **2019**, *9*, 2291. [CrossRef]
309. Kuswanto, D.; Iskandriawan, B.; Mahardhika, P. Power Grip Exoskeleton Design as Rehabilitation Devices for Post-Stroke Survivors. In Proceedings of the 2018 IEEE International Conference on Biomedical Robotics and Biomechatronics (BIOMIC), Bali, Indonesia, 26–29 August 2018; pp. 1–6. [CrossRef]
310. Dragusanu, M.; Iqbal, M.Z.; Lisini, T.; Prattichizzo, D.; Malvezzi, M. Design, Development, and Control of a Hand/Wrist Exoskeleton for Rehabilitation and Training. *IEEE Trans. Robot.* **2022**, *38*, 1472–1488. [CrossRef]
311. De la Cruz Sánchez, B.; Arias-Montiel, M.; Lugo, E. EMG-Controlled Hand Exoskeleton for Assisted Bilateral Rehabilitation. *Biocybern. Biomed. Eng.* **2022**, *42*, 596–614. [CrossRef]
312. Yap, H.K.; Kamaldin, N.; Lim, J.; Nasrallah, F.; Cho, J.; Yeow, R.C.-H. A Magnetic Resonance Compatible Soft Wearable Robotic Glove for Hand Rehabilitation and Brain Imaging. *IEEE Trans. Neural Syst. Rehabil. Eng.* **2016**, *25*, 782–793. [CrossRef]
313. Heung, H.; Tong, R.K.-Y.; Lau, A.; Li, Z. Robotic Glove with Soft-Elastic Composite Actuators for Assisting Activities of Daily Living. *Soft Robot.* **2019**, *6*, 289–304. [CrossRef]
314. Ang, B.; Yeow, R.C.-H. Print-it-Yourself (PIY) Glove: A Fully 3D Printed Soft Robotic Hand Rehabilitative and Assistive Exoskeleton for Stroke Patients. In Proceedings of the 2017 IEEE/RSJ International Conference on Intelligent Robots and Systems (IROS), Vancouver, BC, Canada, 24–28 September 2017; pp. 1219–1223. [CrossRef]
315. Haghshenas-Jaryani, M.; Carrigan, W.; Nothnagle, C.; Wijesundara, M. Sensorized Soft Robotic Glove for Continuous Passive Motion Therapy. In Proceedings of the 2016 IEEE International Conference on Biomedical Robotics and Biomechatronics (BIOROB), Singapore, 26–29 June 2016; pp. 815–820. [CrossRef]

316. Yap, H.K.; Lim, J.; Nasrallah, F.; Low, F.-Z.; Cho, J.; Yeow, R.C.-H. MRC-Glove: A fMRI Compatible Soft Robotic Glove for Hand Rehabilitation Application. In Proceedings of the 2015 IEEE International Conference on Rehabilitation Robotics (ICORR), Singapore, 11–14 August 2015; pp. 735–740. [CrossRef]
317. Serpelloni, M.; Tiboni, M.; Lancini, M.; Pasinetti, S.; Vertuan, A.; Gobbo, M. Preliminary Study of a Robotic Rehabilitation System Driven by EMG for Hand Mirroring. In Proceedings of the 2016 IEEE International Symposium on Medical Measurements and Applications (MeMeA), Benevento, Italy, 15–18 May 2016; pp. 1–6. [CrossRef]
318. Sasaki, D.; Noritsugu, T.; Takaiwa, M.; Yamamoto, H. Wearable Power Assist Device for Hand Grasping Using Pneumatic Artificial Rubber Muscle. In Proceedings of the 2004 IEEE International Conference on Robotics and Biomimetics (ROBIO), Shenyang, China, 22–26 August 2004; pp. 655–660. [CrossRef]
319. Tadano, K.; Akai, M.; Kadota, K.; Kawashima, K. Development of Grip Amplified Glove Using Bi-Articular Mechanism with Pneumatic Artificial Rubber Muscle. In Proceedings of the 2010 IEEE International Conference on Robotics and Automation (ICRA), Anchorage, AK, USA, 3–8 May 2010; pp. 2363–2368. [CrossRef]
320. Toya, K.; Miyagawa, T.; Kubota, Y. Power-Assist Glove Operated by Predicting the Grasping Mode. *J. Syst. Des. Dyn.* **2011**, *5*, 94–108. [CrossRef]
321. Iqbal, J.; Ahmad, O.; Malik, A. HEXOSYS II—Towards Realization of Light Mass Robotics for the Hand. In Proceedings of the 2011 IEEE International Conference on Robotics and Biomimetics (ROBIO), Sanya, China, 7–10 December 2011. [CrossRef]
322. Tang, Z.; Sugano, S.; Iwata, H. Design and Evaluation of an One DOF Finger Rehabilitation Device. In Proceedings of the 2013 IEEE/ASME International Conference on Advanced Intelligent Mechatronics (AIM), Wollongong, NSW, Australia, 9–12 July 2013; pp. 822–827. [CrossRef]
323. Yap, H.K.; Lim, J.; Cho, J.; Yeow, R.C.-H. Design of a Soft Robotic Glove for Hand Rehabilitation of Stroke Patients With Clenched Fist Deformity Using Inflatable Plastic Actuators. *J. Med. Devices* **2016**, *10*, 044504. [CrossRef]
324. Iqbal, J.; Caldwell, D.; Tsagarakis, N. Four-Fingered Lightweight Exoskeleton Robotic Device Accommodating Different Hand Sizes. *Electron. Lett.* **2015**, *51*. [CrossRef]
325. Irimia, D.C.; Poboroniuc, M.S.; Hartopanu, S.; Sticea, D.; Paicu, G.; Ignat, B.E. Post-Stroke Hand Rehabilitation Using a Hybrid FES-Robotic Glove. In Proceedings of the 2016 International Conference and Exposition on Electrical and Power Engineering (EPE), Iasi, Romania, 20–22 October 2016; pp. 356–359. [CrossRef]
326. Wang, B.; McDaid, A.; Biglari-Abhari, M.; Aw, K. Design and Development of a Glove for Post-Stroke Hand Rehabilitation. In Proceedings of the 2017 IEEE International Conference on Advanced Intelligent Mechatronics (AIM), Munich, Germany, 3–7 July 2017; pp. 1047–1051. [CrossRef]
327. Lee, H.; Kang, B.; In, H.; Cho, K.-J. Design Improvement of a Polymer-Based Tendon-Driven Wearable Robotic Hand (Exo-Glove Poly). In Proceedings of the Wearable Robotics: Challenges and Trends, Segovia, Spain, 18–20 October 2016; pp. 95–99. [CrossRef]
328. Low, J.-H.; Ang, M.H.; Yeow, R.C.-H. Customizable Soft Pneumatic Finger Actuators for Hand Orthotic and Prosthetic Applications. In Proceedings of the 2015 IEEE International Conference on Rehabilitation Robotics (ICORR), Singapore, 11–14 August 2015; pp. 380–385. [CrossRef]
329. Agarwal, P.; Yun, Y.; Fox, J.; Madden, K.; Deshpande, A. Design, Control, and Testing of a Thumb Exoskeleton with Series Elastic Actuation. *Int. J. Robot. Res.* **2017**, *36*. [CrossRef]
330. Yi, J.; Shen, Z.; Song, C.; Wang, Z. A Soft Robotic Glove for Hand Motion Assistance. In Proceedings of the 2016 IEEE International Conference on Real-time Computing and Robotics (RCAR), Angkor Wat, Cambodia, 6–10 June 2016. [CrossRef]
331. Lemerle, S.; Nozaki, T.; Ohnishi, K. Design and Evaluation of a Remote Actuated Finger Exoskeleton Using Motion-Copying System for Tendon Rehabilitation. *IEEE Trans. Ind. Inf.* **2018**, *14*, 5167–5177. [CrossRef]
332. Heo, P.; Kim, S.; Kim, J. Powered Finger Exoskeleton Having Partially Open Fingerpad for Flexion Force Assistance. In Proceedings of the 2013 IEEE/ASME International Conference on Advanced Intelligent Mechatronics (AIM), Wollongong, NSW, Australia, 9–12 July 2013; pp. 182–187. [CrossRef]
333. Jiang, Y.; Chen, D.; Liu, P.; Jiao, X.; Ping, Z.; Xu, Z.; Li, J.; Xu, Y. Fishbone-Inspired Soft Robotic Glove for Hand Rehabilitation with Multi-Degrees-of-Freedom. In Proceedings of the 2018 IEEE International Conference on Soft Robotics (RoboSoft), Livorno, Italy, 24–28 April 2018. [CrossRef]
334. Yi, J.; Chen, X.; Wang, Z. A 3D-Printed Soft Robotic Glove with Enhanced Ergonomics and Force Capability. *IEEE Robot. Autom. Lett.* **2017**, *3*, 242–248. [CrossRef]
335. Yun, Y.; Dancausse, S.; Esmatloo, P.; Serrato, A.; Merring, C.; Agarwal, P.; Deshpande, A. Maestro: An EMG-Driven Assistive Hand Exoskeleton for Spinal Cord Injury Patients. In Proceedings of the 2017 IEEE International Conference on Robotics and Automation (ICRA), Singapore, 29 May–3 June 2017; pp. 2904–2910. [CrossRef]

336. Guo, S.; Zhang, F.; Wei, W.; Zhao, F.; Wang, Y. Kinematic Analysis of a Novel Exoskeleton Finger Rehabilitation Robot for Stroke Patients. In Proceedings of the 2014 IEEE International Conference on Mechatronics and Automation (ICMA), Tianjin, China, 3–6 August 2014; pp. 924–929. [CrossRef]
337. Ullah, M.; Hafeez, U.; Shehzad, M.; Awais, M.N.; Elahi, H. A Soft Robotic Glove for Assistance and Rehabilitation of Stroke Affected Patients. In Proceedings of the 2019 International Conference on Frontiers of Information Technology (FIT), Islamabad, Pakistan, 16–18 December 2019; pp. 110–1105. [CrossRef]
338. Mohammadi, A.; Lavranos, J.; Choong, P.; Oetomo, D. Flexo-Glove: A 3D Printed Soft Exoskeleton Robotic Glove for Impaired Hand Rehabilitation and Assistance. In Proceedings of the 2018 Annual International Conference of the IEEE Engineering in Medicine and Biology Society (EMBC), Honolulu, HI, USA, 17–21 July 2018; pp. 2120–2123. [CrossRef]
339. Kim, Y.-J.; Jeong, Y.-J.; Jeon, H.-S.; Lee, D.-W.; Kim, J.-I. Development of a Soft Robotic Glove with High Gripping Force Using Force Distributing Compliant Structures. In Proceedings of the 2017 IEEE/RSJ International Conference on Intelligent Robots and Systems (IROS), Vancouver, BC, Canada, 24–28 September 2017; pp. 3883–3890. [CrossRef]
340. Cao, H.; Zhang, D. Soft Robotic Glove with Integrated sEMG Sensing for Disabled People with Hand Paralysis. In Proceedings of the 2016 IEEE International Conference on Robotics and Biomimetics (ROBIO), Qingdao, China, 3–7 December 2016; pp. 714–718. [CrossRef]
341. Nuckols, R.; Hohimer, C.; Glover, C.; Lucena, D.; Moyo, W.; Wagner, D.; Cloutier, A.; Lin, D.; Walsh, C. Effects of a Soft Robotic Glove Using a High Repetition Protocol in Chronic Stroke: A Pilot Study. In Proceedings of the 2020 IEEE International Conference on Biomedical Robotics and Biomechatronics (BioRob), New York, NY, USA, 29 June–2 July 2020; pp. 428–433. [CrossRef]
342. El-Agroudy, M.; Awad, M.; Rehan, A.; Maged, S. Assistive Exoskeleton Hand Glove Using Soft Pneumatic Actuators: Design Optimization. *IOP Conf. Ser. Mater. Sci. Eng.* **2020**, *973*, 012041. [CrossRef]
343. Akgun, G.; Cetin, A.E.; Kaplanoglu, E. Exoskeleton Design and Adaptive Compliance Control for Hand Rehabilitation. *Trans. Inst. Meas. Control* **2019**, 014233121987497. [CrossRef]
344. Dai, Y.; Ji, J.; Yang, G.; Yang, Y. A Novel Robotic Exoskeleton for Finger Rehabilitation: Kinematics Analysis. *Appl. Bionics Biomech.* **2022**, *2022*, 1751460. [CrossRef]
345. Hernández-Santos, C.; Davizón, Y.A.; Said, A.R.; Soto, R.; Félix-Herrán, L.C.; Vargas-Martínez, A. Development of a Wearable Finger Exoskeleton for Rehabilitation. *Appl. Sci.* **2021**, *11*, 4145. [CrossRef]
346. Yang, S.-H.; Koh, C.-L.; Hsu, C.-H.; Chen, P.-C.; Chen, J.-W.; Lan, Y.-H.; Yang, Y.; Lin, Y.-D.; Wu, C.-H.; Liu, H.-K.; et al. An Instrumented Glove-Controlled Portable Hand-Exoskeleton for Bilateral Hand Rehabilitation. *Biosensors* **2021**, *11*, 495. [CrossRef]
347. Li, M.; Jiazhou, C.; He, G.; Cui, L.; Chen, C.; Secco, E.L.; Yao, W.; Xie, J.; Xu, G.; Wurdemann, H. Attention Enhancement for Exoskeleton-Assisted Hand Rehabilitation Using Fingertip Haptic Stimulation. *Front. Robot. AI* **2021**, *8*, 602091. [CrossRef]
348. Yihun, Y.; Miklos, R.; Perez-Gracia, A.; Reinkensmeyer, D.; Denney, K.; Wolbrecht, E. Single Degree-of-Freedom Exoskeleton Mechanism Design for Thumb Rehabilitation. In Proceedings of the 2012 Annual International Conference of the IEEE Engineering in Medicine and Biology Society (EMBC), San Diego, CA, USA, 28 August–1 September 2012; pp. 1916–1920. [CrossRef]
349. Dragusanu, M.; Troisi, D.; Villani, A.; Prattichizzo, D.; Malvezzi, M. Design and Prototyping of an Underactuated Hand Exoskeleton with Fingers Coupled by a Gear-Based Differential. *Front. Robot. AI* **2022**, *9*, 862340. [CrossRef]
350. Sandison, M.; Phan, K.; Casas, R.; Nguyen, L.; Lum, M.; Pergami-Peries, M.; Lum, P. HandMATE: Wearable Robotic Hand Exoskeleton and Integrated Android App for At Home Stroke Rehabilitation. In Proceedings of the 2020 Annual International Conference of the IEEE Engineering in Medicine and Biology Society (EMBC), Montreal, QC, Canada, 20–24 July 2020; pp. 4867–4872. [CrossRef]
351. Lee, J.; Park, W.; Kim, S.; Bae, J. Design of a Wearable Hand Rehabilitation System for Quantitative Evaluation of the Stroke Hand. In Proceedings of the 2016 International Conference on Control, Automation and Systems (ICCAS), Gyeongju, Republic of Korea, 16–19 October 2016; pp. 419–422. [CrossRef]
352. Moreno-SanJuan, V.; Cisnal, A.; Fraile, J.-C.; Pérez-Turiel, J.; Fuente-Lopez, E. Design and Characterization of a Lightweight Underactuated RACA Hand Exoskeleton for Neurorehabilitation. *Robot. Auton. Syst.* **2021**, *143*, 103828. [CrossRef]
353. Malvezzi, M.; Lisini, T.; Villani, A.; Ciccarese, F.; Prattichizzo, D. Design, Development, and Preliminary Evaluation of a Highly Wearable Exoskeleton. In Proceedings of the 2020 IEEE International Conference on Robot and Human Interactive Communication (RO-MAN), Naples, Italy, 31 August–4 September 2020; pp. 1055–1062. [CrossRef]
354. Du, J.; Tian, Y.; Zhang, D.; Wang, H.; Zhang, Y.; Cheng, B.; Niu, J. Mechanism Design and Performance Analysis of a Wearable Hand Rehabilitation Robot. *Machines* **2022**, *10*, 1211. [CrossRef]
355. Nycz, C.; Butzer, T.; Lambercy, O.; Arata, J.; Fischer, G.; Gassert, R. Design and Characterization of a Lightweight and Fully Portable Remote Actuation System for Use With a Hand Exoskeleton. *IEEE Robot. Autom. Lett.* **2016**, *1*, 976–983. [CrossRef]

356. Ockenfeld, C.; Tong, R.K.; Susanto, E.A.; Ho, S.K.; Hu, X.L. Fine Finger Motor Skill Training with Exoskeleton Robotic Hand in Chronic Stroke: Stroke Rehabilitation. In Proceedings of the 2013 IEEE International Conference on Rehabilitation Robotics (ICORR), Seattle, WA, USA, 24–26 June 2013. [CrossRef]
357. Wege, A.; Kondak, K.; Hommel, G. Mechanical Design and Motion Control of a Hand Exoskeleton for Rehabilitation. In Proceedings of the 2005 IEEE International Conference on Mechatronics and Automation (ICMA), Niagara Falls, ON, Canada, 29 July–1 August 2005; pp. 155–159. [CrossRef]
358. Kladovasilakis, N.; Kostavelis, I.; Sideridis, P.; Koltzi, E.; Piliounis, K.; Tzetzis, D.; Tzovaras, D. A Novel Soft Robotic Exoskeleton System for Hand Rehabilitation and Assistance Purposes. *Appl. Sci.* **2023**, *13*, 553. [CrossRef]
359. Connelly, L.; Jia, Y.; Toro, M.L.; Stoykov, M.E.; Kenyon, R.V.; Kamper, D.G. A Pneumatic Glove and Immersive Virtual Reality Environment for Hand Rehabilitative Training After Stroke. *IEEE Trans. Neural Syst. Rehabil. Eng.* **2010**, *18*, 551–559. [CrossRef]
360. Yap, H.K.; Lim, J.H.; Nasrallah, F.A.; Goh, J.C.H.; Yeow, R.C.H. A soft exoskeleton for hand assistive and rehabilitation application using pneumatic actuators with variable stiffness. In Proceedings of the 2015 IEEE International Conference on Robotics and Automation (ICRA), Seattle, WA, USA, 26–30 May 2015; pp. 4967–4972. [CrossRef]
361. Ryu, D.; Moon, K.W.; Nam, H.; Lee, Y.; Chun, C.; Kang, S.; Song, J.B. Micro hydraulic system using slim artificial muscles for a wearable haptic glove. In Proceedings of the 2008 IEEE/RSJ International Conference on Intelligent Robots and Systems (IROS), Nice, France, 22–26 September 2008; pp. 3028–3033. [CrossRef]
362. Polygerinos, P.; Galloway, K.C.; Savage, E.; Herman, M.; O'Donnell, K.; Walsh, C.J. Soft robotic glove for hand rehabilitation and task-specific training. In Proceedings of the 2015 IEEE International Conference on Robotics and Automation (ICRA), Seattle, WA, USA, 26–30 May 2015; pp. 2913–2919. [CrossRef]
363. Zaid, A.M.; Chean, T.C.; Sukor, J.A.; Hanafi, D. Development of hand exoskeleton for rehabilitation of post-stroke patient. *AIP Conf. Proc.* **2017**, *1891*, 020103. [CrossRef]
364. Ridremont, T.; Singh, I.; Bruzek, B.; Jamieson, A.; Gu, Y.; Merzouki, R.; Wijesundara, M.B.J. Pneumatically Actuated Soft Robotic Hand and Wrist Exoskeleton for Motion Assistance in Rehabilitation. *Actuators* **2024**, *13*, 180. [CrossRef]
365. Rudd, G.; Daly, L.; Jovanovic, V.; Cuckov, F. A Low-Cost Soft Robotic Hand Exoskeleton for Use in Therapy of Limited Hand–Motor Function. *Appl. Sci.* **2019**, *9*, 3751. [CrossRef]
366. Silva, R.C.; Lourenço, B.G.; Ulhoa, P.H.F.; Dias, E.A.F.; da Cunha, F.L.; Tonetto, C.P.; Villani, L.G.; Vimieiro, C.B.S.; Lepski, G.A.; Monjardim, M.; et al. Biomimetic Design of a Tendon-Driven Myoelectric Soft Hand Exoskeleton for Upper-Limb Rehabilitation. *Biomimetics* **2023**, *8*, 317. [CrossRef]
367. Burns, M.K.; Pei, D.; Vinjamuri, R. Myoelectric control of a soft hand exoskeleton using kinematic synergies. *IEEE Trans. Biomed. Circuits Syst.* **2019**, *13*, 1351–1361. [CrossRef] [PubMed]
368. Aruanno, B.; Covarrubias, M. HANDY: Novel hand exoskeleton for personalized rehabilitation. *Comput. Aided Des. Appl.* **2021**, *19*, 405–425. [CrossRef]
369. Chen, X.; Gong, L.; Zheng, L.; Zou, Z. Soft exoskeleton glove for hand assistance based on human-machine interaction and machine learning. In Proceedings of the 2020 IEEE International Conference on Human-Machine Systems (ICHMS), Rome, Italy, 7–9 September 2020; pp. 1–6. [CrossRef]
370. Jamaludin, M.S.; Jamali, A.; Mohamaddan, S. Design and fabrication of finger rehabilitation device for stroke patients-a prototype development. In Proceedings of the 5th Brunei International Conference on Engineering and Technology (BICET 2014), Bandar Seri Begawan, Brunei, 1–3 November 2014. [CrossRef]
371. Han, Y.; Xu, Q.; Wu, F. Design of wearable hand rehabilitation glove with bionic fiber-reinforced actuator. *IEEE J. Transl. Eng. Health Med.* **2022**, *10*, 1–10. [CrossRef]
372. Birlescu, I.; Tohanean, N.; Vaida, C.; Gherman, B.; Neguran, D.; Horsia, A.; Tucan, P.; Condurache, D.; Pisla, D. Modeling and analysis of a parallel robotic system for lower limb rehabilitation with predefined operational workspace. *Mech. Mach. Theory* **2024**, *198*, 105674. [CrossRef]
373. Maldonado-Mejía, J.C.; Múnera, M.; Diaz, C.A.R.; Wurdemann, H.; Moazen, M.; Pontes, M.J.; Vieira Segatto, M.E.; Monteiro, M.E.; Cifuentes, C.A. A fabric-based soft hand exoskeleton for assistance: The ExHand Exoskeleton. *Front. Neurorobot.* **2023**, *17*, 1091827. [CrossRef] [PubMed]
374. Li, M.; Zhuo, Y.; He, B.; Liang, Z.; Xu, Z.; Xie, J.; Zhang, S. A 3D-printed soft hand exoskeleton with finger abduction assistance. In Proceedings of the 2019 16th International Conference on Ubiquitous Robots (UR), Jeju, Republic of Korea, 24–27 June 2019; pp. 319–322. [CrossRef]
375. El-Agroudy, M.N.; Awad, M.I.; Maged, S.A. Soft Finger Modelling and Co-Simulation Control towards Assistive Exoskeleton Hand Glove. *Micromachines* **2021**, *12*, 181. [CrossRef]
376. Le, D.T.G.; Nguyen, L. An efficient force-feedback hand exoskeleton for haptic applications. *Int. J. Intell. Robot Appl.* **2021**, *5*, 395–409. [CrossRef]

377. Zhu, Y.; Gong, W.; Chu, K.; Wang, X.; Hu, Z.; Su, H. A Novel Wearable Soft Glove for Hand Rehabilitation and Assistive Grasping. *Sensors* **2022**, *22*, 6294. [CrossRef]
378. Bressi, F.; Cricenti, L.; Bravi, M.; Pannunzio, F.; Cordella, F.; Lapresa, M.; Miccinilli, S.; Santacaterina, F.; Zollo, L.; Sterzi, S.; et al. Treatment of the Paretic Hand with a Robotic Glove Combined with Physiotherapy in a Patient Suffering from Traumatic Tetraparesis: A Case Report. *Sensors* **2023**, *23*, 3484. [CrossRef]
379. Lucas, L.; DiCicco, M.; Matsuoka, Y. An EMG-Controlled Hand Exoskeleton for Natural Pinching. *J. Robot. Mechatron.* **2004**, *16*, 482–488. [CrossRef]
380. Ramos, O.; Múnera, M.; Moazen, M.; Wurdemann, H.; Cifuentes, C.A. Assessment of Soft Actuators for Hand Exoskeletons: Pleated Textile Actuators and Fiber-Reinforced Silicone Actuators. *Front. Bioeng. Biotechnol.* **2022**, *10*, 924888. [CrossRef]
381. Villoslada, Á.; Rivera, C.; Escudero, N.; Martín, F.; Blanco, D.; Moreno, L. Hand Exo-Muscular System for Assisting Astronauts During Extravehicular Activities. *Soft Robot.* **2019**, *6*, 21–37. [CrossRef]
382. Kadowaki, Y.; Noritsugu, T.; Takaiwa, M.; Sasaki, D.; Kato, M. Development of Soft Power-Assist Glove and Control Based on Human Intent. *J. Robotics Mechatron.* **2011**, *23*, 281–291. [CrossRef]
383. Yurkewich, A.; Kozak, I.; Ivanovic, A.; Rossos, D.; Wang, R.; Hebert, D.; Mihailidis, A. Myoelectric Untethered Robotic Glove Enhances Hand Function and Performance on Daily Living Tasks After Stroke. *J. Rehabil. Assist. Technol. Eng.* **2020**, *7*, 205566832096405. [CrossRef] [PubMed]
384. Jeong, U.; In, H.; Lee, H.; Kang, B.; Cho, K.-J. Investigation on the Control Strategy of Soft Wearable Robotic Hand with Slack Enabling Tendon Actuator. In Proceedings of the 2015 IEEE International Conference on Robotics and Automation (ICRA), Seattle, WA, USA, 26–30 May 2015; pp. 5004–5009. [CrossRef]
385. Polygerinos, P.; Galloway, K.; Sanan, S.; Herman, M.; Walsh, C. EMG Controlled Soft Robotic Glove for Assistance During Activities of Daily Living. In Proceedings of the 2015 IEEE International Conference on Rehabilitation Robotics (ICORR), Singapore, 11–14 August 2015; pp. 55–60. [CrossRef]
386. Kim, B.; In, H.; Lee, D.-Y.; Cho, K.-J. Development and Assessment of a Hand Assist Device: GRIPIT. *J. NeuroEng. Rehabil.* **2017**, *14*, 15. [CrossRef] [PubMed]
387. Mohamaddan, S.; Komeda, T. Wire-Driven Mechanism for Finger Rehabilitation Device. In Proceedings of the 2010 IEEE International Conference on Mechatronics and Automation (ICMA), Xi'an, China, 4–7 August 2010. [CrossRef]
388. Correia, C.; Nuckols, R.; Wagner, D.; Zhou, Y.M.; Clarke, M.; Orzel, D.; Solinsky, R.; Paganoni, S.; Walsh, C. Improving Grasp Function After Spinal Cord Injury With a Soft Robotic Glove. *IEEE Trans. Neural Syst. Rehabil. Eng.* **2020**, *28*, 1407–1415. [CrossRef]
389. Chiri, A.; Giovacchini, F.; Vitiello, N.; Cattin, E.; Roccella, S.; Vecchi, F.; Carrozza, M.C. HANDEXOS: Towards an Exoskeleton Device for the Rehabilitation of the Hand. In Proceedings of the 2009 IEEE/RSJ International Conference on Intelligent Robots and Systems, St. Louis, MO, USA, 10–15 October 2009; pp. 1106–1111.
390. Lee, Y.; Park, H.-S. Design Optimization of a Soft Robotic Rehabilitation Glove Based on Finger Workspace Analysis. *Biomimetics* **2024**, *9*, 172. [CrossRef] [PubMed]
391. Brogi, C.; Secciani, N.; Bartalucci, L.; Di Iorio, F.; Meli, E.; Rinchi, M.; Allotta, B.; Ridolfi, A. An Original Hybrid-Architecture Finger Mechanism for Wearable Hand Exoskeletons. *Mechatronics* **2024**, *98*, 103117. [CrossRef]
392. Iqbal, J.; Tsagarakis, N.; Caldwell, D.G. Human Hand Compatible Underactuated Exoskeleton Robotic System. *Electron. Lett.* **2014**, *50*, 494–496. [CrossRef]
393. Dovat, L.; Lambercy, O.; Gassert, R.; Maeder, T.; Milner, T.; Leong, T.C.; Burdet, E. HandCARE: A Cable-Actuated Rehabilitation System to Train Hand Function After Stroke. *IEEE Trans. Neural Syst. Rehabil. Eng.* **2008**, *16*, 582–591. [CrossRef] [PubMed]
394. Nycz, C.; Delph, M.; Fischer, G. Modeling and Design of a Tendon Actuated Soft Robotic Exoskeleton for Hemiparetic Upper Limb Rehabilitation. In Proceedings of the 2015 IEEE International Conference on Engineering in Medicine and Biology Society (EMBC), Milan, Italy, 25–29 August 2015; pp. 3889–3892. [CrossRef]
395. Tran, P.; Jeong, S.; Wolf, S.; Desai, J. Patient-Specific, Voice-Controlled, Robotic FLEX-otendon Glove-II System for Spinal Cord Injury. *IEEE Robot. Autom. Lett.* **2020**, *5*, 898–905. [CrossRef]
396. Lemerle, S.; Fukushima, S.; Saito, Y.; Nozaki, T.; Ohnishi, K. Wearable Finger Exoskeleton Using Flexible Actuator for Rehabilitation. In Proceedings of the IEEE International Conference on Mechatronics (ICM), Churchill, VIC, Australia, 13–15 February 2017; pp. 244–249. [CrossRef]
397. Ismail, R.; Ariyanto, M.; Hidayat, T.; Setiawan, J. Design of Fabric-Based Soft Robotic Glove for Hand Function Assistance. In Proceedings of the 2019 International Conference on Information Technology, Computer, and Electrical Engineering (ICITACEE), Semarang, Indonesia, 26–27 September 2019; pp. 1–5. [CrossRef]
398. Duanmu, D.; Li, X.; Huang, W.; Hu, Y. Soft Finger Rehabilitation Exoskeleton of Biomimetic Dragonfly Abdominal Ventral Muscles: Center Tendon Pneumatic Bellows Actuator. *Biomimetics* **2023**, *8*, 614. [CrossRef]

399. Yap, H.K.; Lim, J.H.; Nasrallah, F.; Yeow, C.H. Design and Preliminary Feasibility Study of a Soft Robotic Glove for Hand Function Assistance in Stroke Survivors. *Front. Neurosci.* **2017**, *11*, 547. [CrossRef]
400. Yap, H.K.; Khin, P.; Koh, T.; Sun, Y.; Liang, X.; Lim, J.; Yeow, R.C.-H. A Fully Fabric-Based Bidirectional Soft Robotic Glove for Assistance and Rehabilitation of Hand Impaired Patients. *IEEE Robot. Autom. Lett.* **2017**, *2*, 1383–1390. [CrossRef]
401. Koizumi, S.; Shimada, Y.; Chang, T.-H.; Nabae, H.; Endo, G.; Suzumori, K.; Mita, M.; Saitoh, K.; Hatakeyama, K.; Chida, S. Soft Robotic Gloves with Thin McKibben Muscles for Hand Assist and Rehabilitation. In Proceedings of the 2020 IEEE/SICE International Symposium on System Integration (SII), Honolulu, HI, USA, 12–15 January 2020; pp. 93–98. [CrossRef]
402. Takahashi, N.; Takahashi, H.; Koike, H. Soft Exoskeleton Glove Enabling Force Feedback for Human-Like Finger Posture Control with 20 Degrees of Freedom. In Proceedings of the 2019 IEEE World Haptics Conference (WHC), Tokyo, Japan, 9–12 July 2019; pp. 217–222. [CrossRef]
403. Jadhav, S.; Kannanda, V.; Kang, B.; Tolley, M.T.; Schulze, J.P. Soft Robotic Glove for Kinesthetic Haptic Feedback in Virtual Reality Environments. In Proceedings of the IS&T International Symposium on Electronic Imaging: The Engineering Reality of Virtual Reality, Burlingame, CA, USA, 29 January–2 February 2017; pp. 19–24. [CrossRef]
404. Tondu, B.; Lopez, P. Modeling and Control of McKibben Artificial Muscle Robot Actuators. *IEEE Control Syst. Mag.* **2000**, *20*, 15–38. [CrossRef]
405. Sasaki, D.; Noritsugu, T.; Takaiwa, M. Development of Active Support Splint Driven by Pneumatic Soft Actuator (ASSIST). In Proceedings of the IEEE International Conference on Robotics and Automation (ICRA), Barcelona, Spain, 18–22 April 2005; pp. 520–525. [CrossRef]
406. Hand Physical Therapy with the HandMentor™. Available online: http://www.kineticmuscles.com/hand-physicaltherapy-hand-mentor.html (accessed on 12 November 2024).
407. Pisla, D.; Nae, L.; Vaida, C.; Oprea, E.; Pisla, A.; Gherman, B.; Antal, T.; Riessenberger, K.; Plitea, N. Development of a Learning Management System for Knowledge Transfer in Engineering. *Acta Tech. Napoc. Ser. Appl. Math. Mech. Eng.* **2021**, *64*, 361–368.
408. Gopura, R.A.R.C.; Kiguchi, K. Mechanical Designs of Active Upper-Limb Exoskeleton Robots: State-of-the-Art and Design Difficulties. In Proceedings of the IEEE International Conference on Rehabilitation Robotics (ICORR), Kyoto, Japan, 23–26 June 2009; pp. 178–187. [CrossRef]
409. Yuan, J.; Neri, W.; Zakri, C.; Merzeau, P.; Kratz, K.; Lendlein, A.; Poulin, P. Shape Memory Nanocomposite Fibers for Untethered High-Energy Microengines. *Science* **2019**, *365*, 155–158. [CrossRef]
410. Wang, H. Application of Intelligent Materials in the Control System. *J. Comput. Theor. Nanosci.* **2015**, *12*, 2830–2836. [CrossRef]
411. Otsuka, K.; Wayman, C.M. (Eds.) *Shape Memory Materials*; Cambridge University Press: Cambridge, UK, 1999.
412. Mavroidis, C.; Pfeiffer, C.; Mosley, M. Conventional Actuators, Shape Memory Alloys and Electrorheological Fluids. In *Automation, Miniature Robotics and Sensors for Non-Destructive Testing and Evaluation*; Bar-Cohen, Y., Ed.; American Society for Nondestructive Testing: Columbus, OH, USA, 2000; pp. 189–214.
413. Kazeminasab, S.; Hadi, A.; Alipour, K.; Elahinia, M. Force and Motion Control of a Tendon-Driven Hand Exoskeleton Actuated by Shape Memory Alloys. *Ind. Robot* **2019**, *45*, 623–633. [CrossRef]
414. Nilsson, M.; Ingvast, J.; Wikander, J.; von Holst, H. The Soft Extra Muscle System for Improving the Grasping Capability in Neurological Rehabilitation. In Proceedings of the 2012 IEEE-EMBS Conference on Biomedical Engineering and Sciences (IECBES), Langkawi, Malaysia, 17–19 December 2012; pp. 412–417. [CrossRef]
415. Yao, Z.; Linnenberg, C.; Argubi-Wollesen, A.; Weidner, R.; Wulfsberg, J. Biomimetic Design of an Ultra-Compact and Light-Weight Soft Muscle Glove. *Prod. Eng.* **2017**, *11*, 731–743. [CrossRef]
416. Kumar, P.; Lagoudas, D. Introduction to Shape Memory Alloys. In *Shape Memory Alloys*; Springer: Boston, MA, USA, 2008; Volume 1. [CrossRef]
417. Freeman, C.T.; Hughes, A.M.; Burridge, J.H.; Chappell, P.H.; Lewin, P.L.; Rogers, E. Iterative Learning Control of FES Applied to the Upper Extremity for Rehabilitation. *Control Eng. Pract.* **2009**, *17*, 368–381. [CrossRef]
418. Trolier-McKinstry, S.; Zhang, S.; Bell, A.J.; Tan, X. High-Performance Piezoelectric Crystals, Ceramics, and Films. *Annu. Rev. Mater. Res.* **2018**, *48*, 191–217. [CrossRef]
419. Hesse, S.; Schulte-Tigges, G.; Konrad, M.; Bardeleben, A.; Werner, C. Robot-Assisted Arm Trainer for the Passive and Active Practice of Bilateral Forearm and Wrist Movements in Hemiparetic Subjects. *Arch. Phys. Med. Rehabil.* **2003**, *84*, 915–920. [CrossRef]
420. Hesse, S.; Schmidt, H.; Werner, C. Machines to Support Motor Rehabilitation After Stroke: 10 Years of Experience in Berlin. *J. Rehabil. Res. Dev.* **2006**, *43*, 671–678. [CrossRef] [PubMed]
421. Lee, D.W.; Lee, S.J.; Yoon, B.R.; Jho, J.Y.; Rhee, K. Preliminary Study on Analysis of Pinching Motion Actuated by Electro-Active Polymers. *Int. J. Mech. Mechatron. Eng.* **2014**, *8*, 919–921. [CrossRef]

422. Metzger, J.-C.; Lambercy, O.; Gassert, R. High-Fidelity Rendering of Virtual Objects with the ReHapticKnob-Novel Avenues in Robot-Assisted Rehabilitation of Hand Function. In Proceedings of the 2012 IEEE Haptics Symposium (HAPTICS), Vancouver, BC, Canada, 4–7 March 2012; pp. 51–56. [CrossRef]
423. Jo, I.; Bae, J. Design and Control of a Wearable and Force-Controllable Hand Exoskeleton System. *Mechatronics* **2017**, *41*, 90–101. [CrossRef]
424. Bullock, I.M.; Borràs, J.; Dollar, A.M. Assessing Assumptions in Kinematic Hand Models: A Review. In Proceedings of the 2012 4th IEEE RAS & EMBS International Conference on Biomedical Robotics and Biomechatronics (BioRob), Rome, Italy, 24–27 June 2012; Volume 49, pp. 139–146. [CrossRef]
425. Hwang, C.H.; Seong, J.W.; Son, D.-S. Individual Finger Synchronized Robot-Assisted Hand Rehabilitation in Subacute to Chronic Stroke: A Prospective Randomized Clinical Trial of Efficacy. *Clin. Rehabil.* **2012**, *26*, 696–704. [CrossRef] [PubMed]
426. Ang, K.; Guan, C.; Phua, K.S.; Wang, C.; Zhou, L.; Tang, K.Y.; Joseph, G.; Kuah, C.; Chua, K. Brain-Computer Interface-Based Robotic End Effector System for Wrist and Hand Rehabilitation: Results of a Three-Armed Randomized Controlled Trial for Chronic Stroke. *Front. Neuroeng.* **2014**, *7*, 30. [CrossRef] [PubMed]
427. Tohanean, N.; Tucan, P.; Vanta, O.-M.; Abrudan, C.; Pintea, S.; Gherman, B.; Burz, A.; Banica, A.; Vaida, C.; Neguran, D.A.; et al. The Efficacity of the NeuroAssist Robotic System for Motor Rehabilitation of the Upper Limb—Promising Results from a Pilot Study. *J. Clin. Med.* **2023**, *12*, 425. [CrossRef] [PubMed]
428. Kang, B.; In, H.; Cho, K.-J. Modeling of Tendon Driven Soft Wearable Robot for the Finger. In Proceedings of the 2013 10th International Conference on Ubiquitous Robots and Ambient Intelligence (URAI), Jeju, Republic of Korea, 30 October–2 November 2013; pp. 459–460. [CrossRef]
429. Kottink, A.; Nikamp, C.; Buurke, J.; Bos, F.; Sluis, C.; Broek, M.; Onneweer, B.; Stolwijk-Swüste, J.; Brink, S.; Rietman, J.; et al. Six Weeks Use of a Wearable Soft-Robotic Glove During ADL: Preliminary Results of Ongoing Clinical Study. In Proceedings of the 2022 IEEE International Conference on Rehabilitation Robotics (ICORR), Rotterdam, The Netherlands, 25–29 July 2022. [CrossRef]
430. Hesse, S.; Kuhlmann, H.; Wilk, J.; Tomelleri, C.; Kirker, S.G.B. A New Electromechanical Trainer for Sensorimotor Rehabilitation of Paralysed Fingers: A Case Series in Chronic and Acute Stroke Patients. *J. NeuroEng. Rehabil.* **2008**, *5*, 21. [CrossRef] [PubMed]
431. Thielbar, K.O.; Triandafilou, K.M.; Fischer, H.C.; O'Toole, J.M.; Corrigan, M.L.; Ochoa, J.M.; Stoykov, M.E.; Kamper, D.G. Benefits of Using a Voice and EMG-Driven Actuated Glove to Support Occupational Therapy for Stroke Survivors. *IEEE Trans. Neural Syst. Rehabil. Eng.* **2017**, *25*, 297–306. [CrossRef]
432. Akbari, A.; Haghverd, F.; Behbahani, S. Robotic Home-Based Rehabilitation Systems Design: From a Literature Review to a Conceptual Framework for Community-Based Remote Therapy During COVID-19 Pandemic. *Front. Robot. AI* **2021**, *8*, 612331. [CrossRef]
433. Lee, H.C.; Kuo, F.L.; Lin, Y.N.; Liou, T.H.; Lin, J.C.; Huang, S.W. Effects of Robot-Assisted Rehabilitation on Hand Function of People with Stroke: A Randomized, Crossover-Controlled, Assessor-Blinded Study. *Am. J. Occup. Ther.* **2021**, *75*, 7501205020p1–7501205020p11. [CrossRef] [PubMed]
434. Metzger, J.-C.; Lambercy, O.; Chapuis, D.; Gassert, R. Design and Characterization of the ReHapticKnob, a Robot for Assessment and Therapy of Hand Function. In Proceedings of the 2011 IEEE/RSJ International Conference on Intelligent Robots and Systems (IROS), San Francisco, CA, USA, 25–30 September 2011; Volume 10, pp. 3074–3080. [CrossRef]
435. In, H.; Kang, B.B.; Sin, M.; Cho, K.-J. Exo-Glove: A Wearable Robot for the Hand with a Soft Tendon Routing System. *IEEE Robot. Autom. Mag.* **2015**, *22*, 97–105. [CrossRef]
436. In, H.K.; Cho, K.J. Evaluation of the Antagonistic Tendon Driven System for SNU Exo-Glove. In Proceedings of the 2012 9th International Conference on Ubiquitous Robots and Ambient Intelligence (URAI), Daejeon, Republic of Korea, 26–28 November 2012; pp. 507–509. [CrossRef]
437. Du, Q.; Zhao, W.; Cui, X.; Fei, Y. Design, Control and Testing of Soft Pneumatic Rehabilitation Glove. In Proceedings of the 2020 IEEE 3rd World Conference on Mechanical Engineering and Intelligent Manufacturing (WCMEIM), Shanghai, China, 4–6 December 2020; pp. 50–55. [CrossRef]
438. Yang, Y.; Vella, K.; Holmes, D.P. Grasping with Kirigami Shells. *Sci. Robot.* **2021**, *6*, eabd6426. [CrossRef]

technologies

MDPI

Communication

A Dynamic Mechanical Analysis Device for In Vivo Material Characterization of Plantar Soft Tissue

Longyan Wu [1,†], Ran Huang [1,2,3,*,†], Jun Zhu [3] and Xin Ma [1,4,*]

[1] Institute of Biomedical Engineering and Technology, Fudan University, Shanghai 200433, China; 24110860029@m.fudan.edu.cn
[2] Center for Innovation and Entrepreneurship, Taizhou Institute of Zhejiang University, Taizhou 318000, China
[3] Center for Biomedical Engineering, Yiwu Research Institute of Fudan University, Yiwu 322000, China; jzhu_aet@fudan.edu.cn
[4] Shanghai Sixth People's Hospital, Shanghai Jiao Tong University, Shanghai 200233, China
* Correspondence: huangran@fudan.edu.cn (R.H.); xinma_faet@fudan.edu.cn (X.M.)
† These authors contributed equally to this work.

Abstract: Understanding the viscoelastic properties of plantar soft tissue under dynamic conditions is crucial for assessing foot health and preventing injuries. In this work, we document an in vivo device, employing the principles of dynamic mechanical analysis (DMA), which, for the first time, enables in situ, real-time multidimensional mechanical characterization of plantar soft tissues. This device overcomes the limitations of conventional ex vivo and single-DOF testing methods by integrating three sinusoidal mechanism-based multi-DOF dynamic testing modules, providing measurements of tensile, compressive, shear, and torsional properties in a physiological setting. The innovative modular design integrates advanced sensors for precise force and displacement detection, allowing for comprehensive assessment under cyclic loading conditions. Validation tests on volunteers demonstrate the device's reliability and highlight the significant viscoelastic characteristics of the plantar soft tissue. The example dataset was analyzed to calculate the storage modulus, loss modulus, loss factor, and energy dissipation. All design files, CAD models, and assembly instructions are made available as open-source resources, facilitating replication and further research. This work paves the way for enhanced diagnostics and personalized treatments in orthopedic and rehabilitative medicine.

Keywords: plantar soft tissue; dynamic mechanical analysis; in vivo; in situ; viscoelasticity

1. Introduction

The human plantar region consists of specialized soft tissues, predominantly fatty and connective tissues, positioned anatomically between the skin dermis, fascia, and underlying bony structures [1]. The plantar soft tissue demonstrates rate-dependent stress–strain characteristics under large deformations, known as viscoelastic [2]. This behavior can typically be effectively modeled using the Kelvin–Voigt viscoelastic model [3]. The time-dependent viscous properties of plantar soft tissues, particularly in the heel pad and metatarsal head regions, play a crucial role in stress buffering and energy dissipation [4]. These specialized tissues are evolutionarily adapted to provide effective cushioning, absorbing mechanical shocks during weight-bearing activities and thereby protecting underlying skeletal structures from potential injury [5–7]. Changes in the mechanical properties of these tissues may compromise their protective functionality, increasing the risk of injury or pathological conditions due to excessive mechanical loading. Consequently, extensive research efforts, both through in vitro and in vivo approaches, have been dedicated to characterizing and quantifying the mechanical behavior of plantar soft tissues to better understand their functional roles and the implications of their mechanical alterations. In vitro methods for characterizing plantar soft tissues typically involve tests performed on excised specimens, which inherently lack the physiological and biochemical environment present in living tissues [8,9]. To overcome this limitation and capture more realistic mechanical behaviors, several in vivo testing approaches have been explored, including ultrasonic shear wave elastography [10], Shore hardness measurements, indentation testing, and magnetic resonance elastography. Ultrasonic shear wave elastography determines Young's modulus by measuring shear wave propagation speed, assuming linear elasticity and homogeneous, isotropic tissue properties [11]. Shore hardness testing employs a handheld durometer to correlate the resistance of tissues against indentation with their intrinsic stiffness [12]. Nevertheless, these existing methods primarily assess static or quasi-static responses and do not adequately capture the dynamic, viscoelastic properties of plantar soft tissue. Given the importance of time-dependent behavior in accurately evaluating the tissue's response to repetitive physiological loading, comprehensive assessment methods capable of measuring both elastic and viscoelastic properties in dynamic conditions are critically needed [13].

Dynamic mechanical analysis (DMA) is a fundamental technique in materials science and biomechanics used to characterize the viscoelastic properties of materials by assessing their periodic stress–strain responses under controlled temperature and frequency conditions [14–16]. Recent advances have enabled the development of DMA-inspired devices capable of characterizing viscoelastic properties of living human skin in vivo [17]. However, most traditional DMA techniques have primarily been limited to ex vivo analyses of cadaveric tissue samples, lacking the physiological realism of living tissues and resulting in data with inherent limitations [18]. To overcome some of these constraints, recent studies have introduced indentation-based methods, enabling the in vivo measurement of plantar soft tissue properties through the simple application and release of compressive forces [19]. Nevertheless, such indentation approaches typically assess only a limited portion of the tissue's dynamic stress–strain behavior, capturing primarily single-direction loading and unloading cycles. Consequently, these methods fall short of replicating the comprehensive, cyclic, and multidirectional viscoelastic responses characteristic of plantar tissue during real-world dynamic loading conditions, thus emphasizing the need for improved techniques capable of fully capturing the dynamic viscoelastic properties in vivo.

Directly inspired by dynamic mechanical analysis (DMA)—a well-established technique from materials science for characterizing periodic stress–strain responses to assess both elastic and viscous properties of various materials—we have developed an innovative in vivo and in situ DMA-based device specifically designed for assessing the mechanical properties of human plantar soft tissue under physiological conditions. While conventional approaches (e.g., ex vivo testing, indentation, or elastography) are restricted to static or unidirectional measurements, our system uniquely enables simultaneous multidirectional (tensile/compressive, shear, and torsional) and dynamic cyclic mechanical characterization of plantar soft tissue under physiological conditions. Key advantages of our device include the following: (1) high-precision, real-time, in situ measurements without invasive procedures and (2) the integration of multiple loading modes (compression, shear, torsion) for viscoelastic analysis [20]. However, a current limitation is that the three detection modes require repositioning of the foot, which may slightly increase testing time. Despite this, this device offers unparalleled insights into plantar tissue mechanics, with potential applications in clinical diagnostics and biomechanical research. The primary goal of this paper is to thoroughly document the design, assembly, and operational aspects of this device, providing sufficient details for other researchers and clinicians to replicate, adapt, and expand upon this technology, facilitating further innovation and collaboration within the research community.

2. Materials and Methods

To address the existing technological limitations and fulfill the demand for comprehensive in vivo testing, we developed an innovative device specifically designed to perform in situ DMA-like measurements on live soft tissues (Figure 1). This advanced system accurately measures tensile/compressive resistance, shear resistance, and rotational torque properties, effectively overcoming the constraints associated with traditional DMA methods, which are typically restricted to cadaveric samples, as well as the shortcomings of simpler indentation-based approaches. Our device integrates four essential modules—foot fixation, sensor detection, lifting, and probe-to-tissue interaction—combined with a sophisticated control system to facilitate precise, multidirectional, and cyclic viscoelastic evaluations of plantar soft tissue under physiological conditions. To ensure the replicability of this paper, all design files, including CAD models and detailed specifications, have been made freely accessible online. The specifications table, design files summary, and source of materials can be referenced in Appendix A.

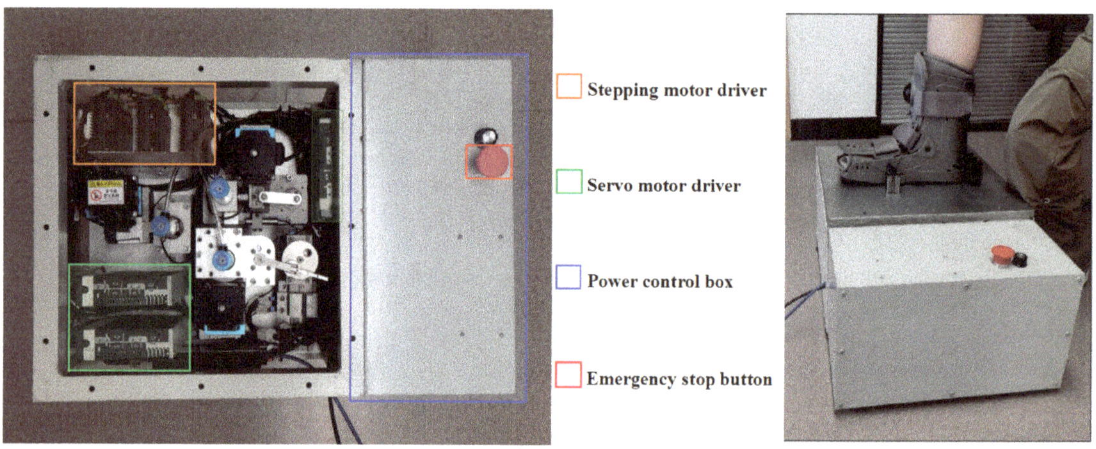

(a) (b)

Figure 1. (**a**) The overview of the device and (**b**) the general act of the in vivo plantar test.

Although plantar soft tissue comprises heterogeneous structures, each exhibiting distinct mechanical properties, it can be approximated as a uniform, single-layer material for analytical simplicity. Consequently, as an initial approach, it is appropriate to analyze the overall mechanical behavior of plantar soft tissue as homogeneous [21]. Extensive previous studies have primarily focused on evaluating tensile and compressive properties; however, limited attention has been given to the characterization of shear and torsional behaviors of plantar tissues, despite their significance in daily functional activities [22]. Considering that plantar soft tissues are continuously subjected to multidirectional forces—such as compression, shear, and torsion—it becomes essential to comprehensively investigate how these directional forces impact tissue integrity and their potential implications for orthopedic and systemic conditions. To address this gap, we designed our testing device to apply sinusoidal displacement stimuli u(t) (in millimeters) along three orthogonal directions (tensile/compressive, shear, and torsion) directly onto the plantar surface using a vacuum composite suction cup attachment, as illustrated in Figure 2. Correspondingly, the induced force responses, F(t), are accurately measured in real-time by integrated force sensors. We simplified the viscoelastic properties of the plantar soft tissue using the Kelvin–Voigt model [23]. In this model, a spring and a dashpot are connected in parallel. The spring corresponds to the elastic response of the material, storing energy, while the dashpot represents the viscous response, dissipating the energy.

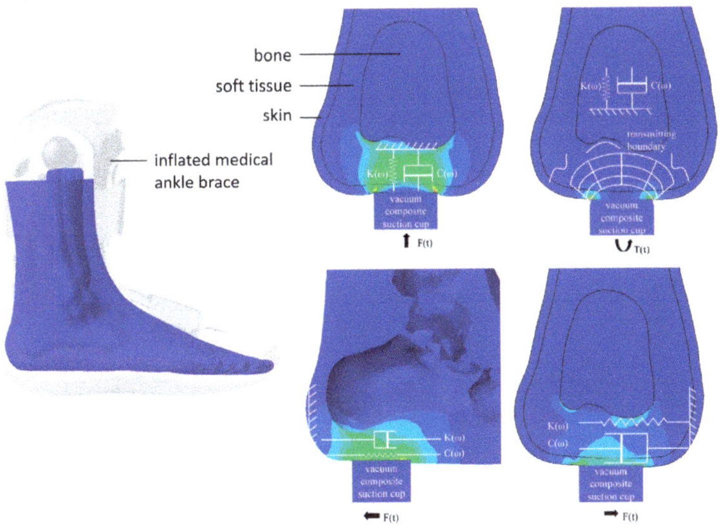

Figure 2. Viscoelastic model of plantar soft tissue in three dimensions.

2.1. Build Instruction of Hardware

As shown in Figure 1, the three stress–strain detection units (tension/compression, shear, and torque) are integrated within a welded support frame. An iron cover plate with three cross-shaped obround holes is secured to the top of the support frame to position the foot. The probes can pass through these holes to contact the testing points on the plantar surface for the respective measurements.

Each unit's detection mechanism is mounted on the sliding table of the lead screw lifting module driven by a stepper motor. This allows the probe head to automatically locate the initial position where it just contacts the plantar surface before testing, thereby avoiding subjective errors caused by the subject actively adjusting foot height to match the probe.

In the tension/compression detection unit, a servo motor is mounted on the slide via a bracket. One end of the connecting rod is eccentrically mounted on a disc at the end of the servo motor, while the other end is connected to the shaft via bearings and a clamping device, with the shaft constrained by linear bearings fixed to the frame. Before each test, the sliding table elevates the servo motor and all components connected to its end as a whole to find the test zero point and then remains stationary throughout the testing process. During detection, the mechanical design of vertical reciprocal motion can be simplified as the crank slider mechanism, as shown in Figure 3a. The servo motor rotates the disc, and through the eccentrically mounted connecting rod, the shaft is driven to perform vertical reciprocating linear motion within the constraints of the linear bearings. The force sensor and probe head are mounted sequentially on the shaft, while the displacement sensor is mounted on a fixed plate.

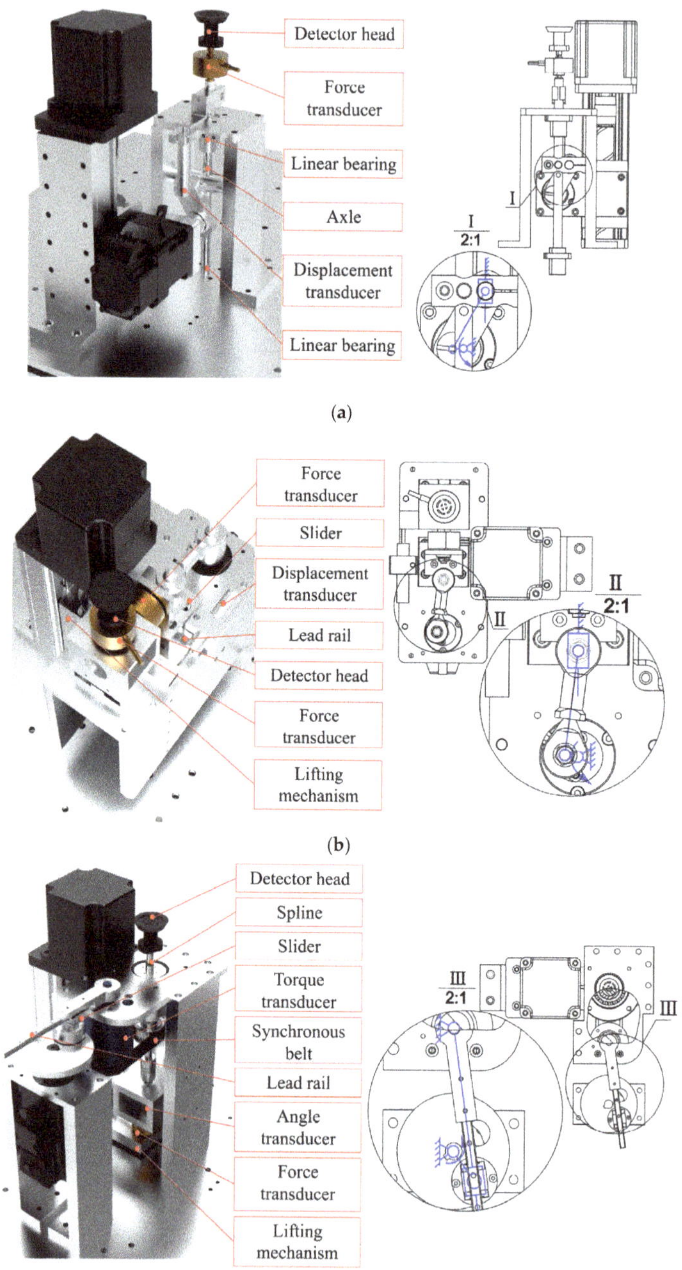

Figure 3. The mechanical structure of the (**a**) tension/compression detection unit; (**b**) the shear detection unit; and (**c**) the torsion detection unit.

In the shear detection unit, the entire testing mechanism is mounted on a horizontally positioned rectangular base plate. One side of the base plate is secured to the sliding table via a vertical bracket, while the other side features a vertical bracket with a rail. This rail, in conjunction with a slide block mounted on the frame, provides vertical guidance. The mechanism of shearing motion can also be simplified as the crank slider, only horizontally, as shown in Figure 3b. The force sensor is mounted below the probe, while the displacement sensor is fixed to one side of the horizontal base plate.

In the torsion testing unit, the L-shaped support plate is attached to the sliding table with screws. The support plate sequentially accommodates the force sensor, angle sensor, coupling, splined shaft, and probe head, with these components moving together as the sliding table is raised or lowered. The splined shaft is guided by splined bearings, which incorporate a self-machined synchronizing belt pulley shaft on their exterior, with rotating bearings mounted on the belt pulley shaft's outer surface and secured to the frame by the bearing block. The motor and the torque sensor housing are also fixed to the frame. The horizontal torsion motion can be realized by the crank rocker mechanism, as shown in Figure 3c. The motor rotates the disk, and a slider eccentrically mounted on the disk via bearings drives a guide rail to oscillate reciprocally about the axis of the torque sensor. The other end of the torque sensor drives a belt pulley via a synchronizing belt, resulting in the reciprocating rotation of the probe.

The mechanical performance and system error of displacement excitation is recorded in Table 1. Notably, each test's standard deviation is remarkably low, indicating the equipment's stability. The difference between set versus measured value comes from minute redundant spaces between components; therefore, we added displacement sensors to preciously measure the true value. Whether through visual observation or relying on the feelings of the subjects, it could be determined that there is no displacement between the composite vacuum suction cup and the plantar tissue.

Table 1. Mechanical performance and system error of displacement excitation.

	Tensile/Compress Displacement (mm)	Longitudinal Shear Displacement (mm)	Transverse Shear Displacement (mm)	Torsion Displacement (degree)
Mean Value	3.63506	3.78726	4.57726	27.27410
Standard Deviation	0.08795	0.00477	0.04109	0.40308

Detailed sensor characteristics are provided in Table 2. These sensors have been demonstrated to effectively meet our testing requirements, offering satisfactory performance in load capacity, response frequency, output sensitivity, repeatability, resolution, etc.

Table 2. Specifics of the sensors.

Sensor	Specifications	Values
Force sensor (DYMH-103)	Capacity	0–5 kg
	Response frequency	10 KHz
	Output sensitivity	1.0–1.5 ± 10% mV/V
	Hysteresis	0.1% F.S.
	Repeatability	0.1% F.S.
	Temperature sensitivity drift	0.1% F.S./10 °C
	Zero temperature drift	0.1% F.S./10 °C

Table 2. *Cont.*

Sensor	Specifications	Values
LVDT (GA09)	Capacity	±5 mm
	Response frequency	1–10 KHz
	Nonlinearity error	±0.5% BFSL
Torque sensor (FYAH)	Capacity	0–1 NM
	Response frequency	200 Hz
	Nonlinearity	±0.25% of R.O.
	Hysteresis	±0.25% of R.O.
	Nonrepeatability	±0.1% of R.O.
Angle sensor (GT-D)	Capacity	0–360°
	Resolution	4096, 12 bits
	independent linearity	0.15% F.S.
	Response frequency	5 KHz

To ensure accurate and reliable test outcomes, it is essential to immobilize the foot to prevent any internal bone displacement during the testing procedure. This immobilization is achieved using an inflated medical ankle brace featuring a flattened, hollowed base, as depicted in Figure 1b. During testing, the foot is sequentially positioned at five predefined measurement locations directly above the three detection probes. After aligning each test site, the foot is securely stabilized in place by four switchable magnets. Additionally, a vacuum composite suction cup is integrated at the detector joint to provide gentle, non-destructive, and non-invasive contact with the plantar surface throughout the inspection process.

2.2. *Operation Instructions*

Prior to testing, it is crucial to ensure the plantar surface of each participant is healthy, with no visible injuries, infections, or pain, and that the participant has not experienced foot trauma in the 12 months preceding data collection. A number of clinical specifics, including gender, age, height, weight, foot length, foot width, foot health, shoe-wearing habits, daily average steps, and exercise habits, are requested of the participant for the records. Due to the substantial structural and mechanical heterogeneity of plantar soft tissues, shear properties can differ significantly depending on the loading direction, reflecting the complex functional characteristics of the foot. Accordingly, our testing protocol incorporates two distinct shear testing orientations—longitudinal and transverse—implemented by rotating the foot 90 degrees around the shear probe head as a pivot point. This approach allows detailed characterization of shear properties in multiple directions at each measurement site. In this study, testing is performed at five critical plantar locations known for high load-bearing capacity or increased susceptibility to ulceration [24], as illustrated in Figure 4. Additional anatomical locations can also be selected for testing as required by specific research or clinical objectives.

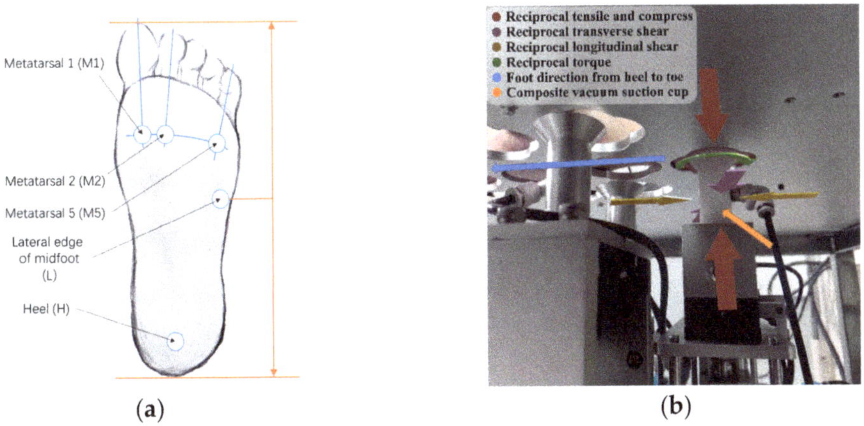

Figure 4. (**a**) The testing spot choices in this study; (**b**) the undercover view of testing on the plantar.

For each measurement, the participant positions the targeted test site precisely over the appropriate detection hole. After each measurement, the magnetic mounts are manually demagnetized by rotating their switches, allowing repositioning of the foot for subsequent testing modes. Upon correct alignment, the lead screw lifting module elevates the probe until it gently contacts the plantar surface. Once the force sensor detects a predefined threshold indicating sufficient contact, the lifting motion ceases, and a vacuum composite suction cup adheres gently to the plantar surface. This ensures non-invasive, stable engagement, allowing the mechanical linkage to induce controlled cyclic displacement synchronized with tissue deformation. For safety, the procedure includes an emergency stop mechanism accessible via the red button on the power supply unit.

The participant is fully informed and signed the consent before trials. The Ethical Review Committee of Huashan Hospital, Fudan University (HIRB), approves the ethical review (see the Supplemental Materials).

3. Results and Discussion

The reciprocal tension/compression and shearing test amplitude is initially set to be ± 2 mm, and the twist range of the torsion test is initially set to be $\pm 14^\circ$, with a frequency of 2 Hz for all tests. The amplitude is chosen based on the regular motion of a healthy plantar pad, and the frequency is determined by the practical upper limit of human foot use, as higher frequencies may cause noticeable discomfort to the participant.

The original data of the in vivo test for the volunteer's plantar soft tissue are shown in Figure 5. To analyze the relationship between load (stimulus) and deformation (response), both FFT and cross-correlation techniques were applied to the corresponding signals. The spectrogram indicates that the peak frequencies of the load and deformation signals are precisely aligned, confirming their frequency synchronization. Cross-correlation analysis produced a maximum coefficient of 0.9559 with a time lag of just 0.003 s, signifying a strong correlation with minimal temporal displacement between the signals. This suggests that the load closely follows the deformation with negligible lag, indicating the soft tissue's prompt response to applied displacement.

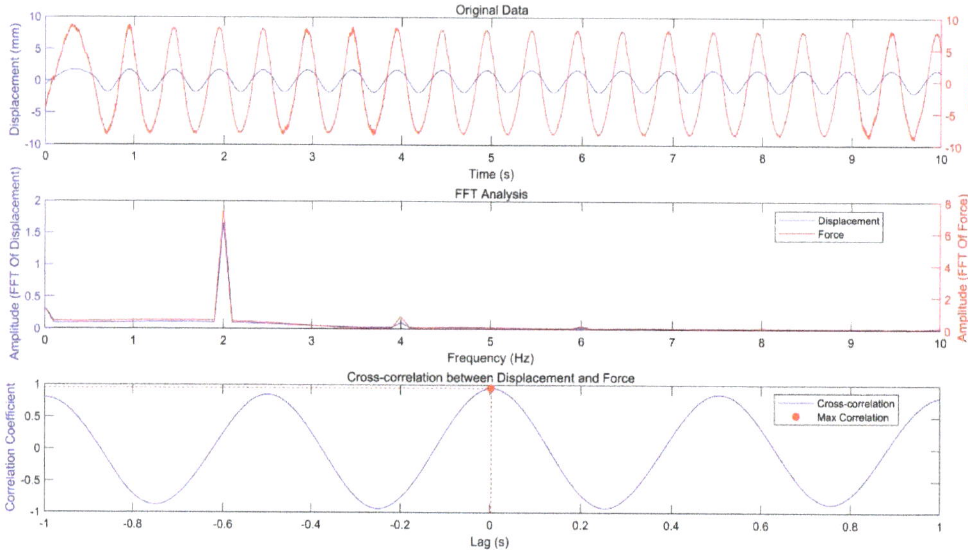

Figure 5. The original data, FFT analysis, and cross-correlation analysis.

The collected raw data were processed and visualized to clearly illustrate key stress–strain relationships, as shown in Figure 6. The figure is organized into four subplots, each depicting distinct mechanical behaviors: tensile/compression, longitudinal shear, transverse shear, and torsion. Measurements were performed at five anatomical plantar locations (M1, M2, M5, L, and H), chosen for their relevance to load bearing or susceptibility to injury. In the presentation of data and graphs, displacement directions were intentionally reversed relative to applied forces to enhance clarity and highlight peak-to-valley variations. (Note: this is likely a manual phase angle adjustment of 180°, which shall be re-adjusted in following data processing and calculations). To ensure clear representation of viscoelastic behaviors, data from a total of sixty loading cycles—comprising twenty cycles per trial over three repeated trials—are superimposed as cloud plots, with the mean values represented by solid lines. These graphical representations effectively capture the distinctive viscoelastic responses of plantar soft tissue under dynamic cyclic loading.

The processed data are presented through force–time and displacement–time curves, clearly illustrating the mechanical response of plantar soft tissue under dynamic cyclic loading conditions. Since the applied displacement remains constant within each testing mode, variations in force magnitude directly reflect differences in the tissue's elastic modulus; a higher force magnitude corresponds to increased stiffness. Furthermore, the viscoelastic properties of the plantar soft tissue are distinctly revealed by the characteristic hysteresis loops obtained from the force–displacement curves. The area enclosed by each hysteresis loop, determined by the phase difference between the applied displacement and the resultant force, quantifies the energy dissipated (ΔW) per loading cycle. A larger hysteresis loop area indicates greater energy dissipation and thus higher tissue viscosity, which significantly influences the damping and shock-absorption capabilities of the tissue. Conversely, a smaller hysteresis area indicates lower viscosity and reduced energy loss.

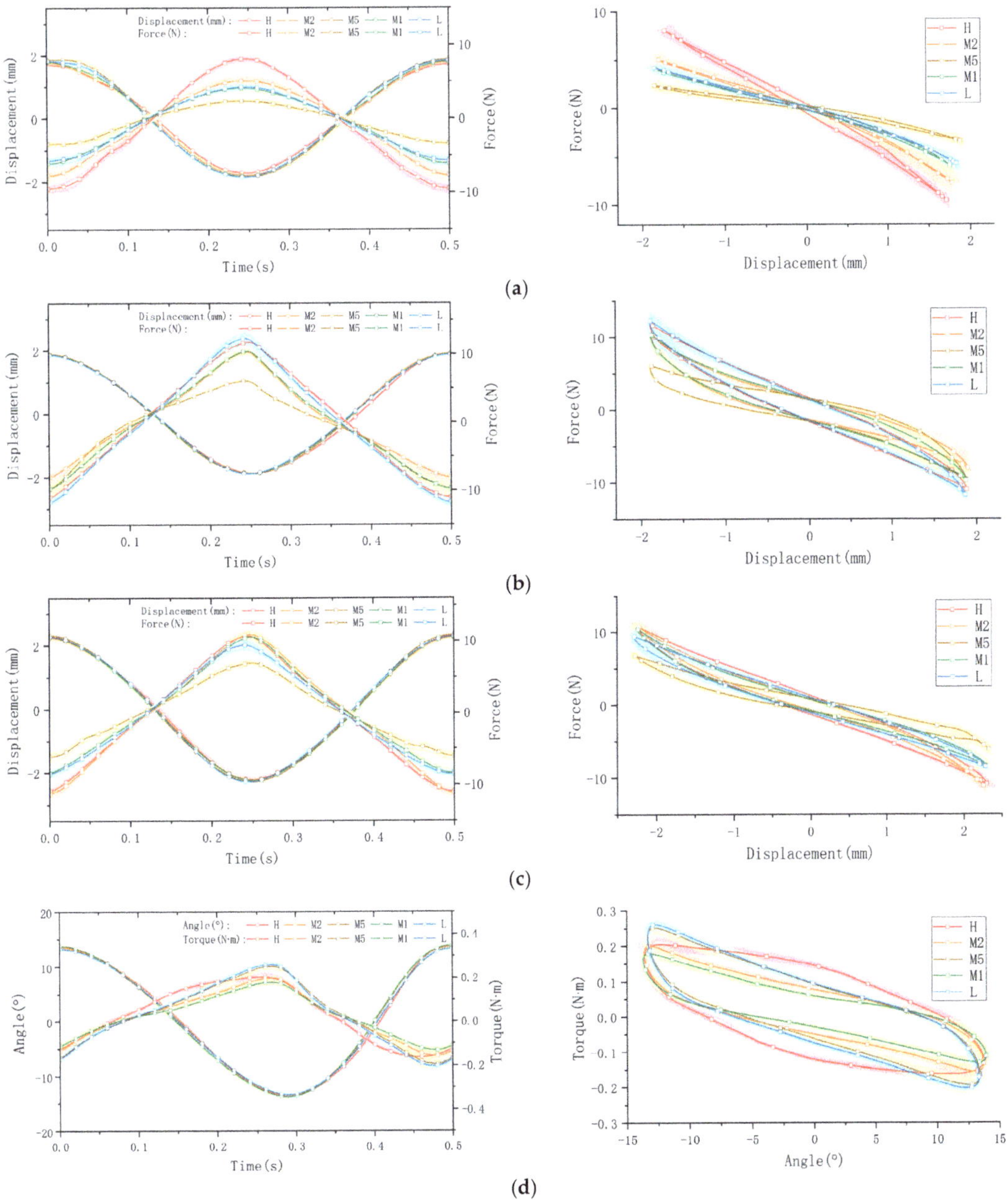

Figure 6. The stress–strain behaviors of a volunteer's plantar soft tissue in four types at 5 various spots: (**a**) the tensile/compression; (**b**) longitudinal shear; (**c**) transverse shear; (**d**) torsion.

Here, we take the longitudinal shear test on the heel spot as one example calculation of viscoelasticity (the red curve in Figure 6b). The viscoelastic characteristics of the tested material were quantified by analyzing experimental data from synchronized cyclic stress–strain measurements. The phase angle can be directly observed in the graph, which is

$11.4^\circ \approx 0.199$ rad. The amplitudes of the stress and strain signals were then determined as $\varepsilon_0 = 1.891245$ mm and $\sigma_0 = 11.738190$ N.

The viscoelastic parameters, namely, the storage modulus (E'), loss modulus (E''), and loss factor (tanδ), were computed using the standard definitions as follows:

$$E' = \frac{\sigma_0}{\varepsilon_0}\cos(\delta) = 6.084\text{N/mm}$$

$$E'' = \frac{\sigma_0}{\varepsilon_0}\sin(\delta) = 1.227\text{N/mm}$$

$$\tan(\delta) = \frac{E'}{E''} = 0.202$$

And the dissipated energy (the energy loss per loading–unloading cycle) calculated from the measured stress–strain hysteresis loop is

$$W_d = \oint \sigma d\varepsilon = 493.16\ \text{N} \cdot \text{mm(mJ)}$$

i.e., the area surrounded by the red hysteresis loop in Figure 6b.

4. Conclusions

In this work, we introduced a novel in vivo dynamic mechanical analysis (DMA) device specifically designed for comprehensive mechanical characterization of plantar soft tissue under realistic physiological conditions. The device effectively addresses critical gaps in current methodologies by providing precise, multidirectional, and dynamic measurements of tensile, compressive, shear, and torsional responses simultaneously. Through validation tests conducted on human participants, we confirmed its capability to reliably capture significant viscoelastic behaviors and accurately quantify tissue stiffness and viscosity. The device demonstrates strong potential for clinical applications, offering critical insights into the mechanical properties and functional health of plantar tissues. Furthermore, by openly sharing detailed CAD models, specifications, and assembly instructions, we aim to facilitate broader adoption, replication, and further innovation within the biomedical and biomechanics research communities. This technology holds substantial promise for improving diagnostic accuracy, personalized therapeutic interventions, and understanding biomechanical dysfunctions in clinical orthopedics and rehabilitation.

While this study provides decent insights into soft tissue material characterization, some limitations should be noted. We examined the effects of biological factors—including tissue composition, sex, age, body mass index (BMI), and body mass—on tissue characterization; however, the potential influence of disease status was not addressed [25]. Future studies should prioritize comparative analyses of healthy and diseased cohorts to elucidate the impact of pathology on plantar soft tissue. A key challenge lies in recruiting sufficient samples with well-documented disease progression.

5. Patents

China Patent ZL2024101221804: multidimensional and broad-spectrum clinical in situ testing equipment for mechanical properties of plantar soft tissue. Ran Huang; Longyan Wu; Jun Zhu; Xinyi Ning; Xin Ma.

U.S. Patent 18/772,135: MULTIDIMENSIONAL BROAD-SPECTRUM CLINICAL IN SITU TESTING EQUIPMENT FOR EVALUATING MECHANICAL PROPERTIES OF PLANTAR SOFT TISSUE. Ran Huang; Longyan Wu; Jun Zhu; Xin Ma.

Netherlands Patent 2034960: In vivo multidimensional stress–strain testing device for plantar soft tissues. Ran Huang; Longyan Wu; Jun Zhu; Xin Ma.

Supplementary Materials: The following supporting information can be downloaded at: https://www.mdpi.com/article/10.3390/technologies13050191/s1, The ethical review form.

Author Contributions: L.W.: Methodology, Investigation, Software, Data curation, Visualization, Writing—Original draft, Validation. J.Z.: Methodology, Resources. X.M.: Supervision, Project administration, Funding acquisition. R.H.: Conceptualization, Methodology, Investigation, Data curation, Validation, Funding acquisition, Supervision, Project administration, Writing—Reviewing and Editing. All authors have read and agreed to the published version of the manuscript.

Funding: This work is financially supported by the National Key Research and Development Program of China (2022YFC2009500), the Fudan-Yiwu Fund (FYX-23-102), and the TZI-ZJU Industrial Program (2023CLG01, 2023CLG01PT).

Institutional Review Board Statement: The ethical review was approved by the Ethical Review Committee of Huashan Hospital, Fudan University (HIRB), (Approval No.: (2022) Temporary Trial No.: (889)) (refer to the Supplemental Materials).

Informed Consent Statement: Informed consent was obtained from all subjects involved in this study.

Data Availability Statement: Data are contained within the article.

Conflicts of Interest: The authors declare no conflicts of interest.

Appendix A

Table A1. Specifications table.

Hardware name	In Situ Plantar Dynamic Mechanical Analysis
Subject area	Medical
Hardware type	Measuring physical properties and in-lab sensors
Closest commercial analog	No commercial analog is available.
Cost of hardware	RMB¥21233–estimated for purchase part
Source file repository	https://data.mendeley.com/datasets/y6nm3pj39r/1 DOI:10.17632/y6nm3pj39r.1

Table A2. Design files summary.

Design File Name	File Type	Location of the File
3D model of the device	STEP file	3D model of a novel in situ dynamic mechanical detection machine for human plantar soft tissue—Mendeley Data
CAD drawings of the device	CAD file	CAD drawing of a novel in situ dynamic mechanical detection machine for human plantar soft tissue—Mendeley Data

The 3D model of the device: A comprehensive mechanical assembly drawing in STEP format, created using SolidWorks 2024, comprising 135 individual components.

CAD drawings of the device: A collection of 49 detailed 2D drawings for the machined components, divided into four sections: frame, tensile/compressive testing unit, shear testing unit, and torsional testing unit.

The equipment is assembled from machined parts and purchased parts. The purchased components mainly include sensors and transmitters, motors and drivers, as well as standard parts such as sliders, guide rails, bearings and so on. In order to achieve precise functionality of the equipment, we also designed and machined some components, such as connecting rods, connectors, brackets, and support plates. Table A3 includes only the purchased components; the custom-designed and machined parts, critical to the assembly, are not individually itemized. Detailed specifications and parameters for these machined components are documented within the CAD drawings.

Table A3. Bill of materials summary.

Component	Number	Cost per Unit-Currency	Total Cost-	Component
Force sensor (DYMH-103)	4	RMB¥171	RMB¥684	1688.com (accessed on 28 August 2024)
LVDT (GA09)	2	RMB¥800	RMB¥1600	1688.com (accessed on 28 August 2024)
Torque sensor (FYAH)	1	RMB¥5960	RMB¥5960	1688.com (accessed on 28 August 2024)
Angle sensor (GT-D)	1	RMB¥202	RMB¥202	1688.com (accessed on 28 August 2024)
Screw lifting module (CB1605-30)	3	RMB¥319	RMB¥957	1688.com (accessed on 28 August 2024)
Stepper motor and driver (57 stepper and DM542)	3	RMB¥86	RMB¥258	1688.com (accessed on 28 August 2024)
Servo motor and driver (Panasonic A6 and MADLT05SF)	3	RMB¥2000	RMB¥6000	1688.com (accessed on 28 August 2024)
Solenoid valve (2V025-08)	3	RMB¥16	RMB¥48	1688.com (accessed on 28 August 2024)
Vacuum pump (G7BL2485S)	1	RMB¥568	RMB¥568	1688.com (accessed on 28 August 2024)
Slider and slide rail (MGN5C)	1	RMB¥42	RMB¥42	1688.com (accessed on 28 August 2024)
Linear sliding table (CHTF-W40-L35)	2	RMB¥235	RMB¥470	1688.com (accessed on 28 August 2024)
Timing belt and pulleys (HTD3M)	1	RMB¥45	RMB¥45	1688.com (accessed on 28 August 2024)
DAQ (USB 3151)	1	RMB¥4399	RMB¥4399	1688.com (accessed on 28 August 2024)

References

1. Natali, A.N.; Fontanella, C.G.; Carniel, E.L. Constitutive formulation and analysis of heel pad tissues mechanics. *Med. Eng. Phys.* **2010**, *32*, 516–522. [CrossRef] [PubMed]
2. Hegde, M.; Karthik, K.; Managuli, V.; Bhat, S.K. A consistent transversely-isotropic hyper-viscoelastic model: Finite element implementation and mechanical characterization of biological tissues. *Int. J. Non-Linear Mech.* **2024**, *160*, 104663. [CrossRef]
3. Haron, A.; Li, L.; Shuang, J.; Lin, C.; Mansoubi, M.; Shi, X.; Horn, D.; Reeves, N.; Bowling, F.; Bradbury, K.; et al. In-shoe plantar temperature, normal and shear stress relationships during gait and rest periods for people living with and without diabetes. *Sci. Rep.* **2025**, *15*, 8804. [CrossRef]
4. Yang, X.; Peng, Z.; Liu, X.; Liu, X.-L.; Lu, S. A narrative review of the measurement methods for biomechanical properties of plantar soft tissue in patients with diabetic foot. *Front. Endocrinol.* **2024**, *15*, 1332032. [CrossRef] [PubMed]

5. Kwan, R.L.C.; Zheng, Y.P.; Cheing, G.L.Y. The effect of aging on the biomechanical properties of plantar soft tissues. *Clin. Biomech.* **2010**, *25*, 601–605. [CrossRef]
6. Cavanagh, P.R. Plantar soft tissue thickness during ground contact in walking. *J. Biomech.* **1999**, *32*, 623–628. [CrossRef]
7. Scott, G.; Menz, H.B.; Newcombe, L. Age-related differences in foot structure and function. *Gait Posture* **2007**, *26*, 68–75. [CrossRef]
8. Ledoux, W.R.; Blevins, J.J. The compressive material properties of the plantar soft tissue. *J. Biomech.* **2007**, *40*, 2975–2981. [CrossRef]
9. Brady, L.; Pai, S.; Iaquinto, J.M.; Wang, Y.-N.; Ledoux, W.R. The compressive, shear, biochemical, and histological characteristics of diabetic and non-diabetic plantar skin are minimally different. *J. Biomech.* **2021**, *129*, 110797. [CrossRef]
10. Tecse, A.; Romero, S.E.; Naemi, R.; Castaneda, B. Characterisation of the soft tissue viscous and elastic properties using ultrasound elastography and rheological models: Validation and applications in plantar soft tissue assessment. *Phys. Med. Biol.* **2023**, *68*, 105005. [CrossRef]
11. Latorre-Ossa, H.; Gennisson, J.L.; De Brosses, E.; Tanter, M. Quantitative imaging of nonlinear shear modulus by combining static elastography and shear wave elastography. *IEEE Trans. Ultrason. Ferroelectr. Freq. Control.* **2012**, *59*, 833–839. [CrossRef] [PubMed]
12. Tonna, R.; Chatzistergos, P.E.; Wyatt, O.; Chockalingam, N. Reliability and Validity of Shore Hardness in Plantar Soft Tissue Biomechanics. *Sensors* **2024**, *24*, 539. [CrossRef]
13. Behforootan, S.; Chatzistergos, P.E.; Chockalingam, N.; Naemi, R. A clinically applicable non-invasive method to quantitatively assess the visco-hyperelastic properties of human heel pad, implications for assessing the risk of mechanical trauma. *J. Mech. Behav. Biomed. Mater.* **2017**, *68*, 287–295. [CrossRef] [PubMed]
14. Macan, J. Application of thermal analysis methods in biology and medicine. *Period. Biol.* **2023**, *125*, 75–100. [CrossRef]
15. Menard, K.P.; Menard, N. *Dynamic Mechanical Analysis*; CRC Press: Boca Raton, FL, USA, 2020.
16. Ginic-Markovic, M.; Choudhury, N.R.; Dimopoulos, M.; Williams, D.R.; Matisons, J. Characterization of elastomer compounds by thermal analysis. *Thermochim. Acta* **1998**, *316*, 87–95. [CrossRef]
17. Yang, G.; Pang, X.; Liu, A.; Li, C.; Zhu, J.; Huang, R.; Ma, X. Design and validation of a DMA-inspired device for in-vivo measurement of human skin mechanics: A finite element analysis approach. In *Journal of Physics: Conference Series, Proceedings of the 7th International Conference on Physics, Mathematics and Statistics, Yichang, China, 23–25 May 2024*; IOP Publishing: Bristol, UK, 2024; Volume 2851, p. 012019.
18. Grigoriadis, G.; Newell, N.; Carpanen, D.; Christou, A.; Bull, A.M.; Masouros, S.D. Material properties of the heel fat pad across strain rates. *J. Mech. Behav. Biomed. Mater.* **2017**, *65*, 398–407. [CrossRef]
19. Negishi, T.; Ito, K.; Kamono, A.; Lee, T.; Ogihara, N. Strain-rate dependence of viscous properties of the plantar soft tissue identified by a spherical indentation test. *J. Mech. Behav. Biomed. Mater.* **2020**, *102*, 103470. [CrossRef]
20. Huang, R.; Ning, X.; Wu, L.; Zhu, J.; Tang, L.; Ma, X. An exploratory in-situ dynamic mechanical analysis on the shearing stress–strain mechanism of human plantar soft tissue. *Sci. Rep.* **2024**, *14*, 11953. [CrossRef]
21. Boyer, G.; Laquièze, L.; Le Bot, A.; Laquièze, S.; Zahouani, H. Dynamic indentation on human skin in vivo: Ageing effects. *Ski. Res. Technol.* **2009**, *15*, 55–67. [CrossRef]
22. Stief, T.; Peikenkamp, K. A new insole measurement system to detect bending and torsional moments at the human foot during footwear condition: A technical report. *J. Foot Ankle Res.* **2015**, *8*, 1–8. [CrossRef]
23. Lewandowski, R.; Chorążyczewski, B. Identification of the parameters of the Kelvin–Voigt and the Maxwell fractional models, used to modeling of viscoelastic dampers. *Comput. Struct.* **2010**, *88*, 1–17. [CrossRef]
24. Pai, S.; Ledoux, W.R. The compressive mechanical properties of diabetic and non-diabetic plantar soft tissue. *J. Biomech.* **2010**, *43*, 1754–1760. [CrossRef] [PubMed]
25. Chavan, R.; Kamble, N.; Kuthe, C.; Sarnobat, S. On Mechanical Behavior and Characterization of Soft Tissues. *Biomed. Eng. Comput. Biol.* **2024**, *15*, 11795972241294115. [CrossRef] [PubMed]

MDPI AG
Grosspeteranlage 5
4052 Basel
Switzerland
Tel.: +41 61 683 77 34

Technologies Editorial Office
E-mail: technologies@mdpi.com
www.mdpi.com/journal/technologies